MARIHUANA AND MEDICINE

MARIHUANA AND MEDICINE

Edited by

GABRIEL G. NAHAS, MD, PhD, DSc

KENNETH M. SUTIN, MD, MS
Department of Anesthesiology
New York University School of Medicine

DAVID HARVEY, PhD

Department of Biochemistry, Oxford University

STIG AGURELL, PhD, PharmD, DSc
Faculty of Pharmacy, University of Uppsala, Sweden

Co-Editors
Nicholas Pace, MD and Robert Cancro, MD

NYU School of Medicine

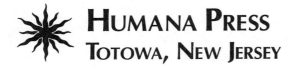 **HUMANA PRESS**
TOTOWA, NEW JERSEY

© 1999 Humana Press Inc.
999 Riverview Drive, Suite 208
Totowa, New Jersey 07512

For additional copies, pricing for bulk purchases, and/or information about other Humana titles,
contact Humana at the above address or at any of the following numbers: Tel: 973-256-1699;
Fax: 973-256-8341; E-mail: humana@humanapr.com

Due diligence has been taken by the publishers, editors, and authors of this book to assure the accuracy of the information
published and to describe generally accepted practices. The contributors herein have carefully checked to ensure that
the drug selections and dosages set forth in this text are accurate and in accord with the standards accepted at the time
of publication. Notwithstanding, as new research, changes in government regulations, and knowledge from clinical
experience relating to drug therapy and drug reactions constantly occurs, the reader is advised to check the product
information provided by the manufacturer of each drug for any change in dosages or for additional warnings and
contraindications. This is of utmost importance when the recommended drug herein is a new or infrequently used drug.
It is the responsibility of the treating physician to determine dosages and treatment strategies for individual patients.
Further it is the responsibility of the health care provider to ascertain the Food and Drug Administration status of each
drug or device used in their clinical practice. The publisher, editors, and authors are not responsible for errors or
omissions or for any consequences from the application of the information presented in this book and make no warranty,
express or implied, with respect to the contents in this publication.

Cover design by Patricia F. Cleary

This publication is printed on acid-free paper. ∞
ANSI Z39.48-1984 (American National Standards Institute) Permanence of Paper for Printed Library Materials.

Printed in the United States of America.   10 9 8 7 6 5 4 3 2 1

Library of Congress Cataloging-in-Publication Data

Marihuana and medicine / edited by Gabriel G. Nahas...[et al.].
          p.   cm.
        Proceedings of a symposium held at New York University School of Medicine, Mar. 20–21, 1998 and papers
        reprinted from various sources.
        Includes index.
        ISBN 0-89603-593-X (alk. paper)
        1. Marijuana—Therapeutic use. 2. Marijuana—Physiological effect. 3. Tetrahydrocannabinol—
        Therapeutic use. 4. Tetrahydrocannabinol—Physiological effect. I. Nahas, Gabriel G., 1920–   .
        RM666'.C266 M356 1999   98-13481
        615'.32345—dc21   CIP

This monograph is dedicated to the memory of
Sir W. D. M. Paton, C.B.E., F.R.S., D.M.
Former Professor of Pharmacology, University of Oxford
and Fellow of Balliol College, Oxford

PREFACE

The curative properties of cannabis were introduced by British physicians, on their return from India, into Western medicine during the second part of the 19th century. The 1854 United States Dispensary described the properties of the drug Indian hemp as follows:

Extract of hemp is a powerful narcotic, causing exhilaration, intoxication, delirious hallucinations, and in its subsequent action, drowsiness and stupor, with little effect upon the circulation. It acts as a decided aphrodisiac, increases the appetite, and occasionally induces the cataleptic state. In morbid states it has been found to produce sleep, to allay spasm, to compose nervous inquietude, and to relieve pain. In these respects it resembles opium in its operation; but it differs from that narcotic in not diminishing the appetite, checking the secretions, or constipating the bowels. It is much less certain in its effects; but may sometimes be preferably employed, when opium is contraindicated by its nauseating or constipating effects. The complaints to which it has been specially recommended are neuralgia, gout, tetanus, hydrophobia, epidemic cholera, convulsions, chorea, hysteria, mental depression, insanity, and uterine hemorrhage. Dr. Alexander Christison, of Edinburgh, has found it to have the property of hastening and increasing the contractions of the uterus in delivery. It acts very quickly, and without anesthetic effect. It appears, however, to exert this influence only in a certain proportion of cases.

The Dispensary also cautioned physicians that alarming side-effects could be observed when large doses were prescribed, and noticed also the marked variability in the potency of the different available commercial preparations.

The drug, in contrast to opium preparations, was not much used during the Civil War. It never seemed to enjoy any great popularity among American physicians; they did not like the slowness of its actions, and the unpredictable potency of its different preparations. Furthermore, its mode of administration by the oral route could not compete with that of opium, or morphine, which could be given by hypodermic injections.

Toward the end of the 19th century the burgeoning pharmaceutical industry attempted to develop more dependable and purified compounds from cannabis, but without much success. Crude cannabis preparations were used with decreasing frequency in the first part of the 20th century, and they were eliminated from the United States Pharmacopeia in 1942; as they were from the British one in 1932.

Marihuana as medicine regained attention in the United States with the discovery of its active ingredient THC, and in the wake of the widespread usage of marihuana as a recreational drug.

The many pharmacological effects produced by THC in experimental animals and humans led investigators to seek some therapeutic application for this drug. The most sought-after applications were for the treatment of disorders of the central nervous system, the primary target of THC. Extensive research programs sponsored by the pharmaceutical industry (Abbott, Squibb, Lilly, Pfizer) and by Federal agencies were initiated to establish the efficacy of THC, its mode of action, and to design related synthetic molecules that would have greater specificity and fewer side-effects.

Its use as an antidepressant, anxiolytic, sedative, hypnotic, and analgesic or for alcohol and opiate withdrawal, proved to be ineffective or inconsistent, especially when compared with the more specific therapeutic molecules that became available at that time. But new and unexpected applications were reported for the original drug, cannabis, in the treatment of glaucoma and of the nausea and vomiting induced by cancer chemotherapy.

In 1972, a new Federal Agency, The National Institute of Drug Abuse was created. It was patterned along the lines of the National Institute of Health, and gives a mandate to investigate all the health and medical aspects of illicit drug use, namely, those of marihuana, the opiates, and cocaine. Each year NIDA is required to issue a special report to Congress on "Marihuana and Health" that summarized the results of studies carried out by the recipients of its research grants and contracts. And NIDA made available to licensed researchers in the field marihuana cigarettes of known THC content or capsules containing 5–10 mg of THC. Some of the research was cosponsored by another Federal agency, the National Institute on Mental Health (NIMH). As a result of this robust US Federal funding, which has been expanding yearly since 1972 (reaching hundreds of millions of dollars), all aspects of the biochemistry, pharmacology, psychology, epidemiology, and psychiatry of marihuana use have been investigated. The results of these studies have been made available in dozens of scientific and medical books and monographs and thousands of articles published over the past 25 years, at a similar expanding pace.

The Research Institute of Pharmaceutical Sciences of the University of Mississippi has collected since 1972 over 10,000 references to scientific studies on cannabis and THC. However, the usefulness of THC as a medication is still debated or even promoted, and the latest report of the NIH (1997) on the subject concluded that additional experimental and clinical research studies were required to assess the therapeutic properties of marihuana.

However, this latest NIH report did not include information on the major advances in molecular biology that have permitted scientists to focus their studies on the molecular mechanism of THC and pinpoint its molecular mode of action, which eluded us so long.

The purpose of the New York University Conference on Marihuana and Medicine held in March of 1998, which was the seed crystal from which the present volume grew, was to review the pharmacological and molecular basis of the therapeutic properties of marihuana and THC, properties which have been debated until this day.

It was not possible for all those on the program to attend and there was such a pressure on the conference time available that some papers were given in much abbreviated form. For this volume, full papers have been used, including articles from scheduled participants unable to attend. In addition, previously published peer-reviewed studies of seminal importance to the subject but difficult to access have been included. The latter articles deal with brain function, reproduction, and cardiovascular function, and provide a pharmacological background to the subsequent molecular studies that they now complement. A historical summary was also included, ending with the 12th century classical Arabic poem "Cannabis and Alcohol," the Green and the Red, translated by Franz Rosenthal.

The current molecular studies reported in this volume indicate that the multiple medical effects of marihuana may be accounted for by an interaction of the drug with basic regulatory signaling mechanisms of the lipid bilayer and integral receptors of the cell membrane. This unique deregulation of cell membrane signaling by THC impairs the function of brain synapses, gametes, and cells of the immune system. Therefore, today the verdict of marihuana in medicine is finally at hand.

Gabriel G. Nahas

ACKNOWLEDGMENTS

The conference on Marihuana and Medicine was held at New York University School of Medicine on March 20–21, 1998. It was organized under the sponsorship of its dean, Saul Farber, and of Associate Dean David Scotch and Robert Soberman of the post graduate Medical School close cooperation with the Department of Anesthesiology and its chairman Dr. Herman Turndorf.

This conference was made possible thanks to an unrestricted grant from the Stuart Mott Foundation. This Foundation also provided an additional grant to defray the cost of publication of the proceedings of the conference. Conference organizers and editors of this monograph are therefore most indebted to the Mott Foundation for its generous support. They also acknowledge the support of the Helen Clay Frick Foundation and of the Jeremiah Millbank Foundation, which provided additional grants to cover the expenses of an expanded edition. Other grants were provided by "Astra Pain Control" and the Swedish Academy of Pharmaceutical Sciences.

Important past contributions in the field have been reprinted with their authors' and editors' permissions, which are acknowledged with thanks.

It is also noted that the editors or authors of *Marihuana and Medicine* will not benefit from the proceeds of its sale.

CONTENTS

PART II. BIOCHEMISTRY AND MOLECULAR MECHANISMS

PART III. PHARMACOLOGY AND PHYSIOPATHOLOGY

PART IV. MARIHUANA AND REPRODUCTIVE FUNCTION

PART V. CANNABINOIDS IN THE TREATMENT OF PAIN

Part VIII. Marihuana and Psychiatry

Part IX. Marihuana and AIDS Management

Part X. Marihuana and Medicine, Public Health, and Public Policy

PART XI. GENERAL CONCLUSIONS

CONTRIBUTORS

PETER ALLBECK, MD • *Department of Social Medicine, Göteborg, Göteborg, Sweden*

RAMONA G. ALMIREZ, MD • *Department of Obstetrics and Gynecology, University of Texas Health Science Center, San Antonio, TX*

G. AMBROSETTO, MD • *Clinica Neurologica di Bologna, Bologna, Italy*

STIG AGURELL, PhD, PharmD, DSc • *Astra Pain Control AB, Jarfalla, Sweden*

HENRI BARUK, MD • *Académie Nationale de Médicine, Paris, France*

HENRI BAYLON, MD • *Académie Nationale de Médicine, Paris, France*

NILS BEJEROT, MD • *The Swedish Carnegie Institute, Stockholm, Sweden*

SANDRA S. BENNETT, MA • *Northwest Center for Prevention and Safety, Portland, OR*

WILLIAM M. BENNETT, MD • *Division of Nephrology, Oregon Health Sciences University, Portland, OR*

KAY BRUNE, MD • *Director, Institute of Experimental and Clinical Pharmacology and Toxicology, University of Erlangen-Nürenberg, Erlangen, Germany*

R. BOURDON, PhD • *School of Pharmacy, Université René Descartes, Paris, France*

LANI J. BURKMAN, MD • *Department of Gynecology and Obstetrics, State University of New York, Buffalo, NY*

GUY A. CABRAL, PhD • *Department of Microbiology and Immunology, Virginia Commonwealth University Medical College, Richmond, VA*

MICHAEL C. CHANG, MD • *Department of Anatomy and Cell Biology, State University of New York, Buffalo, NY*

L. F. CHAPMAN, MD • *Department of Behavioral Biology, University of California Medical School, Sacramento, CA*

JACQUES CHIRAC • *Palais de l'Elysée, Paris, France*

W. CRAWFORD CLARK, PhD • *Columbia University College of Physicians and Surgeons, New York, NY*

PAUL CONSROE, MD, PhD • *Department of Pharmacology and Toxicology, University of Arizona, Tucson, AZ*

DAVID D. COZENS, PhD • *Department of Reproductive Toxicology, Huntingdon Research Center, Huntington, UK*

SUSAN L. DALTERIO, PhD • *Department of Pharmacology, University of Texas Health Science Center, San Antoino, TX*

SANJOY K. DAS, PhD • *Department of Molecular and Integrative Physiology, University of Kansas Medical Center, Kansas City, KS*

W. A. DEVANE, PhD • *NIH, Bethesda, MD*

ORRIN DEVINSKY, MD • *New York University Hospital for Joint Diseases, New York, NY*

EDWARD F. DOMINO, MD • *University of Michigan Medical School, Ann Arbor, MI*

ANDY DRAY, PhD • *Head of Pharmacology, Sandoz Institute, London, UK*

MICHEL DUBOIS, MD • *Director of Pain Management Clinic, New York University School of Medicine, New York, NY*

MAHMOUD A. EL SOHLY, PhD • *School of Pharmacy, University of Mississippi, University, MS*

MAX FORBES, MD • *Edward S. Harkness Eye Institute, Columbia-Presbyterian Medical Center, New York, NY*

GORDON S. FRANCIS, MD • *Medical Director, Serono Laboratories, Inc., Norwell, MA*

HENRY CLAY FRICK, II, MD • *Department of Obstetrics, Columbia University College of Physicians and Surgeons, New York, NY*

ANNA FUGELSTAD, PhD • *Department of Forensic Medicine, Sabbatsberg Hospital, Stockholm, Sweden*

ELIOT L. GARDNER, MD • *Department of Physchiatry, Albert Einstein College of Medicine, Bronx, NY*

S. JOHN GATLEY, PhD • *Medical Department, Brookhaven National Laboratory, Upton, NY*

KATHRYN GILL, MD • *Department of Psychiatry, McGill University, Montreal, Quebec, Canada*

ELISABETH GORDON, MA • *New York University Hospital for Joint Diseases, New York, NY*

RICHARD J. GRALLA, MD • *Ochsner Cancer Institute, New Orleans, LA*

KEITH GREEN, MD • *Department of Ophthalmology, Medical College of Georgia, Augusta, GA*

DAVID J. HARVEY, PhD • *Department of Biochemistry, University of Oxford, Oxford, UK*

WYLIE C. HEMBREE, III, MD • *Department of Obstetrics and Gynecology, Columbia University College of Physicians and Surgeons, New York, NY*

NOBORU HIROI, MD • *Departments of Psychiatry and Neuroscience, Albert Einstein College of Medicine, Bronx, NY*

LEO E. HOLLISTER, MD • *Research Director, University of Texas Health Science Center, San Antonio, TX*

BRUCE T. HOPE, PhD • *Department of Psychiatry, Massachusetts General Hospital, Charlestown, MA*

HOSEA F. S. HUANG, PhD • *Department of Obstetrics and Gynecology, Columbia University College of Physicians and Surgeons, New York, NY*

GEORGE HYMAN, MD • *Department of Medicine, Columbia University College of Physicians and Surgoens, New York, NY*

PAUL JANSSEN, MD • *Janssen Research Foundation, Vosselar, Belgium*

J.-C. JARDILLIER, PhD • *School of Pharmacy, Université de Reims, France*

F. RAÚL JERI, MD • *Neuropsychiatry Department, San Marcos University Medical School, Lima, Peru*

REESE T. JONES, MD • *Department of Psychiatry, University of California, San Francisco, CA*

JEROME P. KASSIRER, MD • *Editor, New England Journal of Medicine, Boston, MA*

JOHN H. KING • *Deputy Assistant Administrator Office of Diversion Control, Drug Enforcement Administration, Arlington, VA*

B. KENNETH KOE, PhD • *Pfizer Central Research, Groton, CT*

C. EVERETT KOOP, MD • *Surgeon General of the United States (1981–1989)*

DONALD P. KOTLER, MD • *Department of Medicine, Columbia University College of Physicians and Surgeons, New York, NY*

COLETTE LATOUR, PhD • *INSERM U26, Hopital Fernand Widal, Paris, France*

PAUL LECHAT, MD • *Académie Nationale de Médecine, Paris, France*

LOUIS LEMBERGER, MD, PhD • *Lilly Laboratories, Indianapolis, IN*

ARON H. LICHTMAN, MD • *Department of Pharmacology and Toxicology, Virginia Commonwealth University, Richmond, VA*

ANNE MARTIN, MD • *Institute of Pharmacology, University of Zürich, Zürich, Switzerland*

BILLY R. MARTIN, PhD • *Department of Pharmacoloy and Toxicology, Virginia Commonwealth University, Richmond, VA*

ALEXANDROS MAKRIYANNIS, PhD • *School of Pharmacy, University of Connecticut, Storrs, CT*

RAPHAEL MECHOULAM, MSc, PhD • *Faculty of Medicine, The Hebrew University of Jerusalem, Jerusalem, Israel*

NANCY K. MELLO, MD • *Alcohol and Drug Abuse Research Center, Harvard Medical School/McLean Hospital, Belmont, MA*

JACK H. MENDELSON, MD • *Alcohol and Drug Abuse Research Center, Harvard Medical School/McLean Hospital, Belmont, MA*

KLAUS A. MICZEK, PhD • *Department of Psychology, Carnegie-Mellon University, Pittsburgh, PA*

LOREN L. MILLER, PhD • *Burroughs Wellcome Co., Research Triangle Park, NC*

JAMES A. MOSS • *Chief of Narcotics Unit, US Attorney's Office for the Southern District of New York, New York, NY*

GABRIEL G. NAHAS, MD, PhD • *Department of Anesthesiology, NYU Medical Center, New York, NY*

JUAN C. NEGRETE, MD • *Addiction Research Foundation, Toronto, Canada*

WILLIAM NOTCUTT, MD • *Consultant Anaesthetist, James Paget Hospital, Great Yarmouth, Norfolk, UK*

NICHOLAS PACE, MD • *Internal Medicine and Rheumatology, New York, NY*

BIBHASH C. PARIA, MD • *Department of Molecular and Integrative Physiology, University of Kansas Medical Center, Kansas City, KS*

STEVEN J. PARKER, MD • *Division of Developmental and Behavioral Pediatrics, Boston City Hospital, Boston, MA*

VICTOR L. PARKER, MD • *Division of Developmental and Behavioral Pediatrics, Boston City Hospital, Boston, MA*

W. D. M. PATON, CBE, FRS, DM • *Late Professor of Pharmacology, University of Oxford, Oxford, UK*

MARIO PEREZ-REYES, MD • *Department of Psychiatry, University of North Carolina at Chapel Hill, Chapel Hill, NC*

ROGER G. PERTWEE, MD • *Department of Biomedical Sciences, Institute of Medical Sciences, University of Aberdeen, Aberdeen, Scotland*

HÉLÈNE PETERS, PhD • *Macalaster College, St. Paul, MN*

ROBERT P. PICONE, PhD • *School of Pharmacy, University of Connecticut, Storrs, CT*

MARIO PRICE, PhD • *Senior Pharmacist, James Paget Hospital, Great Yarmouth, Norfolk, UK*

JOVAN RAJS, MD, PhD • *Department of Forensic Medicine, Karolinska Institute, Stockholm, Sweden*

A. S. RELMAN, MD • *Institute of Medicine, Washington, DC*

NICHOLAS REUTER • *Domestic and International Drug Control, Food and Drug Administration, Washington, DC*

HARRIS ROSENKRANTZ, PhD • *Late Director of Toxicology, EG&G Mason Research Institute, Worcester, MA*

FRANZ ROSENTHAL, PhD • *Professor Emeritus, Near Eastern Literature, Yale University, New Haven, CT*

RONALD G. ROSETTI, MD • *University of Massachusetts Medical Center, Worcester, MA*

E. N. SASSENRATH, PhD • *Department of Behavioral Biology, University of California Medical School, San Francisco, CA*

HERBERT SCHUEL, MD • *Department of Anatomy and Cell Biology, State University of New York, Buffalo, NY*

CAROL GRACE SMITH, PhD • *Department of Pharmacology, Uniformed Services University of the Health Sciences, Bethesda, MD*

JOHN E. STAMBAUGH, MD, PhD • *Thomas Jefferson University, Philadelphia, PA*

RICHARD W. STEGER, PhD • *Department of Pharmacology, University of Texas Health Science Center, San Antonio, TX*

KENNETH M. SUTIN, MS, MD • *Department of Anesthesiology, NYU Medical Center, New York, NY*

DONALD P. TASHKIN, MD • *Department of Medicine, UCLA School of Medicine, Los Angeles, CA*

C. A. TASSINARI, MD • *INSERM U6, Marseille, France*

LARS TERENIUS, PhD • *Department of Clinical Neuroscience, Karolinska Hospital, Stockholm, Sweden*

JOSEPH G. TIMPONE, MD • *Georgetown University Medical Center, Washington, DC*

BRIAN F. THOMAS, PhD • *Research Pharmacologist, Research Triangle Institute, Research Triangle Park, NC*

RENAUD TROUVÉ, PhD • *School of Pharmacy, University of Angers, Angers, France*

J. R. TROUNCE, MD • *Department of Clinical Pharmacology, Guy's Hospital Medical School, London, UK*

H. TUCHMANN-DUPLESSIS, MD • *French National Academy of Medicine, Paris, France*

CARLTON TURNER, PhD • *School of Pharmacy, University of Mississippi, MS*

LASZLO URBAN • *Senior Scientist, Sandoz Institute, London, UK*

NORA D. VOLKOW, MD • *Medical Department, Brookhaven National Laboratory, Upton, NY*

LARRY A. WALKER, PhD • *Department of Pharmacology, School of Pharmacy, The University of Mississippi, MS*

PETER G. WASER, MD • *Institute of Pharmacology, University of Zürich, Zürich, Switzerland*

DAVID J. WRIGHT, MD • *Westat, Inc., Rockville, MD*

ARTHUR M. ZIMMERMAN, PhD • *Department of Zoology, University of Toronto, Toronto, Ontario, Canada*

SELMA ZIMMERMAN, MS • *Division of Natural Science, Glendon College, York University, Toronto, Ontario, Canada*

BARRY S. ZUCKERMAN, MD • *Division of Development and Behavioral Pediatrics, Boston City Hospital, Boston, MA*

ROBERT B. ZURIER, MD • *University of Massachusetts Medical Center, Worcester, MA*

Introduction: Marihuana and Medicine— A Historical Review

I

A BRIEF HISTORY OF FOUR MILLENNIA (B.C. 2000–A.D. 1974)

Hélène Peters and Gabriel G. Nahas

ANCIENT TIMES

Cannabis sativa represents one of humankind's oldest cultivated plants, and possibly one of the oldest plants not grown specifically for its food content. It is an Old World plant, unknown to the Western Hemisphere until the 16th century.

Cannabis sativa seems to have originated in the plains of Central Asia, north of the Himalayas. It was known in China nearly 5000 years ago, where it was cultivated for its fiber and the oil in its seeds. *Cannabis* was never widely used as a psychoactive substance in China except during the first two centuries of our era. Later it became considered as a substance to be avoided because it disturbed the equilibrium of the brain and made one "see devils." In the treatment of pain, the Chinese opted for acupuncture and extracts of medicinal plants devoid of psychoactivity.

From China, *Cannabis* migrated to the Indian subcontinent, where it is mentioned in the *Atharva Veda* (2000 BC) as a sacred plant, and it was used in the performance of rituals in temples. Ancient Hindus also hailed the medicinal properties of the plant, which was credited with curing all major ills and creating "vital energy."

From India, the use of *Cannabis* spread to Persia and Assyria in the 8th century BC, where it was known as "quanabu" or "kanabas." Herodotus (*Historiae III*) reports that the barbarian Scythians of the Caspian and Aral Seas intoxicated themselves with vapors from burning hemp *(1)*.

Cannabis was unknown to the ancient Egyptians; there is no mention of it either in hieroglyphic texts or paintings of the Pharaonic era or in the scriptures of the Old Testament; no cloth made of hemp has been found in the ancient Egyptian tombs. Like the ancient Egyptians, the Greeks and the Romans did not use *Cannabis* as a pleasure-inducing drug as they did beer and wine. However, they cultivated hemp for its fiber, and manufactured ropes and sails. The Greek physicians Dioscorides and Galen described the use of hemp for its medicinal properties, but they neglected to mention its intoxicating effects.

The next widespread use of *Cannabis* after India occurred in the Middle East. It started in the wake of the rise of Islam and met little cultural opposition, since the prophet Muhammad forbids the use of wine but not explicitly the derivatives of *Cannabis*. The Arabic name for the *Cannabis* extract used in the Middle East is hashish, which means "grass."

From: *Marihuana and Medicine*
Edited by: G. G. Nahas et al.   © Humana Press Inc., Totowa, NJ

MIDDLE AGES

The Arab invasions of the ninth through the twelfth centuries introduced *Cannabis* preparations into all of North Africa from Egypt to Tunisia, Algeria, and Morocco. Spain was the only conquered land where the habit was not established *(2)*.

During all these centuries, Muslim physicians describe more medicinal use of *Cannabis* than reported by Galen or Dioscorides. The physician al-Razi (900 AD) recommends its use for the ear, for dissolving flatulence, and to cure epilepsy. Another Arab physician al-Badri (1251 AD) recommends hashish to stimulate the appetite and produce a craving for sweets. A 17th century pharmacopeia prescribed hashish for a large variety of ailments and also mentioned the euphoria and lethargy produced by the drug *(3)*.

Muslim scholars and clerics debated for centuries over the conflicting reports of hashish use by the people and finally decided in the 18th century that *Cannabis* for pleasure should be interdicted to the faithful, except for legitimate medical purposes. They claim that the use of hashish, like that of wine, beclouded the mind and prevented the ritual prayer that all Muslims have to perform five times daily. Today, this religious interdiction still prevails in all Islamic countries under penalty of law, which in some countries include the death sentence *(4)*.

CANNABIS AND MEDICINE IN EUROPE

Cannabis was introduced into British medicine by O'Shaughnessy in 1830 *(1)*. He reported, after observing the medical use of the drug in India, its effectiveness in the treatment of rabies, rheumatism, epilepsy, and tetanus. He found it to be an effective analgesic. In England at that time, *Cannabis* extracts from India were prescribed for scores of different ills. According to the records, dosages given were not strong enough to produce psychoactive effects. Many of the physicians noted the extreme variability in potency of *Cannabis* extracts and the difficulty in obtaining replicable effects. With the advent of the availability of more specific medications (aspirin and barbiturates), hemp preparations were no longer prescribed and were dropped from the British pharmacopeia.

In France, the intoxicating properties of *Cannabis sativa* were observed experimentally in 1840 by Jacques-Joseph Moreau, who is regarded as the father of psychopharmacology. Moreau prepared his own hashish. "The flowering tops of imported plants are boiled in water to which fresh butter has been added. The resulting preparation is sweetened with sugar and scented with fruit." Moreau describes in his book *Hashish Intoxication and Mental Illness (1)* the symptoms and feelings that he experienced after the ingestion of about 30 grams of his preparation. Moreau lists the eight cardinal symptoms that are either observed during hashish intoxication or reported by his mental patients. They are unexplainable feelings of bliss, dissociation of ideas, errors of time and space appreciation, exacerbation of the sense of hearing, fixed ideas, disturbances of the emotions, irresistible impulses, and illusions or hallucinations. By a systematic analysis of the symptoms described by mental patients considered in the light of his own observations during hashish intoxication, Moreau became convinced of the primarily organic nature of mental illness.

Moreau's experiences had no follow-up until over 150 years later when they were duplicated by American physicians. The recreational use of *Cannabis* was not adopted by French society at the time when the medical use of opiates and cocaine, which were also diverted for use as pleasure-producing substances, became possible.

MARIHUANA IN THE AMERICAS

Marihuana smoking came to Brazil in the 17th century via the African slaves who where brought to the New World by the Portuguese merchants. The smoking of "riamba" by the

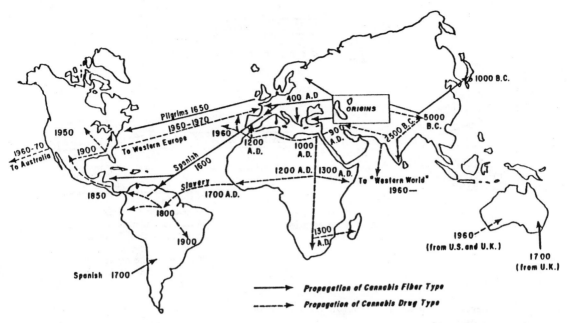

Fig. 1. The propagation of *Cannabis sativa*, drug and fiber type, throughout the ages. (From Fournier [6] 1979, with permission.)

slaves was not adopted by the Portuguese settlers or by the Indians who were disposed to use other, and much more potent, psychoactive substances. It was reported, however, that the last empress of Brazil (1865) was given an extract of *Cannabis* by a devoted black servant to relieve her terminal suffering. By mid century, *Cannabis* use spread beyond Brazil, mostly by sea, along the northern east coast. It reached Central America and Mexico by the end of the 19th century. A century later the use of marihuana as a drug was brought across the border by Mexican workers who settled in Texas and Louisiana.

In the United States, the fiber type of *Cannabis* was cultivated as early as 1720 for manufacture of rope, twine, and sail cloth. The seeds were the source of an oil for soap and paints. But its use for pleasure was unknown.

When "jazz" became popular in New Orleans, marihuana was adopted by black jazz musicians who introduced the drug habit during their concerts along the Eastern seaboard. Otherwise, it was smoked primarily by impoverished black farmers who were singled out as having a "deviant" behavior. In 1937, the Marihuana Tax Act brought *Cannabis* under Federal control, which in effect interdicted its smoking.

Marihuana smoking did not permeate the mainstream of American society until after World War II, during the 1960s, and mostly among university students who used it for its pleasant properties, and not for its medicinal value.

THE MEDICAL USE OF *CANNABIS* EXTRACTS IN THE UNITED STATES

American physicians in the 1850s copied the English in prescribing *Cannabis* for a variety of ills. It was called Tilden's extract of *Cannabis sativa indica*, imported from India. It had the consistency of pitch and an aromatic odor. One to six grains (165–400 mg) were prescribed by physicians for the relief of a variety of ailments ranging from epilepsy, rheuma-

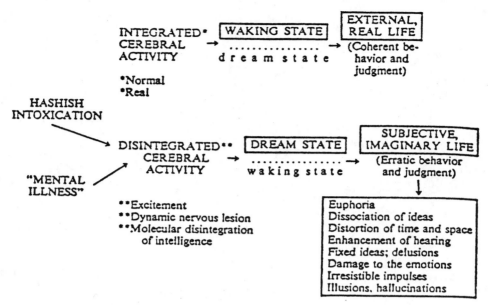

Fig. 2. A schematic representation of Moreau's concept of mental illness, showing its analogy with hashish intoxication. (From ref. *1*.)

tism, menstrual cramps, epidemic cholera, convulsions, chorea, hysteria, depression, insanity, tetanus, gout, neuralgia, and uterine hemorrhage. All of these indications for hemp extract are listed in the 1854 United States dispensary.

It appears that the use of oral medical preparations of hemp was associated with a diversion of its use for its intoxicating properties. Many patent medicines containing Indian hemp were available, and could easily be purchased from local pharmacies or by mail order. One of the most popular elixirs was "a true aphrodisiac made and delivered exclusively by a certain Fred Hollick," a recommendation that led some Americans to experiment on themselves with this remarkable and sought after property ascribed to *Cannabis*. Even Louisa Alcott, the author of *Little Women* describes in *Perilous Play* (1869) the story of a young lady who accepts "sweets" offered by Meredith, who promises they would produce "delicious amusement." She loses her self-control, kisses the doctor and exclaims, "What am I doing? I am mad, for I too have eaten hashish."

Marihuana, in contrast to opiate preparations, was not used during the Civil War, and was used with decreasing frequency during the first part of the 20th century. Marihuana was eliminated from the United States pharmacopeia in 1942.

THE CREATION OF THE NATIONAL INSTITUTE ON DRUG ABUSE (1972)

It was not until the second part of the century that the medical applications of marihuana were investigated as the result of two developments; a renewed vogue of its recreational use and the isolation of the major psychoactive compound present in cannabis, Δ^9-THC *(7,8)*.

This discovery paved the way for scientific investigations of the biological and medical properties of marihuana. In 1972, the U.S. Congress created the National Institute of Drug Abuse (NIDA) to conduct comprehensive health education and training programs for the prevention and treatment of drug abuse. From its inception, NIDA initiated a comprehensive research program to investigate the biological and medical properties of marihuana. NIDA also funded a program of marihuana cultivation to provide researchers with plant material of known THC and cannabinoid content. From this federal plantation in Mississippi, standard marihuana cigarettes and pure cannabinoids were conditioned for scientists in the U.S. and abroad.

THE NIDA SYMPOSIUM OF WILKINSON ISLAND (1974)

NIDA, at the instigation of its director *William Pollin,* organized in the fall of 1974 at Wilkinson Island the largest and most comprehensive medical and scientific symposium on marihuana ever held. Its proceedings were assembled by *Monique Braude* and *Steven Szara,* two of the most seasoned pharmacologists of NIDA, and were reported in two volumes, comprising 863 pages *(9).* The volumes contain 89 papers written by some 300 authors who had all performed experimental or clinical studies with marihuana or THC in the United States, the United Kingdom, Switzerland, Sweden, Greece, and Israel.

Some of the scientists present at this first major symposium on marihuana attended subsequent symposia, and many of their original observations were extended and confirmed. Each contribution was reviewed by the editors and by outside scientists expert in their various disciplines. Most of these studies had either already been published, or appeared subsequently in peer-reviewed journals. The following important contributions from the Wilkinson symposium that are most germane to the subject of the monograph, but that were not reported subsequently in the medical literature, are reported in this monograph.

The following contributions from the Wilkinson symposium that are most germane to the subject but which were not reported subsequently in the medical literature are reported in this monograph:

Waser, P., Martin, A. Analgesic Properties of Cannabinoids, pp. 155–161

Tassinari, C., Ambrosetto, G., Peraita-Adrados, M., Gastaut, H. *The Neuropsychiatric Syndrome of D^9-tetrahydrocannabinol and Cannabis Intoxication in Naive Subjects: A Clinical and Polygraphic Study During Wakefulness and Sleep,* pp. 647–664

Miczek, K. *Does THC Induce Aggression? Suppression and Induction of Aggressive Reactions by Chronic and Acute D^9-Tetrahydrocannabinol Treatment in Laboratory Rats,* pp. 233–241

References

1. Nahas, G. G. (1973) *Marihuana Deceptive Weed.* Raven Press, New York pp. 1–58.
2. Nahas, G. G. Hashish and Islam: 9th to 18th centruy. *Bull. N.Y. Acad. Med.* (1982) **58:**814–831.
3. Rosenthal, F: *The Herb: Hashish versus Medieval Muslim Soceity.* Brill, The Netherlands (1971).
4. Nahas, GG Hashish and Drug Abuse in Egypt during 14th–20th century. *Bull. N.Y. Acad. Med.* (1985) **61:**428–444.
5. Moreau, J: *Hashish and Mental Illness.* Masson, Paris, 1845, translation by Hélene Peters, Raven Press, New York (1973).
6. Nahas, GG: Marihuana in Science and Medicine, in *Botany* Michel Paris, ed. Raven Press, New York (1984), pp. 8–11.
7. Mechoulam, R., and Gaoni, Y. (1965) A total synthesis of *dl*-delta-1tetrahydrocannabinol, the active constituent of hashish. *J. Amer. Chem. Soc.,* **87:**3273–3275.
8. Petrzilka, T., and Sikemeier, C. (1967) Components of hashish II. Synthesis of (-)-delta-6, 1-3, 4 *trans*-tetrahydrocannabinol. *Helv. Chim. Acta.,* **50:**2111–2113.
9. Braude, M and Szara, S: *Pharmacology of Marihuana: A Monograph of the Naitonal Insitute of Drug Abuse,* Raven Press, New York (1976).

II

THE HELSINKI SYMPOSIUM (1975)

The Helsinki Symposium of the Sixth International Congress of Pharmacology held in Helsinki in July of 1975 was organized by Gabriel G. Nahas, William D. M. Paton, and Juhana E. Idanpaan-Heikkila who were editors of the resulting proceedings. This symposium gathered 126 scientists and physicians from the United States, United Kingdom, Canada, France, Sweden, Germany, and Israel who presented 44 papers describing the chemistry, biochemistry, and cellular effects of marihuana. Its proceedings were published in 1976 *(1)*.

WHY ANOTHER MONOGRAPH ON MARIHUANA?

Gabriel G. Nahas

Hasn't this subject been exhausted over the past six years by the publication of the dozen volumes that preceded the present one? After numerous investigations on the acute effects of marihuana smoking in humans described in hundreds of papers, what is left to know? Following the studies of chronic users performed in Boston, Los Angeles, Jamaica, and Greece, hasn't the marihuana question been settled?

Shouldn't we now consider marihuana a "soft drug" to be used for recreational purposes, like alcohol or tobacco, with minimal danger to the user and little damage to society? A number of scientists have already given an affirmative answer to these questions, and their opinions, amplified by the media, seem to be shared by a large section of the lay public. On the other hand, some investigators claim that old empirical observations confirmed by recent scientific evidence indicate that marihuana is a harmful drug. As a result, a great marihuana debate is now raging in the scientific and lay press of the United States. Let us hope that it will not linger as long as the tobacco debate, which was settled only a decade ago.

Meanwhile, the use of marihuana, especially by adolescents, has been spreading exponentially in countries where it was nearly unknown 20 years ago (see Fig. 1). It even seems possible that some countries are prepared to give a new legal status to this drug, thereby eliminating the social stigma attached to its use: marihuana would no longer be considered a "stupefying drug," like opium or coca leaf derivatives, the Single Convention Treaty on Stupefying Drugs would be bypassed, and marihuana products would be made commercially available.

It is against this background that the Helsinki Symposium on Marihuana, which is recorded in this monograph, was organized under the aegis of the Sixth International Congress of Pharmacology. This symposium was called to discuss the biochemical and cellular effects of marihuana products in the general perspective of their long-term use.

Following the work of Agurell, Paton, Lemberger, and Axelrod, investigators established that the fat-soluble cannabinoids remain in tissues for days and weeks.

From: *Marihuana and Medicine*
Edited by: G. G. Nahas et al.   © Humana Press Inc., Totowa, NJ

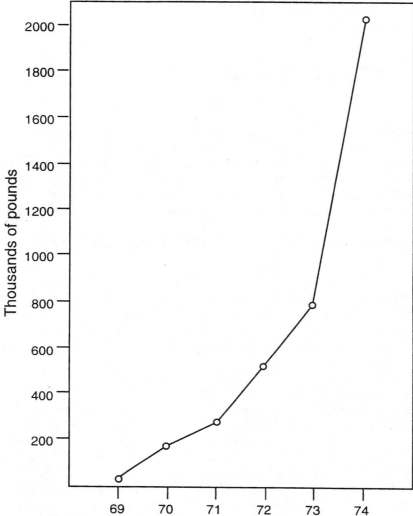

Fig. 1. Removals of marihuana by United States federal authorities. (In order to roughly estimate the amounts consumed, the amounts removed are usually multiplied by six.) From "Hearings of the United States, Senate Committee on the Judiciary (Subcommittee on Internal Security): Marihuana-Hashish Epidemic, Part II, The Continuing Escalation, May 8, 1975," U.S. Government Printing Office, Washington, DC, 1975.

At the same time, Zimmerman, the Leuchtenbergers, Jakubovic, McGeer, Succiu-Foca, Armand, Nahas, and Morishima had independently investigated the effects of marihuana products on cellular anabolism and cell division. A common conclusion emerged from their studies, which employed widely different models: cannabinoids in concentrations of 10^{-6} to 10^{-4} M inhibit the synthesis of DNA, RNA, and proteins in replicating eukaryote cells. Mechoulam's Δ^9-THC and all natural cannabinoids tested–whether psychoactive or not–as well as their metabolites, which accumulated in tissues, inhibited cell anabolism.

These in vitro observations were confirmed in vivo by Rosenkrantz: Rodents given marihuana by ingestion or by inhalation exhibited impairment of growth, spermatogenesis, and the immune system.

A number of investigators reported the inhibitory effect of marihuana in humans on pulmonary macrophages, lymphocyte function, and sperm production.

Although these results await additional confirmation, all of the present experimental evidence tends to corroborate the early in vitro observations, which reported an impairment of cellular anabolism by cannabinoids.

Only longitudinal epidemiological studies of marihuana-smoking populations may document the pathologic effects of long-term *Cannabis* usage. To my knowledge the literature does not contain a single autopsy report on a long-term chronic marihuana smoker. Therefore, the human pathology of marihuana cannot be written before two or three decades. (It took 60 years for investigators to establish the pathology of tobacco smoking.) Meanwhile, on the basis of their present short-term observations and past experience with other drugs, biologists and physicians can only make certain predictions about what this pathology might be.

The papers contained in this monograph, inasmuch as they describe some of the interactions between the biologically active molecules contained in marihuana and the basic components and processes of living cells, might help the biologist and the physician assess the long-term effects of marihuana use on reproduction, embryological development, learning, and growth, as well as on the integrity of physiological functions.

THE IMMUNE RESPONSE AND MARIHUANA

Harris Rosenkrantz

This paper (which is republished on p. 305–316 in this monograph) remains the most thoroughly documented study on the effects of marihuana smoke and of THC on the immune response of rodents. Rosenkrantz was director of the section of pharmacology and toxicology of the Mason Reasearch Institute in Worcester, and performed thoroughly controlled studies on the effects of marihuana on reproductive functions, lung, and immune systems of rodents, under contract with the National Institute on Drug Abuse. References to these papers are given in his paper on the "Immune response and marihuana," and in his paper "Effects of cannabis on fetal development of rodents' (this monograph pp. 411–430).

CONCLUDING SUMMARY

W. D. M. Paton

The analysis of *Cannabis* constituents is far advanced. Even after hearing of an interesting new alkaloid, cannabisativine, one may echo Professor Mechoulam's plea that it may now be time to stop "botanizing," and concentrate instead on the molecular mechanisms of *Cannabis* action. Yet some important analytic problems remain: the chemical genetics of the plant are still not clear, and we still know too little of the pyrolytic changes produced in smoking. These changes may be different if tobacco is or is not mixed with the *Cannabis*, and they could be important biologically.

As to biochemical work and detection and assay in the body, ample reason has been given as to why this is so difficult, from the small quantities present and the multiplicity of metabolites. But there is hope now for a practical radioimmunoassay, which, even if sharp specificity may be hard to achieve, may yet be of great value in clinics, for forensics purposes, or for the research worker wishing to verify claims that *Cannabis* has in fact been taken. Biochemically, if we permute all the possibilities of hydroxylation and subsequent metabolism, we have now almost too many products to disentangle. Yet patterns are beginning to emerge, and we can expect to learn before too long how the choice of metabolic pathway is determined.

The discovery that 3'-hydroxylation of the pentyl side chain gives a highly active product is fascinating–and it makes yet another complication in the correlation of dose and effect. It is interesting, too, that although I recall Professor Mechoulam saying some years ago that he felt the chemists' task was nearly finished, he and his colleagues are as badly needed as ever for preparing authentic samples (labeled or unlabeled) of the putative metabolites. One hopes it will become possible to move from the blood (a vital tissue, but not where the "action" is) to the tissues and to study distribution and kinetics. A technical warning note that the pattern of extracting cannabinoids by different solvents varies with the tissue carries intriguing physicochemical implications.

When one turns to neurochemistry and neuropharmacology, one has–as so often with the pharmacology of the central nervous system–to admit that the field is much less advanced. We have, as it were, too many rather than too few intellectual degrees of freedom. Actions of cannabinoids on the physiology of 5-HT and acetylcholine and on monosynaptic reflex function are now known; but central nervous system changes could also flow indirectly from the effects reported on mitochondria, corticoids, and prostaglandins. Also, there is the question of the relationship to morphine–which is taking on a new aspect with the evidence for "morphinomimetic" peptides in the brain. Patient work is required to distinguish the relative importance of all these substances; perhaps the advances in autoradiography of the brain will help.

The cell biology of *Cannabis*, ranging from toxicology to fundamental molecular mechanisms, is one of the most interesting and most difficult fields. This book has detailed new evidence of effects of *Cannabis* on lymphocytes, fibroblasts and lysosomes, repair mechanisms after radiation, pulmonary macrophages, spermatozoa and the basic histones of sperm and polymorphonuclear leukocytes, cell division in primitive organisms, and the rabbit fetus. As ever, great caution is needed in extrapolating from such studies to consequences for human use; many experiments were performed in vitro; the best evidence must come from much needed epidemiological studies in appropriate communities. But it would be equally rash to ignore this basic work and all its implications.

At the same time, many of these studies in cell biology are taking us toward an understanding of the possible mechanisms of action of THC. *Should one think of a cannabinoid receptor? I prefer the idea of hydrophobic spaces in membranes or macromolecules, the average shape and dimensions of which limit their capacity to accept larger lipophilic molecules. Also, some investigators suspect that the characteristics of the site of action for the more toxic effects may differ from that for psychic effects. In the meantime, there are interesting clues: the variation of potency with small changes in chemical structure and with stereoisomerism; the analogies with some anesthetics, steroids, and vitamin A; and the physiochemical effects on membranes. We can hope that an understanding of the action of* Cannabis *may be more generally applicable and will illuminate lipophilic action on membranes more widely.*

Reference

1. Nahas, G. G., Paton, W. D. M., and Heikkila, I. (1976) *Marihuana: Chemistry and Biological Effects.* Springer, New York.

III

THE REIMS SYMPOSIUM (1978)

The Reims Symposium on marihuana assembled in July of 1978; 127 participants presented 55 papers on the "Biological Effects of Marihuana (Analysis, Metabolism, Cellular Response, Reproduction and Brain)," which were reported in the published proceedings *(1)*. The following papers presented at the symposium have been reprinted in this monograph:

Zimmerman, A., Zimmerman, S. and Raj, A. *Effects of Cannabinoids on Spermatogenesis in Mice.* pp. 347–357.
Huang, H., Nahas, G.G, and Hembree, W.C. *Effects of Marihuana Inhalation on Spermatogenesis of the Rat.* pp. 359–366.
Hembree, W.C., Nahas, G.G., Zeidenberg, P., and Huang H. *Changes in Human Spermatazoa Associated with HIgh-Dose Marihuana Smoking.* pp. 367–378.
Rosenkrantz, H. *Effects of Cannabis on Fetal Development of Rodents.* pp. 411–430.
Dalterio, S., Steger, R., and Bartke A. *Maternal or Paternal Exposure to Cannabinoids Affects Central Neurotransmitter Levels and Reproductive Function in Male Offspring.* pp. 441–447.
Sassenrath, E., Chapman, L.F., and Goo, G.P. *Reproduction in Rhesus Monkeys Chronically Exposed to Delta-9-Tetrahydrocannabinol.* pp. 449–459.
Rosenthal F. *Cannabis and Alcohol—The Green and the Red.* pp. 723–730.

FOREWORD

This symposium, the second satellite symposium on marihuana, like the first satellite meeting in Helsinki in 1975, was the result of international collaboration. Its inclusion as a satellite of the VII Congress of the International Union of Pharmacological Sciences (IUPHAR) was approved following a recommendation of the Congress Programme Committee (J. P. Boissier and P. Lechat). In France, initial grants for the organization of the meeting in Reims were awarded by the Institut National de la Santé et de la Recherche Médicale (INSERM; Camille C. Burg, P. Laudat) and the Ministère de la Santé (Simone Weil, P. Denoix) by the Délégation Générale à la Reserche Scientifique (DGRST) and by the University of Reims (L. Bernard). In the United States, the National Institute on Drug Abuse (NIDA; Robert Dupont, William Pollin) awarded a conference grant to defray the travelling expenses of some of the American participants. The Medical Research Council provided travel expenses from Britain. In addition, grants were provided by the International Business Machines Company, American Telephone and Telegraph Company, Rhodia Incorporated, and the American Council on Marihuana and Other Psychoactive Drugs.

MARIHUANA AND THE CELL

Gabriel G. Nahas

A review of the literature indicates that a great deal of studies on the biological effects of *Cannabis* have been performed since the last symposium held in Helsinki in 1975. Many of

From: *Marihuana and Medicine*
Edited by: G. G. Nahas et al.   © Humana Press Inc., Totowa, NJ

the results that were presented then, have been confirmed and extended in the area of quantitation of cannabinoids, mechanisms of their action, and of their cellular effects on lung, brain, and reproductive organs.

An increasing number of studies have focused on long-term effects of *Cannabis* administration: Because one is dealing with substances with a half-life of the order of one week; their daily consumption should result in tissue levels of the order of the micromole, quite different from the nanomolar concentration required to induce acute intoxication. If cannabinoids have a toxic effect, it would become more apparent as a result of their cumulative storage in the cells.

It is a credit to Harris Rosenkrantz to have established correlation between dosages smoked or ingested by humans and those administered to animals (Table 1). The relevancy of these correlations was proven when blood levels of cannabinoids were measured under such a schedule of administration, and proved to be quite similar in humans and different species studied. *Therefore, one may state that the dosage used in the animal experiments reported in the present monograph are comparable to the doses currently taken by Cannabis users.*

If one wishes to find a common target for all of the multiple effects of cannabinoids described in this volume, one would be tempted to think first of the plasma membrane. The presently accepted view describes this membrane as consisting for the most part of a bimolecular layer of amphipathic lipids and cholesterol overlaid and penetrated by protein molecules, more or less embedded in the lipid matrix. The protein molecules of the membrane are dotted with ion-selective pores and receptor sites with which biologically active molecules will interact.

All pharmacologically active substances must pass through the plasma membrane and thereafter modify intracellular processes in the cytoplasm or some organelles. And many exert their immediate effects by interacting with one of the two major components of the cell membrane envelope: proteins or lipids.

Seeman was one of the first pharmacologists to systematize the way in which the properties of the neuroleptic fat-soluble drugs may be classified into specific and nonspecific, which might be related to their point of impact on the membrane: on the lipid portion or on the protein fraction.

The specific effects of these neuroleptics are based on their stereoselectivity and on their activity recorded with nanomolar concentrations of the drug that will attach to a protein receptor. The nanomolar concentration criterion for specific neuroleptic action refers to the fact that the active concentration of the neuroleptic in plasma water is between 0.1 and 50 nM. Hence, of the many neuroleptic sites proposed, only those affected by nanomolar concentrations (up to 100 nM) would have any likelihood of being truly specific.

Of all the natural cannabinoids, Δ^9 (and perhaps Δ^8-THC) are the only molecules that appear to have a specific activity on or close to a receptor site, for instance, a protein embedded in the lipid matrix of the membrane: They do act in nanomolar concentrations, and stereospecificity is essential for displaying their effects. These specific effects are primarily, if not exclusively, exerted on the neuronal membranes of the brain and of those of the conductive system of the heart.

In addition to these specific effects, neuroleptics also have nonspecific sites of action on the double lipid layer of the plasma membrane. Since neuroleptics are highly fat soluble and surface active, they readily partition into biomembranes. In the case of Δ^9-THC, if the aqueous concentration is 10^{-7} M and the octanol water partition coefficient is 3000, concentration in the plasma membrane phase might be 30 micromolar. It could be expected therefore that such high concentrations within the membrane phase could elicit some nonspecific actions such as membrane expansion and membrane fluidization.

Table 1
Relevancy of Δ^9-Tetrahydrocannabinol Doses and Routes of Administration
Used in Animals as Compared to Humans.

Route[a]	mg/kg Δ^9-THC (marihuana, 1% THC; hashish, 5% THC)		
	Humans[b]	Rat[c]	Mouse[c]
Inhalation, 1 cig/day	0.1–0.5	0.7–3.	5 1–6
3 cigs/day	0.3–1.5	2–10	4–18
6 cigs/day	0.6–3.0	4–20[d]	7–36
Approx. LD_{50}		36–42	40–60[e]
Oral	0.3–1.5	2–10	4–18
	0.9–4.5	6–30	10–54
	1.8–9.0	12–63	20–100
Approx. LD_{50}		800–1200	1400–2200

[a]In human, oral route requires three times the inhalation dose.
[b]Assumes 50 kg mean body weight and 50% loss of THC during smoking.
[c]Dose based on body surface area; conversion factor of 7 and 12 for rat and mouse, respectively.
[d]As a guide, intravenous LD_{50} in monkey was about 100 mg/kg and orally it was estimated to be approximately 15,000 mg/kg.
[e]N value; however, intravenous and inhalation values in rat shown to be nearly identical.
 (Reprinted with permission from: Rosenkrantz, H. [1976] "The immune response and marihuana." In *Marihuana: Chemistry, Biochemistry & Cellular Effects*, Nahas, G., Paton, W. D. M., and J. Idanpaan-Heikkila, eds. Springer Verlag, New York, p. 441.)

Membrane expansion underlies the antihemolytic action of neuroleptics, which in concentrations of 10^{-6} to 10^{-4} M protect erythrocytes from hypotonic hemolysis by increasing the area to volume ratio of the cells. Δ^9-THC and other cannabinoids possess such properties, the concentration of THC required to protect against 50% hemolysis (AH_{50}) is of the order of 10^{-5} M.

Concomitant with membrane expansion, neuroleptics fluidize the membrane, loosening the lipid–protein interactions, increasing the mobility of lipids within the plane of the membrane, as well as permitting water to permeate more readily. As a result, membrane-bound enzyme function may be altered. Several examples of such alterations are included in this monograph. I will present just one instance of a biochemical event that is altered in a similar fashion by neuroleptics: the incorporation of thymidine into cultured lymphocytes. This alteration observed in our laboratory with some cannabinoids and their metabolites was also observed to be a property of other psychotropic drugs (Table 2). The concentration of these drugs required to inhibit by 50% incorporation of thymidine into cultured lymphocytes is well correlated with their octanol water partition coefficient ($p < 0.001$): The more lipophilic a substance, the greater its inhibitory effect. Such a nonspecific effect of these drugs is exerted with micromolar concentrations that may be reached only in daily consumption.

This is especially true for THC and its metabolites that have a prolonged half-life, because of their liposolubility and their enterohepatic recirculation. A daily consumption of 100–400 mg THC equivalent is not uncommon in areas of *Cannabis* cultivation and free availability such as the Blue Hills of Jamaica, the mountains around Ketama in Morocco, or even Ashbury Heights in San Francisco. It would appear that when tolerance develops to psychotropic drugs, the nanomolar concentration required to activate receptor sites is associated with micromolar concentration of these compounds or their metabolites in tissues where they are stored.

Table 2
Daily Dose of Different Psychotropic Drugs, Their Maximal Molar (M)
Plasma Concentration, and Threshold Concentrations Required to Inhibit, in vitro,
Thymidine Incorporation into Cultured Lymphocytes.

	Daily Dose (mg)	Max. Plasma Concentration (M)	"Threshold" IC (M)[a]	IC_{50} (M)[b]	AH_{50} (M)[c]	Log Octanol/ Water Partition Coefficient
Haloperidol	2–30	0.6×10^{-8}	3×10^{-7}	1.1×10^{-5}	2.2×10^{-5}	5.74
Chlorpromazine	200–2000	2.0×10^{-6}	5×10^{-6}	1.3×10^{-5}	1.0×10^{-5}	5.32
Imipramine	50–300	2.5×10^{-6}	3×10^{-5}	4.3×10^{-5}	1.0×10^{-5}	4.62
Δ^9-THC	3.20	4–400	2.0×10^{-7}	5×10^{-6}	3.0×10^{-5}	1.0×10^{-5}
Diazepam	5–30	3.5×10^{-6}	4×10^{-5}	7.8×10^{-5}	4.0×10^{-5}	2.82
Chlordiazepoxide	20–160	6.0×10^{-6}	4×10^{-5}	1.4×10^{-4}	3.0×10^{-4}	2.44
Hydantoin	100–500	9.0×10^{-5}	1×10^{-5}	8.2×10^{-5}	1.5×10^{-3}	2.47
Phenobarbital	30–60	1.3×10^{-4}	8×10^{-4}	1.2×10^{-3}	5.7×10^{-3}	1.42
Meprobamate	400–1200	0.8×10^{-4}	5×10^{-4}	1.7×10^{-3}	–	0.70

[a]"Threshold" inhibiting concentration (producing significant inhibition of thymidine incorporation).
[b]Concentration of drug required to inhibit by 50% incorporation of ^{3}H thymidine.
[c]Concentration of drug to protect against 50% hemolysis.
(Reprinted with permission from *Proc. Soc. Exptl. Biol. Med.* (1979) **160**, 344.)

However, one should not limit the cellular effects of THC (and other cannabinoids) to an inhibition of precursor transport. They are much more far reaching as emphasized in this monograph by Stein, Carchman, and Issidorides who report that the cannabinoids interact with the nucleus, and alter the biosynthesis of chromosomal proteins, such as histones and nonhistones, thereby modifying the expression of the genome. Cannabinoids also interact with hormone-mediated cellular mechanisms.

Such interactions of psychoactive and nonpsychoactive cannabinoids with the fundamental mechanisms of macromolecular synthesis might well account for the biological effects of chronic *Cannabis* administration reported in this monograph: damage to the lung, impairment of spermatogenesis, and alteration of brain ultrastructure.

SUMMARY OF SESSIONS

Quantification of Cannabinoids and Their Metabolites in Body Fluids and Tissues—Pharmacokinetics

D.J. Harvey and R. Bourdon

The high potency of Δ^1-THC and its rapid plasma clearance necessitate the use of highly sensitive methods for quantitation and the most important of these were reviewed briefly. Several specific assays were described in detail. Thin-layer chromatography (TLC) methods were reported to be sensitive and accurate but not always applicable to studies in humans, when, for example, radiolabeled cannabinoids are used. GLC assays can achieve high sensitivity (2 ng/mL) but require extensive purification of the sample. Radioimmunoassay offers the widest scope for rapid results, is sensitive to the low ng/mL range, but is not selective as there is extensive cross reactivity between, for example, Δ^1-THC, other cannabinoids, and several metabolites. This can, however, be advantageous in some clinical and forensic studies where metabolite concentrations are considerable. Where specificity is required, the cannabinoids can be separated by high-performance liquid chromatography (HPLC). A related EMIT assay based on Δ^1-THC antibody inhibition of a THC-mitochondrial malate dehydrogenase complex was described; this was rapid but showed the same limited specificity as the conventional radioimmunoassay. A lower concentration limit of 15 ng/mL was imposed to avoid false positive results. GC-MS methods were reported to be the most specific and sensitive for individual cannabinoids. Although detection limits in the range 0.1–2 ng/mL of plasma are common, extensive sample purification using such techniques as Sephadex LH-20 chromatography limit the number of samples that can be handled. Chemical derivatization is also necessary for high sensitivity with trimethylsilyl derivatives giving the best overall results. Specific assays were presented for Δ^1-THC, CBN, 7-hydroxy-Δ^1-THC, and Δ^1-THC-7-oic acid using deuterated internal standards and 3'-hydroxy-Δ^1-THC using the 7-hydroxy metabolite on a standard. A GC-MS method using an eight-channel peak selector was also described for the semiquantitative measurement of most of the major metabolites of Δ^1-THC present in mouse liver.

Various routes of administration are commonly used for Δ^1-THC but it has been shown that these can lead to widely varying plasma concentrations. This was particularly evident in a study in which plasma levels were studied in the same subject after intravenous, oral, or pulmonary (smoking) administration. Intravenous infusion gives the most reproducible results for acute studies; pulmonary, subcutaneous, and intraperitoneal routes lead to more variable plasma concentrations because of factors such as difficult solubilization and different rates of absorption. The oral route gives the least predictable plasma levels with maximum concentrations considerably lower than those achieved by the other routes. Instability of Δ^1-THC at low pH, variable intestinal absorption, and extensive first-pass metabolism by the liver seem to be the main factors affecting the ultimate plasma levels. Typical maximum plasma levels in human after an intravenous infusion of 4–5 mg of Δ^1-THC are in the range of 50–200 ng/mL. Smoking gives somewhat lower values of around 50–70 ng/mL after two to three minutes for an equivalent dose, whereas after an oral dose of 20 mg, peak plasma levels of only 8–10 ng/mL have been recorded and these occur from 0.5–1.5 hours after administration. Plasma protein binding is extensive, only about 3% of the circulating δ^1-THC is in the free state, the remaining 97% is bound to lipoprotein. 7-Hydroxy-Δ^1-THC binds extensively to albumin.

Plasma levels drop rapidly after the initial peak; for example, in humans a peak concentration of 70 ng/mL measured three minutes after inhaling marihuana smoke had dropped to 5 ng/mL at one hour and 1 ng/mL at four hours. To fit the plasma level-time curves up to five exponentials are needed suggesting at least five body compartments. The terminal elimination phase has a half-life of up to seven days. The 7-hydroxy metabolite shows similar kinetics but its peak plasma concentration is only about 4% of that found for the parent drug. Pharmacokinetic data are lacking for most other metabolites but it appears that δ^1-THC-7-oic acid is eliminated more slowly than the 7-hydroxy metabolite. The observed pharmacokinetics are consistent with rapid uptake of Δ^1-THC into tissues followed by a slow release. Lung, myocardium, adrenal gland, and spleen seem to be the main initial sites for accumulation; fat is also important, but the drug accumulates more slowly, probably because of poor vasculature. Only about 1% reaches the brain, but it has been suggested that higher concentrations of the 7-hydroxy metabolite may be reached although the brain itself does not have the ability to metabolize the drug.

Metabolism of Δ^1-THC by the liver is rapid and complete with several metabolic steps apparently occurring during the first pass. The liver seems to have a high capacity for metabolizing both free and protein-bound drugs. In dogs, the metabolism shows no dose-dependent effects over the range of 0.1–2.0 mg/kg, no saturable metabolic routes, and no enzymic inhibition. In addition, the ratio of metabolites shows little variation with time, consistent with the slow release of Δ^1-THC from tissues. The metabolites are excreted rapidly in feces and urine, but the extensive retention of unmetabolized drug by the tissues results in slow overall elimination. For example, after five days the dog excretes only about 40–45% of an intravenous dose in the feces and a further 15–17% in the urine. Similar patterns have been observed in the rat, monkey, and humans but in the rabbit, the urinary and fecal ratios are reversed. About 10% of the biliary metabolites are enterohepatically recirculated. Only a small percentage of the metabolites appear to be retained by the tissues, for example, in the dog although 16–29% of the administered dose is retained in the tissues after 100 hours, only 11–20% of this has been attributed to metabolites.

Cannabinoids and Cellular Metabolism

J.-C. Jardillier

The effects of different cannabinoids (psychoactive and nonpsychoactive) on several mammalian cells lines are exerted at micromolar concentrations.

ACTION AT THE LEVEL OF THE PLASMA MEMBRANE

These effects are numerous and related in most cases to the lipophilic nature of THC and of its derivatives. Na^+, K^+, and Mg^{++} ATPases are inhibited in vitro with concentration of 10^{-6} M. In vivo, tolerance seems to develop to this effect. The inhibitory mechanism is not the same for all ATPases.

Biosynthesis of membrane phospholipids is also altered as a result of acyltransferase inhibition. The membrane action of cannabinoids is also reflected by their inhibitory effect on intracellular incorporation of the precursors of the biosynthesis of macromolecules such as thymidine, uridine, and leucine. In the case of thymidine inhibition of uptake may be observed within 15 seconds after exposure to 6.5×10^{-5} M THC.

HORMONAL INTERACTIONS AND EFFECTS ON THE NUCLEUS

In vitro, cannabinoids interfere with certain hormone-mediated cellular mechanisms: In Leydig cells, they inhibit testosterone synthesis mediated by choriogonadotropic hormone (HCG) or by dibutyryl cyclic AMP. The inhibitory effect of dexamethasone on the biosynthesis of nucleic acids and proteins is potentiated by cannabinoids. There is no effect of THC at the level of the binding between steroid and cytosol receptor. However, THC facilitates the translocation of the hormone-receptor complex as indicated by a concentration of nuclear material clearly visible in the electron microscope.

At the level of the nucleus, cannabinoids exert certain specific effects in altering the biosynthesis of chromosomal proteins, especially histones and nonhistones.

ACTION ON SPECIALIZED CELLS

The specific functions of certain types of specialized cells may be altered by THC. In neurons, there is a preferential fixation of THC to mitochondria, and a decrease of ribosomes fixed to the nuclear membrane. THC produces biphasic alterations in the neurotransmitters dopamine and norepinephrine, which are related to concentration of the drug: stimulating with nanomolar concentrations, inhibiting with micromolar concentrations.

In myocardial cells cultured in vitro, THC decreases the frequency of contraction and number of "pacemaker" cells. Assorted biochemical changes include alteration of glycolysis and of the activity of several intracellular enzymes.

In micromolar concentrations, which may be reached in chronic consumption, psychoactive and nonpsychoactive cannabinoids alter basic cellular functions including structural and functional properties of the genome. These include condensation of the nucleus and inhibition of chromosomal protein synthesis such as histones.

Cannabis *and Reproduction*

H. Tuchmann-Duplessis

Experimental investigations as well as clinical observations described in the nine papers presented at this session demonstrated the harmful effect of *Cannabis* on the testis, the ovary, and the hypothalamic-pituitary axis. These investigations also describe the developmental effects of cannabis in rodents and primates.

TESTIS

In rodents, Δ^9-THC and cannabidiol significantly decrease testosterone and impair spermatogeneis. Such effects may be related to a direct effect of cannabinoids on the gonads through a decrease in RNA synthesis, and also to an inhibition by THC of the gonadotropin function of the pituitary.

OVARY

Ovarian function is also inhibited. In the female rhesus monkey, THC produces a dose-related depression of ovarian function, with a decrease in gonadotropic function, with a decrease in gonadotropic hormones, LH and FSH. During the luteal phase, THC administration impairs progesterone production and produces anovulatory cycles. In rodents, THC or *Cannabis* extract induces ovarian and uterine atrophy.

PRENATAL DEVELOPMENT

Different cannabinoids are embryotoxic and produce fetal resorptions in rats, mice, and rabbits, but they are not grossly teratogenic. When THC is administered before mating to female rhesus monkeys, the incidence of abortion and neonatal mortality is three to four times higher than in control animals. The offspring from THC-treated mothers present abnormal behavior to sensory stimuli.

CLINICAL OBSERVATION

In humans, one observes a depression of reproductive functions with intermittent decrease of testosterone and presence of morphologic abnormalities of spermatogenesis.

Although considered by some as a soft, if not innocuous drug, *Cannabis* is undoubtedly harmful to humans.

The papers and lively discussions of this session resulted in a clear picture of a problem that had gave rise to contradictory statements.

Cannabis *and the Brain*

In this session, 14 reports were presented on the effects of *Cannabis* on the central nervous system.

Experimental results have shown catecholamine changes in the brains of self-stimulated rats, EEG changes (from deep electrodes in the limbic area) in chronically treated rats and monkeys as well as behavioral changes. Following repeated administration, tolerance and withdrawal can be observed in animals as well as humans.

Clinical results have shown that cannabinoids affect epilepsy. Electroencephalographic studies have placed *Cannabis* in the psychotropic group of "psychodysleptics" according to the classification of Delay and Deniker.

CATECHOLAMINES

Rats with implanted electrodes and stimulated in the reward system described by Olds, showed (one hour after THC administration) a decrease in brain norepinephrine, an increase in brain serotonin, together with a decrease of the rate of self-stimulation. This was followed by a rebound with reversal of the effects and later on by a persistent depression. Mescaline produced the same effects.

ELECTROPHYSIOLOGICAL AND NEUROANATOMICAL EFFECTS

In rats treated for nine months with THC, or monkeys after three months exposure to marihuana via a "smoking machine," permanent subcortial EEG changes can be observed in limbic structures and sensory thalamic nuclei. "Irritative" tracings, with sharp high amplitude waves appear. After five months of marihuana smoking, limbic brain tissues of a monkey, examined by electron microscopy, presented ultrastructural abnormalities.

BEHAVIORAL EFFECTS

Rats, following six months of chronic treatment by THC or ethanol, have presented impairment of learning curves. Following two to three months of THC treatment, monkeys living in a colony became withdrawn and showed immobility and a tendency to isolation. After longer treatment they became very aggressive and were apparently unable to cope with the demand of a new stressful situation.

TOLERANCE AND WITHDRAWAL

Tolerance following *Cannabis* has been observed in mice, rats, pigeons, dogs, and monkeys as well as in humans. A crossed tolerance exists between THC and cannabidiol, THC and diphenylhydantoin or phenobarbital, THC and ethanol, and THC and morphine. A withdrawal symptom can be obtained after three to eight weeks in THC self-injected monkeys and in humans after 10 to 21 days of chronic administration. THC diminishes an experimental withdrawal syndrome induced in rats but this effect is not reversed by naloxone. There is no cross-tolerance between THC and LSD or mescaline. In humans, cutaneous sensitivity to pain is enhanced after THC and the reverse is observed for visceral pain.

EFFECTS IN EPILEPSY

THC can precipitate epileptic fits. In clinical trials cannabidiol showed antiepileptic properties similar to diphenylhydantoin.

EFFECTS ON HUMAN EGG AND MEMORY

Electroencephalographic changes following small doses of THC have revealed quick shifts of vigilance between states of arousal and drowsiness. Subjects have presented body image changes together with visual hallucinations or states of "reverie" associated with intensely vivid imagery. At increasing doses, the psychodysleptic properties of *Cannabis* are enhanced. The quantitative EEG profile of *Cannabis* places it in a subgroup of "euphoriants" within the group of psychodysleptics such as morphinomimetics and hallucinogenic psychotropic drugs. Recall memory was also impaired. Acute and chronic *Cannabis* intoxication is accompanied by abnormal brain function and behavior.

CONCLUDING SUMMARY

W. D. M. Paton

In the three years since the Helsinki meeting, how has knowledge advanced?

1. One can recognize some simplifications. At that meeting, much work was reported on cannabinoid metabolites, and the number of these has further increased. Yet it appears now that, for psychic action in humans at least, it is only Δ^1-THC itself, and perhaps the first metabolite, 7-OH-THC, that contribute significantly; side-chain hydroxylation does not appear to occur in humans. In animals, however, a contribution particularly by the 3′-hydroxyl metabolite must be allowed for. The kinetics of THC in vivo are clearer too. The slow elimination of its metabolites is the result, not of slow metabolism, but because Δ^1-THC (and perhaps 7-OH-THC) is early sequestered and then only gradually released from the deep compartments of the body. Since metabolism is rapid and not rate-limiting, changes in metabolism are unlikely to influence duration of action, although obesity might do so. Daily dosage will lead to body levels 5–10 times higher than a single dose, a "cumulation factor" similar to that estimated from toxicity studies. The clinical assay of urinary or blood cannabinoids is also at last proving accessible; and a relatively simple radioimmunoassay has been proved able to show an association of *Cannabis* with traffic accidents, to distinguish *Cannabis* intoxication from other conditions, and to reveal *Cannabis* use up to 30–50% in addiction treatment clinics. Finally, the "surface-area" rule for calculating equivalent doses in various species, a rule that appeared probable both in principle and from the pharmacological data, has been directly verified by the measurement of cannabinoid blood levels. Rats and mice need, respectively, a dosage by weight about 7 and 12 times higher than humans for equivalent effect, and oral dosage appears about five times less effective than inhalation. These important results confirm the relevance, questioned from time to time on grounds of excessive dosage, of a great deal of experimental work.

2. The question of the "specificity" of the various actions of the cannabinoids remains complicated. Several aspects are involved. Thus any effect that could be strongly correlated with the characteristic psychic activity would be a valuable clue to the mechanism of that action and to a possible "receptor"; on the other hand, effects that correlate simply with partition coefficient into lipid (or some equivalent parameter) could be regarded as strictly nonspecific and comparable to anesthesia. An elegant example of the former is the manner in which Δ^1-THC is 1000 times, and 7-OH-$\Delta^{1(6)}$-THC about 10 times more active in inhibiting lysophosphatidylcholineacyltransferase in mouse brain synaptosomes than predicted from their antihaemolytic potency (a measure of nonspecific action), whereas cannabinol and cannabigerol fell in line with the series of alkanols. In contrast, the ability of the cannabinoids, in higher concentrations, to inhibit the uptake of thymidine in cultured lymphocytes appears to be directly related to fat solubility. Depression of the electrically evoked twitch of the guinea-pig ileum proves to correlate as well with the psychic action of cannabinoids as it does with opiate analgesic action. But with other responses anomalies appear, such as cannabidiol or cannabigerol being unexpectedly active, on dopamine uptake into mouse cortex synaptosomes and on nuclear membrane-attached ribosomes in infant rat brain, respectively. The possibility exists that particular cannabinoids may have their own specific actions, as exemplified by the clear superiority of cannabidiol over other cannabinoids in controlling epilepsy. A difficulty results, therefore, as to what substances to employ as controls for "specificity" of action: CBN, CBD, (+)-Δ^1-THC, (+)-Δ^6-THC, and Δ^7-THC have been used for this purpose. Δ^7-THC, indeed,

may be particularly suitable, since it is especially close to Δ^1-THC instructure, yet it is psychically inactive (an important fact about the THC receptor) and does not form 7-OH-Δ^1-THC. But because other cannabinoids are beginning to reveal characteristic actions, noncannabinoid controls may sometimes be advisable.

3. At the neuronal level, the available evidence about THC action remains tantalizing. It is true that when effects on higher function are studied, as in the discussion of memory and the interaction with the limbic system in this volume, reasonably coherent pictures emerge. The introduction of sensory decision theory into study of the effects of *Cannabis* on pain sense is a useful development, showing (for Hardy-Wolff-type pain) increase both in discriminability and response bias. Tolerance to this pain enhancement develops in parallel with tolerance to the "high." Extension of studies of social behavior from rodents to primates is also welcome; irritability seen in rodents with long-term treatment reappears, alterations in dominance hierarchy develop, and socially adaptive behavior may be impaired. At a simpler level, it appears reasonable to attribute the central stimulant effects of *Cannabis* to generation of hypersynchronous neural discharge, but how this is brought about is still unsettled. Δ^1-THC depresses rewarding self-stimulation behavior, and tolerance develops to this. But we cannot yet reliably link these results to definite neurochemical changes. The curious relation of Δ^1-THC to opiates remains: totally different chemical structures; a number of shared effects; a number of interactions with naloxone; and curious patterns of crosstolerance, never fully reciprocal, and varying with the test used. The suggestions that THC may change the affinity of opiates or of related endogenous peptides for their receptors, or that they release such peptides, deserve detailed study. But we still lack any well-defined type of neurochemical action by Δ^1-THC as a basis for all these effects. Although we must recognize radical differences between THC and general anaesthetics, perhaps it is the case that the actions of both of them are to be defined not in terms of specific transmitters, but in terms of some other characteristic of the components of synapses such as size, geometry, or membrane composition.

4. A notable feature has been the development of work in three interlocking fields: the effects of cannabinoids on spermatogenesis, on endocrine activity, and on fetal development. Three mechanisms for an effect on sperm formation are suggested: in mice the development of abnormal sperm heads, and increased ring and chain chromosomal translocation in spermatocytes, could imply a direct action on germ cells; impairment of testosterone production by isolated Leydig cells stimulated by human chorionic gonadotrophin may be connected with reduced protein synthesis; and there is a reduction of the cytochrome P-450 of rat testis microsomes (required for testosterone synthesis), possibly because of a fall in gonadotrophin level. Chronic high doses of *Cannabis* by inhalation can lead to a fall in sperm count in both rats and man. These effects do not appear to correlate with psychic potency. More work is needed to disentangle the roles of reduced gonadotrophins, directly impaired testosterone production, or direct cellular effects.

An important finding is that reduction by THC of gonadotrophin blood levels, suggested also by the fall in uterine and ovarian weights in Fischer rats after THC treatment, has been demonstrated by radioimmunoassay in the rhesus monkey. This inhibition appears to be at hypothalamic level since it is overcome by luteinizing-hormone-releasing factor. No evidence was found of direct estrogenic or anti-estrogenic activity by THC.

The embryotoxicity of THC and *Cannabis* is now established in the rodent and rhesus monkey, at dose levels corresponding to heavy or moderately heavy chronic marihuana use in the human. Frank teratology was not found in the studies reported here. Midgestational vaginal bleeding in the rodent suggested a direct endometrial effect, with impairment of fetoplacental circulatory development, and gross placental infarction was noted in one instance when a rhesus placenta was obtained; but a failure of endocrinological support also remains a possible cause.

In each field, considerably more endocrinological work is needed, particularly to distinguish actions caused directly by cannabinoids on a target organ from actions of neuroendocrine origin.

5. Two important pulmonary studies were reported in rodents exposed to marihuana smoke. Sustained exposure to doses giving plasma Δ^1-THC levels similar to those found in human users induced a focal pneumonitis progressing to rather serious pathological changes, including focal granulomata and cholesterol clefts; these effects were distinct from those of placebo and tobacco smoke. In the other study, both marihuana and tobacco smoke were shown to impair the lung's antibacterial defenses; the half-time for inactivation of staphylococci in the lung was increased from 3.5 to 4.3 hours by tobacco smoke and to 7.5 hours by marihuana. The latter observation may be related to the immobilization of alveolar macrophages by THC reported at Helsinki. Since deep inhalation and retention of marihuana smoke is necessary for efficient extraction of THC, further pulmonary study is important.

6. Finally, two studies may be mentioned which, like the work on nuclear membrane-attached ribosomes, carry the analysis down to the ultrastructural level. First, at Helsinki, a number of electrophysiological abnormalities were found in recordings from the brains of monkeys chronically exposed to *Cannabis* smoke, and these persisted up to six months after exposure ceased. Ultrastructural abnormalities have now been found to develop under these conditions; these included widening of synaptic gaps, clumping of synaptic vesicles, disorganization of rough endoplasmic reticulum, and nuclear inclusion bodies. Changes were most pronounced in the septal region, next in hippocampus and amygdala, least in cortex. Secondly, at Helsinki, reduction of arginine-rich and increase of lysine-rich histories in leukocytes and spermatozoa of chronic hashish users was reported, with accompanying structural changes. In polymorphs and lymphocytes, abnormal condensation of chromatin and reduction in number of nuclear pores has now been found. Lysine-rich HI histone acts as a condensing factor in somatic cells repressing genomic expression, so that impaired lymphocyte function would be expected. In the spermatozoon, in which arginine-rich protamine replaces the lysine-rich histories and achieves total condensation of the protamine, acrosomes were abnormal or even absent, and chromatin condensation was incomplete. The suggestion is made, therefore, that a single biochemical lesion, arginine-depletion, may be responsible, by cell-specific mechanisms, both for lymphocyte and spermatozoal abnormalities. More generally, interference with cell histories may well underlie the varied chromosomal abnormalities that have now been reported under diverse experimental conditions. The correlation of ultrastructural and functional studies in these ways may be of considerable value.

In conclusion, one may ask what answers may be given to three questions:

How does Δ^1-THC produce its effects? The idea that in low doses it acts on a receptor and in higher doses acts less specifically is becoming probable. High potency and loss of activity with optical isomers or small changes in chemical structure point strongly to some special recognition site, whether it is a conventional receptor or some especially well-fitting hydrophobic site. The less specific actions, now extending over a wide range, are of particular significance for the chronic user.

Does *Cannabis* cause damage to the body? The phrase used in the summary of the session on reproduction, "incontestablement nocif," is justified. Studies with chronic administration reveal long-term damage to lungs, reproductive function, and the immune system. The fact that cannabinoids are cumulative accentuates the risk. Now that structural changes in the central nervous system have been described that outlast exposure to the drug, the reversibility of the effects of long-term use, including that on memory, comes into question. The development of a simple clinical test for cannabinoids in blood and urine should help in quantifying the risks.

Is *Cannabis* addictive? Tolerance occurs to the psychic action, as well as to many other effects. Characteristic withdrawal symptoms develop; these are the more striking in that, because of the slow elimination of *Cannabis* from the body, withdrawal from the tissues must be slow. Psychic dependence is shown by the fact that consumption is not merely to avoid withdrawal symptoms but to maintain the psychic effect: to quote from the study on pain and memory, as tolerance developed, "the subjects were complaining that the cigarettes were no longer producing a high." *Cannabis* satisfies the usual criteria for an addictive drug.

The three fundamental questions concerning the mechanism of action, human toxicity, and addictive property of marihuana were given the proper answers in 1978 by Professor Paton. This monograph, twenty years later, confirms their pertinence and timeliness.

This chapter's excerpts are reprinted with permission from the publisher and the authors.

Reference

1. Nahas, G.G., Paton, W.D.M., Braude, M., Jardillier, J.C., Harvey, D.J. (1979) *Marihuana: Biological Effects (Analysis, Metabolism, Cellular Response, Reproduction and Brain)*. Pergamon Press, New York.

IV

CONFLICTING REPORTS ON MARIHUANA AND HEALTH (1981–1982)

THE AMA AND WHO REPORTS (1981)

During the 1970s, the Research Institute of the University of Mississippi, Pharmacological Sciences, under the direction of Coy Waller and Carlton Turner, undertook the monumental task of collating and annotating all research papers on marihuana published between 1964 and 1979. They assembled 5715 entries in two dictionary-sized volumes. Three independent scientific bodies made a general evaluation of these findings: the Scientific Council of the American Medical Association (AMA, 1981), a task force from both the World Health Organization and the Addiction Research Foundation of Toronto (WHO-ARF, 1981), and the Institute of Medicine (IOM), National Academy of Sciences, 1982.

All three groups expressed their great concern about the extensive use of marihuana, especially among the young, but they reached different conclusions from the documents examined. The most forceful statement came from the Council of the AMA: "Marihuana is a dangerous drug. A growing body of evidence from both animal and human studies and from clinical observations attests to its deleterious effects on behaviour, performance, and functioning of various organ systems (lung, heart, brain, reproductive organs)."

The WHO-ARF report noted in man the respiratory toxicity of cannabis, the development of tolerance and dependence, the vulnerability of adolescents "undergoing rapid developmental changes" and of patients with a variety of diseases such as "various forms of mental illness, cardiovascular disease, and epilepsy." The same report stated that the *Cannabis* effects on the hormonal, reproductive, and immunological states of the users is unclear, but it added, "The results of experimental studies in animals have consistently demonstrated toxicity at doses comparable to those consumed by humans smoking *Cannabis* several times a day. Respiratory Toxicity, CNS (brain) dysfunction, endocrine disturbances, reproductive defects, and suppression of immunity have all been observed after treatment with THC or cannabinoids."

THE INSTITUTE OF MEDICINE (IOM) MARIHUANA AND HEALTH REPORT (1982)

The report of the Institute of Medicine, the most prestigious medical organization in the United States, associated with the National Academy of Sciences, was much more qualified. It stated: "Marihuana has a broad range of psychological and biological effects, some of which (at least under certain conditions) are harmful to human health. Unfortunately, the available information does not tell us how serious this risk may be."

The chairman of the I.O.M. Committee, Arnold Relman, editor of *The New England Journal of Medicine*, concluded in a special editorial the journal *"The verdict of the experts is that*

From: *Marihuana and Medicine*
Edited by: G. G. Nahas et al.   © Humana Press Inc., Totowa, NJ

there is no verdict. Marihuana cannot be exonerated as harmless, but neither can it be convicted of being as dangerous as some have claimed." The text of this editorial follows.

MARIHUANA AND HEALTH

A.S. Relman

Of all the illicit drugs available in this country, marihuana is by far the most widely used and the most controversial.

During the late '60s and early '70s, "pot" was the symbol of the drug counterculture, but its use has increased so much recently, particularly among middle-class adolescents and young adults, that smoking marihuana has become almost a social norm. By 1979 more than 50 million Americans had tried it at least once. In 1981, 7% of the high school seniors surveyed said that they used it daily, and 46% said they had used it at least once during the past 12 months. In 1980, a worldwide survey of United States military personnel on active duty revealed that 5% used marijuana daily and 26% had used it at least once within the past 30 days. Frequent use among high school students is now declining, but there are still more high school seniors who smoke "pot" daily than drink alcohol daily or abuse any substance other than tobacco daily.

Although marihuana is used much more than other illicit psychotropic drugs, the risks associated with it are far less clear. These two facts are probably related. Marihuana has gained popularity in part because it is relatively cheap and available, but the major reason is that there is no consensus about its dangers. Many people believe that marihuana can be used in moderation as a "recreational drug" without risk to health, but there are many others who consider it dangerous. This uncertainty has generated a long-standing debate and continues to pose a difficult problem for public policy. The federal government expends considerable resources in attempting to prevent the entry of marihuana into this country, but state laws against its cultivation, sale, possession, and use vary greatly in their severity, and local enforcement of the laws is uneven. In recent years there have been several authoritative reports on the health effects of marihuana in the United States *(1–3)*, but scientific controversy and public confusion have not abated. Those convinced that marihuana is relatively harmless and that it should therefore be legalized are still in acrimonious debate with those equally persuaded of its hazards and of the necessity for maintaining or strengthening prohibitive laws.

With the hope of providing a fresh and unbiased assessment, the Department of Health and Human Services in 1980 contracted with the Institute of Medicine (IOM) of the National Academy of Sciences for a detailed, critical review of the available scientific information about the health effects of marihuana. The IOM appointed a committee, of which I was a member, to carry out this task and prepare a report that would evaluate and summarize all the evidence in a readable and not overly technical way. The intent was to help private citizens make their own informed decisions about marihuana and to provide a factual basis for future government actions, but not to deal with issues of law or public policy.

After more than a year of study, the IOM's committee has completed its report, called *Marijuana and Health*, which was made public on February 26 by the National Academy of Sciences *(4)*. The verdict of the experts is that there is no verdict. The report concludes that marihuana cannot be exonerated as harmless, but neither can it be convicted of being as dangerous as some have claimed. In its painstaking review of the published data, the committee found much reason to worry about the widespread use of the drug—particularly among the young—but not enough hard evidence to answer many important questions about the extent of the risk.

Some of the findings in the report are the following: Marihuana has acute dose-related effects on mood, perception, and psychomotor coordination. Driving and other machine-operating skills may therefore be seriously affected. It impairs short-term memory and slows learning. Depending on the dose of the drug and the underlying psychological condition of the user, marihuana may cause transient episodes of confusion, anxiety, or even frank toxic delirium. Case reports suggest that it may exacerbate pre-existing mental illness; patients with a history of schizophrenia may be particularly at risk. Although there are no controlled studies, the committee suggests that patients should be warned of this possibility.

The report finds no convincing evidence that prolonged use causes permanent changes in the human nervous system or permanent effects on behavior or brain function. Long-term relatively heavy use may be associated with behavioral disorders and a kind of chronic ennui called the "amotivational syndrome," but the available data do not establish whether use of the drug is a cause or a result of this condition. Tolerance to many of the psychological and physical effects of marihuana develops readily, and relatively mild, transient symptoms occur on withdrawal, indicating that the drug can lead to physical dependence. There is no evidence, however, that marihuana causes addiction to the extent that narcotics do, or that physical dependence has a significant role in the persistent use of the drug.

The committee finds good evidence that marihuana stresses the circulation by increasing heart rate and sometimes blood pressure, but believes that this is likely to be of concern only in patients with underlying cardiovascular disease. Acute exposure to marihuana smoke generally elicits bronchodilation, and prolonged heavy use of the drug causes chronic bronchitis and preneoplastic changes in the airways, similar to the changes produced by tobacco smoke. Since marihuana smoke has many of the components of tobacco smoke, the committee thinks that prolonged heavy smoking of marihuana would probably lead to cancer of the lungs and serious impairment of pulmonary function. The committee carefully points out, however, that there is so far no direct confirmation of this inference.

One of the most important constituents of marihuana, Δ^9-tetrahydrocannabinol, appears to have a small, reversible suppressive effect on the number and motility of human sperm, but there is no proof that it affects male fertility. Although effects on female hormonal function have been reported, the committee says the evidence is not convincing. Marihuana interferes with ovulation in monkeys, but no satisfactory studies of its effects on female fertility and childbearing in human beings have been carried out. Marihuana readily crosses the placental barrier, but there is no evidence as yet of overt teratogenic or other deleterious effects on the fetus. However, the committee cautions that the available data do not exclude the possibility of low-frequency or late-developing effects. Although the evidence is conflicting, the committee concludes that marihuana probably does not break human chromosomes but may affect chromosome segregation during somatic-cell division, resulting in aneuploidy. As yet there is no evidence that this effect is clinically important. The drug may also have a mild immunosuppressant effect, but apparently not enough to be of clinical importance.

The report also examines the evidence on the therapeutic potential of marihuana: Preliminary studies suggest that marihuana, its constituents, or its derivatives may be useful in the acute treatment of glaucoma, in the control of the severe nausea and vomiting caused by cancer chemotherapy, in the treatment of asthma, and possibly also in selected types of seizure disorders and spastic conditions. In all these disorders, the available evidence is incomplete and much more work is needed. The troublesome psychotropic and cardiovascular effects of marijuana and its derivatives limit its therapeutic application, particularly in the elderly. The committee believes that the greater promise probably lies in the development of synthetic analogs that may have greater therapeutic ratios than the marihuana derivatives now available.

In summary, the committee attempted to provide a balanced and careful assessment of what we know and do not know about marihuana and health. It ought to be useful to physicians, the general public, and anyone else interested in the facts. As could almost have been predicted, the report finds the present truth to lie somewhere between the extremes, thus giving no comfort to the zealots on either side of the argument. The IOM committee was not asked to suggest policy but it did come up with numerous suggestions for the kinds of research studies the Federal government may wish to support if it is interested in getting more answers. It is astonishing how few of the really important questions can be answered at present.

In the meantime, as in so many situations in which the hard facts are few and uncertainties prevail, we will have to do the best we can. At present the use of marihuana is prohibited in most states. Even if it become generally legalized, prudence and common sense would dictate that its nontherapeutic use be discouraged.

Reprinted with permission from *The New England Journal of Medicine* **306:**603–605, 1982.

References

1. Tinklenberg, J. R., ed. (1975) *Marijuana and Health Hazards: Methodological Issues in Current Research.* Academic, New York.
2. Department of Health, Education and Welfare, Public Health Service. (1980) *Marijuana and Health. 8th Annual Report to the Congress from the Secretary of Health, Education and Welfare, 1980.* Government Printing Office Washington, DC, (DHEW publication no. [ADM] 80–945).
3. American Medical Association. (1980) *Report of the Council on Scientific Affairs. Marijuana in the '80s.* American Medical Association, Chicago.
4. Committee to study the health-related effects of cannabis and its derivatives. National Academy of Sciences, Institute of Medicine. (1982) *Marijuana and Health.* National Academy Press, Washington, DC.

THE CONTROVERSY LINGERS ON

The three scientific groups (AMA, WHO, IOM) were in agreement that more research was required to document health hazards of marihuana use in humans, mainly in the form of long-term epidemiological studies similar to those performed on tobacco smokers. But recommendations for long-term controlled research, especially on adolescents, raise an ethical dilemma because they imply that *Cannabis* will continue to be used (illegally) at its present rate by millions of young people, and that a significant fraction of them will develop the pathologic lesions necessary for documenting (to the satisfaction of the IOM's criteria, that is) the damaging effects of the drug. Surely modern science might have designed a less arduous task to prove damaging effects in humans of a potentially toxic substance.

As far as the therapeutic potential of marihuana is concerned, the three groups of experts recognized the use of cannabinoids (marihuana chemicals) in the treatment of glaucoma, nausea caused by cancer chemotherapy, and convulsive disorders, but they agreed that a final appraisal of therapeutic usefulness would require more investigation.

Because of the IOM's ambiguous position, the three groups could not speak with one voice on the main issue of marihuana's health hazards. Their conflict raises a crucial question: Is the IOM's required scientific standard of evidence the most appropriate one? Should one discard as anecdotal all historical and clinical evidence that has led the League of Nations and the United Nations to recommend the banning of marihuana from general consumption? Should one overlook the studies on animals and primates that demonstrate toxicity? The FDA has banned scores of drugs, cosmetics, and food additives on the basis of far less experimental evidence.

The scientific controversy could go on for years because the human pathology of mari-huana cannot be written before two or three decades of systematic research: it took 60 years to establish the pathology of tobacco smoking, and only in 1968 was the damaging effect of alcohol on fetal growth established scientifically by Lemoine of the University of Paris who merely confirmed observations made since recorded history. Taking the tobacco story as a precedent, what would happen if and when actual pathological proof of damage ends the sci-entific controversy over marihuana? Will such scientific proof also end the social controversy that has raged since the dawn of mankind, pitting as it does the desires of the individual against the rules of society?

The National Organization for the Reform of Marihuana Laws (NORML) gave the Insti-tute of Medicine Report high marks for its usefulness and objectivity, but many practicing physicians, educators, and parents were disappointed. An important warning in the report's conclusion is, however, a redeeming factor: "What little we know for certain about the effects of marihuana on human health, and all that we have reason to suspect, justifies serious national concern." Dust had barely settled on the controversy created by the IOM's report when an additional document was released by the Committee on "substance abuse and habit-ual behavior" of the National Research Council, an advisory body to the National Academy of Sciences. This committee was heavily weighted with sociologists and legal experts (like John Kaplan, also a member of the advisory committee of NORML), adepts at the Linde-smith philosophy of free access to drugs. Not surprisingly, their report, coming after four years' deliberation, recommended the "decriminalization" of marihuana, based on the "social and law enforcement costs" created by total prohibition, and on the assumption that "decrim-inalization" would not increase consumption. And yet the Committee's own report indicates that during the decade when 11 states formally decriminalized marihuana, and others adopted a policy of *de facto* decriminalization, regular marihuana use tripled among adoles-cents and doubled among young adults. Although careful to analyze the policy costs of law enforcement to prevent marihuana use, the Committee neglected to assess the health costs resulting from marihuana use by millions of adolescents and adults.

After analyzing the report of the National Research Council, the President of the National Academy of Sciences, Frank Press, took the unusual step of publicly stating his personal dis-agreement. Press wrote: "My own view is that the data available to the Committee were insuf-ficient to justify on scientific or analytical grounds changes in current policies dealing with the use of marihuana … I am concerned that the committee may have gone beyond its charge in stating a judgement so value laden that it should have been left to the political process."

THE WARNING OF SURGEON GENERAL C. EVERETT KOOP (1982)

In the midst of these claims and counterclaims, the Surgeon General of the United States Public Health Service, C. Everett Koop, spoke out.

The Surgeon General is the chief medical officer in the nation. One of his responsibilities is to monitor outbreaks of infectious diseases in order to take measures necessary to stop their spread. Besides the control of infectious diseases, he is also concerned about the use of any substance that might be damaging to public health. At his desk "the buck stops" for health-related matters.

For this reason, in 1963 the Surgeon General issued the first warning about the damaging effects of chronic tobacco smoking on the lung and emphasized the risk that smokers had of developing lung cancer. His historical pronouncement ended decades of "scientific" contro-versy and paved the way for a vast campaign that has underscored the health hazards of tobacco smoking.

Thus, in the summer of 1982, after reviewing the evidence concerning marihuana, the Surgeon General issued the following warning: "As Surgeon General, I urge other physicians and professionals to advise parents and patients about the harmful effects of using marihuana and to urge discontinuation of its use.

"The health consequences of marihuana use have been the subject of scientific and public debate for almost 20 years. Based on scientific evidence published to date, the Public Health Service has concluded that marihuana has a broad range of psychological and biological effects, many of which are dangerous and harmful to health.

"Marihuana use is a major public health problem in the United States. In the past 20 years, there has been a 30-fold increase in the drug's use among youth. More than one-quarter of the American population has used the drug. The age at which people first use marihuana has been getting consistently lower and now is most often in the junior high school years. In 1978, nearly 11% of high school seniors used the drug daily, and although this figure declined to 7%, daily use of marihuana is still greater among this age group than that of alcohol. More high school seniors smoke marihuana than smoke cigarettes. The current use (during the previous 30 days) of marihuana is 32%; 29% smoke tobacco.

"On March 24, Secretary Schweiker transmitted to the United States Congress a report reviewing the health consequences of marihuana use. *Marihuana and Health: 1982*, the ninth in a series, is primarily based on two recently conducted comprehensive scientific reviews on the subject: one by the Institute of Medicine of the National Academy of Sciences, and the other by the Canadian Addiction Research Foundation for the World Health Organization. Both independent reviews corroborate the Public Health Service's prior findings of health hazards associated with marihuana use: acute intoxication with marihuana interferes with many aspects of mental functioning and has serious acute effects on perception and skilled performance, such as driving and other complex tasks involving judgment or fine motor skills.

"Among the known or suspected chronic effects of marihuana use are:

Impaired short-term memory and slowed learning;
Impaired lung function similar to that found in cigarette smokers; indications are that more serious effects may ensue following extended use;
Decreased sperm count and sperm motility;
Interference with ovulation and prenatal development;
Impaired immune response;
Possible adverse effects on heart function;
By-products of marihuana remaining in body fat for several weeks with unknown consequences. The storage of these by-products increases the possibilities for chronic effects as well as residual effects on performance even after the acute reaction to the drug has worn off.

"I am especially concerned about the long-term developmental effects of marihuana use on children and adolescents, who are particularly vulnerable to the drug's behavioral and physiological effects. The "amotivational syndrome" has been attributed by some to prolonged use of marihuana by youth. The syndrome is characterized by a pattern of loss of energy, diminished school performance, harmed parental relationships, and other behavioral disruptions. Though more research is required to clarify the course and extent, in recent national surveys, up to 40% of heavy users report that they observe some or all of these symptoms in themselves.

"The Public Health Service review of the health consequences of marihuana supports the major conclusion of the National Academy of Sciences' Institute of Medicine: 'What little we know for certain about the effects of marihuana on human health—and all that we have reason to suspect—justifies serious national concern.'"

Koop's statement echoes the conclusion reached by Professor William Paton at the Reims Symposium, "Undoubtedly, *Cannabis* is harmful to man." It was the first medical warning from the U.S. administration that clearly spelled out the health hazards of marihuana. A warning long overdue to parents, but which the National Institute on Drug Abuse did not give in its 10 reports, *Marihuana and Health*, summarized studies that cost tens of millions of dollars a year. Their conclusions were ambiguous and bland, and declared "the significance of the biological and behavioral changes caused by marihuana in man is uncertain. More research is needed."

After sixteen years, "Just say research" has not solved the basic question of the health hazards of marihuana.

V

THE LOUISVILLE SYMPOSIUM
of the American Society for Pharmacology and Experimental Therapeutics (1982)

This international symposium was organized by William Dewey and Stig Agurell and was held four years after the Reims symposium. Two hundred scientists gathered from the United States, United Kingdom, Sweden, and France to present 59 papers covering all apsects of *Cannabis:* clinical, chemical, metabolic, reproductive, neuropharmacolgical, cellular, and therapeutic *(1)*. The following important contributions were selected for publication in the present monograph and are reprinted with permission of the authors and the publisher:

Miller, L., *Marihuana: Acute effects on human memory.* pp. 227–231
Smith, C., Almirez, R., Scher, P., Asch, R. *Tolerance to the reproductive effects of delta 9 THC.* pp. 374–384
Dalterio, S., Steger, R., Bartke, A. *Maternal or paternal exposure to cannabinoids affect central neurotransmitter levels and reproductive function in male offspring.* pp. 441–447

In addition, this symposium emphasized the health and medical aspects of *Cannabis* use, a topic that had not been discussed at the IUPHAR symposia of previous years. Leo Hollister, who had participated in the Helsinki and Oxford symposia, and achieved unmatched preeminence for his studies of the clinical pharmacology of marihuana, summarized the "Health Aspects of Cannabis Use."

Reference

1. Agurell, S., Dewey, W.L., and Willette, R. E. (1983) *The Cannabinoids: Chemical, Pharmacologic and Therapeutic Apects.* Academic Press, New York.

HEALTH ASPECTS OF CANNABIS USE

Leo E. Hollister

INTRODUCTION

This topic is extremely broad and embraces both the adverse consequences of chronic use of *Cannabis* as well as the potential application of cannabinoids or their homologs as therapeutic agents. Each year the National Institute on Drug Abuse issues a review, *Marijuana and Health*, directed to the United States Congress *(1)*. These comprehensive reviews are more detailed than that which can be presented here. Short reviews of the subject have also been published in the past few years *(2,3)*.

From: *Marihuana and Medicine*
Edited by: G. G. Nahas et al.   © Humana Press Inc., Totowa, NJ

ADVERSE EFFECTS ON HEALTH

General Considerations

The ambiguity currently surrounding the health hazards of *Cannabis* may be attributed to a number of factors besides those which ordinarily prevail. First, it has been difficult either to prove or to disprove health hazards in humans from animal studies. When such studies of *Cannabis* reveal possible harmful effects, the doses used are often large although drug administration is generally short. Second, use of *Cannabis* by humans is still mainly by young persons in the best of health. Fortunately, the pattern of use is more often one of intermittent rather than regular use, the doses of drug usually being relatively small. This factor might lead to an underestimate of the potential impact of *Cannabis* on health. Third, *Cannabis* is often used in combination with tobacco and alcohol, as well as with a variety of other illicit drugs. Thus, potential health hazards from *Cannabis* may be difficult to distinguish from those concomitantly used drugs. Finally, the whole issue of *Cannabis* use is so laden with emotion that serious investigations of the health hazards of the drug have been colored by the prejudices of the experimenter, either for or against the drug as a potential hazard of health.

Chronic Use of Cannabis

The acute effects of *Cannabis*, taken by a variety of routes, have been well described *(4,5)*. The effects of chronic use of *Cannabis* are more to the point when considering the issues of its status as a possible social drug. Three large-scale field trials of *Cannabis* users have been implemented, but the results of these trials have done little to allay apprehensions about the possible ill effects of chronic use. Once again, objections have been made about the small samples used, the sampling techniques and the adequacy of the studies performed.

If field studies fail to provide evidence of harm from prolonged use of *Cannabis*, it is unlikely that experimental studies will do better, and such has been the case.

Experimental studies suggest that tolerance develops rapidly, that a mild withdrawal reaction may occur, and that some acute effects may be reversed (for instance, a slow heart rate with chronic use rather than a rapid one as seen with acute use). Other effects of chronic *Cannabis* use are related in a specific publication of the New York Academy of Sciences on chronic *Cannabis* use *(6)*. On the whole, we must rely heavily on experiments of nature to determine possible adverse effects.

Psychopathology

Cannabis may directly produce an acute panic reaction, a toxic delirium, or an acute paranoid state. Whether it can directly evoke depressive or schizophrenic states, or whether it can lead to sociopathy or even to the "amotivational syndrome" is much less certain. The existence of a specific *Cannabis* psychosis, postulated for many years, is still not established. The fact that users of *Cannabis* may have higher levels of various types of psychopathology does not infer a causal relationship. Indeed, the evidence rather suggests that virtually every diagnosable psychiatric illness among *Cannabis* users began before the first use of the drug. Use of alcohol and tobacco, as well as sexual experience and "acting out" behavior, usually antedated the use of *Cannabis (7)*. Thus, it seems likely that psychopathology may predispose to *Cannabis* use rather than the other way around.

It would seem reasonable to assume that *Cannabis* might unmask latent psychiatric disorders and that this action probably accounts for the great variety that have been described following its use. On the other hand, evidence for a specific type of psychosis associated with its use is still elusive. Needless to say, use of *Cannabis* should be discouraged (as would probably be the case with most socially used psychoactive drugs) in any patient with a history of prior emotional disorder (8).

Whether chronic use of *Cannabis* changes the basic personality of the user so that they become less impelled to work and to strive for success has been a vexing question. As with other questions concerning *Cannabis* use, it is difficult to separate consequences from possible causes of drug use. It has been postulated that the apparent loss of motivation seen in some *Cannabis* users is really a manifestation of a concurrent depression, for which *Cannabis* may have been a self-prescribed treatment (9).

If this syndrome is so difficult to prove, why does concern about it persist? Mainly because of clinical observations. One cannot help being impressed by the fact that promising youngsters change their goals in life drastically after entering the illicit drug culture, usually by way of *Cannabis*. While it is clearly impossible to be certain that these changes were caused by the drug (one might equally argue that the use of drug followed the decision to change life style), the consequences are often sad. With cannabis as with most other pleasures, moderation is the key word. Moderate use of the drug does not seem to be associated with this outcome, but when drug use becomes a preoccupation, trouble may be in the offing.

Brain Damage

The startling report of cerebral atrophy in ten young men who were chronic users of *Cannabis* aroused a great deal of controversy (10). Two studies using computerized tomography have effectively refuted the original claim of brain atrophy (11,12). A model in monkeys chronically smoking *Cannabis* produced EEG abnormalities from deep electrodes and postmortem histopathological alterations of the brain. EEG abnormalities and ultrastructural changes were reported in animals chronically exposed to amount of *Cannabis* consistent with human use (13).

Thus, the issue of brain damage is not totally resolved, although the original observation of brain atrophy seems to have been disproven. The issue is of tremendous importance and probably can only be settled by some suitable animal model, as studies in humans are confounded by too many other variables.

Tolerance/Dependence

The demonstration of tolerance in humans was delayed by ethical restrictions on the amount of exposure permissible to human subjects. For instance, in an early study subjects were exposed only to a test oral dose of 20 mg of Δ^9-tetrahydrocannabinol (THC) and then given the same dose or placebo repeated at bedtime for four more days followed by the same THC dose as a challenge on the fifth day. Using such small doses and relatively infrequent intervals, it was impossible to show tolerance to the psychic effects of the drug, although tolerance to the tachycardia and dizziness produced by the drug was evident (14).

Definite evidence of tolerance to the effects of THC in humans was adduced only when it became permissible to use comparably large doses over longer periods of time. Subjects in one 30-day study were given high oral doses (70–210 mg/day) of THC around the clock. Tachycardia actually became bradycardia and a progressive loss of "high" was noted (15). Similar tolerance to *Cannabis* smoking was observed in a 64-day study in which at least one cigarette daily had to be smoked with smoking as desired later in the same day. Additionally, in this study tolerance developed to the respiratory depressant effect of THC (16).

In humans, mild withdrawal reaction was uncovered after abrupt cessation of doses of 30 mg of THC given every four hours orally for 10 to 20 days. Subjects became irritable, had sleep disturbances, and had decreased appetite. Nausea, vomiting, and occasionally diarrhea were encountered. Sweating, salivation, and tremors were autonomic signs *(15)*. Relatively few reports of spontaneous withdrawal reactions from suddenly stopping *Cannabis* use have appeared, despite the extraordinary amount of drug consumed. Five young persons experienced restlessness, abdominal cramps, nausea, sweating, increased pulse rate, and muscle aches when their supplies of *Cannabis* were cut off. Symptoms persisted for one to three days *(60)*. The rarity of reports of these reactions may reflect the fact that they are mild and seldom is a user completely cut off from additional drug.

Lung Problems

Virtually all users of *Cannabis* in North America take the drug by smoking. As inhaling any foreign material into the lung may have adverse consequences, as is well proven by tobacco, this mode of administration of *Cannabis* might also be suspect.

Young, healthy volunteers in a chronic smoking experiment had pulmonary function tests before and after 47–59 days of smoking approximately five marihuana cigarettes a day. Decreases were found in forced expiratory volume in one second, in maximal midexpiratory flow rate, in plethysomographic-specific airway conductance, and diffusing capacity. Thus, very heavy marihuana smoking for six to eight weeks caused mild but significant airway obstruction *(17)*.

Quite possibly such dramatic early changes are not progressive with continued smoking *(18)*. Compared with tobacco, *Cannabis* smoking yields more residue (tar) but the amount of smoke inhaled is very likely to be considerably less. The study in which five cigarettes daily were consumed represented heavy use of the drug, compared with 20–40 tobacco cigarettes that might be consumed by a heavy tobacco smoker. The issue of damage to lungs from *Cannabis* is also confounded by the fact that many *Cannabis* users also use tobacco. As yet, it is far easier to find pulmonary cripples from the abuse of tobacco than it is to find any evidence of clinically important pulmonary insufficiency from smoking of *Cannabis*.

Cardiovascular Problems

Tachycardia, orthostatic hypotension, and increased blood concentrations of carboxyhemoglobin from *Cannabis* smoking would undoubtedly have deleterious effects on persons with heart disease caused by arteriosclerosis of the coronary arteries or congestive heart failure. A direct test of the effects of marihuana smoking in exercise-induced angina proved this harmful effect of the drug. Smoking one cigarette containing 19 mg of THC decreased the exercise time until angina by only 9%. Thus, smoking marihuana increased myocardial oxygen demand and decreased myocardial oxygen delivery *(19)*.

Clearly, smoking of any kind is bad for patients with angina, but the particular effect of *Cannabis* in increasing heart rate makes this drug especially bad for such patients. Fortunately, few angina patients are devotees of *Cannabis*.

Endocrine and Metabolic Effects

Changes in male sex hormones have been a source of controversy ever since the first report of a decreased serum testosterone level. Decreased levels were associated with morphological abnormalities in sperm and with decreased sexual functioning *(20)*. One possible cause for the lowered serum testosterone levels might be an impairment of synthesis of testosterone in the testis *(21)*. Another possibility might be an increased conversion of testosterone peripherally to estrogens, a factor that might be pertinent to other endocrine side effects.

Data on the effects of *Cannabis* on the female reproductive system are sparse. Preliminary unpublished data indicate that women who use *Cannabis* four times a week or more have more anovulatory menstrual cycles than do nonusers of the same age. Animal work tends to support this observation. THC administered to rats suppressed the cyclic surge of LH secretion and ovulation *(22)*.

The endocrine changes may be of relatively little consequence in adults, but they could be of major importance in the prepubertal male who may use *Cannabis*. If the pattern of hormonal changes that induce puberty is altered by *Cannabis* use, then permanent alterations in bodily and psychosexual development could ensue. Should use of *Cannabis* in early adolescence delay physical growth, could this lead to adverse psychosocial consequences? The questions are not academic, as recent surveys of *Cannabis* use indicate that some boys (and girls) may be exposed to it even as early as the prepubertal years.

Pregnancy and Fetal Development

This is another area of great uncertainty about the meaning of data. Virtually every drug that has been studied for dysmorphogenic effects has been found to have them, if the doses are high enough or if enough species are tested or if treatment is prolonged. The placenta is no barrier to the passage of most drugs, so the assumption should be made that they will reach the fetus if taken during pregnancy.

Studies in primates, still unpublished, indicate that "reproductive efficiency" is reduced when one or both parents have been treated chronically with *Cannabis*, that is, the number of completed pregnancies per mating is reduced. Only variable and nonspecific abnormalities have been found in the aborted offspring, and these were not much different from the findings in spontaneously aborted offspring.

It is still good practice in areas of ignorance, such as the effects of drugs on fetal development, to be prudent. The current admonition against using *Cannabis* during pregnancy is based more on ignorance than on definite proof of harm. Whereas no clinical association has yet been made between *Cannabis* use during pregnancy and fetal abnormalities, such events are likely to be rare at best and could easily be missed. The belated recognition of the harmful effects on the fetus of smoking tobacco and drinking alcoholic beverages indicates that the same caution with *Cannabis* is wise.

Miscellaneous Problems

CELL METABOLISM

Virtually all the changes reported have been in vitro and tend to indicate both slowing of the cell cycle as well as increased mitotic activity *(22,23)*. These conflicting findings are difficult to relate to clinical findings.

CHROMOSOMAL ABNORMALITIES

A slight increase (3.4% versus 1.2%) of chromosomal abnormalities was reported in marihuana users as compared with nonusers *(24)*. The clinical significance of such changes is unknown.

IMMUNITY

Impaired cellular immunity was reported early on in chronic users of marihuana, but later studies have failed to confirm this observation *(25,26)*. Once again, the clinical significance of such impairment is questionable.

CONTAMINANTS

Contamination of *Cannabis* with insecticides, fungi, bacteria, and insects is entirely possible, given the conditions of its growth. A few cases of pulmonary disease have resulted from such contamination, although the frequency is rare.

POSSIBLE ACCUMULATION OF DRUG

Being highly lipophilic, THC should be expected to be sequestered in fatty tissues. Metabolites of the drug are excreted in urine long after exposure to the last dose. The excretion of these metabolites is not associated with any *Cannabis*-like effects, however. No recognized health hazard has been attributed to such accumulation.

Summary of Adverse Reactions

It has been remarked facetiously that the most adverse consequence of *Cannabis* use is getting caught up in the criminal justice system because of such use. That observation may still be true. Yet, it is reasonable to assume that drug-taking, especially by young persons, may seriously interfere with their maturation process. Further, evidence from all drugs, both social as well as therapeutic, indicates that side effects of consequence are inevitable. One will have to make risk-benefit judgements in the case of *Cannabis* just as one does with other drugs.

THERAPEUTIC ASPECTS

The therapeutic aspects of *Cannabis* have been the subject of two reviews in recent years *(27,28)*. In this review, we shall consider some potential uses of *Cannabis* currently under investigation, somewhat in order of their importance and promise.

Antiemetic for Patients in Cancer Chemotherapy

Nausea and vomiting that accompany the use of cancer chemotherapeutic agents are extremely difficult to treat with ordinary antiemetic drugs, such as prochlorperazine. This drug, as well as many others, acts specifically at chemoreceptor trigger zones in the medulla sensitive to chemical stimuli that induce vomiting, e.g., apomorphine. For reasons still not clear, the vomiting induced by anticancer drugs does not always respond to such antiemetics even though it is chemically induced.

The first serious trial of THC as an antiemetic was a controlled comparison of this drug with placebo in 20 patients undergoing cancer chemotherapy. Doses of 15 mg of THC every four hours were given orally as gelatin capsules in which THC was dissolved in sesame oil. Doses were started two hours before chemotherapy and repeated two and six hours later. Results were outstanding. Fourteen of 20 patients in whom an evaluation could be made had an antiemetic effect from THC, whereas none was observed from placebo during 22 courses *(29)*.

These favorable findings have been largely, but not totally, confirmed. An open study in 53 patients refractory to other treatments, revealed that 10 had complete control of vomiting by THC administered prior to chemotherapy and for 24 hours after, 28 had 50% or more reduction in vomiting, and only 15 had no therapeutic effect. Four patients were dropped from the study because of adverse effects *(30)*. A controlled crossover trial comparing doses of 15 mg of THC versus 10 mg of prochlorperazine in 84 patients was done by the original group who proposed THC as treatment. Response was complete to THC in 36 of 79 courses but to prochlorperazine in only 16 or 78 courses. Of 25 patients who received both drugs, 20 preferred THC. However, of the 36 courses of THC that resulted in a complete antiemetic response, 32 were associated with a "high" *(31)*. Additional controlled studies have confirmed the antiemetic efficacy. One hundred sixteen patients were randomized to receive 15 mg of THC, 10 mg of prochlorperazine, or placebo. Many patients given THC found it to be unpleasant *(32)*. Fifteen patients were treated with courses of either THC or placebo, patients acting as their own controls. The THC regimen produced more relief of nausea and vomiting than placebo in 14 of these 15 patients who had received high-dose methotrexate *(33)*. Plasma concentrations of greater than 10 mg/mL of THC were associated with best results. A crossover controlled trial of THC, thiethylperazine, and metoclopramide found no difference in the antiemetic effect of the three agents. Adverse effects of THC were sufficiently greater than those of the other two drugs to question its utility (34). A comparison of THC, prochlorperazine, and placebo found the latter two treatments not to differ, THC being superior to either (35).

Nabilone, a synthetic homolog of THC developed in 1972, has been tested for antiemetic activity. One hundred thirteen patients were treated in a crossover study with either nabilone or prochlorperazine. Response rates were significantly greater with nabilone therapy, but side effects were also more common (36). This drug has not succeeded in totally eliminating the objectionable mental effects of cannabinoids. Two other synthetic THC homologs, levonantradol and BRL 4664 have been found in open studies to have antiemetic effects (37,38). It remains to be seen whether any of these synthetics will be appreciably better than THC itself. In the meantime, extremely promising results have been obtained with intravenous doses, somewhat larger than usually given, of metoclopramide. A comparison of this drug with prochlorperazine and placebo showed it to be more effective than either, the only disturbing side effect being sedation (39). Using doses of 1 mg/kg of metoclopramide intravenously before and several times after treatment with cisplatin (perhaps the most emetic anticancer drug), protection was total in 48% of courses and "major" in another 23% (40).

Thus, the present situation is that although THC and some of its homologs are undoubtedly antiemetics, they have drawbacks, particularly the mental effects so desired by social users. The advent of newer antiemetics with few mental effects, such as metoclopramide and maybe domperidone, may make the issue moot.

Glaucoma

A survey of possible ocular effects of *Cannabis* was added to a multifaceted study of the effects of chronic smoking of large amounts of the drug. Decreases of intraocular pressure up to 45% were found in nine of 11 subjects after 30 minutes of smoking (41). This effect lasted for four to five hours after smoking a single cigarette. Its magnitude was unrelated to the total number of cigarettes smoked. Thus, it appeared that a maximal effect was produced by the amount of THC absorbed from a single cigarette containing 19 mg of THC. In patients with ocular hypertension or glaucoma, seven of 11 patients showed a fall in intraocular pressure of 30%. The effect is real, for it has been confirmed. Intravenous injection of THC in doses of 22 mcg/kg and 44 mcg/kg produced an average fall in intraocular pressure of 37%, with some decreases as much as 51% (42). Similar experiments in rabbits, using several routes of administration have also confirmed the reduction in pressure.

Smoking *Cannabis* or taking it intravenously are hardly reasonable recommendations to make for patients with glaucoma, many of whom are elderly. If the drug could be administered topically, however, any impediments to its use would be overcome. Thus far, all experiments have been done in rabbits, a traditional animal model for studying topical eye medications. The problem of high lipid solubility of THC has been overcome by developing mineral oil as the vehicle for instillation in the eye. The degree of lowering of pressure is at least as great as with the conventional eye drops, such as pilocarpine, and the duration of effect is often longer. A minimal systemic absorption of the drug occurs when it is applied to the conjunctivae, but it is of no consequence in producing mental effects. Besides THC, other cannabinoids, such as cannabinol or THC metabolites, such as 8-alpha- and 8-beta-II-dihydroxy-Δ^9-THC have shown this effect in rabbits (43,44). As these agents have no mental effects, they are of considerable interest for this purpose.

An extract prepared from the nonpsychoactive components of *Cannabis* has been used alone and in combination with timolol eye drops with success. The effects of the two agents are additive and are said to be effective when other measures have failed. The composition of this extract is still uncertain *(45)*. A synthetic THC homolog, BW 146Y, was given orally to treat glaucomatous patients. Although intraocular pressures were reduced, mild orthostatic hypotension and subjective effects were noted *(46)*.

The outlook for this exploitation of cannabinoids in treatment is still promising. It will take a considerable amount of further developmental work to be sure that whichever cannabinoid is selected for clinical use will be lastingly effective and well tolerated. Nonetheless, the potential benefit will be great, for glaucoma treatment still does not prevent blindness as often as it might. Further, the effects of cannabinoids may be additive with those of other drugs, so that the overall benefit to patients may be greater than is currently possible.

Analgesia

THC in single oral doses of 10 and 20 mg was compared with codeine (60 and 120 mg) in patients with cancer pain. The larger THC dose was comparable to both doses of codeine, but the smaller dose, which was better tolerated, was less effective than either dose of codeine *(47)*. When the THC was given intravenously in doses of 44 mcg/kg to patients undergoing dental extraction, an analgesic effect was demonstrated. It was not as good as that achieved by doses of 157 mcg/kg of diazepam intravenously. Anxiety and dysphoria were produced in these patients, several of whom actually preferred the placebo to the dose of 22 mcg/kg of THC *(48)*.

In the chronic spinal dog model, THC, nantradol, and nabilone shared some properties with morphine. They increased the latency of the skin-twitch reflex and suppressed withdrawal abstinence. These actions were not antagonized by naltrexone, suggesting that they are not mediated through opiate receptors *(49)*. A single clinical study compared intramuscular levonantradol and placebo in postoperative pain and confirmed a significant analgesic action. However, no dose-response was observed and the number of side effects were rather high *(50)*.

Considering the present array of very effective new analgesics of the agonist-antagonist type, as well as the prospect of others that may be even more selective on specific opiate receptors, it seems unlikely that any THC homolog will prove to be the analgesic of choice. But it is really too early to be sure.

Muscle Relaxant

The aroma of *Cannabis* smoke is often found around wards housing patients with spinal cord injuries. Part of the streetlore is that *Cannabis* helps to relieve the involuntary muscle spasms that can be so painful and disabling in this condition. Some confirmation of a muscle relaxant, or antispastic, action of THC came from an experiment in which oral doses of 5 of 10 mg of THC were compared with placebo. The 10 mg dose of THC reduced spasticity by clinical measurement *(51)*. A single small study such as this can only point to the need for more study of this potential use of THC, or possibly of some of its homologs. Presently used muscle relaxants, such as diazepam, cyclobenzaprine, baclofen, and dantrolene have major limitations.

Anticonvulsant

Anticonvulsant activity was one of the first therapeutic uses suggested for *Cannabis* and was documented experimentally many years ago *(52)*. Subsequently, a great many studies in various animal species have validated this action.

Despite all these various lines of evidence supporting an anticonvulsant action of various cannabinoids, clinical testing has been rare. A single case report of better control of seizures following regular marihuana smoking was not very convincing *(53)*. A clinical trial in 15 patients not adequately controlled by anticonvulsants added cannabidiol in doses of 200 or 300 mg/day or placebo to their treatment. Control of seizures was somewhat better in those patients receiving cannabidiol *(54)*. As this cannabinoid has little psychoactivity, it would be the obvious one to try in future clinical studies.

Miscellaneous Uses

BRONCHIAL ASTHMA

Bronchodilation from marihuana smoke was discovered during a general study of the effects of the drug on respiration. Normal volunteer subjects were exposed to marihuana smoke calculated to deliver 85 mcg/kg or 32 mcg/kg. The high-dose group showed a fall of 38% in airway resistance and an increase of 44% in airway conductance *(55)*. Ten stable asthmatic patients were treated in another study with aerosols of placebo-ethanol, of THC 200 mcg in ethanol, or of salbutamol 100 mcg. Forced expiratory volume in one second, forced vital capacity, and peak flow rate were measured on each occasion. Salbutamol and THC significantly improved ventilatory function. Improvement was more rapid with salbutamol but the two treatments were equally effective at the end of one hour *(56)*. Whether effective doses of THC delivered by aerosol would be small enough to avoid the mental effects is uncertain. The fact that THC increases airway conductance by a mechanism of action that may be different from the usual beta-adrenergic stimulants makes further inquiry necessary.

Insomnia

Although early speculation had suggested that THC might differ from conventional hypnotics in not reducing rapid eye movement (REM) sleep, study of the drug in the sleep laboratory showed that it did *(57)*. Another sleep laboratory study showed that a dose of 20 mg of THC given orally decreased REM sleep. Abrupt discontinuation of THC after four to six nights of use produced a mild insomnia but no marked REM rebound. The lack of effect on REM rebound seen with low doses of THC was not apparent when very high doses (70–210 mg) were given orally. REM was reduced during treatment and marked REM rebound was observed after withdrawal *(58)*.

These studies indicate that the sleep produced by THC does not differ much from that of most currently used hypnotics. The side effects of the drug before sleep induction as well as the hangover effects make the drug less acceptable than the currently popular benzodiazepines, such as flurazepam. As many other effective hypnotics are currently being developed, it seems unlikely that THC will find a place in treatment of insomnia.

HYPERTENSION

THC itself occasionally produces orthostatic hypotension *(5)*. The development of effective antihypertensive drugs has been one of the outstanding achievements of pharmacology over the past 30 years. The prospect of a new antihypertensive based on orthostatic hypotension, perhaps the least desirable mode of lowering blood pressure, is hardly very enticing *(59)*. Further, it is by no means certain that the mental effects of any homolog of THC can be completely eliminated without losing many of the desired pharmacological actions as well. The issue seems hardly worth pursuing.

Prospects as a Therapeutic Agent

Cannabis and THC homologs should be treated like any other investigational new drug as the search for a clinical use in medicine goes on. We should expect neither less nor more in regard to safety and efficacy than we would from other new agents. At present, *Cannabis* has not yet made its way back into the formularies. It is unlikely that it ever will. The ingenuity of pharmaceutical chemists in developing THC analogs may yet find a way to exploit some of these potential therapeutic uses without the side effects that make *Cannabis* itself undesirable. Modern inquiry into this drug spans less than decades, which is hardly enough time to settle the issue.

SUMMARY

Both the adverse consequences of social use of *Cannabis* as well as the potential therapeutic use of cannabinoids or their homologs are still uncertain. It seems likely that adverse consequences will be fully documented and that therapeutic uses may be found. Only the former concern the chronic user of *Cannabis*, who must still make a personal decision whether the risks outweigh the benefits from the drug.

Reprinted with permission of the author and the publisher.

References

1. Petersen, R. C. (1980) *Marijuana and Health*: 1980, NIDA Research monograph 31, U.S. Government Printing Office, Washington, DC.
2. Nahas, G. G. (1979) Current status of marijuana research. *JAMA* **242**, 2775–2778.
3. Anonymous, AMA Council on Scientific Affairs. (1981) Marijuana: its health hazards and therapeutic potentials. *JAMA* **246**, 1823–1827.
4. Isbell, H., Gorodetsky, C. W., Jasinski, D., Claussen, U., Spulak, F. V. and Korte, F. (1967) Effects of (-)-delta-9-tetrahydrocannabinol in man. *Psychopharmacology* **11**, 184–188.
5. Hollister, L. E., Richards, R. K. and Gillespie, H. K. (1968) Comparison of tetrahydrocannabinol and synhexyl in man. *Clin. Pharmacol. and Ther.* **9**, 783–791.
6. Dornbush, R. L., Freidman, A. F. and Fink, M. (eds.) (1976) Chronic *Cannabis* use. *Ann. N.Y. Acad. Sci.* **282**, 1–430.
7. Halikas, J. A., Goodwin, D. W. and Guze, S. B. (1972) Marijuana use and psychiatric illness. *Arch. Gen. Psych.* **27**, 162–165.
8. Abruzzi, W. (1977) Drug-induced psychosis. *Int. Addict.* **121**, 183–193.
9. Kupfer, D. J., Detre, T., Koral, J. and Fajans, P. (1973) A comment on the "amotivational syndrome" in marijuana smokers, *Am. J. Psych.* **130**, 1319–1321.
10. Campbell, A. M., Thomson, J. L. G. Evans, M., and Williams, M. J. (1972) Cerebral atrophy in young cannabis smokers. *Lancet* 1:743, 202–203.
11. Kuehnle, J., Mendelson, J. H., David, K. R. and New, P. F. J. (1977) Computed tomographic examination of heavy marijuana smokers. *JAMA* **237**, 1231–1232.
12. Co, B. T., Goodwin, D. W., Gado, M., Mikhael, M. and Hill, S. Y. (1977) Absence of cerebral atrophy in chronic cannabis users of computerized transaxial tomography. *JAMA* **237**, 1229–1230.
13. Harper, J. W., Heath, R. G. and Myers, W. (1977) Effects of cannabis sativa on ultrastructure of the synapse on monkey brain. *Neurosci. Res.* **3**, 87–93.
14. Hollister, L. E. and Tinklenbert, J. R. (1973) Subchronic oral doses of marijuana extract. *Psychopharmacology* **29**, 247–252.
15. Jones, R. and Benowitz, N. (1976) The 30-day trip: clinical studies of cannabis tolerance and dependence. In: *Pharmacology of Marijuana*, (Braude, M.C. and Szara, S. eds.) Raven, New York, pp. 627–645.
16. Belleville, J. W., Gasser, J. C. and Miyake, T. (1976) Tolerance to the respiratory effects of marijuana in man. *Pharmacol. Exper. Ther.* **1997**, 326–331.
17. Tashkin, D. P., Shapiro, B. J., Lee, Y. E. and Harper, C. E. (1976) Subacute effects of heavy marijuana smoking on pulmonary function in healthy men. *N. Engl. J. Med.* **294**, 125–129.
18. Vachon, I. (1976) The smoke in marijuana smoking. *N. Engl. J. Med.* **294**, 160–161.
19. Aronow, W. S. and Cassidy, J. (1974) Effect of marijuana and place-marijuana smoking on angina pectoris. *N. Engl. J. Med.* **291**, 65–67.
20. Kolodny, R. C., Masters, W. H., Kolodner, R. M. and Toro, G. (1974) Depression of plasma testosterone levels after chronic intensive marijuana use. *N. Engl. J. Med.* **290**, 872–874.

21. Goldstein, H., Harclerode, J. and Nyquist, S. E. (1977) Effects of chronic administration of delta-9-tetrahydrocannabinol and cannabidiol on rat testicular esterase isozymes. *Life Sci.* **20**, 951–954.
22. Ayalon, D. and Tsafriri, A. (1973) Suppression of the cyclic surge of luteinizing hormone secretion and of ovulation in the rat by delta-l-tetrahydrocannabinol. *Nature* **243**, 470–471.
22. Leuchtenberger, C. and Leuchtenberger, R. (1976) Correlated cytological and cytochemical studies of the effects of fresh smoke from marijuana cigarettes on growth and DNA metabolism of animal and human lung culture. In: *Pharmacology of Marijuana* (Braude, M.C. and Szara, S. eds.) Raven, New York, pp. 595–612.
23. Zimmerman, A. M. and McClean, D. K. (1973) In: *Drugs and Cell Cycle* (Zimmerman, Padilla, and Cameron, eds.) Academic, New York, p. 67.
24. Stencherer, M. A., Kunysz, T. J. and Allen, M. A. (1974) Chromosome breakage in users of marijuana. *Am. J. Obst. Gynecol.* **118**, 106–113.
25. Nahas, G. G., Suciv-Foca, N., Armand, J. P. and Morshima, A. (1974) Inhibition of cellular mediated immunity in marijuana smokers. *Science* **183**, 419–420.
26. Lau, R. J., Tubergen, D. G., Barr, Jr., M., Domino, E. F., Benowitz, W. and Jones, R. T. (1976) Phytohemagglutinin induced lymphocyte transformation in humans receiving delta-9-tetrahydrocannabinol, *Science* **192**, 805–807.
27. Cohen, S. and Stillman, R. C. (eds.) (1976) *The Therapeutic Potential of Marijuana*. Plenum, New York, p. 515.
28. Lemberger, L. (1980) Potential therapeutic usefulness of marijuana. *Ann. Rev. Pharmacol. Toxicol.* **20**, 151–172.
29. Sallan, S. E., Zinberg, N. E. and Frei, E. (1975) Antiemetic effect of delta-9-tetrahydrocannabinol in patients receiving cancer chemotherapy. *N. Engl. J. Med.* **293**, 795–797.
30. Lucas, Jr., V. S. and Laszlo, J. (1980) Tetrahydrocannabinol for refractory vomiting induced by cancer chemotherapy. *JAMA* **243**, 1241–1243.
31. Sallan, S. E., Cronin, C., Zelen, M. and Zinberg, N. E. (1980) Antiemetics in patients receiving chemotherapy for cancer. A randomized comparison of delta-9-tetrahydrcannabinol and prochlorperazine. *N. Engl. J. Med.* **302**, 135–136.
32. Frytak, S., Moertel, C. G., O'Fallon, J. R., Rubin, J., Creagar, E. T., O'Donnell, M. J., Schott, A. J. and Schwartas, N. W. (1979) Delta-9-tetrahydrocannabinol as an antiemetic in patients receiving cancer chemotherapy. A comparison with prochlorperazine and placebo. *Ann. Int. Med.* **91**, 825–830.
33. Chang, A. S., Shiling, D. J., Stillman, R. C., Goldberg, N. H., Seipp, C. A., Barofsky, D., Simon, R. M. and Rosenberg, S. A. (1979) Delta-9-tetrahydrocannabinol as an antiemetic in cancer patients receiving high-dose methotrexate. A prospective, randomized evaluation. *Ann. Int. Med.* **91**, 819–824.
34. Colls, B. M., Ferry., D. G. and Gray, A. J. (1980) The antiemetic activity of tetrahydrocannabinol versus metoclopramide and thiethylperazine in patients undergoing cancer chemotherapy. *N. Zealand Med. J.* **91**, 449–451.
35. Orr, L. L., McKernan, J. F. and Bloome, B. (1980) Antiemetic effect of tetrahydrocannabinol: compared with placebo and prochlorperazine in chemotherapy-associated nausea and emesis, *Arch. Int. Med.* **140**, 1431–1433.
36. Herman, T. S., Einhorn, L. H., Jones, S. E., Nagy, C., Chester, A. B., Dean, J. C., Furnas, B., Williams, S. D., Leigh, S. A., Dorr, R. T. and Moon, T. E. (1979) Superiority of nabilone over prochlorperazine as an antiemetic in patients receiving cancer chemotherapy. *N. Engl. J. Med.* **300**, 1295–1297.
37. Cronin, C. M., Sallan, S. E., Gelber, R., Lucas, V. S. and Laszlo, J. (1981) Antiemetic effect of intramuscular levonantradol in patients receiving anti-cancer chemotherapy. *J. Clin. Pharmacol.* **21**, 43S–50S.
38. Stagret, M., Bron, D., Rosencweig, M. and Kenis, Y. (1981) Clinical studies with a THC analog (BRL 4664) in the prevention of cisplatin-induced vomiting. *J. Clin. Pharmacol.* **21**, 60S–63S.
39. Gralla, R. J., Itri, L. M., Pisko, S. E., Squillante, A. E., Kelsen, D. P., Braunn, Jr., D. W., Bordin, L. A., Braunn, T. J. and Young, C. W. (1981) Antiemetic efficacy of high-dose metoclopramine: randomized trials with placebo and prochlorperazine in patients with chemotherapy induced nausea and vomiting. *N. Engl. J. Med.* **303**, 905–909.
40. Strum, S. B., McDermed, J. E., Opfell, E. W. and Riech, L. P. (1982) Intravenous metoclopramide: an effective antiemetic in cancer chemotherapy. *JAMA* **247**, 2683–2686.
41. Hepler, R. S. and Frank, I. M. (1971) Marijuana smoking and intraocular pressure. *JAMA* **217**, 1392.
42. Cooler, P. and Gregg, J. M. (1977) Effect of delta-9-tetrahydrocannabinol on intraocular pressure in humans. *Southern Med. J.* **70**, 951–954.
43. Green, K. (1975) Marijuana and the eye. *Invest. Opthalmol.* **14**, 261–263.
44. Green, K., Wynn, H. and Bowman, K. A. (1978) A comparison of topical cannabinoids on intraocular pressure. *Exper. Eye Res.* **27**, 239–246.

45. West. M. E. and Lockhart, A. B. (1980) The enhanced effect of the combination of cannasol and timolol and pilocarpine in intraocular pressure. *West Indian Med. J.* **29**, 280.

46. Tiedemann, J. S., Shields, M. P. and Weber, P. A. (1981) Effect of synthetic cannabinoids on elevated intraocular pressure. *Opthalmology* **88**, 270–277.

47. Noyes, R., Brunk, S. F., Aver, D. H. and Canter, A. (1975) The analgesic properties of delta-9-tetrahydrocannabinol and codeine. *Clin. Pharmacol. Ther.* **18**, 84–89.

48. Raft, D., Gregg, J., Ghia, J. and Harris, L. (1977) Effects of intravenous tetrahydrocannabinol on experimental and surgical pain: psychological correlates of the analgesic response. *Clin. Pharmacol. Ther.* **21**, 26–33.

49. Gilbert, P. E. (1981) A comparison of THC, nantradol, nabilone, and morphine in the chronic spinal dog. *J. Clin. Pharmacol.* **21**, 311S–319S.

50. Jain, A. K., Ryan, J. E., McMahon, F. G. and Smith, G. (1981) Evaluation of intra-muscular levonantradol in acute postoperative pain. *J. Clin. Pharmacol.* **21**, 320S–326S.

51. Petro, D. J. and Ellenberger, C. E. (1981) Treatment of human spasticity with delta-9-tetrahydrocannabinol. *J. Clin. Pharmacol.* **21**, 413S–416S.

52. Loewe, S. and Goodman, L. S. (1947) Anticonvulsive action of marijuanna-active substances. *Fed. Proc.* **6**, 352.

53. Consroe, P. F., Wood, G. C. and Guchsbaum, H. (1975) Anticonvulsant nature of marijuana smoking. *JAMA* **234**, 306–307.

54. Carlini, E. A. and Cunnha, J. A. (1981) Hypnotic and antiepileptic effects of cannabidiol. *J. Clin. Pharmacol.* **21**, 417S–427S.

55. Vachon, L., Fitzgerald, M. X., Solliday, N. H., Gould, I. A. and Gaensler, E. A. (1973) Single-dose effect of marijuana smoke: bronchial dynamics and respiratory-center sensitivity in normal subjects. *N. Engl. J. Med.* **288**, 985–989.

56. Williams, S. J., Hartley, J. P. R. and Graham, J. D. P. (1976) Bronchodilator effect of delta-I-tetrahydrocannabinol administered by aerosol to asthmatic patients. *Thorak.* **31**, 720–723.

57. Pivir, R. T., Zarcone, J., Dement, W. C. and Hollister, L. E. (1972) Delta-9-tetrahydrocannabinol and synhexyl: effects on human sleep patterns. *Clin. Pharmacol. Ther.* **13**, 426–425.

58. Feinberg, I., Jones, R. and Walker, J. (1976) Effects of marijuana tetrahydrocannabinol on electroencephalographic sleep patterns. *Clin. Pharmacol. Ther.* **19**, 782–794.

59. Anonymous Editorial. (1978) Cannabis and the cardiovascular system. *Brit. Med. J.* **1**, 450–451.

60. Besusan, S. D. (1971) Marijuana withdrawal symptoms. *Brit. Med. J.* July: 112.

VI

THE OXFORD SYMPOSIUM "MARIHUANA '84"

The Oxford Symposium on marihuana was held under the aegis of the 9th International Meeting of IUPHAR on July 24–26, 1984. It assembled over 120 scientists and physicians from the United Kingdom, United States, France, Sweden, Italy, Switzerland, and Australia who presented 85 papers on chemistry, analysis, cellular properties, endocrine and developmental aspects, neurochemistry and neurophysiology, adverse reactions, and clinical and therapeutic aspects of marihuana *(1)*.

FOREWORD

David J. Harvey and Gabriel G. Nahas

Although only two years had elapsed since the Louisville meeting, it was felt that the time was right for another international meeting to discuss all aspects of *Cannabis* research. Use of the drug in Western countries is still on the increase and yet some fundamental questions regarding the drug's mechanism of action, tissue distribution, and even biological half life have not been resolved. The assembly of a large number of interested pharmacologists in London for the International Congress provided an ideal opportunity for another meeting of those interested in *Cannabis*. Oxford was chosen as the site partly because of its close proximity but mainly to honor the contribution made by Sir William Paton to *Cannabis* research and to mark his retirement as Professor of Pharmacology shortly after the symposium. The symposium was organized by Sir William Paton and D. J. Harvey, Department of Pharmacology, University of Oxford; G. G. Nahas, INSERM, Paris, France; S. Agurell, Astra Lakemedel, Sodertalje, Sweden; C. E. Turner, Special Assistant to the President for Drug Abuse Policy, Washington, DC, M. C. Braude, NIDA, Rockville, MD, and W. L. Dewey, Medical College of Virginia, and was sponsored by the World Health Organization. Special thanks are due to Astra Lakemedel AB and The Lilly Research Centre for financial their financial support, and to the National Institute on Drug Abuse for a grant to cover the expenses of American participants.

SUMMARY OF THE SESSION ON THERAPEUTIC EFFECTS

J. R. Trounce

Scattered throughout the history of pharmacology are a few drugs or families of drugs having several distinct pharmacological actions that have potential therapeutic applications. They also have effects which in certain circumstances might be regarded as adverse rather than therapeutic.

A familiar example is the belladonna alkaloids that have been used therapeutically for their actions on gastric secretion, smooth muscle, the eye, and the central nervous system.

From: *Marihuana and Medicine*
Edited by: G. G. Nahas et al.   © Humana Press Inc., Totowa, NJ

One hopes that these actions, although useful, might in some way be more selective. This hope, however, was not really fulfilled and finally the various therapeutic applications of belladonna and its derivatives were largely taken over by more selective and efficient drugs, for example the H_2 blockers or levodopa.

It seems that *Cannabis* and its derivatives are in very much the same position. It has a number of pharmacological actions, most of which have been known for a very long time. Some of these actions have potential therapeutic applications and indeed *Cannabis* has been widely used over the years for a wide variety of diseases.

This afternoon we have heard about some of the areas where there is reason to believe that it might have some usefulness in treatment.

It would be generally accepted that the best established use of *Cannabis* and cannabinoids at the present time is in the control of nausea and vomiting induced by cytotoxic drugs. Although there have been a large number of trials with *Cannabis*-like drugs, assessment and comparisons are difficult. This is because several variables may influence the efficacy of the antiemetic and the incidence of adverse effects.

Cytotoxic drugs differ in their emetic potential, dosage regimes may vary, and the clinical condition and age of the patient may influence toxicity.

Out of this somewhat confusing picture some general conclusions can be drawn:

1. *Cannabis* and its derivatives are useful antiemetics and are perhaps a little more effective than phenothiazines.
2. The incidence of side effects is appreciable but not unacceptably high, particularly when one remembers the unpleasantness of the symptoms being treated.
3. Vomiting induced by *cis*-platinum still remains a problem and is inadequately controlled by *Cannabis* except in the odd patient. Of interest here is the paper given by Gralla. He has certainly established that high-dose metoclopramide is to be preferred to THC when *cis*-platinum is used. Although the incidence of adverse effects from metoclopramide, particularly dystonia, was lower than experienced by some other observers.
4. There are now several drugs in this group, Δ^9-tetrahydrocannabinol, nabilone, levonantranol, and nonabine, all of which have been tried. There is no clear evidence to indicate the most effective of the group and the drug with the lowest incidence of adverse effects, but it may be significant that work on developing nonabine and levonantranol has now stopped, in the United Kingdom.

In an attempt to try to pinpoint the place of *Cannabis* in the control of cytotoxic-induced vomiting, eight medical oncology units in the United Kingdom were asked for their views. The general opinion was that *Cannabis*, or its derivatives, was useful in a number of patients, but was not the complete answer to drug-induced vomiting. Side-effects were appreciable but not intolerable. There will certainly be further trials with the present group of drugs, but it is doubtful whether at the end of the day we will be able to say much more than this. There is room for trials of cannabinoids in combination with other antiemetics. One of the problems of combining cannabinoids in this way is the cumulative sedative effect which we found unacceptable with nonabine and chlorpromazine. It would be better if a less sedative drug such as domperidone was combined with the cannabinoid.

The place of *Cannabis* and its derivatives in other fields of therapeutics is much more problematic and we have heard some interesting possibilities today. Pars and his colleagues have produced evidence that the derivatives Nabitan and Menabitan have analgesic activity in both animals and humans, albeit with some side-effects. One of the problems facing the physician is the relative lack of analgesics to fill the gap between the minor pain-relieving drugs and the powerful opiates. This gap is now to some degree being closed by the numerous partial opiate agonists such buprenorphine or meptazinol appearing on the market. There is, however, still room in this area for an orally effective analgesic which is nonaddictive and has a low incidence of adverse effects. Whether a cannabinoid could fill this gap is still open to question.

It is a little early to pass judgment on the use of cannabinoids in epilepsy. This is, however, a highly competitive field and although there is always room for improvement, a new anticonvulsant would have to be an impressive drug. It would have to be relatively safe when given over longer periods and preferably nonteratogenic. It was mentioned earlier in this meeting that *Cannabis* reduced muscle spasticity and this is a possible therapeutic use that might be explored. There is a lack of good drugs for this purpose and cerebral palsy and post-stroke spasticity are common conditions.

One of the problems of a review of this type is that it is necessary to discuss subjects about which one has no practical experience. On the face of it, to use a drug like *Cannabis* for glaucoma, a group of disorders in which there seems to be a plethora of treatments, does not seem very promising. However, there may be difficulties with medical treatments, particularly as regards compliance. The results with surgery are not always good and not all patients respond satisfactorily. Merritt has told us about the successful use of *Cannabis* in a rather special group of patients and it seems probable that if this type of medical treatment were to become widely used it would be necessary to produce a derivative with a more specific action on the eye or to design a delivery system that limits systemic effects. In summary, therefore, it is only in the control of cytotoxic-induced vomiting that *Cannabis*, or its derivatives, which are at present available, is clinically useful. There are certainly some signposts that we have heard about today that direct us to other possible therapeutic uses, but it is fair to say that unless new and more specific indications emerge or it is possible by further modification of its structure to isolate one of its potentially useful pharmacological actions, it is unlikely that this group of drugs will play a major role in therapeutics.

FINAL SUMMARY OF THE SESSION ON THERAPEUTIC EFFECTS

D. J. Harvey and W. D. M. Paton

Studies on the mechanism of action of Δ^1-THC have still not resolved the question as to whether the drug acts mainly in a relatively nonspecific way in cell membranes, at a receptor, or both. Much evidence is accumulating, however, to suggest that membranes are the preferred site and this is supported by the drug's effects on a large number of organs and biochemical processes. Interaction does not appear to be of the same type as that of a general anaesthetic as a considerable degree of structural specificity is present. Changes in membrane fluidity have been recorded with an estimated drug to phospholipid ratio as low as 1:20,000 thus emphasizing the potency of cannabinoids as disrupters of membrane structure. It has been proposed that THC may replace cholesterol in membranes as both compounds have a similar structure but an theory proposed at this symposium suggests that THC also competes with tocopherol for membrane sites. Again, similarities between the structures of the compounds are striking. The evidence that the action of THC is specifically linked to release of arachidonic acid may also be relevant.

A property of Δ^1-THC to emerge from several papers on the general effects of the drug was one of general depression of activity; again this supports a mechanism involving membrane disorder. Such effects are the depression of the response to rewarding electrical stimuli, suppression of the generation of neuronal action potentials in the CNS, depression of macromolecular synthesis, suppression of glucose metabolism and consequently of cellular energetics, reduction in sexual activity, and depression of the immune response.

Although many of the actions of Δ^1-THC appear to be caused by membrane interactions, some evidence was presented for drug–receptor interactions. A high-affinity binding site for a quaternary ammonium analogue of Δ^1-THC (TMA) was located in the brain and it was shown that a number of cannabinoids were able to displace TMA from this site in the nanomole range. However, as a number of these cannabinoids were psychically inactive, it is doubtful if this represents the main neuronal receptor for THC, should one exist. There is evidence, however, that Δ^1-THC may act at receptors for several neurotransmitters. Thus the production of hypokinesia by levonantradol in reserpine-pretreated rats in an analogous way to that produced by nicotine has led to the suggestion that the drug acts at central nicotinic cholinergic receptors located in the caudate/putamen, substantia nigra, and dorsomedial thalamus. On the other hand, binding studies have also indicated interaction with adrenergic, dopaminergic, and opiate receptors in the CNS. It seems doubtful that a molecule such as Δ^1-THC would have an affinity for all of these very different receptors. A more likely explanation is that it is interacting at a membrane site in the vicinity of a receptor and that this subsequently has some effect on receptor conformation. These are well documented and include deficiencies of the immune system, learning processes, reproductive function, fetal development, cardiac and pulmonary function, and motor function. The production of an amotivational syndrome and extensive psychopathology are particularly worrying. The extent to which these effects occur in the general population is uncertain because of complications caused by polydrug abuse. Attempts have been made to deconvolute the individual effects of drugs taken simultaneously but this has proved difficult. Analysis of one interesting set of data led to the suggestion that many cases of the "fetal alcohol syndrome" may, in fact be caused, not by alcohol, but by *Cannabis*. Again, however, because of polydrug use it is not clear if *Cannabis* alone can produce the syndrome or whether both *Cannabis* and alcohol are necessary. In studies aimed at comparing the relative potencies of these two drugs in producing performance decrements, it was estimated that oral Δ^1-THC was about 4000 times as potent as alcohol. An equivalent figure for smoked marihuana could not be obtained as dose-response curves were not parallel thus again emphasizing that the *Cannabis* preparation and route of administration must be taken into account in studies with this drug. In another study on the combined effects of alcohol and *Cannabis* it was found that alcohol made little difference to the amount of *Cannabis* consumed to reach a given self-determined social "high," but that in the presence of *Cannabis*, the amount of alcohol was halved. Evidence was presented to the effect that long-term administration of *Cannabis* produces physical and possibly irreversible changes in the brain. One particularly alarming aspect of the occurrence of many of the adverse effects is that they do not seem to be recognized by the majority *Cannabis* users, particularly the young.

The mechanism of action of cannabinoids on organs such as the heart and lung are still unresolved. Tachycardia is well-documented for Δ^1-THC and was demonstrated at the symposium with isolated heart preparations. Contractile force and coronary flow, on the other hand, decrease under the same conditions. Cannabidiol has almost the opposite effect, increasing the contractile force but at the same time having little effect on rate. Studies with 7-hydroxy-Δ^1-THC indicate that the action on the heart does not involve cardiac beta receptors. In humans, one of the most serious cardiovascular effects seems to be postural hypotension.

Considerable emphasis was given to adverse effects on reproduction and associated endocrine systems. *Cannabis* has been shown to produce aberrations in sexual behavior, hormone imbalances, menstrual cycle derangements, inhibition of ovulation, interference with spermatogenesis, embryotoxicity, delayed postnatal development, chromosomal anomalies, and to be weakly teratogenic. Decreased secretion of prolactin and luteinizing hormone appear to be the result of central hypothalamic actions rather than actions on the pituitary. Effects on spermatogenesis, on the other hand, appear to be the result of a direct action on the Sertoli cells. A significant finding is that *Cannabis* not only affects the organism to which it is administered, but that in monkeys, at least, it is able to affect offspring in the form of deficits in both male and female reproductive function. Again, the apparent diversity of effects on reproduction point to a generalized action for the drug such as an interaction with membrane structure.

Reports on the possible clinical usefulness of *Cannabis* were disappointing. Although apparently of some effect in the treatment of vomiting associated with cancer chemotherapy, both natural and synthetic cannabinoids leave much to be desired when it comes to other uses such as the reduction in intraocular pressure, in pain relief, and for the control of epilepsy that looked promising several years ago. Side-effects are mainly to blame and even as an antiemetic, the use of drugs such as nabilone seem to limited by pronounced postural hypotension. Although *Cannabis* preparations might appear to offer something to small, selected groups of patients, other drugs with fewer side-effects are available for treatment of most of the above conditions. The development of compounds with reduced side-effects may yet yield therapeutically useful drugs, but research along these lines appears to be diminishing.

ABOUT SCIENCE AND POLITICS

Carlton Turner

I stand here as a scientist and as a policy maker. My present job was not obtained because of my politics, but because of my of my credentials; credentials as a scientist who also worked with the law enforcement community, the United Nations, the medical community, and with the parents and communities in the United States.

I would like to share some of the problems I face in integrating scientific information into policy matters. What the scientific community has taught me and what the policy maker needs to protect the public health and welfare are not always compatible. This presents a dilemma.

Who lost in these public and policy debates? The scientific community lost. But, that's not unusual. Scientists are usually busy chasing the minutia, forgetting the bigger issue and/or they are so busy making decisions in isolation they do not see the big picture One reason for the isolation could be that scientists talk only to scientists, physicians talk only to physicians, pharmacists talk only to pharmacists, attorneys talk only to attorneys, ministers talk only to ministers, policeofficers talk only to policeofficers, and needed cross fertilization does not occur.

We need cross fertilization to seek the bigger truth. You know the bigger truth is where it has always been. It is in our hearts, our music, our science, our medicine, and our communities. Most importantly to us, it is in the minds of scientists. So let's share what we know with policy makers and the public, but let's also look at the big picture. Let me give you another example of what is happening at the policy level that gives basic scientists a bad name. Let's talk about basic science and marihuana. First, I want to see the hands of those who attended the 1974 meeting in Savannah, Georgia. Within this group lies the true "marihuana mafia"; others are latecomers. But, with this "marihuana mafia" lies some responsibility of the problems we have with the public and marihuana. We knew in 1974 that if we gave labeled Δ^9-THC to a ewe it was transferred to the young lamb via the milk. What else did basic scientists know in 1974? We knew there were 70% more carcinogenic compounds in one marihuana cigarette than in a tobacco cigarette chosen because it contained high levels of carcinogenic compounds. We have known these things for a decade, but what did we do with the knowledge? We certainly didn't communicate it to the public. There is very little known about marihuana that was not known in 1974. Very little, indeed!

From several studies we knew THC and cannabinoids crossed the placenta barrier, but we failed to share these basic scientific findings with policy makers. By failing to communicate, we left our responsibility to prodrug attorneys and the media. We abdicated it to a man by the name of Bob Randell who went around our country saying, "look at me man, I'm smoking marihuana for my glaucoma. I'm getting prescription marihuana." He was not getting prescription marihuana, but participating in an experimental program; thus, lie number one. He did not discontinue taking his regularly prescribed medication in addition to smoking marihuana. Thus, lie number two. As scientists we did not challenge him. We lost! The American National Academy of Sciences has released two reports on marihuana: One said we don't know much about marihuana, but what we do know "creates grave national concern," and the other calls for legalization of marihuana. Do you think that we, as cannabinoid researchers, were extensively consulted and utilized? Well, we know there are over 8500 publications on marihuana, cannabinoids, etc. You wonder where people like those at the Academy have been. All I can say is we let it happen, but our abdication is being reversed. We are beginning to share.

I heard things at this meeting that really made my heart feel good. Yes, we debate internally, but we are developing skills to communicate and share outwardly. This is what science is all about. Because if we don't share and have a desire to help mankind, we are going to evolve into a kind of selfishness and that cold kind of selfishness is going to create a monster. That monster is going to be the public whose kids and families are suffering the effects of marihuana and other drugs. They are going to say, "forget it guys, we are not going to fund you anymore." In fact this is going on now. For example, after President Reagan sent the National Institute on Drug Abuse (NIDA) budget to Congress, the budget was cut. I asked legislators why they did and they said it is the only way to get their attention. So, NIDA received $5 million less than we requested. We should think about that. I think we have failed to bridge the gap between basic and applied research, which in our case is crucial to public health. Until we communicate what we know from basic research to the rest of the world, we are going to continue to have difficulty in getting policies compatible with our knowledge.

Scientific data helps me as a policy maker. But the scientific world is perceived as uninterested in helping policy makers. This, in my opinion, is the reason very few scientists hold positions within the upper echelon of governments, especially in the White House. It reminds me of a scientist who was asked the question, "what is the difference between ignorance and apathy?" and he replied, "I don't know and I don't care." Sometimes I feel like the only pea in the pod until people like Harry Rosencrantz, Monroe Wall, Coy Waller, or Stig Agurell visit, after which I know there is still a place for me.

We need to look at where we go now, and how to change the public's perceptions about us. How do we work together in order to build a better future? What are our needs? Let me use an example to shed some light on this. On July 30, 1984, I addressed the United States Governors' conference, where governors of all states discuss current issues. Representatives from the executive, legislative, and judicial branches of the governments are invited to participate in the discussions.

One question asked was what can you, as a scientist, tell us about marihuana? Because we are under pressure from the public about marihuana, we need some advice. I kept my notes and will read from them. As a scientist I said I feel very comfortable in telling you the following: marihuana retards learning; marihuana affects the reproductive system and production of sex hormones; marihuana has the capacity to affect every organ in the body and can affect individual cells–we have forgotten that in 1974, Gill presented a paper addressing the effects different cannabinoids have on cell wall rigidity; marihuana constituents are stored in fat cells and the brain is one large mass of fat; marihuana affects lung functions; marihuana interferes with psychomotor functions and heart functions; marihuana contains 70% more carcinogenic compounds than a tobacco cigarette; marihuana affects memory; marihuana decreases motivation; and marihuana interferes with the immune system. Their comments were, "we have never heard of anything like this. Is there a possibility of getting this information to us?" That told me I was not doing my job, because if I were doing my job, they would have been better informed. But, I thought where does this put the scientists? Think about that.

We as scientists have been in the trenches and I might add political darkness. We say all politicians are corrupt. In fact, every conceivable risqué word in the world has been used to describe a politician. My grandfather taught me that we have good and bad in all professions. There are no exceptions. We all have problems in life. But regardless of the problem or profession, hindsight is more accurate than foresight; moreover, unless you are willing to sell your ideas and programs to those outside your discipline your foresight will also be myopic.

My grandfather told me a joke that illustrates the careless attitude some have about life. There were two trains; one was going west and one east. They crashed on a sharp curve high in the Rocky Mountains. The railroad company sent its best railroad detective to determine the cause of the accident. Well, the detective studied and studied but couldn't find out why in the world these two trains were on the same track at the same time. One of the brakeman told him there was an old mountain man whose cabin overlooked the track and that he might have seen the crash and might possibly be of help. The old mountain man was visited by the sophisticated detective who looked at him, a simple old mountain man, with a bit of disdain. In his usual detective manner he asked, "sir, did you see the trains on the day the crash occurred?" And, the old man said, "yep." Nothing else. The detective asked, "did you know that the trains were going to crash?" And the old man said, "yep." The detective replied, "well, did you know that people were going to get killed?" And again, the old man said, "yep." Angrily the detective asked, "Well, did it occur to you to go down and stop those two trains?" "Nope," said the old man. At this time the detective was exasperated and he asked, "did anything occur to you?" He said, "yep, yep it did. It occurred to me that that's a hell of a way to run a railroad."

Naturally a little foresight may have yielded better results in that situation and we in the scientific community can learn from that. We are trying to pick up the pieces caused by drug abuse. Unfortunately, those pieces may be members of our own family. We have 14-year-old alcoholics in the United States. The question exists, how do young people become alcoholics? Our young people drink and when they become nauseous, they smoke a joint. Marihuana suppresses the vomiting mechanism and subsequently natural detoxification, vomiting, does not happen. Our scientific foresight did not discover this, our treatment hindsight did. We are picking up the pieces of our young people worldwide.

We have denied the severity of drug abuse at high policy level. I spoke with a very prominent policy maker in this country on Friday. He told me England had no marihuana, hashish, or cocaine problem, only heroin. Yet, I walked on this campus and smelled pot. And I see young people wearing sweaters with *Cannabis* leaf decals and/or prodrug mottos.

Let me leave you with one important thought. As we pick up the pieces on marihuana, we are going to have to pick up some pieces because of cocaine. Yet we have scientists who say we don't know much about cocaine. We do. Have we failed to learn from our history? Have we failed to read the work of Sigmund Freud? If we have, shame on us. And when a media person tells me, "don't you think cocaine is the drug of 80s?" I laugh and say it was: The drug of the 1880s, 1890s, and early 1900s and say where have you guys been for the last 100 years? Let's not let the same be said for scientists in the year 2084.

A FAREWELL TO MY COLLEAGUES

W. D. M. Paton

I would still like to say something by way of welcome. At retirement, one tends to a certain amount of appraisal of the past, and I would like to introduce my first theme by recalling how I came into the *Cannabis* field. It was simply by chance, in September 1966, of attending a meeting on adolescent drug dependence, in the hope that there would be something interesting about the opiates (on which I had been working). That aspect was unproductive. But I heard about two other things. First was a report from New York of an association between the use of heroin and that of *Cannabis*, in 99 of 107 heroin addicts. That was followed by an argument between two British psychiatrists as to the character of young *Cannabis* users. One said that essentially they suffered from depression; but because they were too young to be eligible for treatment of the adult condition, they turned to *Cannabis* for relief. This was flatly contradicted by the other, for whom the users were typically the outgoing and experimental type of youngster. All this seemed rather odd, so I went away, and looked up this peculiar drug. It did not seem to have been studied properly, and I could find no evidence that it had ever, for instance, been subjected to a chronic toxicity test. We were able to obtain supplies of the tincture of *Cannabis*, available at that time for medical use, and Gill extracted from it the active principles with our Craig counter-current machine. So off we went.

At first, I became rather depressed by the polarization that one could recognize in the field. It seemed as though anything one found or said was only looked at for what it might imply for *Cannabis* legislation. But then, as time went on, one began to develop friendships, sometimes quite clearly running across divisions in opinion about general policy. There was, after all, a community of scientific outlook, of belief in a body of knowledge independent of one's prejudices. The scientific ideal, of trying to reach those conclusion that will still be true when the work is done by another man's hands, was still in play. Many of those friends are here tonight. I am very grateful for their friendship, and for what they have shown still to be true about the scientific enterprise. It is a great encouragement for the future.

Professor WDM Paton, CBE, FRS, DM, retired in Oxford and passed away in 1993. The British Pharmacological Society has established a memorial lecture in his honor, the second ever created by the Society.

Reprinted with permission from the publisher and the authors.

References

1. Harvey, D.G., Paton, WDM, and Nahas, G.G., (1985) *Marihuana 84: Proceedings of the Oxford Symposium on Cannabis*. IRL Press, Oxford.

VII

THE PARIS SYMPOSIUM OF THE FRENCH "NATIONAL ACADEMIE DE MEDICINE" (1992)

Between 1990 and 1994, the Mayor of the City of Paris, Mr. Jacques Chirac, sponsored three symposia on the psychopathology of illicit drugs which were held at the French National Academy of Medicine. The second symposium took place in 1992 and was devoted to "cannabis"; 60 physicians and scientists from the United States, United Kingdom, Sweden, The Netherlands, Morocco, and Switzerland presented 40 papers on the physiopathology, detection, and epidemiology of cannabis (1).

The following papers presented at this symposium are reported in this monograph:

Waser, P. *Effects of THC on brain and social organization of ants.* pp. 153–161

Nahas, GG, Latour, C, and Trouve, R. *Distribution of consumption of alcohol and mairhuana.* pp. 731–736

Bejerot, N and Hartelius, J. *The Swedish addiction epidemic in global perspective.* pp. 757–763

FOREWORD

Jacques Chirac

This volume assembles selected proceedings from the Second International Colloquium on the "Physiopathology of *Cannabis* and the Detection of Illicit Drugs," which was held at the National Academy of Medicine with the assistance of the City of Paris.

The physiopathology of *Cannabis* is a subject of major importance for the future of our society. It so happens that the acute impairment of *Cannabis* on mental function was described in 1845 by a French physician Joseph Moreau, the father of modern psychopharmacology. Whereas Moreau described the acute impairing effects of hashish on affective and cognitive functions of the brain, he had no way of assessing the physiopathological effects of this drug.

Today, thanks to the new techniques of medical imaging, it is possible to visualize, as illustrated by the studies of Nora Volkow, the impairment of brain functioning in areas connected with coordination, balance, memory and coherent behavior. Other studies describe the noxious effects of *Cannabis* on reproductive function, and immune surveillance resulting in cancer and leukemia.

The second theme of this colloquium, detection of illicit drugs in body fluids, is also of great importance. We have to protect our communities from the use of substances that impair the integrity of attention, memory, and coordination that are essential for the proper performance of professional tasks. Testing for drugs is already practiced in competitive sports for detection of anabolic substances, and alcohol in road accidents. Unfortunately the present epidemic of drug abuse has resulted in the consumption of other drugs. Like *Cannabis*, they

From: *Marihuana and Medicine*
Edited by: G. G. Nahas et al.   © Humana Press Inc., Totowa, NJ

impair persistently information processing by the brain and prevent it from performing correctly in driving a car, monitoring equipment, or using a computer. It is therefore important to review methods and results already obtained in the detection of illicit drugs in different populations.

At a time when strong voices are advocating the relegalization of illicit drugs, and public health is threatened by the progression of illicit drug consumption, the City of Paris is proud to support outstanding scientific studies that should help to promote prevention programs for our youth. Today, I am eager to listen to scientists who are attempting to evaluate all of the consequences of modern technology on humans and society. The control of the emission of toxic substances that pollute the environment has been initiated thanks to the efforts of concerned scientists. Some of them are now seeking methods to curtail the use and trivialization of substances that pollute the internal milieu of human brains and other vital organs. Our concern today is therefore to preserve mental and physical health, especially that of future generations. Such is our hope and such is our goal.

PREFACE

Henri Baruk

It is quite fitting that this first international colloquium on the Physiopathology of *Cannabis* should have taken place under the aegis of the National Academy of Medicine. Indeed, it was in 1845 that Jacques Joseph Moreau, called Moreau de Tours, the father of psychopharmacology, presented to this Academy his classic treatise *Hashish and Mental Illness*.

This text, which is summarized in this volume, may be considered as the "princeps" experience ever recorded on the clinical pharmacology of marihuana. Moreau, using himself as an experimental subject, was the first physician to study the role of "psychotoxic" substances on the development of acute mental pathology, first ingesting hashish and later inhaling nitrous oxide. He summarizes his experience with hashish as follows: "As the effects of hashish take hold of the brain one experiences profound modification in all aspects of thought processes. A true 'dream-state,' but a dream without sleep does occur." And he added: "It appears that two modes of moral existence, two lives have been imparted to man. Our first life results from our relationship with the external milieu, which we call the great universe. Our second life is but a stored compilation of the first. Sleep is like a barrier separating these two lives. Moreau demonstrated that delirium was a sort of dream. We have made similar observations in our investigations of catatonia that may often be considered as a state of dreaming while being awake. We have also reported a state of mental toxicity and delirium that resulted from bacterial infections, especially with *Enterobacterium coli*. These studies have been reported in the Proceedings of the Society Moreau de Tours, founded 20 years ago.

And today, all the clinical symptomatology of *Cannabis* intoxication described so accurately by Moreau and that has been confirmed by many other psychopharmacologists, is being reinvestigated and correlated with biochemical and neurophysiological markers of the brain. Such studies will be discussed in this colloquium, which should be another landmark in our understanding of the human brain.

INTRODUCTION

Paul Lechat

It is arduous, by definition, either to convince skeptics, or to change the opinion of those who refuse *a priori* to admit the truth. To recognize that the usage of *Cannabis* is damaging contradicts these two attitudes. That is why we must be appreciative of those who have scientifically demonstrated that this drug is neither soft nor harmless, but that its toxicity is manifested in multiple ways among its consumers. The International Colloquium on Illicit Drugs, which was the basis for the present publication, took place in Paris in April of 1992. A number of leading authorities specialized in different aspects of drug dependence, participated in this colloquium and their reports are assembled in this volume. One panel of scientists reported that *Cannabis* impairs psychomotor function, decreases cognitive processes, induces psychiatric disturbances, impairs immunity and reproduction, and facilitates the appearance of certain cancers. The second panel reported that the accurate detection of the metabolites of the elusive cannabinoids is possible, thanks to the very sensitive techniques now available; this detection helps law enforcement authorities and magistrates in their tasks. The third panel discussed recent epidemiological data reporting the usage of *Cannabis* in America and Europe. Society must not capitulate to the destructive forces that are threatening its fabric, and prominent among these must be included drugs of dependence. The greatest help that scientists may offer to save drug addicts from self-destruction is to define and spread, as early as possible, up-to-date information concerning the degradation that threatens their lives. Every type of research must be relentlessly carried out in this field. Indeed, it is only on the basis of unquestionable data that policy makers will be able to make informed decisions in order to define the most adequate measures to fight the bondage of drug dependence.

MESSAGE FROM THE ACADEMY

Henri Baylon

For the second time in two years, the National Academy of Medicine has had the privilege to host a colloquium on the grave problem of public health created by the illicit use of psychotropic substances.

The first colloquium, sponsored like this one, by the City of Paris, was devoted to the Physiopathology of *Cannabis*, Cocaine and Opiates. The present colloquium emphasized problems related more particularly to *Cannabis*.

There are diverging opinions concerning the medical effects of *Cannabis*. Many intellectuals consider it a "soft" drug and advocate its relegalization. On the opposite side, others don't distinguish this addiction from that of "hard drugs" and claim that it is responsible for delinquent behavior. American studies tend to indicate that *Cannabis* consumption is the first step towards the use of heroin or cocaine. Furthermore, it is apparent that the use of *Cannabis* among adolescents occurs more and more precociously, starting at age 12. This early experience with *Cannabis* creates the risk of an escalation in the following years to the consumption of hard drugs.

The responsible leaders of the large cities have realized the grave threat that *Cannabis* smoking represents for their future. In this regard, the City of Paris, which we wish to thank for its generous contribution towards the organization of this colloquium, has expressed an interest in devoting a large part of its scientific reports to *Cannabis*. Internationally recognized scientists have been invited to present the results of their experiments and let us benefit from their special expertise.

The problems raised by *Cannabis* are indeed international, and it is important that different experiences be compared and discussed.

In the first part of this colloquium, the general toxicity and the effects of the consumption of *Cannabis* on behavior, on the genesis of mental illness were reported. Imaging techniques (positron emission tomography) performed on *Cannabis* users illustrated the alterations occurring in brain metabolism, suggesting impairment of neurotransmission.

The second part of the colloquium reported broad surveys and discussions concerning different attitudes towards the use of *Cannabis* in countries of Europe, North and South America. The view point of WHO concluded this discussion.

The third part of the colloquium was devoted to problems of detection of illicit drugs and their consequences in different situations, thus generalizing the theme of the meeting to all of the addiction. Sampling, methods of measurement, interpretation of results were discussed. Consequences of detection in victims of traffic accidents in cars or trucks or railway conductors were reported. Detection in school populations, industry, and the armed forces were discussed. Finally, problems of legislation of illicit drug use were analyzed.

This volume assembles the bulk of the papers presented to the colloquium. In addition, other articles written by specialists of the main subjects under consideration have been included. Older communications of lasting general interest have been reprinted in an appendix.

SCIENTIFIC SUMMARY

The acute and toxic effects of marihuana smoke may be related to its following consitutents:

Delta-9-Tetrahydrocannabinol (THC). This psychoactive ingredient, which binds in nanomolar concentration to specific receptors in the brain, impairs information processing in areas which control pleasure reward, memory, coordination and cognitive function. THC with a half-life of 7 days, will accumulate in tissue.

Nonpsychoactive cannabinoids that like THC inhibit, in micromolar concentraiton, synthesis of DNA, RNA, and protein in fast-dividing cells.

Toxic xenobiotics contained in the gas phase (carbon monoxide, hydrogen cyanide, acetaldehyde) and in the particulate phase (phenols, terpenes, carcinogens) that impair lung and airway.

Marihuana smoke is mutagenic in the Ames test and is carcinogenic in tissue culture. Exposure of animals to marihuna smoke produces symptoms of "neuro behavioral toxicity" in spontaneous and conditioned behavior with residual effects following chronic exposure; disruptive effects on all phases of reproductive function and fetotoxicity in seven different species.

In humans, marihuana smoking produces symptoms of airway obstruction and precancerous "squamous metaplasia"; it impairs a wide range of learned and unlearned behavior including simple motor tasks, complex psychomotor and cognitive tasks.

Clinical manifestations of marihuana physiopathology have now been reported. They include long-term impairment of memory storage in adolescents; prolonged impairment of psychomotor performance, resulting in lethal train and car accidents; residual impairment of plane piloting; a sixfold increase in incidence schizophrenia; cancer of the mouth, jaw, tongue, and lung in 19 to 30 year olds; nonlymphoblastic leukemia in children from marihuana smoking mothers, and fetotoxicity.

GENERAL CONCLUSIONS

Henri Baylon

An international colloquium on illicit drugs organized with the assistance of the City of Paris was held at the National Academy of Medicine in Paris April 8–9, 1992. The program dealt essentially with human effects of *Cannabis* consumption, and the following general conclusions were drawn at the end of the colloquium:

1. The toxicity of *Cannabis* is today well established, experimentally and clinically. This drug adversely effects the central nervous system, the lung, immunity, and reproductive function.
2. Epidemiological studies have reported that the use of hard drugs rarely occurs among subjects who have never consumed *Cannabis*.
3. Consequently, the participants to this colloquium rebut the distinction made between soft and hard drugs.
4. The trivialization ("decriminalization") of *Cannabis* use, where it has occurred, has resulted in a considerable increase of its consumption and of its subsequent damaging effects.
5. It is important to foster a campaign of information and prevention bearing both on the legal aspects and the health consequences of *Cannabis* consumption.

The excerpts in this chapter are reprinted with permission from the publisher and the authors.

Reference

1. Nahas, G.G., and Latour, C. (1993) *Cannabis: Physiopathology, Epidemiology, Detection.* CRC Press, Boca Raton, FL.

VIII

THE 1997 MEDICAL CONTROVERSY OVER THE LEGALIZATION OF MARIHUANA FOR MEDICINE

In November of 1997, following a well financed media campaign, two referenda in Arizona and California were approved, giving a legal status to marihuana for medicine. At that occasion, conflicting positions were formulated by two groups of physicians. One group supported the legal use of marihuana for medicine in smoked or orally administered form, the other objected to the use of smoked marihuana. Their detailed opinions follow: that of Dr. J.P. Kassirer, editor of the *New England Journal of Medicine,* and that of Gabriel Nahas, Kenneth Sutin, William Manger, and George Hyman who expressed their views in the *Wall Street Journal.*

FEDERAL FOOLISHNESS AND MARIHUANA, AN EDITORIAL

Jerome P. Kassirer

The advanced stages of many illnesses and their treatments are often accompanied by intractable nausea, vomiting, or pain. Thousands of patients with cancer, AIDS, and other diseases report they have obtained striking relief from these devastating symptoms by smoking marihuana *(1).* The alleviation of distress can be so striking that some patients and their families have been willing to risk a jail term to obtain or grow the marihuana.

Despite the desperation of these patients, within weeks after voters in Arizona and California approved propositions allowing physicians in their states to prescribe marihuana for medical indications, Federal officials, including the President, the secretary of Health and Human Services, and the Attorney General sprang into action. At a news conference, Secretary Donna E. Shalala gave an organ recital of the parts of the body that she asserted could be harmed by marihuana and warned of the evils of its spreading use. Attorney General Janet Reno announced that physicians in any state who prescribed the drug could lose the privilege of writing prescriptions, be excluded from Medicare and Medicaid reimbursement, and even be prosecuted for a Federal crime. General Barry R. McCaffrey, director of the Office of National Drug Control Policy, reiterated his agency's position that marihuana is a dangerous drug and implied that voters in Arizona and California had been duped into voting for these propositions. He indicated that it is always possible to study the effects of any drug, including marihuana, but that the use of marihuana by seriously ill patients would require, at the least, scientifically valid research.

I believe that a Federal policy that prohibits physicians from alleviating suffering by prescribing marihuana for seriously ill patients is misguided, heavy-handed, and inhumane. Marihuana may have long-term adverse effects and its use may presage serious addictions, but neither long-term side effects nor addiction is a relevant issue in such

From: *Marihuana and Medicine*
Edited by: G. G. Nahas et al.   © Humana Press Inc., Totowa, NJ

patients. It is also hypocritical to forbid physicians to prescribe marihuana while permitting them to use morphine and meperidine to relieve extreme dyspnea and pain. With both these drugs the difference between the dose that relieves symptoms and the dose that hastens death is very narrow; by contrast, there is no risk of death from smoking marihuana. To demand evidence of therapeutic efficacy is equally hypocritical. The noxious sensations that patients experience are extremely difficult to quantify in controlled experiments. What really counts for a therapy with this kind of safety margin is whether a seriously ill patient feels relief as a result of the intervention, not whether a controlled trial "proves" its efficacy.

Paradoxically, dronabinol, a drug that contains one of the active ingredients in marihuana (tetrahydrocannabinol), has been available by prescription for more than a decade. But it is difficult to titrate the therapeutic dose of this drug, and it is not widely prescribed. By contrast, smoking marihuana produces a rapid increase in the blood level of the active ingredients and is thus more likely to be therapeutic. Needless to say, new drugs such as those that inhibit the nausea associated with chemotherapy may well be more beneficial than smoking marihuana, but their comparative efficacy has never been studied.

Whatever their reasons, federal officials are out of step with the public. Dozens of states have passed laws that ease restrictions on the prescribing of marihuana by physicians, and polls consistently show that the public favors the use of marihuana for such purposes (1). Federal authorities should rescind their prohibition of the medicinal use of marihuana for seriously ill patients and allow physicians to decide which patients to treat. The government should change marihuana's status from that of a schedule I drug (considered to be potentially addictive and with no current medical use) to that of a schedule II drug (potentially addictive but with some accepted medical use) and regulate it accordingly. To ensure its proper distribution and use, the government could declare itself the only agency sanctioned to provide the marihuana. I believe that such a change in policy would have no adverse effects. The argument that it would be a signal to the young that "marihuana is OK" is, I believe, specious.

This proposal is not new. In 1986, after years of legal wrangling, the Drug Enforcement Administration (DEA) held extensive hearings on the transfer of marihuana to schedule II. In 1988, the DEA's own administrative-law judge concluded, "It would be unreasonable, arbitrary, and capricious for DEA to continue to stand between those sufferers and the benefits of this substance in light of the evidence in this record" (1). Nonetheless, the DEA overruled the judge's order to transfer marihuana to schedule II, and in 1992 it issued a final rejection of all requests for reclassification (2).

Some physicians will have the courage to challenge the continued proscription of marihuana for the sick. Eventually, their actions will force the courts to adjudicate between the rights of those at death's door and the absolute power of bureaucrats whose decisions are based more on reflexive ideology and political correctness than on compassion.

Reprinted with permission from the New England Journal of Medicine, Jan. 30, 1997.

References

1. Young, F. L. (1988) Opinion and recommended ruling, marijuana rescheduling petition. Department of Justice, Drug Enforcement Administration. Docket 86–22. Washington, DC, Drug Enforcement Administration, Sept. 6, 1988.
2. Department of Justice, Drug Enforcement Administration. (1992) Marijuana scheduling petition: denial of petition: remand. (Docket No. 86–22.) *Fed. Regist.* **57**, 10489–10508.

MARIHUANA IS THE WRONG MEDICINE

Gabriel G. Nahas, Kenneth Sutin, W. Manger, and G. Hyman

The debate over using marihuana as medicine has been distorted by a basic confusion: The implicit assumption that smoking marihuana is a better therapy than the ingestion of its active therapeutic agent THC or a more effective one than approved medications. This assumption is wrong. THC (also known as marinol) is an approved remedy that may be prescribed by physicians for nausea and AIDS wasting syndrome. It is safer than marihuana smoke.

The prestigious *New England Journal of Medicine* added to the confusion with its January 30, 1997 editorial, signed by editor Jerome P. Kassirer, entitled "Federal foolishness and marihuana." Among the editorial's errors:

It underestimates the toxic properties of marihuana smoke. This smoke contains carbon monoxide, acetaldehyde, napthalene, and carcinogens. Inhalation of THC decreases lung defense mechanisms which are already compromised in AIDS patients, who are extremely vulnerable to pulmonary infections and tumors like Kaposi's sarcoma. Thus marihuana smoke is a questionable choice to treat the symptoms of AIDS or cancer, especially when safer and more effective medications are available.

It implies that marihuana smoking relieves pain. THC (or marihuana) does not interfere directly with the basic mechanisms that control pain like opiates or aspirin, which, unlike marihuana, have proven to be effective. Marihuana may even increase the perception of pain. Kassirer declares it hypocritical to forbid a physician to prescribe marihuana yet allow him to prescribe morphine for the relief of pain. If he means to imply that marihuana is analgesic, he is simply wrong. If the implication is that it is hypocritical to prescribe one dependence-producing drug and not another, Kassirer is relying on a spurious analogy that beclouds the basic pharmacological question: What is the effectiveness of a therapeutic substance prescribed by a physician?

It argues that the patient's feelings are the determinant therapeutic criterion. Kassirer deems it hypocritical to demand scientific evidence of therapeutic efficacy. To determine whether marihuana use is an effective therapy, he says, one should rely not on whether a controlled trial proves its efficacy, but on how patients say they feel after the intervention. Marihuana smoking would therefore become a privileged therapeutic procedure, exempted from the general proof of efficacy required for all drugs, and untested in double-blind controlled placebo trials.

It makes implausible claims about the advantages of smoking marihuana over oral THC. Since smoking marihuana produces a rapid increase in the blood level of active ingredients, it is more likely to be therapeutic, Kassirer claims. But based on pharmacology, the opposite should be the case: Plasma THC concentration following oral administration reaches a more sustained, steady level, lasting three to four hours, twice as long as after smoking. Such prolonged concentration should be more effective than a rapid rise and fall of THC concentration after smoking.

It claims the efficacy of new drugs to treat nausea has not been tested. Dr. Kassirer ignores that experimental and clinical studies have clearly established the superiority of substituted benzamide and ondansetron over oral THC, though acknowledges that these drugs may be more beneficial than marihuana.

It dismisses as specious the argument that approving marihuana for medical use would send the wrong signal to the young. Epidemiological surveys, however, indicate that the greater the perception of harm associated with marihuana, the lower the frequency of its use among children and adolescents.

It condemns as misguided, heavy-handed, and inhumane the Drug Enforcement Administration's refusal to reclassify marihuana from schedule I (addictive and illegal) to schedule II (addictive but legal for some medical uses). Yet this refusal was based on a thorough analysis of reports from medical specialists in ophthalmology, oncology, and neurology. None reported evidence that smoking marihuana was more effective than current approved remedies. The DEA's decision was supported by both the Food and Drug Administration and the Public Health Service. A doctor prescribing marihuana to a patient may be courageous in Kassirer's mind—but he is also scientifically misinformed and in violation of Federal law.

Kassirer recommends that the Federal government get into the marihuana business, by declaring itself the only agency sanctioned to provide the marihuana. Thus, the government would ensure its proper distribution and use. In effect, Kassirer is opening the door to the controlled legitimization of marihuana as it exists in the Netherlands—but even the Dutch have not approved marihuana for medical use!

Finally, Kassirer makes the obligatory appeal to compassion for the suffering. He considers the prohibition of marihuana smoking to infringe on the rights of patients at death's door. In this instance, the use of marihuana can no longer be considered a therapeutic intervention but one of several procedures used to ease the ebbing of life of the terminally ill. But for this purpose doctors should prescribe antiemetic and analgesic therapies of proven efficacy, rather than marihuana smoking. This therapeutic course is not based on bureaucratic absolutism, political correctness, or reflexive ideology—but on scientific knowledge and the humane practice of medicine.

In view of such wide differences in opinion concerning the use of marihuana in medicine a conference on this topic was organized at New York University. The purpose of this conference was to review the pharmacological and molecular basis of the therapeutic properties of marihuana and THC, and to evaluate their clinical applications.

The present monograph reports the proceedings of the conference and its conclusions.

Reprinted with permission from the Wall Street Journal, March 11, 1997.

I CHEMISTRY AND PHARMACOKINETICS

1

Cannabinoid Geometry and Biological Activity

Raphael Mechoulam, W. A. Devane, and R. Glaser

Abstract

Since the isolation and structure elucidation of delta-9-THC by our group in 1964, numerous investigations have addressed the structure-activity relationships (SAR) in the cannabinoid series. The rules established in the 1970s have mostly withstood the erosion of time. However, the SAR rules as regards stereochemistry were developed much later. It was shown that in THC-type cannabinoids activity resides exclusively in the (-)cannabinoids with the 6aR, 10aR stereochemistry, as found in natural (-) delta-9-THC. This important observation was one of the factors that led to research that culminated in the identification of cannabinoid receptors. X-ray crystallography and detailed NMR investigation have made possible the establishment of the geometry of the active cannabinoids both in the solid-state and in solution. This geometry is presented now in some detail.

1. INTRODUCTION

Almost all molecules of pharmacodynamic importance in biology—enzymes, receptors, and transmitters—are chiral (asymmetric). Although they possess one or more chiral centers, generally only one enantiomer is formed in the body. This well-defined molecular geometry puts severe restrictions on the structure of compounds (synthetic or natural) interacting with these natural substances. Hence, both structural and stereochemical requirements have to be defined for every group of biologically active products, be they drugs or molecular tools for research investigations. The cannabinoids are no exception. In this review we shall try to summarize the structural and stereochemical requirements for cannabinoid activity; compare the metabolism, biological activity, and receptor binding of those few cannabinoids whose activity has been investigated with both enantiomers; and analyze the geometry of cannabimimetically active compounds.

From: *Marihuana and Medicine*
Edited by: G. G. Nahas et al.   © Humana Press Inc., Totowa, NJ

2. STRUCTURAL AND STEREOCHEMICAL REQUIREMENTS FOR CANNABINOID ACTIVITY

Whereas the structural requirements for cannabimimetic activity are reasonably well-established, the stereochemical ones are still being debated (1–4). The main reason for this discrepancy is technical: although the chemistry of cannabinoids is not complicated by comparison to many other natural products, most cannabinoids are oily materials that are difficult to purify in large amounts; hence, one can reasonably assume that some of the synthetic products of the early syntheses were not completely pure (in particular, as regards the presence of enantiomers). Most of the early cannabinoid tests were performed in vivo. It is quite possible that such tests frequently detected nonspecific activity (5) in addition to activity caused by the presence of enantiomeric impurities.

Nearly 20 years ago we formulated tentative rules for cannabimimetic structure-activity relationships (SAR)(1). Most of these rules have thus far withstood the erosion of time. Over the years, exceptions were noted and refinements were made. In the last few years, synthetic compounds with structures apparently unrelated to those of the classical cannabinoids have shown cannabimimetic activity. Hence, it is possible that in the near future our understanding of cannabimimetic SAR may undergo a revision.

2.1. Methods for Measuring Cannabimimetic Activity

The in vivo and in vitro methods for measuring cannabimimetic activity have been reviewed (5–7); hence, only a short list of methods currently used are presented here. Gratifyingly, the levels of activity measured by any one of the listed methods are reasonably comparable to most of the others.

2.2. Overt Behavior in Rhesus Monkeys or Baboons (1,8)

Active cannabinoids injected intravenously cause a pattern of behavior resembling that of humans under the influence of cannabinoids. The test is semiquantitative. At low doses (0.05 mg/kg), Δ^9-THC (1) causes tranquility, drowsiness, decreased motor activity, occasional partial ptosis, and occasional head drop; at higher doses (0.1–0.25 mg/kg), the drug causes stupor, ataxia, suppression of motor activity, full ptosis, and typical crouched posture (thinker position) maintained for up to 3 hours (the animal may, however, regain normal behavior for short periods of time if external sensorial stimuli are applied); at doses above 0.5 mg/kg, the drug causes severe stupor and ataxia, full ptosis, immobility, crouched posture lasting for more than 3 hours, and absence of reaction to external stimuli. A compound is not considered to be cannabimimetic if, at 5 mg/kg intravenously, it fails to induce the above characteristic syndromes.

2.3. Dog Ataxia (9,10)

This simple, though very sensitive test is also semiquantitative in nature. Δ^9-THC (1) at 0.2 mg/kg injected intravenously causes static ataxia and depressed activity and the tails are typically tucked. This test has been widely used since the beginning of this century. Walton, in his classical book on marihuana published more than 50 years ago (9), presents numerous photographs of dogs under the influence of the crude drug. Walton (9) defined six stages of intensity of effects: a slight depression, a barely recognizable ataxia, an obvious ataxia, a marked ataxia in which the animal frequently pitches forward and barely catches itself, inability to stand alone, and inability to rise and plunge about. The ataxia is chiefly manifested by swaying movements. More recently, Martin's group in Virginia has used the dog ataxia test as one of several routine tests for determining cannabinoid activity (10).

2.4. The Mouse Ring Test (11)

In this simple assay, introduced by Pertwee, a mouse injected subcutaneously with the drug is placed on a horizontal ring and the percentage of time spent immobile during a 5-minute exposure is determined.

2.5. Spontaneous Activity in Rats and Mice (10)

Mice injected intravenously with the drug are placed in a photocell activity chamber. Interruptions of the photocell beams are recorded to quantify the locomotor activity. In a standard variation, rats are used in an open-field test with ambulation, rearing, defecation, grooming, and urination recorded.

2.6. Drug Discrimination (12–14)

Assays based on drug discrimination are at present the most specific in vivo tests available. Rats or pigeons are trained to emit one response when trained with Δ^9-THC and an alternative response when trained without drug. There is no generalization to Δ^9-THC (**1**) from various CNS-active drugs. However, some exceptions have been noted, and it has been suggested that "the discriminative stimulus properties of THC may have some commonality with the effect of diazepam in a subpopulation of rats trained to discriminate THC" *(14)*.

2.7. Binding to the Cannabinoid Receptor (15,16)

The recent discovery of a cannabinoid receptor and the availability of labeled ligands has made possible the efficient screening of compounds for cannabinoid activity. Thus far, however, the binding of only a limited number of cannabinoids has been reported.

2.8. Structural Requirements for Cannabimimetic Activity

In the following discussion, we shall use the benzopyran numbering in order to conform to the rest of the articles in this monograph. For comparative purposes, the terpenoid numbering is indicated in Scheme 1. Although we use statements such as "retains activity," "eliminates activity," and so on, it should be understood that such determinations depend on the sensitivity and specificity of the test. For example, whereas methoxy Δ^9-THC (**2**) is found to be inactive in most tests, *(1,3)* highly sensitive ones have determined a level of activity of approximately 4% compared to that of Δ^9-THC itself *(3)*.

1. A dihydrobenzopyran-type structure, with a hydroxyl group on the C-1 aromatic position and an alkyl group on the C-3 aromatic position, is present in most active cannabinoids, including Δ^9-THC (**1**). Opening of the pyran ring forming cannabidiol (CBD) (**3**) type compounds leads to complete loss of activity.

   However, several major exceptions have been found: Levonantradol (**4**) and some of its derivatives *(17)*: this modification indicates that the benzopyran ring structure may be exchanged with a corresponding tetrahydroquinoline-type structure. Compounds synthesized at Pfizer, numbered CP-47497 (**5**), CP-55940 (**6**), and some of their derivatives *(17!)*: this is a major simplification of the cannabinoid molecule, which indicates that a heterocyclic B ring may not be an absolute requirement for activity *(18,19)*. However, as cannabidiol (a diphenol) has no cannabimimetic activity, and whereas CP-47497 (a monophenol) is cannabimimetic, the exact requirements need further elaboration. It seems that only monophenolic, but not resorcinolic, compounds are active when ring B is missing. The synthesis and testing of additional compounds should be achieved before strict rules can be formulated on the point. Compounds of type **7** and **8** that are not planar:

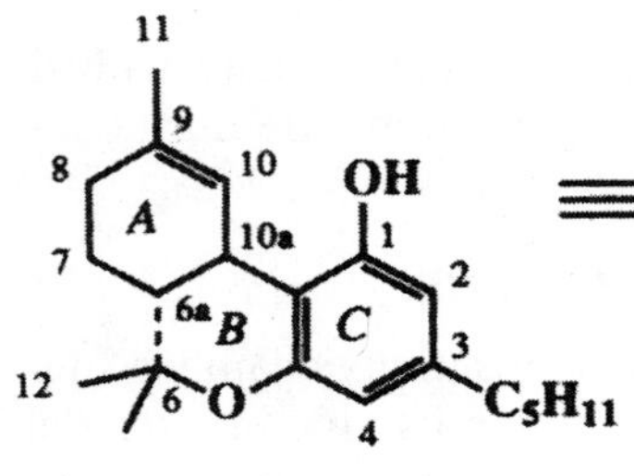

Δ-9-THC (1)

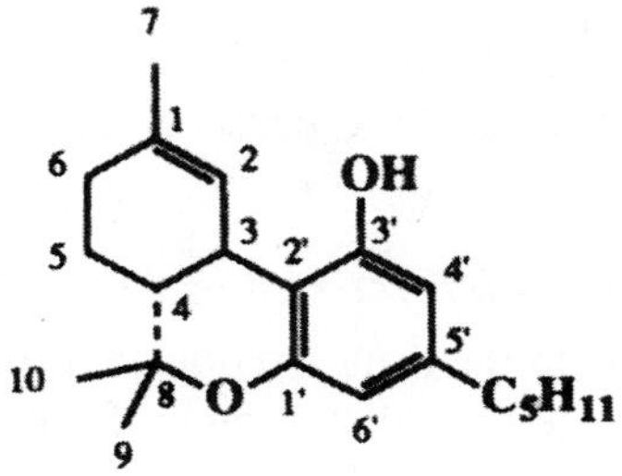

Δ-1-THC
(terpene nemenclature)

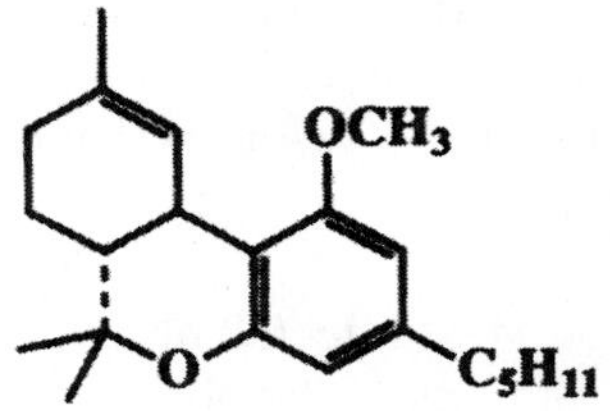

(2)

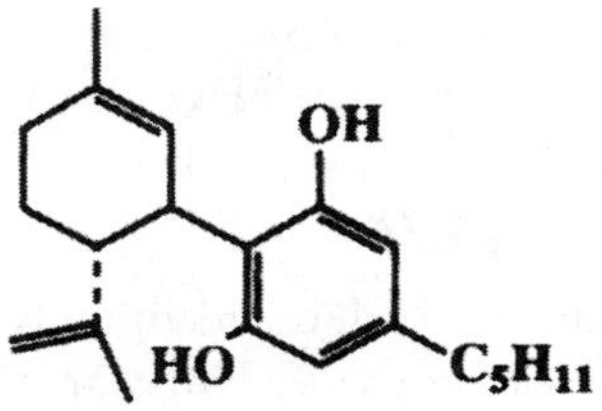

Cannabidiol (3)
(CBD)

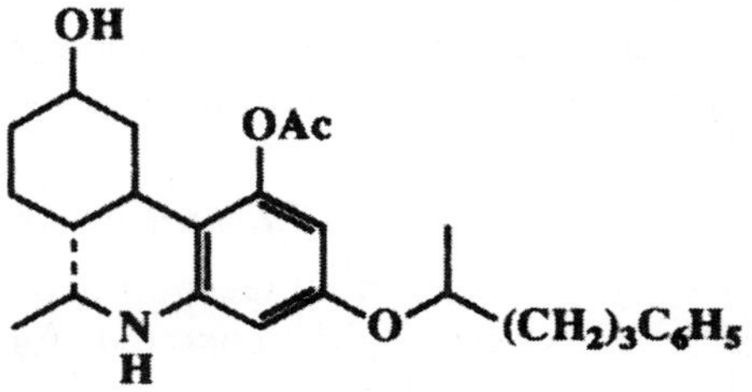

Levonantradol (4)

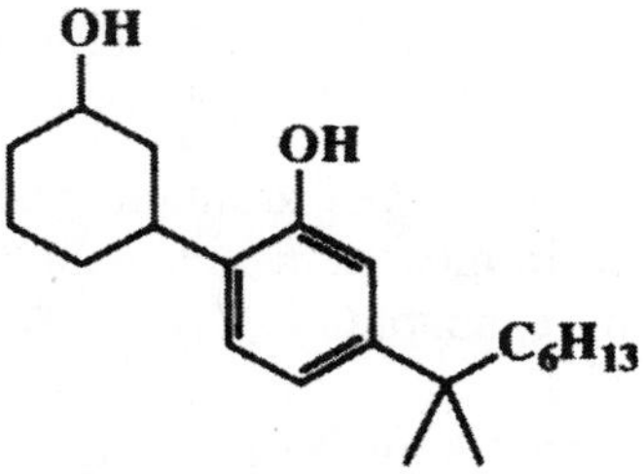

CP-47497 (5)

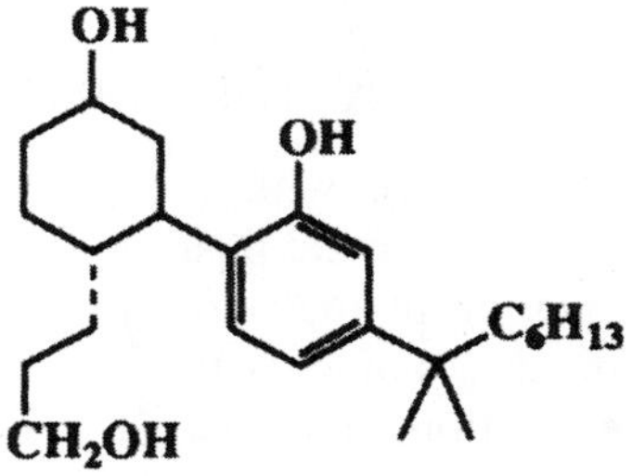

CP-55940 (6)

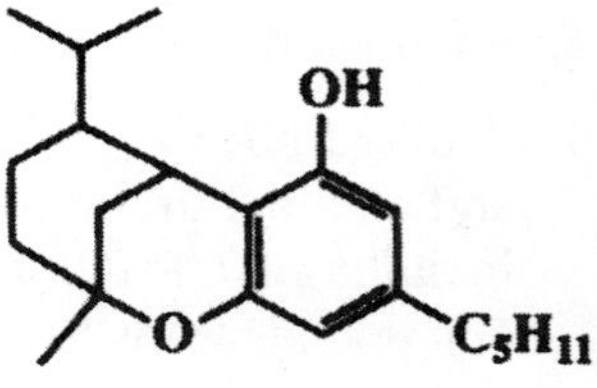

(7)

Scheme 1.

hence, planarity is not an absolute requirement *(18,19)*. Recently, several amino alkyl indoles (AAI) (such as structure **9**) structurally unrelated to the cannabinoids, were found to have a partial cannabimimetic pharmacological profile and bind to the cannabinoid receptor. The SAR in this series remains to be clarified *(20,21)*.

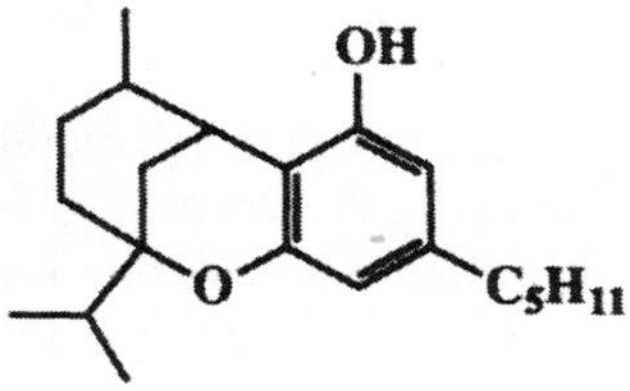

(8) 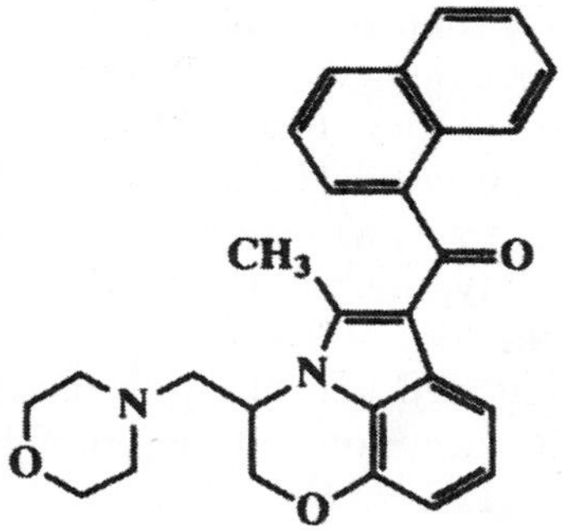 Win-55212-2 (9) 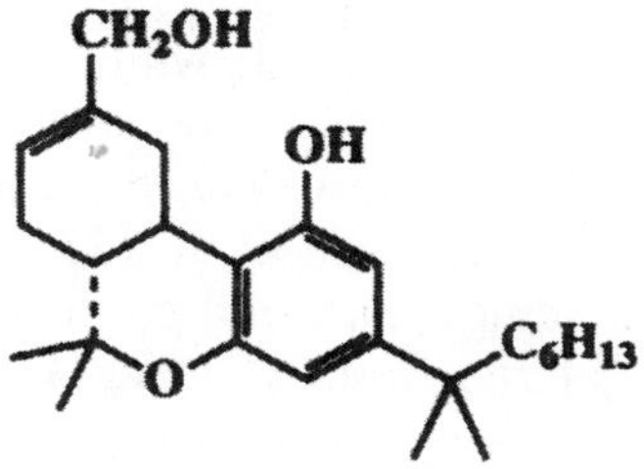 HU-210 (10)

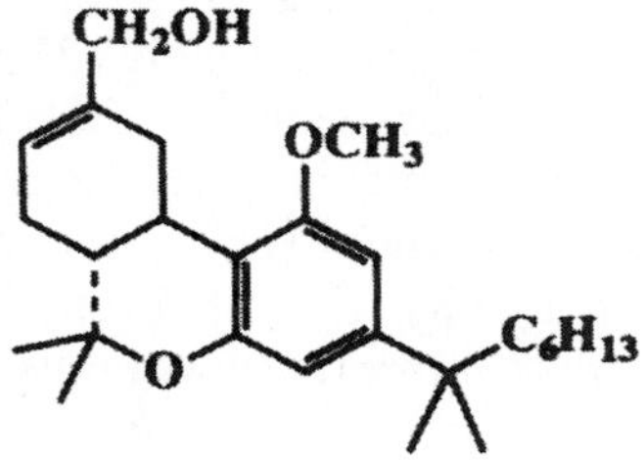

(11) 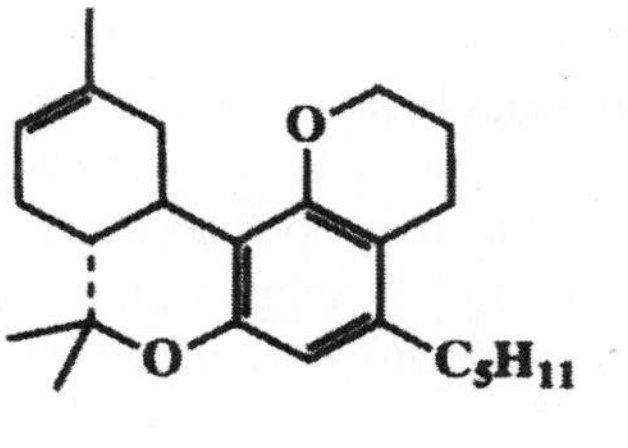 (12) 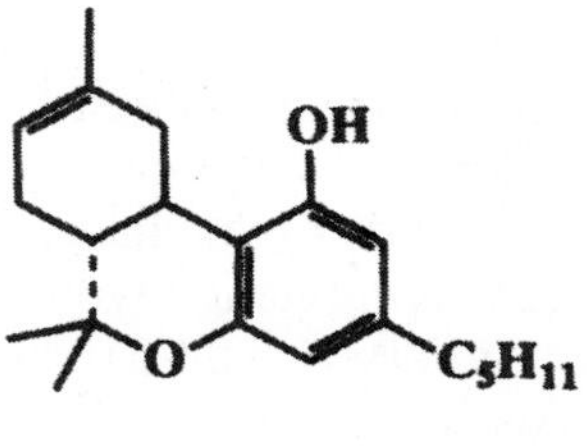 Δ-8-THC (13)

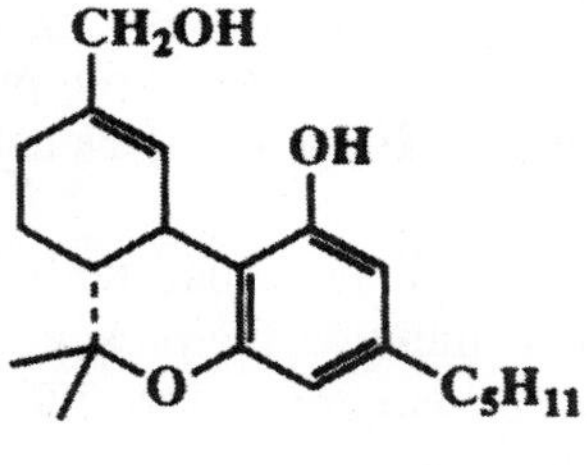

11-OH-Δ-9-THC (14) 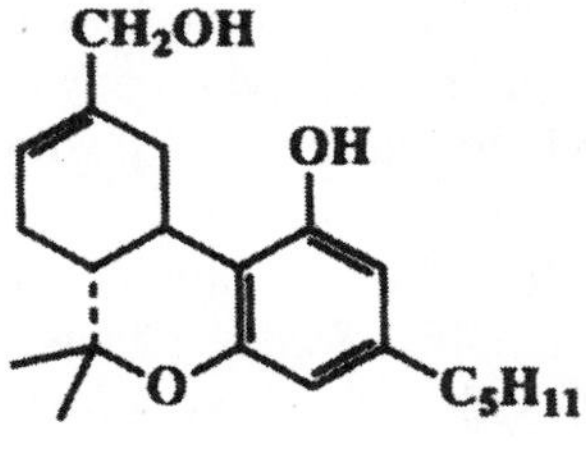 11-OH-Δ-8-THC (15) 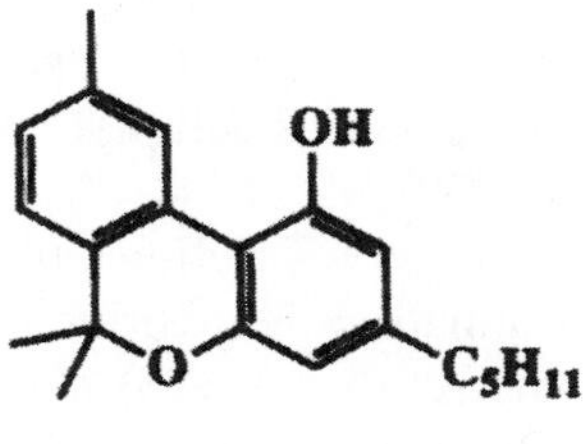 Cannabinol (16)

Scheme 1. (*continued*)

2. The C-1 phenolic group has to be free. Whereas phenol esters exhibit activity in vivo *(1,2)*, this is probably caused by hydrolysis in the body, as no activity has been detected in vitro *(22)*.

Etherification of the phenolic group has been considered to lead to elimination of the activity throughout the cannabinoid series. Recently we observed that etherification (on the phenolic group alone) of the highly potent $(-)$-11-hydroxy-Δ^8-THC-dimethylheptyl leading to compound **11** does not completely abolish binding to the receptor or activity in drug discrimination in the pigeon. The ether (**11**) is considerably less cannabimimetic than the starting material in both tests. The activity is obviously not caused by ether removal which, while possible in vivo , will not be expected in the binding assay. As mentioned above, low levels of activity (approximately 4% of the activity of Δ^9-THC) have been observed for the methyl ether of Δ^9-THC *(3)*.

Seltzman et al. *(23)* have reported that O,2-propano-Δ^8-THC (**12**) depressed rectal temperature and produced antinociception and ring immobility in mice. However, it differed from Δ^9-THC (**1**) *and* Δ^8-THC (**13**) in that it only weakly depressed locomotor activity and failed to substitute for Δ^9-THC in the drug discrimination paradigm. A similar separation of cannabinoid pharmacological effects has not been possible heretofore. These results are of considerable theoretical interest and will be further discussed in subheading 6. Replacement of the phenolic group by an amino group in some cannabinoids retains activity; replacement by a thiol group in all cases tested thus far eliminates activity *(24)*.

3. A major metabolic path in the cannabinoid series involves hydroxylation at C-11 *(25,26)*. Both 11-hydroxy-Δ^9-THC (**14**) and 11-hydroxy-Δ^8-THC (**15**) are cannabimimetic *(27,28)* and somewhat more potent in tests than the parent substances. Further oxidation to the 11-aldehyde or the corresponding carboxylic acid leads to loss of cannabimimetic activity *(28)*, although analgesic activity may be retained *(29)*. Cannabinol (**16**) is weakly cannabimimetic; hydroxylation at C-11 causes an increase in activity *(3)* 11-hydroxy-Δ^8-THC-DMH (HU-210,[**10**]) is apparently the most potent cannabimimetic known thus far (**see** subheading 4.2.) *(31–35)*. The enhancement of activity is caused by the simultaneous introduction of a hydroxyl group at C-11 and the substitution of the pentyl side chain with a 1,1-dimethylheptyl (DMH) one. Surprisingly 11-hydroxy-Δ^9-THC-DMH (**17**) is less active than HU-210 (**10**) *(35,36)*, although Δ^9-THC (**1**) is more active than Δ^8-THC (**13**). Whereas monohydroxylation on the terpene ring usually leads to active derivatives, dihydroxylation generally causes loss of activity *(1,3)*.

Hydroxylation on the side chain has been investigated thoroughly as such compounds are cannabinoid metabolites. Although hydroxylation at the C-1' position leading to (**18**) eliminates activity, a substitution of this type on any one of the other four side-chain positions retains activity. Hydroxylation at the C-3' position leading to (**19**) potentiates activity *(25,37)*.

4. It is now well-established that the Δ^9 isomer is the main, or perhaps the only, cannabimimetic principle in cannabis *(38,39)*. Occasional reports mention the presence of the Δ^8 isomer (**13**), but it is possible that it is actually formed by isomerization *(39,40)*. Other double-bond THC isomers have been prepared by synthesis *(41,42)*. In discrimination tests *(43)* the activity is as follows: Δ^9-THC (**1**) >Δsr8-THC (**13**) >$\Delta^{6a,10a}$-THC (**20**) >$\Delta^{10,10a}$-THC (**21**). Δ^7-THC (**22**), and $\Delta^{9,11}$-THC (**23**) are inactive in animal tests *(41,44)*. However, these compounds have not been extensively tested. $\Delta^{6a,7}$THC (**24**) has not been tested at all.

5. The double bond in the terpene ring is not essential for activity. Reduction of Δ^9-THC leads to the C-9 hexahydrocannabinol epimers, which are both active. Their activity is discussed in subheading 3.

6. The methyl group on position C-9 is not an absolute requirement for activity. 11-norΔ^8-THC (**25**) is active in dogs *(45)*.

7. The alkyl side chain on the aromatic ring is of considerable importance for cannabinoid activity. A side chain of up to three or four carbon atoms apparently is not sufficient for

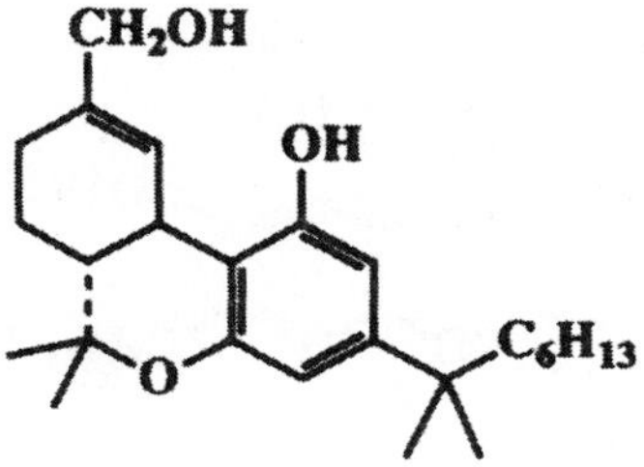

(17)

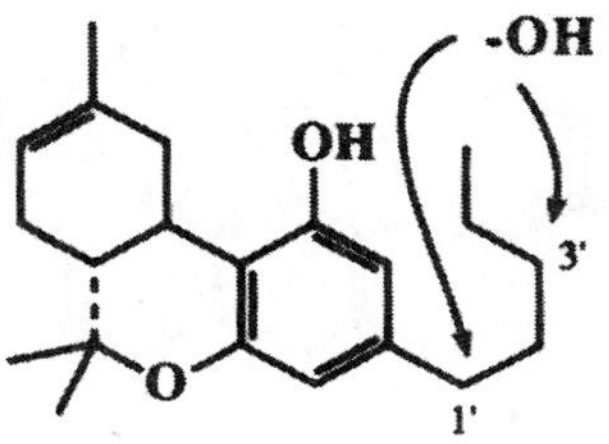

1'-OH-Δ-8-THC (18)
3'-OH-Δ-8-THC (19)

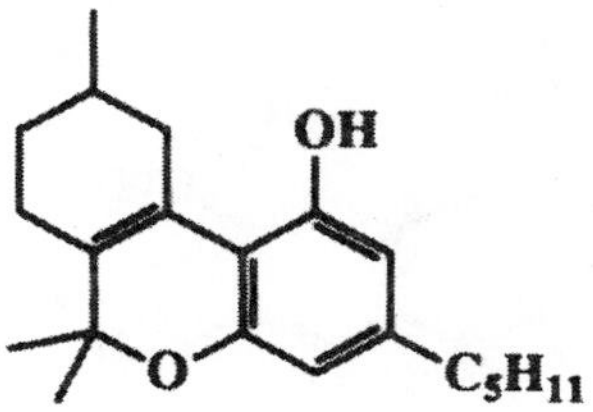

Δ-6a,10a-THC (20)

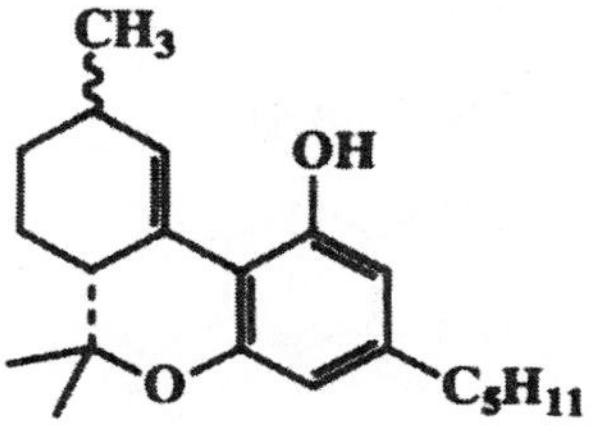

Δ-10,10a-THC (21)

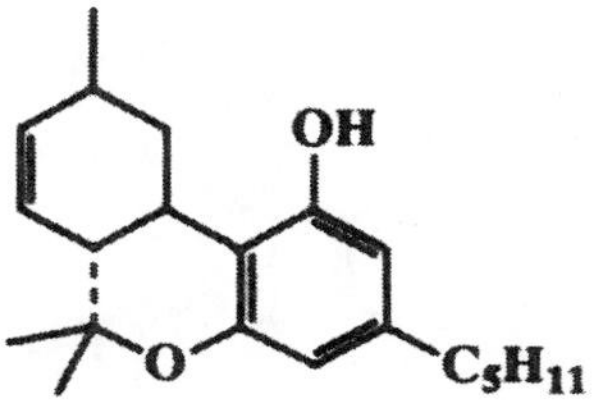

Δ-7-THC (22)

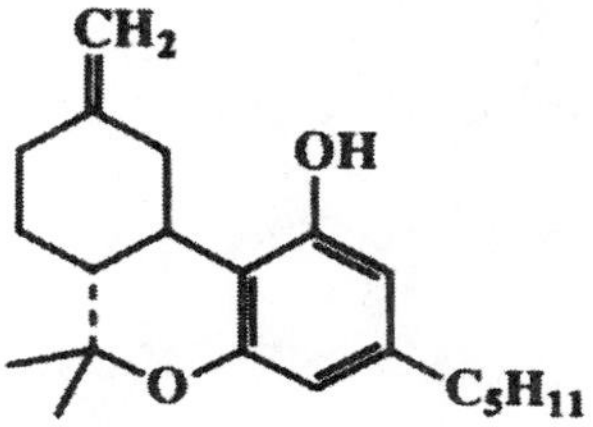

Δ-9,11-THC (23)

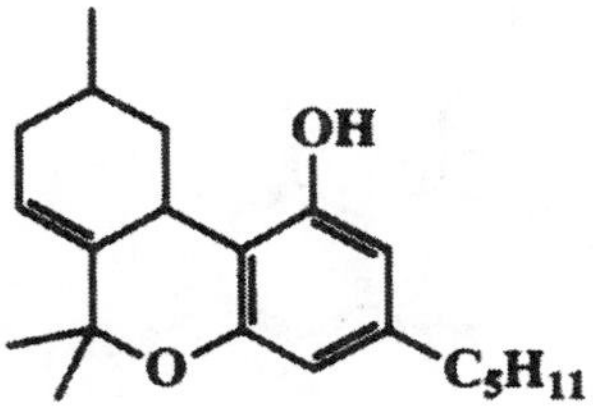

Δ-6a,7-THC (24)

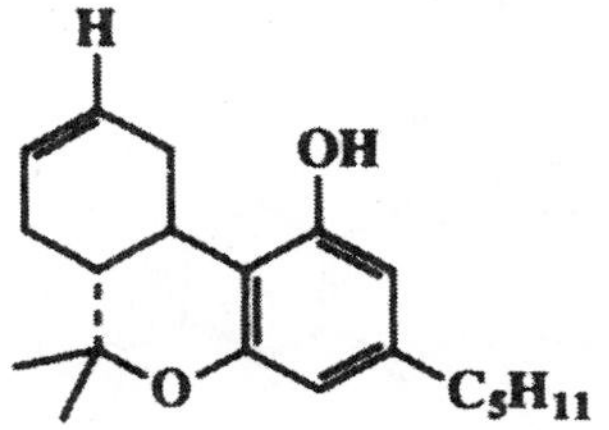

11-Nor-Δ-8-THC (25)

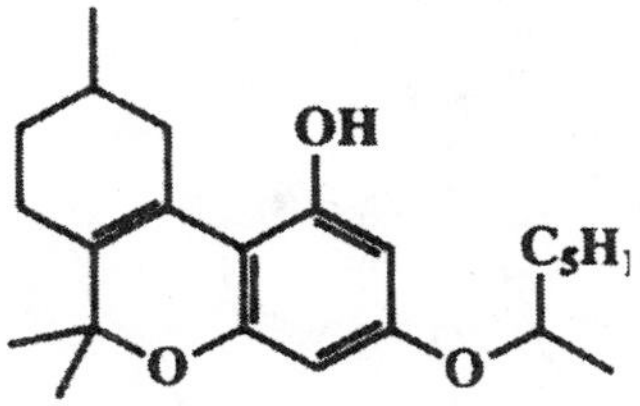

(26)

Scheme 2.

robust activity. The C-5 chain, present in most of the natural cannabinoids, obviously leads to potent compounds. Elongation and branching of the side chain confer potentiation. The most active side chains seem to be the 1,1-dimethylheptyl and 1,2-dimethylheptyl ones *(1,3)*.

An all-carbon side chain may be replaced by one containing an oxygen as an ether; for an example, *see* compound **26.** These modifications do not seem to cause qualitative changes in activity. However, only a few examples have been studied *(17,46,47)*.

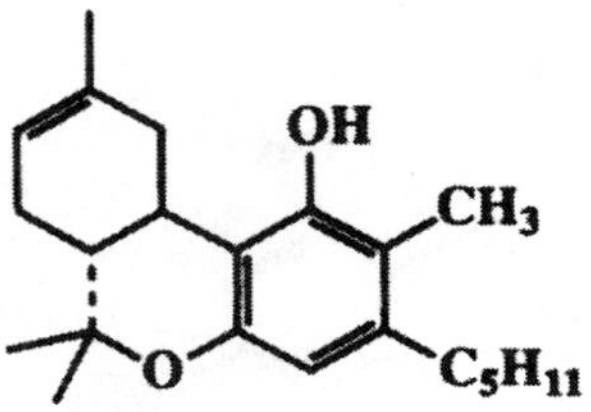

(27) 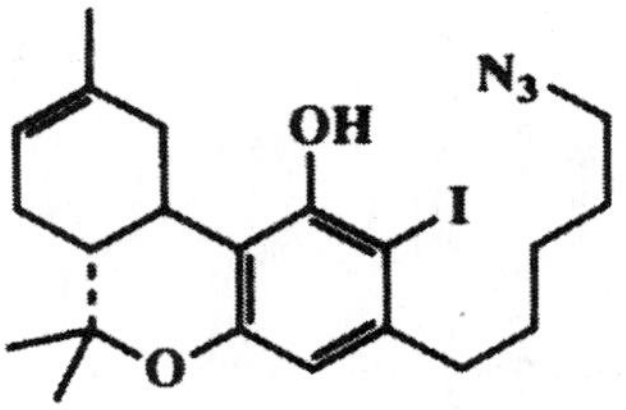   (28) 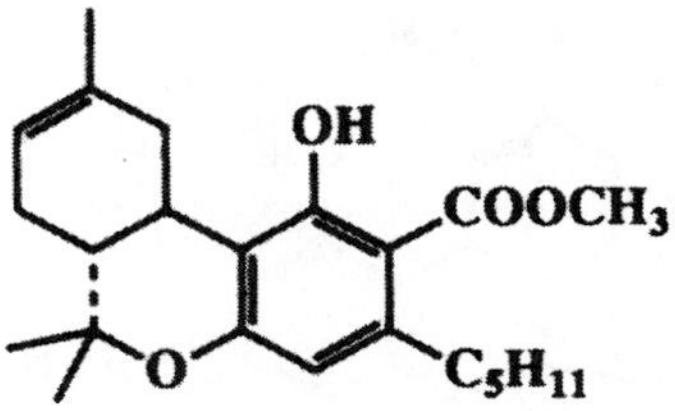   (29)

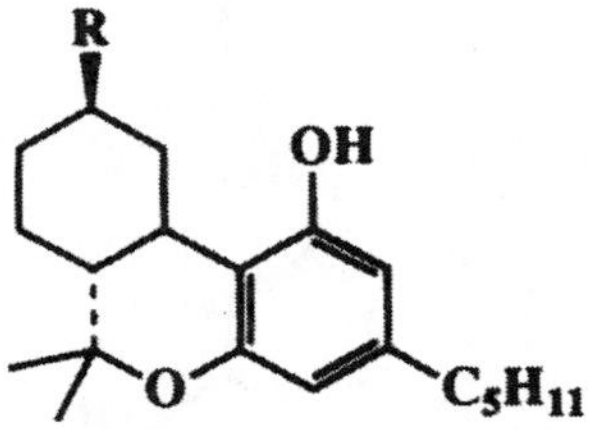

R = CH$_3$ (30a)   R = CH$_3$ (31a)   (32)
R = CH$_2$OH (30b)   R = CH$_2$OH (31b)

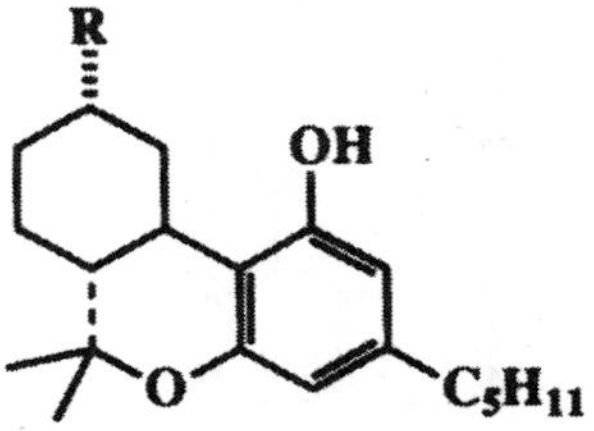

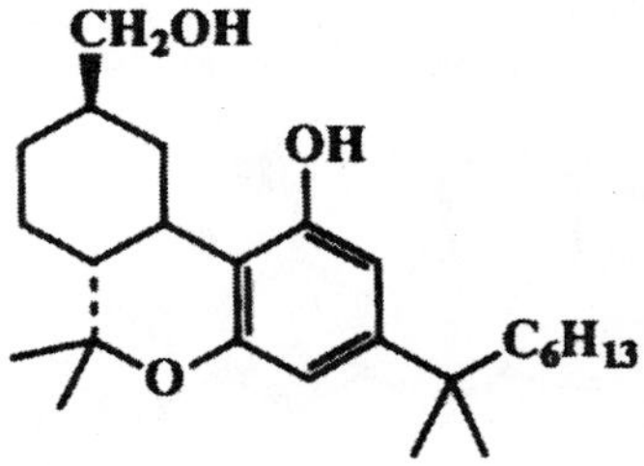

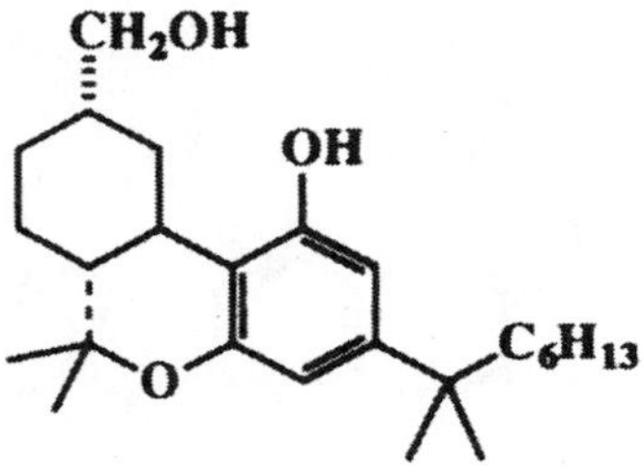

(33) 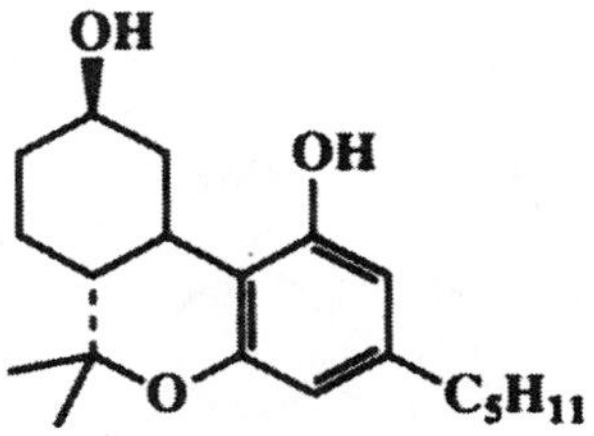   (34) 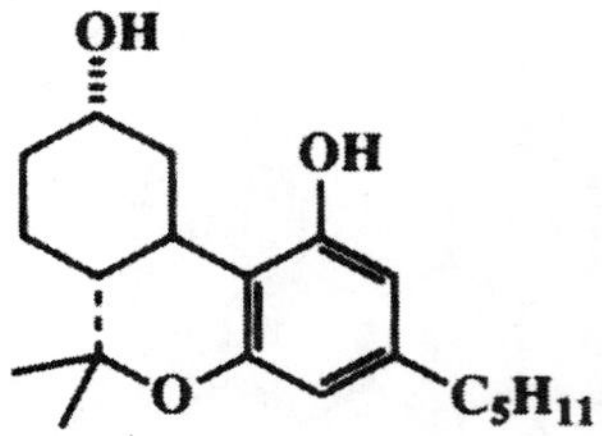   (35)

Scheme 3.

8. Substitution by alkyl groups on C-2 (e.g., compound 27) retains cannabinoid activity, while substitution at C-4 eliminates it *(48)*. Recently, in connection with research on radioactive labeling with iodine, it was reported that 2-iodo-5^1-azido-Δ^8-THC **(28)** showed cannabinoid activity *(49)*. Electronegative groups such as carboxyl (e.g., compound 29), methoxycarbonyl or acetyl at either C-2 or C-4 eliminate activity *(48)*.

A considerable number of additional modifications of the cannabinoid molecule have been prepared and tested, such as replacement of the terpene ring with a heterocyclic one, amino and sulfur substitutions at C-11 and C-12, various esters on the C-1 phenolic group (in order to confer solubility in an aqueous medium), expansion or contraction of the heterocyclic ring, and so on. Many of these compounds are cannabimimetic, but none of them contribute significantly to our understanding of cannabinoid activity. For a detailed listing, *see* ref.*3*.

The above, somewhat sketchy, recapitulation of structural requirements points out that three parts of the cannabinoid molecule are of central importance: the phenolic group, the side chain, and possibly the molecular arrangement around C-9. These requirements fit the classical cannabinoids, represented by the THCs its well as the nonclassical cannabinoids mentioned above (such as CP-47497 [5]), but obviously do not fit the novel cannabimimetic amino alkyl indoles **(9)**.

3. STEREOCHEMICAL REQUIREMENTS FOR CANNNABIMIMETIC ACTIVITY

In this part of our review, we shall look at those cannabinoids in which the configurations of only some of the asymmetric centers have been modified. Pairs of enantiomeric cannabinoids that have been investigated thus far will be discussed in the next section. The reason for this arbitrary separation is that although enantiospecificity (i.e., the specific biological activity of only one of the mirror images of a molecule or enantiomer) is of basic importance to binding to an enzyme or a receptor, the change of configuration at a single asymmetric center and a concomitant change of biological activity may only give us evidence as to the SAR in a particular series of modifications.

1. The stereochemistry at the **6a,10a** in the natural active cannabinoids is *trans* **(6a*R*,10a*R*)** *(50)*. A few *cis* isomers have been tested and have shown very low activity *(2)*. However, *cis* compounds have not been studied over a wide range of tests.
2. As mentioned in the previous section, the double bond in the terpene ring is not essential for activity. Reduction of Δ^9-THC leads to hexahydrocannabinol epimers that are both active, and the equatorial epimer **(30a)** is considerably more active than the axial one **(3la)** *(1,5)*. The same relationship is observed with the 11-hydroxyhexahydrocannabinols **(30b, 31b)** *(52)*. Recently, the corresponding 11-hydroxy compounds with a 1,1-dimethyl heptyl side chain were prepared. The equatorial epimer **(32)** was found to hind to the cannabinoid receptor even better than the highly potent starting material HU-210 **(10)**, while the axial one **(33)** binds considerably less *(53)*. The equatorial epimer has also been tested in a discrimination test and was found to be equipotent to HU-210. It seems that an equatorial substitution (i.e., one in which the methyl or hydroxymethyl group is in the plane of the cyclohexane ring) is preferable to an axial one.
3. In two additional series, an equatorial substituent on C-9 was found to confer greater activity than an axial one. Whereas (9*R*,6a*R*)-$\Delta^{10,10a}$-THC acetate **(21)** (in which the 11-methyl group is equatorial) is active, the corresponding axial epimer is inactive in discrimination tests in pigeons *(43)*. When the methyl group in the hexahydrocannabinols is replaced by a hydroxyl group activity is retained *(54)*. Again, the equatorial epimer **(34)** is much more active than the axial one **(35)** in animal tests.
4. Several hydroxylated metabolites of Δ^9-THC and Δ^8-THC are known in both epimeric forms. Thus 8α and 8β-hydroxy-Δ^9-THC **(36)** and 7α and 7β-hydroxy-Δ^8-THC **(37)** have been identified as relatively minor metabolites. They have been synthesized and tested. Some relatively minor differences in activity were observed *(1,3)*.

4. CANNABINOID ENANTIOMERS: A COMPARISON OF THEIR METABOLISM, BIOLOGICAL ACTIVITY, AND RECEPTOR BINDING

4.1. Metabolism

The metabolism of (–) Δ^9-THC (**1**), (–) Δ^8-THC (**13**), (–) CBD (**3**), and several of the other major natural cannabinoids has been investigated in considerable detail, and numerous reviews are available *(25,26)*. The major primary metabolic pathways are: hydroxylation of the C-11 (in THC), followed by oxidation to the corresponding carboxylic acid; hydroxylation at C-8 (in Δ^9-THC) or C-7 (in Δ^8-THC); and hydroxylation on the side chain, followed by cleavage and oxidation to the corresponding acid. Comparable metabolic pathways are followed for CBD and other natural cannabinoids. The secondary metabolism involves glucuronidation of the carboxylic and phenolic groups. These glucuronides are stored in the body for a relatively long period of time and can be detected frequently in urine several weeks after cannabis consumption.

The unnatural, synthetic (+) enantiomers of the cannabinoids have received much less attention than the natural (–) enantiomers. Only one synthetic route has been reported for these compounds*(55)*. Further routes to the unnatural cannabinoids have been explored and the enantiomeric forms of nabilone, a synthetic antiemetic cannabinoid, have been prepared. However the (+)-THCs have not yet been reported by these routes *(56,57)*.

In (+)-Δ^9-THC (**38**), initial hydroxylation at C-1 is the major in vivo metabolic pathway, followed by oxidation to the carboxylic acid *(58)*. Additional hydroxylation on the side chain occurs. Hence metabolism is very similar to that of the naturally occurring (–) isomers. The main difference observed was the position of the side chain hydroxylation. 1'-Hydroxylation was preferred in (+)-Δ^9-THC, 2'-hydroxylation was mostly observed in (–)-Δ^9-THC. Likewise, less conversion to the carboxylic derivative was noted in the (+) series *(58)*.

A somewhat related picture was observed with (+)-Δ^8-THC (**39**). In vivo , the major metabolic route was again hydroxylation at C-11, followed by side chain hydroxylation, with the C-1' position preferred over the C-2'. In addition, dihydroxylation at positions C-7 and C-11 is much more prominent in (–)-Δ^8-THC than in (+)-Δ^8-THC *(59)*.

The conclusion from these observations was that "the differences in metabolism between the (+) and (–) isomers would not be expected to contribute significantly to the absence of psychoactivity shown by the (+)-isomer" *(58)*.

4.2 Biological Activity

Dewey et al.*(2)* have published a review on the pharmacological effects of cannabinoid stereoisomers that covers most of the work done through the 1980s. Their review compares (+)- with (–)-Δ^9-THC as regards schedule-controlled responding and decreased overt behavior in the monkey, static ataxia in dogs, hypothermia, decreased spontaneous activity and the ring test in the mouse, and action on the isolated ileum of the guinea pig. It also compares the potency of (+)-Δ^8-THC (**39**) with that of (–)-Δ^8-THC (**13**) as regards static ataxia in the dog, analgesia and hypothermia in the mouse, depressed overt behavior in the monkey, drug discrimination, and acetylcholine turnover in the rat. The main conclusion reached was that the (3*S*,4*S*) (+) compounds exhibit sonic cannabimimetic activity, approximately 5–10% of those of the (3*R*,4*R*) (–) compounds. Both types of compounds were found to bind to plasma proteins equally well.

We assume that most of the (+)-THC enantiomers used in the above-reviewed publications were prepared by tile same synthesis *(55)*. Commercial (+)-—pinene (**40**), the starting material for this synthesis, has about 90–95% optical purity and, if intermediates or

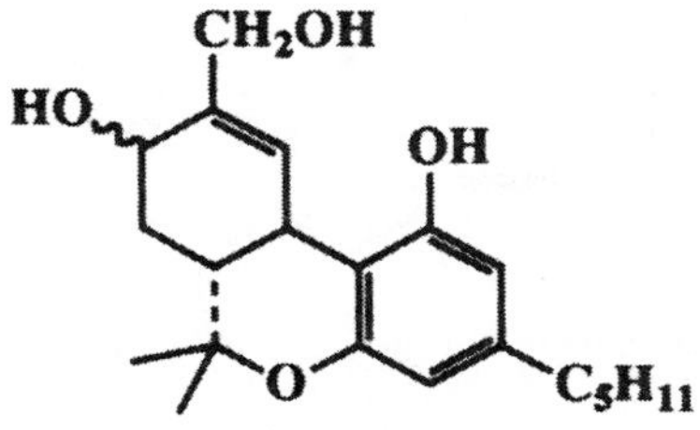

(36)

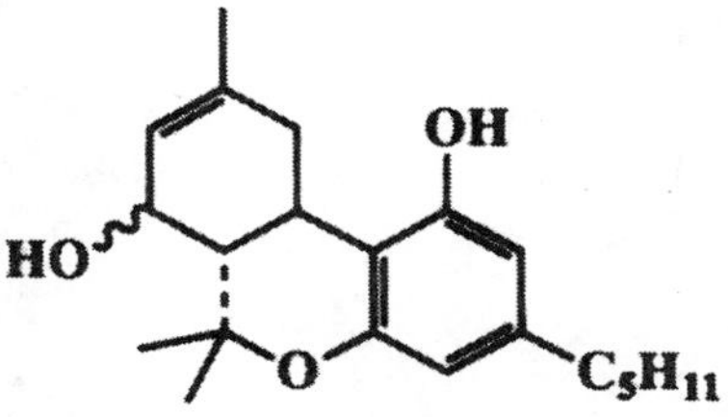

(37)

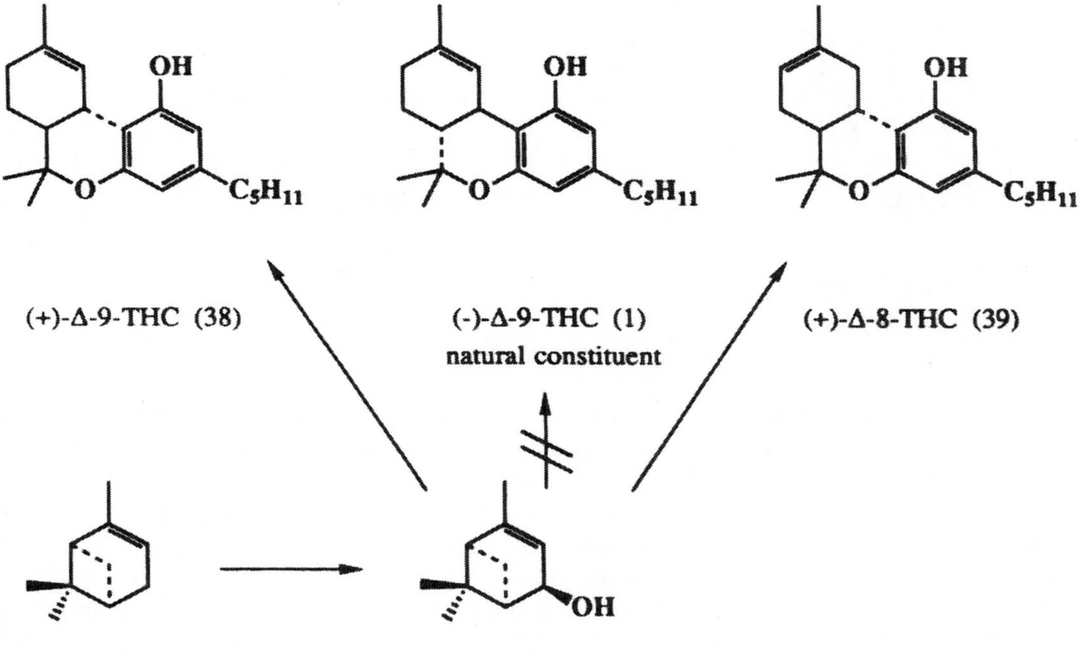

(+)-Δ-9-THC (38)

(-)-Δ-9-THC (1)
natural constituent

(+)-Δ-8-THC (39)

(+)-Pinene (40)

(+)-Verbenol (41)

Scheme 4.

final products are not further purified, THCs with a corresponding level of enantiomeric purity will be obtained. We are not aware that such purifications were indeed performed before the pharmacological tests. Hence. we have to conclude that much, if not all, of the cannabimimetic activity observed may have been caused by contamination by the natural (−)-enantiomers.

We have recently repeated the above synthesis *(60)* The intermediate crystalline *cis* -verbenol **(41)** was recrystallized to 99% optical purity and was further employed in the above synthesis. (+)-Δ^8-THC **(39)** and (+)-Δ^9-THC, **(38)** thus obtained were tested in the mouse ring test, and compared with the corresponding (−)-enantiomers. Natural (−)-THCs showed

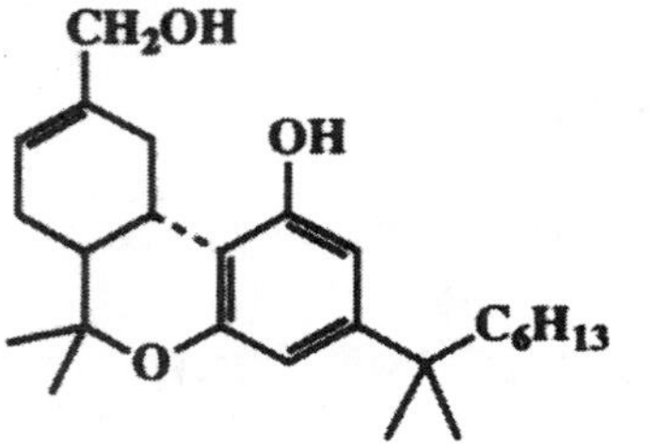

(+)-HU-211 (**42**) 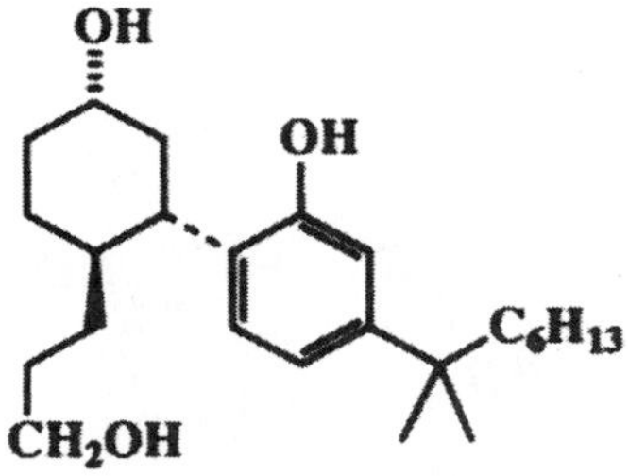   (+)-CP-56667 (**43**) 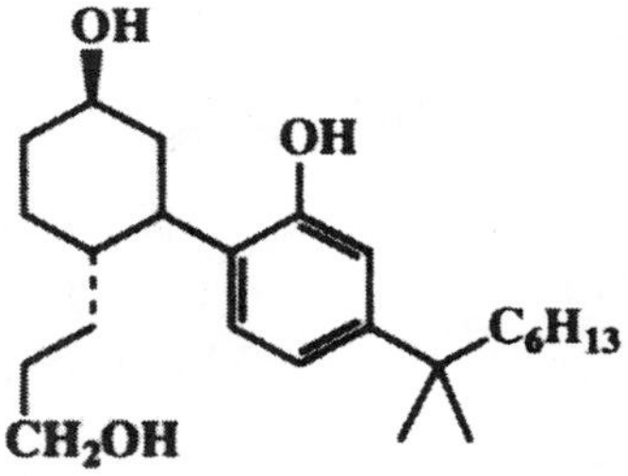   (-)-CP-55940 (**6**)

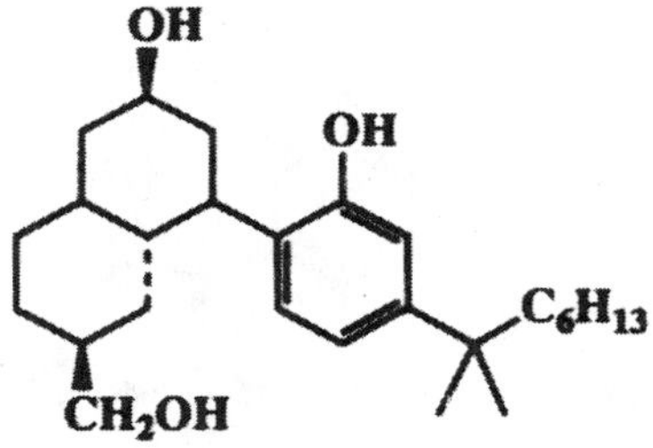

(-)-CP-55244 (**44**) 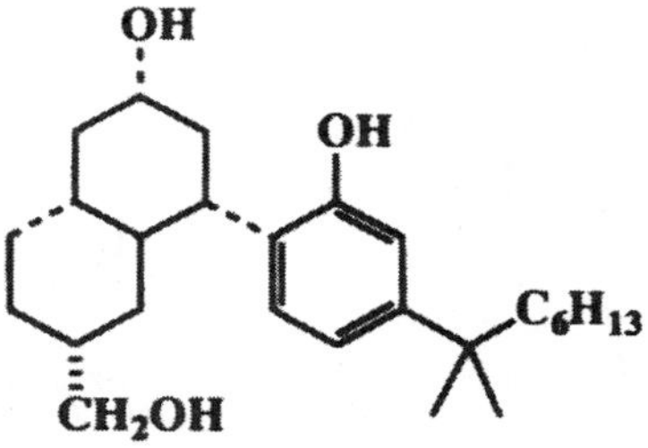   (+)-CP-55243 (**45**)

Scheme 5.

significant activity at 1 mg/kg. No activity was observed with the (+)-enantiomers at 50 mg/kg. However, at 100 mg/kg, definite activity was noted, as would be expected with compounds that are 99% optically pure.

Until further work is reported, we have to assume that complete stereospecificity exists as regards cannabimimetic activity within the THC series. Most of the work done in the past with the (+)-enantiomers has to be reevaluated.

An example of absolute stereospecificity is the case of the enantiomers of the dimethyl-heptyl homologs of 11-hydroxy-Δ^8-THC (**10,42**). The synthesis of these enantiomers has been published *(32)*. It should be pointed out that in this synthesis, both an intermediate and the 11-OH-Δ^8-THC-DMHs themselves are crystalline compounds that can be obtained with absolute enantiomeric purity.

The pharmacological work with these compounds indeed points to the enormous difference in activity between the two enantiomers. As mentioned above, the (−)-enantiomer (HU-210) (**10**) is probably the most active cannabimimetic compound synthesized thus far *(35)*. In drug-stimulus generalization tests, it was found that in the pigeon (−)-11-OH-Δ^8-THC-DMH (HU-210) was about 87 times more active than Δ^9-THC *(33)*. The (+)-11-OH-Δ^8-THC-DMH enantiomer (HU-211) (**42**) was inactive in the pigeon at doses about 4500 higher than the ED$_{50}$ of the (−)-enantiomer; the respective dose in the rat was almost 1000 times higher. Parallel results were obtained in the mouse ring test and in the rotarod test in rats *(31)*.

The effects of the enantiomers of 11-OH-Δ^8-THC-DMH on spontaneous activity, rectal temperature, tail-flick latency, and catalepsy were also studied in mice and in the dog ataxia model *(34)*. The (−)-enantiomer (HU-210) (**10**) was active in all tests at doses between 3 and

Table 1
Relative Potency of Cannabinoid Enantiomeric Pairs

Compound	Potency
$(-)\Delta^9$-THC (1)	1.0
$(-)$HU-210 (10)	100.0
$(+)$HU-211 (42) (estimated)	<0.05
$(-)$-1evonantradol (4)	2.0
$(+)$-Dextronantradol	<0.13
$(-)$-CP-55940 (6)	10.0
$(+)$-CP-56667 (43)	<0. 2
$(-)$-CP-55244 (44)	33.33
$(+)$-CP-55243 (45)	<0. 14

Note. The potency numbers represent an average of various in vivo tests, as compared to that of Δ^9-THC (activity 1.0) *(see also text)*.

100 Ëg/kg, whereas the (+)enantiomer (HU-211) was inactive at 30 mg/kg in the mouse and 1 mg/kg in the dog. Thus, the (−)-enantiomer (HU-210) was 100–800 times more potent than Δ^9-THC in the mouse.

On the basis of the above results, the authors conclude that "the degree of stereoselectivity demonstrated with the enantiomers of 11-OH-Δ^8-THC-DMH greatly exceeded that which had been demonstrated previously for the cannabinoids. The degree of stereoselectivity is on the order of that demonstrated with the opiates, which have a well-defined receptor system. It is likely that the extreme potency of (−)-11-OH-Δ^8-THC-DMH unmasks the true stereoselectivity of the cannabinoids. The stereoselectivity and potency of the (−)-enantiomer is certainly consistent with the existence of a specific receptor for the cannabinoids which is involved in the mediation of some of the pharmacological effects of the cannabinoids"*(34)*. Parallel results were obtained on inhibition of adenylate cyclase and binding to the cannabinoid receptor (see subheading 4.3.) *(61)*.

Other enantiomeric pairs have also been investigated. For example, the nitrogen-containing cannabinoid levonantradol (4), whose stereochemistry parallels that of natural Δ^9-THC, has been compared with its enantiomer dextronantradol *(17,35)*. In a series of analgetic tests, the levo compound was active (MPE$_{50}$) at about 0.2 mg/kg, whereas the dextro compound was not active up to 10 mg/kg. In several tests for cannabimimetic activity (spontaneous activity, hypothermia, and catalepsy), levonantradol was active betweenn 0.123 and 1.5 mg/kg, whereas dextronantradol was inactive.

The same overall picture was seen with the "nonclassical" cannabinoid pairs (−)CP-55940 (6)–(+)CP-56667 (43), and (-)CP55244 (44)–(+)CP55243 (45) *(17,35,36)*. In both series, the (−) enantiomers were found to be highly cannabimimetic in a battery of in vivo tests. The (+)-enantiomers were essentially inactive. The results are presented in Table 1. As the relative ED50 (compared to that of Δ ^{9}-THC) observed for a given drug was similar for all assays, results were averaged to give an estimate of their overall potency, with Δ^9-THC having a potency of 1.0 and HU-210 a potency of 100.0.

The degree of potency and particularly the high enantioselectivity within the four groups of compounds presented above and in Table 1 are strong indications of a molecular mechanism that is highly specific, presumably involving a receptor.

A few other cannabinoid enantiomeric pairs have also been investigated. Less stereospecificity was observed. If the reason for the low specificity is not trivial (the presence of an impurity for example), one can presume that such molecules only partially fit the cannabinoid receptor and the stereochemistry of the active materials is therefore less demanding. The enantiomeric benzofuran cannabinoids **46** and **47** will be further discussed in subheading 6. The ratio of the activity of the more active cannabinoid (**47**) to the less active one (**46**) (in a drug discrimination assay in the pigeon) was only about 20:1 *(620.*

$\Delta^{6a,10a}$-THC (**20**) (as a racemate) was synthesized about 50 years ago by the groups of Roger Adams (United States) and Lord Todd (in the United Kingdom) and was the first identified compound to show hashish-type activity *(63).* Surprisingly, its pure enantiomers were not prepared and tested until a few years ago *(42).* As the racemate had already been administered to humans, the enantiomers were also directly tested intravenously in human volunteers. The cannabimimetic effects observed with one of the enantiomers, $(9S)$-$\Delta^{6a,10a}$-THC, were indistinguishable from those caused by Δ^9-THC. The adjectives used by the volunteers to describe experiences with either drug included "peaceful," "pleasant," "relaxed," "dreamy," "dry mouth," "satisfied," "carefree," "happy," "hungry," "time slowed." The potency of the synthetic drug however was one-third to one-sixth that of the natural Δ^9-THC. No effects were noted with the other enantiomer, $(9R)$-$\Delta^{6a,10a}$-THC *(64).* These enantiomers were later assayed in discrimination tests in pigeons *(43).* In these tests the $(9S)$-enantiomer was found to be only two to three times more active than the $(9R)$-enantiomer. Presumably, the differences between the results in humans and in pigeons are because of the limited range of material administered intravenously to the volunteers. It is quite possible that at higher doses the volunteers on the $(9R)$-enantiomer would have also reported to be "peaceful," "relaxed," and "dreamy."

4.3. Noncannabimimetic Effects

The synthesis of pure cannabinoid enantiomeric pairs has made possible investigations on and comparison of noncannabimimetic compounds and their biological and pharmacological properties.

4.4 CBD

The pharmacological effects of cannabidiol (CBD) (**3**) (and a few of its derivatives) have been well investigated, mostly as regards movement and seizure disorders *(65).* Recently, two groups reported that CBD has an antianxiety effect in rats and mice in the elevated plus-maze at surprisingly low dose levels *(66,67).* These results give support to previous reports that CBD has anxiolytic effects in human volunteers *(65),* as well as in animals *(68).* The (+)enantiomer of CBD (**48**) has not yet been investigated in these tests. In view of the activity of both (−)-CBD (**48**) and (+)-CBD (**49**) in anticonvulsion tests *(69),* work along these lines may be of importance.

Administration of Δ^9-THC to proestrous rats has been shown to suppress the preovulatory luteinizing hormone (LH) surge and ovulation *(70).* (−)-Cannabidiol (**3**) was inactive, but (+)-cannabidiol (**48**) had significant activity at 10 mg/kg. The (+)-CBDDMH homolog (**49**) was considerably more potent than (−)-CBD-DMH (**50**)*71.* These observations have not been followed up. It should be of considerable interest to investigate other members of the (+)-cannabinoid series.

4.5. HU-211

As mentioned above. the (+)-enantiomer of 11-hydroxy-Δ^8-THC-DMH (HU-211) (**42**) is nonpsychotropic *(31–34).* However, HU-211 was found to induce a highly significant inhibition of cisplatin-induced emesis in pigeons, particularly at doses of 2.5 and 3.0 mg/kg ($p < 0.001$) *(72).* In contrast to these results, Δ^9-THC failed to cause a significant antiemetic effect at any of the doses injected. This is in agreement with clinical findings showing only a low inhibition of cisplatin emesis in cancer patients concurrently treated with Δ^9-THC. Cupric salts enhanced the activity of both HU-211 and of Δ^9-THC. These results indicate, for the first time, that separation between the antiemetic and psychotropic activity is possible in the cannabinoid series and may open a new route to antiemetic drugs.

HU-211 induces stereotypy and locomotor hyperactivity in mice and mild tachycardia in rats. These properties are consistent with those of noncompetitive antagonists of the NMDA subclass of glutamate receptors, suggesting that HU-211 might function as an NMDA-receptor antagonist. Indeed, HU-211 protects against the tremorogenic, convulsive, and lethal effects of NMDA in mice. Binding studies indicate that HU-211 blocks NMDA receptors*(73)*. The (–)-enantiomer (HU-210) was inactive.

Recent evidence has indicated that brain damage induced by ischemia is mediated, *inter alia*, by NMDA receptors. In view of the absence of psychotropic or other untoward side effects seen by HU-211 administration at doses that block NMDA effects, this cannabinoid seems to be a suitable candidate for drug development.

4.5 Dextronantradol and (+)-CP-56667

These nonclassical, nonpsychotropic cannabinoids whose (–)-enantiomers, (**4**) and (**6**), respectively, are highly potent cannabimimetics (*see* above) seem to have been only marginally investigated for noncannabinoid activity. However, they have been found to cause changes in the effects ofΔ^9-THC. Thus, CP-56667 reduced the effect of THC on spontaneous activity in mice, but enhanced the catalepsy *(35,36)*.

5. ADENYLATE CYCLASE INHIBITION AND RECEPTOR BINDING

The discovery by Howlett that cannabinoid drugs can inhibit the adenylate cyclase activity of a neuroblastoma cell line led to an extensive biochemical and pharmacological characterization of this response (reviewed in ref. *16* Chapter x). In assessing the ability of cannabinoid drugs to inhibit the secretin-stimulated adenylate cyclase activity of an N18TG2 membrane preparation, a marked enantioselectivity was observed for several compounds (Table 2). The potency ratio of compounds with (–)-TH-like stereochemistry to their corresponding (+)-enantiomers ranges from less than twofold for the simple bicyclic CP-47497 (**5**) ($K_{inh} = 79$ nM) to greater than 1000-fold for the highly potent HLJ-210 ($K_{inh} = 7.2$ nM) and CP-55244 ($K_{inh} = 5$ nM). The great enantioselectivity, as well as the involvement of a G protein in the inhibitory response, suggested that cannabinoid drugs were working through distinct receptors.

Using [^{3}H] CP-55940 (^{3}H-6), a centrifugation binding assay was developed that identified and characterized a cannabinoid receptor in rat brain *(15)*. Because the receptor is coupled to a G protein, its affinity for cannabinoid drugs can be modulated by guanine nucleotides and various ions, similar to the behavior of other G-protein-linked receptors. The assay conditions employed were those that maximized the specific binding of [^{3}H]CP-55940 (^{3}H-6) to a rat cortical membrane preparation. With this centrifugation assay, CP-55940 (**6**) displayed $K_i = 68$ pM and its (+)-enantiomer was 50-fold less potent, with $K_i = 3.4$ nM. HU-210 (**10**) was able to fully compete for the specific binding of [^{3}H]CP-55940 in heterologous displacement studies with $K_i = 234$ pM ; the (+)-enantiomer was 1500-fold less potent. Though CP-55940 (**6**) and HU-210 (**10**) are similarly potent in both the binding studies and the inhibition of adenylate cyclase, it appears that the more rigid structure of the 3-ring HU-210 (**10**) confers a greater enantioselectivity than the bicyclic CP-55940 (**6**).

The identification of a cannabinoid receptor in rat brain was quickly followed by the elegant autoradiographic analyses of Herkenham et al. *(74)* and the cloning of a cannabinoid receptor by Matsuda et al. *(75)*. In addition todetailing the distribution of the cannabinoid

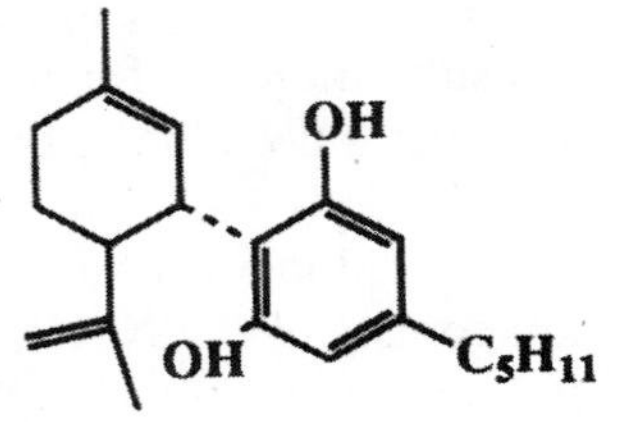

(+)-CBD (48) 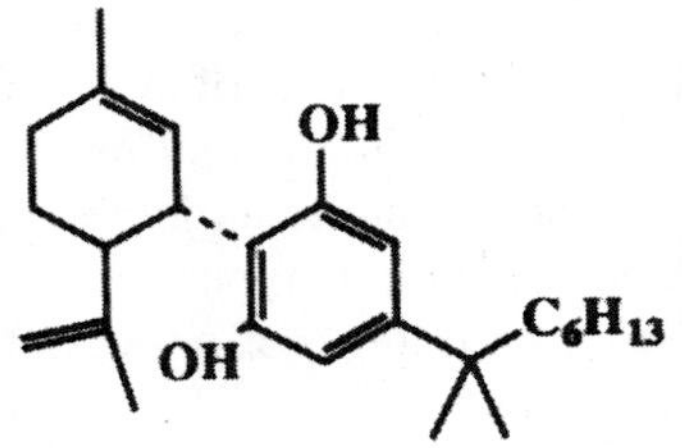   (49) 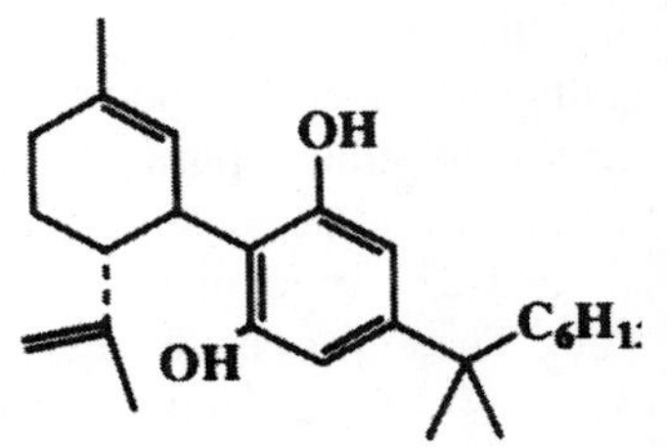   (50)

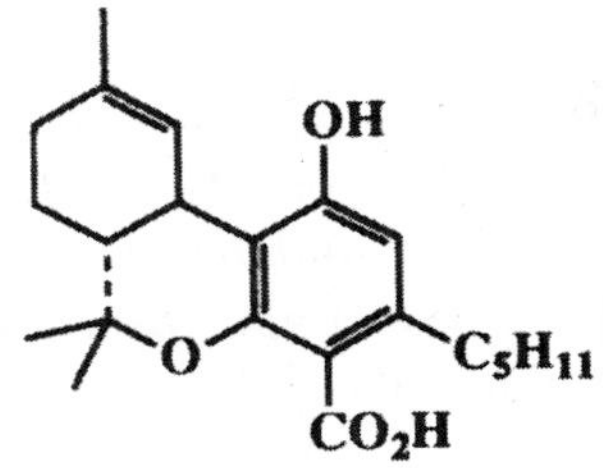

Δ-9-THC acid B (51) 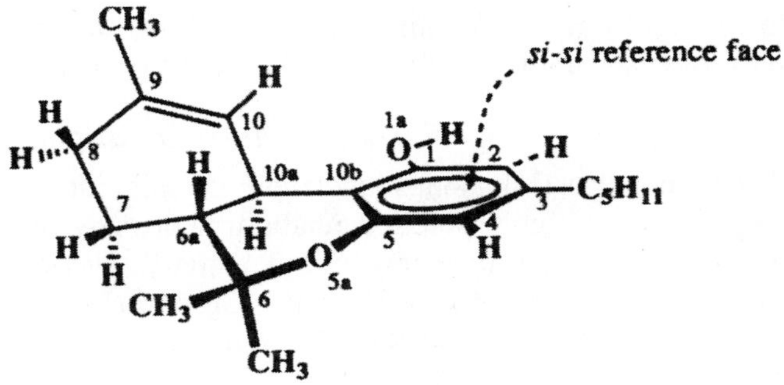   (52)

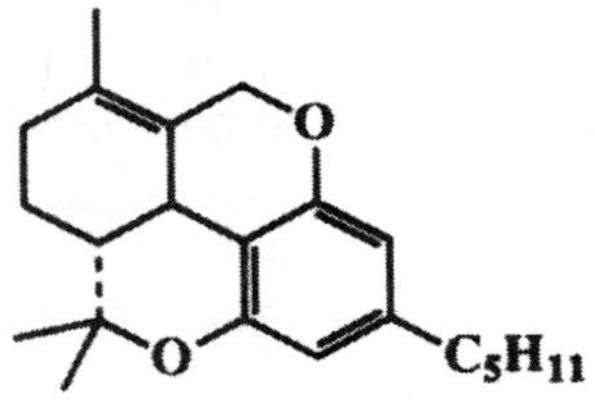

si-si reference face

(53) 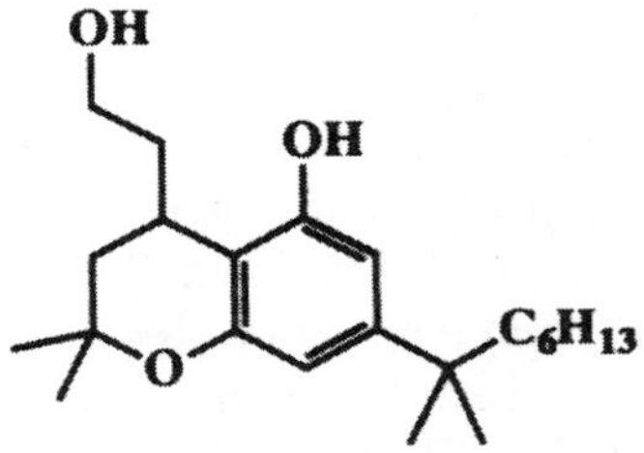   (54)

Scheme 6.

receptor in the brains of several species using classical autoradiography, Herkenham et al. have used slide-mounted sausage sections of whole rat brain to pharmacologically characterize the receptor. The brain preparation and assay conditions are quite different from those used in the previously described centrifugation assay that may account for the 200-fold increase in observed K_i values. The K_i value of CP-55940 (**6**) derived from competitive inhibition studies using the sausage technique was 15 nM vs a K_i = 68 pM using the centrifugation assay. However, the enantiospecificity was similar for both assays: the (+)enantiomer was 30-fold less potent than CP-55940 using the sausage technique, compared with 50-fold

Table 2
Adenylate Cyclase Inhibition and Receptor Binding by Cannabinoid Enantiomeric Pairs

	Inhibition of adenylate cyclase		Binding to cannabinoid receptor	
	K_{inh} $(nM)^a$	IC_{50} $^{(nM)b}$	K_i $(nM)^c$	K_i $(nM)^d$
(−)-CP-55940 (6)	25	0.87	0.068	15
(+)-Enantiomer	>5000	96.3	3.4	470
HU-210 (10)	7.2		0.234	
HU-211 (42)	e		360	
(−)-CP-55244 (44)	5			1.4
(+)-CP-55243 (45)	e			18,000
(−)-Levonantrodal (4)	100			14
(+)-Dextronantrodal	>5000			26,000
(−)-CP-47497 (5)	79			79
(+)-Enantiomer	135			86
(−)Δ^9-THC (1)		13.5		420
(+)Δ^9-THC (38)		773		7,700

[a]Refs. 61 and 77; N18TG2 neuroblastoma cell membranes./tfn [b]Refs. 75; inhibition of cAMP accumulation in transfected CHO-K1 cells.
[c]Refs. 15 and 61; centrifugation assay with rat P2 cortical membranes.
[d]Refs. 74 and 76, sausage sections from whole rat brain.
[e] No significant inhibition at 10 μM.

less potent using the centrifugation assay. They tested several pairs of enantiomers for their ability to inhibit the binding of [³H]]CP-55940 to the sausage sections and the results correlate well with the ability of these drugs to inhibit adenylate cyclase activity in neuroblastoma membranes (Table 2). CP-47497 (5) and its (+)-enantiomer, which exhibited less than a twofold potency ratio in the adenylate cyclase assay, were almost equipotent, with K_i values of 79 and 86 nM, respectively. The most potent compound, CP-55244 (44), had a K_i = 1.4 nM, with its (+)enantiomer (CP-55243) (45) being 12,000-fold less potent. The potency ratio of these (−)- and (+)-enantiomers was greater than 1000-fold in the adenylate cyclase assay.

Using Chinese hamster ovary K1 cells stably transfected with the cDNA for a rat cortical cannabinoid receptor, Matsuda et al. (75) were also able to demonstrate the inhibition of forskolin-stimulated cyclic AMP production by cannabinoid drugs. In this system, CP-55940 exhibited an IC_{50} of 0.87 nM and its (+)-enantiomer was 110-fold less potent. (−)-Δ^9-THC (1) exhibited an IC_{50} of 13.5 nM, whereas (+)-Δ^9-THC (38) was 57-fold less potent.

In both the binding studies and the adenylate cyclase assays, the conformationally more rigid three-ring, highly potent cannabinoids, CP-55244 (44) and HU-210 (10), exhibit the greatest enantioselectivity, followed by the potent but more flexible bicyclic CP-55940 (6). The more simple bicyclic, CP-47497 (5), exhibited little enantioselectivity in either test.

6. THE GEOMETRY OF CANNABIMIMETICALLY ACTIVE CANNABINOIDS

X-ray crystallography has yet to provide us with a solid-state structure of Δ^9-THC (1). However analogs of 1 have been studied by this method; for example. the natural Δ 9-THC acid B (51) (78,79).

Initial ¹H NMR one-dimensional studies provided partial information on the structure of Δ^9-THC in solution (80). Recently, ¹H and ¹³C NMR one- and two-dimensional techniques

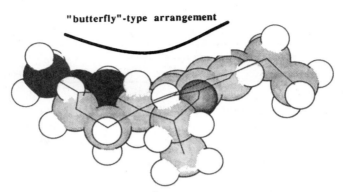

Fig. 1. Space-filling MM2 calculated model of Δ^9-THC (**1**) (with ethyl group instead of *n*-amyl group) looking down the C(6a)-C(10a) bond showing butterfly-type arrangement of rings A and B. C(9)-methyl, C(9), and C(10) colored black.

have been used by Kriwacki and Makriyannis to extensively study the conformation in CDCl$_3$ solution *(81)*. Their analysis clearly shows that the solution-state conformation of Δ^9-THC is very similar to the solid-state conformation of the crystalline carboxylated analog (**51**). Furthermore, both structures are very similar to those calculated by molecular mechanics modeling *(62,80,82)*. This agreement of structural features is really quite reasonable since the Δ^9-THC ring-skeleton is fairly rigid.

The orientation and electronegativity of substituents (e.g., X and Y in a XCH$_2$CH$_2$Y fragment) influence the magnitude of NMR vicinal coupling constants *(83)*. Using Lambert's R-factor method in which the orientation and electronegativity effects on $^3J_{HH}$ are canceled out *(84)* we have calculated a $45 \pm 1°$ value for dihedral angle C(6a)-C(7)-C(8)-C(9) based on the relevant coupling constants of Kriwacki and Makriyannis *(81)* (and estimated standard deviations of 0.2 Hz). This solution-state value compares quite favorably with the $42°$ value determined for crystalline **51**.

The conformation of ring A is that of a chair containing a *synperiplanar* (i.e., circa 0°) torsion angle [C(8)-C(9)-C(l0)-C(10a)]. In this conformation, H(6a) is mutually *antiperiplanar* (i.e., circa 180°) to its H(7A) and H(10a) neighbors, whereas H(8β) and H(6a) have a pseudo *cis*-1,3-diaxial relationship. The equatorial positions at C(6a) and C(10a) provide points of fusion for ring B, thus resulting in a *trans* A,B-ring junction. The conformation of ring B is also that of a chair containing a synperiplanar (circa 0°) torsion angle [O(5a)-C(5)-C(l0b)-C(10a)]. In ring B of the natural (−) (6a*R*, l0a*R*)-Δ^9-THC (**1**), H(6a) is mutually antiperiplanar (circa 180°) to both its H(l0a)and pro-R [axial]methyl C(6)-CH$_3$ (A) neighbors as depicted in structure **52**. As a result of *trans*-fusion, the two flattened-chair rings (A, B) are disposed in a butterfly-type arrangement in which fragment C(10a)-C(9)-CH$_3$ is closer to one of the two *diastereotopic* (i.e., symmetry unrelated) faces of the resorcinol ring (ring C) (*see* Fig. 1). *re,si*-Descriptors *(85)* may be used to define the particular face of the resorcinol ring that is closer to this ring A fragment. Using descriptors for trigonal carbons C(5) and C(10b), the above-mentioned fragment is oriented closer to the *si-si* face of the C(5,10b) double bond reference plane in (−)-Δ^9-THC. Irradiation of the OH afforded only one NOE intensity enhancement [7% into H(2)] and none to H(10), thus testifying to a preferred orientation in CDCl$_3$ solution as shown in **52** *(81)*. In the solid-state, the *n*-amyl side chain of **51** is arranged in an extended staggered-type conformation so that the second carbon of the chain is approximately perpendicular to ring-C *(78)*. Long-range benzylic NMR coupling constants are consistent with such an arrangement, but do not rule out dynamic averaging of other conformations *(81)*.

The importance of the OH group lone pair and its spatial orientation versus the phenoxy proton and its orientation has been the subject of much recent work *(23,86,87)*. Molecular mechanics has shown two low-energy conformations for the phenoxy proton *(86)*. In one of them, it is almost synperiplanar to H(2); the other is almost antiperiplanar to H(2). The lack of cannabimimetic activity of 1-methoxy-Δ^9-THC **(2)** (approximately 20 times less potent than **1**), may be rationalized in terms of either the absence of a phenoxy proton or the inability of the lone pairs of the 1-methoxy oxygen to become oriented into the pharmacologically important conformation. Using the Van der Waal's radii of constituent atoms, volume maps of energy-minimized **1** and **2** were calculated by Semus and Martin *(88)*. Models were made in which the phenoxy proton or the methoxy methyl were located either *syn* or *anti* to C(2). An electropositive atom (hydrogen) 2.8 ^AI from the oxygen atom probed for a hypothetical H bond in which the 1-substition is the acceptor. A lone pair 2.8 ^AI from the phenoxy proton probed for a hypothetical H bond in which the phenolic proton is the donor. Overlap of the cannabinoid volume with the volume of the probing unit (H or lone pair) was considered to be evidence that a hydrogen-bonding interaction between the 1-substituent on the cannabinoid and a receptor/membrane was not possible. Hydrogen bonding involving oxygen lone pairs (using H probe) when either OMe or OH is in an *anti* orientation to C(2) was ruled out since overlap was observed for the OH model and the OMe model does not represent an energy minimum for the cannabinoid. On the other hand, no volume overlap was noted for hydrogen bonding involving oxygen lone pairs when either O*Me* or O*H* is in a *syn* orientation to C(2). Furthermore, no volume overlap was noted for hydrogen bonding involving the phenyl proton (using the lone pair probe) when OH is either *anti* or *syn* to C(2) *(88)*.

Another approach to this problem was taken by preparing rotationally restricted THC ethers **53** and **12** *(23)*. Behavioral and pharmacological evaluations were made for these analogs. Compound **(53)** was completely inactive in all mouse behavioral tests, as well as the rat drug discrimination model *(87)* Compound **12** was found to be similar to Δ^8-THC in that it depressed rectal temperature and produced antinociception and ring immobility in mice. However, it differed from Δ^8-THC in that it only weakly depressed locomotor activity and failed to substitute for Δ^9-THC in the drug discrimination paradigm. On this basis, it was stated that the orientation of the lone pairs of electrons oil the phenolic hydroxyl plays a role in the mediation of some, but not all, behavioral effects of the cannabinoids. Molecular mechanics studies and molecular electrostatic potential maps were calculated for compounds **12** and **53**. Two conformations of the more active **12** were found. These differ primarily in the twist of the O,2-propano moiety, whereby the new pyran ring assumes a chair conformation with a synperiplanar torsion angle. Inversion of the ring torsion angles is possible for this new ring and, thus, two diastereomeric conformations exist.

Recently, enantiomeric bicyclic cannabinoids having a furanyl B ring **(46)** and **(47)** were prepared and tested *(62)* (*see* subheading 4.2.0). NMR spectroscopy together with molecular mechanics modeling studies have shown that the bicyclo[3.1.1]heptyl moiety in the more active (−)-enantiomer of compound **47** contains four carbon atoms (colored black in the stereo view; Fig.2) located in positions similar to those in the C(l0a)-C(10)-C(9)-CH$_3$ fragment of (−)-1. The geminal dimethyl groups on the disubstituted methano bridge in **47** reside in different environments. The methyl group *syn* (on the same side as) to the unsubstituted methano bridge in **47** corresponds spatially to the C(9)-methyl in (−)-1 and to the equatorial C(9)-methyl in hexahydrocannabinol compound **30a**. In saturated ring-A analogs of THC **(30a, 31a)**, the two C(9) epimers show different cannabimimetic activity (*see above*). Molecular mechanics calculations of models for **30a** and **31a** were recently presented by Reggio et al. *(86)*. They discussed the orientation of ring A relative to the resorcinol ring. One of their conclusions was that protrusion of a C(9)-substituent (e.g., the axial C(9)-methyl in **31a**

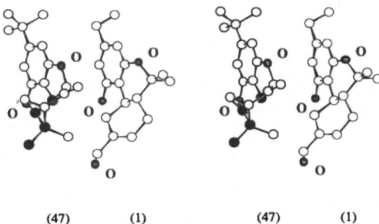

(47)   **(1)**   **(47)**   **(1)**

Fig. 2. Stereo view comparison of MM2 calculated models for **1** (on the right), and **47** (on the left). For the purpose of simplification in the molecular mechanics calculations, a *t*-butyl group has replaced the dimethylheptyl side chain in the model for **47**, and all ethyl group has replaced the *n*-amyl group in the model for **1**. Hydrogen atoms have been omitted for clarity. The four atoms in **47** corresponding to C(10b), C(10), C(9), and CH3 in (**1**) are colored in black.

towards the "bottom" face [i.e., towards the *re-re* reference plane as in **52**]) might hamper or prevent cannabinoid molecules from binding at their site of action. The methyl group *anti* to (on the opposite side of) the unsubstituted methano bridge in the active (−)-*47* molecule corresponds spatially to the axial C(9)-methyl in *31a* and both are located relatively close to the resorcinol ring reference plane. Since *47* shows high cannabimimetic activity, it is probable that the weak activity of *31a* results from in absence of the properly oriented C(9)-substituent (i.e., an equatorial methyl), rather than the presence of the improperly axially oriented C(9)-methyl. However, paradoxically the absence of a substituent at C(9) (i.e., 9-nor-Δ^9-THC, **25**) does not remove all activity *(45,88)*. The overlap of the benzofuran (**47**) and Δ^9-THC [1] is presented in Fig.3. The structures were calculated by molecular mechanics (MM2 program) *(62)*. For simplicity, the *n*-amyl group of **1** was replaced by an ethyl group, and the 1,1-dimethylheptyl group of **47** was replaced by a *t*-butyl group. In this comparison of structures **1** and **47**, the carbon and hydrogen atoms common to the CH₃-C(9)-C(10)-C(10a) fragment in both molecules are highlighted in both molecules. In addition, carbon and hydrogen atoms in **47** that are spatially different than those in rings-A,B of **1** are also highlighted.

The importance of the disposition of C(9)-substituents relative to the resorcinol ring is also demonstrated by compounds **34** and**5** *(17)*. Johnson and Melvin have shown that the relative orientation of the C(9)-OH to the phenolic-OH is similar in molecular mechanics energy minimized models for these two compounds. Compounds **5, 34,** and **54** are all active analgesic agents *(17)*, and all share three common structural features: the aromatic ring, the alkyl chain at C-3, and four atoms corresponding to the CH₃-C(9)-C(10)-C(10a) fragment in Δ^9-THC. As analgesic activity in this series parallels cannabimimetic activity, one can presume that these features are also structurally significant for the latter.

The above results indicate that a simple correlation seems to exist between the relative geometry of rings A and C and cannabimimetic activity. The C(10a), C(10), C(9), C(11) carbon chains attached to the resorcinol ring in compounds **1, 47,** and **10** are reasonably equivalent in terms of the respective distances of the corresponding atoms to the midpoint of the aromatic ring. In addition, these chains of carbon atoms in models for the same compounds (all of which are cannabimimetic) show equivalent signs and magnitudes for their respective

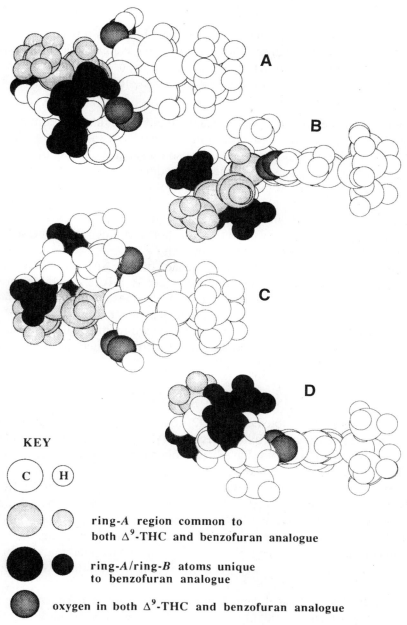

KEY

C H

ring-*A* region common to
both Δ⁹-THC and benzofuran analogue

ring-*A*/ring-*B* atoms unique
to benzofuran analogue

oxygen in both Δ⁹-THC and benzofuran analogue

Fig. 3. Overlay of molecular calculated structures **1** and **47**. View A is looking down upon the *si-si* face of the resorcinol ring. Views A to D represent rotations of 90° in a direction parallel to the C(10a)–C(10b) bond. The CH3-C(9)-C(10)-C(10a) fragment common to both structures is shown. Ring A/ring B atoms unique to **47** are also highlighted.

angles of deviation relative to the *si-si* ('top face of the molecule") face of the plane. The corresponding carbon atoms in the respective enantiomers (which either lack cannabimimetic activity or are much weaker than their enantiomers) show equivalent magnitudes, but opposite signs for the respective angles of deviation.

7. QUO VADIMUS?

The recent identification of a cannabinoid receptor has been a major step forward in our understanding of cannabinoid action. The realization that cannabinoid activity is very highly enantiospecific has contributed much to this advance. We now believe that four major goals are to be accomplished and that their achievement is possible on the basis of the knowledge acquired and the techniques available.

1. Identification of a specific endogenous cannabinoid transmitter. Preliminary work in our laboratory has indicated that such a transmitter(s) exists. It seems to be a lipid.
2. With the help of the natural endogenous transmitter and the accumulated knowledge on SAR (in particular, as regards stereochemical requirements), the tertiary structure of the cannabinoid receptor and the mode of binding of cannabinoids to the receptor could be clarified.
3. We still know very little about the functions of the cannabinoid system in the body. Is it involved in the regulation of movement and in short-term memory as presently presumed? Does it play a role in the modulation of emotions?
4. A major disappointment thus far has been the lack of success in introducing a cannabinoid (synthetic or natural) as a major new drug. Whereas Δ^9-THC and nabilone are very helpful in preventing vomiting during cancer chemotherapy, these compounds do not represent a major therapeutic breakthrough. Let us hope that recent reports on the separation of cannabimimetic from therapeutic activity in synthetic molecules, in particular enantiomers, may revitalize this area and lead to new drugs in neurology (particularly stroke and muscular dystrophy) and against glaucoma.

NOTE ADDED IN PROOF

Since this article was first published in 1992, considerable advances have been reported in the cannabinoid field: a second peripheral receptor (CB2) was identified and cloned *(90)* and 2 types of endogenous cannabinoids have been isolated and their structures were established. Best known are arachidonoylethanolamide and 2-arachidonoyl glycerol *(91,92)*. These endocannabinoids are fatty acid derivatives and obviously differ structurally from the natural plant tricyclic terpeno-phenolic THC. These endocannabinoids even lack an asymmetric center. Yet they bind to the CB1 and CB2 receptors with KD values essentially equivalent to those of THC. Presumably on interaction with the cannabinoid receptors, they take up a conformation close to that of TH. Reggio's group has made excellent analyses of the available data and have produced a receptor-steric map (a binding pocket) that fits the activation of the receptor by tricyclic cannabinoids *(93,94)*.

While the SAR of the classical cannabinoids for CB1 are well-known *(see above)*, those for CB2 have not yet been thoroughly exploited. The few reports published so far indicate that the structural requirements for binding to CB2 differ very much from those of CB1. Gareau et al. have reported that the dimethylheptyl homolog of delta-8-THC binds to both CB1 and CB2 (K_i values of 0.83 and 0.49 nM, respectively); the methyl ether of this compound binds weakly to CB1 (K_i 1585 nM), which is compatible with data for other methyl ethers of cannabinoids. However this methyl ether binds to CB2 with a Ki of 20 nM *(95)*. This selectivity of binding activity may represent an opening to new cannabinoid drugs which act on the periphery only, without CNS side-effects.

As cannabinol has been shown to bind to CB2 with a KD close to that of delta-9-THC *(90)* we recently undertook an SAR study of cannabinol-type cannabinoids. We found that 11-hydroxy-cannabinol, a major primary metabolite, binds potently to both CB1 and CB2, but inhibits only the CB1-mediated adenylyl cyclase; it is actually a specific, though not potent CB2 antagonist (96). The second-stage metabolite, cannabinol-11-oic acid was shown to be inactive, as expected.

Reprinted from : Marijuana/Cannabinoids: Neurobiology and Neuropsychology Edited by Laura Murphy and Andrzej Bartke, CRC Press, Boca Raton, 1992, pp 1–33.

References

1. Mechoulam, R. and Edery, H., Structure-activity relationships in the cannabinoid series, in *Marijuana.- Chemistry, Pharmacology, Metabolism and Clinical Effects,* Mechoulam, R., Ed., Academic Press, New York, 1973.
2. Dewey, W. L., Martin, B. R., and May, E. L., Cannabinoid stereoisomers: pharmacological effects, in *Handbook qf Stereoisoniers: Drugs in Psychchopharmacology,* Smith, D. F., Ed., CRC Press. Boca Raton, FL, 1984, 317.
3. Razdan, R. K., Structure-activity relationships in cannabinoids, *Pharmacol. Rev.,* **38,** 75, 1986.
4. Mechoulam, R., Lander, N., Srebnik, M., Breuer, A., Segal, M., Feigenbaum, J. J., Järbe, T. U. C., and Consroe, P., Stereochernical requirements for cannabirnimetic activity, in *Structure-Activit.y Relationships qf the Cannabinoids,* Rapaka, R. S. and Makriyannis, A., Eds., NIDA Research Monograph 79, Rockville, MD, 1987, 15.
5. Martin, B. R., Cellular effects of cannabinoids, *Pharmacol. Rev.,* **38,** 45, 1996.
6. Dewey, W. L., Cannabinoid pharmacology, *Pharmacol. Rev.,* **38,** 151, 1986.
7. Paton, W. D. M. and Pertwee, R. G., The pharmacology of Cannabis in animals, in *Marijuana: Chemistry, Pharmacology, Metabolism and Clinical Effects,* Mechoulam, R., Ed., Academic Press, New York, 1973.
8. Grunfeld, Y. and Edery, H., Psychopharmacological activity of the active constituents of hashish and some related cannabinoids, *Psycholpharmacologia,* **14,** 200, 1969.
9. Walton, R. P., *Marijuana, America's New Drug Problem,* J.B. Lippincott, Philadelphia, 1938, 168.
10. Martin, B. R., Balster, R. L., Razdan, R. K., Harris, L. S., and Dewey, W. L., Behavior comparisons of the stereoisomers of tetrahydrocannabinols, *Life Sci.,* **29,** 565, 1981.
11. Pertwee, R. G., The ring test: a quantitative method for assessing the cataleptic effect of Cannabis in mice, *Br. J. Pharmacol.,* **46,** 753, 1972.
12. Järbe, T. U. C., Johansson, J. O., and Henriksson, B. G., Characteristics of tetrahydrocannabinol produced discrimination in rats, *Psycholpharmacologia,* **48,** 181, 1976.
13. Järbe, T. U. C., Swedberg, M. D. B., and Mechoulam, R., A repeated tests procedure to assess onset and duration of the cue properties of (-)-delta-9- THC, (-)-delta-8-THC and (+)-delta-g-THC, *Psychopharmacologia,* **75,** 152, 198 1.
14. Mokler, D. J., Nelson, D. B., Harris, L. S., and Rosencrans, J. A., The role of benzodiazepine receptors in the discriminative stimulus properties of delta-9-THC, *Life Sci.,* **38,** 1581, 1986.
15. Devane, W. A., Dysarz, F. A., Johnson, M. R., Melvin, L. S., and Howlett, A. C., Determination and characterization of a cannabinoid receptor in rat brain, *Mol. Pharmacol.,* **34,** 605, 1988.
16. Howlett, A. C., Bidaut-Russell, M., Devane, W. A., Melvin, L. S., Johnson, M. R., and Herkenham, M., The cannabinoid receptor: biochemical, anatomical and behavioral characterization, *Trends Neurosci.,* **13,** 420, 1990.
17. Johnson, M. R. and Melvin, L. S., The discovery of nonclassical cannabinoid analgetics, in *Cannabinoids as Therapeutic Agents,* Mechoulam, R., Ed., CRC Press, Boca Raton. FL, 1986.
18. Houry, S., Mechoulam, R., Fowler, P. J., Macko, E., and Loev, B., Benzoxocin and benzoxonin derivatives: novel groups of terpenophenols with CNS activity, *J. Med. Chem.* **17.** 287, 1974.
19. Houry, S., Mechoulam, R., and Loev, B., Benzoxocin and benzoxonin derivatives: novel groups of terpenophenols with CNS activity, a correction, *J. Med. Chem.,* **18,** 951, 1975.
20. Bell, M. R. et al., Antinociceptive (aminoalkyl) indoles, J. Med. Chem., **34,** 1099, 1991.
21. Haubrich, D. R. et al., Pharmacology of pravadoline: a new analgesic agent, *J.Pharmacol. Exp. Ther.,* **255,** 511, 1990.
22. Banerjee, S. P., Mechoulam, R., and Snyder, S. H., Cannabinoids: influence on neurotransmitter uptake in rat brain synaptosomes, *J. Pharmacol. Exp. Ther.,* **194,** 74, 1975.
23. Seltzman, H. H., Hsieh, Y.-A., Pitt, C. G., and Reggio, P. H., Synthesis of rotationally restricted THC ethers, *J. Org. Chem.,* **56,** 1549, 1991.
24. Matsumoto, K., Stark, P., and Meister, R. G., 1-Amino- and 1-mercapto-7,8,9, 10-tetrahydro-6H-dibenzo[b,d]pyrans, *J. Med. Chem.,* **20,** 17, 1977.

25. Agurell, S., Pharmacokinetics and metabolism of delta-1-THC and other cannabinoidswith emphasis on man, *Pharmacol. Rev.,* **38,** 21, 1986.

26. Harvey, D. J. and Paton, W. D. M., Metabolism of the cannabinoids, *Rev. Biochem. Toxicol.,* **6,** 221, 1984.

27. Lemberger, L., Crabtree, R. E., and Rowe, H.M., 11-Hydroxy-delta-9-THC: pharmacology, disposition and metdbolism of a major metabolite of marihuana in man, *Science,* **177,** 62, 1972.

28. Mechoulam, R., Ben-Zvi, Z., Agurell, S., Nilsson, 1. M., Nilsson, J. L. G., Edery, H.,and Grunfeld, V., Delta-6-THC-7-oic-acid, an urinary delta-6-THC metabolite: isolation and synthesis, *Experientia,* **29,** 1193, 1973.

29. Burstein, S. H., Hull, K., Hunter, S. A., and Latham, V., Cannabinoids and pain responses: a possible role for prostaglandins, *FASEB,* **2,** 3022, 1988.

30. Hollister, L. E., Structure-activity relationships in man of cannabis constituents, and homologs and metabolites of delta-9-THC, *Pharmacol. Rev.,* **11,** 3, 1974.

31. Mechoulam, R., Feigenbaum, J. J., Lander, N., Segal, M., Jiirbe, T. U. C., Hiltunen, A. J., and Consroe, P., Enantiomeric cannabinoids: stereospecificity of psychotropicactivity, *Experientia,* **44,** 762, 1988.

32. Mechoulam, R., Lander, N., Breuer, A., and Zahalka, J., Synthesis of the individual, pharmacologically distinct, enantiomers of a tetrahydrocannabinol derivative, *Tetrahedron: Asymmetry,* **1,** 315, 1990.

33. Järbe, T. U. C., Hiltunen, A. J., and Mechoulam, R., Stereospecificity of the discriminative stimulus functions of the dimethylheptyl homologs of 11-OH-delta-8tetrahydrocannabinol in rats and pigeons, *J. Pharmacol. Exp. Ther.,* **250,** 1000, 1989.

34. Little, P. J., Compton, D. R., Mechoulam, R., and Martin, B., Stereochernical effectsof 11-OH-delta-8-THC-dimethylheptyl in mice and dogs, *Pharmacol. Biochem. Behav.,* **32,** 661,1989.

35. Thomas, B. F., Compton, D. R., and Martin, B. R., Characterization of the lipophilicity of natural and synthetic analogs of delta-9-THC and its relationship to pharmacological potency, *J. Pharmacol. Exp. Ther.,* **255,** 624, 1990.

36. Little, P. J., Compton, D. R., Johnson, M. R., Melvin, L. S., and Martin, B. R., Pharmacology and stereoselectivity of structurally novel cannabinoids in mice, *J. Pharmacol. Exp. Ther.,* **247,** 1046, 1988.

37. Ohlsson, A., Agurell, S., Leander, K., Dahmen, J., Edery, H., Porath, G., Levy, S., and Mechoulam, R., Synthesis and psychotropic activity of side chain hydroxylated delta-6-THC metabolites, *Acta Pharm. Suec.,* **16,** 21, 1979.

38. Gaoni, Y. and Mechoulam, R., Isolation, structure and partial synthesis of an active constituent of hashish, *J. Am. Chem. Soc.,* **86,** 1646, 1964.

39. Turner, C. E., Elsohly, M. A., and Boeren, E. G., Constituents of Cannabis sativa L. XVII. A review of the natural constituents, *J. Nat. Prod.,* **43,** 169, 1980.

40. Gaoni, Y. and Mechoulam, R., Concerning the isomerization of delta-l- to delta-6-tetrahydrocannabinol, *J. Anz. Chem. Soc.,* **88,** 5673, 1966.

41. Mechoulam, R., Ben-Zvi, Z., Varconi, H., and Samuelov, Y., Cannabinoid rearrangements: synthesis of delta-5-tetrahydrocannabinol, *Tetrahedron,* **29,** 1615, 1973.

42. Srebnik, M., Lander, N., Breuer, A., and Mechoulam, R., Base catalysed double bond isomerizations of cannabinoids: structural and stereochemical aspects., *J. Chem. Soc., Perkin Trans.* **1,** 2881, 1984.

43. Järbe, T. U. C., Hiltunen, A. J., Mechoulam, R., Srebnik, M., and Breuer, A., Separation of the discriminative stimulus effects in stereoisomers of delta-2 and delta3-tetrahydrocannabinols in pigeons, *Eur. J. Pharmacol.,* **156,** 361, 1988.

44. Binder, M., Edery, H., and Porath, G., Delta-7-THC, a noripsychotropic cannabinoid: structure activity considerations in the cannabinoid series, in Marihuana: Biological Effect, Nahas, G. G. and Paton, W. D. M., Eds., Pergamon Press, Oxford, 1979, 71.

45. Wilson, R. S. and May, E. L., 9-Nor-delta-8-THC, a cannabinoid of metabolic interest, *J. Med. Chem.,* **17,** 475, 1974.

46. Loev, B., Bender, P. E., Dowalo, F., Macko, E., and Fowler, P. J., Cannabinoids. Structure-activity studies, related to 1,2-dimethylheptyl derivatives., *J. Med. Chem.,* **16,** 2100, 1973.

47. Korbinits, D. et al., Cannabinoids with an ether side chain. Synthesis, solubilization and analgesic properties, *Eur. J. Med. Chem.,* **20,** 492, 1985.

48. Edery, H., Grunfeld, Y., Porath, G., Ben-Zvi, Z., Shani, A., and Mechoulam, R., Structure-activity relationships in the THC series. Modifications on the aromatic ring and on the side chain, *Arzneim. Forsch.,* **22,** 1995, 1972.

49. Burstein, S. H., Audette, C. A., Charalambous, A., Doyle, S. A., Guo, Y., Hunter, S. A., and Makriyannis, A., Detection of cannabinoid receptors by photoaffinit labelling, *Biochem. Biophys. Res. Commun.,* **176,** 492, 1991.

50. Mechoulam, R. and Gaoni Y., The absolute configuration of delta-l-tetrahydrocannabinol, the major active constituent of hashish, *Tetrahedron Lett.,* 1109, 1967.

51. Gaoni, Y. and Mechoulam, R., The isomerization of cannabidiol to tetrahydrocannabinols, *Tetrahedron,* **22,** 1481, 1966.

52. Mechoulam, R., Lander, N., Varkony, T.-H., Kimmel, I., Becker, O., Ben-Zvi, Z., Edery, H., and Porath, G., Stereochemical requirements for cannabinoid activity, *J. Med. Chem.,* **23,** 1068, 1980.

53. Mechoulam, R., Devane, W. A., Breuer, A., and Zahalka, J., A random walk through a cannabis field, *Pharmacol. Biochem. Behav.,* **40,** 461, 1991.

54. Wilson, R. S., May, E. L., Martin, B. R., and Dewey, W. L., 9-Nor-9hydroxyhexahydrocannabinols. Synthesis. Some behavioral and analgesic properties and comparison with the tetrahydrocannabinols,.*J. Med. Chem.,* **19,** 1165, 1976.

55. Mechoulam, R., Braun, P., and Gaoni, Y., Syntheses of delta-1-THC and related cannabinolds. *J. Am. Chem. Soc.,* **94,** 6159, 1972.

56. Archer, R. A., Stark, P., and Lemberger, L., Nabilone, in Cannabinoids as Therapeutic Agents, Mechoulam, R., Ed., CRC Press, Boca Raton, FL, 1986.

57. Huffman, I W., Joyner, H. H., Lee, M. D., Jordan, R. D., and Pennington, W. T., Synthesis of both enantiomers of nabilone from a common intermediate. Enantiodivergent synthesis of cannabinoids, *J. Org. Chem.,* **56,** 2081, 1991.

58. Harvey, D. J., In vivo metabolism of (+)-trans-delta-9-THC in the mouse, *Blomed. Environ. Mass Spectrosc.,* **16,** 117, 1988.

59. Harvey, D.J. and Marriage, H.J., Metabolism of(+)-trans-delta-8-THC in I mouse *in* vitro and *in vivo, Drug Metab. Dispos.,* **15,** 914, 1987.

60. Mechoulam, R., Breuer, A., Feigenbaum, J. J., and Devane, W. A., Noripsychotropic synthetic cannabinoids as therapeutic agents, *Farmaco,* **46** (Suppl. 1), 267, 199 1, and unpublished results.

61. Howlett, A. C., Champion, T. M., Wilken, G. H., and Mechoulam, R., Stereochernical effects of 11-OH-delta-8-tetrahydrocannabinol-dimethylheptyI to inhibit adenylate cyclase and bind to the cannabinoid receptor, *Neuropharrnacology,* **29,** 161, 1990.

62. Mechoulam, R., Breuer, A., Järbe, T. U. C., Hiltunen, A. J., and Glaser R., Cannabimimetic activity of novel enantiomeric benzofuran cannabinoids, *J. Med. Chem.,* **33,**1037,1990.

63. Mechoulam, R., The pharmayohistory of *Cannabis* sativa, in *Cannabinoids* as *Therapeutic Agents,* Mechoulam, R., Ed., CRC Press, Boca Raton, FL, 1986.

64. Hollister, L. E., Gillespie, H. K., Mechoulam, R., and Srebnik, M., Human pharmacology of IS and IR enantiomers of delta-3-THC, *Psychopharmacology,* **92,** 505,1987.

65. Consroe, P. and Snider, S. R., Therapeutic potential of cannabinoids in neurological disorders, in *Cannabinoids as Therapeutic Agents,* Mechoulam, R., Ed., CRC Press, Boca Raton, FL, 1986.

66. Guimaraes, F., Chiaretti, T. M., Graeff, F. G., and Zuardi, A. W., Antianxiety effect of cannabidiol in the elevated plus-maze, *Psychophartnacologia,* **100,** 558, 1990.

67. Onaivi, E. S., Green, M. R., and Martin, B. R., Pharmacological characterization of cannabinoids in the el I evated plus-maze, *J. Phartnacol. Exp. Ther.,* **252,** 1002, 1990.

68. Musty, R. E., Conti, L. H., and Mechoulam, R., Anxiolytic properties of cannabidiol, *in Marihuana '84,* Harvey, D. J., Ed., IRL Press, Oxford, 1985, 1.

69. Leite, J. R., Carlini, E. A., Lander, N., and Mechoulam, R., Anticonvulsant effect of (-) and (+) isomers of CBD and their dimethyl heptyl hornologq, *Pharmacology,* **124,** 141, 1982.

70. Nir, I., Ayalon, D., Tsafriri, A., Cordova, T., and Lindner, H. R., Suppression of the cyclic surge of LH secretion and of ovulation in the rat by delta- 1-THC, *Nature (Londbn),* 243, 470, 1973.

71. Cordova, T., Ayalon, D., Lander, N., Mechoullam, R., Nir, I., Puder, M., and Lindner, H. R., The ovulation blocking effect of cannabinoids: structure-activity relationships, *Psychoneuroendocrinology,* **5,** 53, 1980.

72. Feigenbaum, J. J., Richmond, S. A., Weissman, Y., and Mechoul4m, R., Inhibition of cisplatin induced emesis in the pigeon by a non-psychotropic synthetic cannabinoid, *Eur. J. Pharmacol.,* **169,** 159, 1989.

73. Feigenbaum, J. J., Bergmann, F., Richmond, S. A., Mechoulam, R., Nadler, V., Kloog, Y., and Sokolovsky, M., A non-psychotropic cannabinoid acts as a functional N-methyl-D-asparate (NMDA) receplor blocker, *Proc. Natl. Acad. Sci, U.S.A.,* **86,** 9584, 1989.

74. Herkenham, M. et al., Cannabinoid receptor localization in brain, *Proc. Nad. Acad. Sci. U.S.A.,* **87,** 1932, 1990.

75. Matsuda, L. A., Lolait, S. J., Brownstein, M. J., Young, A. C., and Bonner, T. I., Structure of a cannabinoid receptor and functional expression of the cloned cDNA, *Nature (London),* **346,** 561, 1990.

76. Herkenham, M., Lynn, A. B., Johnson, M. R., Melvin, L. S., de Costa, B. R., and Rice, K. C., Characterization and localization of cannabinoid receptors in rat brain: a quantitative *in vitro* autoradiographic study,./. *Neurosci..* **11,** *563,* 1991.

77. Howlett, A. C., Johnson, M. R., Melvin, L. S., and Milne, G. M., Nonclassical cannabinoid analgetics inhibit adenylate cyclase: development of a cannabinoid receptor model, *Mol. Pharmacol.,* **33,** 297, 1988.

78. Rosenqvist, E. and Ottersen, T., The crystal and molecular structure of delta-9-THC acid B, *Acta Chem. Scand. B.,* **29.** 379, 1975.

79. Mechoulam, R., Ben-Zvi, Z., Vagnitinsky, B., and Shani, A., A new tetrahydrocannabitiolic acid, *Tetrtihedron Lett.,* 2339, 1969.

80. Archer, R. A., Boyd, D. B., Demarco, P. V., Tyminski, I. J., and Allinger, N. L., Structural studies of cannabinoids. A theoretical and proton magnetic resonance study, *J. Am. Chem. Soc.,* **92,** *5200,* 1970.

81. Kriwacki, W. and Makriyannis, A., The conformational analysis of delta-9- and delta-9, 11-THCs in solution using high resolution NMR'spectroscopy, *Mol. Pharmacol.,* **35,** 495,1989.

82. Reggio, P. H. and Mazurek, A. P., A molecular reactivity template for cannabinoid activity, *./. Mol. Struct.,* **149,** 331, 1987.

83. Haasnoot, C. A. G., de Leeuw, F. A. A. M., and Altona, C., The relationship between proton-proton NMR coupling constants and substituent elect ronegativ it ies, *Tetrahedron,* **36,** 2783, 1980.

84. Lambert, J. B., Structural chemistry in solution. The R value, *Acct. Chem. Res* 4, *87,* 1971.

85. Hanson, K. R., Applications of the sequence rule. Narning the paired ligands gg at a tetrahedral atom, *J. Am. Chem. Soc.,* **88,** 2731, 1966.

86. Reggio, P. H., Greer, K. V., and Cox, S. M., The importance of the orientation of the C9 substituent to cannabinoid activity, *J. Med. Clicni.,* **32,** 1630, 1989.

87. Reggio, P. H., Seltzmann, H. H., Compton, D. R., Prescott, W. R., Jr., and Martin, B. R., Investigation of the role of the phenolic hydroxyl in cannabinoid activity, Mol. *Pharmacol.,* **38,** 854. 1990.

88. Semus, S. F. and Martin, B. R., A computergraphic investigation into the pharmacological role of the TFIC-cannabinoid phenolic moiety, *Life Sci.,* **46,** 178 1, 1990.

89. Martin, B. R., Dewey, W. L., Harris, L. S., Bechner, J., Wilson, R. S., and May, E. L., Marihuana-like activity of new synthetic THCs, *Pharmacol. Biochem.Behav.,* **3,** 849, 1975.

90. Munro, S., Thomas, K.L. and Abu-Shaar, M. Molecular characterization of a peripheral receptor for cannabinoids. *Nature,* **365,** 61, 1993.

91. Devane, W.A., Hanus, L., Breuer, A., Pertwee, R.G., Stevenson, L.A., Griffin, G., Gibson, D., Mandelbaum, A., Etinger, A. and Mechoulam, R. Isolation and structure of a brain constituent that binds to the cannabinoid receptor. *Science,* **258,** 1946, 1992.

92. Mechoulam, R., Ben-Shabat, S., Hanus, L., Ligumsky, M., Kaminski, N.E., Schatz, A.R., Gopher, A., Almog, S., Martin, B.R., Compton, D.R., Pertwee, R.G., Griffin, G., Bayewitch, M., Barg, J. and Vogel, Z. Identification of an endogenous 2-monoglyceride, present in canine gut, that binds to cannabinoid receptors. *Biochem. Pharmacol.* **50,** 83, 1995.

93. Lagu, S.G., Varona, A., Chambers, J.D. and Reggio, P.H. Construction of a steric map of the binding pocket for cannabinoids at the cannabinoid receptor. *Drug Des. Discov.* **12,** 179, 1995.

94. Bramblett, R.D., Panu, A.M., Ballesteros, J.A. and Reggio P.H. Construction of a 3D model of the cannabinoid CB1 receptor: determination of helix ends and helix orientation. *Life Sci.* **56,** 1971, 1995.

95. Gareau, Y., Dufresne, C., Gallant, M., Rochette, C., Sawyer, N., Slipetz, D.M., Tremblay, N., Weech, P.K., Metters, K.M. and Labelle, M. Structure activity relationships of tetrahydrocannabinol analogues on human cannabinoid receptors. *Bioorg. Med. Chem. Lett.* **6,** 189, 1996.

96. Rhee, M.-H., Vogel, Z., Barg, J., Bayewitch, M., Levy, R., Hanus, L., Breuer, A. and Mechoulam, R. Canabinol derivative: binding to cannabinoid receptors and inhibition of adenylylcyclase. *J. Med. Chem.* **40,** 3228, 1997.

2

Absorption, Distribution, and Biotransformation of the Cannabinoids

David J. Harvey

Abstract

This paper describes the occurrence, properties, distribution, metabolism, and excretion of the cannabinoids. Over 60 of these compounds have been identified in the plant *Cannabis sativa*, the major ones being the pharmacologically active Δ^9-tetrahydrocannabinol (Δ^9-THC), its biosynthetic precursor, cannabidiol (CBD), and the degradation product, cannabinol (CBN). Once absorbed, usually by smoking, these lipophilic compounds partition into the fatty tissues of the body where they can remain for a considerable time. The half-life of the drug is measured in days or even weeks. Various estimates of the half-life in humans are discussed in the paper.

All cannabinoids are good substrates for the cytochrome P450 mixed function oxidases. Biotransformation of Δ^9-THC and its synthetic isomer, Δ^8-THC, give mono-, di-, and tri-hydroxy metabolites and further oxidation leads to a series of acids, carbonyl compounds, and their hydroxy derivatives. Primary sites of hydroxylation in both isomers are the side-chain and the allylic carbon atoms of the alicyclic ring leading to Δ^9-THC-11-oic acid as the major human metabolite from Δ^9-THC. Lower homologues yield greater proportions of acidic metabolites, whereas higher homologs are metabolized mainly to hydroxy compounds. β-Oxidation and related oxidations of the aliphatic chain lead to a series of chain-shortened metabolites, most of which are additionally hydroxylated in the alicyclic ring or at C-11. Large species-related differences in biotransformation are seen, particularly in the sites of initial hydroxylation. Several of the monohydroxy metabolites, particularly the 11- and 3'-hydroxy THCs show comparable pharmacological activity to that of the parent drug whereas polysubstituted metabolites are inactive. Phase II metabolism is mainly by conjugation with glucuronic acid.

Other cannabinoids are metabolised similarly. CBD yields additional metabolites as the result of hydroxylation and epoxidation of the *iso*-propene group but CBN yields fewer metabolites as the aromatic rings do not appear to be hydroxylated. Cannabichromene and cannabigerol again show extensive, species-related hydroxylation of their alkyl chains.

From: *Marihuana and Medicine*
Edited by: G. G. Nahas et al.   © Humana Press Inc., Totowa, NJ

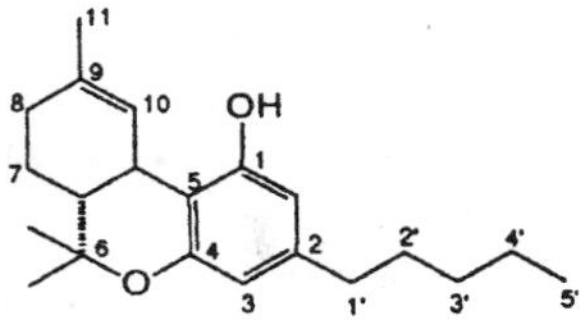

Δ⁹-tetrahydrocannabinol (Δ⁹-THC), I. 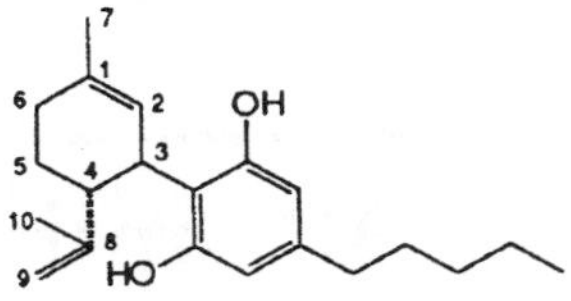   Cannabidiol (CBD), II

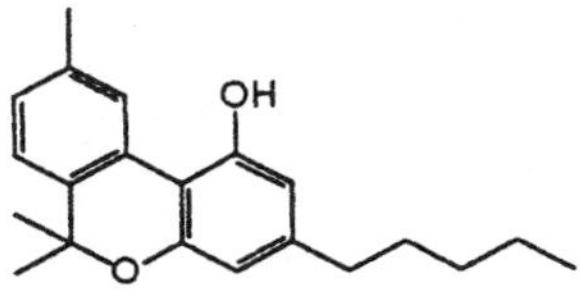

Cannabinol (CBN, III

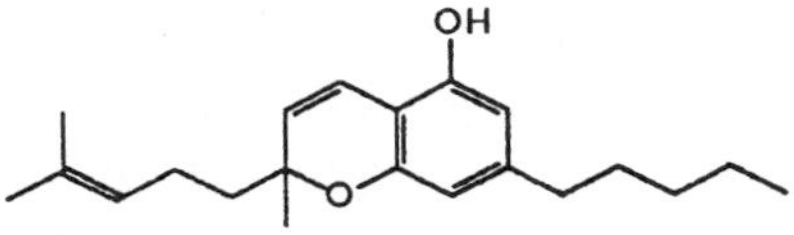

Cannabichromene (CBC), IV 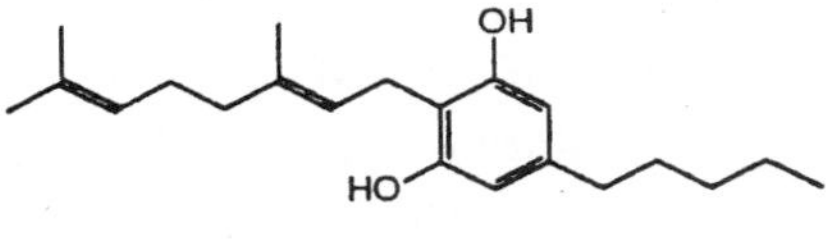   Cannabigerol (GBG), V

Fig. 1. Structures of the major cannabinoids

1. OCCURRENCE OF THE CANNABINOIDS

The cannabinoids are a group of terpene-related compounds produced by the plant *Cannabis sativa* L. and are the major psychoactive constituents of the drug marihuana. Although the drug has been in use for several millennia, the structure of the main active cannabinoid, Δ^9-tetrahydrocannabinol (Δ^9 THC, 1; Fig. 1), was not elucidated until 1964 (*1*). This compound is one of about 60 known cannabinoids (*2*), the others being mainly biosynthetic precursors such as cannabidiol (CBD, II), degradation products (e.g., cannabinol, CBN, III) and lower homologs, particularly those with a propyl chain. The ratio of these compounds, and hence the drug's potency, varies enormously as a function of the age and geographical origin of the plant with specimens grown in hot climates generally producing the most potent drug. Plants from cool climates generally contain much higher proportions of CBD, whereas aged specimens contain increased proportions of the relatively inactive decomposition product, CBN. Many of the natural cannabinoids occur in the plant as the 2- or 4-COOH analogs but are rapidly decarboxylated to the active drug upon smoking (*3*). Δ^8-THC is a synthetic cannabinoid, frequently used in pharmacological studies.

2. PROPERTIES OF THE CANNABINOIDS

The physical, chemical, and pharmacological properties of the cannabinoids are well understood and have been the subject of many reviews. Among the most important are those on botany (4,5), chemistry (6), pharmacology (7,8), cannabinoid receptors (9), adverse effects (10), metabolism (11–13), pharmacokinetics (12), analysis (14–16) and recent research (17).

Unlike many other plant-derived drug substances, the cannabinoids do not contain nitrogen and, thus do not form salts. Many of their pharmacological properties and adverse effects can be attributed to a high lipid solubility that causes rapid transfer through, and accumulation in, biological membranes, causing a change in membrane fluidity (18–20). The octanol:water partition coefficient of Δ^9-THC has been measured at 6000:1 (21) but may well be higher (22). Δ^9-THC is sensitive to heat, light, and atmospheric oxygen, which cause slow decomposition to CBN (23,24), thus accounting for the drug's loss of potency on storage (25,26). Under acidic conditions, but above pH 4.0, Δ^9-THC isomerises to the Δ^8-isomer. Protonation of the double bond with formation of 9-hydroxy-Δ^9-THC has also been found (27). Below pH 4.0, protonation of the pyran ring oxygen also occurs, causing ring cleavage to various substituted CBDs (27,28) with obvious importance for the bioavailability of orally ingested cannabis.

3. ABSORPTION AND BIOAVAILABILITY OF THE CANNABINOIDS

Smoking leads to rapid absorption of cannabinoids with heavy smokers absorbing more of the drug than light smokers. For example, Lindgren et al. (29) recorded absorption values of $10 \pm 7\%$ and $23 \pm 16\%$ for light and heavy smokers, respectively and Ohlsson et al. (30) recorded similar values of $14 \pm 1\%$ and $27 \pm 10\%$ for these two groups. The difference was attributed to more efficient smoking by the experienced (heavy) smokers. Barnett et al. (31) have measured a maximum plasma concentration of 50 ng/mL of Δ^9-THC following the smoking of two cigarettes, each containing 9 mg of the drug. Concentrations of 2 ng/mL are sufficient to produce a "high." Oral administration leads to more erratic uptake (32,33) as the result of degradation of the drug by stomach acids and extensive first-pass metabolism. A value of about one third that absorbed by smoking has been found by Perez-Reyes et al. (34) with peak plasma levels being reached from 60 to 300 minutes after drug administration (33). Blood concentrations of the drug after intramuscular (35) or intraperitoneal (36) administration rise slowly because of retention of the drug in local fat deposits.

The original studies on the pharmacodynamic properties of Δ^9-THC suggested a poor correlation between blood levels and the perceived "high" and effects such as tachydaria, with the effects lagging behind the blood levels by some 15 minutes after smoking (31,33) and by about an hour after oral administration (33). However, later work using continuous blood sampling, has indicated a better correlation (37). The drug produces a "high" at lower blood levels (0.02 ng/mL) after oral administration than after smoking, suggesting a substantial metabolic contribution. On the other hand, such differences may reflect distribution phenomena (38,39).

4. PROTEIN BINDING

Once absorbed into the blood, Δ^9-THC becomes strongly bound to protein; it has been estimated that, at equilibrium, only about 3% of the drug is in the free state (40,41). About 60% of the drug is bound to lipoprotein with the low-density fraction being the major site in humans (42,43). About 9% of the dose is bound to blood cells and the rest to albumin. The major monohydroxy metabolite 11-hydroxy-Δ^9-THC, is even more strongly bound with only 1% remaining in the free state (44).

5. DISTRIBUTION

Because of their high lipophilicity, the cannabinoids rapidly penetrate the tissues and high concentrations are found in the highly vascularized tissues at short times after drug administration as reflected by the high volume of distribution of over 500 liters shown by Δ^9-THC (45). The main distribution sites are liver, heart, lung, gut, kidney, spleen, mammary gland, placenta, adrenal cortex, thyroid, pituitary gland, and brown fat as measured following acute administration of Δ^9-THC (46–51). Lower concentrations are found in brain, testis, and fetus (21,46,52–54).

6. REDISTRIBUTION

At longer times after administration, Δ^9-THC redistributes to fatty tissue. Thus, Agurell et al. (55) found that the spleen and body fat were the major deposition sites after 72 hours. Fat was also identified as the major long-term storage site by Kreuz and Axelrod (56); in a study involving chronic treatment over 24 days, the levels in fat were still rising at the end of the experiment. High concentrations in fat have been found by a number of other investigators (54,57,58); and it appears that the drug takes many weeks to clear this tissue when administration stops (59).

7. PHARMACOKINETICS

In common with other lipophilic drugs, Δ^9-THC rapidly leaves the blood as it distributes between the tissues. However, the extensive deposition in fat results in a long terminal half life. Garrett and Hunt (40) found pentaphasic kinetics in dogs, with a terminal half life of 8.2 ± 0.23 days. A somewhat shorter time of 4 days was found in rabbits after multiple dosing (58) but, as pointed out by Lemberger and Rubin (60) drug half-lives in rabbits tend to be shorter than in other animals. Work with humans has generally been inhibited by the unavailability of assay methods sensitive enough to detect the drug for a sufficient length of time after administration. As analytical methods have become more sensitive, estimates of the drug's half life have increased, but there is still no consensus as to what this may be. Previous estimates have included times of 56 hours (61), 20–29 hours (62), and 4.3 ± 1.6 days (59,63). A mean excretion time of 27 days was reported by Ellis et al. (64) and in one of 27 subjects studied by Cridland et al. (65) a time of 173 days was recorded. Although the terminal half life in man is still unknown with certainty, it is probably safe to say that it averages at least one week and could be considerably longer. The plasma concentration of the major monohydroxy metabolite of Δ^9-THC, 11-hydroxy-Δ^9-THC, is considerably lower than that of Δ^9-THC itself and peaks at the end of smoking (37). Concentrations of its oxidation product, Δ^9-THC-11-oic acid, increase slowly and plateau for extended periods. Pharmacokinetics of CBN (66) and CBD (67) appear to be similar to those of Δ^9-THC.

8. BIOTRANSFORMATION

8.1 Tetrahydrocannabinols

All cannabinoids are good substrates for the cytochrome P450 mixed-function oxidases on account of their high lipid solubility. THCs are hydroxylated at C-11, the allylic positions of the alicyclic ring (C-8 for Δ^9-THC and C-7 for the Δ^8-isomer) and at all positions of the alkyl chain with considerable species variations (68,69) (Fig. 2). C-11 is the preferred hydroxylation site in most species, including man, although hamster and cat prefer alicyclic ring and alkyl-chain hydroxylation, respectively. Species such as the guinea pig hydroxylate several positions of the alkyl chain efficiently, whereas the rat, rabbit, and gerbil essentially use only C-11. Within a given species, patterns of hydroxylation vary between different tissues as shown, for example, by Widman et al. (70) and Halldin et al. (71). Multiple hydroxylation is common. The pattern of hydroxylation reflects the isoform distribution of the P450s (72–74).

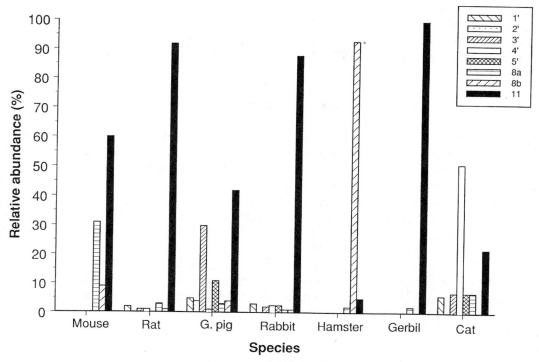

Fig. 2. Percentage hydroxylation at each position of Δ^9-THC in seven species.

In humans, P450 2C9 has been shown to catalyze the formation of the 11-hydroxy metabolite of Δ^9-THC (*75,76*) and P450 3A to be responsible for hydroxylation at the 8β-position (*75*). In monkeys, cytochrome P450RM-A appears to catalyze formation of 11- and 8α-hydroxy-Δ^9-THC and cytochrome P450 JM-C oxidizes the drug in the side chain at position 3′ (*74*). Epoxide formation from the double bond is of minor significance with Δ^9-THC, of more significance with Δ^8-THC with its more exposed bond (*77*) and responsible for the major metabolites from Δ^{11}-THC (*78*), in which the bond is exoclyclic. Although potentially toxic, Δ^1-THC epoxide has been shown to give a negative reaction in the Ames test for mutagenicity (*79*).

Following the initial hydroxylation, many of the hydroxyl groups undergo further oxidation with the major products being the formation of carboxylic acids at C-11 and C-5′ (alkyl chain). The C5′ acid then undergoes β-oxidation and related biotransformations with losses of carbon atoms from the alkyl chain (*80*). As a result of these multiple biotransformations, metabolic profiles are complex and contain a large range of hydroxy and acid metabolites with multiple biotransformations at a number of sites (see refs. 81–83). The lower homologs of the THCs produce simpler metabolic profiles than the naturally occurring pentyl isomers (*84–86*), with most metabolites being relatively simple acids. This simpler profile probably reflects their lower lipophilicity that requires less initial hydroxylation to occur before the molecules are sufficiently soluble to be accessed by the mainly cytosolic enzymes responsible for oxidation to acids. Higher homologs produce metabolites with multiple hydroxylations (*86,87*), again reflecting the need to reduce lipophilicity before further oxidation can occur.

Phase II metabolites appear to be mainly conventional conjugates of the free drug or its phase I metabolites with glucuronic acid (*88,89*). However, an unusual C-glucuronide conjugate, with conjugation to the phenyl ring, has been reported for Δ^8-THC (90). The formation of conjugates with long-chain fatty acids unusually increases rather than decreases lipophilicity (91). These compounds, which resemble membrane constituents, are thought to be the form in which the drug may be retained within tissues for considerable periods of time.

8.2 Cannabidiol

In vitro metabolism of this cannabinoid is complex as hydroxylation can not only occur at the usual allylic positions (6 and 7) and in the side chain, but also on the isopropenyl group by simple hydroxylation and by the epoxide-diol pathway. Eight mono-(92) and eight dihydroxy metabolites (93) were reported in 1976 from rat microsomes and 39 mono-, di-, and trihydroxy metabolites were found in rabbit microsomal preparations by Harvey and Brown in 1990 (94). As with the THCs, considerable species differences occur in the positions of in vitro hydroxylation with 7- or 4'-hydroxylation dominating (69,95). In vivo and urinary metabolites appear to be mainly acids and hydroxy acids. In dogs, 8- rather than 11-hydroxylation is dominant and β-oxidation of the pentyl chain is extensive, particularly after 24 hours, when most of the metabolites lack the terminal four carbon atoms (96). 4',7-Dihydroxy-CBD was the only metabolite found to be conjugated to glucuronic acid in this study, but several other metabolites were found conjugated to glucose (97), a conjugation reaction only rarely seen in mammals. β-Oxidation has been reported to be less significant in man than in dogs (98), but excretion of hydroxy acids is more pronounced. The major metabolite produced by a patient being treated for dystonia was the unusual 2''-hydroxy-3'',4'',6''-tris, nor-CBD-7-oic acid produced by an unknown mechanism. The complexity of CBD metabolism is reflected by the 83 metabolites cataloged by Harvey in 1991 (12).

In addition to being a good substrate for cytochrome P450, CBD also appears to be a microsomal inhibitor (99–102) but does not significantly affect the pharmacokinetics of other cannabinoids (103). The specific isozyme that is inhibited is thought to be cytochrome P450 2C9 (104) although, after prolonged exposure, a second isozyme, immunologically similar to the P-450 induced by phenobarbitone treatment, appears to be involved (105,106). Preincubation of human liver microsomes with CBD has been reported to decrease the formation of THC metabolites catalyzed by cytochrome P450 3A by 60% but to have less effect on the P450 2C9-catalyzed metabolites (107). Both Yamamoto et al. (13) and Bornheim et al. (108) however, report that CBD decreases microsomal production of 11-hydroxy-Δ^9-THC, a metabolite produced by CPY2C9 in mouse liver and it seems to be generally accepted that CBD inhibits both CPY3A and 2C9 (109). After prolonged administration, however, CBD has been reported to induce CPY-2B, -3A, and -2C (110).

8.3 Cannabinol

Metabolism of CBN is simpler than that of the other cannabinoids on account of the absence of allylic hydroxylation of the ring. 11-Hydroxylation is again dominant, in most species both in vitro (111–113) and in vivo (114), but most species produce additional metabolites hydroxylated in various positions of the side-chain. In cat and hamster, 4'-hydroxylation (side chain) is dominant (69,95). Excreted metabolites tend to be mainly 11-hydroxy-CBN, CBN-11-oic acid and its side-chain hydroxylated analogs (115). Conjugation with long-chain fatty acids also occurs (116).

8.4 Minor Cannabinoids

The most abundant minor cannabinoids, other than the homologs discussed above, are cannabichromene (IV, Fig. 1) and cannabigerol (V). Cannabigerol metabolism has only been studied in vitro. Both aliphatic chains are hydroxylated by the seven species investigated with the allylic methyl groups again tending to be preferred (*69,95,117*). In vitro metabolism of cannabichromene is similar (*118*). Dihydroxy metabolites have been found in the rabbit (*119*) and the epoxide-diol route is prominent in hamster, gerbil, and cat, yet insignificant in the other species studied. An in vivo glucuronide conjugate has been reported in mice (*88*).

9. EXCRETION

Both urine and feces are used for the excretion of cannabinoids and, consistent with the drug's high lipophilicity, most material appears as metabolites. Feces are the preferred route in rats (*55,120*) and humans (*121,122*), with about 80% of the excreted dose of Δ^9-THC appearing in the feces. A somewhat higher percentage is excreted in urine by rabbits. Most urinary metabolites are acids. Halldin et al. (*123,124*) have identified 18 acidic metabolites from Δ^9-THC in human urine; most are hydroxylated or β-oxidized analogs of Δ^9-THC-11-oic acid. The major human urinary metabolite, identified by Williams and Moffatt in 1980 (*89*) is the glucuronide of Δ^9-THC-11-oic acid. Huestis et al. (*125*) have measured mean peak urinary concentrations of Δ^9-THC-11-oic acid of 89.8 ± 31.9 ng/mL and 153.4 ± 49.2 ng/mL at 7.7 ± 0.8 and 13.9 ± 3.5 hours after smoking single cigarettes containing 1.75 or 3.55% Δ^9-THC, respectively. The metabolite was detected at a concentration of greater than 15 ng/mL for 33.7 ± 9.2 hours and 88.6 ± 9.5 hours after these two cigarettes. Although there appears to be little correlation between the concentration of Δ^9-THC-11-oic acid in urine and that of Δ^9-THC in blood, the log concentrations have shown a better correlation (*126*). Huestis et al. (*127*) have produced models that claim to be able to predict the time of exposure by measurements of the drug and metabolite concentrations in plasma. Human urinary excretion of CBD shows a similar pattern with acids and glucuronide conjugates dominating the profile (*98*). Unchanged drug also appears in milk (*128*). CBN is similar to CBD in that a greater proportion of the administered dose is excreted unchanged than with the THCs (*129*).

10. CONTRIBUTION OF METABOLITES OF PHARMACOLOGICAL ACTIVITY

Some of the monohydroxy metabolites of Δ^9-THC possess activity similar to that of Δ^9-THC itself, but most of the other metabolites are inactive. The 11-hydroxy-metabolites of Δ^9- and Δ^8-THC appear to be as active or more active than the parent compounds (*130,131*), but cannot alone account for all of the drug's activity (*132*). The equatorial alicyclic hydroxy metabolites are also active, but the corresponding axial metabolites possess little activity (*133*). Hydroxylation of the side chain has variable effects. Hydroxylation at C-1' abolishes activity, yet activity is retained by hydroxylation at other positions, being particularly high for the 3'-hydroxy metabolite (*134,135*). Ohlsson et al. (*33*) have found a good temporal correlation between the cataleptic effects of several hydroxy metabolites of Δ^8-THC and their concentrations in the brain. Only Δ^8-THC and 1'-hydroxy-Δ^8-THC did not fit the pattern. The most active compounds were 3'- and 11-hydroxy-Δ^8-THC with the other side-chain hydroxy metabolites decreasing in potency in the order 5'<4'<2'. The most active compound was the epoxide metabolite. Narimatsu et al. (*136*) have also found a high pharmacological activity for this metabolite in mice in which it had about four times the catalytic effect of the parent drug. It has also been observed that tolerance to locomotor depression can be correlated with the appearance of polar metabolites in the brain (*137*).

11. CONCLUSIONS

The pharmacokinetics and metabolism of the cannabinoids appear to be typical for compounds possessing a high lipophilicity. Biological half-lives are long as the result of extensive accumulation of the drugs by fatty tissue. The compounds are good substrates for cytochrome P450 with more extensive metabolism being shown by the cannabinoids with the highest lipophilicity. CBD has an inhibitory effect on certain P450 isozymes and, thus, marihuana from different sources, which contains variable amounts of CBD would be expected to show variable activity as the result of an altered metabolic profile. As the P450 isozymes also show variability within the human population, marihuana could also exhibit variable effects as the result of altered metabolic ratios.

REFERENCES

1. Gaoni, Y. and Mechoulam, R. (1964) Isolation, structure and partial synthesis of an active constituent of hashish. *J. Am. Chem. Soc.* **86**, 1646–1647.
2. Turner, C. E., ElSohly, M. A., and Boeren, E. G. (1980) Constituents of *Cannabis sativa* L., XVII. A review of the active constituents. *J. Nat. Prods.* **43**, 169–234.
3. Claussen, J. and Korte, F. (1967) Hashish, XIII, behaviour of constituents of *Cannabis sativa L.* during smoking. *Tetrahedron Letts.* 2067–2069.
4. Clarke, R. C. (1981) *Marihuana Botany* And/Or Press, Berkeley, CA.
5. Paris, M. and Nahas, G. G. (1984) Botany: the unestablished species, In: *Marihuana in Science and Medicine* (Nahas, G. G., ed.) Raven, New York, pp. 3–36.
6. Mechoulam, R. (1973) Cannabinoid chemistry, in *Marihuana, Chemistry, Pharmacology, Metabolism and Clinical Effects* (Mechoulam, R., ed.) Academic, New York, pp. 1–99.
7. Paton, W. D. M. (1975) Pharmacology of marihuana. *Annu. Rev. Pharmacol.* **15**, 191–220.
8. Nahas, G. G. (1984) In, *Marihuana in Science and Medicine* (Nahas, G. G., ed.) Raven, New York.
9. Matsuda, L. A. (1997) Molecular aspects of cannabinoid receptors. *Critical Reviews in Neurobiology.* **11**, 143–166.
10. Harvey, D. J. (1985) Summary of the session on the adverse effects of the cannabinoids, In: *Marihuana 84–Proceedings of the Oxford Symposium on Cannabis* (Harvey, D. J., ed.) IRL Press, Oxford, pp. 667–670.
11. Harvey, D. J. and Paton, W. D. M. (1984) Metabolism of the Cannabinoids. *Rev. Biochem. Toxicol.* **6**, 221–264.
12. Harvey, D. J. (1991) Metabolism and pharmacokinetics of the cannabinoids, In: *Biochemistry and Physiology of Substance Abuse.* (Watson, R. R., ed.) CRC Press, Boca Raton, FL pp. 279–365.
13. Yamamoto, I., Watanabe, K., Narimatsu, S., and Yoshimura, H. (1995) Recent advances in the metabolism of cannabinoids. *Int. J. Biochem. Cell Biol.* **27**, 741–746.
14. Harvey, D. J. (1984) Analysis of the cannabinoids, In: *Analytical Methods in Human Toxicology* (Curry, A. S., ed.) MacMillan Press, London, pp. 257–310.
15. Harvey, D. J. (1985) Advances in methods for detection and measurement of the cannabinoids, In: *Marihuana 84–Proceedings of the Oxford Symposium on Cannabis* (Harvey, D. J., ed.) IRL Press, Oxford, pp. 121–136.
16. Harvey, D. J. (1987) Mass spectrometry of the cannabinoids and their metabolites. *Mass Spectrom. Rev.* **6**, 135–229.
17. Musty, R. E., Reggio, P., and Consroe, P. (1995) A review of recent advances in cannabis research and the 1994 International Symposium on Cannabis and the Cannabinoids. *Life Sci.* **56**, 1933–1940.
18. Lawrence, D. K. and Gill, E. W. (1975) The effect of Δ^9-tetrahydrocannabinol and other cannabinoids on spin-labelled liposomes and their relationships to mechanisms of general anaesthesia. *Molec. Pharmacol.* **11**, 595–602.
19. Leuschner, J. T. A., Wing, D. R., Harvey, D. J., Brent, G. A., Demsey, C. E., Watts, A., and Paton, W. D. M. (1984) The partitioning of Δ^9-tetrahydrocannabinol into erythrocyte membranes *in vivo* and its effect on membrane fluidity. *Experientia.* **40**, 866–868.
20. Makriyannis, A., Yang, D. P., Griffin, R. G., and Dasgupta, S. K. (1990) The perturbation of model membranes by (–)-delta-9-tetrahydrocannabinol—studies using solid-state H-2-NMR and C-13-NMR. *Biochim. Biophys. Acta.* **1028**, 31–42.
21. Gill, E. W. and Jones, G. (1972) Brain levels of delta-1-tetrahydrocannabinol and its metabolites in mice-correlation with behaviour and the effect of the metabolic inhibitors SKF 525A and piperonyl butoxide. *Biochem. Pharmacol.* **21**, 2237–2248.

22. Thomas, B. F., Compton, D. R., and Martin, B. R. (1990) Characterization of the lipophilicity of natural and synthetic analogues of delta-9-tetrahydrocannabinol and its relationship to pharmacological potency. *J. Pharmacol. Exptl. Therap.* **255**, 624–630.

23. Harvey, D. J. (1985) Examination of a 140 year old ethanolic extract of *Cannabis*: identification of new cannabitriol homologues and the ethyl homologue of cannabinol, In: *Marihuana 84–Proceedings of the Oxford Symposium on Cannabis* (Harvey, D. J., ed.) IRL Press, Oxford, pp. 23–30.

24. Harvey, D. J. (1990) Stability of cannabinoids in dried samples of cannabis dating from around 1896–1905. *J. Ethnopharmacol.* **28**, 117–128.

25. Turner, C. E., Hadley, K. W., Fetterman, P. S., Doorenbos, N. J., Quimby, M. W., and Waller, C. (1973) Constituents of *Cannabis sativa* L., IV—Stability of cannabinoids in stored plant material. *J. Pharm. Sci.* **62**, 1601–1605.

26. Fairbairn, J. W., Liebmann, J. A., and Rowan, M. G. (1976) The stability of cannabis and its preparations on storage. *J. Pharm. Prarmacol.* **28**, 1–7.

27. Garrett, E. R., Gouyette, A. J., and Roseboom, H. (1978) Stability of tetrahydrocannabinols, II. *J. Pharm. Sci.* **67**, 27–32.

28. Garrett, E. R. and Tsau, J. (1974) Stability of tetrahdrocannabinols, I. *J. Pharm. Sci.* **63**, 1563–1574.

29. Lindgren, J. E., Ohlsson, A., Agurell, S., Hollister, L., and Gillespie, H. (1981) Clinical effects and plasma levels of Δ^9-tetrahydrocannabinol (Δ^9-THC) in heavy and light users of cannabis. *Psychopharmacologia.* **74**, 208–212.

30. Ohlsson, A., Lindgren, J. E., Wahlen, A., Agurell, S., Hollister, L. E., and Gillespie, H. K. (1982) Single-dose kinetics of deuterium-labelled Δ^1-tetrahydrocannabinol in heavy and light cannabis users. *Biomed. Mass Spectrom.* **9**, 6–10.

31. Barnett, G., Chiang, C.-W. N., Perez-Reyes, M., and Owens, S. M. (1982) Kinetic study of smoking marihuana. *J. Pharmacokinetics Biopharmaceut.* **10**, 495–506.

32. Ohlsson, A., Lindgren, J. E., Wahlen, A., Agurell, S., Hollister, L. E., and Gillespie, H. K. (1980) Plasma Δ^9-tetrahydrocannabinol concentration and clinical effects after oral and intravenous administration and smoking. *Clin. Pharmacol. Ther.* **28**, 409–416.

33. Ohlsson, A., Widman, M., Carlsson, S., Ryman, T., and Strid, C. (1980) Plasma and brain levels of Δ^6-THC and seven monohydroxy metabolites correlated to the cataleptic effect in the mouse. *Acta Pharmacol. Toxicol.* **47**, 308–317.

34. Perez-Reyes, M., Lipton, M. A., Timmons, M. C., Wall, M. E., Brine, D. R., and Davis, K. H. (1973) Pharmacology of orally administered tetrahydrocannabinol. *Clin. Pharmacol. Ther.* **14**, 48–55.

35. Litterst, C. L., Flora, K. P., and Cradock, J. C. (1982) Bioavailability of Δ^9-tetrahydrocannabinol-derived radioactivity following intramuscular administration of Δ^9-11-^{14}C-tetrahydrocannabinol to rabbits. *Res. Commun. Substance Abuse.* **3**, 453.

36. Agurell, S., Halldin, M., Lindgren, J.-E., Ohlsson, A., Widman, M., Gillespie, H., and Hollister, L. (1986) Pharmacokinetics and metabolism of Δ^1-tetrahydrocannabinol and other cannabinoids with emphasis on man. *Pharmacol. Rev.* **38**, 21–43.

37. Huestis, M. A., Henningfield, J. E., and Cone, E. J. (1992) Absorption of THC and formation of 11-OH-THC and THCCOOH during and after smoking marihuana. *J. Anal. Toxicol.* **16**, 276–282.

39. Chiang, C. W. N. and Barnett, G. (1984) Marihuana effect and Δ^9-tetrahydrocannabinol plasma level, *Clin. Pharmacol. Ther.* **36**, 234–238.

39. Reeve, V. C., Grant, J. D., Robertson, W., Gillespie, H. K., and Hollister, L. E. (1983) Plasma concentrations of Δ^9-tetrahydrocannabinol and impaired motor function. *Drug Alcohol Dependence* **11**, 167–175.

40. Garrett, E. R. and Hunt, C. A. (1977) Pharmacokinetics of Δ^9-tetrahydrocannabinol in dogs. *J. Pharm. Sci.* **66**, 395–407.

41. Widman, M., Agurell, S., Ehrnebo, M., and Jones, G. (1974) Binding of (+)- and (–)-Δ^1-tetrahydrocannabinols and (–)-7-hydroxy-Δ^1-tetrahydrocannabinol to blood cells and plasma proteins. *J. Pharm. Pharmacol.* **26**, 914–916.

42. Wahlqvist, M., Nilsson, I. M., Sandberg, F., Agurell, S., and Grandstrand, B. (1970) Binding of Δ^1-tetrahydrocannabinol to human plasma proteins. *Biochem. Pharmacol.* **19**, 2579–2589.

43. Klausner, H. K., Wilcox, H. G., and Dingell, J. V. (1975) The use of zonal centrifugation in the investigation of the binding of Δ^9-tetrahydrocannabinol to plasma lipoproteins. *Drug Metab. Dispos.* **3**, 314–319.

44. Widman, M., Nilsson, I. M., Nilsson, J. L. G., Agurell, S., Borg, H., and Grandstrand, B. (1973) Plasma protein binding of 7-hydroxy-Δ^1-tetrahydrocannabinol an active Δ^1-tetrahydrocannabinol metabolite. *J. Pharm. Pharmacol.* **25**, 453–457.

45. Lemberger, L., Axelrod, J., and Kopin, I. J. (1971) Metabolism and distribution of tetrahydrocannabinol in naive and chronic marihuana users. *Ann. NY Acad. Sci.* **191**, 142–154.

46. Ho, B. T., Fritchie, G. E., Kralik, P. M., Englert, F. L., McIsaac, W. M., and Idänpään-Hekkila, J. (1970) Distribution of tritiated Δ⁹-tetrahydrocannabinol in rat tissues after inhalation. *J. Pharm. Pharmacol.* **22**, 538–539.

47. Freudenthal, R. I., Martin, J., and Wall, M. E. (1972) Distribution of Δ⁹-tetrahydrocannabinol in the mouse. *Br. J. Pharmacol.* **44**, 244–249.

48. Burstein, S. H. (1973) Labelling and metabolism of the tetrahydrocannabinols, In: *Marihuana: Chemistry, Pharmacology, Metabolism and Clinical Effects.* (Mechoulam, R., ed.) Academic, New York, pp. 167–190.

49. Ryrfeldt, A., Ramsay, C. H., Nilsson., I. M., Widman, M., and Agurell, S. (1973) Metabolism of cannabis, XIII, Whole body autoradiography of Δ¹-tetrahydrocannabinol in the mouse. Pharmacokinetic aspects of Δ¹-tetrahydrocannabinol and its metabolites. *Acta Pharm. Suec.* **10**, 13–28.

50. Just, W. W., Erdmann, G., Thel, S., Werner, G., and Wiechmann, M (1975) Metabolism and autoradiographic distribution of Δ⁸- and Δ⁹-tetrahydrocannabinol in some organs of the monkey. *Callithrix jaccus, Naunyn Schmiedebergs Arch. Pharmacol.* **287**, 219–225.

51. Erdmann, G., Just, W. W., Thel, S., Werner, G., and Wiechmann, M. (1976) Comparative autoradiographic and metabolic study of Δ⁸- and Δ⁹-tetrahydrocannabinol in the brain of the marmoset. *Callithrix. jaccus. Psychopharmacology* **47**, 53–58.

52. Gill, E. W. and Lawrwnce, D. K. (1973) The distribution of Δ¹-tetrahydrocannabinol and 7-hydroxy-Δ¹-tetrahydrocannabinol in the mouse brain after intraventricular injection. *J. Pharm. Pharmacol.* **25**, 948–952.

53. Martin, B. R., Dewey, W. L., Harris, L. S., and Beckner, J. S. (1977) ³H-Δ⁹-tetrahydrocannabinol distribution in pregnant dogs and their fetuses. *Res. Commun. Chem. Pathol. Pharmacol.* **17**, 457–470.

54. Nahas, G. G., Leger, C., Toque, B., and Hoellinger, H. (1981) The kinetics of cannabinoid distribution and storage with special reference to brain and testis. *J. Clin. Pharmacol.* **21**, 208s–214s.

55. Agurell, S., Nilsson, I. M., Ohlsson, A., and Sandberg, F. (1969) Elimination of tritium-labelled cannabinoids in the rat with special reference to the development of tests for the identification of cannabis users. *Biochem. Pharmacol.* **18**, 1195–1201.

56. Kreuz, D. S. and Axelrod, J. (1973) Δ⁹-Tetrahydrocannabinol localization in body fat. *Science.* **179**, 391–393.

57. Rawich, B., Rohrer, G., and Vardaris, R. M. (1979) Δ⁹-Tetrahydrocannabinol uptake by adipose tissue; preferential accumulation in gonadal fat organs. *Gen. Pharmacol.* **10**, 525.

58. Leuschner, J. T. A., Harvey, D. J., Bullingham, R. E. S., and Paton, W. D. M. (1986) Pharmacokinetics of Δ¹-tetrahydrocannabinol in rabbits following single or multiple intravenous doses. *Drug Metab. Dispos.* **14**, 230–238.

59. Johansson, E., Sjovall, J., Noren, K., Agurell, S., Hollister, L. E., and Halldin, M. M. (1988) Analysis of Δ¹-tetrahydrocannabinol (Δ¹-THC) in human plasma and fat after smoking, In: *Marihuana: An Interdisciplinary Research Report* (Chesher, G., Consroe, P and Musty, R., eds.) National Canpaign Against Drug Abuse, Australian Government Printing Services, Canberra, pp. 291–296.

60. Lemberger, L. and Rubin A. (1975) The physiologic distribution of marihuana in man. *Life Sci.* **17**, 1637–1642.

61. Lemberger, L., Silberstein, S. D., Axelrod, J., and Kopin, I. J. (1970) Marihuana: Studies on the disposition and metabolism of Δ⁹-tetrahydrocannabinol in man. *Science* **170**, 1320–1322.

62. Hunt, C. A. and Jones, R. T. (1980) Tolerance and disposition of tetrahydrocannabinol in man. *J. Pharmacol. Exp. Ther.* **215**, 35–44.

63. Johansson, E., Halldin, M. M., Agurell, S., Hollister, L. E., and Gillespie, H. K. (1989) Terminal elimination plasma half-life of Δ¹-tetrahydrocannabinol (Δ¹-THC) in heavy users of marihuana, *Eur. J. Clin. Pharmacol.* **37**, 273–277.

64. Ellis, G. M., Jr., Mann, M. A., Judson, B. A., Schramm, N. T., and Tashchian, A. (1985) Excretion patterns of cannabinoid metabolites after last use in a group of chronic users. *Clin. Pharmacol. Ther.* **38**, 572–578.

65. Cridland, J. S., Rottanburg, D., and Robins, A. H. (1983) Apparent half-life of excretion of cannabinoids in man. *Human Toxicol.* **2**, 641–644.

66. Agurell, S., Carlsson, S., Lindgren, J.-E., Ohlsson, A., Gillespie, H., and Hollister, L. (1981) Interaction of Δ¹-tetrahydrocannabinol with cannabidiol following oral administration in man—assay of cannabinol and cannabidiol by mass fragmentography. *Experientia* **37**, 1090–1092.

67. Ohlsson, A., Lindgren, J. E., Andersson, S., Agurell, S., Gillespie, H., and Hollister, L. E. (1986) Single-dose kinetics of deuterium-labelled cannabidiol in man after smoking and intravenous administration. *Biomed. Environ. Mass Spectrom.* **13**, 77–83.

68. Burstein, S. and Kupfer, D. (1971) Hydroxylation of trans-Δ¹-tetrahydrocannabinol by hepatic microsomal oxygenases. *Ann. NY Acad. Sci.* **191**, 61–67.

69. Harvey, D. J. and Brown, N. K. (1990) Comparative *in vitro* cannabinoid metabolism in several species. *Life Sci. Adv. Pharmacology* **9**, 763–771.

70. Widman, M., Nordqvist, M., Dollery, C. T., and Briant, R. H. (1975) Metabolism of Δ^1-tetrahydrocannabinol by the isolated perfused dog lung, comparison with *in vitro* liver metabolites. *J. Pharm. Pharmacol.* **27**, 842–848.

71. Halldin, M. M., Isaac, H., Widman, M., Nilsson, E., and Ryrfeldt, A. (1984) A comparison between the metabolism of Δ^1-tetrahydrocannabinol by perfused lung and liver of rat and guinea pig. *Xenobiotica.* **14**, 277–282.

72. Marriage, H. J. and Harvey, D. J. (1986) Metabolism of Δ^1-tetrahydrocannabinol by fractionated isozymes of mouse hepatic cytochrome P-450. *Res. Commun. Substance Abuse.* **7**, 89–97.

73. Narimatsu, S., Watanabe, K., Matsunage, T, Yamamoto, I., Imaoka, S., Funae, Y., and Yoshimura, H. (1992) Cytochrome P-450 isozymes in metabolic activation of Δ^9-tetrahydrocannabinol by liver microsomes of adult female rats. *Drug Metab. Dispos.* **20**, 79–83.

74. Matsunaga, T., Iwawaki, Y., Watanabe, K., Yamamoto, I., Kageyama, T., and Yoshimura, H. (1995) metabolism of Δ^9-tetrahydrocannabinol by cytochrome P-450 isozymes purified from hepatic microsomes of monkeys. *Life Sci.* **56**, 2089–2095.

75. Bornheim, L. M., Lasker, J. M., and Raucy, J. L. (1992) Human hepatic microsomal metabolism of Δ^1-tetrahydrocannabinol. *Drug Matab. Dispos.* **20**, 241–246.

76. Watanabe, K., Matsunaga, T., Yamamoto, I., Funae, Y., and Yoshimura, H. (1995) Involvement of CYP2C in the metabolism of cannabinoids by hepatic microsomes from an old woman. *Biol. Pharm. Bull.* **18**, 1138–1141.

77. Harvey, D. J. and Paton, W. D. M. (1977) The *in vivo* metabolism of $\Delta^{1(6)}$-tetrahydrocannabinol produced by the mouse via the epoxide-diol pathway. *J. Pharm. Pharmacol.* **29**, 498–500.

78. Harvey, D. J., Gill, E. W., Slater, M., and Paton, W. D. M. (1980) Identification of the *in vivo* liver metabolites of (–)-Δ^7-tetrahydrocannabinol produced by the mouse. *Drug Metab. Dispos.* **8**, 439–445.

79. Glatt, H., Ohlsson, A., Agurell, S., and Oesch, F. (1979) Δ^1-Tetrahydrocannabinol and $1\alpha,2\alpha$-epoxytetrahydrocannabinol: mutagenicity investigation in the Ames test. *Mutation Res.* **66**, 329–335.

80. Harvey, D. J. and Leuschner, J. T. A. (1985) Studies on the beta-oxidative metabolism of Δ^1- and Δ^6-tetrahydrocannabinol in the mouse: the *in vivo* biotransformation of metabolites oxidised in the side-chain. *Drug Metab. Dispos.* **13**, 215–219.

81. Nordqvist, M., Lindgren, J. E., and Agurell, S. (1979) Acidic metabolites of Δ^1-tetrahydrocannabinol isolated from rabbit urine. *J. Pharm. Pharmacol.* **31**, 231–237.

82. Nordqvist, M., Agurell, S., Rydberg, M., Falk, L., and Ryman, T. (1979) More acidic metabolites of Δ^1-tetrahydrocannabinol isolated from rabbit urine. *J. Pharm. Pharmacol.* **31**, 238–243.

83. Harvey, D. J. and Paton, W. D. M. (1976) Examination of the metabolites of Δ^1-tetrahydrocannabinol in mouse liver, heart and lung by combined gas chromatography and mass spectrometry, In: *Marihuana: Chemistry, Biochemistry and Cellular Effects* (Nahas, G. G., ed.) Springer-Verlag, New York, pp. 93–109.

84. Brown, N. K. and Harvey, D. J. (1988) *In vivo* metabolism of the methyl homologues of Δ^8-tetrahydrocannabinol, Δ^9-tetrahydrocannabinol and abn-Δ^8-tetrahydrocannabinol in the mouse. *Biomed. Environ. Mass Spectrom.* **15**, 389–398.

85. Brown, N. K. and Harvey, D. J. (1988) *In vivo* metabolism of the *n*-propyl homologues of Δ^8- and Δ^9-tetrahydrocannabinol in the mouse. *Biomed. Mass Spectrom.* **15**, 403–410.

86. Brown, N. K. and Harvey, D. J. (1988) Metabolism of *n*-hexyl homologues of Δ^8-tetrahydrocannabinol and Δ^9-tetrahydrocannabinol in the mouse. *Eur. J. Drug Metab. Pharmacokinetics.* **13**, 165–176.

87. Harvey, D. J. (1985) Identification of hepatic metabolites of *n*-heptyl-Δ^1-tetrahydrocannabinol in the mouse. *Xenobiotica* **15**, 187–197.

88. Harvey, D. J., Martin, B. R., and Paton, W. D. M. (1977) Identification of glucuronides as *in vivo* liver conjugates of seven cannabinoids and some of their hydroxy and acid metabolites. *Res. Commun. Chem. Pathol. Pharmacol.* **16**, 265–279.

89. Williams, P. L. and Moffat, A. C. (1980) Identification in human urine of Δ^9-tetrahydrocannabinol-11-oic acid glucuronide, a tetrahydrocannabinol metabolite. *J. Pharm. Pharmacol.* **32**, 445–448.

90. Levy, S., Yagen, H., and Mechoulam, R. (1978) Identification of a C-glucuronide of Δ^1-tetrahydrocannabinol as a mouse liver conjugate *in vivo*. *Science* **200**, 1391–1392.

91. Leighty, E. G., Fentiman, Jr., A. F., and Foltz, R. L. (1976) Long-retained metabolites of Δ^8- and Δ^9-tetrahydrocannabinol identified as novel fatty acid conjugates. *Res. Commun. Chem. Pathol. Pharmacol.* **14**, 13–28.

92. Martin, B., Nordqvist, M., Agurell, S., Lindgren, J. E., Leander, K., and Binder, M. (1976) Identification of monohydroxy metabolites of cannabidiol formed by a rat liver. *J. Pharm. Pharmacol.* **28**, 275–279.

93. Martin, M., Agurell, S., Nordqvist, M., and Lindgren, J. E. (1976) Dioxygenated metabolites of cannabidiol formed by rat liver. *J. Pharm. Pharmacol.* **28**, 603–608.

94. Harvey, D. J. and Brown, N. K. (1990) *In vitro* metabolism of cannabidiol in the rabbit: identification of seventeen new metabolites including thirteen dihydroxylated in the isopentenyl chain, *Biomed. Environ. Mass Spectrom.* **19**, 559–567.

95. Harvey, D. J. and Brown, N. K. (1990) *In vitro* metabolism of cannabidiol in seven common laboratory mammals. *Res. Commun. Substance Abuse.* **11**, 27–37.

96. Samara, E., Bialer, M., and Harvey, D. J. (1990) Identification of urinary metabolites of cannabidiol in the dog. *Drug Metab. Dispos.* **18**, 571–579.

97. Samara, E. Bialer, M., and Harvey, D. J. (1990) Identification of glucose conjugates as the major urinary metabolites of cannabidiol in the dog. *Xenobiotica* **20**, 177–183.

98. Harvey, D. J. and Mechoulam, R. (1990) Metabolites of cannabidiol identified in human urine, *Xenobiotica.* **20**, 303–320.

99. Paton, W. D. M. and Pertwee, R. G. (1972) Effects of cannabis and certain of its constituents on pentobarbitone sleeping time and phenazone metabolism. *Br. J. Pharmacol.* **23**, 250–261.

100. Fernandes, M., Warning, N., Christ, W., and Hill, R. (1973) Interactions of several cannabinoids with the hepatic drug metabolizing system. *Biochem. Pharmacol.* **22**, 2981–2987.

101. Bornheim, L. M., Borys, H. K., and Karler, R. (1981) Effect of cannabidiol on cytochrome P-450 and hexobarbital sleep time. *Biochem. Pharmacol.* **30**, 503–507.

102. Watanabe, K., Arai, M., Narimatsu, S., Yamamoto, I., and Yoshimura, H. (1987) Self-catalysed inactivation of cytochrome P-450 during microsomal metabolism of cannabidiol. *Biochem. Pharmacol.* **36**, 3371–3377.

103. Hunt, C. A., Jones, R. T., Herning, R. I., and Bachman, J. (1981) Evidence that cannabidiol does not significantly alter the pharmacokinetics of tetrahydrocannabinol in man *J. Pharmacokinetics, Biopharmaceut.* **9**, 245–260.

104. Narimatsu, S., Watanabe, K., Yamamoto, I., and Yoshimura, H. (1988) Mechanism for inhibitory effect of cannabidiol on microsomal testosterone oxidation in male rat liver. *Drug Metab. Dispos.* **16**, 880–889.

105. Bornheim, L. M. and Correia, M. A. (1989) Effect of cannabidiol on cytochrome P-450 isozymes. *Biochem. Pharmacol.* **28**, 2789–2794.

106. Bornheim, L. M. and Correia, M. A. (1989) Purification and characterization of a mouse liver cytochrome P-450 induced by cannabidiol. *Molec. Pharmacol.* **36**, 377–383.

107. Jaeger, W., Benet, L. Z., and Bornheim, L. M. (1996) Inhibition of cyclosporine and tetrahydrocannabinol metabolism by cannabidiol in mouse and human microsomes. *Xenobiotica* **26**, 275–284.

108. Bornheim, L. M., Kim, K. Y., Li, J., Perotti, B. Y., and Benet, L. Z. (1995) Effect of cannabidiol pretreatment on the kinetics of tetrahydrocannabinol metabolites in mouse brain. *Drug. Metab. Dispos.* **23**, 825–831.

109. Bornheim, L. M., Everhart, E. T., Li, J., and Correia, M. A. (1993) Characterization of cannabidiol-mediated cytochrome P-450 inactivation. *Biochem. Pharmacol.* **45**, 1323–1331.

110. Bornheim, L. M., Everhart, E. T., Li, J., and Correia, M. A. (1994) Induction and genetic regulation of mouse hepatic cytochrome P-450 by cannabidiol. *Biochem. Pharmacol.* **48**, 161–171.

111. Yamamoto, I., Kuzuoka, K., Watanabe, K., Narimatsu, S. and Yoshimura, H. (1988) Metabolic formation and pharmacological effects of 11-hydroxy-cannabinol, In: *Marihuana: An Interdisciplinary Research Report* (Chesher, G., Consroe, P. and Musty, R., eds.) National Campaign Against Drug Abuse, Australian Government Printing Services, Canberra, pp. 135–140.

112. Brown, N. K. and Harvey, D. J. (1990) Comparative *in vitro* metabolism of cannabinol in rat, mouse, rabbit, guinea pig, hamster, gerbil and cat. *Eur. J. Drug Metab. Pharmacokinetics* **15**, 253–258.

113. Yisak, W., Widman, M., and Agurell, S. (1978) Acidic *in vivo* metabolites of cannabinol isolated from rat faeces. *J. Pharm. Pharmacol.* **30**, 554–557.

114. Harvey, D. J., Martin, B. R., and Paton, W. D. M. (1977) *In vivo* metabolism of cannabinol by the mouse and rat and a comparison with the metabolism of Δ^1-tetrahydrocannabinol and cannabidiol. *Biomed Mass Spectrom.* **4**, 364–370.

115. Burstein, S. H. and Varanelli, C. (1975) Transformations of cannabinol in the mouse. *Res. Commun. Chem. Pathol. Pharmacol.* **11**, 343–354.

116. Yisak, W., Agurell, S., Lindgren, J. E., and Widman, M. (1978) *In vivo* metabolites of cannabinol identified as fatty acid conjugates. *J. Pharm. Pharmacol.* **30**, 462–463.

117. Harvey, D. J. and Brown, N. K. (1990) *In vitro* metabolism of cannabigerol in the mouse, rat, guinea pig, rabbit, hamster, gerbil and cat. *Biomed. Environ. Mass Spectrom.* **19**, 545–553.

118. Brown, N. K. and Harvey, D. J. (1990) *In vitro* metabolism of cannabichromene in 7 common laboratory animals. *Drug Metab. Dispos.* **16**, 1065–1070.

119. Harvey, D. J. and Brown, N. K. (1991) Identification of cannabichromene metabolites by mass spectrometry–identification of eight new dihydroxy metabolites in the rabbit. *Biological Mass Spectrometry* **20**, 275–285.

120. Klausner, H. K. and Dingell, J. V. (1971) The metabolism and excretion of Δ^9-tetrahydrocannabinol in the rat. *Life Sci.* **10**, 49–59.

121. Lemberger, L., Weiss, J. L., Watanobe, A. M., Galanter, I. M., Wyatt, R. J., and Cardon, P. V. (1972) Δ^9-Tetrahydrocannabinol: temporal correlation of the psychological effects and blood levels after various routes of administration. *New Engl. J. Med.* **286**, 685–688.

122. Hollister, L. E., Kanter, S. L., Moore, F., and Green, D. E. (1972) Marihuana metabolites in urine of man *Clin. Pharmacol. Ther.* **13**, 849–855.

123. Halldin, M. M., Karlsson, S., Kanter, S. L., Widman, M., and Agurell, S. (1982) Urinary metabolites of Δ^1-tetrahydrocannabinol in man. *Arzneim. Forsch.* **32**, 764–768.

124. Halldin, M. M., Andersson, L. K. R., Widman, M., and Hollister, L. E. (1982) Further urinary metabolites of Δ^1-tetrahydrocannabinol in man. *Arzneim. Forsch.* **32**, 1135–1138.

125. Huestis, M. A., Mitchell, J. M., and Cone, E. J. (1996) Urinary excretion profiles of 11-nor-9-carboxy-Δ^9-tetrahydrocannabinol in humans after single smoked doses of marihuana. *J. Anal. Toxicol.* **20**, 441–452.

126. Moody, D. E., Monti, K. M., and Crouch, D. J. (1992) Analysis of forensic specimens for cannabinoids. II. Relationship between blood Δ^9-tetrahydrocannabinol and blood and urine 11-nor-Δ^9-tetrahydrocannabinol-9-carboxylic acid concentrations. *J. Anal. Toxicol.* **16**, 302–306.

127. Huestis, M. A., Henningfield, J. E., and Cone E. J. (1992) Models for the prediction of time of marihuana exposure from plasma concentrations of Δ^9-tetrahydrocannabinol (THC) and 11-nor-carboxy-Δ^9-tetrahydrocannabinol (THCCOOH). *J. Anal. Toxicol.* **16**, 283–290.

128. Yoo, S. D., Fincher, T. K., and Holladay, J. W. (1994) Mammary excretion of cannabidiol in rabbits after intravenous administration. *J. Pharm. Pharmacol.* **46**, 926–928.

129. Hollister, L. E. (1973) Cannabidiol and cannabinol in man. *Experientia* **29**, 825–826.

130. Christensen, H. D., Freudenthal, R. I., Gidley, J. T., Rosenfeld, R., Boegli, G., Testino, L., Brine, D. R., Pitt, C. G., and Wall, M. E. (1971) Activity of Δ^8- and Δ^9-tetrahydrocannabinol and related compounds in the mouse. *Science* **172**, 165–167.

131. Perez-Reyes, M., Timmons, M. C., Lipton, M., Davis, K. H., and Wall, M. E. (1972) Intravenous injection in man of Δ^9-tetrahydrocannabinol and 11-hydroxy-Δ^9-tetrahydrocannabinol. *Science* **177**, 633–635.

132. Jones, G., Widman, M., Agurell, S., and Lindgren, J. E. (1974) Monohydroxylated metabolites of Δ^1-tetrahydrocannabinol in mouse brain. Comparison with *in vitro* liver metabolites. *Acta Pharm. Suec.* **11**, 283–294.

133. Narimatsu, S., Matsubara, K., Shimonishi, T., Watanabe, K., Yamamoto, I. and Yoshimura, H. (1985) Pharmacological activities in the mouse of Δ^9-tetrahydrocannabinol metabolites oxidized in the 8-position. *Chem. Pharm. Bull.* **33**, 392–395.

134. Ohlsson, A., Agurell, S., Leander, K., Dahmen, J., Edery, H., Porath, G., Levy, G., and Mechoulsm, R. (1979) Synthesis and psychotropic activity of side-chain hydroxylated Δ^6-tetrahydrocannabinol metabolites. *Acta Pharm. Suec.* **16**, 21–33.

135. Yamamoto, I., Tanaka, T., Watanabe, K., Narimatsu, S., and Yoshimura, H. (1986) Pharmacological activity of side-chain hydroxylated metabolites of Δ^9-tetrahydrocannabinol in mice. *Res. Commun. Substance Abuse* **7**, 19.

136. Narimatsu, S., Yamamoto, I., Watanabe, K., and Yoshimura, H. (1983) 9a,10a-epoxyhexahydrocannabinol formation from Δ^9-tetrahydrocannabinol by liver microsomes of phenobarbital-treated mice and its pharmacological activities in mice *J. Pharmacobio-Dyn.* **6**, 558–564.

137. Magour, S., Coper, H., and Fahndrich, C. (1977) Is tolerance to Δ^9-tetrahydrocannabinol cellular or metabolic? The subcellular distribution of Δ^9-tetrahydrocannabinol and its metabolites in brain of tolerant and non-tolerant rats. *Psychopharmacology.* **51**, 141–145.

3

Pharmacokinetics of THC in Inhaled and Oral Preparations

Marilyn Huestis

The topic of the pharmacokinetics of THC as illustrated by Harvey is very complex. But it is very important when you study a drug to look at some of the processes involved in its absorption, distribution, and elimination. We can vary drug dosages, and marihuana can be administered in a number of different ways: inhalation, orally and rectally. The drug dosage and the form in which it is administered greatly affects absorption. There are many other processes that determine not only what the free-drug concentration will be in the extracellular fluid, but also drug concentration at the site of drug action, which determines the pharmacodynamic effect. It is a complex situation that includes protein binding, storage in the tissues, metabolism, active and inactive metabolites, as well as mechanisms of excretion through biliary excretion with enterohepatic recirculation, fecal excretion, and renal excretion. The drug is also present in other biological tissues and fluids, including hair, saliva, and sweat (Fig. 1).

I must acknowledge all of the important contributions by colleagues to the field over the years (Table 1), who have pioneered the pharmacokinetics of THC. The present studies express my humble appreciation for all the work that was done before our own.

Most of the early work on marihuana and THC metabolism was done with radiolabeled compounds that have advantages because there is a tremendous amount of sensitivity using this type of study, but there is very low specificity in which analyte you are measuring (Table 2). THC concentrations in plasma and tissue are very low, because of its extensive metabolism, as Harvey has reported. THC is very rapidly distributed throughout the body because of its lipophilic nature and it binds nonspecifically to almost everything. It is very hard to characterize the rapid absorption of THC because it occurs so quickly, and the excretion is difficult to capture because it extends over a very long time period.

---

* This paper is a verbatim transcript of Dr. Huestis' presentation illustrated by the slides of her talk which she graciously provided to the audience.

From: *Marihuana and Medicine*
Edited by: G. G. Nahas et al.   © Humana Press Inc., Totowa, NJ

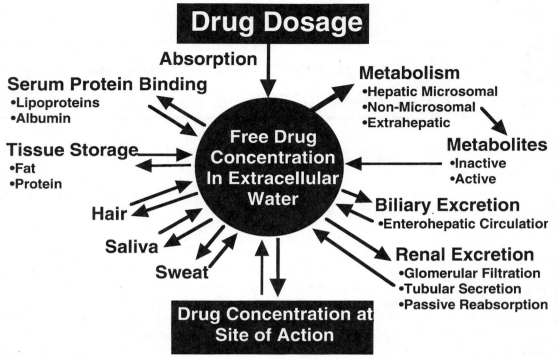

Fig. 1.

One of the real difficulties with studying the inhalation route is the impossibility of determining the exact dose of THC that is absorbed (Fig. 2). One-third to one-half of the drug may be pyrolyzed during the smoking process. Ten to twenty percent can be left in the marihuana cigarette butt that is not actually consumed. There is great variability in individuals' efficiency in smoking the marihuana cigarettes (I worked with human drug users at the Addiction Research Center where we do controlled studies of self-administration); it is incredible to see the variety of techniques that marihuana users employ to smoke their cigarette. We do know that absorption through inhalation is very rapid, with a bioavailability of 18–50% of the THC in the cigarette (Table 3). Many features, such as how long one smoked the cigarette, and how many puffs were inhaled, affect the amount of drug absorbed. A key point is that the inhalation route is a very efficient route of drug absorption, and the resulting rapid delivery of drug to the brain certainly contributes to the abuse liability of smoked drugs.

Oral absorption is a much slower, erratic absorption, is difficult to predict, varies considerably between individuals, and results in a much lower availability (Table 4). The drug is degraded in the gut from the acid environment, and is also metabolized rapidly by a first-pass effect through the liver where efficient metabolism occurs. The pharmacological effects of the drug seem to be higher at lower THC concentrations because following the oral route, there are almost equal concentrations of THC and 11-OH-THC, and 11-OH-THC is nearly as active as THC. Thus you observe a more pronounced effect with lower THC plasma levels. Effects also occur at later times and last a little longer. Monroe Wall's group, comparing oral THC absorption to intravenous administration had very interesting results. Whereas smoking (inhalation route) compares quite favorably with intravenous administration, the oral route is very different.

Table 1

Lemberger Agurell Wall
Ohlsson Perez-Reyes
Mechoulam Harvey Law
Garrett Hunt Jones
Hollister Johansson
Cone Halldin Davis

Table 2

Introduction

Radiolabeled drug for early studies—high sensitivity, low specificity
THC analysis difficult—low levels, extensively metabolized, rapidly
    distributed, highly lipophilic, and nonspecific binding
Time course of very rapid absorption and very slow excretion, difficult
    to capture

Table 3

Absorption: Inhalation

Rapid, peak occurs during smoking
Systemic availablitiy 18–50%
Smoking dynamics important: number of puffs, duration and volume of
    inhalation, hold time, time between puffs, smoking time, experience
    of smoker
Highly efficient route of drug delivery to the brain, similar to intravenous
    route

Table 4

Absorption: Oral

Slow and erratic absorption
Peak levels low, occur at 1–5 h
Systemic availablitiy low 6–20%
Vehicle important, degradation in gut, first pass effect in liver
Effects appear later, last longer, greater effects at lower THC levels
THC $\approx$ 11-OH-THC

Because THC is highly lipophilic, it is rapidly distributed throughout the body (Table 5). The clearance rate is similar to hepatic blood flow, about 1 L/min. It is highly protein bound to lipoproteins and albumin in the blood. The volume of distribution is very large as you would expect for a lipophilic drug. Enterohepatic recirculation will affect the elimination half-life of the drug. Elegant work from Hunt and coworkers showed that the release of THC that is sequestered throughout the body, especially in fat tissues, is the rate-limiting step in the elimination process.

THC Disposition During Marijuana Smoking

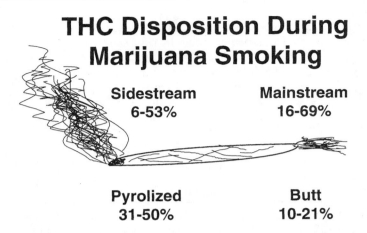

Sidestream
6-53%

Mainstream
16-69%

Pyrolized
31-50%

Butt
10-21%

Fig. 2.

Metabolism is extensive and results in numerous metabolites (Table 6). Oxidation occurring with conversion to the primary metabolites 11-OH-THC, 8-—OH-THC, 8-—OH-THC and THC-COOH. In humans there is much less side-chain oxidation. Very important metabolic reactions result in glucuronidation and sulfation to form the THC-COOH, which is a water-soluble compound readily excreted in the urine. There are no metabolic differences between genders or between frequent or infrequent marihuana users. Most of the metabolism occurs in the liver, but it also can occur in other organs, including the lung and the intestine, and different metabolites predominate by the different routes. Cytochromes CYP2C9, C11, and CYP3A play important roles.

About one-third of the absorbed dose is excreted in the urine, an amount that varies according to different investigators and about two-thirds of the excretion occurs through the feces (Table 7). There are wide individual variations that may be attributed to genetic polymorphism. The half-lives reported in the literature span a wide period of time because determination of half-lives varies according to the time period during which excretion is monitored, sensitivity of assay, its specificity, and how frequently or how high the concentrations are in the individual's body. Probably the best estimated half-lives of THC have been by Johansen and others in humans and which correspond to 4.3 days. In some very heavy chronic users they reported elimination half-lives of up to 12 days.

The reported figures for THC urinary excretion vary considerably, but a period of three days has been well documented, which is a very long excretion time for a substance.

I am reporting the work I have done in conjunction with Dr. Ed Cone at the Addiction Research Center. We were interested in focusing on the rapid absorption phase of marihuana smoking. For this we used a continuous blood-withdrawal pump to take continuous samples during the absorption phase and we monitored the sampling for seven days after marihuana administration. Figure 3 describes the respective plasma concentrations of THC, 11-OH-THC, and the carboxy metabolite. Each arrow represents a single puff on a marihuana cigarette. One can see how rapidly the THC concentration increases, and also that there is significant drug concentration even after a single puff. The mean concentrations after a low-dose cigarette (1.75% THC) was 7 ng/mL, and after the high-dose cigarette (3.25 mg) the mean concentration was 18 ng/mL.

Looking at mean data collected on six subjects, there is a beautiful dose response with the low-dose THC and the high-dose THC (Fig. 4). Looking at individual results after the high-

Table 5

Distribution

Lipophilic, rapid distribution to tissues
Clearance ≈ hepatic blood flow 0.8 L/min
Highly protein bound in blood ≈ 97%
Volume of distribution ≈ 10 L/Kg
Enterohepatic circulation
Slow release of sequestered drug from tissues rate limiting step in
    elimination

Table 6

Metabolism

Rapid and extensive metabolism
Phase 1: oxidation, primary metabolites 11-OH-THC, 8α and 8β-OH-
    THC, THCCOOH, little side chain oxidation
Phase 2: glucuronidation, sulfation
Cytochrome P450, CYP2C9 and 11, CYP3A
No differences between sexes, frequent and infrequent users
Liver, lung, and intestine

Table 7

Excretion

Urine excretion ≈ 15–30%, fecal 27–65%
Half-lives affected by sampling time, assay sensitivity, and specificity,
    frequency use
Plasma THC $t_{1/2}$ best estimate ≈ 4.3 d
Urine THCOOH $t_{1/2}$ best estimate ≈ 3.0 d

dose cigarette, there is tremendous variability between subjects. Sampling was performed with a computer-controlled, paced smoking program. The number of puffs were controlled, as were the dose of THC in the marihuana cigarette, the time between puffs, the retention time in the lungs, and the resting time between puffs. However, we did not control the depth of inhalation; individuals were able to titrate the dose inhaled according to the feeling that they wanted to have, as the onset of effects is very rapid and subjects could titrate the amount of drug that they took by controlling their smoking.

A comparison of the three different primary analyses illustrates the different shapes of the plasma concentration–time curve. There is a rapid and very high concentration of THC that peaks before the end of smoking. We were able to demonstrate this distribution because we collected all samples during the absorption phase. There is a very low concentration of 11-OH-THC metabolite. The THC-COOH does not reach the height of the maximum concentrations of THC, but displays a plateau curve for a fairly long period of time before decreasing slowly (Fig. 5). We have collected every urine sample from subjects over a four week time period and they were analyzed by GC/MS and immunoassay. We were able to detect the THC-COOH in urine for seven days when all samples were still positive at a 0.5 ng/mL level.

Mean THC, 11-OH-THC & THCCOOH
During Marijuana Smoking (3.55% THC)

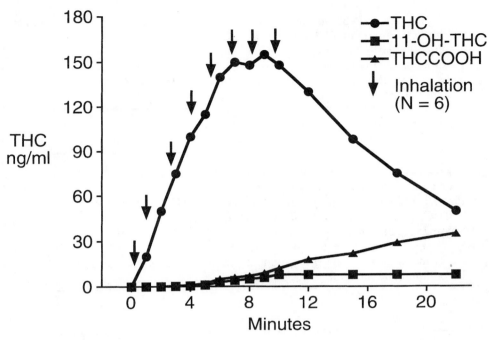

Fig. 3.

THC Dose Response

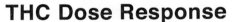
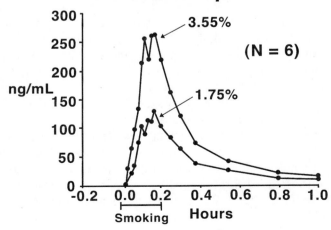

Fig. 4.

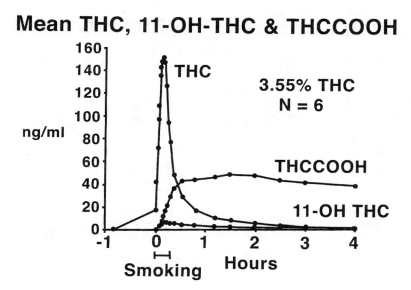

Fig. 5.

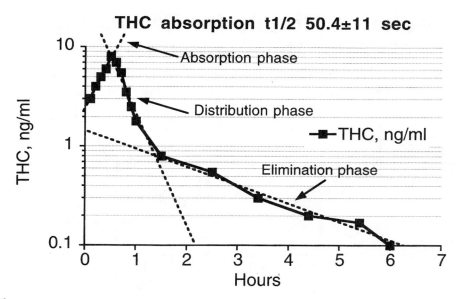

Fig. 6.

Pharmacokinetic modeling was utilized and we developed a pharmacokinetic model for our data. We looked at a two-compartment model. Using a linear/nonlinear representation, we modeled it as if each puff the individual took corresponded to a separate THC dose. We observed that the absorption half-life was about 50 seconds (Fig. 6). There is a very rapid absorption and delivery of this drug to the brain, which again, contributes to its abuse liability.

We are interested in pharmacodynamic effects as well. It had been suggested that plotting THC on a constant-effect time curve would get a counterclockwise hysteresis. Figure 7

Mean Concentration Effect Curves

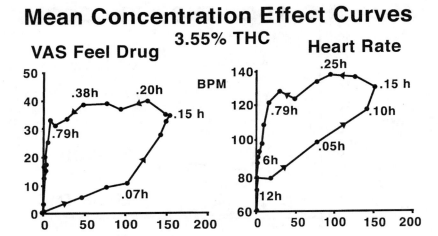

Fig. 7.

Predictive Models for Estimating Time of Marijuana Usage

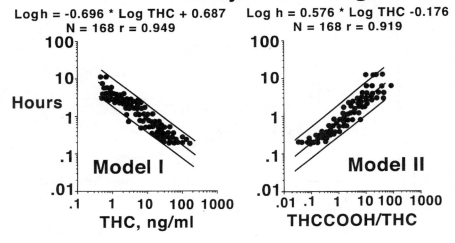

Fig. 8.

demonstrates two counterclockwise hysteresis for THC, one corresponds to the subjective effects and represents a mood scale (how strongly the individual feels the effect of the drug), and the other corresponds to the increase in heart rate. What is important about these hysteresis curves is that if you look at a particular concentration in plasma, such as 100 ng/mL, you have very little effect at one point in time, but at the same drug concentration at a later time one observes very strong effects. We were able to show that in most studies measurements started at a time when this entire portion of the time curve was missed. Our rapid sampling

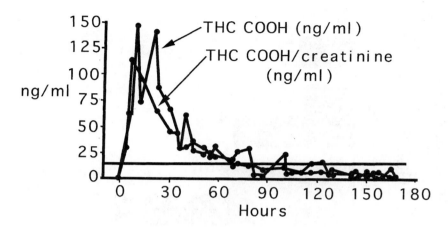

Urinary Excretion Profile
Subject B 3.55% THC

Fig. 9.

indicated to us that there was almost a linear absorption of the drug, followed by a very long period when the distribution and equilibrium is occurring, there is a linear excretion and a reduction of the effects. Because of this type of occurrence and thanks to the many forensic drug samples we examine, we were able to develop models that predict the elapsed time after marihuana smoking, on the basis of a single plasma cannabinoid level. We have two models, one based on the THC concentration, and one based on the ratio of THC-COOH to THC. We can predict within a 95% confidence interval the time a subject smoked and this measurement is used around the world in accidents to determine driving under influence of the drug (Fig. 8).

Figure 9 represents the excretion of THC-COOH in the urine. If one looks at just the concentration in ng/mL, one has a saw-tooth pattern, and especially around immunoassay or GC/MS cutoff it becomes very difficult to interpret results. That is one of the factors we try to understand. It is not just how accurate the quantitative numbers are, but what they mean. In this case you would get a positive, a negative, a positive, a negative, and a positive result. So you do not know whether the individual smoked the drug again or whether there is residual drug excretion. One of the things we have done is to normalize to the urine creatinine concentration. We have actually worked up models based on the concentrations in two urine specimens that should help predict whether a subject has used the drug again or whether you have residual drug excretion.

The cutoff that one uses affects tremendously the detection time of last use and how long one can detect the marihuana use by measurement of the drug in the urine (Fig. 10). A big take-home message is that at 50 ng/mL concentration, which is the current federally mandated urine cutoff level, one only detects the drug for one to two days after a high or low dose, and this is in infrequent marihuana users or occasional marihuana users. It is a different story in chronic users.

Although there is a tremendous variation in the amount of THC-COOH that is excreted by different individuals, we have observed that the percentage of the total drug excreted was very similar across subjects, so about 50% of the THC-COOH is excreted in the first day and decreases over time, and also according to doses (Figs. 11 and 12).

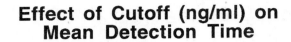

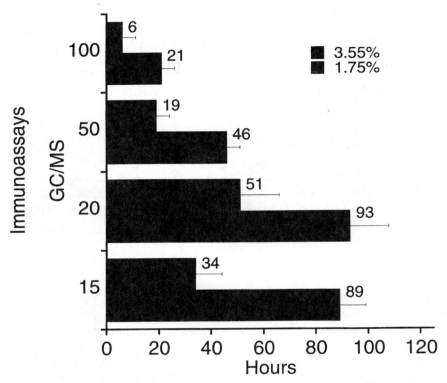

Fig. 10.

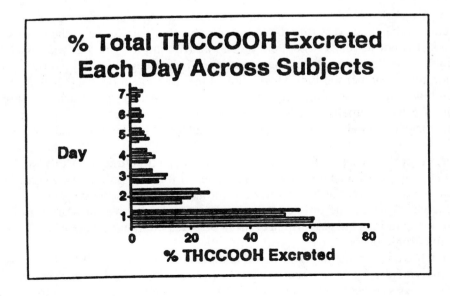

Fig. 11.

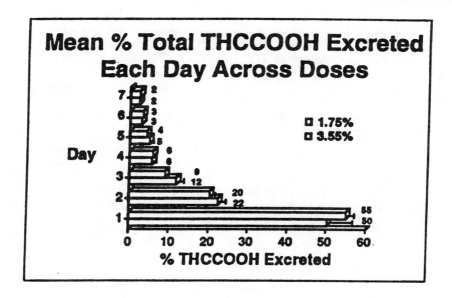

Fig. 12.

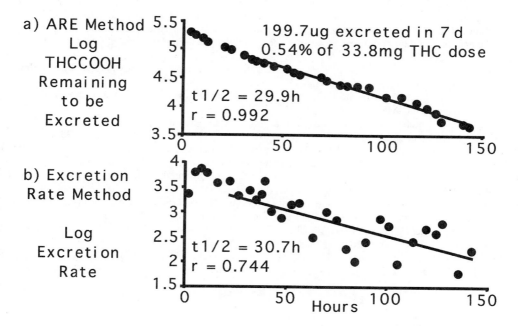

Fig. 13. The two methods of measurements of THC COOH elimination in the urine.

There are two different ways of measuring elimination half-lives in urine: by the amount remaining to be excreted method (ARE), or by signal-minus method; and by the excretion-rate method (Fig. 13). Certainly the ARE method has a lot of advantages, but it requires collection of every urine sample, which is what we did. You can see that there is much less variability when the ARE method is used. Figure 13 illustrates the drug excretion in six individuals indicating that the half-life is about 30 hours. Figure 8 describes the results of our predictive models to estimate time of marihuana usage.

Table 8

Normalize to creatinine to distinguish new use from residual excretion
Significant concentrations of THC and 11-OH-THC in urine when E coli
   β glucuronidase
Suggest that urinary THC and 11-OH-THC useful for predicting elapsed
   time after smoking
High concentrations of THC and 11-OH-THC found in DUI cases

One important new observation is that there is a lot of THC and 11-OH-THC excreted in the urine. This is because of the enzyme that is used for separating the compound in the analytical procedure. We are also finding extremely high concentrations of THC and 11-OH-THC in cases of driving under the influence. Another important distinction obtained is to differentiate oral use from smoked marihuana. It is not yet a validated method, and it is not yet developed, but it appears that it can be done (Table 8).

References

1 . Cone, E.J. (1997) New developments in biological measures of drug prevalence. NIDA *Res. Monogr.* **167,** 108–129.
2. Cone, E.J., and Huestis, M.A. (1993) Relating blood concentrations of tetrahydrocannabinol and metabolites to pharmacologic effects and time of marijuana usage. *Therapeutic Drug Monitoring.* **15,** 527–532.
3. Giardino, N.J. (1997) An indoor air quality-pharmacokinetic simulation of passive inhalation of marijuana smoke and the resultant buildup of 11-nor-delta-9-tetrahydrocannabinol-9-carboxylic acid in urine. *J. Forensic Sci.* **42,** 323–325.
4. Giardino, N.J. (1996) Stability of 11-nor-delta 9-tetrahydrocannabinol in negative human urine in high-density polyethylene (Nalgene) [letter]. *J. Anal. Toxicol.* **20,** 275–276.
5. Huestis, M.A., Mitchell, J.M., and Cone, E.J. (1995) Detection times of marijuana metabolites in urine by immunoassay and GC-MS. *J. Anal. Toxicol.* **19,** 443–449.
6. Huestis, M.A., Mitchell, J.M., and Cone, E.J. (1996) Urinary excretion profiles of 11-nor-9 carboxy-delta 9-tetrahydrocannabinol in humans after single smoked doses of marijuana. J *Anal Toxicol.* **20,** 441–452.
7. Jaeger, W., Benet, L.Z., and Bornheim, L.M. (1996) Inhibition of cyclosporine and tetrahydrocannabinol metabolism by cannabidiol in mouse and human microsomes. *Xenobiotica.* **26,** *275–284.*
8 Jenkins., A.T., Darwin, W.D., Huestis, M.A., Cone, E.J., and Mitchell, J.M. (1995) Validity testing of the accuPINCH THC test. *J. Anal. Toxicol.* **19,** 5–12.
9. Moore, C., Lewis, D., Becker, J., and Leikin, J. (1996) The determination of 11-nor-delta 9tetrahydro-cannabinol-9-carboxylic acid (THCCOOH) in meconium. *J. Anal. Toxicol.* **20,** 50–51.
10. Szirmai, M., Beck, O., Stephansson, N., and Halldin, M.M. (1996) A GC-MS study of three major acidic metabolites of delta 1-tetrahydrocannabinol. *J. Anal. Toxicol.* **20,** 573–578.
11. Wilkins, D., Haughey, H., Cone, E., Huestis, M., Foltz, R., Rollins, D. (1995) Quantitative analysis of THC, 11-OH-THC, and THCCOOH in human hair by negative ion chemical ionization mass spectrometry. *J. Anal. Toxicol.* **19,** 483–491.

4

Pharmacokinetics and Mechanisms of Action of Analgesics in Clinical Pain

John E. Stambaugh

Abstract

Because of recent interest in the development of drug assay techniques, the pharmacokinetics of many analgesics have been defined. In addition, mechanisms of action of the commonly used analgesics have been partly delineated, and currently accepted analgesic regimens and usages are being questioned. By considering both the pharmacokinetics and the mechanism of action of each of these analgesics, it would appear that only a few of the currently available agents are needed for the treatment of acute and chronic pain. Newer agents with reduced toxicity have been introduced but have resulted in little expansion of novel ways to interfere with pain. The recent discovery of the β-endrophin system, the re-evaluation of older agents, and the development of new agents that work at pain pathways other than the classical sites hold out the promise of alternative means of control of certain types of pain. An agent that has analgesic efficacy equivalent to morphine but with reduced toxicity is especially exciting in the development of new analgesics. An agent that, in addition, does not lead to intolerable psychomimetic reactions but instead addresses multiple aspects of treating the fear, pain, and tension triad of pain will be beneficial in acute pain but will especially enhance the spectrum of the control of chronic pain such as cancer, neuralgia, and arthralgia.

Pain is one of the most common symptoms treated by physicians, and yet in too many instances it is treated with a "routine" analgesic regimen, with little or no consideration of the intensity or chronicity of the symptom. With proper attention, a better degree of analgesia is achievable, since scriptors for the evaluation of clinical pain have been described and relative potency of most of the commonly used analgesics has been defined. By defining the intensity of pain and/or pain relief as none (0), mild (1), moderate (2), severe (3), and very severe (4), the initial pain and subsequent treatment results can be evaluated. The duration of analgesia can be determined by repeated evaluation of pain intensity and pain relief from minutes to hours to days, depending on the duration of pain and duration of analgesia.

From: *Marihuana and Medicine*
Edited by: G. G. Nahas et al.   © Humana Press Inc., Totowa, NJ

Table 1
Comparison of Analgesics. Mechanism of Action and Efficacy

Analgesic	Mechanism of action	Duration of action (h)	Equianalgesic ratio to morphine (mg/mg)
Acetylsalicylic acid	Prostaglandin inhibition (peripheral)	4	650/5*
Acetaminophen	Midbrain–spinothalamic tract	4	650/5*
Morphine and congeners	Opiate-receptor agonist		
Morphine	Cerebral cortex	4 (euphoria)	10/10**
Codeine		4	120/10**
Oxycodone		4	20/10*
Meperidine		2	100/10**
Metadone		4	10/10**
Narcotic antagonists	Opiate-receptor		
Butorphanol	agonist and antagonist	4	2/10**
Nalbuphine	action	4	10/10**
Hydroxyzine	Unknown (not cerebral cortex)	4–6	100/10**
Zomepirac	Prostaglandin inhibition (peripheral)	4	100/10**
Propoxyphene napsylate	Possibly opiate receptor	4	200/5*

* Oral.
** Parenteral.

The evaluation of new analgesics, including progenitors of new classes such as levonantradol, should present no problem with respect to relative efficacy evaluation, because both acute and chronic pain models have been described and predicted responses for most currently available analgesics have been reported. Single versus repeat dosage studies can lead to extensive information regarding analgesic efficacy and/or toxicity. Evaluations of side effects, overall impressions of analgesia, and the need for concomitant or additional medication are also important parameters to monitor during studies of clinical pain. Although developed as a research tool for the evaluation of new analgesics, the methods described and information obtained should be applied, at least in part, in the routine management of all patients with clinical pain.

Comparison of an oral analgesic to acetylsalicylic acid or acetaminophen or to an oral narcotic alone or in combination should define the relative efficacy of the analgesic (Table 1). Morphine remains the standard of comparison for parenteral analgesics, but comparison to the narcotic agonist-antagonist group of analgesics is now also necessary. Since the goal of any new analgesic is at least an efficacy as good as one of the reference compounds but with either less toxicity and/or an alternate mechanism for pain relief, such a goal may lead to a different therapeutic approach to analgesia (such as low-dose combination formulations). Compounds with a potential for more than one clinical use offer the potential of management of a clinical symptom complex by a single agent. Recent studies with hydroxyzine have

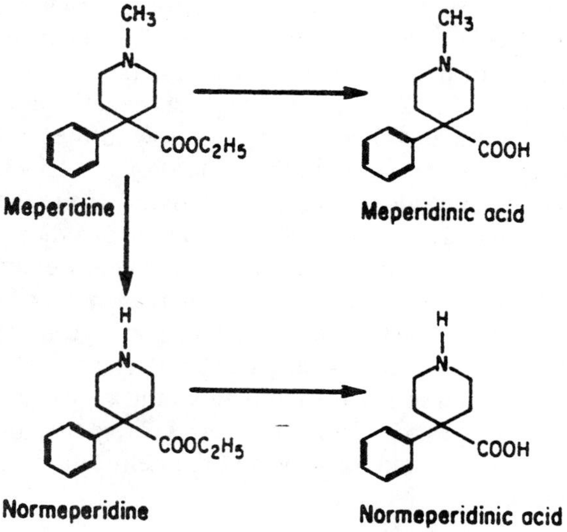

Fig. 1. Metabolites of meperidine.

shown that in addition to the antianxiety activity, both analgesic and antinauseant activity can result. As pain is associated with the triad of fear, pain, and tension, and because many clinical syndromes involve several symptomatologies, a single agent with several actions may be indicated.

In an attempt to control associated symptoms caused by the disease process and/or symptoms resulting from the analgesic, multiple analgesic regimens have become customary in clinical practice. All of the combination therapies used with the analgesics such as phenothiazines, antihistamines, sedatives, tranquilizers, and soon, have resulted from clinical use but often offer no increase in analgesic efficacy and a marked increase in toxicity. With the exception of hydroxyzine, none of these agents have analgesic activity, and few, if any, add any increased spectrum of pain relief.

Only recently have the pharmacokinetics of the analgesics been described (1–10), and only with the case of meperidine have the efficacy and toxicity of the analgesic been correlated with the pharmacokinetic data. In order to delineate the usefulness of the evaluation of pharmacokinetic data in patients and volunteers while simultaneously determining efficacy and/or toxicity of the drug, a summary of the meperidine studies is presented. Meperidine is metabolized as shown in Fig. 1 (11). The serum kinetics of meperidine and its toxicity have been described recently (7). Identification of urinary excretion products versus time is needed to define toxic metabolites and to delineate alterations of meperidine metabolism by concomitant medications. Such studies led to the conclusions that the combination of phenobarbitol and meperidine can result in alterations in metabolism and the enhanced production of normeperidine, a toxic metabolite (13).

Similar studies have demonstrated that combination with the phenothiazines increases cardiovascular and CNS toxicity both directly at the receptor and perhaps alternatively through a change in hepatic biotransformation (14). The MAO inhibitors, when used in combination with meperidine, are potentially lethal; the contraceptives can alter meperidine metabolism (15); and many other analgesic combinations with tranquilizers lead to increased toxicity without an increase in efficacy.

Hydroxyzine leads to a tolerable increase in CNS toxicity when used with meperidine *(16)*, but with additive analgesia since hydroxyzine alone is an analgesic *(17)*. A study determining the pharmacokinetics of meperidine and hydroxyzine showed no change in serum or urinary pharmacokinetics *(18)*. The kinetics of both drugs exactly parallel onset and duration of pain relief *(19)*. Because the above series of studies with meperidine combined kinetic data with analgesic efficacy and/or toxicity in the same subjects, conclusions regarding those serum levels of drug needed to produce analgesia and toxicity were made.

In summary, it appears that the methods for evaluation of efficacy and toxicity of new classes of analgesics such as levonantradol are clearly defined. Relative potency to standard analgesic regimens should be readily resolved in the management of mild to severe pain of acute or chronic duration. It is suggested for all such new analgesics that simultaneous comparisons of kinetic data with observed efficacy and toxicity should form an important and early component of their evaluation since such data would be extremely useful in defining adequate serum levels for analgesia and serum levels for toxicity. In addition, kinetic data may parallel duration of analgesia and toxicity, and the delineation of metabolites may help explain observed discrepancies.

Reprinted with permission from The Journal of Clinical Pharmacology, 21 (8 & 9), Supplement, 295S–298S, 1981.

REFERENCES

1. Graham, G. G., Champion, G. D., Day, R. O., and Paull, P. D. (1977) Patterns of plasma concentrations and urinary excretions of salicylate in rheumatoid arthritis. *Clin. Pharm. Ther.* **22**, 410–420.
2. Gram, L. F., Schou, J., Way, W. L., Heltberg, J., and Bodin, N. O. (1979) d-Propoxyphene kinetics after single oral and intravenous doses in man. *Clin. Pharm. Ther.* **26**, 473–482.
3. Olsen, G. D., Wendel, H. A., Livermore, B. A., Leger, R. M., Lynn, R. K., and Gerber, N. (1976) Clinical effects and pharmacokinetics of racemic methadone and its optical isomers. *Clin. Pharm. Ther.* **21**, 147–157.
4. Holmstrand, J., Anggard, E., and Gunne, L. M. (1978) Methadone maintenance: plasma levels and therapeutic outcome. *Clin. Pharrn. Ther.* **23**, 175–180.
5. Inaba, T., Stewart, D. J., and Kalow, W. (1978) Metabolism of cocaine in man. *Clin. Pharm. Ther.* **23**, 547–552.
6. Findlay, J. W. A., Butz, R. F., and Welch, R. M. (1977) Codeine kinetics as determined by radioimmunoassay. *Clin. Pharm. Ther.* **22**, 439–446.
7. Stambaugh, J. E., Wainer, I. W., Sanstead, J. K., and Hemphill, D. M. (1976) The clinical pharmacology of meperidine-comparison of routes of administration. *J. Clin. Pharmacol.* **16**, 245–256.
8. Findlay, J. W. A., Jones, E. C., Butz, R. F., and Welch, R. M. (1978) Plasma codeine and morphine concentrations after therapeutic oral doses of codeine-containing analgesics. *Clin. Pharm. Ther.* **24**, 60–68.
9. Stanski, D. R., Greenblatt, D. J., and Lowenstein, E. (1978) Kinetics of intravenous and intramuscular morphine. *Clin. Pharm. Ther.* **24**, 52–59.
10. Berkowitz, B. A., Asling, J. H., Schnider, S. M., and Way, E. L. (1969) Relationship of pentazocine plasma levels to pharmacologic activity in man. *Clin. Pharm. Ther.* **10**, 320–328.
11. Burns, J. J., Berger, B. L., Lief, P. A., Nollack, A., Papper, E. M., and Brodie, B. B. (1955) The physiologic disposition and fate of meperidine (Demerol) in man and a method for its estimation in plasma. *J. Pharmacol. Exp. Ther.* **114**, 289–298.
12. Stambaugh, J. E., and Wainer, I. W. (1975) The bioavailability of meperidine using urine assays for meperidine and normeperidine. *J. Clin. Pharmacol.* **15**, 269–271.
13. Stambaugh, J. E., Wainer, I. W., and Schwartz, I. (1978) The effect of phenobarbitol on the metabolism of meperidine in normal volunteers. *J. Clin. Pharmacol.* **18**, 482–490.
14. Stambaugh, J. E., and Wainer, I. W. (1981) Drug interactions: meperidine and chlorpromazine, a toxic combination. *J. Clin. Pharmacol.* **21**, 140–146.
15. Stambaugh, J. E., and Wainer, I. W. (1975) Drug interactions 1: meperidine and oral contraceptives. *J. Clin. Pharmacol.* **15**, 46–51.
16. Stambaugh, J. E., and Wainer, I. W. (1976) Drug interactions II: meperidine and hydroxyzine hydrochloride. Proceedings of the First World Congress, International Association for the Study of Pain.

17. Beaver, W. T., and Feise, G. (1976) Comparison of the analgesic effects of morphine, hydroxyzine and their combination in patients with postoperative pain. In: *Advances in Pain Research and Therapy*, vol. 1. Raven, New York, pp 553–557.
18. Stambaugh, J. E., and Wainer, I. W. (1976) Metabolic studies of hydroxyzine and meperidine in human subjects. In: *Advances in Pain Research and Therapy*, vol. 1. Raven, New York, pp. 559–565.
19. Stambaugh, J. E., and Lane, C. Analgesic efficacy and pharmacokinetic evaluation of meperidine and hydroxyzine, alone and in combination. *Cancer Invest.* **1**(2):111–117. (in press).

5

Δ⁹-THC Hemisuccinate in Suppository Form as an Alternative to Oral and Smoked THC

Larry A. Walker, Ernest C. Harland,
Allyson M. Best, and Mahmoud A. ElSohly

Abstract

Although Δ⁹-tetrahydrocannabinol (THC) has demonstrated utility for several medicinal applications, several studies have reported the inconsistent bioavailability of the oral soft gelatin capsule formulation, because of erratic absorption and variable first-pass metabolism of THC. This problem limits the utility of THC for its approved indications, and also prevents efficient assessment of other potential therapeutic applications. In an effort to overcome these pharmacokinetic limitations, we have explored the utility of various ester prodrugs of THC in suppository formulations as alternatives for effecting the systemic delivery of THC. Studies designed to characterize the bioavailability and efficacy of these preparations are reviewed here. In addition, studies designed to confirm the behavior of THC-hemisuccinate (THC-HS) as a prodrug were conducted. In rodents and dogs, intravenous administration of THC and THC-HS produced identical pharmacological responses (hypothermia and potentiation of thiamylal sleep times in mice; bradycardia in dogs) except at very high doses. Pharmacokinetic evaluations after intravenous and rectal administration of THC-HS also showed that the parent ester could not be detected in plasma, but that THC and its metabolite were detected in a fashion consistent with the immediate hydrolysis of THC-HS to THC in the absorption process or in the plasma. Administration of the THC-HS via suppositories resulted in excellent bioavailability, sustained plasma levels of THC, and improved efficacy as compared to the oral formulations, suggesting the feasibility of this route for the delivery of THC in various therapeutic applications.

From: *Marihuana and Medicine*
Edited by: G. G. Nahas et al.   © Humana Press Inc., Totowa, NJ

1. INTRODUCTION

Δ^9-tetrahydrocannabinol (THC) is the primary psychoactive constituent in marihuana (*Cannabis sativa* L.), and is likely responsible for marihuana's other interesting pharmacological actions. THC has been approved by the Food and Drug Administration (FDA) for the control of nausea and vomiting associated with chemotherapy and, more recently, for appetite stimulation in AIDS patients suffering from the wasting syndrome. Cannabinoids, however, also possess pharmacologic attributes that have led to proposed use for symptomatic treatment in several other disorders, such as glaucoma *(1)*, migraine headache *(2,3)*, and other pain syndromes *(4)*, spasticity *(4)*, anxiety *(5,6)*, and depression *(4,7)*. It is because of these promising therapeutic applications that public debate has arisen over the legalization of marihuana for medicinal purposes. Balancing the therapeutic use of a drug against its abuse potential is often a delicate issue. This is particularly true in regard to marihuana smoking, for which the purported medicinal uses are used to justify legalization and of marihuana. Thus, there are legal, political, and social, as well as medical issues to be addressed.

One point well argued by the medicinal marihuana proponents is the fact that the legally available THC, prepared as a soft gelatin capsule formulation and sold as Marinol®, is very expensive and lacks consistency in its effects. The latter point could be explained by the fact that oral THC has erratic absorption from the gastrointestinal tract, and is subject to a marked first-pass effect in the liver, resulting in extensive metabolism *(8,9)*. This results in the formation of high levels of 11-OH-THC, which may have undesirable side effects. Pharmacokinetic studies indicate bioavailability is only 10–20% in healthy adults *(9)*, and this may be further decreased by emetic episodes in patients. A recent meta-analysis revealed a poor or partial response in approximately 65% of 750 courses of oral therapy *(10)*.

In an effort to overcome problems with the consistent delivery of THC, we have devoted a considerable effort to identifying a formulation and route of administration with improved bioavailability. An evaluation of several different esters as prodrugs of THC demonstrated that the hemisuccinate ester (THC-HS) afforded substantial bioavailability from a suppository base *(11)*, whereas THC itself totally lacks bioavailability from suppositories *(12)*.

The formulation of THC as the hemisuccinate ester in suppositories appears to overcome all the problems associated with the oral preparation and shows consistent bioavailability in animal studies *(11,13)*. Preliminary clinical investigations show promise for this formulation *(14–16)*.

The purpose of this report is to review the bioavailability studies carried out on the hemisuccinate ester (THC-HS) and to establish whether THC-HS is truly acting as a prodrug of THC. We therefore compared the pharmacological and toxicological effects of intravenous THC-HS and THC, in dogs and rodents, in addition to the evaluation of the blood levels of THC, and its major metabolite (THC-COOH) after iv administration in monkeys.

METHODS

2.1. Comparison of the Toxicity and Pharmacology of THC and THC-HS in Mice

ICR Swiss mice weighing 25–30 g were housed in group boxes of five each, and two boxes were allocated to each study group. On the day of the experiment, each mouse was temporarily restrained in a plastic cylinder to allow access to a tail vein for iv injections. Immediately after injection, the mice were returned to their home cages. The groups received the vehicle (ethanol:Alkamuls [Rhone-Poulenc, Research Triangle Park, NC] saline, 1:1:8),

200 µL, or various doses of THC or THC-HS in the same volume. Doses are expressed as THC equivalents, accounting for the molecular weight of the ester.

For comparative toxicity assessment of THC and THC-HS, the dose range was adjusted for each compound to span the range from no deaths (10 and 30 mg/kg, respectively) to 100% dead (100 and 200 mg/kg, respectively). Four hours was used as the cutoff point. All deaths occurred within 2 hours, and most within minutes of injection. The 95% confidence limits for the LD50 were determined by probit analysis.

For comparative assessment of the hypothermic effects, the dose range evaluated was 0.3, 1.0, 3.0, and 10.0 mg/kg iv. Body temperature was measured with a Yellow Springs Instruments recorder fitted with a mouse rectal probe. Measurements were made before and at 60 minutes after dosing (determined in preliminary experiments to be the time of peak response). Responses were assessed by comparison of the absolute change in body temperature between the two drugs.

The effects of THC and THC-HS on barbiturate-induced sleep times were also compared. The dose range evaluated was 0.3, 1.0, 3.0, and 10.0 mg/kg iv. Thirty minutes after administration of THC or THC-HS, mice received an intraperitoneal injection of thiamylal, 45 mg/kg. This dose of thiamylal alone produces sleep times of 2 minutes or less. Onset of sleep was defined as the point of loss of righting reflex. End of sleep was defined as the point at which the animal could right itself three consecutive times.

2.2 Comparison of the Pharmacological Effects of THC and THC-HS in Dogs

Four beagle dogs (Marshall Farms, Kensington PA) weighing 10–12 kg were utilized in these studies. Dogs were acclimated to handling over a period of several weeks, being trained to sit or lie quietly on an examination table with electrocardiographic chest leads and a rectal temperature probe in place. They were studied once weekly, in a crossover design, with each dog receiving iv ethanol (0.5 mL), THC (0.5 mg), or THC-HS (equivalent to 0.5 mg THC) in a random sequence. Heart rate was monitored for 2 hours following drug administration, then the dogs were returned to their cages. At various times up to 8 hours, body temperature was monitored by removing the animals from their cages, placing them on the examination table, and inserting the rectal probe. Data were analyzed by one-way ANOVA, repeated measures design, with a significance limit of $p < 0.05$.

2.3. Bioavailability of D9-THC from Suppositories Containing the Hemisuccinate Ester in Monkeys (13)

Four male cynomolgus monkeys were used in a randomized 4×4 crossover design with a two-week washout period between administrations. Animals were fasted overnight prior to treatment, and ketamine was used at 10 mg/kg intramuscularly to anesthetize the animals prior to testing. Four treatments were used: Δ^9-THC IV (0.5 mg/kg), Δ^9-THC -hemisuccinate IV (0.5 mg/kg equivalent), Δ^9-THC oral (10 mg/animal), and Δ^9-THC-hemisuccinate (10 mg equivalent in Witepsol H-15 suppositories). Blood samples were collected at 0, 5, 15, 30, 60, and 90 minutes and at 2, 3, 4, 6, 8, and 24 hours. Plasma from all blood samples was analyzed for Δ^9-THC and its carboxylic acid metabolite using gas chromatography/mass spectrometry (GC/MS).

2.4. Bioavailability of D9-THC from Suppositories Containing the Hemisuccinate Ester in Dogs (11)

The bioavailability of Δ^9-THC from suppositories containing the hemisuccinate ester was carried out in dogs trained to accept suppositories without anesthesia. Four dogs were used

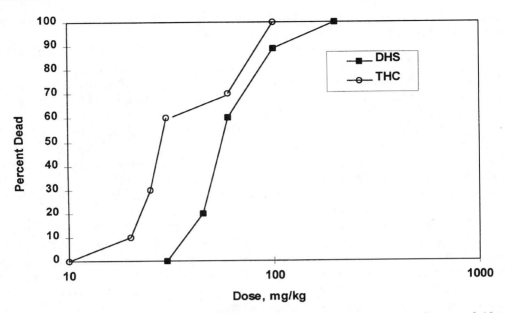

Fig. 1. Comparative toxicity of intravenously administered THC and THC-HS. Groups of 10 mice received various doses of either drug, and lethality wasc assessed at 4 hours after dosing.

and were administered Δ^9-THC-hemisuccinate (equivalent of 2 mg Δ^9-THC per dog) in 0.5 mL ethanol. Blood samples were collected at 0, 5, 10, 15, 30, 60, and 90 minutes, and then at 2, 4, and 6 hours. After a 2-week washout period the dogs were administered one suppository each containing the equivalent of 10 mg Δ^9-THC as the hemisuccinate ester in Witepsol H-15 base, and blood samples were collected at 0, .5, 1, 2, 4, 6, and 8 hours. Plasma from all blood samples was analyzed by GC/MS for Δ^9-THC.

RESULTS AND DISCUSSION

3.1. Comparison of the Toxicity and Pharmacology of THC and THC-HS in Mice

THC and THC-HS exhibited slightly but significantly different LD$_{50}$ values when given by the intravenous route in mice (Fig. 1). The THC-HS appeared to be less toxic at the lower doses, but the separation was less distinct as the dose was increased. THC demonstrated an LD$_{50}$ of 34.4 mg/kg (95% C.L., 27.1–45.6); for THC-HS, the LD$_{50}$ was 59.7 mg/kg (95% C.L., 49.6–75.4). The vehicle showed no measurable toxicity.

Pharmacological evaluations of the two drugs utilized the well established hypothermic and sedative effects of cannabinoids. THC and THC-HS elicited virtually identical hypothermic responses (Fig. 2), except for the highest dose (10 mg/kg) at which there was a slight but significant difference. The hypothermia proved to be the most sensitive of the pharmacological endpoints evaluated, with 1 mg/kg eliciting a drop in body temperature of 2°C. Vehicle administration did not have any effect on body temperature.

The potentiations of barbiturate-induced sleep were also virtually identical at doses from 0.3–3 mg/kg (Fig. 3), with sleep times increased up to 60 minutes or greater from the 2-minute sleep times with thiamylal alone. There was a significant difference between the two drugs in this parameter only at the highest dose.

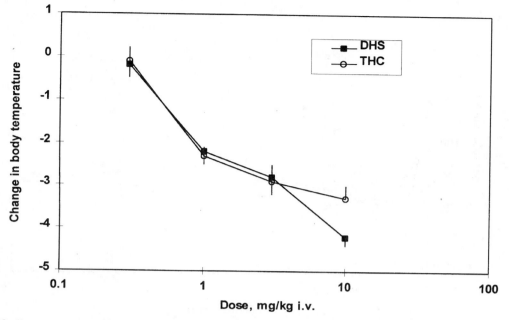

Fig. 2. Comparison of the hypothermic effects of THC and THC-HS after iv administration in mice. Body temperatures were recorded at 60 minutes after drug administration, n = 10.

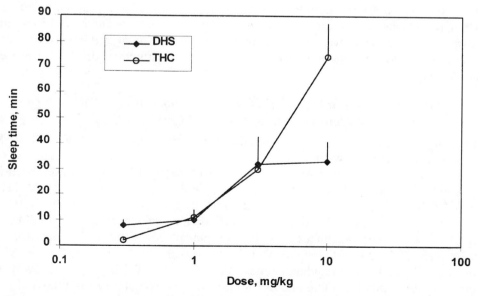

Fig. 3. Comparison of the effects of THC and THC-HS on potentiation of thiamylal-induced sleep in mice. Thirty minutes after iv administration of the drugs, thiamylal was administered intraperitoneally at 45 mg/kg.

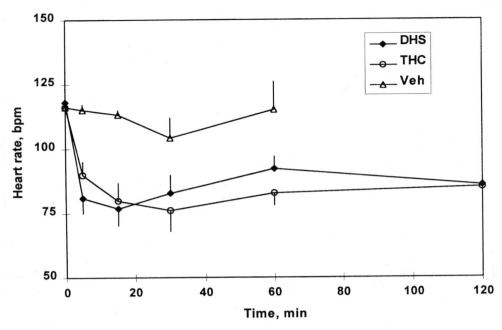

Fig. 4. Comparison of the heart rate responses to THC and THC-HS after iv administration of 0.5 mg THC equivalents in conscious dogs.

3.2. Comparison of the Pharmacological Effects of THC and THC-HS in Dogs

The two drugs were further evaluated in dogs for comparison of heart rate and body temperature responses to iv administration. Both THC and THC-HS at 0.5 mg-THC equivalents (approximately 0.05 mg/kg) iv caused an immediate, pronounced bradycardia, reducing heart rate by about 30 beats per minute (bpm) (Fig. 4). Peak responses occurred at 15–30 minutes after dosing. Some recovery was observed by the 1 hour time point, but the effects were still evident at 2 hours. No hypothermic effects were observed with either drug at this dose level (data not shown).

3.3. Bioavailability of Δ^9-THC from Suppositories Containing the Hemisuccinate Ester in Monkeys (13)

Figure 5 shows the plasma THC concentration versus time curves for THC iv, THC-HS iv, and THC-HS suppositories, whereas Fig. 6 shows the curves for the acid metabolite (THC-COOH). This study showed that Δ^9-THC was approximately 13% bioavailable from a suppository formulation using Witepsol H-15 as the lipophilic base. In addition, the Δ^9-THC and Δ^9-THC-COOH profiles following the i.v. administration of either Δ^9-THC or the Δ^9-THC-hemisuccinate were similar, indicating that Δ^9-THC-hemisuccinate behaves in blood as a true prodrug for Δ^9-THC. The area under the curves for plasma concentrations vs time for the two treatments were 925 ng/hr/mL for the Δ^9-THC IV versus 926.1 ng/h/mL for the Δ^9-THC-hemisuccinate IV, with mean residence times of 3.4 ± 1.8 and 2.7 ± 1.1, respectively. It was also noticed in this study that there was essentially zero bioavailability from the oral route.

The relatively low bioavailability from the suppositories in the monkeys might be because the monkeys were anesthetized, or caused by poor retention and leakage.

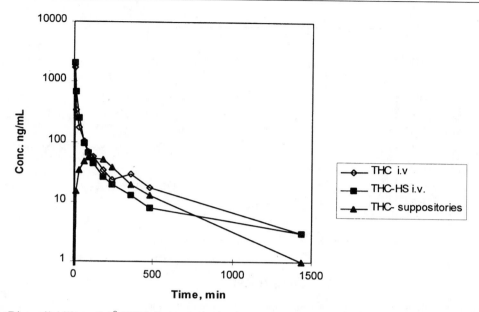

Fig. 5. Bioavailability of Δ^9-THC from suppositories containing the hemisuccinate ester in monkeys, mean plasma concentrations of Δ^9-THC following the administration of 0.5mg/kg THC iv, 0.5 mg/kg equivalent THC as THC-HS iv, and 10 mg equivalent THC as THC-HS suppositories.

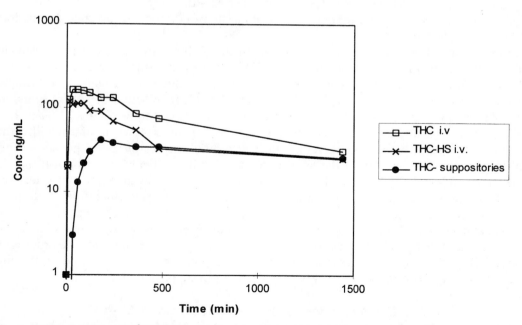

Fig. 6. Bioavailability of Δ^9-THC from suppositories containing the hemisuccinate ester in monkeys, mean plasma concentrations of 11-NOR- Δ^9-THC -9-COOH following the administration of 0.5 mg/kg THC iv, 0.5 mg/kg equivalent THC as THC-HS iv and 10 mg equivalent THC as THC-HS suppositories.

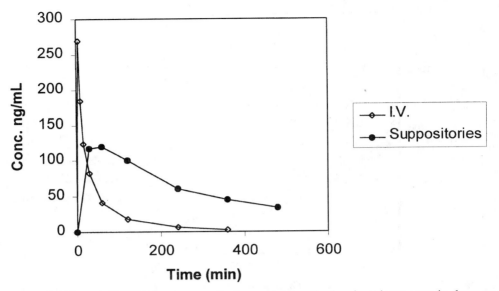

Fig. 7. Bioavailability of Δ^9-THC from suppositories containing the hemisuccinate ester in dogs: mean plasma concentration of Δ^9-THC following the administration of 2 mg equivalent THC as THC-HS iv and 10 mg equivalent THC as THC-HS in suppositories per dog.

3.4. Bioavailability of Δ^9-THC from Suppositories Containing the Hemisuccinate Ester In Dogs (11)

Figure 7 shows the plasma THC concentration versus time curves for the iv and suppository doses of THC-HS. The bioavailability from this experiment was calculated to be 67.3%, which shows promise of the ester derivative from a suppository base as a viable dosage form to deliver Δ^9-THC.

Subsequent to this first study in dogs, different lipophilic formulations were investigated for further improvement on the bioavailability. Witepsol H-15 (Huls america Systems, Bristol, PA) was compared with Hydrokote (Capital City Products, Columbus, OH), Kaomel (Durkee Foods, Rockville Center, NY), and Suppocire AIML (Gattefosse Corp., Elmsford, NY). The mean bioavailability from these four bases was found to be 60.9 + 21.9%, 51.9 + 30%, 57.8 + 14.3%, and 57.8 + 24.2%, respectively. There was no significant difference among the lipophilic bases, and, therefore, the selection of the best base for the dosage form will be based on the stability of the hemisuccinate ester in the final formulation. It must be added that, although hydrophilic bases provided enhanced bioavailability, the ester form hydrolyzed fairly quickly after preparation of the dosage form and, therefore, hydrophilic bases were unacceptable. In addition, other esters of Δ^9-THC such as the hemiglutarate, the N-formylalaninate, the N-methyl carbamate, and methoxyacetate esters were investigated and were found to either produce much lower bioavailability or did not behave as true prodrugs of Δ^9-THC. Therefore, the hemisuccinate ester in a lipophilic base was selected as the final dosage form for effecting bioavailability of Δ^9-THC from suppositories.

3.5. The Concentration of Δ^9-THC in Plasma in Dogs from Hemisuccinate Suppositories is Dose Dependent (11)

Dogs were administered either 5, 10, 20, or 40 mg equivalent of Δ^9-THC as the hemisuccinate in suppositories, and blood samples were collected over a period of 8 hours. Figure 8

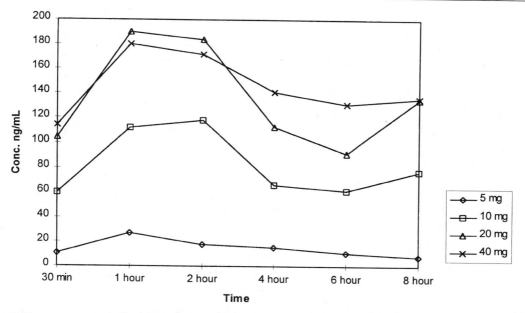

Fig. 8. Concentration of Δ^9-THC in plasma following administration of various does (5, 10, 20, or 40 mg THC as THC-HS) of the hemisuccinate ester in suppositories in dogs.

shows that the concentration of Δ^9-THC in plasma is dose-dependent at the different data points; however, there was no difference between the 20- and 40-mg doses in the first 2 hours postdosing, but a significant difference was observed beginning with the 4-hour period.

3.6. The Bioavailability of Δ^9-THC from Suppositories Containing the Hemisuccinate Ester is Demonstrated in Humans

Several studies were carried out to demonstrate the utility of suppositories containing the hemisuccinate ester in delivering Δ^9-THC in humans.

In the first study *(14)*, each of three subjects was administered a single suppository containing 11.8 mg of the hemisuccinate ester (equivalent to 9 mg Δ^9-THC). Plasma Δ^9-THC concentration as well as Δ^9-THC-COOH (major metabolite) were determined using GC/MS analysis, and the results are shown in Figs. 9 and 10. The data were compared with those obtained for the same subjects after oral administration of a 10 mg dose. The results of this study showed that the area under the curve for plasma THC following the suppository dosage form was more than 30-fold higher than that obtained after oral dosing. In addition, it was also shown that the plasma levels of THC were sustained in nature.

In the second study *(15)*, six subjects were each administered 2.5 mg Δ^9-THC as the hemisuccinate in suppositories twice daily for 3 days, and the blood levels as well as the effect of this dose on caloric intake was compared with those values obtained after oral ingestion of an equivalent dose of Δ^9-THC. Figure 11 shows the area under the curve data from this study over the 72-hour period. The results of this study show the enhanced blood levels of Δ^9-THC from the suppositories over the equivalent oral dose.

In the third study *(16)*, one subject was administered one suppository containing the equivalent of 5 mg Δ^9-THC as the hemisuccinate ester daily for 4 days, and another subject was administered the equivalent of 2.5 mg dose daily for 4 days. Again, plasma samples were

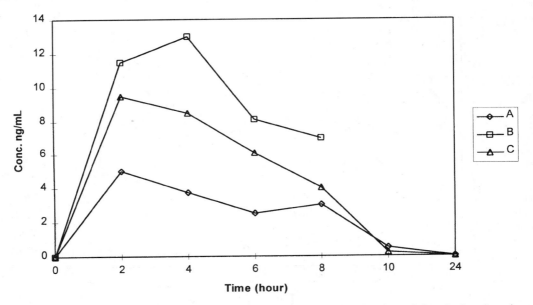

Fig. 9. Plasma levels of D^9-THC following administration of a suppository containing the hemisuccinate ester (equivalent to 9 mg Δ^9-THC) to three subjects (A–C).

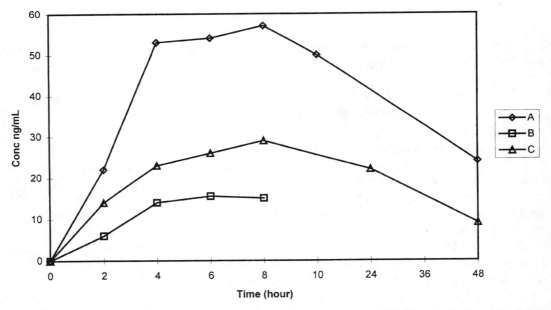

Fig. 10. Plasma levels of Δ^9-THC acid metabolite following administration of a suppository containing the hemisuccinate ester (equivalent to 9 mg Δ^9-THC) to three subjects (A–C).

analyzed from these subjects over the course of the study, and the results were consistent with those obtained in the previous studies.

These studies demonstrated that Δ^9-THC is consistently available through administration of suppositories containing the hemisuccinate ester. In all cases, as in the animal studies, the

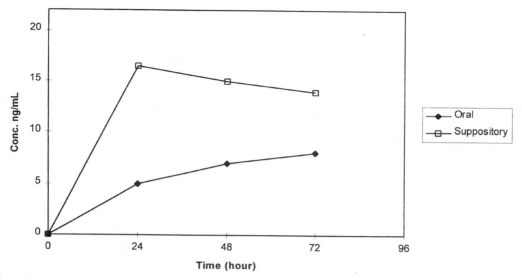

Fig. 11. AUC data for oral and suppository THC. Six subjects dosed twice daily with 2.5 mg Δ^9-THC orally or 2.5 mg equivalent THC as THC-HS in suppository dosage form.

blood levels of Δ^9-THC following suppository administration were of sustained duration, suggesting the feasibility of using a once- or twice-daily regimen in humans.

3.7. Preliminary Evidence of Efficacy of Δ^9-THC when Administered in Suppositories Containing the Hemisuccinate Ester

3.7.1. APPETITE STIMULATION

In one of the studies cited above *(15)*, the caloric intake of the subjects administered 2.5-mg doses of Δ^9-THC as the hemisuccinate suppositories was compared to the caloric intake after oral dosing (single and multiple dose) and after acute inhalation with the following conclusions:

1. The mean caloric intake during suppository treatment in the multiple-dose study was substantially greater than after oral dosing (4835 kcal vs 4390 kcal) over three days.
2. Mean caloric intake during suppository treatment was significantly higher in the single-dose study (3726 + 341 kcal) than oral dosing (2680 + 114 kcal, p = 0.026) or placebo (2542 + 232, p = 0.017).
3. Mean caloric intake during suppository treatment was substantially, although not statistically, higher compared to intake after inhalation in the multi-route study (2778 + 385, p = 0.084).

3.7.2. MANAGEMENT OF SPASTICITY

Brenneisen, et al. *(16)*, examined the effects of Δ^9-THC-HS suppositories on spasticity. Two subjects were used. Subject A, a 40-year-old male with multiple dystrophy with cervical myelopathy and progressive spastictetraparesis, was administered a 5-mg dose suppository. Subject B, a 64-year-old male with multiple sclerosis and light cervical myelopathy, was administered a 2.5 mg suppository dose. In addition to the collection of blood samples and analysis for Δ^9-THC and its acid metabolite as described above, the subjects were monitored for several neurological, psychological, and vegetative responses to the drug.

Whereas there was no change in mood, *miction* frequency, blood pressure, heart rate, or body temperature, there was an improved passive motility and walking ability for both subjects, with reduced rigidity for Subject A and no change in rigidity for Subject B. There was reduced or no pain with no need for analgesia in both subjects while under treatment with the suppositories. Whereas similar effects were achieved with oral Δ^9-THC, the required oral dose was 2–6 times higher than the suppository dose. A 15 mg oral dose of THC given to Subject B resulted in temporary exacerbation of the rigidity with deterioration of concentrating ability, and mood.

4. CONCLUSION

The data presented in this report showed that THC-HS behaves as a true prodrug for Δ^9-THC in the sense that it serves to effect systemic delivery of Δ^9-THC, without detectable systemic levels of the parent ester. This ester has the distinct advantage of providing substantial and consistent bioavailability from a suppository dosage form. This is exhibited by the almost identical biological effects following administration of either THC or THC-HS and the equivalent blood levels of THC following iv administration of either form of the drug. The suppository dosage form was developed to overcome problems associated with oral THC and exhibits effects similar to those following smoked THC, with the exception of avoiding the psychological effects associated with the initial surge of the drug following inhalation. The following are distinct advantages of the developed suppository dosage form:

1. It avoids the first-pass metabolism associated with oral dosing.
2. Plasma levels are shown to be dose-dependent in both animals and humans.
3. Absorption is efficient enough to rapidly achieve therapeutic blood levels.
4. The blood levels are sustained in duration allowing a once or twice-a-day dosing schedule.
5. The bioavailability is established in human subjects.
6. Suppositories are easily self-administered.
7. This dosage form is more suitable for patients suffering from nausea and vomiting.

REFERENCES

1. ElSohly, M. A., Harland, E., and Waller, C. W. (1984) Cannabinoids in glaucoma II: the effect of different cannabinoids on the intraocular pressure of the rabbit. *Curr. Eye Res.* **3(6)**, 841–850.
2. El-Mallakh, R. S. (1987) Marihuana and migraine. *Headache* **27(8)**, 442–443.
3. Volfe, Z., Dvilansky, A., and Nathan. I. (1985) Cannabinoids block release of serotonin from platelets induced by plasma from migraine patients. *Intl. Clin. Pharmacol. Res.* **5(4)**, 243–246.
4. Maurer, M., Henn, V., Dittrich, A., and Hofmann, A. (1990) Delta-9-tetrahydrocannabinol shows antispastic and analgesic effects in a single case double-blind trial. *Eur. Arch. Psychiatry Clin. Neurosci.,* **240 (1)**, 1–4.
5. Musty, R. E. (1984) Possible anxiolytic effects of cannabidiol, In: *The Cannabinoids: Chemical, Pharmacologic and Therapeutic Aspects.* (Agurell, S., Dewey, W. L., and Willette, R. E., eds.) Academic, Orlando, FL, pp. 795–813.
6. McLendon, D. M., Harris, R. T., and Maule, W. F. (1976) Suppression of the cardiac conditioned response by delta-9-tetrahydrocannabinol: a comparison with other drugs. *Psychopharmacology,* **50(2)**, 159–163.
7. Regelson, W., Butler, J. R., Schultz, J., Kirk, T., Peck, L., Green, M. L., and Zalis, M. O. (1976) *The Pharmacology of Marihuana,* vol.2, (Braude, M. C. and Szara, S.) Raven, New York, pp. 763–776.
8. Agurell, S., Halldin, M., Lindgren, J., Ohlsson, A., Widman, M., Gillespie, H., and Hollister, L. (1986) Pharmacokinetics and metabolism of delta-l-tetrahydrocannabinol and other cannabinoids with emphasis on man. *Pharmacol. Rev.* **38,** 21–43.
9. Wall, M. E., Sadler, B. M., Brine, D., Taylor, H., and Parez-Reyes, M. (1983) Metabolism, disposition, and kinetics of delta-9-tetrahydro-cannabinol in men and women. *Clin. Pharmacol. Ther.* **34,** 352–363.
10. Plasse, T. F., Gorter, R. W., Krasnow, S. H., Lane, M., Shepard, K. V., and Wadleigh, R. G. (1991) Recent clinical experience with Dronabinol. *Pharmacol. Biochem Behav.* **40,** 695–700.

11. ElSohly, M. A., Little, T. L., Hikal, A., Harland, E., Stanford, D. F., and Walker, L. (1991) Rectal bioavailability of delta-9-tetrahydrocannabinol from various esters. *Pharmacol. Biochem Behav.* **40,** 497–502.
12. Perlin, E., Smith, C. G., Nichols, A. J., Almirez, R., Flora, K. P. Craddock, J. C., Peck, C. C. (1985) Disposition and Bioavailability of various formulation of tetrahydrocannabinol in the rhesus monkey. *J. Pharm. Sci.* **74,** 171–174.
13. ElSohly M. A., Stanford, D. F., Harland, E. C., Hikal, A. H., Walker, L.A., Little, T. H., Jr., Rider, J. N., and Jones, A. B. Rectal bioavailability of delta-9-tetrahydrocannabinol from the hemisuccinate ester in monkeys. *J. Pharm. Sci.* **80,** 942–945.
14. Mattes, R. D., Shaw, L. M., Edling-Owens, J., Engelman, K., and ElSohly, M. A. (1993) Bypassing the first-pass effect for the therapeutic use of cannabinoids. *Pharmacol. Biochem. Behav.* **44(3),** 745–747.
15. Mattes, R. D., Engelman, K., Shaw, L. M., and ElSohly, M. A. (1994) Cannabinoids and appetite stimulation. *Pharmacol. Biochem. Behav.* **49(1),** 187–195.
16. Brenneisen, R., Egli, A., ElSohly, M. A., Henn, V., and Speiss, Y. (1996) The effect of orally and rectally administered delta-9-tetrahydrocannabinol on spasticity: a pilot study with 2 patients. *Intl. J. Clin. Pharmacol. Therap.* **34(10),** 446–452.

6 Composition and Stability of a Standard Marihuana Cigarette

Brian F. Thomas, Victor L. Parker,
Lillian W. Caddell, Larry V. Jones,
Surinder K. Sabharwal, Andy I. McDaniel,
Alison R. Keimowitz, Nicole M. Scheffler,
E. Dale Hart, John M. Mitchell,
and Kenneth H. Davis, Jr.

The recorded use of *Cannabis* dates back well over 3000 years, with use as an intoxicant and as a medicinal formulation contributing to its considerable historical presence. Despite the recognition and use of *Cannabis* as a medicinal natural product by many cultures, its use in Western medicine began to decrease early in this century. With the passing of the Marihuana Tax Act of 1937, its use was effectively prohibited and its cultivation was disallowed in the United States. In 1942, the U.S. Pharmacopeia removed marihuana from its listings. In the 1960s, however, whereas the medicinal and industrial use of marihuana continued to decrease in the United States, the use of marihuana as an illegal intoxicant increased dramatically. By the early 1990s, the only legal therapeutic application of *Cannabis* in the United States was to a small number of individuals (less than 20) who still received marihuana through a compassionate use program that was terminated in 1992. So it was remarkable when, despite numerous efforts to discourage marihuana use in the United States, grassroots organizations in Arizona and California were able to pass proposals to legalize the prescription and use of medicinal marihuana in 1997.

The United States government has been controlling the distribution of marihuana for medicine and research since 1975 when the Investigational New Drug Compassionate Access Program was established, enabling some patients to receive medicinal marihuana from the government. Despite the fact that, in 1992, the Bush administration closed the program to all new applicants, and, in 1994, the Clinton administration decided against reopening the program, it remains in operation for the eight surviving individuals with previously approved use. To control the manufacture and distribution of marihuana, the government provided

From: *Marihuana and Medicine*
Edited by: G. G. Nahas et al. © Humana Press Inc., Totowa, NJ

funding through the National Institutes of Health for a central facility for the controlled growth of marihuana, and a facility to process the plant material and manufacture and distribute marihuana cigarettes and cannabinoid formulations. Thus, for the last 23 years, Research Triangle Institute (RTI) has been subcontracted by the National Institute on Drug Abuse (NIDA) to serve as a central facility for the manufacture and distribution of standardized marihuana cigarettes and cannabinoid preparations. This work effort involves the production of marihuana cigarettes of varying potencies (including placebo marihuana cigarettes), and their characterization, storage, and distribution. Whereas the majority of their distribution has been to a relatively small number of individuals receiving marihuana cigarettes through the Compassionate Access Act, government-approved research programs are also authorized to receive this material.

The cigarette manufacturing procedures that have been developed at RTI have been used to prepare over 1.3 million cigarettes of varying potencies. The equipment required for this process is contained within a central facility that was specifically built for this purpose and includes large-capacity mixers, an apparatus used to remove unwanted material (e.g., seeds and stems) from the bulk material received from the University of Mississippi, and a cigarette-rolling machine. The AMF cigarette-making machine and the Bonsack feeder have been highly modified to allow for the smooth handling of a variety of *Cannabis* potencies, including the resinous and sticky high potency plant material. At peak operation, this equipment can produce approximately 800 cigarettes per minute and allows the preparation of standardized marihuana cigarettes.

Typically, production runs involve over 100 kg of *Cannabis* plant material. This material is usually grown from a Mexican seed stock at the University of Mississippi and provided to RTI in a dried and somewhat manicured condition (e.g., large stems and the primary stalk of the plants have been removed). Prior to processing this material, the material is sampled for cannabinoid content so that selective blending of various *Cannabis* batches can be used to control the final potency of the cigarettes. The plant material is sprayed with the necessary amount of distilled water in a large-capacity mixer to bring the moisture content of the plant material, after equilibration, to approximately 18%. This humidified plant material is thus made more suitable for the next stage of the manufacturing process, which involves an apparatus that has been custom-made to remove fine particles, stems, seeds, and foreign matter. After the plant material is humidified, cleaned, and homogenized, it is rolled in paper to a diameter of approximately 8.5 mm and cut to a length of approximately 85 mm, yielding individual cigarettes weighing approximately 0.8–1.0 g each. A typical flow diagram of the plant material as it undergoes the processing and rolling procedures is provided in Fig. 1. The finished cigarettes are allowed to dry to a moisture content that is less favorable for mold, mildew, or microorganism growth (< 13% humidity). Because of the need to lower the humidity for storage, these cigarettes are often rehumidified immediately prior to use to provide a less harsh smoke and a lower burning temperature. Finally, the finished cigarettes are packaged by weight to contain 300 cigarettes per can, sealed with freezer tape, labeled with permanent labels, encased in clear plastic bags, and stored in freezers.

During the manufacturing process, clean room apparel is used to minimize exposure of personnel as well as contamination of the plant material. We are in the process of conducting exposure studies to determine the extent of the dermal and inhalation exposure to personnel during the humidification, homogenization, and manicuring procedures. The manufacturing process is typically monitored by an RTI quality-assurance officer to ensure that standard operating procedures are adhered to and that adequate records are kept. All instruments and equipment are calibrated prior to, during, and after a manufacturing run so that cigarettes of

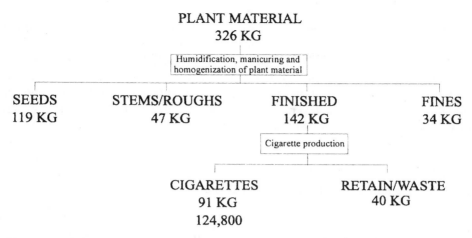

Fig. 1. Flowchart of marihuana plant material as it is formulated into cigarettes.

consistent moisture content, weight, particle size, length, diameter, paper, and glue type are obtained.

Once the marihuana cigarettes are produced, whether they are to be used as research products in laboratory animals or as human dosage formulations, they require additional quality assurance procedures and analytical methods to identify and monitor the concentration and stability of the active constituents. Δ^9-Tetrahydrocannabinol (Δ^9-THC), and its congeners, particularly the carboxylic acid forms that are pyrolyzed to give Δ^9-THC during smoking, are primary compounds of interest to pharmacologists because of their correlation to psychoactivity in man. However, there are cannabigerols, cannabidiols, cannabichromenes, Δ^8s and side-chain analogs of endogenous cannabinoids that are present in differing concentrations in different varieties of *Cannabis* that may also interact with the receptors for cannabinoid compounds. At the present time, there are well over 50 natural constituents of *Cannabis* that have been identified as cannabinoids based on their molecular structure (i.e., terpenophenols, for review see ref. *1*). This diversity in the constituents of *Cannabis* suggests that it is not sufficient to equate the pharmacological activity of marihuana to the presence of one cannabinoid, specifically, Δ^9-THC, and that the profile of cannabinoid compounds in marihuana more accurately describes its potency and pharmacological activity.

A widely used analytical procedure for the qualitative and quantitative analysis of *Cannabis* constituents is gas chromatography, particularly when combined with an electron-impact ionization mass spectrometer *(2–4)*. This approach allows for comparisons to be made between components and spectral databases for peak identification purposes. Peak purity can be assessed using extracted ion-current profiles and selected ion monitoring can be used for trace analysis. Cannabinoids can be derivatized with a number of reagents that provide further characterization of the complex mixture of components present in *Cannabis*. A specific example of this is the use of trimethylsilyl-derivative extracts to separate and quantitate some carboxylic acid forms, which as discussed previously, thermally decompose to form Δ^9-THC if not gas chromatographed as the TMS derivatives.

A concentrated ethanolic extract of *Cannabis*, prepared by Soxhlet extraction for 8 hours, can be used to characterize the principal cannabinoids contained within marihuana cigarettes or plant material. These extracts can be chromatographed on a wide variety of analytical columns. However, when the gas chromatograph (GC) is interfaced with a mass spectrometer, capillary columns are frequently used because of their high resolution and low helium flow rates. Typical total ion-current profiles obtained with plant material of relatively high Δ^9-THC content (< 3.0 %) are shown in Fig. 2. One can see from this figure that there is consistency in the profile of primary components of each chromatogram, which might be expected when all of the material was grown at the same location, using the same seed, and harvested at the same time. However, close inspection of the chromatograms also shows the variability in these components because of individual plant variations and variations in the extraction and recovery of minor components.

The predominant peak in these profiles is that of Δ^9-THC, as indicated by the mass spectra recorded during its elution (Fig. 3). Other peaks of interest in these chromatograms are also identifiable using mass spectral matching, and include cannabidiol and cannabinol. These compounds' concentrations may vary significantly in marihuana samples, and Carlini and colleagues (5) reported that marihuana containing varying levels of these compounds produced markedly different effects. Karniol and Carlini (6,7) further suggested that increasing the amount of CBD or CBN in relation to THC led to potentiation of some of the effects of Δ^9-THC and antagonism of others. Therefore, we have chosen to monitor the concentration of these compounds in the marihuana cigarettes and other *Cannabis* preparations maintained within the NIDA inventory. The analytical data is provided in a data sheet that is included with any shipment of these products, along with instructions for their proper storage and rehumidification. This information is also filed with NIDA for inclusion within their drug master file for marihuana cigarettes.

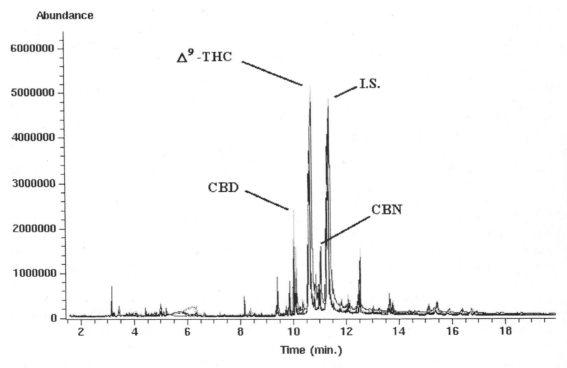

Fig. 2. Overlay of six total-ion chromatograms recorded for ethanolic extracts (8 hour Soxhlet extraction) of samples obtained from six barrels of Mexican plant material. The peak labeled I.S. is the internal standard (androst-4-ene-3,17-dione) used for quantitation when flame-ionization detection is used. Other abreviations used are CBD, cannabidiol; and CBN, cannabinol.

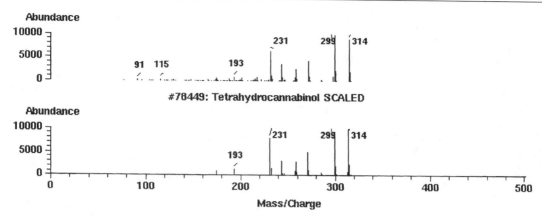

Fig. 3. Comparison of the mass spectrum recorded for the primary chromatographic peak (*see* Fig. 2, peak labeled Δ^9-THC) in an ethanolic extract of Mexican marihuana (top) to the Wiley mass spectral databases entry #78449, Tetrahydrocannabinol (bottom). Note the library spectrum has been filtered to contain only 20 ions.

It is well-documented that the constituents of *Cannabis* can undergo chemical rearrangements (e.g., conversion of Δ^9-THC to Δ^8-THC) and decomposition (e.g., conversion of Δ^9-THC to CBN) when exposed to certain environments, including prolonged exposure to heat, oxygen, and light *(1,8)*. If these chemical changes are not avoided through the proper storage and handling of the plant material, the content of Δ^9-THC can fall to levels where some pharmacological activity is lost. Thus, it is important that stability studies monitor a *Cannabis* formulation's principal active constituents. We have maintained retainer samples of *Cannabis* cigarettes dating back over 20 years under various storage conditions in order to characterize the long term stability of these dosage formulations. For these studies, we typically quantitate each sample for its CBN, CBD and Δ^9-THC, and frequently use TMS-derivatization to differentiate between the carboxylic acid forms and the non-carboxylated species. As others have reported (*see* ref. *9*), we have found that the decomposition of *Cannabis* occurs relatively slowly, particularly when stored at temperatures below 0°C (Fig. 4). Indeed, when stored at -18°C, we found only a modest decrease in the Δ^9-THC content (approx 33% decrease from the initial value) in high potency cigarettes over a 16 year period.

Smoking *Cannabis* cigarettes involves risks associated with the tars produced in the combustion process. These tars decrease the efficiency of macrophages in the lung and also decrease airway conductance *(10,11)*. In addition, marihuana cigarettes can harbor inhalable pathogenic bacteria and fungi *(12–15)*. Furthermore, *Cannabis* smoke is harmful to the bronchial mucosa and may promote lung cancer and chronic bronchitis *(11)*. However, different mechanisms of inhalation (e.g., water pipes) and filtration devices may reduce lung injury yet allow adequate volatilization and transfer of active cannabinoids *(16)* and cigarette sterilization may reduce the risk of infection *(13)*. Clearly, there remain many important questions regarding the therapeutic utility of a *Cannabis* cigarette dosage form that must be placed into context with the existence of specific hazards associated with the inhalation of smoke from plant materials. It should also be noted that in addition to the naturally occurring cannabinoid constituents, extremely potent synthetic cannabinoid agonists and antagonists of a variety of structural classes have now been identified. Thus, with the pharmacological targets known, and a wide variety of cannabinoid structural classes to work with, there is reason to believe that therapeutic *Cannabis* preparations or cannabinoid formulations in addition to Marinol will be identified and successfully marketed.

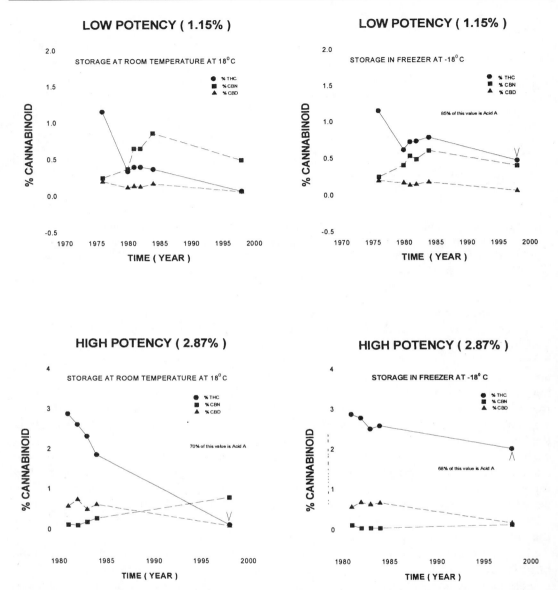

Fig. 4. Stability studies of two batches of marihuana cigarettes, a low-potency and a high-potency formulation, when stored in the dark at room temperature and when stored in the dark at −18°C.

REFERENCES

1. Turner, C. E., Hadley, K. W., Fetterman, P. S., Doorenbos, N. J., Quimby, M. W., and Waller, C. (1973) Constituents of *Cannabis sativa* L. IV: stability of cannabinoids in stored plant material. *J. Pharm. Sci.* **62,** 1601–1605.
2. Farmilo and Lerner (1963)
3. Lerner and Zeffert (1968)
4. Davis, K. H., Jr., Martin, N. H., Pitt, C. G., Wildes, J. W., and Wall, M. E. (1970) The preparation and analysis of enriched and pure cannabinoids from marihuana and hashish. *Lloydia* **33,** 453–460.
5. Carlini, E. A., Santos, M., Claussen, U., Bieniek, D., and Korte, F. (1970) Structure-activity relation of four tetrahydocannabinols and the pharmacological activity of five semipurified extracts of *Cannabis* sativa. *Psychopharmacology* **18,** 82–93.

6. Karniol, I. G. and Carlini, E. A. (1973) Pharmacological interaction between cannabidiol and Δ^9- tetrahydrocannabinol. *Psychopharmacology.*. **33**: 53–70.
7. Karniol, I. G. and Carlini, E. A. (1973) Comparative study between semipurified extracts of marihuana obtained in Fermany and Brazil. Possible interference of cannabidiol and/or canabinol on the effect of D9-trans-tetrahydrocannabinol. *Cienc. Cult.* **25**, 749–751.
8. Fairbairn, J. W., Liebmann, J. A., and Rowan, M. G. (1976) The stability of *Cannabis* and its preparations on storage. *J. Pharm. Pharmac.* **28**, 1–7.
9. Harvey (1990)
10. Sherman et al. (1991)
11. Hollister (1986)
12. Chusid, M. J., Gelfand, J. A., Nutter, C., and Fauci, A. S. (1975) Pulmonary aspergillosis, inhalation of contaminated marihuana smoke, chrnic granulomatous disease. *Ann. Int. Med.* **82**, 682–682.
13. Ungerleider, J. T., Andrysiak, T., Tashkin, D. P., and Gale, R. P. (1982) Contamination of marihuana cigarettes with pathogenic bacteria – possible source of infection in cancer patients. *Cancer Treat. Lett.* **66**, 589–592.
14. Kagen, S. L., Kurup, V. P., Sohnle, P. G., and Fink, J. N.(1983) Marihuana smoking and fungal sensitizatioin. *J. Allergy Clin. Immunol.* **71**, 389–393.
15. Karup, V. P., Resnick, A., Kagen, S. L., Cohen, S. H., and Fink, J. N. (1983) Allergenic fungi and actinomycetes in smoking materials and their health implications. *Mycopathologia* **82**, 61–64.
16. Perez-Reyes, M. (1990) Marihuana smoking: factors that influence the bioavailability of tetrahydrocannabinol, In: (Chiang, N.C. and Hawks R., eds.), *Research Findings on Smoking of Abused Substances,* NIDA Research Monograph vol. 99, pp. 42–61.

7

Study Design Considerations in Clinical Trials with Marihuana

Reese T. Jones

Abstract

Political and social pressures exist to make smoked marihuana available for treatment of a variety of seemingly unrelated medical disorders. Efficacy of smoked marihuana for any disorder remains unproven by scientifically valid techniques. Study design considerations for clinical trials with marihuana are considered.

Marihuana is a plant with great variability. Although the clinical pharmacology of THC is well studied, relatively little medication development efforts have been devoted to marihuana itself. Control of delivered cannabinoid dose from smoked marihuana will be difficult. Protocols that require multiple dose levels and placebos will present problems. The availability of illicit marihuana may pose compliance problems in controlled trials, particularly with patients assigned to low-dose or placebo conditions. Some patients may consider the diversity of marihuana effects, particularly cognitive and cardiovascular effects, as adverse or unwanted. Decisions about the ultimate usefulness of marihuana should be based on relative benefits and risks. The risks of smoked marihuana for some medical applications may be greater than the risks posed by typical nonmedical use because of more frequent and regular dosing. Marihuana's utility as a medicine should be determined by generally accepted principles guiding medication development. Standards for determining the efficacy and safety of marihuana as a therapeutic agent should be equivalent to those used in other medication trials. Problematic study design issues are a consequence of the need to evaluate the therapeutic efficacy and safety of a smoked, crude natural product. Clinical trials with marihuana will be difficult, and fairly expensive to execute, but not impossible.

1. INTRODUCTION

I will mostly consider clinical trial design issues relevant to the use of smoked marihuama. Clinical trials with isolated cannabinoids administered in pills or capsules have more traditional and, in general, less complicated design considerations. For most medications, drug

From: *Marihuana and Medicine*
Edited by: G. G. Nahas et al.   © Humana Press Inc., Totowa, NJ

delivery by routes other than cigarette smoking are preferable. However, there is great social and political pressure to evaluate medical applications of smoked marihuana itself, not just the utility of individual cannabinoids in marihuana (1). If clinical researchers and funding agencies respond to social pressures, many clinical trials with marihuana will include smoked marihuana as a drug delivery system.

2. PROBLEMS WITH USE OF NATURAL PRODUCTS FOR PHARMACOTHERAPY

When planning or evaluating clinical trials of smoked marihuana, it is important to keep mind that marihuana is not a single drug (2–4). Marihuana comes from the plant *Cannabis sativa*. It is a mixture of leaves and flowers: a natural product. The clinical pharmacology of any natural product is complicated, particularly when smoked. Smoking marihuana delivers a variable mix of hundreds of pharmacologically active substances to the lungs (2,3). Consider the pharmacology and toxicology of smoked tobacco and nicotine. Marihuana pharmacology is no less complex. Although the inherently variable potency of *Cannabis* plant material can be decreased and even standardized to some extent by cultivation and processing under controlled conditions, problems remain if the plant material is to be used for medical treatments (2).

Much of the current debate about the utility of marihuana as a medicine arises from claims that smoked marihuana offers significant advantages over oral doses of Δ^9-tetrahydrocannabinol (THC) or other isolated and standardized cannabinoids for treating an enormous variety of seemingly unrelated diseases and medical conditions (5,6). Unfortunately, no questions have been definitively answered about the efficacy of smoked marihuana in any disorder using scientifically valid techniques. At this time adequate information remains to be established as to optimal therapeutic dose and dose frequency, side effects, safety, and patient acceptability when smoked marihuana is used as a medicine. In 1982 an extensive Institute of Medicine (IOM) review of marihuana pharmacology suggested more research is needed (7). Another million-dollar IOM review that is more focused on medical applications is in progress. My guess is that report, when issued early in 1999, will conclude that more research is needed.

3. WHY MIGHT SMOKED MARIHUANA BE USEFUL? CANNABINOID CONTENT OR PHARMACOKINETICS?

Much is known about the pharmacology of THC. However demonstration that the pharmacology of a marihuana cigarette is *entirely* determined by the amount of THC it contains remains elusive. Proponents of marihuana's therapeutic applications emphasize possible, even plausible, but not always well-documented differences between the effects of the crude marihuana plant and THC (5,6). Proponents argue that availability of THC or other cannabinoids in oral-dose formulations do not satisfy the need to evaluate the medical utility of marihuana itself (8). Although it is well established that THC is the principal *psychoactive* component of cannabis plant material (3), other cannabinoids in marihuana, for example cannabidiol (CBD), also have pharmacologic activity (9,10) and might have useful therapeutic properties. In addition, it is well established that the pharmacokinetics of THC from smoked marihuana differ substantially from oral THC (3). It is argued the pharmacokinetics of smoked marihuana offers therapeutic advantages over other routes (8).

4. HOW TO SPECIFY THE DOSE OF MARIHUANA?

When researching or prescribing a medication, it is useful to be able to specify the dose. Some would say it is essential. Unfortunately, a problem with smoked marihuana, as with any smoked drug, is difficulty in controlling or measuring dose. With tobacco and nicotine this problem is well characterized. Cigarettes smoked per day or number of puffs per cigarette do not adequately specify nicotine dose actually absorbed (11,12). Even well-motivated tobacco smokers in research studies individually adjust their delivered nicotine dose to suit their own needs, mostly by smoking behaviors not under volitional control (13). The same is true for marihuana smoking (14).

Whether a one-gram marihuana cigarette contains 2 or 8% THC, the cigarette will generally be smoked so as to deliver the smoker's desired cannabinoid dose, not necessarily the dose specified by a research protocol. By varying puff and inhalation volume and other aspects of smoking behavior, smokers adjust their dose of cannabinoids (14). Inexperienced smokers tend to overdose or underdose. Smoking behavior is difficult to control in a laboratory. Control is probably impossible in an outpatient clinical trial. Inexperienced smokers in a clinical trial will have to be taught how to smoke. Acquired tolerance will make for changes in self-administered dose over the course of a study. If cannabinoid dose is considered important, for example in a protocol that specifies multiple dose levels, absorbed dose of cannabinoids will have to be verified, ideally in plasma or by metabolites in urine; not a simple undertaking. THC is a very potent drug and small differences in dose may be important.

5. WHAT SHOULD BE MEASURED TO CHARACTERIZE DOSE?

For treatment trials what in marihuana should be the compound(s) of greatest interest; THC, CBD, cannabinol (CBN), or something else in marihuana? In past research THC alone has been the primary index of dose. In fact most of what is known about the pharmacology of marihuana is based more on studies of the pharmacology of THC than on the pharmacology of marihuana. However, for treating some disorders, CBD doses maybe more relevant than THC. CBD does not have THC's dramatic psychoactive and cardiovascular effects but it is an anticonvulsant (10) and drug-metabolizing-enzyme inducer (15). Anticonvulsants without prominent psychoactive effects are now popular "mood stabilizers" or "regulators" and are used in the treatment of pain disorders suggesting that CBD's therapeutic utility might be reconsidered.

6. GENERAL STUDY DESIGN ISSUES

The essentials of any clinical study with a psychopharmacologic agent are well-established. A specific diagnosis and determination of severity of the disorder being treated may seem so obvious as to hardly warrant mention. But for many of the conditions mentioned as appropriate for treatment with marihuana, diagnosis is sometimes imprecise and severity varies, for example, headache, nausea, depression, pain, appetite disorders, epilepsy, movement disorders, multiple sclerosis, and tremor.

As in any clinical trial, random assignment and some control over concurrent pharmacologic and nonpharmacologic therapies is needed. Well-defined, ideally objective, outcome measures are important. Particularly if subjective assessments or self-reports are involved, they should be made under double-blind conditions. Unfortunately, the use of smoked plant material and the nature of smoking makes the use of placebo groups or high- vs low-dose designs more problematic than with other drug delivery routes.

Adequate informed consent is necessary. However, one consequence of marihuana's history and controversy as an illicit drug is that a balanced description and discussion of risks versus benefits in a clinical trial is more challenging than would be the case with a new, relatively unknown, pharmaceutical just appearing on the research scene. Marihuana's history creates a risk of investigators to either overemphasize or underemphasize certain risks and benefits.

Research questions asked of clinical trials should be presented as testable hypotheses. In occasional studies, the basic question might be does smoked marihuana have greater efficacy than no pharmacologic treatment? However with most disorders, more relevant questions will be whether smoked marihuana offers any significant advantages over other, safer cannabinoid dosage forms or other pharmacotherapies or does smoked marihuana have additive therapeutic effects when combined with standard therapies? Hypotheses might also address relative benefits for patients already found unresponsive to standard therapies or relative benefits for marihuana-experienced patients as compared to patients who have had little or no prior experience with marihuana.

7. RISKS

Decisions about the ultimate usefulness of any medication are based on determination of relative benefits and risks. Decisions about marihuana's utility as a medicine should follow this generally accepted principle. Whatever its benefits may turn out to be, many of marihuana's risks are already well established, particularly risks of smoking marihuana.

When treating disorders like glaucoma or wasting, are marihuana's expected perceptual and cognitive alterations to be considered a risk or a benefit? Cognitive effects that a marihuana-dependent user seeks in a nonmedical situation would, if experienced by many patients in a clinical trial, be considered an adverse psychological effect. Obtaining informed consent might be a lengthy procedure if all the risks described in National Institute on Drug Abuse warnings about the hazards of marihuana use are fully addressed (16,17). If those risks are downplayed in treatment trials, is a prospective research patient fully informed? People will disagree.

The special risks of smoked marihuana described in other chapters must be considered. For the treatment of many medical disorders, much more frequent and prolonged dosing will be likely than is the norm for most nonmedical marihuana use. Thus not only immediate adverse effects but also long-term risks for patients with chronic diseases may be greater.

Age, immune status, and concomitant illnesses must be considered in the determination of risks. A possibility that frequent and prolonged marihuana use might lead to clinically significant impairments of immune-system function exists. Appropriate studies should be part of any marihuana medication development research, particularly when patients with compromised immune systems will be treated with marihuana (18).

Development of inhalation devices or dosage forms for pulmonary delivery of cannabinoids free of dangerous combustion byproducts would be useful. However cannabinoid chemistry, particularly water insolubility, makes it unlikely this goal will be accomplished quickly. The tobacco industry's vast resources have so far failed to provide a satisfactory smoke-free inhaled nicotine delivery system. If adequate cannabinoid delivery from ground marihuana administered in baked goods or by sublingual ethanol tinctures of plant extracts was possible, then many design considerations including risks of smoking would be simpler. Cannabis tinctures were used in medicine a 100 years ago, but have not been well researched.

Risks will vary with the disease and the patient populations. For example, the use of relatively few smoked doses over a relatively short time (days or weeks) in the management of nausea associated with chemotherapy presents less potential risk than the use of marihuana for treating glaucoma, epilepsy, spastic motor disease or chronic pain. For treating some disorders, four to eight cigarettes daily might be required for many years. Immune-suppressant effects associated with the treatment of conditions where patients are already immune-compromised might present more risk than with other patients.

As with many other psychoactive drugs, the risks of adverse behavioral or cardiovascular events are greater early in a clinical trial and would likely decrease as tolerance is acquired. Thus, for some clinical trials, particularly those requiring higher doses, marihuana-experienced individuals with some degree of acquired tolerance might be at less risk of behavioral toxicity than would marihuana-naive individuals entered into the same clinical trial.

8. DRUG INTERACTIONS

Many prospective patients are likely to be using other treatment drugs when they enter a marihuana trial. THC and CBD inhibit the metabolism of drugs metabolized by hepatic mixed-function oxidase enzymes (15,19,20). Absorption may be decreased because of changes in intestinal motility (21). THC is highly bound to plasma proteins, so interactions from competition for binding sites are likely (22). Drug interactions can also occur at a functional (neural) level (23). Recent or concurrent THC or CBD exposure alters the pharmacokinetics or effects of ethanol, barbiturates, nicotine, amphetamines, cocaine, phencyclidine, opiates, atropine, and clomipramine (7). Most past marihuana research has been with healthy volunteers not taking other prescribed drugs. Adequate drug interaction information will be needed before beginning trials with patients on concurrent therapies.

9. PATIENT SELECTION

The patients studied, particularly inclusion/exclusion criteria, will alter perceived benefits from marihuana and the profile of adverse effects. Selection alternatives include all patients who present with the disorder of interest or subsets of patients:

1. Nonresponders or incomplete responders to existing therapies.
2. Marihuana-experienced patients selected from uncontrolled trial patients who responded to marihuana.
3. Naive versus experienced marihuana smokers who have not already tried self-medication for their disorder.

Patients thought to be responsive to marihuana from an open uncontrolled trial, i.e., "enrichment designs," could be withdrawn from their own marihuana use and assigned to experimental marihuana or other study drugs or control groups and evaluated in a prospective study. Of course it would be difficult to generalize results to a different or larger population. An important consideration is that any marihuana-experienced patients in a protocol who find themselves randomly assigned to a less-than-adequate experimental treatment or dose would be more likely to revert to self-administration of illicit marihuana than would patients who have never used marihuana.

10. EXCLUSIONS

What exclusions or precautions might be in a future *Physician's Desk Reference* entry for smoked marihuana? Precautions listed on a Marinol package insert mention pregnancy, mental illness, cardiac disease, concurrent medications, drug abuse or dependence, risky occupations, and elderly people. Unfortunately, almost everything we know about marihuana pharmacology from controlled clinical studies is mainly from healthy male volunteers under the age of 30 given one or two doses in a laboratory. Pharmacokinetics and cardiovascular toxicity in elderly patients is completely unstudied.

Persons who smoke marihuana and have cardiovascular diseases, respiratory diseases, and schizophrenia, probably have increased risk of precipitating or worsening symptoms of their diseases, concluded a recent Australian government sponsored literature review *(24)*. People who are or have been dependent upon alcohol or other drugs, may have an increased risk of developing dependence on cannabis.

Choice of outcome measures for evaluation of potential efficacy should include objective clinically relevant measures whenever possible. For example the number of vomiting episodes associated with chemotherapy, intraocular pressure in glaucoma trials, body weight and changes in body composition in AIDS-wasting syndrome studies. Unfortunately, many disorders said to respond to marihuana therapy offer less than objective endpoints.

11. CONCLUSIONS

There is political pressure to fast-track marihuana because it is allegedly needed for treatment of "life-threatening" diseases. Standards for determining the efficacy and safety of marihuana as a therapeutic agent should be equivalent to those used in other medication trials. Problematic study-design issues are a consequence of the need to evaluate the therapeutic efficacy and safety of a smoked crude natural product. Control of dose and the diversity of marihuana's multisystem effects will pose problems in large-scale clinical trials. Clinical trials with smoked marihuana will be difficult, will likely be expensive, but will not be impossible.

REFERENCES

 1. United States. Congress. Senate. Committee on the Judiciary. (1997) Prescription for addiction? The Arizona and California medical drug use initiatives: hearing before the Committee on the Judiciary, United States Senate, One Hundred Fourth Congress, second session, on examining the newly adopted initiatives that modify Arizona and California law by decriminalizing drug use in some circumstances, December 2, 1996. United States Government Printing Office, Washington, DC.
 2. Graham, J. D. P. (1976) *Cannabis and Health*, Academic, New York.
 3. Agurell, S., Dewey, W. L., and Willette, R. E. (1984) *The Cannabinoids: Chemical, Pharmacologic, and Therapeutic Aspects*. Academic, New York.
 4. Mechoulam, R. and Burstein, S. H. (1973) *Marihuana: Chemistry, Pharmacology, Metabolism and Clinical Effects*. Academic Press, New York.
 5. Grinspoon L, and Bakalar JB. (1997) *Marihuana: the Forbidden Medicine*. Yale University Press, New Haven.
 6. Rosenthal E, Mikuriya TH, and Gieringer DH. (1997) *Marijuana Medical Handbook*: *A Guide to Therapeutic Use*. Quick American Archives, Oakland, CA.
 7. Institute of Medicine (U.S.) (1982) Division of Health Sciences Policy. Marijuana and health: report of a study. National Academy Press, Washington, D.C.
 8. Zimmer LE and Morgan JP. (1997) *Marijuana Myths, Marihuana Facts: A Review of the Scientific Evidence*. Lindesmith Center, New York.
 9. Mechoulam, R. and Carlini, EA. Toward drugs derived from cannabis. *Naturwissenschaften* **65(4)**, 174–179.
10. Turkanis, S. A., Cely, W., Olsen, D. M., and Karler, R. (1974) Anticonvulsant properties of cannabidiol. *Research Communications in Chemical Pathology and Pharmacology* **8(2)**, 231–246.
11. Benowitz, N. L. and Jacob, P. (1984) Daily intake of nicotine during cigarette smoking. *Clin. Pharmacol. Therap.* **35(4)**, 499–504.
12. Herning, R. I., Jones, R. T., Benowitz, N. L., and Mines, A. H. (1983) How a cigarette is smoked determines blood nicotine levels. *Clin. Pharmacol. Therap.* **33(1)**, 84–90.
13. Benowitz, N. L. and Jacob, P. (1984) Nicotine and carbon monoxide intake from high- and low-yield cigarettes. *Clin. Pharmacol. Therap.* **36(2)**, 265–270.
14. Herning RI, Hooker WD, and Jones RT. (1986) Tetrahydrocannabinol content and differences in marihuana smoking behavior. *Psychopharmacology* **90(2)**, 160–162.
15. Benowitz NL, Nguyen TL, Jones RT, Herning RI, and Bachman J. (1980) Metabolic and psychophysiologic studies of cannabidiol-hexobarbital interaction. *Clin. Pharmacol. Therap.* **28(1)**, 115–120.
16. National Institute on Drug Abuse. (1995) *Marijuana, Facts for Teens*, Bethesda, Md.: National Institute on Drug Abuse National Institutes of Health.
17. National Institute on Drug Abuse. (1995) *Marihuaja, Facts Parents Need to Know*, National Institute on Drug Abuse National Institutes of Health, Bethesda, MD.

18. Friedman H, Klein TW, Newton C, and Daaka Y. (1995) Marijuana, receptors and immunomodulation. *Adv. Exper. Med. Biol.* **373,** 103–113.
19. Hollister LE. (1986) Interactions of cannabis with other drugs in man. *NIDA Research Monograph* **68,** 110–116.
20. Benowitz NL and Jones RT. (1977) Effects of delta-9-tetrahydrocannabinol on drug distribution and metabolism. Antipyrine, pentobarbital, and ethanol. *Clin. Pharmacol. Ther.* **22(3),** 259–268.
21. Adams AJ, Brown B, Haegerstrom-Portnoy G, Flom MC, and Jones RT. (1978) Marijuana, alcohol, and combined drug effects on the time course of glare recovery. *Psychopharmacology* **56(1),** 81–86.
22. Hunt CA and Jones RT. (1980) Tolerance and disposition of tetrahydrocannabinol in man. *J. Pharmacol. Exp.Ther.* **215(1),** 35–44.
23. Adams IB and Martin BR. (1996) Cannabis: pharmacology and toxicology in animals and humans. *Addiction* **91(11),** 1585–1614.
24. Hall W, Solowij N, and Lemon J. (1994) The health and psychological consequences of cannabis use. Australian Government Publishing Service, Canberra, Australia

II BIOCHEMISTRY AND MOLECULAR MECHANISMS

8

Effects of THC on Brain and Social Organization of Ants

Peter Waser

Abstract

After a single dose of ^{3}H-LSD or THC (100 µg/ml), the maximum brain concentration of LSD reached 150 pg after 12 hours and that of THC reached 800 pg after 36 hours. Ants fed sugar water containing 100 µg/mL LSD or 1 mg/mL THC (the maximum that could be solubilized in water-Tween) presented impairment of social behavior. Behavioral reactions or the performance of individual ants were likewise altered.

1. INTRODUCTION

In humans, social factors such as group formation among children and adolescents, broken home situation, educational system, and subculture, either separately or in combination are determinants for the development of drug addiction. Group influences are also seen in behavioral manifestations of the drug effects themselves. Altogether, the role of human society in the manifestation of drug abuse is very important.

This is the main reason to test hallucinogenic substances in animals living together in highly organized communities—namely in insect societies. We selected ants for these investigations, because they live in high numbers in a limited space and because their reduced flying capacity allows experiments under controlled laboratory conditions.

We wish to point out here that human society and an ant colony are completely different in their structural organization. But as Edward O. Wilson (1) mentioned in his prospect for a "unified sociobiology," there are some functional similarities between them. Both societies are characterized by an extensive division of labor, which needs a good coordination of activities. The members of cooperative groups have to communicate among one another using signals perceptible by the existing sensory channels: Humans have unique languages with enormous potential and plasticity transmitted through generations by learning. In contrast, the communication system of ants is genetically fixed and highly stereotyped.

The social behavior of ants is well-known and was summarized, e.g., by Sudd (2), Wilson and Dumpert (3). However, pharmacological experiments on the behavior of ants are scarce.

From: *Marihuana and Medicine*
Edited by: G. G. Nahas et al.   © Humana Press Inc., Totowa, NJ

Kostowski and his group (*4–8*) investigated the actions of many substances on the aggressive behavior of ants against beetles.

We examined:

1. The behavioral and toxic effects of lysergic acid diethylamide tartrate (LSD) and Δ^9-tetrahydrocannabinol (THC) in individual ants (*9*).
2. We investigated the uptake of LSD and THC into the ants' brain (*10*).
3. We established their effects on the social behavior of ants, which is discussed herein (*11*).

2. ANTS

All our investigations were done with ants of the species *Formica pratensis* Retz. They were taken out of a colony 13 km southeast of Zurich and kept in a formicary equipped with their genuine nesting material. During this period in our laboratory, we made sugar-water (250 mg/mL sucrose) available to them.

3. DRUGS: APPLICATION AND DOSAGE

In all experiments reported here, the drugs were administered to the ants orally in the food.

First, we evaluated in individual ants the suitable drug concentrations to be used in the food, according to the toxicities. LSD was mixed with sugar water containing 250 mg/mL sucrose. A drug concentration of 100 µg/mL sugar water seemed to be reasonable. A single uptake of this food caused typical LSD effects in a good many ants. These ants often displayed fumbling movements with their forelegs in the air at each step. The head was kept elevated and the antennae were stretched out and agitated. In addition, these ants often avoided the approach or touch with a probe instead of showing threat posture and seizing. These drug effects eventually disappeared in almost all ants. Even in ants having free access to this diet for 10 days, the mortality rate was increased only slightly. Because of the low water solubility of THC, we suspended this drug in sugar water containing 10 vol% of Tween-80 as an emulsifier. The uptake of a solution containing 1 mg/mL THC was very good. But subsequently, no distinct changes in the individual behavior of ants could be observed, not even after repeated drug administrations. Because of increasing difficulties to dissolve the drug in higher concentrations, we used 1 mg/mL THC for further experiments.

4. DRUG LEVELS IN ANT BRAINS

A fundamental question for a centrally acting drug is its rate of uptake into the brain and the accumulation in the central nervous system. These mechanisms have not been examined before in ants. Similar investigations in other species, e.g., small laboratory mammals, are not compatible because of the morphological differences in the anatomy of the alimentary tract and of the blood–brain barrier.

At increasing time intervals from a single feeding with [^{3}H]LSD, or (^{3}H)THC, ants were taken for analysis of incorporated radioactivity. The brains were dissected and their radioactive content evaluated by means of a liquid scintillation counter. To obtain comparable results, all values were normalized to one brain and a drug concentration of 100 µg/mL food. The results of these experiments are shown in Fig. 1.

The [^{3}H]LSD content in the brain increased gradually during 12 hours after feeding to about 150 pg/brain. After 42 hours however, the drug content decreased to one-third of its maximum value. After feeding with [^{3}H]THC, the drug content in the brain increased steeply during 24 hours. The maximum, corresponding to about 800 pg THC per brain was not reached before 24–48 hours. Subsequently, the drug content decreased to about one-third only after 6 days.

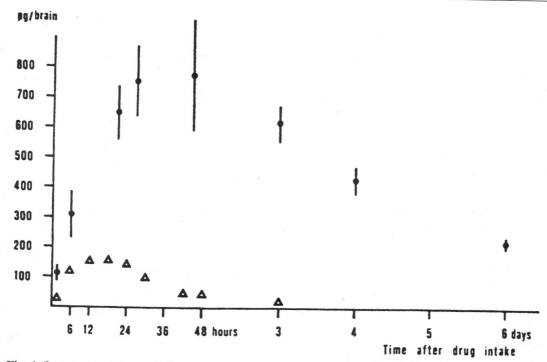

Fig. 1. Drug contents in ant brains at different times after a single intake of food containing 100µg/ml of either ^{3}H·LSD ($\Delta \bar{x} n = 10$), or ^{3}H·THC ($\phi \bar{x} \pm$ s.e.m., $n = 6$, or 8).

THC is taken up by the nervous system of ants to a larger extent than LSD and remains there for a longer time. This finding corresponds with results in mammals. The THC molecules are lipophilic and cross the blood–brain barrier much more easily than LSD molecules with their polar carboxy and amino groups. But it should be noted that a strikingly long time is required for the peak levels of drug concentration in the ant's brain to be reached. This might be connected to some peculiarities of the ants' intestinal tracts.

5. ACUTE DRUG EFFECTS ON INTERACTIONS OF ANTS

Taking account of these findings, we started our investigations on the social behavior of ants under the influence of LSD and THC. In a first series of experiments, we always introduced one drug or control-fed ant to 10 hungry nestmates and noted its interactions for 10 minutes. The following patterns of social behavior were observed: aggressive behavior (threat, seizing, and biting), social grooming, food-sharing behavior (frequency and duration), and the number of social interactions per encounter. At the beginning, we used sugar water alone and sugar water containing 100 µg/mL LSD. At intervals of 2, 9, 18, 24 and 48 hours from feeding, 10 drug and 10 control experiments were done.

After introducing a control-fed ant to 10 hungry nestmates, aggressive elements were scarce and limited to the first encounters. Soon the test ants calmed and began to share food among the hungry nestmates. In experiments up to 24 hours after feeding, each foodsharing behavior took generally more than 10 seconds. Subsequently, the acceptors often groomed the donors. Later on, many acceptors proceeded in secondary food-sharing behavior as donors.

Table 1 shows the effects of feeding the introduced test ant with sugar water containing 100 µg/mL LSD, compared to sugar water alone, on their social interactions with hungry

Table 1
Differences in social interactions between an ant fed with sugar water containing 100 µg/mL
LSD and 10 hungry nestmates. Compared to sugar water controls (n = 10)

Behavioral elements	Time after food intake				
	2 hours	9 hours	18 hours	24 hours	48 hours
Agressive behavior					
Threat	n.s.	n.s.	n.s.	n.s.	n.s.
Biting	n.s.	n.s.	n.s.	n.s.	n.s.
Social Grooming	n.s.	n.s.	n.s.	n.s.	n.s.
Food sharing					
Exchange < 10 s	↑↑	n.s.	n.s.	↑	n.s.
Exchange > 10 s	n.s.	n.s.	↓↓	↓↓↓	n.s.
Duration of	n.s.	↓↓↓	↓↓	↓↓↓	n.s.
Interactions per meeting	n.s.	↓↓↓	↓	↓↓	↓

Significant differences (Wilcoxon-Test) at p < 0.1, 0.05, 0.01: ↑↓, ↑↑↓↓, ↑↑↑↓↓↓.

nestmates: 2 hours after drug intake, food-sharing behavior of short duration was increased. At 9, 18, and 24 hours after drug feeding, the ants often moved irritatedly and showed the typical LSD effects in locomotion mentioned before. In addition, these ants often ceased, or even avoided social touchings. This resulted at 18 and 24 hours after drug feeding in a decrease of food-sharing behavior lasting more than 10 seconds. Likewise the duration of food-sharing behavior and the number of interactions per meeting were diminished at 9, 18, and 24 hours after drug intake. Forty-eight hours after LSD feeding, the drug effects faded, showing just a slightly decreased number of interactions per meeting.

The period of most intense drug effects (9–24 hours after LSD feeding) coincided with the period of highest LSD content in the brain. The predominant alterations in social behavior of worker ants included a diminished food flow among nestmates and a reduced number of interactions per meeting. Aggressive behavior toward nestmates was not changed. In another series of experiments, LSD-fed ants likewise adopted queens from their own nest, from which they were isolated 2–3 months ago. At 9, 24, and 48 hours after intake of food containing 100 µg/mL LSD, the adoptions were even less dramatic compared to the corresponding controls. This point contrasts with findings of Floru, Ishay and Gitter (12) in hornets, in which LSD in a concentration of 10 µg/ml glucose solution not only impaired locomotion and decreased social activities, but also increased aggression toward members of the same colony and toward foreign wasps. Kostowski, Wysokowski, and Tarchalska (8), however, after injecting LSD (30 µg/g) into the abdominal cavity of ants, could not find any significant changes in intraspecific aggression, whereas attacks towards beetles were decreased at 1 and 3 hours following drug administration.

In an analogous series of experiments, where one fed worker ant was added to 10 hungry nestmates, we used THC in a concentration of 1 mg/mL, and the solvent, sugar water with 10 vol. % of Tween-80 as a control. The occurrence of aggressive elements, social grooming, food-sharing behavior, and the number of interactions per meeting were not altered at 2, 9, 24, and 48 hours after a single feeding with THC, compared to their corresponding controls. Likewise at 2, 9, 24, and 48 hours after intake of food containing 1 mg/mL THC, all adoptions of queens in groups of worker ants were successful.

6. ACUTE DRUG EFFECTS ON GROUP FORMATION

In a next series of experiments, we investigated the distribution and group formation of ants in bipartite formicaries, holding 50 worker ants in either half. The ants in one compartment had free access to control food (i.e., sugar water, or sugar water with 10 vol % Tween) for 1 hour, whereas those in the other half were fed with drugged food containing 100 µg/mL LSD, or 1 mg/mL THC. At 2, 9, 24, and 48 hours after food intake, photographs were taken. To evaluate the localization of ants, either compartment was subdivided into 16 squares.

With all four food qualities the ants preferred the four corner squares compared to the four center squares. Significant differences between control and drug compartments were rare: 2 hours after THC intake the gathering of ants in the corner squares was increased compared to the controls, and 9 hours after LSD feeding, the accumulation of ants in the center squares was lower than with sugar water. The mean number of neighbors in the same square decreased from 9–24 hours after LSD intake and at 48 hours it was reduced compared to the sugar-water controls. Altogether, LSD diminished the tendency of group formation 1 and 2 days following drug intake, whereas THC had little influence on the distribution of worker ants in a formicary.

7. EFFECTS OF MULTIPLE DRUG APPLICATION TO LARGE GROUPS OF ANTS

Our next experiments concerned multiple-drug application to large groups of ants, consisting of several hundreds of worker ants and a few queens. These investigations were done in a special arrangement in which the nest was spatially separated from the feeding place in the excursion area. Between these compartments two connecting tubes existed. Because of their construction (wide entrances laterally and narrow exits at the cover) a well-functioning one-way traffic flow took place. Photocells were fitted immediately before the exits to count ants interrupting the light beam. Repeated readings from the counters yielded activity diagrams between nest and excursion area and vice versa.

In a first experiment, during period I of four weeks, the ants had free access to sugar water with 10 vol % of Tween-80. Then, during period II of three weeks, the food contained 1 mg/mL THC in addition, and during period III of four weeks, the ants were fed again with control solution. Fresh food was supplied daily at 9:00 A.M., except for weekends. Observations of behavior and activity measurements were obtained from 10 and 15 days of each test period.

The daily activity back to the nest from 8:00 A.M. to 5:00 P.M. was significantly increased during drug feeding, compared to the preceding and succeeding control periods. Similar differences were found from readings on the photocell between nest and feeding place. Figure 2 illustrates the diurnal activity of ants obtained by hourly readings from the counter of the photocell between the excursion area and the nest. To compare activities during control period I and III and during drug feeding (II), the total activity from 8:00 A.M. to 5:00 P.M. was taken as 100% and the relative activities per hour are shown. During either control period I and III, the relative activities/hour increased gradually from 8:00 A.M. to 12:00 P.M.. With THC (II), a large increase of activity above control levels was found for 1 and 2 hours following the supply of fresh food. In the afternoon, the relative activities per hour were slightly decreased during drug feedings. From observations of the ants' movements it became clear that foraging workers returned very promptly to the nest after uptake of THC-solution. However, these ants lacked distinct behavioral impairments and the domestic workers nursed eggs, larvae, and pupae even after a drug period of four weeks.

FEEDING PROCEDURE

I Sugar-water   (4 weeks. 16 experimental days)
II Sugar-water + 100 μg/ml LSD   (2 weeks. 8 experimental days)

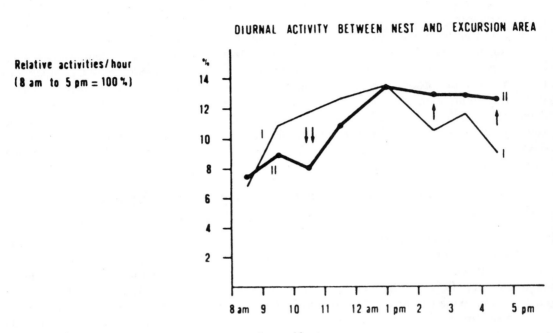

DIURNAL ACTIVITY BETWEEN NEST AND EXCURSION AREA

Relative activities/hour
(8 am to 5 pm = 100 %)

Significant Differences at P ≤ 0.1. 0.05 ↑ ↓. ↑↑ ↓↓ (Wilcoxon–Test)

Fig. 2.

In a similar experiment, during period I of four weeks, the ants had free access to sugar water. Afterwards, during period II of two weeks, the food contained 100 μg/mL LSD in addition. Behavior and activities were observed for 16 and 8 days.

The daily total activity from 8:00 A.M. to 5:00 P.M. was not altered by changing from sugar water to drugged food. The distribution of the relative activities per hour in the daytime however, showed a distinct shift: during control feeding (I), the activity increased by steps from 8:00 A.M. to 12:00 P.M., and in the afternoon the activity decreased. In contrast, during LSD-feeding (II) the activity did not increase before 11:00 A.M., and no distinct decrease from maximum occurred in the afternoon. Behavioral observations showed that domestic workers proceeded to care for the queens and the brood during the LSD feeding period. Foraging workers however, in the excursion area, often showed distinct drug effects. The locomotion of these ants exhibited sporadic periods of unsteadiness and sometimes they displayed fumbling movements with their forelegs in the air at each step. Foraging workers with extremely filled gasters in part isolated themselves socially and didn't return to the nest. Altogether, a distinct gradient of LSD effects was found from foraging to domestic worker ants. The following reasons might account for this observation: Domestic workers do not procure their food themselves, but receive it by food-sharing behavior from foraging ants. Our experiments suggest that LSD influenced some foraging workers to return no more to the nest, and LSD decreased food-sharing behavior among worker ants. Either effect prevented an equal distribution of the drug among the whole colony. Nevertheless, feeding with sugar water containing 100 µg/mL LSD has detrimental effects for the entire colony. The amount of food available to the queens, larvae, and domestic workers decreased. This deficiency has to be made good by recruiting additional foraging workers, which is achieved only by depleting the number of nursing ants. This shift in group population stunts an ant colony, even if their existence is not immediately endangered.

Reprinted with permission from Cannabis: Physipathology, Epidemiology, Detection (Nahas, G.G.; Latour, C., eds.) CRC Press, Boca Raton, 1993, pp. 359–367.

REFERENCES

1. Wilson, E. O. (1971) *The Insect Societies* Belknap Press, Cambridge, MA.
2. Sudd, J. H. (1967) *An Introduction to the Behaviour of Ants* Arnolds, London.
3. Dumpert, K. (1978) *Das Sozialleben der Ameisen*. Paul Parey, Berlin.
4. Kostowski, W. A. (1966) A note on the effects of some psychotropic drugs on the aggressive behaviour in the ant, *Formica rufa. J. Pharm. Pharmacol.* **18**, 747–749.
5. Kostowski, W. (1968) A note on the effect of some cholinergic and anticholinergic drugs on the aggressive behaviour and spontaneous electrical activity of the central nervous system in the ant, *Formica rufa. J. Pharm. Pharmacol.* **20**, 381–384.
6. Kostowski, W., Beck, J., and Meszaros, J. (1965) Drugs affecting the behaviour and spontaneous bioelectrical activity of the central nervous system in the ant, *Formica rufa. J. Pharm. Pharmacol.* **17**, 253–254.
7. Kostowski, W., Tarchalska, B., and Wanchowicz, B. (1975) Brain catecholamines, spontaneous bioelectrical activity and aggressive behaviour in ants (*Formica rufa.*) *Pharmacol. Biochem. Behav.* **3**, 337–342.
8. Kostowski, W., Wysokowski, J., and Tarchalska, B. (1972) The effect of some drugs modifying brain 5-hydroxytryptamine on the aggressiveness and spontaneous bioelectrical activity of the central nervous system of the ant *Formica rufa. Dissert. Pharm. Pharmacol.* **24**, 233–240.
9. Frischknecht, H. R. and Waser, P. G. (1978) Actions of hallucinogens on ants (*Formica pratensis*) II. Effects of amphetamine, LSD and delta-9-tetrahydrocannabinol. *Gen. Pharmacol.* **9**, 375–380.
10. Frischknecht, H. R. and Waser, P. G. (1978) Actions of hallucinogens on ants (*Formica pratensis*) I. Brain levels of LSD and THC following oral administration. *Gen. Pharmacol.* **9**, 369–373.
11. Frischknecht, H. R. and Waser, P. G. (1980) Actions of hallucinogens on ants (*Formica pratensis*) III. Social behavior under the influence of LSD and tetrahydrocannabinol. *Gen. Pharmacol.* **11**, 97–106.
12. Floru, L., Ishay, J., and Gitter S. (1969) The influence of psychotropic substances on hornet behaviour in colonies of *Vespa orientalis* (Hymenoptera). *Psychopharmacology* **14**, 323–341.

9

Studies of the Brain Cannabinoid System Using Positron and Single-Photon Emission Tomography

S. John Gatley, Nora D. Volkow,
and Alexandros Makriyannis

1. INTRODUCTION

Studies using radiolabeled cocaine in conjunction with positron emission tomography (PET) have been conducted since 1989 to image cocaine-binding sites in the human brain *(1)*. Among other findings, they have demonstrated that the concentration of these sites is decreased in chronic cocaine abusers *(2)*, and that > 50% of the binding sites in striatum must be occupied for subjects to experience a high *(3)*. Similar studies of marihuana were for many years hampered by the unsuitability of radiolabeled forms of THC for PET studies *(4–5)*, and the unavailability of other in vivo imaging agents for cannabinoid receptors. However, recent developments in medicinal chemistry have made new agonists and antagonists available with high affinity for the cannabinoid receptor. This has led to the synthesis of [^{123}I]AM 281, the first radioligand able to visualize the brain cannabinoid CB$_1$ receptor by *ex vivo* autoradiography and single-photon emission computed tomography (SPECT) *(6–8)*. Other radiotracers for cannabinoid receptor imaging with SPECT and PET will probably soon become available. This chapter briefly reviews these developments, together with the results of PET studies of the effects of marihuana and other abused drugs on brain blood flow and metabolism.

2. DRUGS OF ABUSE

The mechanisms of action of most abused drugs involve their binding to various classes of neurotransmitter receptors that are involved in the operation of the brain. The drugs may be either receptor agonists or antagonists (Table 1). Receptor stimulation may be either direct, as for cannabinoid and opioid receptors, or indirect, as exemplified by cocaine, which blocks clearance of the neurotransmitter dopamine from the synaptic cleft between nerve cells and

From: *Marihuana and Medicine*
Edited by: G. G. Nahas et al. © Humana Press Inc., Totowa, NJ

Table 1
Some Abused Drugs, Neurotransmitter Binding Sites, and Radioligands

Drug of abuse	Target	Endogenous ligand	PET/SPECT agent
Agonists			
Cocaine	Dopamine transporter	Dopamine	[^{11}C]cocaine *(1)*
Nicotine	Nicotinic acetylcholine receptor	Acetylcholine	[^{18}F]NFEP *(13)*
Marihuana (THC)	Cannabinoid receptor	Anandamide?	[^{123}I]AM281 *(8)*
Morphine	Opioid receptors	Endorphins	[^{11}C]carfentanil *(14)*
Valium	Benzodiazepine receptor	Unknown, steroid(s)?	[^{123}I]iomazenil *(15)*
LSD	Serotonin receptor	Serotonin	[^{11}C]NMS *(16)*
Antagonists			
Caffeine	Adenosine receptor	Adenosine	none *(17,18)*
Phencyclidine	Glutamate receptor	Existence uncertain	none *(19,20)*

thus increases signaling at neurons containing dopamine receptors *(9)*. The abuse of the compounds shown in Table 1 involves self-administration of small amounts of the drugs, ranging from about 50 µg of LSD to about 50 mg of cocaine. Drugs such as alcohol or nitrous oxide that are abused in larger quantities are exceptions to this picture, and probably alter subjective states via effects on neuronal membranes. Until quite recently many investigators held the opinion that THC also exerted its effects through relatively nonspecific membrane effects. During the last 10 years, however, achievements such as in vitro autoradiographic imaging of binding sites using high-affinity labeled cannabinoids *(10)*, the cloning of genes for cannabinoid receptors *(11)*, and the development of the CB^1 cannabinoid receptor antagonist SR141716A *(12)*, which blocks biological effects of THC have provided evidence that THC acts (certainly predominantly) through specific receptors.

The right-hand column in Table 1 gives one example of a PET or SPECT tracer, where these have been developed. None are yet available for adenosine or glutamate receptors, though the references cited indicate that progress is being made in these areas. Note that THC is the rule and cocaine is an exception in that labeled forms of abused drugs usually do not have acceptable properties as in vivo imaging radiotracers.

3. ABUSED AND THERAPEUTIC DRUGS

Substances that interact with neurotransmitter systems can have medically beneficial effects as well as permit abuse. Often, as for example with valium or morphine, the same drug can be viewed as belonging to either category depending on the circumstances of their administration. Often, too, the same binding site may be the target of both abused and therapeutic drugs. For example, cocaine, which appears to have uniquely addictive properties, acts by blocking the dopamine transporters. However, methylphenidate, which blocks the dopamine transporter with a similar affinity to cocaine, is prescribed to millions of American children to treat attention deficit disorder *(21)*. The divergent characteristics of these two drugs may result from different routes of administration, different kinetics at the dopamine transporter, different affinities for other binding sites, or conceivably because they interact with the dopamine transporter in distinct ways. As another example, hallucinogens such as LSD act via stimulation of serotonin receptors *(22)*. However, elevation of brain serotonin by administration of drugs such as tricyclic antidepressants or selective serotonin-reuptake inhibitors does not produce hallucinations.

In addition to helping understand mechanisms of addiction, PET studies of drugs of abuse may help our understanding of mental diseases, and produce useful leads for the development of drug therapies for these illnesses. A better understanding of the cannabinoid-receptor system might produce useful drugs with, for example, antiemetic or analgesic properties, but with minimal abuse potential *(23)*.

4. RADIOLIGAND STUDIES

Compounds that have been radiolabeled to high specific radioactivities, and which bind with high affinity to neurotransmitters receptors and transporters ("radioligands") are important tools in neuroscience. The development of tritium- and iodine-125-labeled radioligands, and of autoradiographic techniques, have enabled the mapping of receptor and transporter distributions in the brains of experimental animals, and in postmortem human brains *(24)*. These labeled compounds have also greatly facilitated molecular pharmacological studies of receptor/neurotransmitter interactions, as well as the screening of compounds with potential pharmacological properties.

5. EMISSION TOMOGRAPHY (PET AND SPECT)

PET and SPECT are nuclear medicine imaging techniques that are able to measure the regional and temporal concentrations of positron-emitting nuclides in small volumes of the human body *(25,26)*. They therefore allow the extension of radioligand binding studies to the living human and nonhuman primate brains, provided that suitable labeled compounds are available *(27,28)*. For use in PET, carbon, nitrogen, and oxygen all have positron-emitting isotopes that in principle can be used to label organic compounds, including drugs of abuse, without altering their pharmacological behavior. In practice, nitrogen-13 (half-life 10 minutes) and oxygen-15 (half-life 2 minutes) are rarely used except in the form of simple inorganic radiotracers. In contrast, organic compounds that incorporate atoms of carbon-11 (half-life 20 minutes) and also fluorine-18 (half-life 110 minutes) are frequently employed as PET radiotracers. Over the last 20 years the chemistry of these positron emitters has evolved to the point at which many radioligands are available in major PET centers, in spite of problems stemming from their very short half-lives. Their use is associated with reasonably benign radiation dosimetry that often allows repeated studies on the same subject. Thus longitudinal studies as well as test-retest studies involving administration of pharmacologically active drugs are possible. The 20-minute half-life of carbon-11 allows repeated studies in a single scanning session. SPECT cameras offer poorer resolution than PET scanner (7 vs 4 mm), but are far more widely available because they have been designed for clinical uses. Among the available radionuclides, iodine-123 (half-life 13 hours) has the best properties for labeling low-molecular-weight organic compounds yet retaining biological activity *(28)*.

PET can be used to study drugs of abuse in several ways. Firstly, abused substances can be labeled with carbon-11. This permits the distribution of drugs in the brain to be directly measured following intravenous administration. Furthermore, if a very low mass of the labeled drug is administered (so that only a small fraction of the binding sites is occupied) and the drug has suitable properties *(see below)*, then PET images will reflect local concentrations of drug-binding sites. Since few drugs contain iodine atoms, SPECT cannot be used in this way. Secondly, however, the ability of an abused drug to compete with or to displace a different radioligand for the same binding sites can be measured with either PET or SPECT. It may

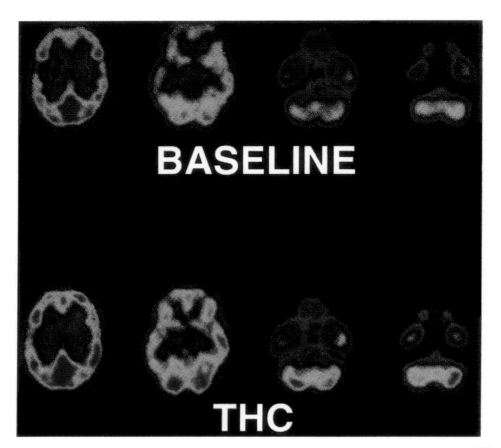

Plate 1. PET/FDG images of the human brain. Top images represent FDG accumulation in four different slices of the brain of a representative marihuana-abusing subject, measured using PET. A rainbow color scale was used, where red>orange>yellow, and so on. Images at the bottom are the same brain slices 30–40 minutes after intravenous administration of THC (2 mg.) THC increased metabolism in the cerebellum (normalized to whole-brain metabolism) in all eight subjects tested. The mean increase was 7%. (Volkow et al. [1991] *Psychiatr. Res.* **40,** 69–78.)

then be possible to measure the degree of receptor occupancy achieved by the abused drug and to compare the occupancy with behavioral and subjective changes caused by the drug. Thirdly, by using radioligands that bind to different sites it may be possible to examine effects of abused drugs on other neurotransmitter systems. For example, the in vivo binding of the dopamine D_2 receptor radioligand [^{11}C]raclopride, and the muscarinic cholinergic radioligand [^{11}C]benztropine, have both been shown to be sensitive to alterations in levels of endogenous neurotransmitters (dopamine and acetylcholine, respectively) *(29–31)*. Fourthly, in addition to receptor and transporter radioligand studies, PET may be used to measure local values of cerebral blood flow (lCBF) *(32)* and of cerebral metabolic rate for glucose (lCMR-glu) *(33)*. The most common radiotracers are oxygen 15-labeled water (for lCBF) and fluorine 18-labeled 2-deoxy-2-fluoro-D-glucose (FDG; for lCMRglu). These radiotracers allow effects of abused drugs on overall brain physiology to be evaluated, since flow and metabolism depend on nerve-terminal activity. No equivalent of FDG is available for SPECT, studies *(34)*, but perfusion changes can be measured with radiopharmaceuticals such as [^{99m}Tc]HMPAO *(35)*. Both acute and chronic effects of abused drugs may be examined using these four general approaches.

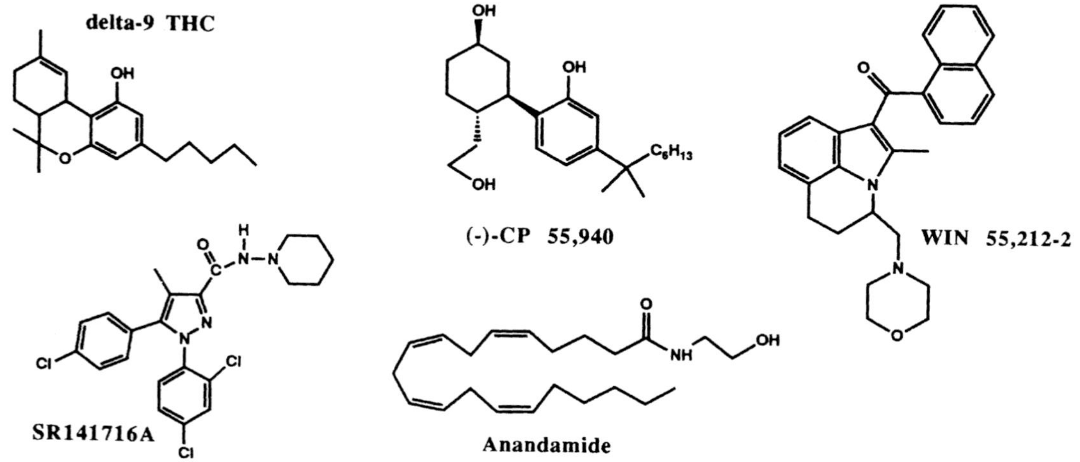

Fig. 1. Chemical structures of some natural and synthetic compounds that bind to cannabinoid receptors.

6. CANNABINOID RECEPTORS

Autoradiographic studies with tritiated CP 55,940 *(10,36)* have demonstrated high concentrations of cannabinoid receptors in the basal ganglia and (especially in its outflow nuclei the globus pallidus and substantia nigra.) High concentrations are also found in hippocampus and cerebellum. The cerebral cortex also contains appreciable concentrations of cannabinoid receptors, the highest being the cingulate gyrus. Some other regions including most of the brainstem and the thalamus contain low or negligible concentrations. The pattern of distribution of cannabinoid receptors in many brain regions is similar to that of dopamine D_1 receptors, which has led to the suggestion that a function of the cannabinoid system may be to indirectly modulate brain dopaminergic activity *(36)*.

7. COMPOUNDS THAT BIND TO CANNABINOID RECEPTORS

The major psychoactive ingredient of marihuana, Δ^9-THC, binds to cannabinoid receptors with moderate affinity, as do several related compounds. In recent years, synthetic molecules with higher affinities have been developed. These include the cannabinoid receptor agonists CP 55,244 *(37)* and the structurally dissimilar WIN 55,212-2 *(38)* (Fig. 1). Even more recently, a high-affinity cannabinoid receptor antagonist, SR141716A, has been synthesized *(40)*. It can be expected that these new ligands will allow the design of experiments that will greatly expand our knowledge of the role that the cannabinoid receptor plays in normal brain functions. Additionally, they will facilitate studies of the effects of chronic stimulation of the cannabinoid receptor, and of withdrawal from marihuana intoxication.

8. PROGRESS TOWARDS PET AND SPECT RADIOLIGANDS FOR CANNABINOID RECEPTORS

A logical starting point for development of such a ligand is to incorporate an atom of an appropriate radionuclide into the structure of one of the molecules shown in Fig.1. In fact, THC has been modified by labeling with fluorine-18 in the hydrocarbon side chain. Unfortunately, this compound did not produce PET images that showed any particular regional pat-

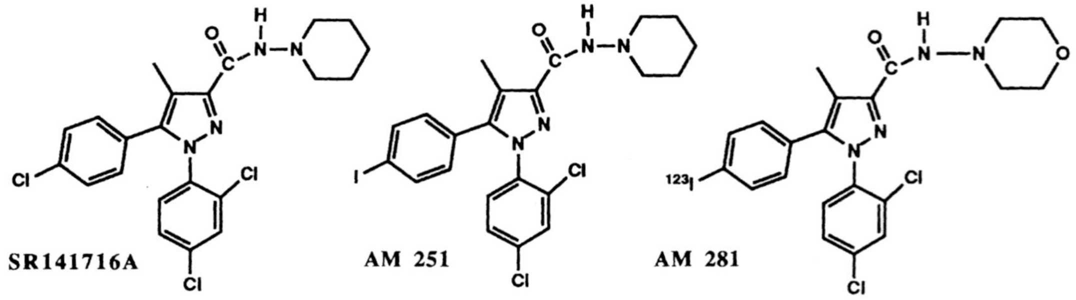

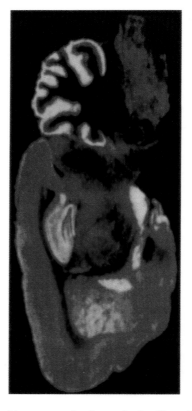

Fig. 2. Chemical structures of the prototypic cannabinoid CB_1-receptor antagonist SR141716A and iodine-substituted congeners evaluated as SPECT imaging radiotracers.

Plate 2. Distribution of cannabinoid receptors in the rat brain. Cannabinoid receptors in a slide-mounted sagittal section of a rat brain were visualized using the high-affinity cannabamimetric drug CP 55,940, labled with tritium. The color scale is hot metal where orange>red>black. (Courtesy of Miles Herdenham, NIMH.)

tern of brain localization when injected into a baboon *(5)*. It showed poor uptake, but was widely distributed in the brain with a relatively higher concentration in the cerebellum. Furthermore, uptake of radioactivity in the skull was apparent, which suggested in vivo decomposition producing labeled fluoride ion. It is therefore likely that the PET images represented

Table 2
Dopamine Transporter Radioligands Based on Cocaine and Methylphenidate

Radioligand	K_i in vitro, nM	log p	Peak ST, nCi/cc/mCi	ST/CB	T_{max},min	$B_{max}/K_{d'}$,mL/g
RTI-55	1.5	1.6	130	12+	>1200	6.7
WIN 35,428	12	0.8	150	4+	>120	5
dtMP	40	1.4	100	2.3	30–40	1.6
Cocaine	100	1.3	85	1.7	5-7	0.6

RTI-55 and WIN 35,428 are, respectively, the I-123 labeled 3β-iodophenyl and the C-11 3β-fluorophenyl analog of cocaine *(43,44)*. dtMP is C-11 d-threomethylphenidate, the active isomer of methylphenidate *(27,28)*. log p is lipophilicity measured using an HPLC method *(47)*. Peak ST is the fraction of administered radioactivity localizing in the striatum. ST/CB is the ratio of concentration of radioactivity in striatum to that in the cerebellum. T^{max} is the time after injection of radioligand at which striatal accumulation of radioactivity is at a maximum. $B^{max}/K_{d'}$ is the ratio of binding parameters in vivo estimated from the radioligand distribution volume *(48)*.

only nonspecific uptake of the tracer with a negligible component because of specific binding to cannabinoid receptors. Further developments in this area necessitated the synthesis of compounds with a combination of higher affinity for the cannabinoid receptor to increase specific binding, and of lower lipophilicity, to decrease nonspecific binding. The structures of CP 55,940, WIN 55,212-2, and SR141716A (Fig. 1) may in principle serve as lead compounds for these efforts. Our recent studies with the SR141716A congeners AM251 and AM281 *(6–8)* confirm that this class of molecules is capable of producing in vivo imaging radiotracers.

The structure of SR141716A contains three chlorine atoms. In initial work, one of these was replaced with an atom of iodine-123 (half-life 13 hours) which, as mentioned above, can be imaged using SPECT. Although this compound (AM251) gave promising results in mice *(6)*, and in in vitro autoradiography *(7)*, it failed to enter the brains of baboons used in SPECT experiments *(8)*. A further change was therefore made in the structure, namely the insertion of an oxygen atom into the piperidine ring, in the anticipation that it would reduce the lipophilicity of the molecule. This molecule, [^{123}I]AM281, although possessing a somewhat lower affinity for CB_1 receptors than SR141716A or AM 251, was able to penetrate the baboon blood–brain barrier *(8)*. It also clearly localized in rat brain in an *ex vivo* autoradiographic experiment, giving a distribution essentially identical to earlier in vitro autoradiographic experiments *(see* color plates). Work continues to evaluate the full potential of the SR141716A class of molecules as SPECT and PET radiotracers.

Other molecular skeletons might also serve as the starting point for PET and SPECT tracers. For example, as outlined in Fig. 3, CP 55,940 might be a good option, since it possesses the highest affinity *(37)*. However, the structure is such that labeling with carbon-11 would probably be quite difficult. Incorporation of a fluorine-18 atom into the alkyl side-chain might be a more fruitful approach, since the labeling chemistry would be easier, and in addition the longer half-life of fluorine-18 would allow more time in imaging experiments for nonspecific binding to clear. Naturally, there is no guarantee that the fluorine-containing analog of CP 55,940 would retain the same affinity for the cannabinoid receptor.

Our experience with AM281 suggests that dealing with the issue of excessive lipid solubility is probably key to the successful in vivo direct imaging of THC-binding sites. The importance of lipophilicity may be illustrated by the experience of the last few years in imaging cocaine-binding sites. Table 3 shows several compounds, including [^{11}C]cocaine, which suc-

AM251　　　　　AM281

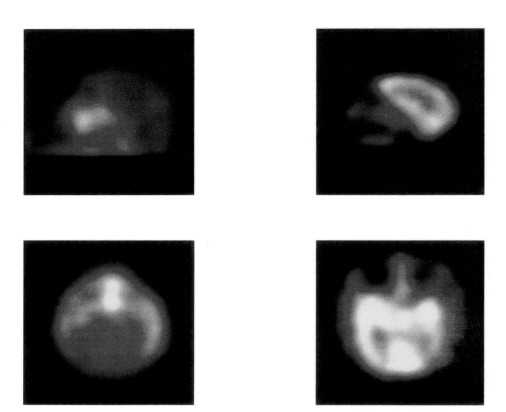

Plate 3. SPECT images. Baboons were injected intravenously over a 1-minute period with 8–10 mC of [^{123}I]AM281 or [^{123}I]AM251 blood plasma (prepared from the same animal immediately before the imaging study) plus 4 mL of which had been dissolved in 1 mL of 0.9% saline. Scanning was commenced at the beginning of the injection period. The impages show the average concentration of radioactivity between 0 and 60 minutes. Top images are sagittal views, bottom images are transaxial views. (Gatley et al. [1998] *J. Neurochem.* **70,** 417–423.

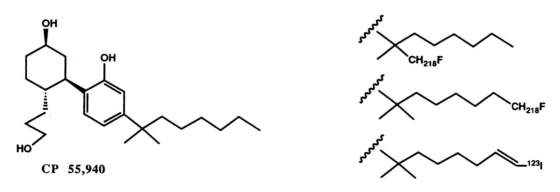

Fig. 3. Possible approaches to labeling synthetic, high-affinity cannabinoid-receptor ligands with suitable radionuclides for PET or SPECT imaging.

Table 3
PET Studies of Glucose Metabolism Involving Drugs of Abuse

Drug	MR	OFC	OC	BG	TH	CB	Resp.	Recovery
Acute								
Heroin	↓							
Cocaine	↓						—	—
Amphetamine	↓						—	—
Alcohol	↓		↓		↑	↓	—	—
marihuana	NC.	[b]2				↑	—	—
Diazepam	↓		↓		↑low↓high		—	—
Chronic								
Cocaine	↑	↑early↓late		↑ ↓↓↓late			ND	≈6d(early)
Alcohol	↓	↓early		↓			↑	≈30d(partial)
Alcohol[a]							↓	
Marihuana	NC.	↑		↑		↓		

MR, global metabolic rate; OFC, orbital frontal cortex; OC, occipital cortex; BG, basal ganglia; TH, thalamus; CB, cerebellum; Resp., response to administration of drug; NC, no change; ND, not determined.
[a]Alcoholics responded to a diazepam challenge with lower responses in BG, OFC, and TH *(61)*.
[b]Marihuana abusers only, not normal controls.

cessfully visualize the dopamine transporter. These four tracers give essentially identical results, when their different affinities for the transporter are accounted for. However, two other positron-emitting compounds with very high affinity for the dopamine transporter, fluorine-18-labeled GBR 13119 and GBR 12909 *(40,41)*, with lipophilicities more similar to that of THC (log p >3), were much less satisfactory PET radioligands. This is probably because of widespread brain uptake, followed by extremely slow clearance from tissue lipid pools in all brain areas. When these problems have been overcome for cannabinoid-receptor radioligands, PET studies similar to those now underway with C-11 cocaine and its congeners, and with C-11 methylphenidate will become possible. Studies in cocaine abusers have shown that although there are increases in measures of dopamine-transporter density shortly after withdrawal begins, there are decreases or no changes with protracted withdrawal *(2)*. Other drugs of abuse also alter transporter availability. For example, a preliminary study done in violent alcoholics showed significant elevations of DAT when compared with nonalcoholic subjects *(42)*. In contrast nonviolent alcoholics had lower DAT levels than controls.

9. EFFECTS OF THC ON BRAIN GLUCOSE METABOLISM

Effects of acute intravenous injection of THC on lCMRglu have been investigated in both chronic marihuana abusers and in normal control subjects *(49,50)*. The experimental design involved a baseline scan on day 1 and a second scan on day 2, 30–40 minutes after administration of 2 mg of THC. The most consistent observation in both normal controls and habitual marihuana users was an increase in relative metabolic rate in the cerebellum. This increase was positively correlated both with concentrations of THC in the plasma and with the intensity of the subjective sense of intoxication. However, the average increase in cerebellar metabolism after THC administration was less in marihuana users than in controls. Addition-

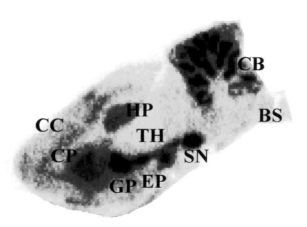

Plate 4. *Ex vivo* autoradiography in rat brain. A rat (150 g) was injected intravenously with 800 MCi of [^{123}I]AM281 and sacrificed after 2 hours. The carcass was frozen in liquid nitrogen and 50-micron sections cut using a whole-body cryotome. Dessicated sections were left in contact with a phosphor-imaging plate overnight. Abbreviations: BS, brian stem; CB, cerebellum; CC, cerebral cortex; CP, caudate-putamen; EP, entopendunclar nucleus; GP, globus pallidus; HP, hippocampus; SN, substantia nigra; TH, thalamus. (Gatley et al. [1998] *J. Neurochem.* **70** 417–423.)

ally, the marihuana users had lower cerebellar metabolism than the controls during the baseline scans. Thus it appears that the brain area showing the greatest metabolic increase in response to acute THC, the cerebellum, responds to chronic marihuana exposure with a decrease in baseline metabolic rate. The FDG PET studies also demonstrated that marihuana users responded to THC administration with increased metabolic activity in the prefrontal cortex, orbitofrontal cortex and basal ganglia. These increases were not seen in controls. In contrast to the robust effects of THC on relative metabolic rates, absolute global changes in CMRglu in response to THC were quite variable. In approximately one-third of the subjects metabolism increased by more than 10%, and in another third metabolism decreased by more than 10%. There was also variability in subjective response to marihuana; most subjects reported the experience as pleasant, but some reported only minimal effects, and a few became anxious or paranoid.

The involvement of the cerebellum in the psychoactive effects of marihuana and in changes in cerebral metabolic rate is consistent with the view that THC interacts with the high concentration of cannabinoid receptors in this brain area. Decreased cerebellar metabolic rates in habitual marihuana users may reflect the effects of chronic exposure to the drug. Functions known to be associated with the cerebellum, such as motor coordination, proprioception and learning, have been documented to be adversely affected both during acute marihuana intoxication and in habitual users of the drug (51). The PET scanner used in these investigations lacked sufficient resolution to examine metabolic rates in other brain areas, such as hippocampus, substantia nigra, and caudate nucleus, which contain high concentrations of cannabinoid receptors. PET cameras with improved performance will allow further studies of the changes in brain metabolic rates induced by acute and chronic THC. Development of a PET radioligand for cannabinoid receptors will allow changes in metabolism to be related to local receptor concentrations.

In a recent PET/[^{15}O]water study with 32 abusers (52), THC dose-dependently increased CBF in the frontal regions, insula, cingulate gyrus, and subcortical structures with somewhat greater effects in the right hemisphere. Self-ratings of THC intoxication were correlated most markedly with the right-frontal region.

10. EFFECTS OF OTHER ABUSED DRUGS ON BRAIN GLUCOSE METABOLISM

The effects of acute admistration of cocaine, alcohol, morphine, amphetamine, and benzodiazepines have also been evaluated in PET experiments in normal subjects (53–58). A decrease in global brain metabolism was noted in each of the cited studies, in spite of the different mechanisms of action of these drugs. Thus, THC apparently behaved dissimilarly to these other abused drugs, in that single acute administration did not reduce overall metabolic rates (49–50). However, it should be noted that recent studies with amphetamine have failed to find a consistent decrease in global metabolic rate, perhaps because results of imaging studies with stimulants may depend on the attentional state of the subjects and other factors (59,60). Findings that have been reported in terms of local drug-induced changes in glucose metabolism are summarized in Table 3. For alcohol, activity in the thalamus is decreased relatively less than in other brain areas (61), whereas occipital cortex and cerebellum show larger decreases; for diazepam, low doses do not change whereas high doses markedly decrease thalamic metabolic rates (56). Activity in occipital cortex is also markedly decreased by benzodiazepines (62).

Chronic cocaine abusers and alcoholics, like marihuana abusers, show metabolic abnormalities in the orbito frontal cortex (OFC) and basal ganglia. Cocaine abusers have increased metabolic activity in the OFC and basal ganglia, relative to normal controls, during early detoxification. Later (>6 days) in detoxification, activity in the OFC is decreased relative to controls (40). Alcoholics, on the other hand, show decreased activity in the OFC and basal ganglia during detoxification (43). By 30 days after withdrawal, the decrements in activity in these areas have been partially restored, relative to controls. Thus, patterns of metabolic rates after cessation of drug self-administration are time dependent.

11. CONCLUSIONS

Compared with PET investigations of cocaine-binding sites, imaging researches into the brain cannabinoid system of the living human brain are still in their infancy. The first in vivo radioligand for cannabinoid CB_1 receptors, [^{123}I]AM281 has recently been developed, and work is proceeding on other labeled compounds for PET as well as SPECT. Studies of the effects of THC on cerebral glucose metabolic rates have been conducted, and have shown that in contrast to other drugs of abuse THC increases metabolism in the cerebellum, in both habitual marihuana users and normal controls. The relationship between this increase and the high concentration of cannabinoid receptors in the cerebellum seen in postmortem and animal brains may become clear as radioligands are developed that allow PET studies of these receptors in human subjects.

Several other avenues of investigation will be opened up by the ability to measure cannabinoid-receptor density in the human brain. These may include measurement of long-term alterations of binding-site densities in conditions such as disease states, withdrawal from habitual marihuana use, and treatment with therapeutic drugs, and of relationships between receptor occupancies and the subjective and physiological effects of marihuana and related compounds.

ACKNOWLEDGMENTS

This work was carried out at Brookhaven National Laboratory under contract DE-AC02-76CH00016 with the U.S. Department of Energy and supported by its Office of Health and Environmental Research. The research was also supported by the National Institute on Drug Abuse (DA03801, DA 06278, DA07515, DA09158)

REFERENCES

1. Fowler, J. S., Volkow, N. D., Wolf, A. P., Dewey, S. L., Schlyer, D. J., and MacGregor, R. R. (1989) Mapping cocaine binding sites in human and baboon brain in vivo. *Synapse* **4,** 371–377.
2. Volkow, N. D., Wang, G. J., Fowler, J. S., Logan, J., Hitzemannn, R., Gatley, S. J., MacGregor, R. R., and Wolf, A. P. (1996) Cocaine uptake is decreased in the brain of detoxified cocaine abusers. *Neuropsychopharmacology* **14,** 159–168.
3. Volkow, N. D., Wang, G. J., Fischman, M. W., Foltin, R. W., Fowler, J. S., Abumrad, N. N., Vitkun, S., Logan, J., Gatley, S. J., Pappas, N., Hitzemann, R., and Shea, C. E. (1997) Relationship between subjective effects of cocaine and dopamine transporter occupancy. *Nature* **386,** 827–830.
4. Marciniak, G., Charalambous, A., Shiue, C. Y., Dewey, S. L., Schlyer, D. J., Makriyannis, A., and Wolf, A. P. (1991) Fluorine-18 labeled tetrahydrocannabinol: synthesis and PET studies in a baboon. *J. Label Cmpds.* **30,** 413–415.
5. Charalambous, A., Marciniak, G., Shiue, C. Y., Dewey, S. L., Schlyer, D. J., Wolf, A. P., and Makriyannis, A. (1991) PET studies in the primate brain and biodistribution in mice using (-)-5'-18F-delta 8-THC. *Pharmacol. Biochem. Behav.* **40.** 503–507.
6. Gatley, S. J., Gifford, A. N., Volkow, N. D, Lan, R., and Makriyannis, A. (1996) Iodine-123 labeled AM251: a radioiodinated ligand which binds in vivo to the mouse brain CB1 cannabinoid receptor. *Eur. J. Pharmacol.* **307,** 301–308.
7. Gatley, S. J., Lan, R., Volkow, N. D., and Makriyannis, A. (1997) Binding of the non-classical cannabinoid CP 55,940 and the diarylpyrazole AM251 to rodent cannabinoid receptors. *Life Sci.* **61,** 191–197.
8. Gatley, S. J., Lan, R., Volkow, N. D., Pappas, N., King, P., Wong, C. T., Gifford, A. N., Pyatt, B., Dewey, S. L., and Makriyannis, A. (1998) Imaging the brain marihuana receptor—development of a radioligand that binds to cannabinoid cb1 receptors in-vivo. *J. Neurochem.* **70,** 417–423.
9. Ritz, M. C., Lamb, R. J., Goldberg, S. R., and Kuhar, M. J. (1987) Cocaine receptors on dopamine transporters are related to self administration of cocaine. *Science* **237,** 1219–1223.
10. Herkenham, M., Lynn, A. B, Little, M. D., Johnson, M. R., Melvin, L. S., DeCosta, B. R., and Rice, K. C. (1990) Cannabinoid receptor localization in brain. *Proc. Natl. Acad. Sci. USA* **87,** 1932–1936.
11. Matsuda, L. A., Lolait, S. J., Brownstein, M. J., Young, A. C., and Bonne, T. I. (1990) Structure of a cannabinoid receptor and functional expression of the cloned cDNA. *Nature* **346,** 561–564.
12. Rinaldicarmona, M., Barth, F., Heaulme, M., Shire, D., Calandra, B., Congy, C., Martinez, S., Maruani, J., Neliat, G., Caput, D., Ferrara, P., Soubrie, P., Breliere, J. C., and Lefur, G. (1994) SR141716A, a potent and selective antagonist of the brain cannabinoid receptor. *FEBS Lett.* **350,** 240–244.
13. Ding, Y.-S., Gatley, S. J., Fowler, J. S., Volkow, N. D., Aggarwal, N., Logan, J., Dewey, S. L., Liang, F., Carroll, F. I., and Kuhar, M. J. (1996) Mapping Nicotinic Acetylcholine Receptors with PET. *Synapse* **24,** 403–407.
14. Frost, J. J., Mayberg, H. S., Sadzot, B., Dannals, R. F., Lever, J. R., Ravert, H. T., Wilson, A. A, Wagner, H. N., Jr., and Links, J. M. (1990) Comparison of [11C]diprenorphine and [11C]carfentanil binding to opiate receptors in humans by positron emission tomography. *J. Cereb. Blood Flow Metab.* **10,** 484–492.
15. Zoghbi, S. S., Baldwin, R. M., Seibyl, J. P., al-Tikriti, M. S, Zea-Ponce, Y., Laruelle, M., Sybirska, E. H., Woods, S. W., Goddard, A. W., Malison, R. T., et al. (1992) Pharmacokinetics of the SPECT benzodiazepine receptor radioligand [^{123}I]iomazenil in human and non-human primates. *Nucl. Med. Biol.* **19** 881–888.
16. Wang, G. J., Volkow, N. D., Logan, J., Fowler, J. S., Schlyer, D., MacGregor, R. R., Hitzemann, R. J., Gjedde, A., and Wolf, A. P. (1995) Serotonin 5-HT2 receptor availability in chronic cocaine abusers. *Life Sci.* **56,** PL299–303.
17. Holschbach, M. H., Fein, T., Krummeich, C., Lewis, R. G., Wutz W., Schwabe, U., Unterlugauer, D., and Olsson, R. A. (1998) A1 adenosine receptor antagonists as ligands for positron emission tomography (PET) and single-photon emission tomography (SPET). *J. Med. Chem.* **41,** 555–563.
18. Orita, K., Sasaki, S., Maeda, M., Hashimoto, A., Nishikawa, T., Yugami, T., and Umezu, K. (1993) Synthesis and evaluation of 1-(1-[5-(2'-[18F]fluoroethyl)-2-thienyl]- cyclohexyl)piperidine as a potential in vivo radioligand for the NMDA receptor-channel complex. *Nucl. Med. Biol.* **20,** 865–873.
19. Ouyang, X., Mukherjee, J., and Yang, Z. Y. (1996) Synthesis, radiosynthesis, and biological evaluation of fluorinated thienylcyclohexyl piperidine derivatives as potential radiotracers for the NMDA receptor-linked calcium ionophore. *Nucl. Med. Biol.* **23,** 315–324.
20. Stone-Elander, S., Thorell, J. O., Eriksson, L., Fredholm, B.B., and Ingvar, M. (1997) In vivo biodistribution of [N-11C-methyl]KF 17837 using 3-D-PET: evaluation as a ligand for the study of adenosine A2A receptors. *Nucl. Med. Biol.* **24,** 187–191.

21. Volkow, N. D., Ding, Y.- S., Fowler, J. S., Wang, G.-J., Logan, J., Gatley, S. J., Dewey, S., Ashby, C., Lieber-mann, J., Hitzemann, R., and Wolf, A. P. (1995) Is methylphenidate like cocaine? Studies on their pharmaco-kinetics and distribution in human brain. *Arch. Gen. Psychiatry* **52,** 456–463.

22. Glennon, R. A., Titeler, M., and McKenney, J. D. (1984) Evidence for 5-HT2 involvement in the mechanism of action of hallucinogenic agents. *Life Sci.* **24,** 2505–2511.

23. Hollister, L. E. (1986) Health aspects of cannabis. *Pharmacol. Rev.* **38,** 1–20.

24. Young, W. S. and Kuhar, M. J. (1979) A new method for receptor autoradiography: [³H]opioid receptors in rat brain. *Brain Res.* **179,** 255–270.

25. Phelps, M. E. (1991) PET: a biological imaging technique. *Neurochem. Res.* **16.** 929–940.

26. Todd-Pokropek, A. E. (1992) Functional imaging of the brain using single photon emission computerized tomography (SPECT). *Brain Topogr.* **5,** 119–127.

27. Fowler, J. S. and Wolf, A. P. (1991) Recent advances in radiotracers for PET studies of the brain. In:(Diksic, M. and Reba, R. C., eds.) *Radiopharmaceuticals and Brain Pathology Studied with PET and SPECT.* CRC Press, Boca Raton, FL.

28. Gatley, S. J. (1993) Drug standards for iodine-123 radiopharmaceuticals. *Pharmacopeial Forum* **19,** 5850–5853.

29. Dewey, S. L., Smith, G. S., Logan, J., Brodie, J. D., Fowler, J. S., and Wolf, A. P. (1993) Striatal binding of the PET ligand ¹¹C-raclopride is altered by drugs that modify synaptic dopamine levels *Synapse* **13,** 350–356.

30. Dewey, S. L., Smith, G. S., Logan, J., and Brodie, J. D. (1993) Modulation of central cholinergic activity of GABAergic and serotonergic drugs: PET Studies with ¹¹C-benztropine in Primates *Neuropsychopharmacol-ogy* **8,** 371–376.

31. Volkow, N. D., Wang, G.-J., Fowler, J. S., Logan, J., Schlyer, D. J., Hitzemann, R., Lieberman, J., Angrist, B., Pappas, N., MacGregor, R. R., Burr, G., Cooper, T., Dewey, S. L., and Wolf, A. P. (1994) Imaging endogenous dopamine competition with [¹¹C]raclopride in the human brain. *Synapse* **16,** 255–262.

32. Holden, J. E., Gatley, S. J., Hichwa, R. D., Ip, W. R., Shaughnessy, W. J., Nickles, R. J., and Polcyn, R. E. (1981) Cerebral blood flow using PET measurements of fluoromethane kinetics. *J. Nucl. Med.* **22,** 1084–1088.

33. Reivich, M., Kuhl, D. E., Wolf, A. P., Greennberg, J., Phelps, M. E., Ido, T., Casella, V., Fowler, J. S., Hoff-man, E., Alavi, A., Som, P., and Sokoloff, L. E. (1979) The [¹⁸F]fluorodeoxyglucose method for the measure-ment of local cerebral glucose utilization in man. *Circ. Res.* **44** 127–137.

34. Gatley, S. J. (1995) Iodine-123-labeled glucose analogs — prospects for a single-photon-emitting analog of fluorine-18-labeled deoxyglucose. *Nucl. Med. Biol* **22,** 829–835.

35. Iyo, M., Namba, H., Yanagisawa, M., Hirai, S., Yui, N., and Fukui, S. (1997) Abnormal cerebral perfusion in chronic methamphetamine abusers: a study using 99MTc-HMPAO and SPECT. *Prog. Neuropsychopharma-col. Biol. Psychiatry* **21** 789–796.

36. Biegon, A. and Kerman, I. (1995) Quantitative autoradiography of cannabinoid receptors in the human brain post mortem. In:(Biegon, A. and Volkow, N. D., eds.) *Sites of Drug Action in the Human Brain.* CRC Press, Boca Raton, FL, pp. 65–74.

37. Compton, D. R., Johnson, M. R., Melvin, L. S., and Martin, B. R. (1992) Pharmacological profile of a series of bicyclic cannabinoid analogs: classification as cannabimimetic agents. *J. Pharmacol. Exp. Ther.* **260,** 201–209.

38. Compton, D. R., Gold, L. H., Ward, S. J., Balster, R. L., and Martin, B. R. 1992) Aminoalylindole analogs: cannabimimetic activity of a class of compounds structurally distinct from delta-9 tetrahydrocannabinol. *J. Pharmacol. Exp. Ther.* **263,** 1118–1126.

39. Rinaldicarmona, M., Barth, F., Heaulme, M., Shire, D., Calandra, B., Congy, C., Martinez, S., Maruani, J., Neliat, G., Caput, D., Ferrara, P., Soubrie, P., Breliere, J. C., and Lefur, G. (1994) SR141716A, a potent and selective antagonist of the brain cannabinoid receptor. *FEBS Lett.* **350.** 240–244.

40. Kilbourn, M. R. (1988) In vivo binding of [¹⁸F]GBR 13119 to the brain dopamine uptake system. *Life Sci.* **42,** 1347–1351.

41. Koeppe, R. A., Kilbourn, M. R., and Frey, K. A. (1990) Imaging and kinetic modeling of [¹⁸F]GBR 12909, a dopamine uptake inhibitor. *J. Nucl. Med.* **31,** p720.

42. Tihonen, J., Kuikka, J., Bergstrom, K., Hakola, P., Karhu, J., Ryynanen, O. P., and Fohr, J. (1995) Altered stri-atal dopamine re-uptake site densities in habitually violent and non-violent alcoholics. *Nature Med.* **1,** 654–657.

43. Boja, J. W., Mitchell, W. M., Patel, A., Kopajtic, T. A., Carroll, F. I., Lewin, A., Abraham, P., and Kuhar, M. J. (1992) High-affinity binding of [¹²⁵I]RTI-55 to dopamine and serotonin transporters in rat brain. *Synapse* **12,** 27–36.

44. Madras, B. K. (1994) 11C-WIN 35,428 for detecting dopamine depletion in mild Parkinson's disease. *Ann. Neurol.* **35,** 376–377.

45. Ding, Y. S., Fowler, J. S., Volkow, N. D., Logan, J., Gatley, S. J., and Sugano, Y. (1995) [^{11}C]d-threo-methylphenidate: a new PET ligand for the dopamine transporter. I. Characterization of its binding in the baboon brain. *J. Nucl. Med.*

46. Gatley, S. J., Ding, Y. S., Volkow, N. D., Chen, R. Y., Sugano, and, Y., Fowler, J. S. (1995) Binding of d-threo-[C-11]methylphenidate to the dopamine transporter in-vivo-insensitivity to synaptic dopamine. *Eur. J. Pharmacol.* **281,** 141–149.

47. Stathis, M., Scheffel, U., Lever, S. Z., Boja, J. W., Carroll, F. I., and Kuhar, M. J. (1995) Rate of binding of various inhibitors at the dopamine transporter in vivo. *Psychopharmacol.* **119,** 376–384.

48. Logan, J., Fowler, J. S., Volkow, N. D., Wolf, A. P., Dewey, S. L., Schlyer, D. J., MacGregor, R. R., Hitze-mann, R., Bendirem, B., Gatley, S. J., Christman, D. R. (1990) Graphical analysis of reversible radioligand binding from time activity measurements applied to [N-^{11}C-methyl]- (-)cocaine PET studies in human subjects. *J. Cereb. Blood. Flow. Metab.* **10,** 740–747.

49. Volkow, N. D., Gillespie, H., Mullani, N., Tancredi, L., Grant, C., Ivanovic, M., and Hollister, L. (1991) Cerebellar metabolic activation by delta-9-tetrahydrocannabinol in human brains. A study with positron emission tomography and ^{18}F-2-deoxy-2-fluoro-D-glucose. *Psych. Res.* **40,** 69–80.

50. Volkow, N. D., Gillespie, H., Tancredi, L., and Hollister, L. (1995) The effects of marihuana in the human brain measured with regional brain glucose metabolism. In: (Biegon, A. and Volkow, N. D., eds.) *Sites of Drug Action in the Human Brain.* CRC Press, Boca Raton, FL, pp.75–86.

51. Varma, V. K., Malhorta, A. K., Dang, R., Das, K., and Nehra, R. (1988) Cannabis and cognitive functions: a prospective study. *Drug Alcohol Depend.* **21,** 147–158.

52. Mathew, R. J., Wilson, W. H., Coleman, R. E., Turkington, T. G., and DeGrado, T. R. (1997) Marihuana intoxication and brain activation in marihuana smokers. *Life Sci.* **60,** 2075–2089.

53. deWit, H., Metz, J. T., Wagner, N., and Cooper, M. D. (1990) Behavioral and subjective effects of alcohol: relationship to cerebral metabolism using PET. *Alcohol Clin. Exp. Res.* **14,** 482–489.

54. London, E. D., Cascella, N. G., Wong, D. F., Phillips, R. L., Dannals, R. F., Links, J. M., Herning, R., Grayson, R., Jaffe, J. H., and Wagner, H. N. J. (1990) Cocaine-induced reduction of glucose utilization in human brain. A study using positron emission tomography and [fluorine 18]-fluorodeoxyglucose. *Arch. Gen. Psychiat.* **47,** 567–574.

55. London, E. D., Broussolle, E. P., Links, J. M., Wong, D. F., Cascella, N. G., Dannals, R. F., Sano, M., Herning, R., Snyde, F. R., and Rippetoe, L. R. (1990) Morphine-induced metabolic changes in human brain. Studies with positron emission tomography and [fluorine 18]fluorodeoxyglucose. *Arch. Gen. Psychiat.* **47,** 73–81.

56. Volkow, N. D., Hitzemann, R., Wolf, A. P., Logan, J., Fowler, J., Christman, D., Dewey, S., Schlyer, D., Burr, G., Vitkun, S., and Hirschowitz, J. (1990) Acute effects of ethanol on regional brain glucose metabolism and transport. *Psychiatry Res.* **35,** 39–48.

57. Volkow, N. D., Fowler, J. S., Wolf, A. P., Hitzemann, R., Dewey, S. L., Bendriem, B., Alpert, R., and Hoff, A. (1991) Changes in brain glucose metabolism in cocaine dependence and withdrawal. *Am. J. Psychiat.* **148,** 621–626.

58. Wolkin, A., Angrist, B., Wolf, A., Brodie, J., Wolkin, B., Jaeger, J., Cancro, R., and Rotrosen, J. (1987) Effects of amphetamine on local cerebral metabolism in normal and schizophrenic subjects as determined by positron emission tomography. *Psychopharmacology* **92,** 241.

59. Ernst, M., Zametkin, A. J., Matochik, J., Schmidt, M., Jons, P. H., Liebenauer. L. L., Hardy, K. K., and Cohen, R. M. (1997) Intravenous dextroamphetamine and brain glucose metabolism. *Neuropsychopharmacology* **17,** 391–401.

60. Ernst, M., Zametkin, A. J., Matochik, J. A., Liebenauer, L., Fitzgerald, G. A., and Cohen, R. M. (1994) Effects of intravenous dextroamphetamine on brain metabolism in adults with attention-deficit hyperactivity disorder (ADHD). Preliminary findings. *Psychopharmacol. Bull.* **30,** 219–225.

61. Volkow, N. D., Wang, G. J., Hitzemann, R., Fowler, J. S., Pappas, N., Lowrimore, P., Burr, G., Pascani, K., Overall, J., and Wolf, A. P. (1995) Depression of thalamic metabolism by lorazepam is associated with sleepiness. *Neuropsychopharmacol.* **12,** 123–132.

62. deWit, H., Metz, J. T., and Cooper, M. D. (1994) The effects of drugs of abuse on regional cerebral metabolism and mood. In:(Dhawan, B. N, Srimal, R. C., Raghubir, R., and Rapaka, R. S., eds.) *Recent Advances in the Study of Neurotransmitter Receptors.* Central Drug Research Institute, Lucknow, pp.482-489.

63. Volkow, N. D., Wang, G.-J., Hitzemann, R., Fowler, J. S., Burr, G., and Wolf, A. P. (1995) Recovery of Brain Glucose Metabolism in Detoxified Alcoholics. *Am. J. Psychiatry* **151,** 178–183.

10 Cannabinoid Receptors and Their Ligands in Brain and Other Tissues

Roger G. Pertwee

Abstract

Mammalian tissues contain two types of cannabinoid receptor, CB_1 and CB_2, both coupled to their effector systems through $G_{i/o}$ proteins. CB_1 receptors are present in the central nervous system as well as in certain neuronal and nonneuronal peripheral tissues. Some CB_1 receptors occur at nerve terminals where they modulate transmitter release when activated. CB_2 receptors are found mainly in cells of the immune system. The possibility that mammalian tissues express additional cannabinoid receptor types of physiological significance cannot be excluded. Indeed, preliminary pharmacological evidence supporting this possibility already exists. Endogenous ligands for cannabinoid receptors have also been discovered, the most important being arachidonoylethanolamide and 2-arachidonoyl glycerol. These ligands and their receptors constitute the endogenous cannabinoid system. The discovery of this system has important physiological, pathophysiological, pharmacological, and therapeutic implications. Already selective CB_1- and CB_2-receptor agonists and antagonists have been developed and two cannabinoid receptor agonists, Δ^9-tetrahydrocannabinol and nabilone, are used clinically as antiemetics or to boost appetite. Additional therapeutic uses of cannabinoid receptor agonists may include the suppression of some multiple sclerosis and spinal injury symptoms and the management of glaucoma, bronchial asthma, pain, and inflammatory disorders. One possible therapeutic strategy for the future is the development and use of drugs that activate cannabinoid receptors indirectly by modulating extracellular levels of endogenous cannabinoids. CB_1-receptor agonists that do not cross the blood-brain barrier or whose potency is determined more by affinity than efficacy may also have clinical potential.

1. THE ENDOGENOUS CANNABINOID SYSTEM

There is now conclusive evidence for the existence of at least two types of cannabinoid receptors in mammalian tissues, CB_1 and CB_2 (1). Both these receptor types are negatively coupled to adenylate cyclase through $G_{i/o}$ proteins and positively coupled to mitogen activated protein kinase. In addition, CB_1 receptors are positively coupled to inwardly rectifying

From: *Marihuana and Medicine*
Edited by: G. G. Nahas et al.   © Humana Press Inc., Totowa, NJ

and A-type potassium channels and negatively coupled to N-type and P/Q-type calcium channels, again through $G_{i/o}$ proteins. Other effector systems for the CB_1 receptor have also been proposed (1,2).

CB_1 receptors are present in the brain and spinal cord and in certain peripheral tissues (1). The distribution pattern of these receptors within the central nervous system is heterogeneous and can account for several prominent pharmacological properties of CB_1-receptor agonists: the ability to impair cognition and memory, to alter motor function, and to relieve pain. Organs and tissues outside the central nervous system that contain CB_1 receptors include neurons, leukocytes, spleen, some endocrine glands, heart, and parts of the reproductive, urinary and gastrointestinal tracts (1). Some central and peripheral CB_1 receptors are located at nerve terminals (1,3) where they probably modulate neurotransmitter release when activated (4–13). The concentration of CB_1 receptors is considerably less in peripheral tissues than in the central nervous system. This does not necessarily imply that peripheral CB_1 receptors are unimportant as some tissues may contain high concentrations of CB_1 receptors, localized in discrete regions such as nerve terminals that form only a small part of the total tissue mass. CB_2 receptors are expressed primarily by immune tissues, for example leukocytes, spleen, and tonsils (1). There is markedly more mRNA for CB_2 than CB_1 receptors in the immune system, the level of CB_2 mRNA in human tonsils matching that of CB_1 mRNA in the brain. Levels of CB_1 and CB_2 mRNA in human leukocytes have been shown to vary with cell type (B cells > natural killer cells > monocytes > polymorphonuclear neutrophils, T4, and T8 cells) (14). Although CB_2 mRNA has not been detected in human or rat brain (14,15), there is one report of its presence together with CB_1 mRNA both in primary cultures of cerebellar granule neurons obtained from 7- to 8-day-old mice and in cerebellar tissue taken from 4-week-old mice (16).

The discovery of CB_1 and CB_2 receptors was followed by the demonstration of the existence of endogenous cannabinoid-receptor agonists (1,17). The most important of these are arachidonoylethanolamide (anandamide) and 2-arachidonoyl glycerol, and there is evidence that both these compounds can serve as neuromodulators or neurotransmitters. This comes from demonstrations that they are synthesized by neurons, that they can undergo depolarization-induced release from neurons and that once released they are rapidly removed from the extracellular space (17,18). For anandamide, such removal seems to depend on a carrier-mediated, saturable uptake process present in neurons and astrocytes (19). Once within the cell, anandamide is presumably hydrolyzed to arachidonic acid and ethanolamine by fatty acid amide hydrolase (17,18). This is a microsomal enzyme, found both in neurons and in some nonneuronal tissues, that seems to serve as a general fatty acid amide hydrolase. Enzymic hydrolysis of 2-arachidonoyl glycerol has been detected in cytoplasmic and microsomal fractions of $N_{18}TG_2$ mouse neuroblastoma cells (20). The presence of an uptake process for 2-arachidonoyl glycerol in neurons remains to be established. However, such a process has been detected in RBL-2H3 (basophilic) cells (21). Cannabinoid receptors and their endogenous ligands together constitute what is now often referred to as "the endogenous cannabinoid system."

2. CANNABINOID-RECEPTOR LIGANDS

2.1. CB₁-Selective Ligands

The availability of CB_1 and CB_2 receptor-binding assays has facilitated the development of ligands with significant selectivity for CB_1 or CB_2 receptors (1,17). Among the former are the agonists (R)-(+)-arachidonoyl-1'-hydroxy-2'-propylamide (methanandamide), arachidonoyl-(2'-fluoroethyl)amide (O-585), and 2-methylarachidonoyl-(2'-fluoroethyl)amide (O-689).

These have 40.8-, 37.7-, and 23.2-fold greater affinity for CB_1 than CB_2 receptors respectively. They are all structural analogs of anandamide that also have in common the property of being more resistant to enzymatic hydrolysis than anandamide (17). Other important ligands are SR141716A and LY320135, both of which behave as competitive, surmountable, CB_1-selective antagonists (1,17). Methyl arachidonyl fluorophosphonate is also of interest as it behaves as a competitive, insurmountable, CB_1-receptor antagonist (22). Whether this agent also has significant affinity for CB_2 receptors remains to be established.

When administered by itself, SR141716A produces effects in some bioassay systems that are opposite in direction to those produced by cannabinoid-receptor agonists (1,4,5,8–10, 13,17,23). This presumably reflects the presence of "cannabimimetic tone" in these bioassay systems that is susceptible to reversal by SR141716A. Such tone could arise from ongoing production of an endogenous cannabinoid-receptor agonist. Alternatively (or in addition), it could stem from the presence of constitutively active cannabinoid receptors. Thus, like certain other G-protein-coupled receptors (24), it may be possible for cannabinoid receptors to exist in at least two interchangeable states, one precoupled to and the other uncoupled from the effector system. It could then be that SR141716A shows activity by itself because it is an inverse agonist rather than a pure antagonist, binding preferentially to the receptors in the uncoupled state and so shifting the equilibrium away from the receptors in the precoupled state. There is some evidence from binding experiments with [^{35}S]GTPγS for the presence of precoupled cannabinoid receptors both in certain CB_1-transfected cell lines (23,25) and in rat cerebellar membranes (26). However, whether precoupled cannabinoid receptors occur *in vivo* at concentrations that are sufficient to produce significant cannabimimetic tone remains to be established.

2.2. CB_2-Selective Ligands

CB_2-selective ligands include JWH-015 and JWH-051, SR144528, and L-759633 and L-759656 (17,27,28). These have been reported to have 27.8-, 37.5-, 728-, 793- and >1000-fold greater affinity for CB_2 than CB_1 receptors, respectively. JWH-015 and JWH-051 may both be CB_2-receptor agonists (29). Whether the Merk-Frosst compounds, L-759633 and L-759656, behave as agonists or antagonists has yet to be announced. The same applies to a range of other CB_2-selective ligands that have been developed by Merk-Frosst (28,30). SR144528 is a potent antagonist with a dissociation constant of 0.6 nM as determined by its ability to displace [^{3}H]CP55940 from specific CB_2-binding sites (27). There is evidence that SR144528 resembles the CB_1-selective antagonist, SR141716A Subheading 2.1), in being an inverse agonist rather than a pure antagonist. Thus experiments with Chinese hamster ovary cells transfected with human CB_2 receptors indicate that by itself, SR144528 augments forskolin-stimulated cyclic AMP production (27), an effect opposite in direction to that of CB_2-receptor agonists.

One compound that merits further investigation is palmitoylethanolamide. This has been shown by Facci et al. (31) to displace [^{3}H]WIN55212-2 readily from specific binding sites on the membranes of RBL-2H3 cells, which they have found to contain CB_2 but not CB_1 mRNA. In spite of these data, the identity of the sites to which palmitoylethanolamide binds in this cell line is not clear, there being evidence that this fatty acid amide has little affinity for CB_2 (or CB_1) receptors (17).

2.3. Other Cannabinoid-Receptor Ligands

Some commonly used cannabinoid-receptor agonists differ little in their affinities for CB_1 and CB_2 receptors (17). For example, Δ^9-tetrahydrocannabinol and CP55940 have each been shown in binding assays to have approximately equal affinity for these two receptor types, whereas anandamide has only marginal selectivity for CB_1 receptors and the aminoalkylindole, WIN55212-2, has only marginal selectivity for CB_2 receptors (17). In view of their binding properties, it is interesting to note that Δ^9-tetrahydrocannabinol and anandamide seem to be significantly less effective in activating CB_2 than CB_1 receptors. More specifically, there are reports that both compounds are effective inhibitors of cyclic AMP production in cell lines expressing CB_1 receptors (32–36), but produce negligible inhibition in cell lines containing only CB_2 receptors (36–38). Indeed, in one set of experiments, CB_2-receptor-mediated inhibition of adenylate cyclase was found to be antagonized by Δ^9-tetrahydrocannabinol (36). In other experiments with CB_2 receptor-containing cell lines, however, Δ^9-tetrahydrocannabinol and anandamide have been found to behave as agonists; the measured response again being inhibition of cyclic AMP production (33,39). The reason for this discrepancy remains to be established. However, one possibility is that it stems from intertissue differences in CB_2-receptor density. Thus, if Δ^9-tetrahydrocannabinol and anandamide do indeed have relatively low CB_2 efficacies, they may well elicit detectable CB_2 receptor-mediated responses only in biological systems that are particularly highly populated with this receptor type.

3. OTHER TYPES OF CANNABINOID RECEPTORS

One important question still to be resolved is that of whether mammalian tissues contain any as yet undiscovered cannabinoid receptor types or subtypes that are of physiological or clinical importance. Already, a spliced variant of CB_1 cDNA ($CB_{(1a)}$) has been isolated from a human lung cDNA library (40). However, any significant differences between the distribution pattern or pharmacological properties of CB_1 and $CB_{(1a)}$ receptors have yet to be identified (1,40). Although other evidence for novel types/subtypes of cannabinoid receptors in mammalian tissues is beginning to emerge, this is still tantalizingly incomplete and inconclusive. Consider, for example, results we have obtained with 6-iodopravadoline (AM630) in experiments using the mouse isolated vas deferens (41). This is a tissue in which cannabinoids can potently inhibit the amplitude of electrically evoked contractions, an effect that seems to depend on cannabinoid-induced inhibition of contractile neurotransmitter release and to be mediated by cannabinoid receptors located on prejunctional neurons (1,17). In these experiments, AM630 behaved as a competitive, surmountable antagonist of Δ^9-tetrahydrocannabinol, CP55940, WIN55212-2, methanandamide, and anandamide. Unexpectedly, these cannabinoid-receptor agonists did not all show the same susceptibility to antagonism by AM630, the dissociation constant (K_D) values of this compound against these agents being 14, 17.3, 36.5, 85.9, and 278.8 nM respectively (41). Such agonist-dependent variations in K_D could indicate the presence of more than one type of cannabinoid receptor in this tissue. Even though Δ^9-tetrahydrocannabinol, CP55940, and WIN55212-2 are all readily antagonized in the vas deferens by the CB_1-selective antagonist, SR141716A, (K_D = 2.66, 0.64, and 2.4 nM respectively (42)), there are some reasons for believing that AM630 may not antagonize these three cannabinoids in this tissue by binding to CB_1 receptors. First, methanandamide, which is the most CB_1-selective of the agonists we investigated (Subheading 2.1), was less susceptible than Δ^9-tetrahydrocannabinol, CP55940, or WIN55212-2 to antagonism by AM630. Second, AM630 showed markedly greater potency against WIN55212-2-induced inhibition of electrically evoked contractions of the vas deferens than against WIN55212-2-induced stimulation of [^{35}S]GTPγS binding in mouse and guinea-pig brain tissue (43,44), an effect that presumably is CB_1 receptor-mediated. More specifically, the K_D values of AM630 in the [^{35}S]GTPγS binding experiments were calculated to be 3.1 and 9.3 μM respectively and these are notably higher than its K_D value against WIN55212-2 in the vas deferens. Finally, the value of the dissociation constant of AM630 we obtained from our experiments with the vas deferens is closer to the CB_2 dissociation constant of AM630 (11.2 nM), as measured by its ability to compete with [^{3}H]CP55940 for specific CB_2 binding sites in mouse spleen, than to the CB_1 dissociation constant of AM630 (710nM), as measured by its ability to compete with [^{3}H]CP55940 for specific CB_1-binding sites in guinea-pig forebrain membranes (R. Ross and R. Pertwee, unpublished). In view of the relatively high affinity of AM630 for CB_2 receptors, it is noteworthy that in addition to CB_1 receptors, prejunctional neurons of the mouse vas deferens may contain CB_2-like receptors that can mediate inhibition of electrically evoked contractions (29). However, it is unlikely that AM630 acted through these putative receptors. Thus, even at a concentration of 316.2 nM, AM630 failed to attenuate the presumed ability of the CB_2-selective ligand, JWH-015, to activate the CB_2-like receptors of the vas deferens (29). Moreover, although the CB_2-selective antagonist, SR144528, has been shown to antagonize CP55940 in the mouse vas deferens (27), its dissociation constant for this interaction (501 nM) is closer to its CB_1 dissociation constant (437 nM) than to its CB_2 dissociation constant (0.6 nM) as measured in binding experiments with human CB_1- and CB_2-transfected Chinese hamster ovary cells. When taken together, these data raise the possibility that the mouse vas deferens contains one or more types of non-CB_1, non-CB_2 cannabinoid receptor capable of mediating inhibition of electrically evoked contractions.

4. THERAPEUTIC ASPECTS

Our present knowledge of the physiology and pathophysiology of the endogenous cannabinoid system is still at an early stage. Even so, there is already evidence that it can be modulated to therapeutic advantage. Indeed, two cannabinoid-receptor agonists are already used clinically to suppress nausea and vomiting provoked by anticancer drugs or to boost the appetite of AIDS patients (45). These are Δ^9-tetrahydrocannabinol (dronabinol), which is the main psychoactive constituent of cannabis, and its synthetic analog, nabilone (1). Possible additional therapeutic uses of cannabinoid receptor agonists include the relief of postoperative pain, cancer pain, and/or neuropathic pain; the suppression of some of the symptoms associated with multiple sclerosis or spinal injury (e.g., muscle spasms, pain, tremor, and bladder dysfunction); and the management of glaucoma, bronchial asthma, and inflammatory disorders (45–50). The CB_1 receptor antagonist, SR141716A, may also have therapeutic potential, for example in reducing memory deficits associated with aging or neurological diseases (45,46).

One important goal in the search for novel therapeutic agents is to devise strategies that will minimize the incidence of unwanted effects without also producing significant reductions in the abilities of the agents under development to produce their sought-after effect(s). For the endogenous cannabinoid system, one approach would be to seek out alternatives to centrally active CB_1-receptor agonists as these have the disadvantage of maximizing the incidence of adverse effects by producing indiscriminate activation of all CB_1 receptors. One strategy would be to develop drugs that activate the endogenous cannabinoid system indirectly by selectively inhibiting the tissue uptake or metabolism of endogenous cannabinoids so as to increase their concentrations at cannabinoid receptors. This strategy relies on the likelihood that these drugs will not affect all parts of the endogenous cannabinoid system at one time but rather produce effects only at sites where there is ongoing production of endogenous cannabinoids. As detailed elsewhere (17,18), some drugs that inhibit one or other of the processes responsible for the removal of endogenous cannabinoids from the extracellular space already exist.

As far as direct activation of CB_1 receptors is concerned, it may be possible to minimize the resulting unwanted central effects by administering a high-affinity, low-efficacy CB_1-receptor agonist (affinity-driven agonist) rather than a high-efficacy agonist (efficacy-driven agonist). This is because it is to be expected that the ability of an agonist to elicit a response will be much more affected by intertissue variations in receptor concentration or coupling efficiency when this agonist is affinity-driven than when it is efficacy-driven. Because significant regional variations within the brain both in the concentration and in the coupling efficiency of cannabinoid receptors are known (1,51), it could well be that the effects produced by an affinity-driven cannabinoid receptor agonist in vivo are fewer in number and some of them also less intense than those produced by an efficacy-driven agonist. Consequently, it might be possible to develop an affinity-driven agonist for CB_1 receptors that possesses fewer unwanted properties and yet is still capable of producing its sought-after effect(s). Current knowledge about the structural features of CB_1- or CB_2-receptor agonists that determine efficacy as opposed to receptor affinity or overall potency is still somewhat sparse. However, the recent development of the GTPγS binding assay (51,52) should help to change this situation. Indeed results obtained with this assay have already provided evidence that the relative efficacies at the CB_1 receptor of the cannabinoids CP55940, anandamide, and Δ^9-tetrahydrocannabinol are 1, 0.39, and 0.27, respectively (53). One compound that exhibits the expected properties of an affinity-driven agonist, at least in functional in vitro bioassays, is the high-affinity CB_1 receptor ligand 6'-cyanohex-2'-yne-D^8-tetrahydrocannabinol (O-823) (54). This behaves as a cannabinoid-receptor agonist in the mouse isolated vas deferens, a tissue that appears to be relatively well-populated with cannabinoid receptors, but as a cannabinoid-receptor antagonist in the myenteric plexus-longitudinal muscle preparation of guinea-pig small intestine, a tissue that seems to be less well populated with these receptors.

Another approach that could have therapeutic advantages would be the development of CB_1 receptor agonists that do not readily cross the blood-brain barrier, but that can still gain access to cannabinoid receptors in peripheral tissues. These drugs might, for example, be effective in treating disorders of gastrointestinal tract, urinogenital tract, or cardiovascular system, all of which appear to contain CB_1 receptors that modulate neurotransmitter release when activated (1,17). The probability that such agents could be designed is high, as the development of an effective CB_1-receptor antagonist that does not seem to cross the blood brain–barrier has already been reported (55).

5. CONCLUSIONS

The recent discovery of the endogenous cannabinoid system has sparked renewed interest in the therapeutic potential of cannabinoids by providing important new targets for drugs. Already a number of novel compounds has been developed that can modulate this system either directly, by selectively activating or blocking CB_1 and/or CB_2 receptors, or indirectly, by inhibiting the tissue uptake or enzymic hydrolysis of endogenous ligands for these receptors. The possible therapeutic advantages of developing CB_1-receptor agonists that do not readily cross the blood–brain barrier or that are affinity-driven have yet to be explored. Further research is also required to obtain a more complete understanding of the production, release and fate of endogenous cannabinoids and to establish the physiological roles of the endogenous cannabinoid system in greater detail than has happened to date. Knowledge about the roles of CB_2 receptors is particularly scant at present. Even so, it is tempting to speculate that one important function of both established types of cannabinoid receptor is to regulate the release of chemical messengers, the CB_1 receptor serving to modulate the release of a range of transmitters from central and peripheral neurons (Subheading 1.), and the CB_2

receptor to modulate the release of cytokines and other chemical messengers from immune cells *(56)*. Finally, the possible existence of further types or subtypes of cannabinoid receptors or of additional endogenous cannabinoids merits investigation as does the possibility that inappropriately high or low levels of cannabinoid receptor expression or of endogenous cannabinoid release may give rise to some disease states or be responsible for some of their signs and symptoms.

ACKNOWLEDGMENTS

Parts of this work were supported by grants 034924, 039538 and 047980 from the Wellcome Trust and by grant DA9158 from the National Institute on Drug Abuse.

REFERENCES

1. Pertwee, R. G. (1997) Pharmacology of cannabinoid CB_1 and CB_2 receptors. *Pharmacol. Ther.* **74,** 129–180.
2. Stefano, G.B., Liu, Y., and Goligorsky, M.S. (1996) Cannabinoid receptors are coupled to nitric oxide release in invertebrate immunocytes, microglia, and human monocytes. *J. Biol. Chem.* **271,** 19,238–19,242.
3. Tsou, K., Brown, S., Sañudo-Peña, M. C., Mackie, K., and Walker, J. M. (1998) Immunohistochemical distribution of cannabinoid CB_1 receptors in the rat central nervous system. *Neuroscience,* **83,** 393–411.
4. Gifford, A. N. and Ashby, C. R. (1996) Electrically evoked acetylcholine release from hippocampal slices is inhibited by the cannabinoid receptor agonist, WIN 55212-2, and is potentiated by the cannabinoid antagonist, SR 141716A. *J. Pharmacol. Exp. Ther.* **277,** 1431–1436.
5. Gifford, A. N., Samiian, L., Gatley, S. J., and Ashby, C. R. (1997) Examination of the effect of the cannabinoid receptor agonist, CP 55,940, on electrically evoked transmitter release from rat brain slices. *Eur. J. Pharmacol.* **324,** 187–192.
6. Shen, M., Piser, T. M., Seybold, V. S., and Thayer, S. A. (1996) Cannabinoid receptor agonists inhibit glutamatergic synaptic transmission in rat hippocampal cultures. *J. Neurosci.* **16,** 4322-4334.
7. Cadogan, A.-K., Alexander, S. P. H., Boyd, E. A., and Kendall, D. A. (1997) Influence of cannabinoids on electrically evoked dopamine release and cyclic AMP generation in the rat striatum. *J. Neurochem.* **69,** 1131–1137.
8. Schlicker, E., Timm, J., and Göthert, M. (1996) Cannabinoid receptor-mediated inhibition of dopamine release in the retina. *Naunyn-Schmiedeberg's Arch. Pharmacol.* **354,** 791–795.
9. Schlicker, E., Timm, J., Zentner, J., and Göthert, M. (1997) Cannabinoid CB_1 receptor-mediated inhibition of noradrenaline release in the human and guinea-pig hippocampus. *Naunyn-Schmiedeberg's Arch. Pharmacol.* **356,** 583–589.
10. Coutts, A. A. and Pertwee, R. G. (1997) Inhibition by cannabinoid receptor agonists of acetylcholine release from the guinea-pig myenteric plexus. *Br. J. Pharmacol.* **121,** 1557–1566.
11. Ishac, E. J. N, Jiang, L., Lake, K. D., Varga, K., Abood, M. E., and Kunos, G. (1996) Inhibition of exocytotic noradrenaline release by presynaptic cannabinoid CB_1 receptors on peripheral sympathetic nerves. *Br. J. Pharmacol.* **118,** 2023–2028.
12. Stefano, G. B., Salzet, B., Rialas, C. M., Pope, M., Kustka, A., Neenan, K., Pryor, S., and Salzet, M. (1997) Morphine- and anandamide-stimulated nitric oxide production inhibits presynaptic dopamine release. *Brain Res.* **763,** 63–68.
13. Pertwee, R. G., Fernando, S. R., Nash, J. E., and Coutts, A. A. (1996) Further evidence for the presence of cannabinoid CB_1 receptors in guinea-pig small intestine. *Br. J. Pharmacol.* **118,** 2199–2205.
14. Galiègue, S., Mary, S., Marchand, J., Dussossoy, D., Carrière, D., Carayon, P., Bouaboula, M., Shire, D., Le Fur, G., and Casellas, P. (1995) Expression of central and peripheral cannabinoid receptors in human immune tissues and leukocyte subpopulations. *Eur. J. Biochem.* **232,** 54–61.
15. Munro, S., Thomas, K. L., and Abu-Shaar, M. (1993) Molecular characterization of a peripheral receptor for cannabinoids. *Nature* **365,** 61–65.
16. Skaper, S. D., Buriani, A., Dal Toso, R., Petrelli, L., Romanello, S., Facci, L., and Leon, A. (1996) The ALIAmide palmitoylethanolamide and cannabinoids, but not anandamide, are protective in a delayed postglutamate paradigm of excitotoxic death in cerebellar granule neurons. *Proc. Nat. Acad. Sci. USA.* **93,** 3984–3989.
17. Pertwee, R. G. (1998) Advances in cannabinoid receptor pharmacology, In: *Cannabis* (Brown, D., ed.) Harwood Academic Publishers, in press.

18. Pertwee, R. G. (1998) Pharmacological, physiological and clinical implications of the discovery of cannabinoid receptors. *Biochem. Soc. Transact.* **26**, 267–272.
19. Di Marzo, V., Fontana, A., Cadas, H., Schinelli, S., Cimino, G., Schwartz, J.-C., and Piomelli, D. (1994) Formation and inactivation of endogenous cannabinoid anandamide in central neurons. *Nature* **372**, 686–691.
20. Bisogno, T., Sepe, N., Melck, D., Maurelli, S., De Petrocellis, L., and Di Marzo, V. (1997) Biosynthesis, release and degradation of the novel endogenous cannabimimetic metabolite 2-arachidonoylglycerol in mouse neuroblastoma cells. *Biochem. J.* **322**, 671–677.
21. Di Marzo, V., De Petrocellis, L., Bisogno, T., Melck, D., and Sepe, N. (1997) Cannabimimetic fatty acid derivatives: biosynthesis and catabolism, In: *Proc. 4th Int. Congress on Essential Fatty Acids and Eicosanoids, Edinburgh 20–24 July*, in press.
22. Fernando, S. R. and Pertwee, R. G. (1997) Evidence that methyl arachidonyl fluorophosphonate is an irreversible cannabinoid receptor antagonist. *Br. J. Pharmacol.* **121**, 1716–1720.
23. Bouaboula, M., Perrachon, S., Milligan, L., Canat, X., Rinaldi-Carmona, M., Portier, M., Barth, F., Calandra, B., Pecceu, F., Lupker, J., Maffrand, J.-P., Le Fur, G., and Casellas, P. (1997) A selective inverse agonist for central cannabinoid receptor inhibits mitogen-activated protein kinase activation stimulated by insulin or insulin-like growth factor 1. Evidence for a new model of receptor/ligand interactions. *J. Biol. Chem.* **272**, 22,330–22,339.
24. Milligan, G. and Bond, R. A. (1996) Inverse agonism and the regulation of receptor number. *Trends Pharmacol. Sci.* **18**, 468–474.
25. Landsman, R. S., Burkey, T. H., Consroe, P., Roeske, W. R., and Yamamura, H. I. (1997) SR141716A is an inverse agonist at the human cannabinoid CB_1 receptor. *Eur. J. Pharmacol.* **334**, R1–R2.
26. Petitet, F., Jeantaud, B., Capet, M., and Doble, A. (1997) Interaction of brain cannabinoid receptors with guanine nucleotide binding protein. A radioligand binding study. *Biochem. Pharmacol.* **54**, 1267–1270.
27. Rinaldi-Carmona, M., Barth, F., Millan, J., Derocq, J.-M., Casellas, P., Congy, C., Oustric, D., Sarran, M., Bouaboula, M., Calandra, B., Portier, M., Shire, D., Brelière, J.-C., and Le Fur, G. (1998) SR144528, the first potent and selective antagonist of the CB2 cannabinoid receptor. *J. Pharmacol. Exp. Ther.* **284**, 644–650.
28. Gareau, Y., Dufresne, C., Gallant, M., Rochette, C., Sawyer, N., Slipetz, D. M., Tremblay, N., Weech, P. K., Metters, K. M., and Labelle, M. (1996) Structure activity relationships of tetrahydrocannabinol analogues on human cannabinoid receptors. *Bioorg. Med. Chem. Letts.* **6**, 189–194.
29. Griffin, G., Fernando, S. R., Ross, R. A., MacKay, N. G., Ashford, M. L. J., Shire, D., Huffman, J. W., Yu, S., Lainton, J. A. H., and Pertwee, R. G. (1997) Evidence for the presence of CB_2-like cannabinoid receptors on peripheral nerve terminals. *Eur. J. Pharmacol.* **339**, 53–61.
30. Gallant, M., Dufresne, C., Gareau, Y., Guay, D., Leblanc, Y., Prasit, P., Rochette, C., Sawyer, N., Slipetz, D. M., Tremblay, N., Metters, K. M., and Labelle, M. (1996) New class of potent ligands for the human peripheral cannabinoid receptor. *Bioorg. Med. Chem. Letts.* **6**, 2263–2268.
31. Facci, L., Dal Toso, R., Romanello, S., Buriani, A., Skaper, S. D., and Leon, A. (1995) Mast cells express a peripheral cannabinoid receptor with differential sensitivity to anandamide and palmitoylethanolamide. *Proc. Natl. Acad. Sci. USA* **92**, 3376–3380.
32. Felder, C. C., Briley, E. M., Axelrod, J., Simpson, J. T., Mackie, K., and Devane, W. A. (1993) Anandamide, an endogenous cannabimimetic eicosanoid, binds to the cloned human cannabinoid receptor and stimulates receptor-mediated signal transduction. *Proc. Natl. Acad. Sci. USA* **90**, 7656–7660.
33. Felder, C. C., Joyce, K. E., Briley, E. M., Mansouri, J., Mackie, K., Blond, O., Lai, Y., Ma, A. L., and Mitchell, R. L. (1995) Comparison of the pharmacology and signal transduction of the human cannabinoid CB_1 and CB_2 receptors. *Mol. Pharmacol.* **48**, 443–450.
34. Vogel, Z., Barg, J., Levy, R., Saya, D., Heldman, E., and Mechoulam, R. (1993) Anandamide, a brain endogenous compound, interacts specifically with cannabinoid receptors and inhibits adenylate cyclase. *J. Neurochem.* **61**, 352–355.
35. Barg, J., Fride, E., Hanus, L., Levy, R., Matus-Leibovitch, N., Heldman, E., Bayewitch, M., Mechoulam, R., and Vogel, Z. (1995) Cannabinomimetic behavioral effects of and adenylate cyclase inhibition by two new endogenous anandamides. *Eur. J. Pharmacol.* **287**, 145–152.
36. Bayewitch, M., Rhee, M.-H., Avidor-Reiss, T., Breuer, A., Mechoulam, R., and Vogel, Z. (1996) (-)-Δ^9-Tetrahydrocannabinol antagonizes the peripheral cannabinoid receptor-mediated inhibition of adenylyl cyclase. *J. Biol. Chem.* **271**, 9902–9905.
37. Bayewitch, M., Avidor-Reiss, T., Levy, R., Barg, J., Mechoulam, R., and Vogel, Z. (1995) The peripheral cannabinoid receptor: adenylate cyclase inhibition and G protein coupling. *FEBS Letts.* **375**, 143–147.
38. Slipetz, D. M., O'Neill, G. P., Favreau, L., Dufresne, C., Gallant, M., Gareau, Y., Guay, D., Labelle, M., and Metters, K. M. (1995) Activation of the human peripheral cannabinoid receptor results in inhibition of adenylyl cyclase. *Mol. Pharmacol.* **48**, 352–361.

39. Shire, D., Calandra, B., Rinaldi-Carmona, M., Oustric, D., Pessègue, B., Bonnin-Cabanne, O., Le Fur, G., Caput, D., and Ferrara, P. (1996) Molecular cloning, expression and function of murine CB2 peripheral cannabinoid receptor. *Biochim. Biophys. Acta* **1307,** 132–136.

40. Shire, D., Carillon, C., Kaghad, M., Calandra, B., Rinaldi-Carmona, M., Le Fur, G., Caput, D., and Ferrara, P. (1995) An amino-terminal variant of the central cannabinoid receptor resulting from alternative splicing. *J. Biol. Chem.* **270,** 3726–3731.

41. Pertwee, R., Griffin, G., Fernando, S., Li, X., Hill, A., and Makriyannis, A. (1995) AM630, a competitive cannabinoid receptor antagonist. *Life Sci.* **56,** 1949–1955.

42. Pertwee, R. G., Griffin, G., Lainton, J. A. H., and Huffman, J. W. (1995) Pharmacological characterization of three novel cannabinoid receptor agonists in the mouse isolated vas deferens. *Eur. J. Pharmacol.* **284,** 241–247.

43. Hosohata, K., Quock, R. M., Hosohata, Y., Burkey, T. H., Makriyannis, A., Consroe, P., Roeske, W. R., and Yamamura, H. I. (1997) AM630 is a competitive cannabinoid receptor antagonist in the guinea pig brain. *Life Sci.* **61,** PL115–118.

44. Hosohata, Y., Quock, R. M., Hosohata, K., Makriyannis, A., Consroe, P., Roeske, W. R., and Yamamura, H. I. (1997) AM630 antagonism of cannabinoid-stimulated [^{35}S]GTPγS binding in the mouse brain. *Eur. J. Pharmacol.* **321,** R1–R3.

45. Pertwee, R. G. (1997) Cannabis and cannabinoids: pharmacology and rationale for clinical use. *Pharmaceut. Sci.* **3,** 539–545.

46. Pertwee, R. G. (1996) Cannabinoid receptor ligands: clinical and neuropharmacological considerations relevant to future drug discovery and development. *Exp. Opin. Invest. Drugs* **5,** 1245–1253.

47. Hollister, L. E. (1986) Health aspects of cannabis. *Pharmacol. Rev.* **38,** 1–20.

48. Pertwee, R. G. (1995) Pharmacological, physiological and clinical implications of the discovery of cannabinoid receptors: an overview, In: *Cannabinoid Receptors* (Pertwee, R. G., ed.), Academic Press, London, pp. 1–34.

49. Finnegan-Ling, D. and Musty, R. E. (1994) Marinol and phantom limb pain: a case study. *Proc. Int. Cannabinoid Res. Soc.* p. 53.

50. Herzberg, U., Eliav, E., Bennett, G. J., and Kopin, I. J. (1997) The analgesic effects of *R*(+)-WIN 55,212-2 mesylate, a high affinity cannabinoid agonist, in a rat model of neuropathic pain. *Neurosci. Letts.* **221,** 157–160.

51. Sim, L. J., Selley, D. E., and Childers, S. R. (1995) *In vitro* autoradiography of receptor-activated G proteins in rat brain by agonist-stimulated guanylyl 5'-[γ-[^{35}S]thio]-triphosphate binding. *Proc. Natl. Acad. Sci. USA* **92,** 7242–7246.

52. Selley, D. E., Stark, S., Sim, L. J., and Childers, S. R. (1996) Cannabinoid receptor stimulation of guanosine-5'-O-(3-[^{35}S]thio)triphosphate binding in rat brain membranes. *Life Sci.* **59,** 659–668.

53. Burkey, T. H., Quock, R. M., Consroe, P., Ehlert, F. J., Hosohata, Y., Roeske, W. R., and Yamamura, H. I. (1997) Relative efficacies of cannabinoid CB$_1$ receptor agonists in the mouse brain. *Eur. J. Pharmacol.* **336,** 295–298.

54. Pertwee, R. G., Fernando, S. R., Griffin, G., Ryan, W., Razdan, R. K., Compton, D. R., and Martin, B. R. (1996) Agonist-antagonist characterization of 6'-cyanohex-2'-yne-Δ^8-tetrahydrocannabinol in two isolated tissue preparations. *Eur. J. Pharmacol.* **315,** 195–201.

55. Pério, A., Rinaldi-Carmona, M., Maruani, J., Barth, F., Le Fur, G., and Soubrié, P. (1996) Central mediation of the cannabinoid cue: activity of a selective CB1 antagonist, SR 141716A. *Behav. Pharmacol.* **7,** 65–71.

56. Berdyshev, E. V., Boichot, E., Germain, N., Allain, N., Anger, J.-P., and Lagente, V. (1997) Influence of fatty acid ethanolamides and Δ^9-tetrahydrocannabinol on cytokine and arachidonate release by mononuclear cells. *Eur. J. Pharmacol.* **330,** 231–240.

11

Cannabinoid Interaction with Brain Reward Systems

Eliot L. Gardner

Abstract

With few exceptions, addicting drugs enhance electrical brain-stimulation reward and act as direct or indirect dopamine agonists in the reward-relevant dopaminergic projections of the medial forebrain bundle. These dopaminergic projections constitute a crucial drug-sensitive link in the brain's reward circuitry, and addictive drugs derive significant abuse liability from enhancing these circuits. Furthermore, basal aberrations in dopaminergic function within these circuits appear to constitute a major neurobiological vulnerability factor for drug addiction. Marihuana was long considered an "anomalous" addictive drug, lacking pharmacological interaction with these brain reward substrates. However, it is now clear–from more than 10 years of consistent research findings–that Δ^9-tetrahydrocannabinol (THC), marihuana's principal psychoactive constituent, acts on these brain reward substrates in strikingly similar fashion to noncannabinoid addictive drugs. Specifically, THC enhances MFB electrical brain-stimulation reward, and enhances both basal and stimulated dopamine release in reward-relevant MFB projection loci. THC's actions on these mechanisms is tetrodotoxin-sensitive, calcium-dependent, and naloxone-blockable. Furthermore, THC modulates brain μ and δ opioid receptors. Also, withdrawal from THC produces neurophysiological and neurochemical sequelae that are strikingly similar to those seen in withdrawal from other addictive drugs. Mechanistically, THC appears to act on brain reward substrates by inhibiting the reuptake of dopamine from the synaptic cleft in reward-relevant synapses of the nucleus accumbens. Behaviorally, THC enhances reward-related behaviors and incentive motivation. This paper reviews these data, and suggests that marihuana's interaction with brain reward systems is fundamentally similar to that of other addictive drugs. This paper concludes that persistent claims that cannabinoids do not interact with brain reward mechanisms must be dismissed–on the basis of more than 10 years of consistent published findings–as either uninformed or biased pleadings.

From: *Marihuana and Medicine*
Edited by: G. G. Nahas et al.   © Humana Press Inc., Totowa, NJ

1. INTRODUCTION

The reward/reinforcement circuitry of the mammalian brain consists of synaptically inter-connected neurons associated with the medial forebrain bundle (MFB), linking the ventral tegmental area, nucleus accumbens, and ventral pallidum. Electrical stimulation of this circuit supports intense self-stimulation in animals, and intense pleasure/euphoria in humans. This circuit is strongly implicated in the neural substrates of drug addiction, and in such addiction-related phenomena as withdrawal dysphoria and craving. This circuit is also implicated in the pleasures produced by natural rewards (e.g., food, sex). Cannabinoids are euphorigenic in humans and have addictive liability in vulnerable persons, but were long considered anomalous addictive drugs, lacking pharmacological action on these brain reward substrates. However, it is now clear that cannabinoids activate these brain substrates and influence reward-related behaviors in a manner strikingly similar to that of other addictive drugs.

1.1. Neuroanatomy, Neurophysiology, and Neurochemistry of Brain Reward

The brain-reward-relevant MFB-associated neuronal tracts consist of first-stage, second-stage, and third-stage reward-related neurons in series with one another (1). The first-stage neurons originate diffusely within the anterior ventral limbic forebrain–in the anterior bed nuclei of the medial forebrain bundle (anterior lateral hypothalamus, horizontal limb of the diagonal band of Broca, interstitial nucleus of the stria medullaris, lateral preoptic area, magnocellular preoptic nucleus, olfactory tubercle, substantia innominata, and ventral pallidum), presumably constituting an anatomic convergence of disparate neurally encoded information critical to the set point of hedonic tone. These first-stage reward neurons run posteriorly within the medial forebrain bundle in a myelinated moderately fast-conducting pathway of unknown neurotransmitter type, and synapse on dopamine (DA) cells in the ventral tegmental area (VTA) of the ventral mesencephalon. The second-stage DA neurons project anteriorly within the MFB to the nucleus accumbens (NAcb), where they synapse on a variety of cell types. Only a small subset of these DA neurons appear specialized for carrying reward-relevant information. From NAcb, third-stage reward-relevant neurons carry the rewarding neural signal further. This third-stage pathway uses the endogenous opioid peptide enkephalin as its primary neurotransmitter and projects anatomincally to the ventral pallidum (VP). This third-stage output pathway appears critical for the expression of reward-related and incentive-related behaviors. Mutually reciprocal anatomic interconnections exist between VP, NAcb, and VTA, important to the set-point of reward functions and reward-driven behaviors. Another NAcb output pathway–the medium spiny output neurons which use γ-aminobutyric acid (GABA) as a neurotransmitter, and especially that portion in which the opioid neuropeptide enkephalin is colocalized–may constitute another brain reward output path. Additional circuits synapse onto the first-stage, second-stage, or third-stage elements of this brain reward system, to regulate the overall hedonic set-point. The neurotransmitters of some of these regulatory circuits are known–including opioid peptides, serotonin, glutamate, and GABA. The reward-related neurons in these pathways may be functionally heterogeneous–with some neurons encoding reward magnitude per se, whereas others encode expectancy of reward, errors in reward-prediction, prioritized reward, and other more complex aspects of reward-driven learning and reward-related incentive motivation (2–5). Amongst this complexity, however, one of the primary functions of those reward substrates is to compute hedonic tone and neural payoffs. These brain circuits appear to have evolved to subserve natural, biologically significant rewards (6–9).

1.2. Actions of Addictive Drugs on Brain Reward Mechanisms

Whereas the first-stage reward neurons are preferentially activated by electrical brain stimulation reward (BSR), it is on the second-stage DA convergence–with its DA cell bodies in VTA and DA axon terminals in NAcb–that addictive drugs act to enhance brain reward functions and produce the pleasurable/euphoric effects that constitute the high or rush sought by drug addicts. Thus, this DA component appears to be the crucial convergence upon which addictive drugs (regardless of chemical structure or pharmacological category) act to enhance neural reward functions, subjective experience of reward, and reward-related behaviors. Drug reward *per se* and drug potentiation of electrical brain stimulation reward appear to have common substrates within these reward circuits. BSR and the pharmacological rewards of addicting drugs appear to hijack these reward circuits to produce their habit-forming effects *(10)*. Also, aberrations within these brain reward circuits appear to confer vulnerability to drug addiction and dependence *(11–14)*.

2. CANNABINOID EFFECTS ON BRAIN REWARD SUBSTRATES

Although marihuana and other cannabinoids have clear addictive potential *(15–21)*, they have been considered by some to be anomalous drugs of abuse, lacking interaction with brain reward substrates *(see, e.g., ref22)*. That position is absolutely untenable, in view of more than 10 years of research that shows clearly that marihuana and other cannabinoids have potent augmenting effects on brain reward mechanisms.

2.1. Cannabinoids Enhance Electrical Brain Stimulation Reward

As early as 1988, my research group showed that Δ^9-tetrahydrocannabinol (THC), the psychoactive and addictive constituent of marihuana and hashish, enhances electrical BSR (i.e., lowers brain reward thresholds) in the MFB of laboratory rats *(23)*. For these experiments, a titrating threshold electrical BSR procedure was used in which the animal indicates its threshold for brain reward on a minute-to-minute basis. This is accomplished by using test chambers containing two response levers. Each response by an animal on the primary or stimulation lever delivers BSR, the intensity of which (in μA) decrements by a fixed percentage at every third press of the primary lever. At any point during the ensuing decremental BSR, the animal can reset the current back up to maximum by pressing a "reset" lever (which does not itself deliver BSR). The mean self-determined reset level is operationally defined as the brain reward threshold. Whereas neither saline nor the 20% polyvinylpyrrolidone (PVP) vehicle had any effect, 1.5 mg/kg (intraperitoneally) THC significantly lowered MFB BSR thresholds *(23–25)* (Fig. 1). We have also examined the effects of THC on BSR thresholds using a rate-frequency curve-shift quantitative electrophysiological brain-reward-threshold paradigm *(26,27)*. Animals were trained to lever press for a series of 16 different pulse frequencies, ranging from 25 to 141 Hz, presented in descending order. At each pulse frequency, animals responded for two 30-second time periods (bins), following which the pulse frequency was decreased by 0.05 log units. Two measures of reward threshold were recorded: M_{50}–the pulse frequency at which the animals responded at half-maximum; and Θ_0–the frequency at which animals ceased to respond for rewarding stimulation. Both are reliable indices of reward efficacy. Reward thresholds were considered stable when M_{50} and Θ_0 were within 0.01 log units of their respective previous values for three consecutive days. Animals were then injected with the vehicle solution and tested in the brain reward procedure. The next day, animals were injected with 1.0 mg/kg THC (intraperitoneally) and tested in the brain reward procedure. On each test day, testing began 20 minutes after vehicle or THC injection. THC significantly enhanced BSR (i.e., lowered reward thresholds) *(26,27)*.

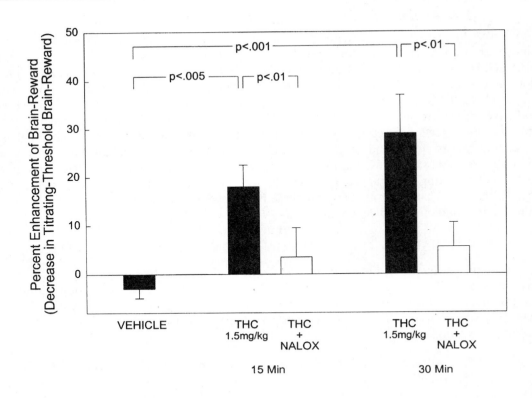

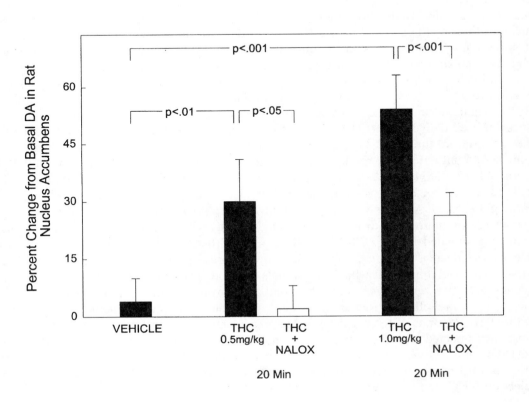

Fig. 1 (left). Enhanced brain-stimulation reward (top) and enhanced nucleus accumbens extracellular dopamine overflow (bottom) following acute systemic administration of Δ^9-tetrahydrocannabinol (THC), the psychoactive and addictive constituent of marihuana and hashish, and attenuation of resulting enhancements by acute naloxone (NALOX). Top: Enhanced brain reward (decreased electrical brain-stimulation reward thresholds, measured by titrating-threshold quantitative electrophysiological brain reward procedure through electrodes implanted in the medial forebrain bundle) produced by THC at 15 and 30 minutes postinjection, and attenuation of THC's brain-reward enhancement by naloxone. Bottom: Enhanced extracellular dopamine overflow (measured by in vivo brain microdialysis in brain-reward-relevant nucleus accumbens dopamine axon terminals) produced by THC over a 20 minute microdialysis sampling period post-THC, and attenuation of THC's nucleus accumbens dopamine enhancement by naloxone. Probability values are for the comparisons shown.

2.2 Cannabinoids Enhance Extracellular DA Overflow in Brain Reward Loci

2.2.1 IN VIVO BRAIN MICRODIALYSIS STUDIES

As early as 1986, my research group showed that THC enhances extracellular DA overflow in reward-relevant brain loci, as measured by in vivo brain microdialysis *(28)* (Fig. 1). Subsequent work, both by my group *(29–32)* and others *(33)*, has amply confirmed those original reports. The DA-enhancing effect is tetrodotoxin-sensitive and calcium-dependent *(24,25,32)*, and is seen not only in NAcb *(32)* but also in other reward-relevant forebrain DA terminal projection loci, including medial prefrontal cortex *(31)* and neostriatum *(28,29,33)*. Very recently, Tanda, Pontieri, and Di Chiara published a complete confirmation of the previous demonstrations from my research group of an enhancing effect of cannabinoids on extracellular NAcb DA *(34)*. Tanda et al. found that the DA-enhancing effect occurs selectively within NAcb shell–not unexpected, given that the shell seems specialized for mediating drug-enhanced brain reward *(1,35–38)*. Also, Tanda et al. extended the previous demonstrations from my group of cannabinoid-induced DA augmentation to include the synthetic cannabinoid agonist WIN55212–2, and showed that the effects on DA were blocked by the selective cannabinoid antagonist SR141716A.

2.2.2. IN VIVO BRAIN VOLTAMMETRIC ELECTROCHEMISTRY STUDIES

As early as 1988, my research group showed THC-induced synaptic DA enhancement in reward-relevant forebrain loci using yet another in vivo method–voltammetric electrochemistry *(29)*. Thus, despite one negative report *(39)*, the overwhelming evidence from several different labs and using two different in vivo neurochemical techniques is that cannabinoids enhance extracellular DA in the reward-relevant forebrain. Therefore, persistent claims that cannabinoids do not interact with DA brain reward substrates (e.g., ref.22) must be dismissed as either uninformed or biased pleadings.

2.3. Cannabinoids May Enhance DA Neuronal Firing in Brain Reward Circuits

Some addictive drugs enhance DA functions in reward-relevant brain loci by enhancing DA release or inhibiting DA reuptake (e.g., amphetamines, cocaine) *(1)*. Other compounds (e.g., opioids, nicotine) act by stimulating the firing rate of the second-stage reward-relevant DA neurons *(1,40,41)*. The question arises as to whether cannabinoids augment DA function in the DA reward system by augmenting *neuronal firing* within that system. My colleagues and I could find no evidence for such an effect by THC, using single-neuron electrophysiological recording techniques in the VTA *(42)*. On the other hand, French *(43)* recently reported finding that THC *does* augment the firing of single VTA DA neurons, and that this effect is blocked by the cannabinoid antagonist SR141716A. Given the similar methods used, the dissimilar findings are not readily explicable. But given French's positive finding, it must be concluded that cannabinoids may well augment DA neuronal firing in at least a subset of the reward-relevant DA projections from VTA to NAcb.

2.4. Cannabinoid Enhancement of Brain Reward Substrates Occurs at Doses Relevant to Human Marihuana Use

We have consistently seen the above-outlined effects of THC on brain reward and on extracellular DA overflow in brain reward loci at doses ranging from 0.5 to 2.0 mg/kg (23–32). The question arises as to the relevance of such doses to human marihuana use. Rosenkrantz and colleagues (44) translated THC oral doses in rats to inhalation doses in humans by correcting for 7:1 differences in body surface area, 50% pyrolysis, and a 3:1 difference in oral: inhalation dose. Taking these assumptions, one marihuana cigarette per day weighing 1 g with 2% THC would result in absorption of 0.2 mg/kg THC. Marihuana smoking of one to three cigarettes per day is well within the range of human use. After converting oral to intraperitoneal doses, these calculations indicate that the robust effects we see with THC in the 0.5–2.0 mg/kg range correspond to human use of as few as one to two marihuana cigarettes of moderate THC content, and thus relevant to human marihuana use.

2.5. Cannabinoid Enhancement of Brain Reward Substrates Shows Genetic Variation

Genetic differences are known to influence both addictive drug preference and propensity to self-administer (11,45–50), and some animal strains that show high ethanol preference and self-administration generalize this drug-seeking behavior to other addictive drugs such as nicotine and opiates (46,48,51,52). This suggests that generalized vulnerability to the rewarding effects of addictive drugs may have at least a partial genetic basis. The Lewis rat strain is particularly intriguing. Lewis rats appear to be inherently drug-seeking and drug-preferring–they work harder for opiate and cocaine self-administration, cue-condition more readily to opiates and cocaine, and voluntarily drink ethanol more readily, than other rat strains (11,47–49,53). To see if cannabinoid effects on brain reward are subject to similar genetic variation, my research group compared the effects of THC on brain reward substrates in addictive-drug-preferring Lewis rats, addictive-drug-neutral Sprague-Dawley

Fig. 2 (right). Genetic variation in enhanced brain-stimulation reward (top) and enhanced nucleus accumbens extracellular dopamine overflow (bottom) following acute systemic administration of Δ^9-tetrahydrocannabinol (THC), the psychoactive and addictive constituent of marihuana and hashish. Top: Enhanced brain reward (decreased electrical brain-stimulation reward thresholds, measured by rate-frequency curve-shift quantitative electrophysiological brain reward procedure through electrodes implanted in the medial forebrain bundle) produced by THC in rats of the drug-seeking Lewis strain, the drug-neutral Sprague-Dawley strain, and the drug-rejecting Fischer 344 strain. In Lewis rats, THC significantly shifted the brain-reward function curve to the left (enhanced brain reward), as indicated by significant leftward shifts in both M_{50} and Θ_0 points (see text). In Sprague-Dawley rats, THC enhanced brain stimulation reward only in terms of a significant leftward shift in the Θ_0 point (see text). In Fischer 344 rats, THC did not significantly affect the brain stimulation reward function curve. Bottom: Enhanced extracellular dopamine overflow (measured by in vivo brain microdialysis in brain-reward-relevant nucleus accumbens dopamine axon terminals) produced by THC in rats of the drug-seeking Lewis strain, the drug-neutral Sprague-Dawley strain, and the drug-rejecting Fischer 344 strain. In Lewis rats, THC significantly enhanced nucleus accumbens dopamine at both 1.0 mg/kg and 0.5 mg/kg THC. In Sprague-Dawley rats, THC significantly enhanced nucleus accumbens dopamine only at 1.0 mg/kg THC. In Fischer 344 rats, THC did not significantly affect nucleus accumbens dopamine at either 1.0 mg/kg or 0.5 mg/kg THC.

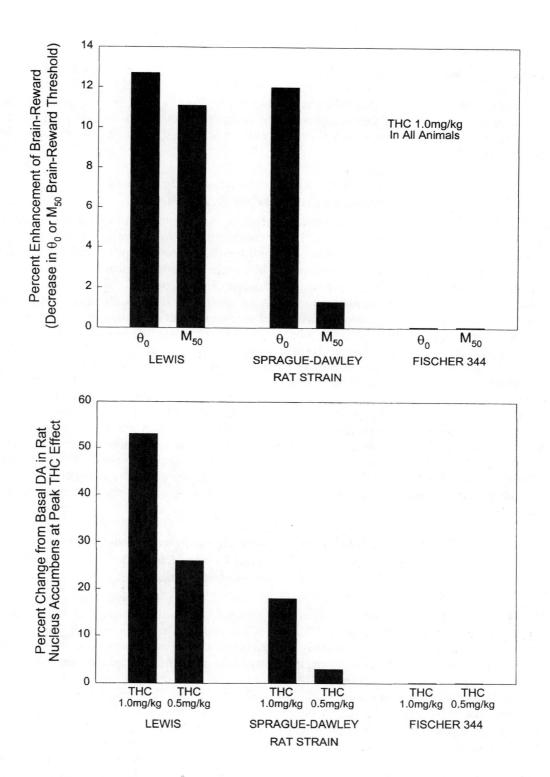

rats, and addictive-drug-resistant Fischer 344 rats. Using quantitative electrophysiological brain-stimulation techniques, we found that THC produces robust enhancement of BSR in drug-preferring Lewis rats, moderate enhancement in drug-neutral Sprague-Dawley rats, and no change in drug-resistant Fischer 344 rats (26,27,54,55) (Fig. 2). We further found, using in vivo brain microdialysis, that THC produces robust enhancement of NAcb DA in drug-preferring Lewis rats, moderate enhancement in drug-neutral Sprague-Dawley rats, and no change in drug-resistant Fischer 344 rats (55,56) (Fig. 2). We suggest that the behavioral vulnerability of Lewis rats to cannabinoids and other addicting drugs arises, at least partly, from this augmented vulnerability of brain reward substrates to enhancement by addicting drugs.

2.6. Cannabinoid Enhancement of Brain Reward Substrates is Naloxone Reversible

The DA brain reward system is interconnected with endogenous opioid peptide neural systems in VTA, NAcb, and VP (1). These endogenous opioid peptide systems appear important for the set-point of hedonic tone, and for the expression of reward-related and incentive-related behaviors (1). Furthermore, the brain reward enhancement produced by all well-studied addictive drugs (including nonopiates such as ethanol, barbiturates, benzodiazepines, phencyclidine, amphetamines, and cocaine) is blocked or attenuated by opiate antagonists (1), implicating endogenous opioid mechanisms in mediating the euphorigenic action of such drugs. The question thus arises as to the possible role of endogenous opioid mechanisms in cannabinoid effects on brain reward systems. As early as 1989, my research group addressed this question, using both BSR and in vivo microdialysis techniques. We reported almost 10 years ago that the opiate antagonist naloxone attenuates THC-induced BSR enhancement (24,25,57) (Fig. 1). We also found that naloxone attenuates THC-induced enhancement of NAcb DA (24,25,30,32,58) (Fig. 1). Very recently, Tanda et al. (34) have independently confirmed these results from my research group. They also report that the selective μ_1 opiate antagonist naloxonazine duplicates the naloxone effect, implicating the μ_1 opiate receptor subtype in mediating cannabinoid effects on brain reward. These findings by my group and the confirmation by Tanda et al. are congruent with an older report that naloxone attenuates THC-enhanced DA synthesis in brain, as measured by in vitro biochemistry (59).

2.7. Cannabinoid Enhancement of Brain Reward Substrates Within the MFB-Associated Reward Circuitry May Be Localized in the Nucleus Accumbens

Different addictive drugs enhance brain reward by acting at different sites within the MFB-associated reward circuitry. Nicotine, ethanol, benzodiazepines, and barbiturates appear to act (primarily transsynaptically) in VTA; cocaine, amphetamines, and dissociative anesthetics appear to act primarily in NAcb (1). Opiates act on reward substrates in VTA, NAcb, and VP (1). As early as 1992, my colleagues and I examined the effects of local cannabinoid microinjection on DA overflow in reward-relevant brain loci (60). THC microinfusions into NAcb dose-dependently enhanced NAcb DA, whereas THC microinjections into VTA dose-dependently increased VTA DA. However, VTA THC microinjections did not alter NAcb DA. This suggests that local VTA THC does not alter local DA neuronal firing. We surmise that the elevated NAcb DA and augmented electrical BSR produced by systemic THC result from local actions by THC at or near the reward-relevant DA axon terminals in NAcb (60). On the other hand, Tanda et al. have reported that local microinjections of the μ_1 opioid antagonist naloxonazine into VTA attenuate cannabinoid-enhanced NAcb DA, which they interpret as implicating a VTA site of action for cannabinoid effects on brain reward substrates (34).

2.8. *Cannabinoid Enhancement of Brain Reward Resembles That of a DA Reuptake Blocker*

Different addictive drugs enhance brain reward by acting through different mechanisms within the reward circuitry. Amphetamines (and probably some phencyclidine-like dissociative anesthetics) act as presynaptic DA releasers, cocaine as a presynaptic DA reuptake blocker, opiates and nicotine as transsynaptic enhancers of DA neuronal firing, and other addictive drugs by yet other mechanisms (1). As early as 1988, my research group began to explore the mechanism(s) by which cannabinoids enhance DA function in the reward circuitry of the brain. As noted in the previous paragraph, our studies using local intracerebral THC microinjections led us to surmise that THC's principal site of action is in the vicinity of the reward-relevant NAcb DA axon terminals (60). This in itself narrows the field of possible mechanisms, as it eliminates opiate-like or nicotine-like transsynaptic augmentation of neuronal firing (albeit with the caution of French's findings, noted above, ref. 43). Also, as noted above, we found that THC-induced NAcb DA augmentation is calcium-dependent and tetrodotoxin-sensitive (24,25,32), implicating an action-potential-dependent mechanism. We also found–using in vivo voltammetric electrochemistry to study THC-induced synaptic DA overflow in forebrain DA terminal projection fields–that the THC-induced electrochemical signature resembles that of a DA reuptake blocker rather than that of a presynaptic DA releaser (29) (Fig. 3). To further explore the hypothesis that cannabinoids may act (possibly indirectly or transsynaptically) to inhibit presynaptic DA reuptake, we carried out additional experiments. First, we explored the effects of various combinations of THC and the DA-receptor blocker haloperidol on NAcb DA using in vivo brain microdialysis (61). The rationale for this is that impulse-induced facilitation of DA release underlies a synergistic effect between DA receptor blockers and DA-reuptake inhibitors (62). We found that pretreatment with the DA-receptor blocker haloperidol (0.1 mg/kg) has a synergistic effect on THC's enhancement of NAcb DA, and that THC (1.0 mg/kg) pretreatment before haloperidol has a similar synergistic effect on haloperidol's enhancement of NAcb DA (61). Tetrodotoxin perfused locally into NAcb abolished the synergism between THC and haloperidol (61). Since this type of synergistic effect on DA is highly characteristic of the effect seen with coadministration of a DA antagonist such as haloperidol and a DA-reuptake blocker such as GBR12909 (62,63), we suggest that the synergistic enhancement of haloperidol-induced increase in NAcb DA by THC is consistent with the notion that THC's enhancing action on NAcb DA results from DA reuptake blockade (possibly indirect or transsynaptically mediated) at NAcb DA terminals (24,25,61). Second, we also explored this hypothesis using in vivo microdialysis of the DA metabolite 3-methoxytyramine (3-MT) (64). Whereas only a small portion of released DA is metabolized to it, 3-MT is believed to be a sensitive index of enhanced extracellular DA (65) and–most importantly–a sensitive marker for distinguishing DA releasing agents from DA reuptake blockers since DA releasers such as amphetamine and methamphetamine increase 3-MT levels, whereas DA-reuptake blockers such as bupropion and nomifensine do not (66). We therefore examined the effects of amphetamine, cocaine, nomifensine, and THC on extracellular NAcb 3-MT levels using in vivo microdialysis. We found that the DA releaser amphetamine significantly increased both DA and 3-MT in NAcb, whereas the DA-reuptake blockers cocaine and nomifensine increased only DA (64). THC increased only DA, resembling the DA reuptake blockers (64). These in vivo findings are congruent with older in vitro studies showing that cannabinoids have DA reuptake blockade actions in brain tissue (67–69).

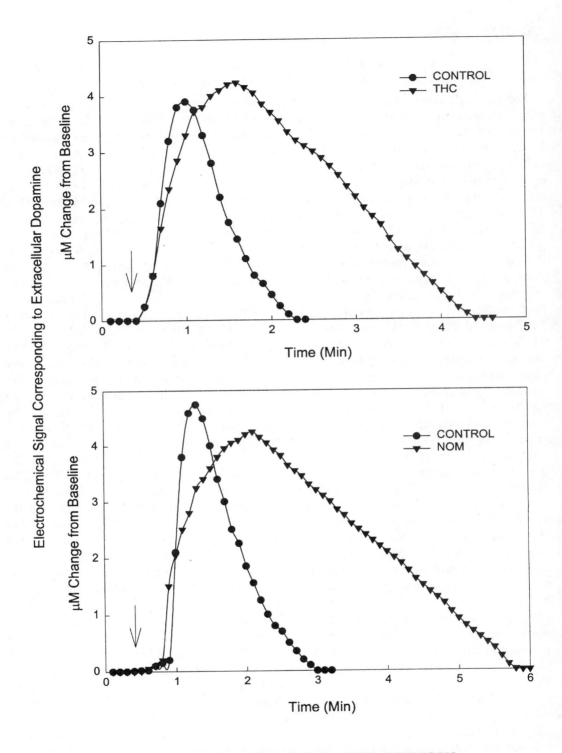

3. CANNABINOID EFFECTS ON ENDOGENOUS BRAIN OPIOID SYSTEMS

As noted, the opiate antagonist naloxone antagonizes THC's effects on electrical BSR and on DA in brain reward loci. On these grounds alone, one may hypothesize an important interaction between endogenous brain opioid systems and the neural substrates through which

Fig. 3 (left). Enhanced extracellular dopamine overflow in forebrain dopamine axon terminals following acute systemic administration of (top) Δ^9-tetrahydrocannabinol (THC), the psychoactive and addictive constituent of marihuana and hashish, or (bottom) the presynaptic dopamine reuptake blocker nomifensine (NOM), as measured by in vivo voltammetric brain electrochemistry. Top: Effect of THC (0.5 mg/kg, ip) on K$^+$-evoked voltammetric electrochemical signals corresponding to extracellular dopamine. The arrow indicates the timing of the localized intracerebral micropressure K$^+$ applications. Bottom: Effect of NOM (5.0 mg/kg, ip) on K$^+$-evoked voltammetric electrochemical signals corresponding to extracellular dopamine. The arrow indicates the timing of the localized intracerebral micropressure K$^+$ applications. The time-dynamic profile of the THC-enhanced extracellular dopamine signal is identical to that of the NOM-enhanced extracellular dopamine signal, raising the possibility that THC may act on reward-relevant forebrain dopamine neurons by inhibiting presynaptic DA reuptake. (Reprinted from *Brain Research*; vol. 451; J.M. Ng Cheong Ton, G.A. Gerhardt, M. Friedemann, A.M. Etgen, G.M. Rose, N.S. Sharpless, and E.L. Gardner; The effects of Δ^9-tetrahydrocannabinol on potassium-evoked release of dopamine in the rat caudate nucleus: an in vivo electrochemical and in vivo microdialysis study; pp. 59–68; Copyright 1988; with permission from Elsevier Science).

cannabinoids act on brain reward. Other findings also support the concept that at least some cannabinoid effects on the brain are mediated by endogenous opioid systems: pharmacological effects of THC other than those on reward mechanisms are also blocked by opiate antagonists *(70,71)*; THC ameliorates naloxone-precipitated opiate withdrawal *(72,73)*; and THC's effects on luteinizing hormone releasing hormone and prolactin are naloxone-blockable *(74)*. In addition, endogenous opioid peptide mechanisms appear to be crucial for the set-point of hedonic tone within the reward circuits of the forebrain and for expression of reward-related and incentive-related behaviors *(1)*. We and others have therefore studied interactions of cannabinoids with endogenous brain opioid systems.

3.1. Cannabinoids Modulate Brain Opioid Receptors

As early as 1985, my colleagues and I examined the in vitro effects of THC and other cannabinoids on brain opioid receptors, as well as on cholinergic (muscarinic) and DA receptors *(75)*. We found that THC produced a dose-dependent inhibition of μ and δ opioid receptor binding (decreased receptor density; no change in receptor affinity) in both membrane-bound and solubilized partially purified brain opioid receptor preparations *(75)*, but failed to alter κ, σ, DA, or muscarinic binding. We proposed that cannabinoids produce a direct allosteric modulation of the opioid receptor complex *(75)*. We also compared the potencies of a large number of cannabinoids to inhibit μ-receptor binding, and found a good correlation with psychoactive potencies in humans *(75)*. In an analogous experiment (but with significant methodological differences), Ali et al. were unable to find any cannabinoid effects on opioid-receptor binding in rat brain *(76)*.

3.2. Cannabinoids Modulate Brain Opioid Neurotransmitters

In studies of cannabinoid effects on endogenous opioid neurotransmitters, a reasonably consistent pattern emerges–chronic THC treatment during adulthood or perinatally results in significantly elevated levels of methionine enkephalin and β-endorphin in virtually all brain areas sampled, and in significantly elevated methionine enkephalin-like and β-endorphin-like immunoreactivity in the preoptic area and medial basal hypothalamus *(74,77–79)*.

4. CANNABINOID WITHDRAWAL EFFECTS ON REWARD-RELATED BRAIN MECHANISMS

As noted, addictive drugs enhance BSR and augment DA in brain reward loci. Conversely, *withdrawal* from addictive drugs produces *inhibition* of BSR and *depletion* of DA in brain

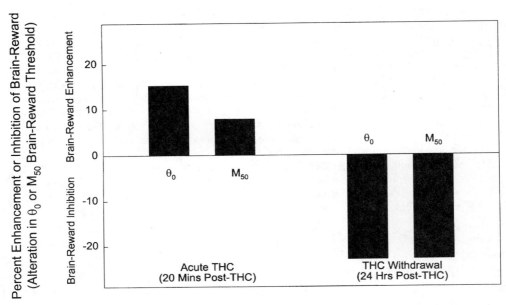

Fig. 4. Enhanced brain-stimulation reward following acute systemic administration of 1.0 mg/kg i.p. Δ^9-tetrahydrocannabinol (THC), the psychoactive and addictive constituent of marihuana and hashish (left two bars) and *diminished* brain-stimulation reward during withdrawal from an acute 1.0 mg/kg dose of THC (right two bars). Enhanced brain-reward is experimentally defined as a left-shift, and diminished brain-reward as a right-shift, in mean quantitative electrophysiological rate-frequency curve-shift electrical brain stimulation reward functions from brain-reward electrodes in the medial forebrain bundle (*see* text). THC significantly shifted the brain-reward function curve to the left (enhanced brain reward), as indicated by significant leftward shifts in the Θ_0 and M_{50} points (left two bars). *Withdrawal* from THC significantly shifted the brain-reward function curve to the right (diminished brain reward), as indicated by significant rightward shifts in the M_{50} and Θ_0 points (right two bars).

reward loci (*80–86*). Recently, Koob and colleagues have proposed yet another common feature of withdrawal from addictive drugs–elevations of corticotropin-releasing factor (CRF) in the central nucleus of the amygdala (*87–89*). This is provocative, as the amygdala has been implicated in mediating neural substrates of an emotional memory system that facilitates drug-seeking behavior (*90–94*). It may thus be asked whether cannabinoid withdrawal mimics withdrawal from other addicting drugs, either in regards to BSR thresholds or amygdaloid CRF. With respect to BSR, my research group has reported (*95*) that withdrawal from as little as a single 1.0 mg/kg dose of THC produces significant elevation in brain reward threshold (Fig. 4), identical to that seen in withdrawal from other addictive drugs. With respect to amygdaloid CRF, Rodríguez de Fonseca and colleagues have recently shown that cannabinoid withdrawal is accompanied by marked elevation in extracellular amygdaloid CRF similar to that seen in withdrawal from other addictive drugs (*96*).

4. CANNABINOID EFFECTS ON REWARD-RELATED BEHAVIORS

4.1. Cannabinoid Effects on Conditioned Taste Preference/Aversion

Conditioned taste preference/aversion is used for inferring drug appetitiveness/aversiveness. Conditioned taste preference is the learned approach and consumption of a substance, if followed by reward. Conditioned taste aversion (CTA) is the learned avoidance of a substance, if followed by an aversive state. Cannabinoids produce CTAs *(97–102)*. But many drugs produce CTAs at doses that are *clearly rewarding* when assessed by other techniques. This paradox is seen even when the same drug produces CTAs *and* conditioned place *prefer-ence(103)*, *avid* intravenous drug self-administration *(104)*, or *enhanced* speed of running to a goal box where the drug is given *(105)*. Thus, many drugs with rewarding/addicting proper-ties serve as compound stimuli, evoking both reward and aversion *(104)*, and the CTA para-digm appears uniquely sensitive to the aversive properties.

4.2. Cannabinoid Effects on Conditioned Cue or Place Preference/Aversion

Conditioned cue or place preference/aversion is also used for inferring drug appetitive-ness/aversiveness *(106)*. Several groups have reported that cannabinoids appear aversive in this paradigm *(101,102,107,108)*. On the other hand, my research group has found that THC produces robust conditioned place *preferences (109,110)*. We found that timing and dose were critical, as is the case for other addicting drugs *(25,111–113)*. In humans, a parallel phe-nomenon is seen–low THC doses produce a high; high doses are aversive *(114–116)*. Provocatively, Rubio et al. report that adult rats exposed pre- and perinatally to THC show enhanced morphine place preference *(117)*.

4.3. Cannabinoid Effects on Natural Reward-Related Behaviors

In general, cannabinoids augment the consumption of sweet foods and solutions (which are presumably naturally rewarding) *(118–120)*, and increase the reward value of ingested foods and solutions as assessed by a progressive-ratio break-point reinforcement schedule *(121)*. Provocatively, Arnone and colleagues have recently reported *(122)* that sucrose con-sumption is *inhibited* by a cannabinoid *antagonist*, suggesting that basal activity within cen-tral endogenous cannabinoid circuits is important for the central reward processes activated by such natural rewards, and may act to augment their incentive-reward value. Noncannabi-noid addicting drugs share this property of augmenting consumption and increasing reward value of naturally rewarding substances *(120)*.

4.4. Cannabinoid Self-Administration in Animal Model Systems

Peculiarly, cannabinoids are not reliably self-administered in animals *(123–132)*. Many plausible reasons can be adduced for this, including genetic differences between animal strains *(25)*, cannabinoid-induced stress effects *(133,134)*, and technical difficulties in work-ing with insoluble natural cannabinoids. Recently, Fratta and colleagues reported robust intra-venous self-administration of the synthetic cannabinoid agonist WIN55212–2 in drug-naive mice, and reported that this effect was blocked by the cannabinoid antagonist SR141716A *(135)*. Additional studies are clearly needed to resolve the issue of cannabinoid self-adminis-tration in animal models.

4. CONCLUSIONS

Cannabinoids activate the reward circuitry of the mammalian brain, as measured electro-physiologically and biochemically, in a manner akin to that of other addicting drugs. Withdrawal phenomena characteristic of other addicting drugs are also seen both electro-physiologically and biochemically in cannabinoid withdrawal. Cannabinoids are euphorigenic in humans and have addictive liability in vulnerable persons, but were long considered anom-alous drugs of abuse, lacking pharmacological action on brain reward substrates. On the basis of more than 10 years of highly consistent work with many different brain-reward-related paradigms, it is clear that such a presumption is no longer tenable, and persistent claims to the contrary must be dismissed as uninformed or biased pleadings.

5. ACKNOWLEDGEMENTS

Work from the author's laboratory cited in this paper was supported the U.S. National Institutes of Health (grant RR05397), National Institute on Drug Abuse (grants DA02089, DA03622), National Institute on Alcohol Abuse and Alcoholism (grant AA09547), National Science Foundation (grant BNS-86–09351); and by the Natural Sciences and Engineering Research Council of Canada, the New York State Office of Alcoholism and Substance Abuse Services, and the Aaron Diamond Foundation of New York.

REFERENCES

1. Gardner, E. L. (1997) Brain reward mechanisms. In *Substance Abuse: A Comprehensive Textbook, 3rd ed.* (Lowinson, J. H., Ruiz, P., Millman, R. B. and Langrod, J. G., eds.), Williams & Wilkins, Baltimore, MD, pp. 51–85.
2. Gardner, E. L. and Lowinson, J. H. (1993) Drug craving and positive/negative hedonic brain substrates activated by addicting drugs. *Sem. Neurosci.* **5**, 359–368.
3. Di Chiara, G. (1995) The role of dopamine in drug abuse viewed from the perspective of its role in motivation. *Drug Alc. Depend.* **38**, 95–137.
4. Schultz, W., Dayan, P. and Montague, P. R. (1997) A neural substrate of prediction and reward. *Science* **275**, 1593–1599.
5. Wickelgren, I. (1997) Getting the brain's attention. *Science* **278**, 35–37.
6. Kornetsky, C. and Bain, G. (1992) Brain-stimulation reward: a model for the study of the rewarding effects of abused drugs. *Natl. Inst. Drug Abuse Res. Monogr. Ser.* **124**, 73–93.
7. Kornetsky, C. and Duvauchelle, C. (1994) Dopamine, a common substrate for the rewarding effects of brain stimulation reward, cocaine, and morphine. *Natl. Inst. Drug Abuse Res. Monogr. Ser.* **145**, 19–39.
8. Shizgal, P. (1997) Neural basis of utility estimation. *Curr. Opinion Neurobiol.* **7**, 198–208.
9. Wise, R. A. (1996) Addictive drugs and brain stimulation reward. *Annu. Rev. Neurosci.* **19**, 319–340.
10. Goldstein, A. (1994) *Addiction: From Biology to Drug Policy.* W. H. Freeman, New York.
11. Nestler, E. J. (1993) Molecular mechanisms of drug addiction in the mesolimbic dopamine pathway. *Sem. Neurosci.* **5**, 369–376.
12. Self, D. W. and Nestler, E. J. (1995) Molecular mechanisms of drug reinforcement and addiction. *Annu. Rev. Neurosci.* **18**, 463–495.
13. Blum, K., Cull, J. G., Braverman, E. R. and Comings, D. E. (1996) Reward deficiency syndrome. *Amer. Scientist* **84**, 132–145.
14. Koob, G. F. and Le Moal, M. (1997) Drug abuse: hedonic homeostatic dysregulation. *Science* **278**, 52–58.
15. Kozel, N. J. and Adams, E. H. (1986) Epidemiology of drug abuse: an overview. *Science* **234**, 970–974.
16. Goldstein, A. and Kalant, H. (1990) Drug policy: striking the right balance. *Science* **249**, 1513–152.
17. MacCoun, R. and Reuter, P. (1997) Interpreting Dutch cannabis policy: reasoning by analogy in the legalization debate. *Science* **278**, 47–52.
18. Kleber, H. D. (1988) Introduction–cocaine abuse: historical, epidemiological, and psychological perspectives. *J. Clin. Psychiat.* **49(suppl)**, 3–6.
19. Crowley, T. J., Macdonald, M. J., Whitmore, E. A. and Mikulich, S. K. (1998) Cannabis dependence, withdrawal, and reinforcing effects among adolescents with conduct symptoms and substance use disorders. *Drug Alc. Depend.* **50**, 27–37.
20. Anthony, J. C., Warner, L. A. and Kessler, R. C. (1994) Comparative epidemiology of dependence on tobacco, alcohol, controlled substances and inhalants: basic findings from National Comorbidity Study. *Exp. Clin. Psychopharmacol.* **2**, 244–268.
21. Hall, W., Solowij, N. and Lemon, J. (1994) The Health and Psychological Consequences of Cannabis Use (National Drug Strategy Monograph Series No. 25). Australian Government Publishing Service, Canberra.
22. Felder, C. C. and Glass, M. (1998) Cannabinoid receptors and their endogenous agonists. *Annu. Rev. Pharmacol Toxicol.* **38**, 179–200.
23. Gardner, E. L., Paredes, W., Smith, D., Donner, A., Milling, C., Cohen, D. and Morrison, D. (1988) Facilitation of brain stimulation reward by Δ^9-tetrahydrocannabinol. *Psychopharmacology* **96**, 142–144.

24. Gardner, E. L. and Lowinson, J. H. (1991) Marijuana's interaction with brain reward systems: update 1991. *Pharmacol. Biochem. Behav.* **40**, 571–580.

25. Gardner, E. L. (1992) Cannabinoid interaction with brain reward systems–the neurobiological basis of cannabinoid abuse. In: *Marijuana/Cannabinoids: Neurobiology and Neurophysiology* (Murphy, L. L., Bartke, A., eds), CRC Press, New York, pp. 275–335.

26. Gardner, E. L., Liu, X., Paredes, W., Savage, V., Lowinson, J. and Lepore, M. (1995) Strain-specific differences in Δ^9-tetrahydrocannabinol (THC)-induced facilitation of electrical brain stimulation reward (BSR). *Soc. Neurosci. Abstr.* **21**, 177.

27. Lepore, M., Liu, X., Savage, V., Matalon, D. and Gardner, E. L. (1996) Genetic differences in Δ^9-tetrahydrocannabinol-induced facilitation of brain stimulation reward as measured by a rate-frequency curve-shift electrical brain stimulation paradigm in three different rat strains. *Life Sci. (Pharmacol. Lett.)* **58**, PL365–PL372.

28. Ng Cheong Ton, J. M. and Gardner, E. L. (1986) Effects of delta-9-tetrahydrocannabinol on dopamine release in the brain: intracranial dialysis experiments. *Soc. Neurosci. Abstr.* **12**, 135.

29. Ng Cheong Ton, J. M., Gerhardt, G. A., Friedemann, M., Etgen, A. M., Rose, G. M., Sharpless, N. S. and Gardner, E. L. (1988) The effects of Δ^9-tetrahydrocannabinol on potassium-evoked release of dopamine in the rat caudate nucleus: an in vivo electrochemical and in vivo microdialysis study. *Brain Res.* **451**, 59–68.

30. Chen, J., Paredes, W., Li, J., Smith, D. and Gardner, E. L. (1989) In vivo brain microdialysis studies of Δ^9-tetrahydrocannabinol on presynaptic dopamine efflux in nucleus accumbens of the Lewis rat. *Soc. Neurosci. Abstr.* **15**, 1096.

31. Chen, J., Paredes, W., Lowinson, J. H. and Gardner, E. L. (1990) Δ^9-Tetrahydrocannabinol enhances presynaptic dopamine efflux in medial prefrontal cortex. *Eur. J. Pharmacol.* **190**, 259–262.

32. Chen, J., Paredes, W., Li, J., Smith, D., Lowinson, J. and Gardner, E. L. (1990) Δ^9- Tetrahydrocannabinol produces naloxone-blockable enhancement of presynaptic basal dopamine efflux in nucleus accumbens of conscious, freely-moving rats as measured by intracerebral microdialysis. *Psychopharmacology* **102**, 156–162.

33. Taylor, D. A., Sitaram, B. R. and Elliot-Baker, S. (1988) Effect of Δ-9-tetrahydrocannabinol on release of dopamine in the corpus striatum of the rat. In: *Marijuana: An International Research Report* (Chesher, G., Consroe, P. and Musty, R., eds.), Australian Government Publishing Service, Canberra, pp. 405–408.

34. Tanda, G., Pontieri, F. E. and Di Chiara, G. (1997) Cannabinoid and heroin activation of mesolimbic dopamine transmission by a common μ_1 opioid receptor mechanism. *Science* **276**, 2048–2050.

35. Pontieri, F. E., Tanda, G. and Di Chiara, G. (1995) Intravenous cocaine, morphine, and amphetamine preferentially increase extracellular dopamine in the "shell" as compared with the "core" of the rat nucleus accumbens. *Proc. Natl. Acad. Sci. USA* **92**, 12304–12308.

36. Johnson, P. I., Goodman, J. B., Condon, R. and Stellar, J. R. (1995) Reward shifts and motor responses following microinjections of opiate-specific agonists into either the core or shell of the nucleus accumbens. *Psychopharmacology* **120**, 195–202.

37. Carlezon, W. A. Jr. and Wise, R. A. (1996) Rewarding actions of phencyclidine and related drugs in nucleus accumbens shell and frontal cortex. *J. Neurosci.* **16**, 3112–3122.

38. Carlezon, W. A. Jr. and Wise, R. A. (1996) Microinjections of phencyclidine (PCP) and related drugs into nucleus accumbens shell potentiate medial forebrain bundle brain stimulation reward. *Psychopharmacology* **128**, 413–420.

39. Castañeda, E., Moss, D. E., Oddie, S. D. and Whishaw, I. Q. (1991) THC does not affect striatal dopamine release: microdialysis in freely moving rats. *Pharmacol. Biochem. Behav.* **40**, 587–591.

40. Gysling, K. and Wang, R. Y. (1983) Morphine-induced activation of A10 dopamine neurons in the rat. *Brain Res.* **277**, 119–127.

41. Grenhoff, J., Aston-Jones, G., Svensson, T. H. (1986) Nicotinic effects on the firing pattern of midbrain dopamine neurons. *Acta Physiol. Scand.* **128**, 351–358.

42. Gifford, A. N., Gardner, E. L. and Ashby, C. R. Jr. (1997) The effect of intravenous administration of delta-9-tetrahydrocannabinol on the activity of A10 dopamine neurons recorded in vivo in anesthetized rats. *Neuropsychobiology* **36**, 96–99.

43. French, E. D. (1997) Δ^9-Tetrahydrocannabinol excites rat VTA dopamine neurons through activation of cannabinoid CB1 but not opioid receptors. *Neurosci. Lett.* **226**, 159–162.

44. Rosenkrantz, H., Sprague, R. A., Fleischman, R. W. and Braude, M. C. (1975) Oral Δ^9-tetrahydrocannabinol toxicity in rats treated for periods up to six months. *Toxicol. Appl. Pharmacol.* **32**, 399–417.

45. Cannon, D. S. and Carrell, L. E. (1987) Rat strain differences in ethanol self-administration and taste aversion. *Pharmacol. Biochem. Behav.* **28**, 57–63.

46. George, F. R. (1987) Genetic and environmental factors in ethanol self-administration. *Pharmacol. Biochem. Behav.* **27**, 379–384.

47. Suzuki, T., George, F. R. and Meisch, R. A. (1988) Differential establishment and maintenance of oral ethanol reinforced behavior in Lewis and Fischer 344 inbred rat strains. *J. Pharmacol. Exp. Ther.* **245**, 164–170.

48. George, F. R. and Goldberg, S. R. (1989) Genetic approaches to the analysis of addiction processes. *Trends Pharmacol. Sci.* **10**, 78–83.

49. Guitart, X., Beitner-Johnson, D., Marby, D. W., Kosten, T. A. and Nestler, E. J. (1992) Fischer and Lewis rat strains differ in basal levels of neurofilament proteins and their regulation by chronic morphine in the mesolimbic dopamine system. *Synapse* **12**, 242–253.

50. Kosten, T. A., Miserendino, M. J., Chi, S. and Nestler, E. J. (1994) Fischer and Lewis rat strains show differential cocaine effects in conditioned place preference and behavioral sensitization but not in locomotor activity or conditioned taste aversion. *J. Pharmacol. Exp. Ther.* **269**, 137–144.

51. George, F. R. and Meisch, R. A. (1984) Oral narcotic intake as a reinforcer: genotype x environment interaction. *Behav. Genetics* **14**, 603.

52. Khodzhagel'diev, T. (1986) Formirovanie vlecheniia k nikotinu u myshei linii C57B1/6 i CBA [Development of nicotine preference in C57B1/6 and CBA mice]. *Biull. Eksp. Biol. Med.* **101**, 48–50.

53. Miserendino, M. J. D., Kosten, T. A., Guitart, X., Chi, S. and Nestler, E. J. (1992) Individual differences in vulnerability to drug addiction: behavioral and biochemical correlates. *Soc. Neurosci. Abstr.* **18**, 1078.

54. Gardner, E. L., Paredes, W., Smith, D., Seeger, T., Donner, A., Milling, C., Cohen, D. and Morrison, D. (1988) Strain-specific sensitization of brain stimulation reward by Δ^9-tetrahydrocannabinol in laboratory rats. *Psychopharmacology* **96(suppl)**, 365.

55. Gardner, E. L., Chen, J., Paredes, W., Li, J. and Smith, D. (1989) Strain-specific facilitation of brain stimulation reward by Δ^9-tetrahydrocannabinol in laboratory rats is mirrored by strain-specific facilitation of presynaptic dopamine efflux in nucleus accumbens. *Soc. Neurosci. Abstr.* **15**, 638.

56. Chen, J., Paredes, W., Lowinson, J. H. and Gardner, E. L. (1991) Strain-specific facilitation of dopamine efflux by Δ^9-tetrahydrocannabinol in the nucleus accumbens of rat: an *in vivo* microdialysis study. *Neurosci. Lett.* **129**, 136–140.

57. Gardner, E. L., Paredes, W., Smith, D. and Zukin, R. S. (1989) Facilitation of brain stimulation reward by Δ^9-tetrahydrocannabinol is mediated by an endogenous opioid mechanism. *Adv. Biosci.* **75**, 671–674.

58. Gardner, E. L., Chen, J., Paredes, W., Smith, D., Li, J. and Lowinson, J. (1990) Enhancement of presynaptic dopamine efflux in brain by Δ^9-tetrahydrocannabinol is mediated by an endogenous opioid mechanism. In: *New Leads in Opioid Research* (van Ree, J. M., Mulder, A. H., Wiegant, V. M. and van Wimersma Greidanus, T. B., eds.), Elsevier Science Publishers, Amsterdam, pp. 243–245.

59. Bloom, A. S. and Dewey, W. L. (1978) A comparison of some pharmacological actions of morphine and Δ^9-tetrahydrocannabinol in the mouse. *Psychopharmacology* **57**, 243–248.

60. Chen, J., Marmur, R., Pulles, A., Paredes, W. and Gardner, E. L. (1993) Ventral tegmental microinjection of Δ^9-tetrahydrocannabinol enhances ventral tegmental somatodendritic dopamine levels but not forebrain dopamine levels: evidence for local neural action by marijuana's psychoactive ingredient. *Brain Res.* **621**, 65–70.

61. Gardner, E. L., Paredes, W. and Chen, J. (1990) Further evidence for Δ^9-tetrahydrocannabinol as a dopamine reuptake blocker: brain microdialysis studies. *Soc. Neurosci. Abstr.* **16**, 1100.

62. Westerink B. H., Tuntler, J., Damsma, G., Rollema, H. and de Vries, J. B. (1987) The use of tetrodotoxin for the characterization of drug-enhanced dopamine release in conscious rats studied by brain dialysis. *Naunyn Schmiedeberg's Arch. Pharmacol.* **336**, 502–507.

63. Shore, P. A., McMillen, B. A., Miller, H. H., Sanghera, M. K., Kiserand, R. S. and German, D. C. (1979) The dopamine neuronal storage system and non-amphetamine psychotogenic stimulants: a model for psychosis. In: *Catecholamines: Basic and Clinical Frontiers* (Usdin, E., Kopin, I. J. and Barchas, J., eds.), Pergamon, New York, pp. 722–735.

64. Chen, J., Paredes, W. and Gardner, E. L. (1994) Δ^9-Tetrahydrocannabinol's enhancement of nucleus accumbens dopamine resembles that of reuptake blockers rather than releasers–evidence from in vivo microdialysis experiments with 3-methoxytyramine. *Natl. Inst. Drug Abuse Res. Monogr. Ser.* **141**, 312.

65. Wood, P. L. and Altar, C. A. (1988) Dopamine release in vivo from nigrostriatal, mesolimbic, and mesocortical neurons: utility of 3-methoxytyramine measurements. *Pharmacol. Rev.* **40**, 163–187.

66. Heal, D. J., Frankland, A. T. J. and Buckett, W. R. (1990) A new and highly sensitive method for measuring 3-methoxytyramine using HPLC with electrochemical detection: studies with drugs which alter dopamine metabolism in the brain. *Neuropharmacology* **29**, 1141–1150.

67. Banerjee, S. P., Snyder, S. H. and Mechoulam, R. (1975) Cannabinoids: influence on neurotransmitter uptake in rat brain synaptosomes. *J. Pharmacol. Exp. Ther.* **194**, 74–81.

68. Hershkowitz, M., Szechtman, H. (1979) Pretreatment with Δ^1-tetrahydrocannabinol and psychoactive drugs: effects on uptake of biogenic amines and on behavior. *Eur. J. Pharmacol.* **59**, 267–276.

69. Poddar, M. K. and Dewey, W. L. (1980) Effects of cannabinoids on catecholamine uptake and release in hypothalamic and striatal synaptosomes. *J. Pharmacol. Exp. Ther.* **214**, 63–67.

70. Tulunay, F. C., Ayman, I. H., Portoghese, P. S. and Takemori, A. E. (1981) Antagonism by chlornaltrexamine of some effects of Δ^9-tetrahydrocannabinol in rats. *Eur. J. Pharmacol.* **70**, 219–224.

71. Wilson, R. S. and May, E. L. (1975) Analgesic properties of the tetrahydrocannabinols, their metabolites, and analogs. *J. Med. Chem.* **18**, 700–703.

72. Bhargava, N. M. (1976) Inhibition of naloxone-induced withdrawal in morphine dependent mice by 1-trans-Δ^9-tetrahydrocannabinol. *Eur. J. Pharmacol.* **36**, 259–262.

73. Hine, B., Friedman, E., Torrelio, M. and Gershon, S. (1975) Morphine-dependent rats: blockage of precipitated abstinence by tetrahydrocannabinol. *Science* **187**, 443–445.

74. Kumar, M. S. and Chen, C. L. (1983) Effect of an acute dose of delta-9-THC on hypothalamic luteinizing hormone releasing hormone and met-enkephalin content and serum levels of testosterone and corticosterone in rats. *Subst. Alcohol Actions Misuse* **4**, 37–43.

75. Vaysse, P. J. -J., Gardner, E. L. and Zukin, R. S. (1987) Modulation of rat brain opioid receptors by cannabinoids. *J. Pharmacol. Exp. Ther.* **241**, 534–539.

76. Ali, S. F., Newport, G. D., Scallet, A. C., Gee, K. W., Paule, M. G., Brown, R. M. and Slikker, W. Jr. (1989) Effects of chronic delta-9-tetrahydrocannabinol (THC) administration on neurotransmitter concentrations and receptor binding in the rat brain. *Neurotoxicology* **10**, 491–500.

77. Kumar, M. S., Patel, V. and Millard, W. J. (1984) Effect of chronic administration of Δ^9-tetra- hydrocannabinol on the endogenous opioid peptide and catecholamine levels in the diencephalon and plasma of the rat. *Subst. Alcohol Actions Misuse* **5**, 201–210.

78. Kumar, A. M., Solomon, J., Patel, V., Kream, R. M., Drieze, J. M. and Millard, W. J. (1986) Early exposure to $\Delta9$-tetrahydrocannabinol influences neuroendocrine and reproductive functions in female rats. *Neuroendocrinology* **44**, 260–264.

79. Kumar, A. M., Haney, M., Becker, T., Thompson, M. L., Kream, R. M., Miczek, K. (1990) Effect of early exposure to $\Delta9$-tetrahydrocannabinol on the levels of opioid peptides, gonadotropin-releasing hormone and substance P in the adult male rat brain. *Brain Res.* **525**, 78–83.

80. Schaefer, G. J. and Michael, R. P. (1986) Changes in response rates and reinforcement thresholds for intracranial self-stimulation during morphine withdrawal. *Pharmacol. Biochem. Behav.* **25**, 1263–1269.

81. Frank, R. A., Martz, S. and Pommering, T. (1988) The effect of chronic cocaine on self-stimulation train-duration thresholds. *Pharmacol. Biochem. Behav.* **29**, 755–758.

82. Schulteis, G., Markou, A., Gold, L. H., Stinus, L. and Koob, G. F. (1994) Relative sensitivity of multiple indices of opiate withdrawal: a quantitative dose-response analysis. *J. Pharmacol. Exp. Ther.* **271**, 1391–1398.

83. Wise, R. A. and Munn, E. (1995) Withdrawal from chronic amphetamine elevates baseline intracranial self-stimulation thresholds. *Psychopharmacology* **117**, 130–136.

84. Parsons, L. H., Smith, A. D. and Justice, J. B. Jr. (1991) Basal extracellular dopamine is decreased in the rat nucleus accumbens during abstinence from chronic cocaine. *Synapse* **9**, 60–65.

85. Pothos, E., Rada, P., Mark, G. P. and Hoebel, B. G. (1991) Dopamine microdialysis in the nucleus accumbens during acute and chronic morphine, naloxone-precipitated withdrawal and clonidine treatment. *Brain Res.* **566**, 348–350.

86. Rossetti, Z. L., Hmaidan, Y. and Gessa, G. L. (1992) Marked inhibition of mesolimbic dopamine release: a common feature of ethanol, morphine, cocaine and amphetamine abstinence in rats. *Eur. J. Pharmacol.* **221**, 227–234.

87. Koob, G. F., Markou, A., Weiss, F. and Schulteis, G. (1993) Opponent process and drug dependence: neurobiological mechanisms. *Sem. Neurosci.* **5**, 351–358.

88. Merlo Pich, E., Lorang, M., Yeganeh, M., Rodríguez de Fonseca, F., Raber, J., Koob, G. F. and Weiss, F. (1995) Increase in extracellular corticotropin-releasing factor-like immunoreactivity levels in the amygdala of awake rats during restraint stress and ethanol withdrawal as measured by microdialysis. *J. Neurosci.* **15**, 5439–5447.

89. Koob, G. F. (1996) Drug addiction: the yin and yang of hedonic homeostasis. *Neuron* **16**, 893–896.

90. Cador, M., Robbins, T. W. and Everitt, B. J. (1989) Involvement of the amygdala in stimulus-reward associations: interaction with the ventral striatum. *Neuroscience* **30**, 77–86.

91. Everitt, B. J., Cador, M. and Robbins, T. W. (1989) Interactions between the amygdala and ventral striatum in stimulus-reward associations: studies using a second-order schedule of sexual reinforcement. *Neuroscience* **30**, 63–75.

92. Gaffan, D. (1992) Amygdala and the memory of reward. In: *The Amygdala: Neurobiological Aspects of Emotion* (Aggleton, J. P., ed.), Wiley, New York, pp. 471–483.

93. Hiroi, N. and White, N. M. (1991) The lateral nucleus of the amygdala mediates expression of the amphetamine conditioned place preference. *J. Neurosci.* **11**, 2107–2116.

94. White, N. M. and Hiroi, N. (1993) Amphetamine conditioned cue preference and the neurobiology of drug-seeking. *Sem. Neurosci.* **5**, 329–336.

95. Gardner, E. L. and Lepore, M. (1996) Withdrawal from a single dose of marijuana elevates baseline brain-stimulation reward thresholds in rats. Paper presented at meetings of the Winter Conference on Brain Research, Aspen, CO, January 1996.

96. Rodríguez de Fonseca, Carrera, M. R. A., Navarro, M., Koob, G. F., Weiss, F. (1997) Activation of corticotropin-releasing factor in the limbic system during cannabinoid withdrawal. *Science* **276**, 2050–2054.

97. Elsmore, R. F. and Fletcher, G. V. (1972) Δ⁹-Tetrahydrocannabinol: aversive effects in rats at high dosages. *Science* **175**, 911–912.

98. Kay, J. (1975) Aversive effects of repeated injections of THC in rats. *Psychol. Rep.* **14**, 89–92.

99. Fischer, G. J. and Vail, B. J. (1980) Preexposure to delta-9-THC blocks THC-induced conditioned taste aversion in rats. *Behav. Neural Biol.* **30**, 191–196.

100. Switzman, L., Fishman, B. and Amit, Z. (1981) Pre-exposure effects of morphine, diazepam and Δ⁹-THC on the formation of conditioned taste aversions. *Psychopharmacology* **74**, 149–157.

101. Parker, L. A. and Gillies, T. (1995) THC-induced place and taste aversions in Lewis and Sprague-Dawley rats. *Behav. Neurosci.* **109**, 71–78.

102. McGregor, I. S., Issakidis, C. N. and Prior, G. (1996) Aversive effects of the synthetic cannabinoid CP 55,940 in rats. *Pharmacol. Biochem. Behav.* **53**, 657–664.

103. Reicher, M. and Holman, E. (1977) Location preference and flavor aversion reinforced by amphetamine in rats. *Animal Learning Behav.* **5**, 343–346.

104. Wise, R. A., Yokel, R. A. and DeWit, H. (1976) Both positive reinforcement and conditioned aversion from amphetamine and from apomorphine in rats. *Science* **191**, 1273–1275.

105. White, N., Sklar, L. and Amit, Z. (1977) The reinforcing action of morphine and its paradoxical side effect. *Psychopharmacology* **52**, 63–66.

106. van der Kooy, D. (1987) Place conditioning: a simple and effective method for assessing the motivational properties of drugs. In *Methods for Assessing the Reinforcing Properties of Abused Drugs* (Bozarth, M. A., ed), Springer-Verlag, New York, pp. 229–240.

107. Goett, J. M. and Kay, E. J. (1981) Lithium chloride and delta-9-THC lead to conditioned aversions in the pigeon. *Psychopharmacology* **72**, 215–216.

108. Sañudo-Peña, M. C., Tsou, K., Delay, E. R., Hohman, A. G., Force, M. and Walker, J. M. (1997) Endogenous cannabinoids as an aversive or counter-rewarding system in the rat. *Neurosci. Lett.* **223**, 125–128.

109. Lepore, M., Lowinson, J. and Gardner, E. L. (1994) Δ⁹-Tetrahydrocannabinol produces conditioned place-preference in laboratory rats. Paper presented at meetings of the International Cannabis Research Society, Esterel, Quebec, July 1994.

110. Lepore, M., Vorel, S. R., Lowinson, J. and Gardner, E. L. (1995) Conditioned place preference induced by Δ⁹-tetrahydrocannabinol: comparison with cocaine, morphine, and food reward. *Life Sci.* **56**, 2073–2080.

111. Fudala, P. J., Teoh, K. W. and Iwamoto, E. T. (1985) Pharmacologic characterization of nicotine-induced conditioned place preference. *Pharmacol. Biochem. Behav.* **22**, 237–241.

112. Jorenby, D. E., Steinpreis, R. E., Sherman, J. E. and Baker, T. B. (1990) Aversion instead of preference learning indicated by nicotine place conditioning in rats. *Psychopharmacology* **101**, 533–538.

113. Fudala, P. J. and Iwamoto, E. T. (1990) Conditioned aversion after delay place conditioning with amphetamine. *Pharmacol. Biochem. Behav.* **35**, 89–92.

114. Noyes, J. R., Brunk, S. F., Avery, D. H. and Canter, A. (1975) The analgesic properties of delta-9 -tetrahydrocannabinol and codeine. *Clin. Pharmacol. Ther.* **18**, 84–89.

115. Raft, D., Gregg, J., Ghia, J. and Harris, L. (1977) Effects of intravenous tetrahydrocannabinol on experimental and surgical pain. Psychological correlate of the analgesic response. *Clin. Pharmacol. Ther.* **21**, 26–33.

116. Laszlo, J., Lucas, V. S., Hanson, D. C., Cronin, C. M., Sallan, S. E. (1981) Levonantradol for chemotherapy-induced emesis: phase I-II oral administration. *J. Clin. Pharmacol.* **21**, 51S–56S.

117. Rubio, P., Rodríguez de Fonseca, F., Muñoz, R. M., Ariznavarreta, C., Martín-Calderón, J. L. and Navarro, M. (1995) Long-term behavioral effects of perinatal exposure to Δ⁹-tetrahydrocannabinol in rats: possible role of pituitary-adrenal axis. *Life Sci.* **56**, 2169–2176.

118. Sofia, R. D. and Knoblock, L. C. (1976) Comparative effects of various naturally occurring cannabinoids on food, sucrose and water consumption by rats. *Pharmacol. Biochem. Behav.* **4**, 591–599.

119. Brown, J. E., Kassouny, M. and Cross, J. K. (1977) Kinetic studies of food intake and sucrose solution preference by rats treated with low doses of delta-9-tetrahydrocannabinol. *Behav. Biol.* **20**, 104–110.

120. Milano, W. C., Wild, K. D., Hui, Y. Z., Hubbell, C. L. and Reid, L. D. (1988) PCP, THC, ethanol, and morphine and consumption of palatable solutions. *Pharmacol. Biochem. Behav.* **31**, 893–897.

121. McGregor, I. S., Saharov, T., Dielenberg, R. A., Arnold, J. C., Booker, S. L. and Topple, A. N. (1997) The effects of cannabinoids on beer and sucrose consumption in rats. Paper presented at meetings of the International Cannabinoid Research Society, Stone Mountain, Georgia June 1997.

122. Arnone, M., Maruani, J., Chaperon, F., Thiébot, M.-H., Poncelot, M., Soubrié, P. and Le Fur. G. (1997) Selective inhibition of sucrose and ethanol intake by SR 141716, an antagonist of central cannabinoid (CB1) receptors. *Psychopharmacology* **132**, 104–106.

123. Kaymakçalan, S. (1972) Physiology and psychological dependence on THC in Rhesus monkeys. In *Cannabis and its Derivatives* (Paton, W.D.M. and Crown, J., eds.), Oxford Univ. Press, London, pp. 142–149.

124. Corcoran, M. E. and Amit, Z. (1974) Reluctance of rats to drink hashish suspensions: free-choice and forced consumption, and the effects of hypothalamic stimulation. *Psychopharmacologia* **35**, 129–147.

125. Leite, J. R. and Carlini, E. A. (1974) Failure to obtain "cannabis directed behavior" and abstinence syndrome in rats chronically treated with cannabis sativa extracts. *Psychopharmacologia* **36**, 133–145.

126. Harris, R. T., Waters, W. and McLendon, D. (1974) Evaluation of reinforcing capability of Δ^9-tetrahydrocannabinol in monkeys. *Psychopharmacologia* **37**, 23–29.

127. Carney, J. M., Uwaydah, I. M. and Balster, R. L. (1977) Evaluation of a suspension system for intravenous self-administration of water insoluble substances in the rhesus monkey. *Pharmacol. Biochem. Behav.* **7**, 357–364.

128. Takahashi, R. N. and Singer, G. (1981) Cross self-administration of delta 9-tetrahydrocannabinol and D-amphetamine in rats. *Braz. J. Med. Biol. Res.* **14**, 395–400.

129. Pickens, R., Thompson, T. and Muchow, D. C. (1973) Cannabis and phencyclidine self-administered by animals. In: *Psychic Dependence [Bayer-Symposium IV]* (Goldfarb, L. and Hoffmeister, F., eds.), Springer-Verlag, Berlin, pp. 78–86.

130. Deneau, G. A. and Kaymakçalan, S. (1971) Physiological and psychological dependence to synthetic Δ^9-tetrahydrocannabinol (THC) in rhesus monkeys. *Pharmacologist* **13**, 246.

131. Takahashi, R. N., Singer, G. (1979) Self-administration of Δ^9-tetrahydrocannabinol by rats. *Pharmacol. Biochem. Behav.* **11**, 737–740.

132. Takahashi, R. N. and Singer, G. (1980) Effects of body weight levels on cannabis self-administration. *Pharmacol. Biochem. Behav.* **13**, 877–881.

133. Onaivi, E. S., Green, M. R. and Martin, B. R. (1990) Pharmacological characterization of cannabinoids in the elevated plus-maze. *J. Pharmacol. Exp. Ther.* **253**, 1002–1009.

134. Rodríguez de Fonseca, F., Rubio, P., Menzaghi, F., Merlo-Pich, E., Rivier, J., Koob, G. F. and Navarro, M. (1996) Corticotropin-releasing factor (CRF) antagonist [D-Phe^{12}, Nle^{21,38}, C$^\alpha$MeLeu^{37}]CRF attenuates the acute actions of the highly potent cannabinoid receptor agonist HU-210 on defensive-withdrawal behavior in rats. *J. Pharmacol. Exp. Ther.* **276**, 56–64.

135. Fratta, W., Martellotta, M. C., Cossu, G. and Fattore, L. (1997) WIN 55, 212–2 induces intravenous self-administration in drug-naive mice. *Soc. Neurosci. Abstr.* **23**, 1869.

12 Dependence, Tolerance, and Alteration in Gene Expression

Noboru Hiroi

Abstract

The rewarding effects of drugs of abuse such as stimulants, opiates, and cannabinoids appear to depend on the mesolimbic dopamine pathway and related brain regions in the basal ganglia. Activation of dopamine receptors causes induction of various genes. One such gene, *fos*B, plays a critical role in the rewarding effects of stimulants. This transcription factor may be a mediator of a drug's abusive properties.

1. INTRODUCTION

There is an overwhelming body of evidence that dopamine is critically involved in the abusive properties of drugs *(1,2)*. The mesolimbic dopamine pathway is a neural substrate through which most drugs of abuse alter behavior. This pathway originates from the ventral tegmental area in the midbrain and projects to the nucleus accumbens, a ventral part of the striatum in the forebrain. The mesolimbic dopamine pathway is a part of a functionally connected neuronal system, including the amygdala *(3,4)* and the ventral pallidum *(5,6)*. These regions collectively constitute limbic components of the basal ganglia, and, thus, drugs of abuse preferentially target limbic systems of the brain.

2. NEUROBIOLOGY OF CANNABINOIDS

Recent studies have included cannabinoids in a class of drugs that act on the mesolimbic dopamine system *(7)*. Δ^9-tetrahydrocannabinol (Δ^9-THC), the psychoactive component of cannabinoids, increases dopamine release in the midbrain and in the nucleus accumbens *(8–10)* as do most drugs of abuse. Δ^9-THC also induces behavioral changes that drugs of abuse establish. Lepore et al. *(11)* demonstrated that Δ^9-THC, at low doses (2 and 4 mg/kg), induces conditioned place preference, a behavioral paradigm that measures the rewarding and abusive properties of drugs *(12)*. It is important to note, however, that Δ^9-THC induces conditioned place aversion at a high dose (15 mg/kg) *(13)*. Thus, Δ^9-THC induces a biphasic action at differ-

From: *Marihuana and Medicine*
Edited by: G. G. Nahas et al.   © Humana Press Inc., Totowa, NJ

ent doses in the place-conditioning paradigm. On the other hand, Δ^9-THC fails to support intravenous self-administration *(14)*, or establishes self-administration only after physical dependence has been established *(15)*. Nonetheless, a significant fraction of users of hashish, a high-dose cannabis preparation, meet the criteria for substance dependence *(see* ref. *7)*.

The receptors for cannabinoids in the brain are termed CB_1 *(16)* and CB_{1A}, a N-terminus-modified isoform of CB_1 *(17)*. Both CB_1 and CB_{1A} inhibit adenylate cyclase activity via G_i *(17–20)*, but agonists have less affinity for CB_{1A} than for CB_1 *(20)*.

The cannabinoid receptor is distributed abundantly in the basal ganglia *(21–26)*. Given that CB_1 mRNA is not reliably detected in the substantia nigra or the globus pallidus *(23–25)*, the localization of CB_1-binding sites in these structures *(22,26)* is likely to be located on striatonigral and striatopallidal terminals. Also, there is evidence that CB_1 is not localized on the dopamine neurons and their terminals *(21,23)*. The relative distribution of CB_1 and CB_{1A} varies considerably among different brain regions. CB_1/CB_{1A} ratios are higher in the cerebellum and the frontal cortex than in the brainstem, hippocampus, temporal and occipital cortexes, striatum, and substantia nigra in the adult rat *(17)*.

In the striatum, the CB_1 receptor is likely to be colocalized with dopamine D_1-like and D_2-like receptors *(21)* and there is interaction between CB_1 and striatal dopamine receptors. Stimulation of CB_1 receptors inhibits cAMP accumulation evoked by activation of dopamine D_1 receptors *(27)*. On the other hand, stimulation of either D_2 receptors or CB_1 receptors alone inhibits forskolin-stimulated accumulation of cAMP in vitro *(28,29)*, but concurrent stimulation of CB_1 and D_2 dopamine receptors enables the accumulation of cAMP by forskolin *(29)*. This stimulatory action is dependent on the G_s pathway *(29)*. Because systemic injections of Δ^9-THC activate CB_1 and induce dopamine release in the nucleus accumbens, the stimulatory effect on striatal cAMP pathway could occur in response to cannabinoids *in vivo*.

3. GENE ALTERATION AND DRUG DEPENDENCE

Stimulation of a neuron by extracellular signals activates a set of genes, some of which encode proteins that act as transcription factors. Transcription factors are proteins that regulate the transcription of other genes. By activating or suppressing the transcription of other genes, transcription factors could alter the neurochemical phenotype of a neuron. For example, transcription factors could alter the levels of receptors, neurotransmitters, and intracellular molecules in a neuron and change a neuron's responsiveness to external signals.

The *fos* family proteins are the best known transcription factors. There are at least five members in the *fos* family, c-Fos, FosB, ΔFosB, Fra1 and Fra2. These proteins dimerize with Jun family proteins and achieve different degrees of transcriptional activation and suppression *(30,31)*. c-Fos activates the transcription of other genes when combined with c-Jun, but acts as a repressor when combined with JunB. Thus, Fos and Jun family proteins achieve complex regulation of genes.

Recent studies have demonstrated that drugs of abuse such as amphetamine and cocaine induce a set of genes in the nucleus accumbens through activation of dopamine receptors. Cocaine and amphetamine induce Fos family proteins in the nucleus accumbens. Their activation occurs, at least partially, through activation of dopamine D_1-like receptors *(32–35)*. Given that the D_1 dopamine receptor is linked to the cAMP pathway, it is likely that drugs of abuse interact with the cAMP pathway to activate Fos family member proteins.

*fos*B has been shown to be induced in the accumbens after acute and chronic treatments with cocaine, amphetamine, and morphine *(36–40)*. Little had been known about its functional significance in a drug's behavioral actions, but we recently demonstrated that cocaine induces more behavioral activation in *fos*B mutant mice, compared to their wild-type littermates *(41)*. Moreover, *fos*B mutant mice exhibited a higher level of conditioned place preference to cocaine at a low dose, compared to their wild-type littermates *(41)*. These findings suggest that induction of *fos*B by cocaine represents a compensatory adaptation that opposes cocaine's behavioral actions. Because behavioral activation and its sensitization have been hypothesized to predict a drug's abusive potency *(42,43)*, the level of *fos*B gene products may determine an individual's susceptibility to drug dependence: individuals who have low levels of *fos*B or *fos*B with a mutation might experience unusually strong rewarding effects when they encounter drugs of abuse.

The induction of *fos*B gene products is heterogeneous and follows a compartmental organization of the striatum. The nucleus accumbens, a ventral extension of the striatum, is divided into two compartments, the core and the shell. These two compartments differ in their neurotransmitter distributions and their connections with other brain regions. *fos*B gene products are preferentially expressed in the core division of the nucleus accumbens *(41)*. ΔFosB, a splicing variant of the *fos*B gene, has been shown to act as a transcriptional repressor in vitro *(44,45)*, and a major role of ΔFosB in neurons of the core division of the nucleus accumbens might be to reduce the rate of transcriptional regulation of genes, thereby reducing the functional activation of these neurons. Our finding that the absence of *fos*B in the accumbens core facilitates the rewarding and motor activating actions of cocaine is consistent with this hypothesis. In more general terms, our findings are consistent with the suggestion that the brain is equipped with molecules that oppose the formation of neuronal plasticity *(46)*.

Another Fos family protein, c-Fos, is induced in the nucleus accumbens by acute and chronic treatments with cocaine, amphetamine, methamphetamine, and morphine *(32,33,36,37,47–51)* and its expression also follows the compartmental organization of the striatum *(32,51)*. However, c-*fos*-mutant mice do not show abnormality in cocaine-induced locomotor activity or locomotor sensitization *(41)*.

Fos family proteins become functional only after they dimerize with Jun family proteins. Indeed, these drugs of abuse also induce c-*jun (37,39,49)* and *jun*B *(35–37,39,47,51,53)*. Moreover, JunD is the predominant Jun family protein present in the striatum after chronic cocaine treatment *(54)*. It remains unclear what roles these gene products play in many behavioral effects drugs of abuse induce. Given that *fos*B gene products function together with *jun* family proteins, it is likely that the behavioral phenotype *fos*B-mutant mice show is also seen in mice that lack *jun* family gene(s).

We have just begun to understand the role of intracellular molecules in drug dependence and tolerance. A future challenge is to decipher intracellular molecules that convey signals initiated by drugs of abuse such as cannabinoids and nicotine. Moreover, the rewarding effects of cannabinoids vary widely among different rat strains *(55)*, which is likely to reflect the difference in their genomic composition *(56)*. Gene regulation could thus be an important determinant for a wide range of normal and abnormal behavioral traits.

ACKNOWLEDGEMENT

I thank Drs. Eliot L. Gardner and Marino Lepore for their comments on an early draft of this manuscript.

REFERENCES

1. Koob, G. F. and LeMoal, M. (1997) *Science* **278**, 52–58.
2. Nestler, E. J. and Aghajanian, G. K. (1997) *Science* **278**, 58–62.
3. Hiroi, N. and White, N. M. (1991) *J. Neurosci.* **11**, 2107–2116.

4. Rodriguez de Fonesca, F., Carrera, M. R. A., Navarro, M., and Koob, G. F. Weiss, F. (1997) *Science* **276**, 2050–2054.
5. Hiroi, N. and White, N. M. (1993) *Neurosci. Lett.* **156**, 9–12.
6. Hubner, C. B. and Koob, G. F. (1990) *Brain Res.* **508**, 20–29.
7. Gardner, E. L. and Vorel, S. R. (1998) *Seminars in the Neurosci.* in press.
8. Chen, J., Paredes, W., Li, J., Smith, D., Lowinson, J., and Gardner, E. L. (1990) *Psychopharmacol.* **102**, 156–162.
9. Chen, J., Marmur, R., Pulles, A., Paredes, W., and Gardner, E. L. (1993) *Brain Res.* **621**, 65–70.
10. Tanda, G., Pontieri, F. E., and DiChiara, G. (1997) *Science* **276**, 2048–2050.
11. Lepore, M., Vorel, S. R., Lowinson, J., and Gardner, E. L. (1995) *Life Sci.* **56**, 2073–2080.
12. White, N. M. and Hiroi, N. (1993) *Sem. Neurosci.* **5**, 329–336.
13. Sanudo-Pena, M. C., Tsou, K., Delay, E. R., Hohman, A. G., Force, M., and Walker, J. M. (1997) *Neurosci. Lett.* **223**, 125–128.
14. Harris, R. T., Waters, W., and McLendon, D. (1974) *Psychopharmacology* **37**, 23–29.
15. Kaymakcalan, S. (1972) In: *Cannabis and its Derivatives* (Paton, W. D. M., and Cowan, J. eds.) Oxford, London, UK, pp. 142–149.
16. Matsuda, L. A., Lolait, S. J., Brownstein, M. J., Young, A. C., and Bonner, T. I (1990) *Nature* **346**, 561–564.
17. Shire, D., Carillon, C., Kaghad, M., Calandra, B., Rinaldi-Carmona, M., Le Fur, G., Caput, D., and Ferrara, P. (1995) *J. Biol. Chem.* **270**, 3726–3731.
18. Howlett, A. C. (1985) *Mol. Pharmacol.* **27**, 429–436.
19. Howlett, A. C., Qualy, J. M., and Khachatrian, L. L. (1986) *Mol. Pharmacol.* **29**, 307–313.
20. Rinaldi-Carmona, M., Calandra, B., Shire, D., Bouaboula, M., Oustric, D., Barth, F., Casellas, P., Ferrara, P., and Le Fur, G. (1996) *J. Pharmacol. Exp. Ther.* **278**, 871–878.
21. Herkenham, M., Lynn, A. B., de Costa, B. R., and Richfield, E. K. (1991) *Brain Res.* **547**, 267–274.
22. Herkenham, M., Lynn, A. B., Johnson, M. R., Melvin, L. S., deCosta, B. R., and Rice, K. C. (1991) *J. Neurosci.* **11**, 563–583.
23. Mailleux, P. and Vanderhaeghen, J. J. (1992) *Neurosci.* **48**, 655–668.
24. Matsuda, L. A., Bonner, T. I., and Lolait, S. J. (1993) *J. Comp. Neurol.* **327**, 535–550.
25. Westlake, T. M., Howlett, A. C., Bonner, T. I., Matsuda, L. A., and Herkenham, M. (1994) *Neurosci.* **63**, 637–652.
26. Herkenham, M., Lynn, A. B., Little, M. D., Johnson, M.R., Melvin, L. S., deCorta, B. R., Rice, K.C. (1990) *Proc. Natl. Acad. Sci. USA* **87,** 1932–1936.
27. Bidaut-Russell, M. and Howlett, A. (1991) *J. Neurochem.* **57**, 1769–1773.
28. Felder, C. C., Veluz, J. S., Williams, H. L., Briley, E. M., and Matsuda, L. A. (1992) *Mol. Pharmacol.* **42**, 838–845.
29. Glass, M. and Felder, C. C. (1997) *J. Neurosci.* **17**, 5327–5333.
30. Sheng, M. and Greenberg, M. E. (1990) *Neuron* **4,** 477–485.
31. Morgan, J. I. and Curran, T. (1991) *Ann. Rev. Neurosci.* **14**, 421–451.
32. Graybiel, A. M., Moratalla, R., and Robertson, H. A. (1990) *Proc. Natl. Acad. Sci. USA* **87**, 6912–6916.
33. Young, S. T., Porrino, L. J., and Iadarola, M. J. (1991) *Proc. Natl. Acad. Sci. USA* **88**, 1291–1295.
34. Nye, H. E., Hope, B. T., Kelz, M. B., Iadarola, M. J., and Nestler, E. J. (1995) *J. Pharmacol. Exp. Ther.* **275**, 1671–1680.
35. Moratalla, R., Xu, M., Tonegawa, S., and Graybiel, A. M. (1996) *Proc. Natl. Acad. Sci. USA* **93**, 14928–14933.
36. Cole, A. J., Bhat, R. V., Patt, C., Worley, P. F., and Baraban, J. M. (1992) *J. Neurochem.* **58**, 1420–1426.
37. Hope, B. T., Kosofsky, B., Hyman, S. E., and Nestler, E. J. (1992) *Proc. Natl. Acad. Sci. USA* **89**, 5764–5768.
38. Hope, B. T., Nye, H. E., Kelz, M. B., Self, D. W., Iadarola, M. J., Nakabeppu, Y., Duman, R. S., and Nestler, E. J. (1994) *Neuron* **13**, 1235–1244.
39. Persico, A. M., Schindler, C. W., O'Hare, B. F., Brannock, M. T., and Uhl, G. R. (1993) *Mol. Brain Res.* **20**, 91–100.
40. Nye, H. E. and Nestler, E. J. (1996) *Mol. Pharmacol.* **49**, 636–645.
41. Hiroi, N., Brown, J. R., Haile, C. N., Ye, H., Greenberg, M. E., and Nestler, E. J. (1997) *Proc. Natl. Acad. Sci. USA* **94**, 10397–10402.
43. Robinson, T. E. and Berridge, K. C. (1993) *Brain Res.* **18**, 247–291.
43. Koob, G. F. (1996) *Neuron* **16**, 893–896.
44. Mumberg, D., Lucibello, F. C., Schuermann, M., and Muller, R. (1991) *Genes Dev.* **5**, 1212–1223.
45. Nakabeppu, Y. and Nathans, D. (1991) *Cell* **64**, 751–759.
46. Abel, T., Martin, K. C., Bartsch, D., and Kandel, E. R.(1998) *Science* **279**, 338–341.
47. Liu, J., Nickolenko, J., and Sharp, F. R. (1994) *Proc. Natl. Acad. Sci. USA* **91**, 8537–8541.

48. Couceyro, P. and Douglass, J. (1995) *Mol. Pharmacol.* **47,** 29–39.
49. Kosofsky, B. Geneva, L. M., and Hyman, S. E. (1995) *J. Comp. Neurol.* **351,** 41–50.
50. Wang, J. Q., Smith, A. J. W., and McGinty, J. F. (1995) *Neurosci.* **68,** 83–95.
51. Moratalla, R., Elibol, B., Vallejo, M., and Graybiel, A. M. (1996) *Neuron* **17,** 147–156.
52. Couceyro, P., Pollock, K. M., Drews, K., and Douglass, J. (1994) *Mol. Pharmacol.* **46,** 667–676.
53. Moratalla, R., Vickers, E. A., Robertson, H. A., Cochran, B. H., and Graybiel, A. M. (1993) *J. Neurosci.* **13,** 423–433.
54. Chen, J. S., Nye, H. E., Kelz, M. B., Hiroi, N., Nakebeppu, Y., Hope, B. T., and Nestler, E. J. (1995) *Mol. Pharmacol.* **48,** 880–889.
55. Lepore, M., Liu, X., Savage, V., Matalon, D., and Gardner, E. L. (1996) *Life Sci.* **58,** PL365–PL372.
56. Brodkin, T. and Nestler, E. J. (1998) *The Neuroscientist*, in press.

13

Cocaine and a Mechanism for Long-Term Changes in Gene Expression

Bruce T. Hope

1. INTRODUCTION

The intensity and persistence of drug-craving behavior in the human addict suggests that the difficulty people experience in overcoming addiction is far more complex than a simple lack of will power. Drugs of abuse, such as cocaine, also appear to cause long-term physical alterations in the brain that may make it very difficult for them to merely change their minds about using drugs. In a discussion of these kinds of physical alterations at the molecular level, there is a great deal of detail and jargon. Added detail and extra jargon were saved for the figure legends and bracketed comments and can be ignored by those uninterested in the details.

2. COCAINE AND THE MESOLIMBIC DOPAMINE SYSTEM

The rat has been the most frequently employed animal model for investigating the effects of cocaine at the behavioral, physiological, and molecular level. Rats display many of the same behaviors as humans in response to acute and repeated cocaine use *(1)*. One of the most important aspects of the animal model is that biochemical studies of the effects of cocaine on the brain require brain tissue, which cannot be obtained from humans under normal circumstances. Investigations using the rat animal model have shown that the neurotransmitter dopamine and the mesolimbic dopamine system play a major role in regulating the rewarding effects of cocaine and other drugs of abuse *(2,3)*. The mesolimbic dopamine system includes the dopamine-producing cells in the ventral tegmental area (VTA) of the brainstem that send fibers to a large number of target regions in the forebrain (Fig. 1).

One of the most important target regions is the nucleus accumbens (NAc), which appears to mediate many of the rewarding effects of drugs of abuse. It is for this reason that researchers have focused on biochemical and physiological changes in the VTA and the NAc following cocaine administration.

From: *Marihuana and Medicine*
Edited by: G. G. Nahas et al.   © Humana Press Inc., Totowa, NJ

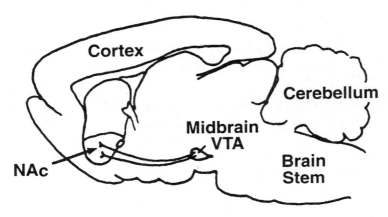

Fig. 1. Schematic drawing of brain showing the mesolimbic dopamine pathway. Within the midbrain region, there is an area called the ventral tegmental area (**VTA**). These neurons produce the neurotransmitter dopamine that send fibers through the medial forebrain bundle to many forebrain regions (arrows). One the most important forebrain regions for the rewarding effects of cocaine is the nucleus accumbens (**NAc**).

3. ACUTE COCAINE TREATMENT

Within the NAc, dopaminergic fibers release dopamine from nerve endings called synaptic boutons (Fig. 2). The dopamine crosses the synaptic cleft and either binds to dopaminergic receptor molecules on the receptive neuron or is rapidly removed from the synaptic cleft by the dopamine transporter protein. The rewarding effects of acute cocaine correlate best with cocaine's ability to block these dopamine transporter proteins *(4)*. The result is a large increase of dopamine in the cleft, leading to a powerful activation of the dopaminergic receptors.

The dopaminergic receptors then use what is called a second-messenger pathway to indicate to the inside of the cell that there are high levels of dopamine present in the cleft (for more detail *see* Fig. 2) *(1,5)*. The most important second-messenger pathway regulated by dopamine receptors is the cyclic adenosine monophosphate (cAMP) pathway. cAMP regulates the activity of a large number of proteins via protein kinase A (PKA) and a process called protein phosphorylation. Phosphorylation of proteins is generally rapid and persists for a relatively short time after cocaine is eliminated from the synapse. cAMP-dependent protein phosphorylation alters the activity of many different proteins involved in a great variety of cellular processes, including regulation of the electrical activity of the neuron, its responsiveness to other neural input, and gene expression. Furthermore, pharmacological regulation of cAMP in the NAc has been shown to regulate the reinforcing behavior of acute cocaine administration *(6)*. This is consistent with the cAMP pathway mediating at least some aspects of the rewarding behavior of cocaine.

4. CHRONIC COCAINE TREATMENT

In contrast to the behavioral effects associated with acute cocaine administration, addictive behavior develops gradually with repeated usage and persists long after the last administration of cocaine *(1,5)*. The difference in time courses is important for understanding the mechanisms underlying them. Although the biochemical and cellular mechanisms underlying the acute effects of cocaine have been extensively studied, relatively little effort has been made to understand the mechanisms underlying chronically induced alterations that appear to be more relevant to drug craving.

It is often assumed that alterations within the same mesolimbic dopamine system and target brain regions that regulate acute cocaine reward also underlie the development of drug craving during repeated cocaine administration. Thus again, most research investigating the biochemical changes induced by chronic cocaine treatment has focused on the VTA and the NAc. Chronic administration of cocaine gradually produces long-term changes in the levels of proteins involved in neuronal signaling within the NAc and VTA. These molecular changes are likely to underlie the physiological changes in neurotransmitter release and receptor responsiveness observed long after the elimination of the drug from the nervous system. For example, the laboratory of Eric Nestler has performed biochemical studies on rat brains that were exposed to twice-daily intraperitoneal injections of 15 mg/kg cocaine *(5)*. Within the NAc, there were increases in the protein levels of AC, PKA, and a number of cAMP-regulated phosphoproteins (Fig. 2). As well, there was a decrease in the level of G_i proteins. The results indicate an overall increase in the cAMP second-messenger pathway by which dopamine, and thus cocaine, act in the NAc. There are three important points to consider:

1. For each protein, the overall amount of protein was altered and not merely modified by phosphorylation.
2. The alterations were gradually induced by chronic cocaine treatment, and not by acute cocaine treatment.
3. The alterations persist long after the last cocaine treatment.

Alterations in the levels of neurotransmitters and intracellular messengers or modifications of receptors and other proteins are relatively short-lived after the elimination of cocaine and therefore do not, by themselves, sustain long-lasting physiological or behavioral changes. Thus, the most likely mechanism underlying the long-lasting behavioral features of chronic cocaine treatment appears to be alteration of protein levels.

5. REGULATION OF GENE EXPRESSION

Although there are a number of cellular mechanisms to achieve gradual long-lasting alterations in protein levels, one of the most important is by regulating the expression of these genes which encode these proteins *(7)*. Gene expression has often been implicated in the gradual induction of long-lasting alterations at the biochemical, cellular, and higher levels. It is an important mechanism by which cells adapt to a new environment, such as repeated cocaine exposure. Before continuing it is important to define the term gene expression in detail (Fig. 3).

First of all, the blueprint for producing proteins is encoded by DNA sequences within genes found within the nucleus of a neuron. This poses a problem because the translation apparatus for making proteins based on this blueprint is found not in the nucleus but in the surrounding cytoplasm. To circumvent this problem, the DNA sequence of a gene is copied into a messenger RNA (mRNA) sequence by a process called transcription. Unlike DNA, the copies of mRNA can then be translocated to the cytoplasm where it is translated into the amino acid sequence of a protein. This whole process of producing a specific protein from a specific gene is called gene expression and can include degradation of the mRNA message or the protein itself. Regulation of gene expression can occur at any step along the way.

One of the most important mechanisms for regulating gene expression is at the transcription step. RNA polymerase and a large number of associated proteins form the general transcription apparatus that transcribe mRNA from all genes (Fig. 3) *(8)*. The activity of this general transcription apparatus on any given gene is tightly controlled by a large class of pro-

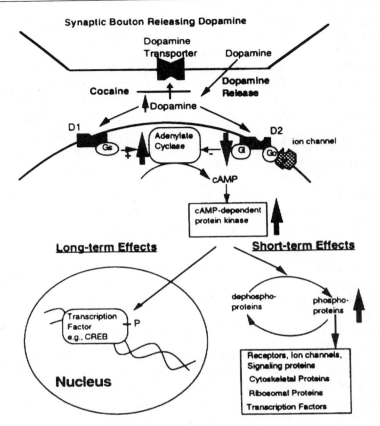

Fig. 2. Schematic drawing of a dopaminergic synapse releasing dopamine onto a neuron in the NAc. The dopaminergic fibers release dopamine from synaptic boutons. Dopamine crosses the synaptic cleft and binds to dopamine receptor molecules (D_1 and D_2) on the receptive neuron. Once dopamine is released into the synaptic left it is rapidly removed by the dopamine transporter protein. *Acute* cocaine blocks this removal of dopamine from the synapse (indicated by thick line blocking dopamine removal). The result is a large increase (indicated by small arrow in synaptic cleft) of dopamine in the cleft leading to a powerful activation of the dopaminergic receptors. These receptors activate G proteins that can either activate or repress the activity of an enzyme called adenylate cyclase (AC). The D_1 class of dopamine receptors in the NAc use stimulatory G proteins (G_s) to activate AC, whereas the D_2 class of dopamine receptors use inhibitory G proteins (G_i) to inhibit AC activity. The overall effect of cocaine in the NAc is to increase AC activity which produces the second-messenger molecule, cAMP. The only way for cAMP to have its effects is by activating PKA. PKA can add phosphate chemical groups to specific proteins, called phosphoproteins, and in so doing alters their activity. These phosphoproteins are involved in many aspects of controlling cellular activity, including short-term effects such as altering the electrical activity of the neuron or altering its responsiveness to other neural input, or long-term effects such as altering gene expression in the nucleus. Chronic cocaine treatment alters the levels of some of the proteins along this second-messenger pathway. These alterations are indicated in the figure by large arrows. These alterations result in an overall increase in the activity of the cAMP pathway. Modified from ref. *1*.

teins called transcription factors. Many specific transcription factors bind to DNA in the promoter (regulatory region) of a gene, usually found upstream of the start site for transcription. The action of any transcription factor depends on all other transcription factors present at that same promoter; all the transcription factors on a given promoter interact to either up- or downregulate transcription.

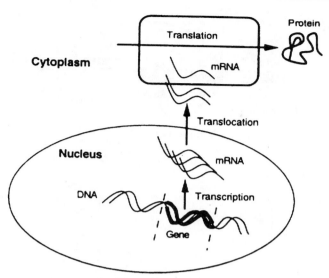

Fig. 3. Schematic drawing of gene expression within a neuron. A gene encodes the blueprint for producing specific proteins. Each gene is only a very small part of the total DNA sequence within a cell. It is transcribed (transcription) into multiple copies of mRNA within the nucleus which can then translocate (translocation) to the cytoplasm. Ribosomes are the site of translation in the cytoplasm. The ribosomes translate the mRNA message from the nucleus into the amino acid sequence of a protein.

6. AP-1, FRAS, AND IEGS: WHAT ARE THEY?

There has been a great deal of interest in a class of transcription factors encoded by the immediate early genes (IEGs), which are induced in neurons by a variety of extracellular stimuli *(9)* (Fig. 4A).

These IEGs are thought to link acute extracellular stimuli with subsequent changes in gene expression by acting as "third messengers" during signal transduction. Fos, the protein product of the prototypical IEG, *c-fos*, forms a heterodimer with another IEG protein product called Jun (Fig. 4B). The resulting AP-1 complex binds to a specific DNA consensus sequence called an AP-1 DNA site, found in the promoter region of many important neuronal genes, to activate or repress their transcription. There are several known Fos-related proteins called Fos-related antigens (Fras) as well as several different Jun-related proteins capable of forming AP-1 DNA-binding complexes. Because AP-1 complexes regulate gene expression, any changes in the regulation or composition of the AP-1 complex following chronic cocaine treatment is likely to produce changes in the pattern of gene expression in brain, including genes important for neuronal signaling. In addition, if these genes are altered in the NAc, they are also likely to play a role in long-term alterations in the rewarding behavior of cocaine.

7. REGULATION OF IEGS BY COCAINE

We have begun an investigation of how transcription factors may regulate long-term changes in gene expression and alterations in protein levels by examining the regulation of the AP-1 transcription factor in the NAc following chronic, versus acute, cocaine treatment. Previously, the IEGs encoding AP-1 proteins were shown to be induced rapidly following acute cocaine treatment, leading the investigators to suggest that these acutely induced IEGs may be involved in the long-term effects of cocaine treatment *(10,11)*. In contrast, we had observed [using Northern blots] that these same IEG's are no longer induced by an acute

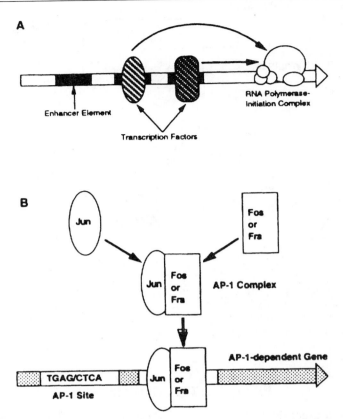

Fig. 4. Transcription regulation within a neuron. **(A)** Transcription factor proteins bind to specific sequences of DNA called enhancers in the regulatory region of a gene called the promoter. These transcription factors interact directly or indirectly to either up or downregulate formation of the RNA polymerase-initiation complex. Formation of this complex initiates transcription and forms the rate-limiting step in the transcription of almost all genes. **(B)** The proteins Jun [there are several types (isoforms) of Jun] and Fos [there are several types of Fos-related isoforms called Fras] combine to form an AP-1 complex. The AP-1 complex can be formed by many different combinations of the Jun, Fos, or Fra proteins. The AP-1 complex binds to the enhancer called the AP-1 DNA site encoded by the specific DNA sequence indicated. This AP-1 complex then interacts with the other transcription factors on the same promoter to regulate transcription of the AP-1-dependent gene.

challenge following chronic cocaine treatment *(12)*. Other investigators have shown similar loss of induction of *c-fos* and *c-jun* as well as their protein products following chronic cocaine, chronic electroconvulsive seizure, and chronic amphetamine treatments *(13–15)*. The lack of induction of these acutely induced transcription factors following chronic cocaine treatment, in addition to their short time courses, makes it unlikely that they are involved in the gradual and sustained changes in gene expression following chronic treatments. One might imagine that the IEGs are important for adapting to *acute* stimuli such as cocaine, whereas other substrates are required for adapting to *chronic* cocaine use.

8. REGULATION OF THE AP-1 TRANSCRIPTION FACTOR BY COCAINE

When DNA binding by the AP-1 complex was examined in the NAc [using the gel-shift assay] there was a maximal induction of AP-1 DNA binding two hours after acute cocaine, which returned to baseline 18 hours later *(12)*. Surprisingly, AP-1 DNA binding remained at maximal acute levels 18 hours after the chronic cocaine treatment even though the IEGs encoding the known AP-1 proteins were not induced. Whereas acute cocaine induced a transient increase in AP-1 DNA binding, chronic cocaine gradually induced a long-lasting AP-1 DNA-binding complex, called the chronic AP-1 complex, with a half-life of approximately seven days following the last chronic treatment *(16)*. This time course corresponds well with previous observations of a gradual induction of long-term biochemical and behavioral changes following chronic cocaine treatment.

The AP-1 complexes induced by acute and chronic cocaine treatment also appear to have a different composition. [This is shown by a difference in their relative mobilities in gel-shift assays. "Supershift" experiments and Western blots with the anti-Fra antibody indicated that the chronic AP-1 complex contained 35–37 kDa Fras that are gradually induced by chronic, but not acute, cocaine treatment. This anti-Fra antibody recognizes a peptide sequence, called the M-peptide, common to all known Fras. Two-dimensional Western blots indicate there are at least four chronically induced Fras.] Four different Fos-related proteins are induced by chronic, but not acute, cocaine treatment. One or all of these chronic Fras could be responsible for the long-lasting AP-1 DNA-binding complex observed following chronic cocaine treatment.

The same chronic Fras induced by chronic cocaine are also induced by other chronic treatments, such as haloperidol, tranylcypromine, electroconvulsive seizures, and apomorphine in specific brain regions unique to each treatment *(17,18)*. Thus, the induction of chronic Fras and the chronic AP-1 complex appears to be a general phenomenon in regions that are repeatedly activated by a wide variety of chronic treatments. We hypothesize that in those cells receiving repeated or continuous stimulation by cocaine, there are initially insignificant levels of chronic Fras *(16; see* Fig. 5).

However, because of the long half-life of chronic Fras, there is a gradual accumulation of chronic Fras with repeated stimuli. The increasing levels of chronic Fras would result in the gradual induction of significant levels of a long-lasting AP-1 complex following chronic, but not acute, treatment.

We have shown previously that the AP-1-binding complexes induced by acute and chronic treatment have different affinities for some AP-1-like DNA sites *(17)*. This suggests that the chronic AP-1 complex could produce "qualitatively" different types of gene expression relative to those induced by acute treatment, in the pattern of expression of those genes containing AP-1 sites in their promoters (Fig. 6).

This is in addition to the differences in gene expression caused by the longer-lasting effects of a chronic, versus acute, AP-1 complex. Finally, the difference in the composition for the chronic, versus acute, AP-1 complexes suggests different transcriptional-regulating abilities upon binding to a given AP-1 site. Even if the chronic AP-1 complex does not directly activate or repress transcription, it is still capable of occupying the AP-1 DNA site to block the activity of more transcriptionally active transcription factors.

9. SUMMARY

It should be repeated that there are many other transcription factors that are regulated by cocaine and there are several nontranscriptional mechanisms of regulating protein levels as well. However, the induction of the chronic AP-1 complex and the chronic Fras provides a mechanism capable of underlying long-lasting alterations in gene expression following chronic cocaine treatment. We hypothesize that, while the well-known acute effects of cocaine are occurring, the second-messenger pathways are also inducing two general types of

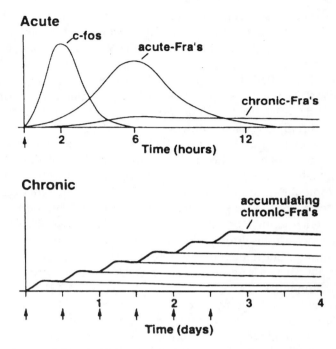

Fig. 5. Hypothetical scheme of the gradual accumulation of the chronic-Fras versus the rapid and transient induction of c-Fos and the acute-Fras. **(A)** There are several waves of Fras induced by each acute stimulus. c-Fos is induced rapidly and degraded within several hours of the acute stimulus, whereas the acute-Fras are induced somewhat later and persist somewhat longer than c-Fos. The chronic-Fras are also induced following a single acute stimulus but persist for many days at low levels (with a half-life of seven days). In a complex with Jun-like proteins, these waves of Fra's form AP-1 binding complexes with shifting composition over time. **(B)** With repeated (e.g., twice daily) stimulation, each acute stimulus induces a low level of chronic Fras. This is indicated by the lower set of overlapping lines, which indicate chronic Fras induced by each acute stimulus. The result is a gradual increase in the total level of chronic Fras with repeated stimuli during a course of chronic treatment. This is indicated by the increasing stepped line in the graph. The increasing levels of chronic Fras with repeated stimulation would result in the gradual induction of significant levels of a long-lasting AP-1 complex. From ref. *16*.

alterations in gene expression. The acutely induced alterations in gene expression are rapidly induced and relatively short-lived. This would allow the cell to rapidly adapt to cocaine in its environment without committing to long-term changes.

In contrast, the alterations induced by chronic cocaine treatment are gradually induced and long-lasting. This could be produced by long-lasting changes in gene expression induced by each acute treatment during chronic administration. The level of induction of these long-lasting changes in gene expression would be relatively small and insignificant compared to the rapidly induced acute alterations in gene expression. However, these small changes would accumulate with each acute administration during chronic cocaine treatment, similar to the gradual induction of the chronic AP-1 complex (Fig. 5). The cumulative changes would eventually reach a level where they produce significant and long-lasting alterations in gene expression different from those induced acutely. This incremental induction of long-lasting alterations in gene expression would allow the cell to gradually commit to long-term alterations for the purpose of adapting more appropriately to repeated long-term exposure to cocaine in its environment. The

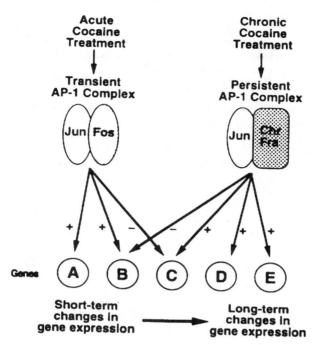

Fig. 6. Scheme illustrating the regulation of AP-1-binding proteins by acute and chronic cocaine. Acute cocaine administration transiently induces several AP-1-binding proteins in the NAc and striatum, including c-Fos, c-Jun, FosB, and JunB. Induction of these transcription factors could mediate some of the rapid stimulatory (+) and inhibitory (-) effects of cocaine on the expression of neural genes (A–E) that contain AP-1-binding sites. In contrast, chronic cocaine administration results in the persistent induction of AP-1-binding activity which is accounted for by the chronic Fras. Such chronic, persistent AP-1 complexes of altered composition might be expected to exert different transcriptional effects compared to the acute AP-1 complexes, and could mediate some of the long-term effects of cocaine on gene expression. From ref. *1*.

long-lasting alterations in gene expression may underlie the gradual induction of persistent changes in protein levels, neuronal signaling, and related behaviors.

We hope these investigations provide ideas for specific pharmacological blockade or reversal of the long-term vs short-term alterations in gene expression that lead to addiction, without interfering with the animal's or human's ability to experience reward. This would be important for ensuring both efficacy and compliance.

Reprinted with permission from Drug Abuse in the Decade of the Brain (Nahas, G.G.; Burks, T.F., eds.), IOS Press, Amsterdam, Netherlands, 1997, pp. 213–221.

REFERENCES

1. Nestler, E. J., Hope, B. T., and Widnell, K. L. (1993) *Neuron* **11**, 995–1006.
2. Fibiger, H. C., Phillips, A. G., and Brown, E. E. (1992) *Ciba Found. Symp.* **166**, 96–124.
3. Koob, G. F. (1992) *Trends Pharmacol. Sci.* **13**, 177–184.
4. Kuhar, M. J., Ritz, M. C., and Boja, J. W. (1991) *Trends Neurosci.* **14**, 299–302.
5. Nestler, E. J. (1992) *J. Neurosci.* **12**, 2439–50.
6. Self, D. W. and Nestler, E. J. (1995) *Ann. Rev. Neurosci.* **18**, 463–95.
7. Hyman, S. E. And Nestler, E. J. (1993) The Molecular Foundations of Psychiatry American Psychiatric Press, Washington, D.C.

8. Tjian, R. and Maniatis, T. (1994) *Cell* **77,** 5–8.
9. Morgan, J. I. and Curran, T. (1991) *Ann. Rev. Neurosci.* **14,** 421–451.
10. Graybiel, A. M., Moratalla, R., and Robertson, H.A. (1990) *Proc. Natl. Acad. Sci. USA* **87,** 6912–6916.
11. Young, S. T., Porrino, L. J., and Iadarola, M. J. (1991) *Proc. Natl. Acad. Sci. USA* **88,** 1291–1295.
12. Hope, B.T., Kosofsky, B., Hyman, S.E., and Nestler, E.J. (1992) *Proc. Natl. Acad. Sci. USA* **89,** 5764–5768.
13. Ennulat, D. J., Babb, S. M., and Cohen, B. M. (1994) *Mol. Brain Res.* **26,** 106–112.
14. Gerfen, C. R. Steiner, H. (1993) *J. Neurosci.* **13,** 5066–81.
15. Winston, S. M., Hayward, M. D., Nestler, E. J., and Duman, R. S. (1990) *J. Neurochem.* **54,** 1920–1925.
16. Hope, B. T., Nye, H. E., Kelz, M. B., Self, D. W., Iadarola, M. J., Nakabeppu, Y., Duman, R. S., and Nestler, E. J. (1994) *Neuron* **13,** 1235–1244.
17. Hope, B. T., Kelz, M. B., Duman, R. S., and Nestler, E. J. (1994) *J. Neurosci.* **14,** 4318–4328.
18. Nye H. E., Hope B. T., Kelz M., Iadarola M. J., Nestler E. J. (1995) *J. Pharmacol. Exp. Ther.* (in press).

14

Cannabinoids and the Cholinergic System

Edward F. Domino

Abstract

Δ^9-Tetrahydrocannabinol (THC) decreases EEG activation and causes slow waves in the cat. The EEG slow-wave activity is accompanied by a concomitant decrease in acetylcholine release from the neocortex. The findings suggest that THC depresses the brainstem-activating system. Large doses of Δ^8- and Δ^9-THC increase brain acetylcholine levels in rodents such as the mouse and rat, but this effect is not seen with minimal doses of the cannabinoids that show behavioral effects. The most dramatic change produced by THC is that brain acetylcholine utilization is reduced, primarily in the hippocampus.

1. INTRODUCTION

It is still far from clear how cannabinoids produce their remarkable pharmacologic effects. The cannabinoids interact with many different neuronal and biochemical systems *(1,2)*, but which action is the most important in relation to therapeutic effects is still unknown. Marihuana and Δ^9-tetrahydrocannabinol (THC) have remarkable effects on human memory and cognition *(3–5)*. Recently, Ferraro *(6)* has reviewed the extensive literature on this subject. Although marihuana's acute effects on memory vary, he concluded that they are always detrimental to the marihuana user. Our animal neurochemical research suggests that these undesirable side effects of *Cannabis* and probably other synthetic cannabinoids are related to a decrease in the release of neuronal acetylcholine (ACh) and its turnover in certain regions of the brain. This report summarizes these results from our laboratory. It should be pointed out that at least three other laboratories in the United States have been active in this field *(7–9)*. The results from all four laboratories differ in details, but all agree that *Cannabis* preparations interact with the cholinergic system. Cannabinoids, especially the 7-OH derivatives, inhibit the twitch response of the guinea pig ileum to electric-field stimulation *(10)*, a finding consistent with an ACh antirelease effect either indirectly or directly. There are a number of prominent side effects of cannabinoids in humans that also suggest an interaction with the cholinergic system, including dry mouth, tachycardia and bradycardia, drowsiness, sedation, and short-term memory loss.

From: *Marihuana and Medicine*
Edited by: G. G. Nahas et al.   © Humana Press Inc., Totowa, NJ

2. METHODS

Mice, rats, and cats have been used in this research; details of the methods employed have been published elsewhere *(11–16)*. Briefly, a large variety of ACh assay techniques have been used including bioassays such as the frog rectus abdominus and the leech muscle, and chemical assays including the enzymatic choline kinase method, pyrolysis and chemical demethylation, gas chromatography-flame ion detection (GC-FID), gas chromatography-nitrogen detection (GC-ND), and gas chromatography-mass spectrometry (GC-MS). Current results, obtained using chemical demethylation and GC-ND or GC-MS, are fully consistent with the results obtained using bioassay and chemical assay techniques.

3. RESULTS

3.1 Effects of Cannabinoids on Neocortical Acetylcholine Release in the Cat

Inasmuch as wakefulness involves a brainstem-activating mechanism in the reticular formation and hypothalamus which has widespread neocortical and limbic system effects, it was postulated that THC would affect these systems. Both EEG and ACh-release data were obtained to indicate that this indeed is the case *(13)*. It is known that the level of spontaneous release of ACh from the neocortex varies with the degree of anesthesia and level of brainstem transection. In order to assure a high level of spontaneous release, pretrigeminal brainstem transected preparations were used. Usually, the mean of three assays before and after drug administration was obtained. In our animals, the range in baseline release varied from a low of 8.0 to a high of 51.4 ng/cm^2/10 min, with a mean ± SE for 24 animals before drug of 22.9 ± 2.2 ng/cm^2/10 min three hours after halothane anesthesia and brainstem transection. The factors involved in the wide range observed in baseline release of ACh probably include residual anesthesia and postsurgical brain trauma.

THC in intravenous doses of 0.5 to 11.0 mg/kg produced high-voltage slow waves in the EEG of the neocortex of pretrigeminal midpontine transected cats. EEG high-voltage slow waves were more prominent in the frontal than the occipital cortical leads. The left frontal cortical lead which contained the bathing solution for collecting ACh showed EEG spikes and slow waves typical of the local effects of physostigmine. Small doses of THC tended to exaggerate these effects, but in larger doses they were reduced. The administration of (+)-amphetamine in intravenous doses of 2.5 mg/kg dramatically antagonized most of the effects induced by THC. Small doses of THC in the order of 0.5 mg/kg produced variable effects on ACh release. Some animals showed a definite increase in Ach release, whereas others showed a slight decrease. However, larger doses of THC produced consistent and progressively greater depression of ACh release. These effects are antagonized by (+)-amphetamine.

The mean ± SE acetylcholine concentration in rat brain for 12 control animals given no injection was 25.3 ± 0.8 nmole/g. Thirty minutes after Tween vehicle alone was given to 11 rats, brain ACh was 26.4 ± 1.3 nmole/g. This value was not significantly different from that achieved after no injection. After 1 μg acetylseco HC-3 (ASHC-3) was administered intraventricularly in 13 animals, brain ACh was significantly reduced to 20.3 ± 0.9 nmole/g ($p < 0.001$). When THC was given alone in doses of 3.2, 10, and 32 mg/kg intraperitoneally 30 minutes later, only the largest dose caused a significant increase in brain ACh above control ($p < 0.05$). Doses of THC of 5 mg/kg intravenously and 10 mg/kg intraperitoneally one hour later also did not significantly affect total brain ACh. On the other hand, in animals pretreated with ASHC-3, doses of 10 and 30 mg/kg THC intraperitoneally significantly elevated brain ACh to control levels ($P < 0.001$), indicating that ACh utilization was reduced.

Similar findings were observed in mouse brain in which 3.2 µg ASHC-3 was given intraventricularly. None of the control vehicles had any significant effect on mouse brain ACh 30 minutes later, whereas ASHC-3 reduced brain ACh levels significantly ($p < 0.001$). Both Δ^8- and Δ^9-THC significantly reduced mouse brain ACh utilization just as Δ^9-THC did in the rat.

3.2 Effects of THC on Regional Rat Brain Acetylcholine Levels and Utilization

Inasmuch as whole-brain ACh utilization was reduced by THC, it seemed important to localize this effect. Because the method involves the intraventricular injection of ASHC-3, brain areas close to the ventricles (hippocampus, hypothalamus, thalamus, and caudate) were studied. Male Holtzman rats (six per group) without intraventricular cannulation were given either THC (10 mg/kg, intraperitoneally) or vehicle and were sacrificed one hour later by microwave irradiation. Only slight, insignificant changes were found in the regional levels of ACh. In view of the lack of any dramatic effects of THC on regional brain ACh levels, its effects on regional brain ACh utilization were examined. Male Holtzman rats (six per group) were given intraperitoneally 1.0–32 mg/kg THC suspended in 4% Tween-20–0.9% NaCl and sacrificed one hour later by focused microwave irradiation. The procedure differed from that when using normal animals in that polyethylene cannulas (PE10) were implanted under light ether anesthesia 48 hours prior to drug administration. Each rat was implanted with an intraventricular cannula 4.5 mm below the cranial surface. Two days later, on the experimental day, 30 minutes before sacrifice, ASHC-3 (3.2 mg) was injected into the left lateral ventricle through the cannula. Acetylcholine levels in the hypothalamus, thalamus, hippocampus, and the caudate nucleus were then assayed. No significant alteration of ACh utilization was found in the hypothalamus, thalamus, or caudate nucleus. However, the previously depleted hippocampal levels of ACh increased in a dose-effect manner, ranging from 123 (1.0 mg/kg) to 243% (32 mg/kg).

4. DISCUSSION

Among the many neurochemical actions of the cannabinoids is their effect on the release and turnover of acetylcholine. Whether any of the potential therapeutic effects of cannabinoids are related to a cholinergic mechanism is certainly questionable. However, some of the potential undesirable side effects of cannabinoids are almost certainly related to a decrease in ACh release and turnover.

Large doses of 10 mg/kg or more of THC elevate rat-brain ACh and reduce its turnover. Inasmuch as doses of 3.2 mg/kg THC already depress acquisition of rat shuttle-box behavior, the failure of this dose to affect total rat brain ACh indicates a dissociation of total brain ACh and THC behavioral effects. Regional brain ACh studies indicate that THC, in doses of 3.2 mg/kg intraperitoneally in rats, produces localized hippocampal ACh effects.

Our finding of a decreased rat-brain hippocampal ACh turnover by THC suggests that at least this neurochemical effect may be related to an unwanted side effect of cannabinoid administration. It would be of great interest to examine other synthetic cannabinoids such as nabilone and levonantradol for similar effects. If these agents also reduce short-term memory, they may be of special interest therapeutically to anesthesiologists. If indeed these new cannabinoids do affect short-term memory, it would be of value to study their effects on brain ACh release, content, utilization, and turnover.

Reprinted with permission from The Journal of Clinical Pharmacology, Vol. 21, Nos. 8 & 9, Supplement, pp. 249S–255S, 1981.

REFERENCES

1. Koe, B. K. and Weissman, A. (1981) Facilitation of benzodiazepine binding by levonantradol. *J. Clin. Pharmacol.* **21**, 397S–405S.
2. Nahas, G. G., Paton, W. D. M. and IdanpaanHeikkila, J. E., eds. (1976) *Marihuana: Chemistry, Biochemistry, and Cellular Effects.* Springer-Verlag, New York, pp. 1–556.
3. Domino E. F., Rennick P. and Pearl J. H. (1974) Dose-effect relations of marijuana smoking on various physiological parameters in experienced male users. *Clin. Pharm. Therap.* **15**, 514–520.
4. Pearl, J. H., Domino, E. F. and Rennick, P. (1973) Short-term effects of marijuana smoking on cognitive behavior in experienced male users. *Psychopharmacologia* **31**, 13–24.
5. Domino, E. F., Rennick, P. and Pearl, J. H. (1976) Short term neuropsychopharmacological effects of marijuana smoking in experienced male users. In: *Pharmacology of Marijuana* (Braude, M. C. and Szara, S., eds) Raven, New York, pp. 393–412.
6. Ferraro, D. P. (1980) Acute effects of marijuana on human memory and cognition. In: *Marijuana Research Findings*: 1980, NIDA Monograph 31 (Petersen, R.C., ed.) Rockville, MD, June 1980, pp. 98–119.
7. Askew, W. E., Kimball, A. P. and Ho B. T. (1974) Effect of tetrahydrocannabinols on brain acetylcholine. *Brain Res.* **69**, 375–378.
8. Cheney, D. L. and Costa E. (1977) Pharmacological implications of brain acetylcholine turnover measurements in rat brain nuclei. *Ann. Rev. Pharmacol. Toxicol.* **17**, 369–386.
9. Tripathi, H. L., Vocci F. J. and Dewey, W. L. Effects of cannabinoids on levels of acetylcholine and choline, and on turnover rate of acetylcholine, in various regions of mouse brain. *J. Pharmacol. Exp. Therap.* (in press).
10. Rosell, S. Agurell, S. and Martin, B. (1976) Effects of cannabinoids on isolated smooth muscle preparations. In: *Marihuana: Chemistry, Biochemistry, and Cellular Effects.* (Nahas G. G., Paton W. D. M., Idanpaan-Heikkila J. E., eds.), Springer-Verlag, New York, pp. 397–406
11. Domino, E. F. (1971) Neuropsychopharmacologic studies of marijuana: some synthetic and natural THC derivatives in animals and man. *Ann. NY Acad. Sci.* **191**, 166–191.
12. Domino, E. F. and Wilson, A. E. (1972) Psychotropic drug influences on brain acetylcholine utilization. *Psychopharmacologia* **25**, 291–298.
13. Domino, E. F. and Bartolini, A. (1972) Effects of various psychotomimetic agents on the EEG and acetylcholine release from the cerebral cortex of brainstem transected cats. *Neuropharmacology* **11**, 703–713.
14. Domino, E. F., Mohrman, M. E., Wilson A. E. and Haarstad, V. B. (1973) Acetylseco hemicholinium-3, a new choline acetyltransferase inhibitor useful in neuropharmacological studies. *Neuropharmacology* **12**, 549–561.
15. Domino, E. F. Effects of Δ^9-tetrahydrocannabinol and cannabinol on rat brain acetylcholine. In: *Marihuana: Chemistry, Biochemistry, and Cellular Effects.* (Nahas G. G., Paton, W. D. M., Idanpaan-Heikkila, J. E., eds.) Springer-Verlag, New York, pp. 407–413.
16. Domino, E. F., Donelson, A. C. and Tuttle, T. (1979) Effects of Δ^9-tetrahydrocannabinol on regional brain acetylcholine. In: *Cholinergic Mechanisms and Psychopharmacology.* (Jenden, D. F., ed.) Plenum, New York, pp. 673–678.

15

Marihuana
Acute Effects on Human Memory

Loren L. Miller

1. INTRODUCTION

The single most consistently reported behavioral effect of cannabinoids in humans is an alteration in memory functioning *(1)*. Interest in the effects of *Cannabis* on memory stemmed from anecdotal reports of the effects of *Cannabis* on mood and thinking. In 1845, the French psychiatrist de Tours Moreau *(2)* provided an elegant characterization of the effects of hashish on human mental functioning. Moreau stated that one of the more prominent effects of hashish was a "gradual weakening of the power to direct thoughts at will." Ideas extraneous to the focus of an individual's attention appeared to enter the mind producing a loosening of associations. Other early investigators such as Bromberg *(3)* and Ames *(4)* employing less potent *Cannabis* preparations than those used by Moreau and his followers also noted fragmentation of thought and confusion on attempting to remember recent occurrences.

Objective substantiation of some of these observations has been gained in studies employing known doses of Δ^9-tetrahydrocannabinol (THC). Tinklenberg et al. *(5)* found that orally administered THC (20,40,60 mg) impaired immediate memory for digits recalled in forward or reverse order with peak impairment at 1.5 and 3.5 hours, respectively. Memory impairment was intermittent and not dependent on dose. The transient nature of the memory loss was reminiscent of the waxing and waning effect following marihuana intoxication described by Clark et al. *(6)*. Oral THC has also been found to induce "temporal disintegration," which is defined as a difficulty in retaining, coordinating, and serially indexing those memories, perceptions, and expectations that are relevant to the attainment of some goal *(7,8)*. The measure of temporal disintegration was the Goal Directed Serial Alternation Test (GDSA) that required a subject to subtract and add numbers from each other until some specified number was reached. The dose-related disruption found on this task was thought to be related to impaired time perception. Also, the inability to temporally coordinate recent memories with intentions might account for disorganized speech patterns found by Weil and Zinberg *(9)* following marihuana intoxication. Since words and phrases are hierarchically ordered in a goal-directed fashion, speech may become disorganized under the drug and a person is likely to

From: *Marihuana and Medicine*
Edited by: G. G. Nahas et al.   © Humana Press Inc., Totowa, NJ

lose his or her train of thought. Whereas the GDSA has proven to be an interesting measure with which to assess the effects of cannabinoids, Abel *(10)* has questioned its reliability. Studies by Rafaelsen et al. *(11)* and Tinklenberg et al. *(12)* have found some difficulty in replicating their original findings with the GDSA. This lack of replicability appears to be caused partly by limited drug session employment of the GDSA task that resulted in an abbreviated sampling of the behavior in question.

In order to determine a specific locus of action of marihuana on memory, it has been suggested that testable models of human memory be employed so that any selective impairment caused by intoxication might be determined *(1,13)*. One such model has been proposed by Shiffrin and Atkinson *(14)*. The model is based on psychological evidence as well as neurophysiological and anatomical observations that suggest that memory might be best conceptualized as a two-component process containing a short-term and long-term storage component. The short-term memory store is an individual's working memory. It is responsible for holding the trace of the external stimulus and at the same time matching the memory trace of the stimulus with a previously encoded representative of the stimulus from the long-term storage component. The short-term store and long-term store differ in terms of both information capacity and duration. Only a small number of items can be maintained in the short-term store at any given time. Maintenance of memory can be achieved by various control processes including rehearsal, imagery, or use of mnemonics. When information resides in short-term storage for a reasonable period of time, it is automatically transferred to long-term memory. The long-term store is a permanent repository for information.

A number of studies have investigated the actions of marihuana on different stages of memory employing this model. The experimental paradigm usually consists of a free recall task involving lists of words. The dependent variable is the probability of recall or number of words recalled as a function of position of word in a list or its "serial position." A bimodal U-shaped function relating probability of recall to serial position of an item can be plotted. Since the beginning and end of the serial position curve respond differently to a range of experimental variables, the positions are thought to represent output from different storage mechanisms. The probability of recall for both early and late items is higher than for middle items. These two effects are termed, respectively, the primacy and recency effects.

A study by Darley et al. *(15)* demonstrated the effects of orally administered THC (20 mg) on the different stages of memory proposed by this model. Subjects were presented with 10 lists of 20 words, each of which was followed by an immediate recall test. Immediately following the last list, half the subjects ingested a 20 mg dose of THC, the other half placebo. One hour later, subjects were given a delayed recall and recognition test. Then, the whole sequence of list presentation, immediated, delayed recall, and recognition was repeated. The results indicated that if THC was administered after list presentation but before delayed recall, no effects were noted that were different from placebo, suggesting that retrieval processes were not influenced.

When THC was administered prior to list presentation, performance during immediate recall testing was depressed except for those items in the terminal list positions, suggesting that some aspect of long-term storage was disrupted. However, items appeared to enter the sensory register and short-term store equally well. Since the memory of THC-treated subjects was lower for both delayed recall and recognition, it was suggested that transfer of information from short-term to long-term memory did not take place. One possible reason for the lack of transfer is that subjects did not rehearse incoming information, a process necessary for transfer to occur *(16)*. However, Darley and Tinklenberg *(13)* found that drugged subjects still displayed impaired recall when amount of rehearsal was fixed in both groups. It was felt that there was a reduced level of attention to list items probably because of increased competition during the intoxicated state from the subjects' own thoughts, which might have accounted for the inadequate transfer. Another possibility was that items residing in the short-term store were lost more quickly and this resulted in the transfer deficit.

Although the results of the Darley et al. study suggested that storage of information rather than retrieval of information was affected by THC or marihuana intoxication, this view is still open to speculation. The lack of definitiveness has arisen because of methodological and theoretical considerations. These issues are discussed in a later portion of this paper.

Research efforts in our laboratory concerning the effects of marihuana on memory have centered mainly on assessing the actions of the drug on free recall. This paradigm was employed because of its strong theoretical underpinnings and because of the consistency with which marihuana produces reliable effects across studies using this technique. The research to be described took place over a period of four years in an effort to define and analyze the effects of marihuana on human memory.

2. MARIJUANA AND MEMORY–AN INTEGRATIVE ASSESSMENT

Recently, a method for analyzing impaired memory, termed the "restricted reminding technique," has been developed (17). This method provides for the assessment and simultaneous analysis of storage, retention, and retrieval during a verbal memory task. In the restricted reminding task, an individual must recall information spontaneously without presentation. The usual free-recall paradigm analysis of memory is confounded because of interference produced by the immediate recall of items that were recently presented. According to Bushke and Fuld (17), an item can be considered to be in long-term memory only when it is recalled without repeated presentation. Recall is assessed independently of confounding by continued presentation of stimuli on each trial.

The data to be described are strikingly similar (in pattern of effects on memory but not magnitude) to those found with patients experiencing amnesia caused by herpes simplex encephalitis (18), Korsakoff syndrome (19,20), or Alzheimer's disease (21). Herpes simplex and Alzheimer's disease are thought to affect the limbic system via disruption of muscarinic limbic pathways (18,22,23), whereas Korsakoff syndrome may be caused by lesions in the hippocampus, mamilliary bodies, and/or dorsalmedial nucleus of the thalamus (24).

The task employed was a free recall task in which words in a list are presented individually until recall of the word occurs once. Following initial recall, words are not presented again so that eventually recall trials occur without any further presentation of items. All words are recalled on each trial. Buschke has argued that storage and retrieval of items in memory cannot be evaluated when all items are presented before every recall attempt because immediate recall of items does not demonstrate that an item resides in long-term memory (17). The dependent variables in this paradigm are long-term storage, which consists of the number of items encoded on a given trial, whereas retrieval consists of the number of items recalled on each trial that are considered to be in long-term storage.

Miller et al. (25), employing the restricted-reminding technique, ran 16 male volunteers in a crossover design with each receiving both smoked marijuana (10.5 mg THC) or placebo in successive sessions separated by one week. In each session, a different 30-item word list was employed with words being presented at a three-second rate. Recall testing occurred for 12 trials. Only the most salient features will be emphasized.

It can be seen that the number of items eventually encoded under marihuana and placebo were essentially the same although it took more recall trials for the same number of items to be encoded under drug. However, retrieval of items from long-term storage was significantly impaired under drug and this was because of the fact that more memory lapses or recall failures took place following intoxication. That is, intoxicated subjects displayed an inconsistency in recall. For example, under marihuana, an encoded word might be retrieved on a given trial following which a three to four trial lapse in recall would occur before the word would be recalled again. Intrusion error rates were significantly elevated in the drug condition in comparison to placebo. Intrusions consisted of the number of different extra list words which were emitted. What intoxicated subjects tended to do was commit an intrusion error, encode the word and repeat it on the majority of recall trials or if they committed one error, they might drop that word and substitute another. Thus, extraneous words from long-term memory were introduced which may have interfered with recall.

These data suggest that the mechanism of impaired recall in the intoxicated individual may be in his capacity to integrate material in some meaningful fashion for recall to occur. Buschke suggests that when items of information are consistently retrieved in memory they are integrated with the retrieval of other items in the list. Thus, items in memory are encoded within a given context. Information about a target item and its relationship to other words in the semantic system provides a basis of organization. That is, the learner imposes structure on information already in long-term memory. Marihuana may affect an individual's capacity to make use of information in his semantic memory to employ efficient recall strategies. Thus, the depth to which information is processed following cannabis intoxication may be an important mechanism by which recall is impaired. Intrusion errors may be seen as being secondary to organizing and integrating deficiencies since information from long-term memory, which is the basis for semantic organization intrudes on the recall process.

These data are consistent with the interpretation of Adam (26) for the effect of anesthetic gases on memory processes. These agents may make memory traces temporarily inaccessible, a form of anterograde amnesia. Impaired retrieval of information occurs because encoding processes are not consistent with efficient retrieval.

In conclusion, the deleterious effect of *Cannabis* on free-recall memory is a reliable and consistent finding. The pattern of memory deficits are similar to those found in neurally compromised patients with memory disorders thought to be mediated by cholinergic limbic dysfunction. These memory deficiencies are characterized by: lapses in recall, inconsistent retrieval of information, and memory intrusions.

Reprinted with permission from The Cannabinoids: Chemical, Pharmacologic, and Therapeutic Aspects (Agurell, S.; Dewey, W. and Willette, R., eds.), Academic Press, New York, 1984, pp. 21–46.

REFERENCES

1. Miller, L. L. (1976) Marijuana and human cognition: a review of laboratory investigations. In: *The Therapeutic Potential of Marijuana* (Cohen, S. and Stillman, R. C., eds.). Plenum, New York.
2. Moreau, J. J. (1845) Du hachish et de l'alienation mentale: E´tudes psychologiques, 34, Pacis: Libraire de Roxten, Maison Paris.
3. Bomberg, W. (1934) Marijuana intoxication. *Am. J. Psych.* **91**, 303–330.
4. Ames, F. A. (1958) A clinical and metabolic study of acute intoxication with cannabis sativa and its role in the model psychoses. *J. Mental Sci.* **104**, 972–999.
5. Tinklenberg, J. R., Kopell, B. S., Melges, F. T. and Hollister, L. E. (1972) Marijuana and alcohol: time production and memory functions. *Arch. Gen. Psych.* **27**, 812–815.
6. Clark, L. D., Hughes, R. and Nakashima, E. N. (1970) Behavioral effects of marijuana: experimental studies. *Arch. Gen. Psych.* **23**, 193–198.
7. Melges, F. T., Tinklenberg, J. R., Hollister, L. E. and Gillespie, H. K. (1970) Marijuana and temporal disintegration. *Science* **168**, 1118–1120.

8. Melges, F. T., Tinklenberg, J. R., Hollister, L. E. and Gillespie, H. K. (1971) Marijuana and temporal span of awareness. *Arch. Gen. Psych.* **24**, 564–567.

9. Weil, A. T. and Zinberg, N. E. (1969) Acute effects of marijuana on speech. *Nature* **222**, 434–437.

10. Abel, E. I. (1975) Marijuana, learning and memory. In *International Review of Neurobiology* (Pfeiffer, C. and Smythies, J., eds.). Academic, New York.

11. Rafaelsen, L., Christup, A., Bech, P. and Rafaelesen, O. J. (1973) Effects on cannabis and alcohol on psychological tests. *Nature* **242**, 117–118.

12. Tinklenbert, J. R., Kopell, B. S., Melges, F. T. and Hollister, L. E. (1972) Marijuana and alcohol: time production and memory functions. *Arch. Gen. Psych.* **27**, 812–815.

13. Darley, C. F. and Tinklenberg, J. R. (1974) Marijuana and memory. In: *Marijuana: Effects on Human Behavior* (Miller, L. L., ed.). Academic, New York.

14. Shiffrin, W. and Atkinson, R. E. (1969) Storage and retrieval processes in long-term memory. *Psychol. Rev.* **76**, 179–193.

15. Darley, C. F., Tinklenberg, J. R., Roth, W. T., Hollister, L. E. and Atkinson, R. C. (1973) Influence of marijuana on storage and retrieval processes in memory. *Memory Cognition* **1**, 196–200.

16. Abel, E. L. (1971) Marijuana and memory: acquisition or retrieval? *Science* **173**, 1038–1040.

17. Buschke, H. (1974) Retrieval in verbal learning. *Trans. Acad. Sci.* **236**, 721–729.

18. Peters, B. H. and Levin, H. S. (1977) Memory enhancement after physostigmine treatment in the amnesic syndrome. *Arch. Neurol.* **34**, 215–219.

19. Kovner, R., Mattis, S., Goldmeier, E., and Davis L. (1981) Korsakoff amnesic syndrome: the result of simultaneous deficits in several independent processes. *Brain Language* **12**, 23–32.

20. Fuld, P. A. (1976) Storage, retention and retrieval in Korsakoff's syndrome. *Neuropsychologica* **14**, 225–236.

21. Davis, K. L. et al., Cholinomimetic agents and human memory: clinical studies in Alzheimer's disease and scopolamine dementia. Pharmacological strategies in aging and dementia and the cholinergic hypothesis. In *Strategy for the Development of an Effective Treatment for Senile Dementia* (Cook, T. and Gershon, S., eds.). Mark Powley Associates, New Canann, CT., 1981.

22. Davies, P. and Maloney, A. J. F. (1976) Selective loss of central cholinergic neurons in Alzheimers disease. *Lancet* **2**, 1043.

23. Whitehouse, P. J., Price, D., Struble, R. G., Clark, A. W., Gayle, J. T. and DeLong, M. R. (1982) Alzheimer's disease and senile dementia: loss with neurons in the basal forebrain. *Science* **215**, 1237–1239.

24. Meissner, W. W. (1968) Learning and memory in the Korsakoff syndrome. *Int. J. Neuropsych.* **4**, 6–20.

25. Miller, L. L., Cornett,, T. and McFarland, D. (1978) Marijuana: an analysis of storage and retrieval deficits in memory with the technique of restricted reminding. *Pharmacol. Biochem. Behav.* **8**, 327–332.

26. Adam, U. (1979) Disruption of memory functions associated with general anesthetics. In: *Functional Disorders of Memory* (Kihlstrom, J. F. and Evans, F. J. eds.). Lawrence Erlbaum Press, Hillsdale, N J.

16   Does THC Induce Aggression?

Suppression and Induction of Aggressive Reactions by Chronic and Acute Δ⁹-Tetrahydrocannabinol Treatment in Laboratory Rats

Klaus A. Miczek

1. INTRODUCTION

With a few exceptions all laboratory investigations on the relationship between *Cannabis* and aggression were performed within the last five years. It has been reported that cannabis extracts and Δ^9-tetrahydrocannabinol (THC) may induce or facilitate as well as strongly and specifically suppress aggressive reactions. There are also indications that *Cannabis* does not alter aggressive behavior significantly. The array of seemingly contradictory observations from the animal laboratory has been summarized in Tables 1 and 2. In addition to the systematic studies included in Tables 1 and 2 there are a number of anecdotal remarks on the relationship between cannabinoids and certain aggressive reactions *(1)*.

Among the many important differences in the methodological details, which contribute to the inconsistent pattern of results, the schedule of drug administration appears to be particularly important in determining the direction of the drug effect. *Cannabis* extracts or THC has been found consistently to suppress intra- and interspecies aggressive behavior in all species and situations studied so far, when administered *acutely* (Table 1). On the other hand, *chronic* administration appears to induce or facilitate some nonspecific abnormal aggressive reactions and possibly predatory behavior in certain strains of rats exposed to aversive conditions (Table 2).

A further important source for discrepancies in the literature is the ambiguous conceptualization and behavioral analysis of aggressive behavior. In summarizing the literature on *Cannabis* and aggressive behavior in animals, a scheme was followed that differentiates between intra-, inter-, and nonspecific aggression. Particularly important is the distinction between intraspecific attack and threat, typically shown by a dominant animal, and defense, submission, and flight, which constitute the behavior pattern of a subordinate animal. This classificatory scheme is built on the ethological analysis of aggressive behavior, emphasizing the species-specific acts and postures characteristic of the various forms of attack, defense,

From: *Marihuana and Medicine*
Edited by: G. G. Nahas et al.   © Humana Press Inc., Totowa, NJ

Table 1

Effects of Acute Administration of Marihuana (Extracts; Δ^9-tetrahydrocannabinol) on Aggression in Animals

Intraspecies aggression		Interspecies aggression (predatory behavior)	Nonspecific aggression (irritability, indiscriminate biting, etc.)
Attack, threat	Defense, submission, flight		
Santos, Sampaio, Fernandes, and Carlini (1966) Suppression of isolation-induced attack in mice (extract, i.p.) Dubinsky, Robichaud, and Goldberg (1973) Suppression of isolation-induced attack in mice (5.0–20.0 mg/kg Δ^9-THC, ip) Siegel and Poole (1969). Reduction of attack in large colonies of mice (2.0–10.0 mg/kg Δ^9-THC, extracts, ip) Kilbey, Fritchie, McLendon, and Johnson (1972). Suppression of attack in mice (0.6–2.5 mg/kg Δ^9-THC, ip) Miczek and Barry (1974) Suppression of attack in rats (1–4 mg/kg Δ^9-THC, ip) Gonzalez, Matsudo, and Carlini (1971) Suppression of aggressive displays in Betta Splendens (extract) Cherek and Thompson (1972); Cherek, Thompson, and Heistad (1972) Suppression of attack in pigeons (0.125–1.0 mg/kg Δ^9-THC, im)	Dubinsky et al. (1973) Suppression of hypothalamically elicited defensive hissing in cats (5–20 mg/kg Δ^9-THC, ip) Miczek and Barry (1974) Impairment of defense; facilitation of immobility in rats Δ^9-THC, ip) Cutler, Mackintosh, and Chance (1975) Facilitation of immobility and flight in mice (extract, ip)	McDonough, Manning, Jr., and Elsmore (1972) Suppression of turtle attack in rats (6.4 mg/kg Δ^9-THC, ip) Kilbey, Moore, Jr., and Hall (1973) Suppression of frog kill in rats (0.25–2.5 mg/kg Δ^9-THC, iv) Dubinsky et al. (1973) Suppression of mouse kill in rats (5.0 mg/kg Δ^9-THC, ip). Suppression of hypothalamically elicited attack of rats by cats (5.0–20.0 mg/kg Δ^9-THC, ip) Alves and Carlini (1973) Suppression of mouse killing in rats (200 mg/kg, extract, ip)	Carlini and Gonzalez (1972) Facilitation of morphine withdrawal aggression in rats (5.0 mg/kg Δ^9-THC, ip) Alves, Goyos, and Carlini (1973) Induction of aggression in REM deprived rats (20–40 mg/kg Δ^9-THC, extract, ip) Carder and Olson (1972). Facilitation of foot-shock aggression in naive rats (0.25–0.5 mg/kg Δ^9-THC in extract, ip). Suppression of foot-shock aggression in rats (1.0–2.0 mg/kg Δ^9-THC in extract, ip) Manning and Elsmore (1972) No effect on foot-shock aggression in rats (0.064–6.4 mg/kg Δ^9-THC, ip) Dubinsky et al. (1973) Suppression of foot-shock aggression in rats and mice (15–22 mg/kg Δ^9-THC, ip)

Table 2

Effects of Chronic Administration of Marihuana (Extracts; Δ^9-tetrahydrocannabinol) on Aggression in Animals

Intraspecies aggression		Interspecies aggression (predatory behavior)	Nonspecific aggression (irritability, indiscriminate biting, etc.)
Attack, threat	Defense, submission, flight		
Carlini (1968) No effect on isolation-induced aggression in mice (28days, extract, ip) ten Ham and van Noordwijk (1973) Prolonged suppression of isolation-induced aggression in mice and "spontaneous" aggression in hamsters (30 days, 5 mg/kg Δ^9-THC, 50 mg/kg Δ^9-THC, ip) ten Ham and de Jong (1974) Prolonged suppression of isolation-induced aggression in mice (3–5days, 10 mg/kg/day Δ^9-THC, 25 mg/kg/dayΔ^9-THC)		Ueki, Fujiwara, and Ogawa (1972) Induction of mouse killing in rats (1–16 days, 6 mg/kg Δ^9-THC, ip) Alves and Carlini (1973) Induction of mouse killing in rats (starting day 10, 20 mg/kg, extract, ip)	Carlini and Masur (1969, 1970) Facilitation of foot-shock aggression; induction of aggressive reactions in Wistar rats (15–18 days, extract, 2.5–20.0 mg/kg Δ^9-THC, ip) Carlini, Hamaoui, and Martz (1972) Facilitation of foot-shock aggression; induction of aggressive reactions in Wistar rats (ca. 11–25 days, extract, ip) Palermo Neto and Carlini (1972) Induction of aggressive reactions in Wistar rats (ca. 7 days, extract, ip) Palermo Neto and Carvalho (1973) Induction of aggressive reactions in Wistar rats (ca. 5–15 days, extract, ip) Rosenkrantz and Braude (1973) "Fighting" in female and male Fischer rats (2.1 or 4.2 mg/kg/day Δ^9-THC inhaled from cannabis cigarettes for ca. 15–25 days)

submission, and flight, which have been amply described by students of animal aggression (2–4). Anthropomorphic terms such as "aggressiveness … hostility," "viciousness," and so on, are avoided, because they are misleading and confusing, and no precise definition of such terms seems to be generally agreed upon. Usage of such terms varies considerably from laboratory to laboratory. Especially when the significance of drug-induced behaviors needs to be assessed, the species-specific behavior patterns serve as guiding standards for comparison. The evidence for *Cannabis* inducing aggressiveness in animals under certain conditions should therefore be evaluated very cautiously by comparing carefully *Cannabis*-induced aggressive reactions with the species-specific patterns of fighting or killing behavior, and by describing precisely the physical characteristics of unusual and potentially pathological *Cannabis*-induced behaviors.

The present experiments attempted to compare the effects of acute and chronic THC administration on several kinds of aggressive and nonaggressive activities, focusing on intra- and interspecies aggressive behavior. It was of particular interest to identify the conditions under which chronic THC induces aggressive reactions and to describe the nature of the *Cannabis*-induced aggressive behavior.

2. GENERAL METHOD

In all experiments adult male albino rats of the Sprague-Dawley strain (Zivic-Miller, Pittsburgh, PA) were used, weighing between 300 and 400 g. The animals were kept in a colony with controlled temperature, humidity, and photo-cycle (12 hours light/12 hours dark).

The THC was administered in a suspension of propyleneglycol (10%) in 1% polysorbate-Tween-80-isotonic saline. The control fluid was the vehicle for the THC. Injections were given intraperitoneally in a volume of 1 mL/kg.

3. ACUTE THC AND FIGHTING BEHAVIOR (INTRASPECIES AGGRESSION) IN RATS

There is consistent evidence that low doses, sometimes less than 1 mg/kg, of THC suppress intraspecies attack behavior in mice, pigeons, and fighting fish (5–8). In the absence of a satisfactory experimental paradigm for intraspecies attack behavior in rats, several experimenters have resorted to the electric foot-shock situation, which generates the mutual upright posture accompanied by front paw movements. This shock-elicited behavior in a pair of rats is primarily defensive and submissive in nature (9) and should not be confused with attack behavior. THC has been found to have inconsistent effects on shock-elicited upright postures (6,10,11).

In the present experiment fighting episodes were generated between pairs of rats in which one animal showed characteristic sequences of species-specific attacks, threat displays, and other aggressive acts and postures, and thereby established its dominance; the subordinate opponent typically exhibits a pattern of defense, submission, and flight. The salient elements of species-specific fighting behavior have been extensively documented (2,3). The details of the training and testing procedure have been described previously (12). THC was administered 30 minutes prior to the 15-minute test to either the dominant ($n = 9$) or the subordinate rat ($n = 11$) at the different dose levels according to a Latin square sequence.

The main effects of THC on the various components of fighting behavior by the THC-treated rat and its nondrugged opponent are depicted in Fig. 1. When THC was administered to the dominant rat (solid lines in Fig. 1), it attacked less frequently and showed fewer threats, and consequently, the nondrugged subordinate opponent exhibited fewer submissive and defensive behaviors. On the other hand, administration of THC to the subordinate rat

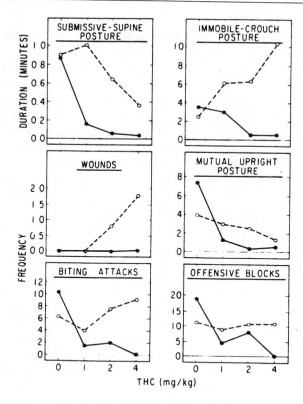

Fig. 1. Effects of acute THC (1, 2, 4 mg/kg) and control vehicle injected in the dominant rat (solid lines and dots) and in the subordinate rat (o–o) on duration of submissive-supine and immobile-crouch postures and number of wounds (in the subordinate rat), duration of mutual upright posture (by both rats), and frequency of biting attacks and offensive blocks (by the dominant rat). (From ref.*18*, with permission by Academic Press)

(dashed lines in Fig. 1) drastically increased the immobile-crouch reaction and decreased the display of the submissive-supine posture. The nondrugged dominant opponent attacked and injured the THC-treated subordinate rat more frequently. The display of the mutual upright posture is sometimes referred to as the fighting behavior; however, most students of rodent aggression attribute to it offensive as well as defensive functions. In the present experiment, the frequency of this posture was decreased when either opponent was drugged.

It is noteworthy that most drug effects were already significant at the 1.0 mg/kg dose level, showing a high degree of behavioral specificity for the antiaggressive properties of THC. These results show clear differential effects of THC on various components of species-specific fighting behavior, emphasizing the complex structure of intraspecies aggression and the necessity for a multiresponse analysis.

4. CHRONIC THC AND INTRASPECIES AGGRESSION IN RATS

Several reports indicate that chronic administration of *Cannabis* extracts or THC in certain strains of rats and circumstances can induce aggressive reactions (e.g., refs.*1,13,14*). Unfortunately, no accurate topographic description of the *Cannabis*-induced aggressive reactions is available, but all indications are that the drug-induced behavior differs clearly from species-specific patterns of aggression and involves primarily prolonged maintenance of upright postures and indiscriminate biting reactions. Two series of experiments were conducted to determine whether or not chronic. THC induces aggressive interactions between pairs of rats and, if so, to assess the nature of these drug-induced behaviors.

In the first experiment 36 rats, single housed and maintained on a restricted feeding regimen (about 20 g/day), were assigned to one of three treatment groups: 2 mg/kg/day of THC for 5 weeks ($n = 8$); 10 mg/kg/day of THC for 8 weeks ($n = 16$); and propylene glycol (10%)-Tween-80-isotonic saline vehicle ($n = 12$). Once a week pairs of rats of each treatment group were observed for 15 minutes in a neutral test area, and all social interactions as well as self-directed activities were recorded by two observers. There were no signs of any aggressive, defensive, or submissive behaviors evident in any of the rats treated with either dose of THC. The most predominant activities observed were crouching and self-grooming.

In a second experiment 30 rats, maintained in double housing and on a restricted feeding schedule, behavior in rats and cats (6,15–17), at dose levels that have little or no effect on neuromuscular capacities (Table 1). The present experiments purported to replicate this finding and extend it to male Sprague-Dawley rats which, in contrast to other strains of rats such as Long-Evans, show a very low percentage of "spontaneous" mouse killing behavior.

Twelve adult male albino rats were housed singly in regular sized ($18 \times 24 \times 18$ cm) wire cages during the first part of the experiment and transferred into larger cages ($64 \times 24 \times 18$ cm) for the second part. All rats had *ad libitum* access to water and were maintained on a restricted feeding regimen so that their weight stabilized between 300 and 400 g during the course of the experiment. Eight of the rats were induced to kill by chronic pilocarpine treatment (25 mg/kg/day for three weeks) two months prior to the start of the present experiments; the other four rats were natural mouse killers. All rats had extensive experience with mouse killing before the start of the experiment. Tests for mouse killing were conducted at least five days apart. One hour before an adult albino mouse was introduced into the home cage of the rat, each rat was administered intraperitoneally with one of four doses of THC (5, 10, 20, 40 mg/kg) or the vehicle (propylene glycol-Tween-80-saline). Drug administrations were scheduled according to a Latin square sequence. After completion of the five tests in the regular-sized home cages all rats were transferred into larger cages and a second series of tests under the five drug conditions was completed. Each test was maximally 10 minutes long or terminated by the mouse kill. If the rats did not kill within 10 minutes, further 10-minutes tests were conducted in consecutive hours. Attack and kill latency, anatomical site of kill bites, and whether or not the rat started to devour the mouse were recorded.

Table 3 summarizes the results of both series of experiments. There was little evidence for inhibition of mouse killing, even after doses as high as 40 mg/kg, in the regular-sized wire cages. In spite of the considerable sedation produced by the higher doses of THC, there was no were assigned to one of the following treatments: 10 mg/kg/day for eight weeks ($n = 10$); 20 mg/kg/day for eight weeks ($n = 10$); and propylene glycol-Tween-80-saline for eight weeks ($n = 10$). Each pair of rats, housed together, was subjected to the same drug treatment and observed three times per day for 10 minutes each: 30 minutes prior to injection, immediately following the injection, and 30 minutes after the injection. All interactions between the rats and self-directed behaviors were recorded.

Again, there was no evidence for increased aggressive activities in the THC-treated rats at any point in the drug treatment. In two pairs of rats administered with the control vehicle, mutual upright postures with accompanying front paw movements were seen immediately following the injection from the first week of treatment on; however, no attack bites or threat displays were noticed. Two further pairs in the control condition showed fighting behavior at least once during the 60-day treatment schedule. Similarly, three pairs of the 10-mg-THC and three pairs of the 20-mg-THC groups exhibited mutual upright postures and neck-grooming

Table 3
Effects of Acute Δ^9-Tetrahydrocannabinol on Mouse Killing

Dose (mg/kg)	Regular size cage (18 × 24 × 18 cm)		Large cage (64 × 24 × 18 cm)	
	n	Percent mouse killing	n	Percent mouse killing
Vehicle	12	100	11	100
5	12	100	11	72.7
10	12	100	11	63.6
20	12	72.7	11	63.6
40	12	72.7	11	54.5

during the 60-day treatment period, but these behaviors were not seen on more than five occasions and were of low intensity when compared with normal fighting behavior in rats. One pair of rats treated with 10 mg/kg/day displayed a very peculiar pattern of behavior from the third to seventh week of treatment. Immediately after the injection both rats assumed the mutual upright posture, leaped toward each other and away from each other, maintaining the upright position, and began to chew their forelimbs. Eventually, these two rats self-mutilated their entire front paws. This pattern of behavior was clearly different from species-specific fighting behavior and can probably be considered "pathological."

5. ACUTE THC AND MOUSE KILLING IN "KILLER" RATS

There is consistent evidence that acutely administered THC suppresses predatory attack and killing significant difference in attack and kill latencies in those animals that continued to kill under all doses (12.4-second average kill latency under vehicle condition; 38.0-second average kill latency under 40 mg/kg THC). Even in the larger cages, which required more active and coordinated pursuit of the mouse, only 40 mg/kg THC produced close to 50% inhibition of mouse killing.

6. CHRONIC THC AND MOUSE KILLING IN "NONKILLER" RATS

Ueki et al. (19) reported that three to four female Wistar rats out of groups of six began to kill mice either on the first (single-housed condition) or sixteenth day (group-housed condition) of chronic THC administrations (6 mg/kg/day, intraperitoneally), whereas none of the vehicle-treated rats showed any mouse killing. The present experiment attempted to investigate THC-induced killing behavior in larger groups of male Sprague-Dawley rats and to establish a dose-response relationship.

Eighty-three rats of the Sprague-Dawley strain were tested for mouse killing prior to any drug treatment. All "nonkiller" rats were then assigned to the following chronic drug administrations: 2 mg/kg/day of THC for five weeks (n = 8), 10 mg/kg/day of THC for eight weeks (n = 27), 20 mg/kg/day of THC for eight weeks (n = 10), vehicle control (propylene glycol-Tween-80-saline) for eight weeks (n = 22), and 25 mg/kg/day of pilocarpine hydrochloride for three weeks (n = 16). Ten rats of the 10 and 20 mg/kg THC and of the vehicle condition were maintained in double housing and the rest of the animals were maintained in the single-housed conditions. Mouse-killing tests were performed once a week in the home cage of the rat for maximally 10 minutes. Attack and kill latencies, anatomical site(s) of kill bites, and

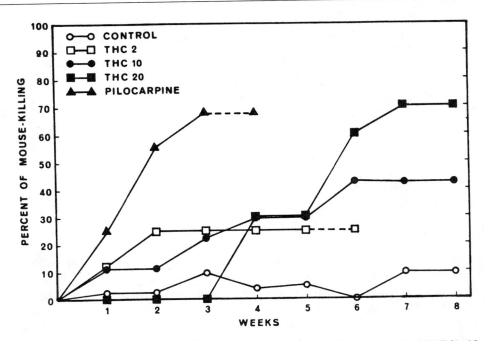

Fig. 2. Effects of daily intraperitoneal injections of THC at three dose levels, 2 mg/kg (THC 2), 10 mg/kg (THC 10), and 20 mg/kg (THC 20) and 25 mg/kg of pilocarpine hydrochloride (pilocarpine) and vehicle control on mouse killing in previously nonkiller rats. The daily administrations of 2 mg/kg THC were discontinued after five weeks and those of 25 mg/kg of pilocarpine were terminated after three weeks. The percentage of mouse killing was also assessed in the week after termination of the treatment; the results of these tests are depicted by dashed lines and the corresponding symbol for the drug treatment.

whether or not eating of the prey occurred were recorded. In the week immediately following the termination of the drug treatment all rats were subjected to a final mouse-killing test.

The results of this experiment are depicted in Fig. 2. More than half of all rats treated daily with 25 mg/kg pilocarpine started to kill mice after two weeks of drug administrations. At the end of the injection schedule (three weeks), two-thirds of all pilocarpine-treated rats killed mice. Those rats which had started to kill during pilocarpine administrations continued to do so after the end of the treatment. Chronic THC administration induced dose-dependent mouse-killing behavior over a much more prolonged time course than pilocarpine administrations. Daily injections of 2 mg/kg THC generated mouse killing in 25% of the animals after two weeks, and this percentage did not change during the remainder of the administration schedule. The same percentage of killing behavior was also evident in the posttreatment test. Administration of 10 mg/kg/day of THC induced more than 40% of the rats to kill mice. It is noteworthy that killing behavior did not appear suddenly at some fixed time in the treatment; rather, there was a gradual increase in the number of rats starting to kill mice from the second to the sixth week of the administrations. An even higher percentage of mouse-killing behavior was observed in the group of rats receiving 20 mg/kg/day of THC; after the seventh week of daily administrations 70% of these rats killed mice. Again, no starting point for this change in behavior can be fixed for the 20-mg-THC group. Beginning at the third week of treatment a gradual increasing number of rats became mouse killers.

The topography of mouse killing in pilocarpine- or THC-induced killer rats differed clearly from that of natural mouse killing. The initial pursuit of the mouse was mostly unsuccessful, showing signs of disorientation. Kill biting was not confined to the neck region of the mouse, but directed to almost all regions of the mouse's body, and occurred repeatedly, even after the mouse's spine was broken, and constant chewing and gnawing followed the kill. However, after three to four mouse-killing experiences there were no clearly detectable differences between a THC- or pilocarpine-induced and a natural mouse-killing rat.

The different housing conditions for some of the animals in the 10-mg-THC and vehicle control group had no influence on the percentage of mouse-killing in the respective groups. The percentages of mouse killing in single-housed and double-housed rats administered with 10 mg/kg/day of THC were not significantly different from each other and are depicted combined in Fig. 2.

Reprinted with permission from The Pharmacology of Marihuana (M. C. Braude and S. Szara, eds.) Raven Press, New York, 1976, pp. 499–514.

REFERENCES

1. Rosenkrantz, H. and Braude, M. C. (1974) Acute, subacute and 23-day chronic marihuana inhalation toxicities in the rat. *Toxicol. Appl. Pharmacol.* **28**, 428–441.
2. Barnett, S. A. (1963) *The Rat: A Study in Behavior.* Aldine, Chicago.
3. Grant, E. C. and Mackintosh, J. H. (1963) A comparison of the social postures of some common laboratory rodents. *Behaviour* **21**, 246–259.
4. Chance, M. R. A. and Silverman, A. P. (1964) The structure of social behavior and drug action. In: *Animal Behaviour and Drug Action*, (Steinberg and De Reuck, A. V. S. eds.) Churchill, London, pp. 65–79.
5. Kilbey, M. M., Fritchie, G. E., McLendon, D. M. and Johnson, K. M. (1972) Attack behavior in mice inhibited by Δ^9-tetrahydrocannabinol. *Nature* **238**, 463–465.
6. Dubinsky, B., Robichaud, R. C. and Goldberg, M. E. (1973) Effects of (–)^9-trans-tetrahydrocannabinol and its selectivity in several models of aggressive behavior. *Pharmacology*, **9**, 204–216.
7. Gonzales, S. C., Matsudo, V. K. R. and Carlini, E. A. (1971) Effects of marihuana compounds on the fighting behavior of siamese fighting fish (Betta Splendens). *Pharmacology*, **6**, 186–190.
8. Cherek, D. R., Thompson, T. and Heistad, G. T. (1972) Effects of Δ^1-tetrahydrocannabinol and food deprivation level on responding maintained by the opportunity to attack. *Physiol. Behav.* **9**, 795–800.
9. Reynierse, J. H. (1971) Submissive postures during shock-elicited aggression. *Anim. Behav.* **19**, 102–107.
10. Manning, F. J. and Elsmore T. F. (1972) Shock-elicited fighting and Δ^9-tetrahydrocannabinol. *Psychopharmacologia* **25**, 218–228.
11. Carder, B. and Olson, J. (1972) Marihuana and shock-induced aggression in rats. *Physiol. Behav.* **8**, 599–602.
12. Miczek, K. A. (1974) Intraspecies aggression in rats: effects of d-amphetamine and chlordiazepoxide. *Psychopharmacologia* **39**, 275–301.
13. Carlini, E. A. and Masur, J. (1969) Development of aggressive behavior in rats by chronic administration of *Cannabis sativa* (marihuana). *Life Sci.* **8**, 607–621.
14. Carlini, E. A. and Masur, J. (1970) Development of fighting behavior in starved rats by chronic administration of (–)^9-trans-tetrahydrocannabinol and cannabis extracts. *Commun. Behav. Biol.* **5**, 57–61.
15. McDonough, J. H., Jr., Manning, F. J. and Elsmore T. F. (1972) Reduction of predatory aggression of rats following administration of Δ^9-tetrahydrocannabinol. *Life Sci.* **11**, 103–111.
16. Kilbey, M. M. and Moore, J. W., Jr. (1973) Effects of Δ^9-tetrahydrocannabinol on appetitive- and aggressive-rewarded maze performance in the rat. *Physiol. Psychol.* **1**, 174–176.
17. Kilbey, M. M., Moore, J. W., Jr. and Hall, M. (1973): Δ^9-tetrahydrocannabinol induced inhibition of predatory aggression in the rat. *Psychopharmacologia* **31**, 157–166.
18. Miczek, K. A. and Barry, H., III (1974) Δ^9-tetrahydrocannabinol and aggressive behavior in rats. *Behav. Biol.* **11**, 261–267.
19. Ueki, S., Fujiwara, M. and Ogawa, N. (1972) Mouse-killing behavior (muricide) induced by Δ^9- tetrahydrocannabinol in the rat. *Physiol. Behav.* **9**, 585–587.

III PHARMACOLOGY AND PHYSIOPATHOLOGY

17

The Psychologic and Physiologic Effects of Active Cannabinoids

Mario Perez-Reyes

Abstract

This communication reviews the pharmacologic effects observed when Δ^9-THC and other cannabinoids were administered to humans by different routes of administration. Active cannabinoids, regardless of the route of administration, produced a temporary euphoric state with diversely perceived affective, sensory, somatic, and cognitive changes. Δ^9-THC produced heart rate increase, dry mouth, conjunctival congestion, and reduction of intraocular pressure. Larger doses of Δ^9-THC produced dysphoric reactions, postural hypotension, and occasionally myoclonic jerks. The magnitude of the psychologic and physiologic effects paralleled the temporal increase of Δ^9-THC plasma concentrations. Δ^8-THC produced milder psychologic effects and was as effective as Δ^9-THC in decreasing intraocular pressure. This cannabinoid therapeutic application merits further investigation.

1. INTRODUCTION

This communication reviews the pharmacologic effects observed when Δ^9-tetrahydrocanabinol (Δ^9-THC) and other cannabinoids were administered to humans by different routes of administration. The characteristics of the volunteers, experimental protocols, methods of procedure, and chemical analytical techniques used in the studies are summarized. Precise descriptions can be found in the papers cited.

Briefly, ratings of the magnitude of "high" were measured at frequent intervals in a 0–100 analog scale, and the heart rate was recorded continuously from electrodes placed on the chest wall. For their oral administration, Δ^9-THC, Δ^8-THC, or cannabinol were dissolved in sesame oil and placed in gelatin capsules. A microsuspension of Δ^9-THC, Δ^8-THC, or 11-OH-Δ^9-THC in human serum albumin was infused intravenously at the rate of 0.2 mg/min until the subjects reached their desired level of "high." The dose infused per minute was increased for less active cannabinoids (e.g., cannabinol, cannabidiol). Standard NIDA marihuana cigarettes of different Δ^9-THC content were used in the smoking studies. The data

From: *Marihuana and Medicine*
Edited by: G. G. Nahas et al.   © Humana Press Inc., Totowa, NJ

reported was obtained from healthy, male volunteers familiar with the use of marihuana. All of the studies were approved by the Committee on the Rights of Human Subjects of the University of North Carolina at Chapel Hill.

2. PSYCHOLOGIC EFFECTS

The major psychologic effect of Δ^9-THC (the most active psychoactive compound of marihuana) was a temporary euphoric state with diversely perceived affective, sensory, somatic, and cognitive changes that are commonly described as a "high." Subjects often reported that maximal psychologic effects fluctuate in intensity, called a "rush." The quality of psychologic effects varied between subjects and within the same subject when retested and were influenced by personality characteristics, emotional state prior to testing, and the experimental setting.

The prominent psychologic manifestations that have been observed include the following:

1. Affective: elation and easy laughing.
2. Sensory: increased exteroception (sound and visual stimuli were more sharp and vivid) and increased proprioception (subjects reported feeling the blood being drawn distantly from their shoulders when blood samples were taken from an antecubital vein)
3. Somatic: The subjects reported feeling their body floating in the air or sinking in the bed
4. Cognitive: distortion in the perception of time, memory lapses, difficulty in concentration, grandiose ideation, and loss of the ability to evaluate ideas and judgements critically (1).

An example of the impairment of cognitive function was the inability of many of the volunteers to continue reading material (whether serious books, magazines, or newspapers) that they brought with them to occupy their time during the experiments. In addition, psychomotor performance was decreased. Thus, marihuana smoking produced a significant reduction in accuracy and prolongation of reaction time in a difficult divided attention visual task (2).

The quality of psychologic effects was similar whether Δ^9-THC was administered orally, intravenously, or by smoke inhalation, but their magnitude depended on the dose administered. When infused intravenously (11-OH-Δ^9-THC, Δ^8-THC, cannabinol) (1,3) or when administered orally (Δ^8-THC, cannabinol) (4), these active cannabinoids have similar psychologic effects as those produced by Δ^9-THC. The magnitude of these effects, however, differed for each of these cannabinoids. The 11-OH-metabolite was as potent as its parent compound (5), but Δ^8-THC was 50% and cannabinol only 5% as potent as Δ^9-THC (1,3).

Large doses of Δ^9-THC, whether infused intravenously or administered orally, frequently induced dysphoric effects characterized by apprehension, fear, panic, and paranoid ideation. These dysphoric reactions were not ameliorated by reassurance but were rapidly controlled by the intravenous injection of 10 mg of diazepam (6).

3. PHYSIOLOGIC EFFECTS

The major consistent physiologic effect of Δ^9-THC and other active cannabinoids was a marked increase in the heart rate, which paralleled subjective ratings of "high" over time. This tachycardic effect was probably because of vagal inhibition, which leaves sympathetic cardioacceleratory activity unrestrained. Thus, in experiments in which atropine was intravenously injected (0.2 mg), the tachycardic effect produced was similar to that produced by the smoke inhalation of marihuana cigarettes of 1.3 and 4.6% THC content (Fig. 1). The unrestrained cardiacceleratory sympathetic activity of THC was counteracted by intravenous injection of the beta-blocking agent propranolol (6).

MEAN PERCENT HEART RATE INCREASE

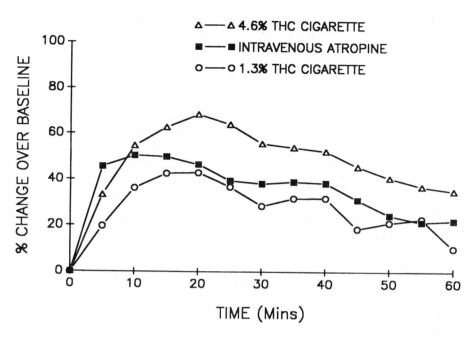

Fig. 1. The data shown derives from a study in which four subjects smoked in a crossover design NIDA marihuana cigarettes containing 1.3 or 4.6% Δ^9-THC. In a third experiment the subjects were injected intravenously with 0.2 mg of atropine sulfate.

Other cardiovascular effects of Δ^9-THC were measured by impedance cardiography using the techniques and instrumentation recommended by Sherwood et al. (7) The results of this study in which subjects smoked marihuana showed that the heart rate and the cardiac output were increased, and the stroke volume and the systemic vascular resistance were decreased. There were no significant changes in blood pressure although the systolic pressure showed a tendency to fall and the diastolic pressure to rise (Fig. 2).

Other physiologic effects consistently observed were dryness of the mouth and conjunctival congestion. Occasionally, large doses of Δ^9-THC, whether administered intravenously, orally, or by the inhalation (high potency marihuana) produced severe postural hypotension and bradycardia (vasovagal syndrome). In some individuals, large oral or intravenous doses of Δ^9-THC produced the occurrence of myoclonic movements of the lower extremities, sometimes extending throughout the body, even to the facial muscles (6). Myoclonic jerking was unnoticed by the subjects and did not trigger dysphoric reactions. The intrinsic mechanism of these abnormal movements is not known, but suggests the presence of cannabinoid receptors in the motor pathways.

Of therapeutic importance was the finding that active cannabinoids decreased intraocular pressure. Thus, in a study in which cannabinoids were infused intravenously, the mean reduction of intraocular pressure produced by Δ^9-THC was 33%; by 11-OH-Δ^9-THC, 34%; and by Δ^8-THC, 37% (Fig. 3). In this study, although the dose of Δ^8-THC was twice the dose of Δ^9-THC or its 11-hydroxylated metabolite, the psychologic effects produced were less intense (8).

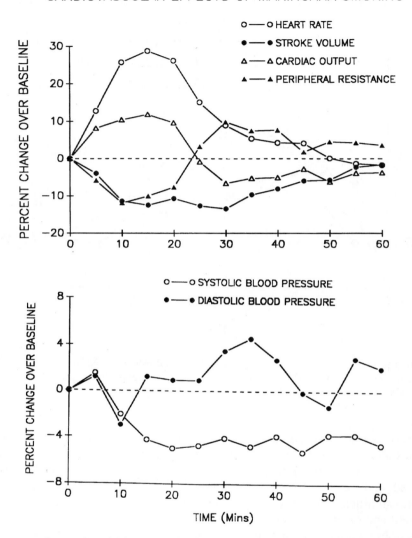

Fig. 2. Shown are the results of 28 experiments in which subjects smoked NIDA marihuana cigarettes containing 2.8% Δ^9-THC. The heart rate, stroke volume, and cardiac output were recorded continuously with a Hutcheson Impedance Cardiograph; the blood pressure was measured using an Accutracker (Suntech Medical Instruments); and the systemic peripheral resistance was calculated from simultaneous determinations of the cardiac output and the blood pressure.

4. Δ^9-THC PLASMA CONCENTRATION AND EFFECTS

A description of the pharmacologic effects of Δ^9-THC would be incomplete without discussing the temporal relationship with the plasma concentration. The rate at which Δ^9-THC reached the blood compartment and maximal concentration was influenced by the route of administration.

When administered orally, Δ^9-THC was absorbed slowly and reached maximal plasma concentration approximately two hours after ingestion. Psychologic effects and heart rate

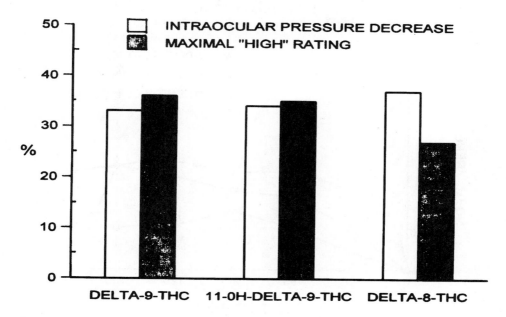

Fig. 3. Shown are the mean percent reduction of intraocular pressure from baseline values. In this study six subjects were intravenously infused at the rate of 0.2 mg/min with Δ^9-THC, 11-OH-Δ^9-THC, or Δ^8-THC. The total dose infused in micrograms/kg was 51, 42, and 85, respectively. Measurements of intraocular pressure were made with a Schiotz tonometer.

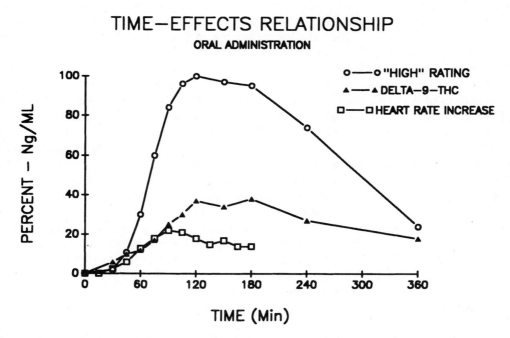

Fig. 4. Mean pharmacologic effects obtained from a study in which six subjects ingested gelatin capsules containing 20 mg of Δ^9-THC dissolved in sesame oil.

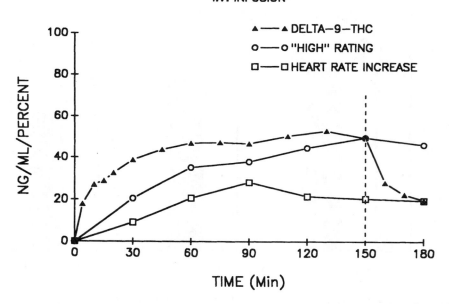

Fig. 5. Mean pharmacologic effects obtained from a study in which six subjects were intravenously infused at a rate of 0.074 mg/min with Δ^9-THC continuously for 150 minutes. The vertical dotted line marks the end of infusion.

increase also peaked at approximately the same time (Fig. 4). In comparison to the intravenous infusion or smoke inhalation of the drug, the plasma concentrations of Δ^9-THC after oral administration were significantly lower, but the magnitude of the psychologic effects was equal or greater. This discrepancy between the magnitude of drug plasma concentrations and effects may be explained partially by the higher plasma concentration of the equipotent 11-hydroxylated metabolite associated with Δ^9-THC oral administration (9). After oral administration of Δ^9-THC, the plasma concentration of 11-OH-Δ^9-THC was 43% of that of Δ^9-THC, compared to only 6% after intravenous infusion or smoke inhalation.

The temporal relationship between Δ^9-THC plasma concentration and effects after intravenous infusion are shown in Fig. 5. In this study, Δ^9-THC was intravenously infused continuously for 150 minutes at a rate of 0.074 mg/min. The plasma concentrations of Δ^9-THC increased steadily for as long as the infusion lasted and then rapidly declined. Psychologic effects and heart rate increase paralleled drug plasma concentrations.

Studies in which NIDA marihuana cigarettes of different Δ^9-THC contents were smoked have been reported elsewhere (*11,12*). These studies showed that regardless of marihuana potency, drug plasma concentrations peaked very rapidly (approximately seven minutes after the beginning of smoking). Maximal Δ^9-THC plasma concentrations invariably occurred several minutes before peak subjective and heart rate effects (Fig. 6). This consistent relationship indicates that when Δ^9-THC reaches the blood compartment rapidly, it requires time to access a deeper compartment (presumably brain) for its pharmacologic effects to reach maximal values.

In conclusion, Δ^9-THC, regardless of the route of administration, produced similar psychologic and physiologic effects. The magnitude of these effects was dose related. Δ^9-THC

TIME EFFECTS RELATIONSHIP

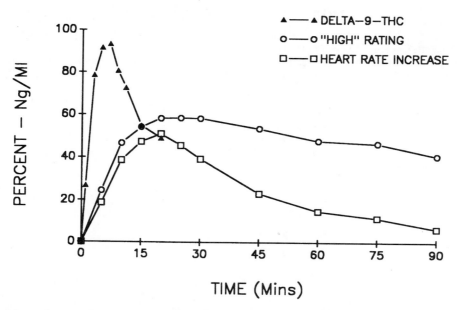

Fig. 6. Mean pharmacologic effects measured on 43 separate experiments in which NIDA marihuana cigarettes of different Δ^9-THC contents were smoked in the subjects customary manner.

invariably increased the heart rate and the cardiac output, but occasionally produced postural hypotension and bradycardia (vasovagal syndrome) after large doses or in susceptible individuals. These effects must be considered when Δ^9-THC is administered for therapeutic purposes to the elderly or debilitated patients. Δ^8-THC produced milder subjective effects and was as effective as Δ^9-THC in decreasing intraocular pressure. Therefore, this cannabinoid therapeutic applications merits further investigation.

REFERENCES

1. Perez-Reyes, M. (1985) Pharmacodynamics of certain drugs of abuse, in *Pharmacokinetics and Pharmacodynamics of Psychoactive Drugs* (Barnett, G. and Chiang, C. N., eds.), Biomedical Publications, Maryland, p. 287.
2. Perez-Reyes, M., Hicks, R. E., Bumberry, J., Jeffcoat, A. R., and Cook, C. E. (1988) Interaction between marihuana and ethanol: effects on psychomotor performance. *Alcoholism: Clin. Exp. Res.* **12**, 268–276.
3. Perez-Reyes, M., Timmons, M. C., Lipton, M. A., Davis, K. H., and Wall, M. E. (1972) Intravenous injection in man of D-9-tetrahydrocannabinol and 11-OH-D-tetrahydrocannabinol. *Science* **197**, 633–635.
4. Perez-Reyes, M. and Wall, M. E. (1981) Pharmacology of delta-9-tetrahydrocannabiol and other cannabinoids: clinical implications, In: *Treatment of Cancer Chemotherapy-Induced Nausea and Vomiting* (Poster, D. D., Penta, J. S. and Bruno, S., eds.) Masson Publishing New York, pp. 75–92.
5. Perez-Reyes, M., Timmons, M. C., Lipton, M. A., Christensen, H. D., Davis, K. H., and Wall, M. E. (1973) A comparison of the pharmacological activity of D-9-tetra-hydrocannabinol and its monohydroxylated metabolites in man. *Experientia* **29**, 1009–1010.
6. Perez-Reyes, M., Timmons, M. D., Lipton, M. A., Brine, D. R., Davis, K. H., and Wall, M. E. (1973) The clinical pharmacology of orally administered D-9-tetra-hydrocannabinol. *Clin Pharmacol and Therap.* **14**, 48–55.
7. Sherwood A., Allen, M. T., Kelsey, R. M., Lovallo, W. R., and van Doornen, L. J. P. (1990) Methodological Guidelines for Impedance Cardiography. *Psychophysiology* **27**, 1–23.

8. Perez-Reyes, M., Wagner, D., Wall, M. E., and Davis, K. H. (1976) Intravenous administration of cannabinoids and intraocular pressure, In: *Pharmacology of Marihuana*, vol. 2 (Braude, M. D. and Szara, S., eds.), Raven, New York, pp. 829–832.
9. Wall, M. E., Salder, B. M., Brine D., Taylor, H., and Perez-Reyes, M. (1983) Metabolism, disposition, and kinetics of delta-9-tetrahydrocannabinol in men and women. *Clin. Pharmacol. and Therap.* **34**, 353–363.
10. Perez-Reyes, M., DiGuiseppi, S., and Owens, S. M. (1981) The clinical pharmacology and dynamics of marihuana cigarette smoking. *J. Clin. Pharmacol.* **21**, 201S-207S.
11. Perez-Reyes, M., DiGuiseppi, S., Davis, K. H., Schindler, V. H., and Cook, C. E. (1982) The clinical pharmacology of three potencies of marihuana cigarettes, a comparative study. *Clin. Pharmacol. and Therap.* **31**, 617–724.

18

Physiological and Pharmacological Interactions of Marihuana (THC) with Drugs and Anesthetics

Kenneth M. Sutin and Gabriel G. Nahas

Abstract

THC is one of the 60 natural cannabinoids contained in the marihuana plant, which is psychoactive. It is a long-acting agent with multiple pharmacological effects. THC produces bronchodilation, but can also cause airway irritation. Marihuana smoke possesses toxic components, including carbon monoxide, tar, and carcinogens, which cause significant adverse pulmonary effects. THC causes a dose-dependent tachycardia, which is exacerbated by chronotropes and antagonized by β-blockers, diazepam, and clonidine. Increases of blood pressure can occur, but orthostatic hypotension is also observed. Marihuana exacerbates angina pectoris in patients with exercise-inducible myocardial ischemia. Some patients report relief of neuropathic pain and discomfort after smoking marihuana or ingesting THC. However, in a controlled study on healthy volunteers who were studied by using the sensory decision theory to account for the psychoactive drug effects, marihuana smoking caused hyperalgesia. As an antiemetic, THC is much less effective than metoclopramide or 5-HT$_3$ receptor antagonists, and it often causes unwanted psychoactive effects. THC is not effective as a premedication for anesthesia, and preoperative marihuana smoking exacerbates perioperative tachycardia. THC interacts with other drugs: it increases the depressant effects of sedatives and mitigates the effects of stimulants. In addition, severe adverse psychoactive side-effects have been observed when this agent is combined with barbiturates. In combination with opiates or ethanol, THC increases sedation and respiratory depression. The existing data indicate that marihuana or THC is not an acceptable adjunct to anesthesia.

1. INTRODUCTION

Cannabinoids are a group of C_{21} compounds naturally occurring in the *Cannabis sativa* plant (which has about 60 different cannabinoids). Delta^9-THC (THC) is one of the naturally occurring cannabinoid molecules, which is psychoactive and is biotransformed into

From: *Marihuana and Medicine*
Edited by: G. G. Nahas et al.   © Humana Press Inc., Totowa, NJ

mostly nonpsychoactive but still biologically active metabolites. Cannabinoid pharmacology has been reviewed recently *(3,25,46)*. THC is highly lipophilic (octanol:water coefficient of 6000:1) and highly protein-bound, and has the potential to displace other extensively protein-bound drugs. Cannabinoids are optically active, and the (–) enantiomers are much more potent than the (+) ones. Especially with repeated administration, THC accumulates in tissues, mostly in neutral fat, from which it is slowly released, a factor that contributes to its prolonged terminal elimination half-life of 3–5 d in humans. THC undergoes enterohepatic recirculation and is extensively metabolized by the hepatic cytochrome P-450 system. Of all the cannabinoids and their metabolites (over 100 for THC alone), only Δ^8-THC and Δ^9-THC and their hydroxy metabolites possess psychoactive properties in nanomolar concentration. Acutely, cannabinoids, and especially cannabidiol, cause inhibition of microsomal function in the liver *(93)*, which can slow the metabolism of drugs dependent on hepatic elimination. Chronic use causes induction of the cytochrome oxidase system, which may increase the clearance of other drugs (e.g., barbiturates and aminophylline). Less than 1% of the drug crosses the blood–brain barrier. Unchanged THC is excreted in the bile (approximately 80%), while most THC metabolites, the first being COOH, are excreted in the urine (approximately 20%). Genetic polymorphism accounts for the marked variability of effects in different subjects, as well as the concentration of other cannabinoids, like cannabidiol.

2. PHYSIOLOGICAL INTERACTIONS OF THC

2.1 Pulmonary System

2.1.1 MARIHUANA SMOKING

In addition to natural cannabinoids, marihuana smoke contains the same respiratory irritants and toxins found in tobacco smoke (gas phase: carbon monoxide, acetaldehyde, acrolein, toluene, nitrosamine, and vinyl chloride; insoluble particulate or tar phase: phenol, benzanthracene, benzapyrene, cresol, and naphthalene), some of which are carcinogens, e.g., the polycyclic aromatic hydrocarbons. Exogenous contaminants such as viable fungal spores have also been reported *(45,51,66,121)*. A marihuana cigarette causes a fivefold greater increase in blood carboxyhemoglobin and one-third more insoluble particles (tar) are retained in the respiratory tract than tobacco smoking does *(138)*. Cigarette smoking is a substantial etiologic factor in respiratory disorders, including chronic bronchitis, bronchial asthma, chronic obstructive pulmonary disease, and lung cancer. Chronic marihuana smoking has similar adverse effects *(118,119)*. Marihuana smoke impairs pulmonary antibacterial defenses *(53)*, is mutagenic in the Ames Salmonella/microsome test *(14)*, and causes DNA damage in human alveolar macrophages *(110)*. One preliminary epidemiological study reported that marihuana smoking was not an independent risk factor for cancer in humans *(112)*. Of particular concern is the observed synergy between tobacco and marihuana smoking on pathology of the respiratory mucosa *(29)* and reports of head and neck cancer in young marihuana smokers *(26)*.

2.1.2 RESPIRATORY CONTROL

Studies report inconsistent findings regarding the effects of marihuana or THC on respiration. Minute ventilation has been observed to either increase *(141)* or decrease *(137)*. In normal subjects, smoking marihuana either had no effect on the respiratory response to carbon dioxide *(129)* or produced slight respiratory depression *(8,9)*. In one study in which respiratory depression was observed *(8)*, tolerance to this effect was observed after daily marihuana smoking for 90 d.

Smoking marihuana at typical doses causes at most a mild, transient respiratory depression. Perhaps more important, marihuana increases the effects of other respiratory depressant drugs (see below). Depression of respiration and consciousness and airway obstruction also occur in children after ingestion of cannabis resin or following exposure to marihuana smoke *(13,49,57,72,106,133)*.

In eight healthy subjects who had previously used marihuana, Zwillich et al. *(141)* reported increases in minute ventilation (40%), ventilatory response to CO_2 (from 2.7 to 5.4 L/min per mm Hg), and oxygen consumption (21%) after inhalation of marihuana smoke (22 mg THC). In contrast, Wu et al. *(137)* did not observe any effect of marihuana smoking (THC 17.7 or 35.8 mg) on either minute ventilation or mouth occlusion pressure (at 0.1 s) in response to hypercapnia or isocapnic hypoxia in habitual marihuana smokers. They also did not observe any changes in resting minute ventilation, oxygen consumption, or CO_2 production *(137)*. It is possible that habitual use induces tolerance or decreases drug-associated anxiety and concomitant sympathetic activation.

2.1.3 CHRONIC MARIHUANA SMOKING AND RESPIRATORY PATHOLOGY

Chronic smoking of tobacco or marihuana causes airway inflammation and symptoms of acute and chronic bronchitis. Marihuana smokers consistently report a higher incidence of respiratory symptoms (chronic cough, sputum production, wheezing, and infections of the upper and lower respiratory tract) than nonsmokers *(12,111,121)*. In humans, smoking THC may cause or exacerbate respiratory disorders including rhinopharyngitis, uvulitis, bronchitis, pneumonia, and bronchial asthma *(47,74,127)*.

The most consistent pulmonary function abnormality described in chronic marihuana users is impairment of large airway function (increased airflow resistance and decreased specific airway conductance) with relative sparing of small airway function *(120,121,126)*. Others, however, have reported a significant abnormality of small airway function in chronic marihuana smokers *(12,111)*. Thus, it is uncertain if regular marihuana smoking increases the risk of developing chronic obstructive pulmonary disease (primarily a small-airways disease). An additive negative effect on FEV_1 of combined tobacco and marihuana smoking has also been observed *(111)*.

In habitual marihuana smokers, significant histopathologic abnormalities have been described in bronchial biopsy specimens. These include premalignant lesions such as metaplasia and cell nucleus abnormalities *(29,47)*. In a study of heavy marihuana smokers examined bronchoscopically, Gong and others *(38)* observed airway hyperemia and increased secretions. Subsequent histopathologic examination of bronchial biopsy specimens in 15 subjects revealed multiple epithelial changes including squamous metaplasia (53%), goblet and basal cell hyperplasia (80%), cellular disorganization (53%), nuclear variation (26%), and inflammation (93%), in addition to basement membrane thickening (47%) and submucosal inflammation (93%). These abnormalities were uncommon in nonsmokers. Many findings were similar to those observed in tobacco smokers, except that cellular disorganization occurred twice as often in marihuana users.

In a case report, smoking marihuana prior to general anesthesia and tracheal intubation was associated with postextubation airway obstruction from severe uvular edema, which has been associated with particularly heavy marihuana or hashish use *(43,75,127)*. It usually resolves in 12–24 h, and is perhaps caused by the high temperature of marihuana combustion compared with conventional (filtered) tobacco cigarettes.

2.1.4 BRONCHODILATION

Both Δ^8-THC and Δ^9-THC possess bronchodilating activity, but this is not observed with cannabinol or cannabidiol *(39)*. This effect does not appear to be caused by direct sympathomimetic activation, parasympatholysis, or prostaglandin inhibition *(40,63)*. In healthy, experienced marihuana smokers, smoked marihuana (10 or 20 mg THC) and oral THC (10, 15, or 20 mg) decreased airway resistance (R_{aw}) for 1 h and 6 h, respectively *(123)*. In asthmatic subjects, aerosolized Δ^1-THC 200 µg caused bronchodilation and an increase in FEV_1 equivalent to 100 µg of aerosolized salbutamol without causing cardiac or mood-altering effects *(136)*. In stable asthmatics, exercise- or methacholine-induced bronchospasm caused a decrease in specific airway conductance ($SG_{aw} = R_{aw}-1/TGV$, where TGV = thoracic gas volume) and an increase in thorac gas volume (hyperinflation) that was reversed by either smoked marihuana (20 mg THC) or aerosolized isoproterenol (1.25 mg) *(124)*. Salbutamol *(136)* or isoproterenol *(124)* exhibited a more rapid onset of effect than THC, but all three agents were equally efficacious. In other studies, however, aerosolized THC caused chest discomfort, cough, and severe bronchoconstriction in subjects with asthma; this airway irritant effect "may make it unsuitable for therapeutic use" *(122)*. Even oral THC has been reported to cause severe paradoxical bronchoconstriction *(1)*. After 47–59 d of daily marihuana smoking (mean 5.2 marihuana cigarettes/day), there was marked diminution of the bronchodilating activity indicating tachyphylaxis, and evidence of mild airway obstruction (decreased FEV_1, FEF_{25-75}, and airway conductance), which improved following cessation of smoking *(125)*.

Smoked marihuana is a suboptimal means of THC delivery because noxious gases and irritant particles can exacerbate coughing, airway irritation, and bronchospasm. Bronchodilation is usually observed at THC doses, which also cause tachycardia and psychologic manifestations. Further clinical evaluation of low-dose metered inhalers of THC has been suggested *(40)*. However, since there are many effective antiasthmatic drugs (e.g., inhaled β_1-agonists, inhaled and parenteral corticosteroids, inhaled anticholinergics, methylxanthines, and leukotriene inhibitors), THC will probably never become a mainstay of therapy for bronchospasm. Furthermore, smoking is contraindicated in asthmatics.

2.2 Cardiovascular System

2.2.1 TACHYCARDIA

Smoked marihuana, in fact THC delivered by any route, produces a dose-related tachycardia in normal adults *(58,104)* and in subjects with coronary artery disease *(5)*. Tachycardia correlates with the drug "high" *(16)* and is such a consistent finding that it is often used as a surrogate marker of THC effect in clinical studies. Tachycardia reaches a maximum after 30 min and usually lasts for more than 90 min; its duration is dose-dependent *(58)*. Propranolol given prior to smoking marihuana prevents tachycardia *(7,117)*, while pretreatment with clonidine blunts the chronotropic response *(20)*. In contrast, atropine and epinephrine exacerbate marihuana-induced tachycardia *(7)*. Following chronic THC exposure, marihuana smoking (20 mg THC) fails to increase heart rate *(10)*. THC has a mild sympathomimetic effect, which is not associated with a significant incidence of cardiac dysrhythmias or premature ventricular contractions in young healthy men *(105)*. It has been proposed that arachonidyl ethanolamine (AEA) is an endothelium-derived hyperpolarizing factor (EDHF) and causes vasorelaxation in mesenteric and coronary circulations of the rat *(102,103)*. By contrast to humans, the major cardiovascular effects of THC in most animal species studied are bradycardia and hypotension *(24,41)*.

2.2.2. MYOCARDIAL ISCHEMIA

The effects of THC on the normal heart may be clinically insignificant; however, consequential adverse effects can occur in individuals with coexistent coronary artery disease, valvular pathology (e.g., mitral stenosis), or myocardial disease (e.g., hypertrophic car-

Table 1

Exercise Tolerance in Patients with Coronary Artery Disease[a]

	Exercise Time Onset to Angina (min)	Heart Rate (beats/sec)	Blood Pressure (S/D, mm Hg)	Product of Systolic Blood Pressure × Heart Rate
Baseline	244.3±16	129.1±2.3	150±1.2	19,363±391
			81.3±1.1	
After Smoking Marihuana	129.4±13.6*	124.6±2.4*	147.8±1.3*	18,406±394*
			81.5±1.2*	

[a]Exercise time on a bicycle ergometer was measured in 10 habitual tobacco cigarette smokers with documented chronic stable angina pectoris. Table shows exercise time required to provoke anginal symptoms at baseline and after smoking a marihuana cigarette (19.8 mg THC). Also shown is peak heart rate, blood pressure, and pressure-rate product (data are means of 10 subjects). * = significantly different from control, and $p < 0.05$. The clinically important difference is that marihuana smokers were able to exercise only about one-half as long as those that did not smoke the drug (adapted from *ref. 5*).

diomyopathy). Aronow and Cassidy *(5)* measured the duration of bicycle exercise required to provoke anginal symptoms in 10 cigarette smokers with stable angina pectoris. After smoking a marihuana-containing cigarette (19.8 mg THC), the duration until onset of angina was reduced by about 50% (Table 1). Marihuana had a greater adverse effect on exercise time to onset of angina than a high-nicotine cigarette *(6)*. In persons with inducible myocardial ischemia, smoking marihuana can lead to an oxygen supply–demand imbalance because of the increase in blood carboxyhemoglobin and heart rate *(138)*.

2.2.3. Blood Pressure and Blood Flow

Marihuana has been observed to cause both hypotension *(10)* and hypertension *(58)*; however, orthostatic hypotension is the most consistent finding *(10,42)*. Presyncopal and syncopal episodes may result from orthostatic hypotension or vasovagal reactions *(134)*. Marihuana smoking inhibits the normal reflex bradycardia observed during the forced exhalation phase following a Valsalva maneuver *(104)*, and increases the tachycardia normally observed when rising to a standing position *(78)*. During chronic marihuana exposure, tolerance develops to orthostatic hypotension *(10)*. When the dose of smoked marihuana exceeds 10 mg THC, a slight but significant increase in systolic and diastolic blood pressure is observed *(58)*. During a 14-d exposure to marihuana (maximum 210 mg THC per os), both systolic and diastolic blood pressures decreased slightly, and returned to baseline following discontinuance of the agent *(10)*.

Marihuana also increases cardiac output and muscle blood flow *(7)*. In normal adults, following IV administration of 134 µ/kg THC, the cardiac index increased from 4.04±0.62 to 6.92±2.34 L/min/m² *(73)*.

2.3. Nervous and Muscular Systems

Marihuana is often smoked to produce mood altering effects *(92)*; however, it also alters neuromuscular and psychomotor functions (e.g., reaction time, motor and hand–eye coordination), cognition (e.g., attentiveness), and the sense of time; this impairs the ability to fly or drive *(16,37)*. THC causes conjunctival injection and at times pupillary dilation *(48,92,113)*. Marihuana smoking may also decrease salivary flow by as much as 35% *(60)* and cause dry mouth *(73)*. Several studies have reported antiseizure activity of cannabidiol *(15,69)*. In fact, low doses of THC possess anticonvulsant and high-dose proconvulsant activity, which precludes its routine use in seizure therapy *(21,28)*. Following marihuana smoking, global cerebral blood flow (CBF) decreased in inexperienced volunteers *(79)*. Baseline CBF was significantly lower in habitual marihuana users than in the inexperienced group, and it increased in the left and right frontal regions and the left temporal region after exposure to marihuana *(79)* In experienced users, the CBF increase was correlated with the perceived drug "high," pulse rate, and plasma THC level *(77)*. After smoking marihuana, cerebral glucose utilization as measured by PET scan increases most consistently in the cerebellum *(36)*. In habitual users, glucose utilization also increases in the prefrontal cortex, orbitofrontal cortex, and basal ganglia.

THC does produce significant effects on the autonomic ganglia deregulating the baroreflex; however, it inhibits parasympathetic effects in the gastrointestinal system and to slow gastric and intestinal motility *(11,70,94)* probably as a result of reduced acetylcholine release at postganglionic parasympathetic nerve endings *(65)*.

In an animal model, THC decreased presynaptic acetylcholine release and, in addition, elicited a potent inhibitory effect at the neuromuscular junction *(62)*. THC also decreased sodium and potassium conductance in skeletal muscle. This can account for the mild muscular weakness and ptosis *(52,84)*. THC has been used to relieve the muscular spasticity of multiple sclerosis *(100)*. There is no indication that THC can provide adequate muscle relaxation for surgery.

2.4. Immune System

A large number of studies in animals and humans indicate that, especially after chronic use of marihuana, cellular and humoral immunity are impaired, in addition to natural killer cell, macrophage, and leukocyte functions. The proinflammatory cytokines IL-6 and TNF-a are suppressed and IL-1 is enhanced. In animal models, this is associated with increased susceptibility to infection with *Listeria*, *E. coli*, *Salmonella*, and *Legionella (61)*. These adverse immune effects may have deleterious consequences in immunocompromised patients *(33)*.

3. INTERACTIONS OF THC WITH OTHER DRUGS

Marihuana generally increases the depressant effects of alcohol and sedative agents, and mitigates the effects of stimulants. THC interacts with several commonly used drugs (Table 2) *(87)*. This has been clearly demonstrated in experimental animals *(34,55,56,114)*, and human studies support this conclusion. These interactions are dose-related and vary between individuals owing to differences in sensitivity and in drug disposition and metabolism.

3.1. Inhalational Anesthetics

In rats, THC was observed to decrease the MAC (minimum alveolar concentration) of cyclopropane; the effect did not vary following chronic THC administration *(132)*. In a dog study, intravenous THC produced a dose-dependent decrease in halothane MAC that diminished over time *(115)*. Large doses (THC = 0.5–2.0 mg/kg IV) were required to produce this effect. This should be compared to the typical dose, about 0.05 mg/kg, of inhaled THC required to produce a "high" in humans. It is not known if this effect can be extrapolated to humans.

3.2. Sedatives/Hypnotics

When combined with secobarbital, smoked marihuana enhanced symptoms of CNS depression and impaired psychomotor performance in an additive fashion *(23,67)*. In a detailed study by Johnstone et al. *(59)* involving healthy adult men, pentobarbital (100 mg/70 kg IV) alone caused no change in blood pressure, heart rate, cardiac index, or peripheral vascular resistance (Table 3). When this dose of pentobarbital was followed by incremental

Table 2
Summary of Drug Interactions with THC

Drug Given with THC	Clinical Interaction
Aminophylline	Increased dose required due to enhanced hepatic drug elimination. Aminophylline clearance increased most in smokers of marihuana and tobacco (60a).
Anti-Cholinesterases	Physostigmine antagonizes marihuana intoxication and reduces tachycardia and conjunctival injection. In marihuana users, physostigmine may induce severe depression and psychomotor retardation (25a,32a).
Anti-Cholinergics: atropine,scopolamine	Possible additive drowsiness. Atropine may blunt or enhance marihuana-induced tachycardia (7,7a,10).
Anti-Depressants-Selective Serotonin Reuptake Inhibitors: fluoxetine	Case report of severe mania with psychosis in patient on fluoxetine shortly after smoking marihuana. THC may inhibit serotonin reuptake and increase its synthesis (115a)
Anti-Depressants-Tricyclics; e.g. amitriptyline	Additive tachycardia, hypertension, and drowsiness. Transient delirium and severe cognitive problems observed in four children with attention deficit disorder on nortriptyline or desipramine. One adult developed disorientation, restlessness, dizziness, palpitations and tachycardia (60b,135a).
Anti-Psychotics: chlorpromazine	In schizophrenic patients on neuroleptic therapy, marihuana may induce acute psychosis (possibly due to antagonism of neuroleptic activity) (61a).
Barbiturates	THC enhances drowsiness and CNS depression in a dose-dependent manner. Low-dose barbiturate induced increases in ventilation cancels mild respiratory depression of THC. Combination increases heart rate. Increased incidence of anxiety and hallucinations. Acutely cannabis decreases hepatic clearance of pentobarbital. After chronic cannabis is discontinued, metabolism of pentobarbital is enhanced (11,23,59,67).
Benzodiazepines	THC enhances drowsiness, and respiratory and CNS depression in a dose-dependent manner. Diazepam may be used (cautiously and in titrated doses) to sedate a patient with agitation due to acute THC intoxication.
β-blockers: propranolol	Blunts marihuana-related tachycardia (7,10).
Cocaine	Marihuana-induced dilation of nasal mucosa increases absorption of intranasal cocaine and the peak plasma cocaine level. Marihuana combined with cocaine causes additive tachycardia but increases in blood pressure are due mostly to cocaine (31,71).
Disulfiram	In a study evaluating treatment of alcoholism, no adverse interactions were reported. One case report of extreme confusional state followed by mania, and another case report of hypomania (61a,71a,104a).
Ethanol	Additive drowsiness, tachycardia, and CNS impairment, (perception, cognition and motor performance). Delayed ethanol absorption possibly due to decreased gastric motility. Minimal effect on ethanol metabolism. Increased effect of ethanol is not related to an increase in ethanol blood level (11,70,76,96).

(Table continues)

Table 2 (Continued)

Drug Given with THC	Clinical Interaction
Inhalational Anesthetics: (e.g. Halothane)	High dose THC decreases halothane MAC in rats and dogs *(115,132)*.
Ketamine	Possible additive CNS depression. Increased sleep time in mice *(34)*.
Opiates	THC enhances sedation and respiratory depression in a dose-dependent manner. Combination increases cardiac output, heart rate and decreases peripheral vascular resistance *(59)*.
Sympathomimetics: epinephrinc, amphetamines, cocaine	With epinephrine, effect is dose-dependent: at low dose of either causes minimal interaction, at higher dose, additive tachycardia and hypertension. Possible enhancement of cardiotoxicity or arrhythmias. When combined with amphetamines, psychomotor impairment primarily due to marihuana (no additive effect) *(7,7a,27,27a,32,139)*.

Table 3
Cardiovascular Effects of Pentobarbital, and Pentobarbital Followed by THC in Healthy Men[a]

	Cardiac Index $(L/min/m^2)$	Heart Rate (beats/min)	Mean Blood Pressure (mm Hg)	Peripheral Vascular Resistance $(dyn \cdot sec/cm^5)$
Control	4.4 ± 1.5	75 ± 17	102 ± 10	980 ± 290
Pentobarbital 100 mg/70 kg iv	3.8 ± 0.7	76 ± 16	101 ± 8	$1,070 \pm 240$
THC 90 µg/kg iv (Given after Pentobarbital)	5.6 ± 1.9	$130 \pm 32*$	96 ± 4	720 ± 300

[a]* = significantly different from control, and $p < 0.05$. (Adapted from *ref. 59*).

doses of THC (40–134 µg/kg IV), there was no decrease in minute ventilation or the respiratory response to CO_2; however, tachycardia was observed. Four of the seven subjects were unable to tolerate the full dose of THC because of "severe psychological side-effects" including anxiety, while five developed hallucinations. In a different study, when THC (5 mg IV) was followed by incremental doses of diazepam (cumulative dose 5, 10, or 20 mg per 70 kg IV), there was additive respiratory depression, and diazepam also blunted the tachycardia caused by THC in a dose-dependent fashion *(113)*. Severe psychological side-effects have not been reported when benzodiazepines are combined with THC, and, in fact, diazepam is often used to treat THC-induced anxiety or agitation.

In healthy chronic users of marihuana, pentobarbital pharmacokinetics were studied at baseline, during a 10–14-d interval of daily THC administration, and 5–6 d after stopping THC. During THC administration, the plasma half-life and volume of distribution for pentobarbital increased, while its metabolic clearance rate decreased slightly *(11)* Five to six days following the trial, the pentobarbital plasma half-life decreased to slightly less than baseline, while the metabolic clearance rate increased significantly above that observed prior to chronic marihuana exposure. It is likely that during the marihuana exposure, the hepatic elimination of the barbiturate was inhibited, but at the same time there was induction of

Table 4
Cardiovascular Effects of Oxymorphone, and Oxymorphone Followed by THC in Healthy Men

	Cardiac Index (L/min/m²)	Heart Rate (beats/min)	Mean Blood Pressure (mm Hg)	Peripheral Vascular Resistance (dyn • sec/cm⁵)
Baseline	3.5 ± 1.1	68 ± 14	98 ± 5	$1,150 \pm 260$
Oxymorphone 1 mg/70 kg iv	4.1 ± 1.3	66 ± 12	97 ± 9	$1,030 \pm 260$
THC 90 µg/kg iv (Given after Oxymorphone)	$5.6 \pm 2.9*$	$105 \pm 32*$	93 ± 10	$730 \pm 240*$

* = significantly different from control, and $p < 0.05$. (Adapted from *ref. 59*).

hepatic enzymes that produced the accelerated barbiturate metabolism observed after THC was discontinued.

3.3. Opiates

Johnstone et al. *(59)* observed that oxymorphone (1 mg/70 kg IV) followed by THC (27–134 µg/kg IV) produced increased respiratory depression (right-shift and decrease in slope of the ventilatory response curve to CO_2). When given alone, oxymorphone caused no change in hemodynamics (Table 4), but when it was followed by IV THC, there was an increase in cardiac index and heart rate and a decrease in peripheral vascular resistance. Subjectively, the combination of oxymorphone and THC produced excess sedation; three of six subjects could not stay awake without verbal stimulation. With this combination, five of the subjects were nauseated, four vomited, and one retched for 2 h. Contrary to a previous suggestion by Mechoulam et al. *(85)*, there is no evidence in humans that THC enhances the analgesic effects of opiates or decreases their side-effects.

3.4. Ethanol

Following chronic exposure to THC (60–180 mg/day PO for 10–14 d), ethanol clearance from the blood and ethanol metabolic rate decreased slightly, but the results were not statistically significant *(11)*. Marihuana smoking enhances the psychological effects of ethanol. Manno et al. *(76)* observed that at a 0.05% blood alcohol concentration, marihuana smoking (2.5 or 5 mg THC) exacerbated tachycardia and impairment of motor, cognitive, and psychological performance in an additive fashion. Perhaps of greater social importance is the observation that the ethanol-related impairment of automobile driving skills is similarly affected *(96)*.

3.5. Amphetamines

In a study of 10 chronic users of marihuana who were given dextroamphetamine (15 mg per os) or marihuana cigarettes (15 mg THC) alone or in combination, Zalcman et al. *(139)* observed that the pulse rate was increased with marihuana, but there was no further increase with amphetamine. Also, blood pressure increased after amphetamine, but marihuana produced no additional effect. Similarly, Forney et al. *(32)* did not detect any interaction between marihuana smoking (25 µg/kg THC) and dextroamphetamine (10 mg/70 kg PO); the increase in heart rate and the subjective and psychomotor performance effects with the combination of agents was no different from those observed with marihuana smoking alone. When the marihuana (THC) dose was increased to 50 µg/kg THC, Evans et al. *(27)* observed that the drug combination caused impairment of psychomotor performance equal to that of marihuana alone, whereas there was an additive effect on tachycardia and mean systolic blood pressure, and there was a greater than additive effect on the intensity and duration of the subjective effects (assessed by modified Cornell Medical Index). In fact, the intensity of symptoms for the combination was double that observed for marihuana alone.

3.6. Cocaine

Smoking marihuana potentiates the effects of intranasal cocaine. Marihuana causes vasodilation of the nasal mucosa and inhibits cocaine-mediated vasoconstriction. Tachycardia is enhanced, and plasma absorption rate and peak plasma level of cocaine are increased *(71)*. Furthermore, when intravenous cocaine (maximum 32 mg) was combined with smoked marihuana (maximum 27 mg THC), there was an additive effect on tachycardia, but the increase in blood pressure was the same as that due to cocaine alone *(30,31)*.

4. MOLECULAR INTERACTIONS OF THC

4.1. Receptor Mediated

Psychoactive THC exerts primarily its effect on the brain function as it interacts with a stereospecific "cannabinoid" receptor "CB1." This receptor is coupled to a G protein, which inhibits adenylate cyclase. The brain receptor to THC has been cloned and identified *(80,97,98)*. Its endogenous ligand, arachidonyl ethanolamide (anandamide), has been identified *(83)*. In the brain, receptor density is greater in "basal ganglia," molecular layer of the cerebellum, innermost olfactory bulb, hippocampus, the frontal cortex, and least in brain stem and spinal cord *(2,46)*. THC receptors have been localized in pre- and postsynaptic membranes *(98)*. In addition, peripheral receptors to THC (CB2) and their endogenous ligand arachidonyl diacylglycerol have been identified in many cells and tissues. This signaling system is involved with cellular function of the immune, cardiovascular, and reproductive systems.

4.2. Nonreceptor Mediated

Some effects of the THC receptor are not inhibited by THC receptor antagonists or pertussis toxin (which inactivates the alpha subunit of the G-protein complex) *(44,98,131)*. In 1973, Paton and Pertwee *(94)* described biphasic effects of THC and in 1979, Paton *(91)* proposed that THC may change the affinity of an endogenous ligand for its receptor. Since then, there have been observations of receptor-independent *(98)*, dual *(44)*, biphasic high/low dose effects of cannabinoids *(116)*, and direct activity on isolated receptors *(130)*. Perturbation of the lipid bilayer membrane by THC (partial anesthetic property) will also alter the physical property of membrane fluidity and alter the response of other membrane receptors by an allosteric effect.

The major difference between the endogenous ligands, which are derivatives of membrane phospholipids and THC, is that THC has a much longer half-life, has a greater affinity for its receptor protein, and alters fluidity and configuration of the membrane lipid bilayer to a greater extent than arachinodic acid derivatives.

5. PROPERTIES OF MARIHUANA RELEVANT TO ANESTHESIA

5.1. Anesthetic Effect

At nanomolar concentration, THC produces its effects by interaction with cannabinoid receptors; at micromolar concentration, it exerts a nonspecific destabilizing effect on lipid membranes *(91,93)*. At high levels, THC reduces the MAC requirement of inhalational anesthetics *(115,132)*, but does not induce a state of general anesthesia. This condition has been referred to as "partial anesthesia" *(64,95)*, which may result from the limited solubility of THC in cell membrane lipids, resulting in a ceiling on the increase in membrane fluidity *(64)*.

5.2. Analgesic Effect

The analgesic action of THC reported in the experimental animal *(109)* is equivocal in clinical trials. At doses of THC, which also produce psychotropic effects, clinical studies report hyperalgesia *(18,50)*, no analgesia *(101)*, or mild analgesic activity *(54,86,90,99)*. Different cannabinoids have been tested in an attempt to enhance analgesic potency and limit psychotropic side-effects, but none has proven to be clinically effective.

In one of the frequently quoted studies reporting analgesic activity, a single dose of 10 or 20 mg of THC per os was compared to 60 or 120 mg of codeine, for the treatment of cancer pain in 36 patients *(90)*. At the larger dose of THC, this analgesic effect was similar to either dose of codeine. However, there were also more side-effects (dizziness 97%, sedation 94%, blurred vision 64%, mental clouding 53%, and ataxia 44%) and adverse reactions (extreme anxiety 14%) than were seen with high-dose codeine. The lower dose of THC was better tolerated, but was not as effective in relieving pain as either dose of codeine.

Assay of analgesic affect and comparison with opiate analgesia is complicated by the fact that THC intoxication can alter pain perception and/or pain response criteria *(18)*. For example, opiates decrease pain perception by decreasing sensory input (a true analgesic effect), whereas diazepam decreases the pain response criteria by affecting the subjective perception of pain (a psychological effect). A double-blind comparison with opiates is not meaningful, since subjects who receive THC experience its psychotropic effects. The blind becomes transparent, which may alter expectations and pain response.

The analgesic effect of marihuana smoking was evaluated in a rigorously controlled study performed in a hospital environment by Clark et al. *(18)*. The effect on thermal pain was evaluated in 16 heavy marihuana smokers in a controlled environment. They concluded that marihuana causes hyperalgesia. The drug enhances the perception of pain in moderate smokers, while in heavy smokers, it increases the pain report criteria. No similar study using the sensory decision theory has yet been performed with orally administered THC or THC-like compounds in order to assess the analgesic property of the drug. Considering the variety of available analgesics of the opiate or NSAID type that are effective against both acute and chronic pain, smoked marihuana is not recommended for the treatment of pain by pharmacologists or anesthesiologists.

5.3. Antiinflammatory Effect (Chronic Pain)

A nonpsychoactive cannabinoid metabolite of THC, THC-11-oic acid, inhibits cyclooxygenase-2 and has been shown experimentally to be an effective antiinflammatory agent *(140)*.

5.4. Antiemetic Effect

THC and some of its synthetic derivatives (e.g., levonantradol) possess an antiemetic effect *(68)*. The greatest reduction in nausea and vomiting occurs when the plasma THC concentration exceeds 10 ng/mL *(17)*, which also causes psychoactive effects. Most studies have examined the effect of marihuana for the nausea and vomiting caused by antineoplastic therapy *(107,128)*. In this setting, THC has been found to be as effective as prochlorperazine *(35,128)* or metoclopramide *(19)*; however, more side-effects were associated with THC. Other applications such as postoperative nausea and vomiting have not been evaluated. Mechoulam et al. *(82)* suggested that a derivative of THC may be found in which effects of THC may be separable from its psychoactive effects; however, this agent has not been discovered. Since there are several specific and effective antiemetic agents with minimal side-effects (e.g., metoclopramide and the 5-HT$_3$ receptor antagonists odansetron and ganisetron [see Gralla, Chapter 47]), there is no convincing evidence to advocate the use of THC to treat nausea and vomiting *(108)*. It should be noted that dronabinol, the oral form of THC approved by the FDA, is available in 2.5, 5, and 10 mg tablets. FDA indications for dronabinol include nausea and vomiting associated with cancer chemotherapy, which is refractory to conventional therapies, and anorexia or wasting associated with AIDS. In the package insert, a warning states that dronabinol should be used cautiously and with psychiatric monitoring in patients with mania, depression, or schizophrenia, as these disorders can be exacerbated.

5.5. Neurological Disorders

Consroe and Sandyk *(22)* have reviewed the potential therapeutic role of the cannabinoids (THC and its synthetic derivatives, CBD) in epilepsy, dystonia, movement disorders (Huntington's chorea, Tourette's syndrome, Parkinsonism, tardive dyskinesia), spasticity, migraine, and neuropathic pain. They concluded that the available clinical trials did not support the use of THC, its synthetic derivatives, or CBD to treat these conditions.

5.6. Sedation, Sleep and Anxiolysis

THC increases sleep time in experimental animals and humans *(92)*. THC, however, is not an anxiolytic, and in clinical studies, diazepam is the drug of choice to prevent anxiety *(42,88,101)*. Although some users describe the marihuana "high" as "mellowing out," well-described adverse psychologic sequelae are observed frequently in marihuana-naive subjects. These include anxiety and panic reactions, acute delirium, and dysphoria. These may have significant adverse consequences and preclude the use of marihuana as a preoperative medication *(89)*. Schizophreniform reactions and chronic psychosis have been described in chronic marihuana users *(4)*.

5.7. Effect on Glaucoma

Marihuana or THC reduces intraocular pressure and causes untoward side-effects (such as hypotension and dysphoria). THC may not be used topically to lower intraocular pressure, and it is much less effective than current medications, especially the local application of prostaglandin F$_2$-alpha.

6. MARIHUANA AND ANESTHESIA

6.1. Studies on Marihuana and Anesthesia

There are surprisingly few studies on preoperative use of marihuana and its interaction with anesthesia. In 10 subjects, Raft et al. *(101)* compared the "analgesic" activity of diazepam (0.157 mg/kg IV), THC (22 or 44 µg/kg IV), or placebo for premedication of patients scheduled for extraction of a third molar under local anesthesia (lidocaine 2% with epinephrine 1:100,000). Subjects rated high-dose marihuana as the worst premedication, associated with the most pain, whereas, much less pain was experienced by patients receiving diazepam. In 3 of 10 subjects, low-dose THC was better than placebo, but inferior to diazepam. In the same 10 patients, Gregg et al. *(42)* reported that the heart rate after 44 µg/kg THC increased to 69% above baseline, but cardiac dysrhythmias were not observed. Anxiety scores on State-Trait Anxiety Inventory were elevated significantly in the group that received marihuana. The investigators concluded that "THC has no particular advantage over diazepam … [and it may] compromise to some degree the surgical patient's adaptivity to stress and interact unfavorably with other anesthetic medications."

This study is the only one that has investigated the effects of THC on general anesthesia in a series of patients. Ten patients received atropine 0.4 mg, fentanyl 100 µg, diazepam 15 mg, O_2/N_2O-30:70%, and methohexital titrated to effect; they were not intubated. Following surgery, 5 of 10 patients admitted to smoking marihuana within 72 h prior to surgery. The significant difference between groups was observed in the postoperative period. In marihuana smokers, the heart rate increased postoperatively to 65% over preoperative baseline and remained elevated for about 40 min, while in patients who did not smoke marihuana, HR increased 40% above the preoperative baseline.

6.2. Marihuana and Management of Anesthesia

Marihuana discontinuance following habitual drug usage produces a generally mild withdrawal syndrome (change in sleep or appetite, or feeling nervous, tense, or restless) *(135)*. It is unnecessary to continue its use perioperatively in the habitual marihuana user; diazepam or oral dronabinol will control withdrawal symptoms if they occur. During acute intoxication, diazepam can be used to treat acute anxiety or excitation. In the chronic or heavy marihuana user, one should be aware of possible pulmonary concerns and the rare possibility of uvular edema.

Tachycardia associated with THC is exacerbated by atropine and other chronotropic agents (e.g., epinephrine added to local anesthetics). This may be especially problematic in patients with cardiac pathology including coronary artery disease *(7)*. Diazepam, β-blockers, or clonidine will decrease tachycardia; however, they may exacerbate orthostatic hypotension. If the patient is at risk for coronary disease, it may be prudent to delay surgery until the acute chronotropic effects of marihuana wane, ideally for more than 72 h, to help prevent postoperative tachycardia.

7. CONCLUSIONS

The current trend in anesthesia is to minimize the hospital stay. The preferred anesthetic agents are highly specific, do not possess active metabolites, and have a short duration of action. Smoking marihuana is neither a practical nor a harmless mode of drug delivery, especially in the hospital where smoking is prohibited and an open flame is unsafe. Marihuana is slowly eliminated, has active metabolites, is inadequate as an anesthetic agent, and has adverse interactions with other drugs administered in the perioperative period. It has multiple pharmacological effects and causes adverse psychoactive effects at the dose level required to achieve a therapeutic endpoint. Especially with an aging surgical population and the high incidence of cardiac disease, the use of THC imposes a high risk for perioperative tachycardia and myocardial ischemia. The anesthesiologist has a variety of highly selective, short-acting drugs that effectively produce analgesia, amnesia, sedation, sleep, anxiolysis, muscle relaxation, antiemesis, bronchodilation, antihypertension, and antisialosis with minimal side-effects. These data do not support the perioperative use of marihuana or THC.

ACKNOWLEDGMENTS

The authors would like to acknowledge with thanks the editorial corrections contributed by their colleague Dr. Sanford M. Miller. Excellent editorial assistance was also provided by D. Michael Taylor and Montimer Mason.

REFERENCES

1. Abboud, T. T. and Sanders, H. D. (1976) Effect of oral administration of delta-9-tetrahydrocannabinol on airway mechanics in normal and asthmatic subjects. *Chest*, **70**, 480–485.
2. Abood, M. E. and Martin, B. R. (1996) Molecular neurobiology of the cannabinoid receptor. *Int. Rev. Neurobiol.* **39**, 197–221.
3. Adams, I. B. and Martin, B. R. (1996) Cannabis: pharmacology and toxicology in animals and humans. *Addiction* **91**, 1585–1614.
4. Andreasson, S. and Allebeck, P. (1987) Cannabis and schizophrenia: A longitudinal study of Swedish conscripts. *Lancet* **2**, 1483.
5. Aronow, W. S. and Cassidy, J. (1974) Effect of marihuana and placebo-marihuana smoking on angina pectoris. *N. Engl. J. Med.* **291**, 65–67.
6. Aronow, W. S. and Cassidy, J. (1975) Effect of smoking marihuana and of a high-nicotine cigarette on angina pectoris. *Clin. Pharmacol. Ther.* **17**, 549–554.
7. Beaconsfield, P., Ginsburg, J. and Rainsbury, R. (1972) Marijuana smoking: cardiovascular effects in man and possible mechanisms. *N. Engl. J. Med.* **287**, 209–212.
7a. Beaconsfield, P. (1974) Some cardiovascular effects of cannabis (Editorial). *Am. J. Heart.* **87**, 143–146.
8. Bellville, J. W., Gasser, J. C., Miyake, T. and Aqleh, K. (1976) Tolerance to the respiratory effects of marijuana in man. *J. Pharmacol. Exp. Ther.* **197**, 326–331.
9. Bellville, J. W., Swanson, G. D., Halderman, G., Aqleh, K. and Sato, T. (1974) Respiratory effects of tetrahydrocannabinol, pentobarbital and alcohol. *Proc. West. Pharmacol. Soc.* **17**, 215–218.
10. Benowitz, N. L. and Jones, R. T. (1977) Cardiovascular effects of prolonged delta-9-tetrahydrocannabinol ingestion. *Clin. Pharmacol. Ther.* **22**, 287–297.
11. Benowitz, N. L. and Jones, R. T. (1977) Effects of delta-9-tetrahydrocannabinol on drug distribution and metabolism: antipyrene, pentobarbital and ethanol. *Clin. Pharmacol. Ther.* **22**, 259–268.
12. Bloom, J. W., Kaltenborn, W. T., Paoletti, P., Camilli, A. and Lebowitz, M. D. (1987) Respiratory effects of non-tobacco cigarettes. *Brit. Med. J.* **295**, 1516–1518.
13. Bro, P. and Schou, J. (1975) Cannabis poisoning with analytical verification. *N. Engl. J. Med.* **293**, 1049–1050.
14. Busch, F. W., Seid, D. A. and Wei, E. T. (1979) Mutagenic activity of marihuana smoke condensates. *Cancer Lett.* **6**, 319–324.
15. Carlini, E. A. and Cunha, J. H. (1981) Hypnotic and antiepileptic effects of cannabidiol. *J. Clin. Pharmacol.* **21**, 417S–427S.
16. Chait, L. and Pierri, J. (1992) Effects of smoked marijuana on human performance: a critical review, in *Marijuana/Cannabinoids: Neurobiology and Neurophysiology* (Murphy, L., Bartke, A., eds.), CRC Press, Boca Raton, FL, pp. 387–424.
17. Chang, A. E., Shiling, D. J., Stillman, R. C., Goldberg, N., Seipp, C., Barofsky, I., Simon, R. and Rosenberg, S. (1979) Delta-9-tetrahydrocannabinol as an antiemetic agent in cancer patients receiving high-dose methotrexate: a prospective, randomized evaluation. *Ann. Intern. Med.* **91**, 819–824.
18. Clark, W. C., Janal, M. N., Zeidenberg, P. and Nahas, G. G. (1981) Effects of moderate and high doses of marihuana on thermal pain: a sensory decision theory analysis. *J. Clin. Pharmacol.* **21**, 299S–310S.
19. Colls, B. M., Ferry, D. G., Gray, A. J., Havey, A. J. and McQueen, E. G. (1980) The antiemetic activity of tetrahydrocannibinol versus metoclopramide and thiethylperazine in patients undergoing cancer chemotherapy. *N. Z. Med. J.* **91**, 449–451.
20. Cone, E. J., Welch, P. and Lange, W. R. (1988) Clonidine partially blocks the physiologic effects but not the subjective effects produced by smoking marijuana in male human subjects. *Pharmacol. Biochem. Behav.* **29**, 649–652.
21. Consroe, P., Jones, B., Laird, H. I. and Reinking, J. (1976) Anti-convulsant and convulsant effects of delta-9-tetrahydrocannabinol, in *The Therapeutic Potential of Marijuana* (Cohen, S., Stillman, R. C., eds.), Plenum Medical Book Company, NY, pp. 363–382.
22. Consroe, P. and Sandyk, R. (1992) Potential role of cannabinoids for therapy of neurological disorders, in *Marihuana/Cannabinoids: Neurobiology and Neurophysiology* (Murphy, L., Bartke, A., eds.), CRC Press, Boca Raton, FL, pp. 459–524.
23. Dalton, W. S., Martz, R., Lemberger, L., Rodda, B. E. and Forney, R. B. (1975) Effects of marijuana combined with secobarbital. *Clin. Pharmacol. Ther.* **18**, 298–304.
24. Dewey, W., Yonle, L., Harris, L., Reavis, W. M., Griffin, E. D. J. and Newby, E. V. (1970) Some cardiovascular effects of trans-delta-9-THC. *Pharmacologists* **12**, 259.
25. Dewey, W. L. (1986) Cannabinoid pharmacology. *Pharmacol. Rev.* **38**, 151–178.
25a. El-Yousel, M. K., Janowsky, D.S., Davis, J. M., and Rosenblatt, J. E. (1973) Induction of severe depression by physostigmine in marihuana intoxicated individuals. *Br. J. Addict.* **68,** 321–325.

26. Endicott, J. N., Skipper, P. and Hernandez, L. (1993) Marijuana and head and neck cancer. *Adv. Exp. Med. Biol.* **335**, 107–113.

27. Evans, M. A., Martz, R., Rodda, B. E., Lemberger, L. and Forney, R. B. (1976) Effects of marijuana-dextroamphetamine combination. *Clin. Pharm. Ther.* **20**, 350–358.

27a. Evans, M. A. R., Martz, L., Lemberger, L., Rodda, B. E., and forney, R. B. (1974) clinical effects of marihuana dextroamphetamine combination [Abstract #519]. *The Pharmacologist.* **16**, 281.

28. Feeney, D. M. (1979) Marihuana and epilepsy: paradoxical anticonvulsant and convulsant effects, in *Marihuana: Biological Effects. Analysis, Metabolism, Cellular Responses, Reproduction and Brain* (Nahas, G. G., Paton, W. D. M., eds.), Vols. 22–23, Pergamon Press, Elmsford, New York. pp. 643–657.

29. Fligiel, S. E. G., Roth, M. D., C., K. E., Barsky, S. H., Simmons, M. S. and Tashkin, D. P. (1997) Tracheobronchial histopathology in habitual smokers of cocaine, marijuana and/or tobacco. *Chest*, **112**, 319–326.

30. Foltin, R. W. and Fischman, M. W. (1993) Behavioral effects of cocaine alone and in combination with ethanol or marijuana in humans. *Drug Alcohol. Depend.* **32**, 93–106.

31. Foltin, R. W., Fischman, M. W., Pedroso, J. J. and Pearlson, G. D. (1987) Marijuana and cocaine interactions in humans: cardiovascular consequences. *Pharmacol. Biochem. Behav.* **28**, 459–464.

32. Forney, R. B., Martz, R., Lemberger, I. and Rodda, B. (1976) The combined effect of marihuana and dextroamphetamine. *Ann. NY Acad. Sci.* **281**, 162–170.

32a. Freemon, F. R., Rosenblatt, J. E., and K, E. L.-Y. M. (1975) Interaction of physostigmine and delta-9-tetrahydrocannabinol in man. *Clin. Pharmacol. Ther.* **17**, 121–126.

33. Friedman, H. (1997) Neuroimmunology and marijuana, in *Drug Abuse in the Decade of the Brain* (Nahas, G. G., Burks, T. F., eds.), IOS Press, Amsterdam, Netherlands, pp. 145–151.

34. Frizza, J., Chesher, G. B., Jackson, D. M., Malor, R. and Starmer, G. A. (1977) The effect of delta-9-tetrahydrocannabinol, cannabidiol, and cannabinol on the anaesthesia induced by various anaesthetic agents in mice. *Psychopharmacology (Berl.)* **55**, 103–107.

35. Frytak, S., Moertel, C. G., O'Fallon, J. R., Rubin, J., Creagan, E. T., O'Connell, M. J., Schutt, A. J. and Scharttau, N. W. (1979) Delta-9-tetrahydrocannabinol as an antiemetic for patients receiving cancer chemotherapy: a comparison of prochlorperazine and a placebo. *Ann. Intern. Med.* **91**, 825–830.

36. Gatley, S. J. and Volkow, N. D. (1997) Studies of the brain cannabinoid system using positron emission tomography, in *Drug Abuse in the Decade of the Brain* (Nahas, G. G., Burks, T. F., eds.), IOS Press, Amsterdam, Netherlands, pp. 127–138.

37. Gieringer, D. H. (1988) Marijuana, driving, and accident safety. *J. Psychoactive Drugs* **20**, 93–101.

38. Gong, H., Fligiel, S., Tashkin, D. P. and Barbers, R. G. (1987) Tracheobronchial changes in habitual, heavy smokers of marijuana with and without tobacco. *Am. Rev. Resp. Dis.* **136**, 142–149.

39. Gong, H., Tashkin, D. P., Simmons, M. S., Calvarese, B. and Shapiro, B. J. (1984) Acute and subacute bronchial effects of oral cannabinoids. *Clin. Pharmacol. Ther.* **35**, 26–32.

40. Graham, J. D. P. (1986) The bronchodilator action of cannabinoids, in *Cannabinoids as Therapeutic Agents* (Mechoulam, R., ed.), CRC Press, Boca Raton, FL, pp. 147–158.

41. Graham, J. D. P. and Li, D. M. F. (1973) Cardiovascular and respiratory effects of cannabis in cat and rat. *Br. J. Pharmacol.* **49**, 1–10.

42. Gregg, J. M., Campbell, R. L., Levin, K. J., Ghia, J. and Elliott, R. A. (1976) Cardiovascular effects of cannabinol during oral surgery. *Anesth. Analg.* **55**, 203–213.

43. Guarisco, J. L., Cheney, M. L., LeJeune, F. E., Jr. and Reed, H. T. (1988) Isolated uvulitis secondary to marijuana use. *Laryngoscope* **98**, 1309–1312.

44. Hampson, A. J., Bornheim, L. M., Scanziani, M., Yost, C. S., Gray, A. T., Hansen, B. M., Leonoudakis, D. J. and Bickler, P. E. (1998) Dual effects of anandamide on NMDA receptor-mediated responses and neurotransmission. *J. Neurochem.* **70**, 671–676.

45. Harvey, D. J. (1984) Chemistry, metabolism, and pharmacokinetics of the cannabinoids, in *Marihuana in Science and Medicine* (Nahas, G. G., Harvey, D. J., Paris, M., Brill, H., eds.), Raven Press, New York. pp. 37–107.

46. Harvey, D. J. (1997) Pharmacokinetics, metabolism, and brain distribution of the cannabinoids, in *Drug Abuse in the Decade of the Brain* (Nahas, G. G., Burks, T. F., eds.), IOS Press, Amsterdam, Netherlands, pp. 111–125.

47. Henderson, R. L., Tennant, F. S. and Guerry, R. (1972) Respiratory manifestations of hashhish smoking. *Acta Otolaryngol.* **95**, 248–251.

48. Hepler, R. S., Franks, I. M. and Ungerleider, J. T. (1972) Pupillary constriction after marijuana smoking. *Am. J. Ophthalmol.* **74**, 1185–1190.

49. Hervás, J. A., Fiol, M., Vidal, C. and Masip, M. C. (1987) [Poisoning by hashish ingestion in children (letter)]. *Med. Clin. (Barc.)* **88**, 563.

50. Hill, S. Y., Schwin, R., Goodwin, D. W. and Powell, B. J. (1974) Marihuana and pain. *J. Pharmacol. Exp. Ther.* **188**, 415–418.

51. Hoffman, D., Brunneman, D. K. and Gori, G. B. (1975) On the carcinogenicity of marijuana smoke. *Recent Adv. Phytochem.* **9**, 63–81.

52. Hollister, L. E., Richard, R. K. and Gillespie, H. K. (1968) Comparison of tetrahydrocannabinol and synhexyl in man. *Clin. Pharmacol. Ther.* **9**, 783–791.

53. Huber, G. L., Pochay, V. E., Pereira, W., Shea, J. W., Hinds, W. C., First, M. W. and Sornberger, G. C. (1980) Marijuana, tetrahydrocannabinol, and pulmonary antibacterial defenses. *Chest* **77**, 403–410.

54. Jain, A. K., Ryan, J. R., McMahon, F. G. and Smith, G. (1981) Evaluation of intramuscular levonantradol and placebo in acute postoperative pain. *J. Clin. Pharmacol.* **21**, 320S–326S.

55. Jandhyala, B. S. (1978) Effects of prolonged administration of delta-9-tetrahydrocannabinol on the autonomic and cardiovascular function and regional hemodynamics in mongrel dogs. *Res. Commun. Chem. Pathol. Pharmacol.* **20**, 489–508.

56. Jandhyala, B. S., Malloy, K. P. and Buckley, J. P. (1976) Effects of chronic administration of delta-9-tetrahydrocannabinol on the heart rate of mongrel dogs. *Res. Commun. Chem. Pathol. Pharmacol.* **14**, 201–204.

57. Johnson, D., Convadi, A. and McGuigan, M. (1991) Hashish ingestion in toddlers [Abstract]. *Vet. Hum. Toxicol.* **33**, 393.

58. Johnson, S. and Domino, E. F. (1971) Some cardiovascular effects of marijuana smoking in normal volunteers. *Clin. Pharmacol. Ther.* **12**, 762–768.

59. Johnstone, R. E., Lief, P. L., Kulp, R. A. and Smith, T. C. (1975) Combination of delta-9-tetrahydrocannabinol with oxymorphone or pentobarbital: Effects on ventilatory control and cardiovascular dynamics. *Anesthesiology* **42**, 674–684.

60. Jones, R. T. (1971) Marihuana-induced "high": influence of expectation, setting and previous drug experience. *Pharmacol. Rev.* **23**, 359–369.

60a. Jusko, W. J., Gardner, M. J., Mangione, A., Schentag, J. J., Koup, J. R., and Vance, J. W. (1979) Factors affecting theophylline clearances: age, tobacco, marijuana, cirrhosis, congestive heart failure, obesity, oral contraceptives, benzodiazepines, barbiturates, and ethano. *J. Pharm. Sci.* **68**, 1358–1366.

60b. Kizer, K. W. (1980) Possible interaction of TCA and marijuana [letter]. *Ann. Emerg. Med.* **9**, 444.

61. Klein, T. W., Newton, C., Zhu, W., Daaka, Y. and Friedman, H. (1995) delta-9-Tetrahydrocannabinol, cytokines, and immunity to Legionella pneumophila. *Proc. Soc. Exp. Biol. Med.* **209**, 205–212.

61a. Knudsen, P. and Vilmar, T. (1984) Cannabis and neuroleptic agents in schizophrenia. *Acta Psychiatr. Scand.* **69**, 162–174.

62. Kumbarachi, N. M. and Nastuk, W. L. (1980) Effects of Δ^9-tetrahydrocannabinol on excitable membranes and neuromuscular transmission. *Mol. Pharmacol.* **17**, 344–345.

62a. Lacoursiere, R. B. and Swateck, R. (1983) Adverse interaction between disulfiram and marijuana: a case report. *Am. J. Psychiatry.* **140**, 242–244.

63. Laviolette, M., Bèlanger, J. (1986) Role of prostaglandins in marihuana-induced bronchodilation. *Respiration* **49**, 10–15.

64. Lawrence, D. K. and Gill, E. W. (1975) The effects of $\Delta1$-tetrahydrocannabinol and other cannabinoids on spin-labeled liposomes and their relationship to mechanisms of general anesthesia. *Mol. Pharmacol.* **11**, 595–602.

65. Layman, J. M. and Milton, A. S. (1971) Some actions of Δ^1-tetrahydrocannabinol and cannabidiol at cholinergic junctions. *Br. J. Pharmacol.* **41**, 379P–380P.

66. Lee, M. L., Novotny, M. and Bartle, K. D. (1976) Gas chromatography/mass spectrometric and nuclear magnetic resonance spectrometric studies of carcinogenic polynuclear aromatic hydrocarbons in tobacco and marijuana smoke condensates. *Anal. Chem.* **48**, 405–416.

67. Lemberger, L., Dalton, B., Martz, R., Rodda, B. and Forney, R. (1976) Clinical studies on the interaction of psychopharmacologic agents with marihuana. *Ann. NY Acad. Sci.* **281**, 219–228.

68. Levitt, M. (1986) Cannabinoids as antiemetics in cancer chemotherapy, in *Cannabinoids as Therapeutic Agents* (Mechoulam, R., ed.), CRC Press, Boca Raton, FL, pp. 71–83.

69. Loewe, S. and Goodman, L. S. (1947) Anticonvulsant action of marijuana-active substances. *Fed. Proc.* **6**, 352.

70. Lukas, S. E., Benedikt, R., Mendelson, J. H., Kouri, E., Sholar, M. and Amass, L. (1992) Marihuana attenuates the rise in plasma ethanol levels in human subjects. *Neuropsychopharmacology* **7**, 77–81.

71. Lukas, S. E., Sholar, M., Kouri, E., Fukuzako, H. and Mendelson, J. H. (1994) Marihuana smoking increases plasma cocaine levels and subjective reports of euphoria in male volunteers. *Pharmacol. Biochem. Behav.* **48**, 715–721.

71a. Mackie, J. and Clark, D. (1994) Cannabis toxic psychosis while on disulfiram [letter]. *Br. J. Psychiatry.* **164**, 421.

72. Macnab, A., Anderson, E. and Susak, L. (1989) Ingestion of cannabis: a cause of coma in children. *Pediatr. Emerg. Care.* **5**, 238–239.

73. Malit, L. A., Johnstone, R. E., Bourke, D. I., Kulp, R. A., Klein, V. and Smith, T. C. (1975) Intravenous delta-9-tetrahydrocannabinol: Effects of ventilatory control and cardiovascular dynamics. *Anesthesiology* **42**, 666–673.

74. Mallat, A., Roberson, J. and Brock-Utne, J. G. (1996) Preoperative marijuana inhalation–an airway concern. *Can. J. Anaesth.* **43**, 691–693.

75. Mallat, A. M., Roberson, J. and Brock-Utne, J. G. (1996) Preoperative marijuana inhalation–an airway concern. *Can. J. Anaesth.* **43**, 691–693.

76. Manno, J. E., Kiplinger, G. F., Scholz, N. and Forney, R. B. (1971) The influence of alcohol and marihuana on motor and mental performance. *Clin. Pharmacol. Ther.* **12**, 202–211.

77. Mathew, R. J. and Wilson, W. H. (1993) Acute changes in cerebral blood flow after smoking marijuana. *Life Sci.* **52**, 757–767.

78. Mathew, R. J. and Wilson, W. H. (1992) The effects of marijuana on cerebral blood flow and metabolism, in *Marijuana/Cannabinoids: Neurobiology and Neurophysiology* (Murphy, L., Bartke, A., eds.), CRC Press, Boca Raton, FL, pp. 337–386.

79. Mathew, R. J., Wilson, W. H. and Tant, S. R. (1989) Acute changes in cerebral blood flow associated with marijuana smoking. *Acta Psychiatria Scand.* **79**, 118–128.

80. Matsuda, L. A. (1997) Molecular aspects of cannabinoid receptors. *Crit. Rev. Neurobiol.* **11**, 143–166.

81. McPartland, J. M. and Pruitt, P. L. (1997) Medical marijuana and its use by the immunocompromised. *Altern. Ther. Health Med.* **3**, 39–45.

82. Mechoulam, R., Breuer, A., Feigenbaum, J. J. and Devane, W. A. (1991) Nonpsychotropic synthetic cannabinoids as therapeutic agents. *Farmaco.* **46 (Suppl 1)**, 267–276.

83. Mechoulam, R., Devane, W. A. and Glaser, R. (1992) Cannabinoid Geometry and Biological Activity, in *Marijuana/Cannabinoids: Neurobiology and Neuropsychology* (Murphy, L., Bartke, A., eds.), CRC Press, Boca Raton, FL, pp. 1–33.

84. Mechoulam, R. and Edery, H. (1972) Structure-activity relationships in the cannabinoid series, in *Cannabis and its Derivatives: Pharmacology and Experimental Psychology* (Paton, W. D. M., Crown, J., eds.), Oxford University Press, Oxford, UK, pp. 101–136.

85. Mechoulam, R., Lander, N., Srebnik, M., Zamir, I., Breuer, A., Shalita, B., Dikstein, S., Carlini, E. A., Leite, J. R., Edery, H. and Porath, G. (1984) Recent advances in the use of cannabinoids as therapeutic agents, in *The Cannabinoids: Chemical, Pharmacologic and Therapeutic Uses* (Agurell, S., Dewey, W. L., Willette, R. E., eds.), Academic Press, New York. pp. 777–793.

86. Milstein, S. L., MacCannell, K., Karr, G. and Clark, S. (1975) Marijuana-produced changes in pain tolerance. Experienced and non-experienced subjects. *Int. Pharmacopsychiatry* **10**, 177–182.

87. Nahas, G. G. (1984) Toxicology and Pharmacology, in *Marihuana in Science and Medicine* (Nahas, G. G., Harvey, D. J., Paris, M., Brill, H., eds.), Raven Press, New York, pp. 109–246.

88. Nakano, S., Gillespie, H. K. and Hollister, L. E. (1978) A model for evaluation of antianxiety drugs with the use of experimentally induced stress: comparison of nabilone and diazepam. *Clin. Pharmacol. Ther.* **23**, 54–62.

89. Negrete, J. C., Knapp, P. W. and Douglas, D. E. (1986) Cannabis affects the severity of schzophrenic symptoms: results of a clinical survey. *Psychological Medicine* **16**, 515.

90. Noyes, R., Jr., Brunk, S. F., Avery, D. A. H. and Canter, A. C. (1975) The analgesic properties of delta-9-tetrahydrocannabinol and codeine. *Clin. Pharmacol. Ther.* **18**, 84–89.

91. Paton, W. D. M. (1979) Concluding summary, in *Marihuana: Biological Effects. Analysis, Metabolism, Cellular Responses, Reproduction and Brain* (Nahas, G. G., Paton, W. D. M., eds.), Vols. 735–738, Pergamon Press, Elmsford, NY, pp. 643–657.

92. Paton, W. D. M. and Pertwee, R. G. (1973) The actions of cannabis in man, in *Marijuana: Chemistry, Pharmacology, Metabolism, and Clinical Effects* (Mechoulam, R., ed.), Academic Press, New York, pp. 287–333.

93. Paton, W. D. M. and Pertwee, R. G. (1972) Effect of cannabis and certain of its constituents on phenobarbital sleeping time and phenazone metabolism. *Br. J. Pharmacol.* **44**, 250–261.

94. Paton, W. D. M. and Pertwee, R. G. (1973) The pharmacology of cannabis in animals, in *Marijuana: Chemistry, Pharmacology, Metabolism, and Clinical Effects* (Mechoulam, R., ed.), Academic Press, New York, pp. 191–285.

95. Paton, W. D. M., Pertwee, R. J. and Temple, D. M. (1972) The general pharmacology of cannabinoids, in *Cannabis and its Derivatives: Pharmacology and Experimental Psychology* (Paton, W. D. M., Crown, J., eds.), Oxford University Press, Oxford, pp. 50–74.

96. Perez-Reyes, M., Hicks, R. E., Bumberry, J., Jeffcoat, A. R. and Cook, C. E. (1988) Interaction between marihuana and ethanol: effects on psychomotor performance. *Alcohol Clin. Exp. Res.* **12**, 268–276.

97. Pertwee, R. (1993) The evidence for the existence of cannabinoid receptors. *Gen. Pharmacol.* **24**, 811–824.

98. Pertwee, R. G. (1997) Pharmacology of cannabinoid CB1 and CB2 receptors. *Pharmacol. Ther.* **74**, 129–180.

99. Petro, D. J. (1980) Marijuana as a therapeutic agent for muscle spasm or spasticity. *Psychosomatics* **21**, 81.

100. Petro, D. J. and Ellenberger, C. E. (1981) Treatment of human spasticity with delta-9-tetrahydrocannabinol. *Clin. Pharmacol.* **21**, 413S–416S.

101. Raft, R., Gregg, J., Ghia, J. and Harris, L. (1977) Effects of intravenous tetrahydrocannbinol on experimental and surgical pain: psychological correlates of the analgesic response. *Clin. Pharmacol. Ther.* **21**, 26–33.

102. Randall, M. D., Alexander, S. P., Bennett, T., Boyd, E. A., Fry, J. R., Gardiner, S. M., Kemp, P. A., McCulloch, A. I. and Kendall, D. A. (1996) An endogenous cannabinoid as an endothelium-derived vasorelaxant. *Biochem. Biophys. Res. Commun.* **229**, 114–120.

103. Randall, M. D. and Kendall, D. A. (1997) Involvement of a cannabinoid in endothelium-derived hyperpolarizing factor-mediated coronary vasorelaxation. *Eur. J. Pharmacol.* **335**, 205–209.

104. Renault, P. F., Schuster, C. R., Heinrich, R. and Freeman, D. (1971) Marijuana: standardized smoke administration and dose effect curves on heart rate in humans. *Science* **174**, 589–591.

104a. Rosenberg, C. M., Gerrein, J. R., and Schnell, C. (1978) Cannabis in the treatment of alcoholism. *J. Stud. Alcohol.* **39**, 1955–1958.

105. Roth, S. H. (1978) Stereospecific presynaptic inhibitory effect of delta9-tetrahydrocannabinol on cholinergic transmission in the myenteric plexus of the guinea pig. *Can. J. Physiol. Pharmacol.* **56**, 968–975.

106. Rubio, F., Quinbtero, S. and Hernandez, A. (1993) Flumazenil for coma reversal in children. *Pediatr. Emerg. Care* **5**, 238–239.

107. Sallan, S. E., Zinberg, N. E. and Frei, E. (1975) Antiemetic effect of delta-9-tetrahydrocannabinol in patients receiving cancer chemotherapy. *N. Engl. J. Med.* **293**, 795–797.

108. Schwartz, R. H., Voth, E. A. and Sheridan, M. J. (1997) Marijuana to prevent nausea and vomiting in cancer patients: a survey of clinical oncologists. *South Med. J.* **90**, 167–172.

109. Segal, M. (1986) Cannabinoids and analgesia, in *Cannabinoids as Therapeutic Agents* (Mechoulam, R., ed.), CRC Press, Boca Raton, FL, pp. 105–120.

110. Sherman, M. P., Aeberhard, E. E., Wong, V. Z., Simmons, M. S., Roth, M. D. and Tashkin, D. P. (1995) Effects of smoking marijuana, tobacco or cocaine alone or in combination on DNA damage in human alveolar macrophages. *Life Sci.* **56**, 2201–2207.

111. Sherrill, D. L., Krzyzanowski, M., Bloom, J. W. and Lebowitz, M. D. (1991) Respiratory effects of nontobacco cigarettes: a longitudinal study in general population. *Int. J. Epidemiol.* **20**, 132–137.

112. Sidney, S., Quesenberry, C. P., Jr., Friedman, G. D. and Tekawa, I. S. (1997) Marijuana use and cancer incidence (California, United States). *Cancer Causes Control* **8**, 722–728.

113. Smith, T. C. and Kulp, R. A. (1976) Respiratory and cardiovascular effects of delta-9-tetrahydrocannabinol alone and in combination with oxymorphine, pentobarbital and diazpeam, in *The Therapeutic Potential of Marijuana* (Cohen, S., Stillman, R. C., eds.), Plenum Medical Book Co., New York, pp. 123–135.

114. Sofia, R. D. and Barry, H. (1973) Interactions of chronic and acute Δ^1-tetrahydrocannabinol pretreatment with zoxazolamine and barbiturates. *Res. Commun. Chem. Pathol.* **5**, 91–98.

115. Stoelting, R. K., Martz, R. C., Gartner, J., Creasser, C., Brown, D. J. and Forney, R. B. (1973) Effects of delta-9-tetrahydrocannabinol on halothane MAC in dogs. *Anesthesiology* **38**, 521–524.

115a. Stoll, A. L., Cole, J. O., and Lukas, S. E. (1991) A case of mania as a result of fluoxetine-marijuana interaction [letter]. *J. Clin. Psychiatry.* **52**, 280–281.

116. Sulcova, E., Mechoulam, R. and Fride, E. (1998) Biphasic effects of anandamide. *Pharmacol. Biochem. Behav.* **59**, 347–352.

117. Sulkowski, A., Vachon, I. and Rich, E. S. (1977) Propranalol effects on acute marihuana intoxication in man. *Psychopharmacology* **52**, 47–53.

118. Tashkin, D. P. (1998) Marihuana and the lung, in *Marihuana and Medicine* (Nahas, G. G., ed.), Humana Press, Inc., Totowa, NJ.

119. Tashkin, D. P. (1990) Pulmonary complications of smoked substance abuse. *West. J. Med.* **152**, 525–530.

120. Tashkin, D. P., Calvarese, B. M., Simmons, M. S. and Shapiro, B. J. (1980) Respiratory status of seventy-four habitual marijuana smokers. *Chest* **78**, 699–706.

121. Tashkin, D. P., Coulson, A. H., Clark, V. A., Simmons, M., Bourque, L. B., Duann, S., Spivey, G. H. and Gong, H. (1987) Respiratory symptoms and lung function in habitual heavy smokers of marijuana alone, smokers of marijuana and tobacco, smokers of tobacco alone and nonsmokers. *Am. Rev. Resp. Dis.* **135**, 209–216.

122. Tashkin, D. P., Reiss, S., Shapiro, B. J., Calvarese, B., Olsen, J. L. and Lodge, J. W. (1977) Bronchial effects of aerosolized D-9-tetrahydrocannabinol in healthy and asthmatic subjects. *Am. Rev. Respir. Dis.* **115**, 57–65.

123. Tashkin, D. P., Shapiro, B. J. and Frank, I. M. (1973) Acute pulmonary physiologic effects of smoked marijuana and oral delta-9-tetrahydrocannabinol in healthy men. *N. Engl. J. Med.* **289**, 336–341.

124. Tashkin, D. P., Shapiro, B. J., Lee, Y. E. and Harper, C. E. (1975) Effects of smoked marijuana in experimentally induced asthma. *Am. Rev. Respir. Dis.* **112**, 377–386.
125. Tashkin, D. P., Shapiro, B. J., Lee, Y. E. and Harper, C. E. (1976) Subacute effects of heavy marijuana smoking on pulmonary function in healthy men. *N. Engl. J. Med.* **294**, 125–129.
126. Tashkin, D. P., Simmons, M. S., Sherrill, D. L. and Coulson, A. H. (1997) Heavy habitual marijuana smoking does not cause an accelerated decline in FEV1 with age. *Am. J. Respir. Crit. Care Med.* **155**, 141–148.
127. Tennant, F. S., Jr. and Prendergast, T. J. (1971) Medical manifestations associated with hashish. *JAMA* **216**, 1965–1969.
128. Ungerleider, J. T., Andrysiak, T., Fairbanks, L., Goodnight, J., Sarna, G. and Jamison, K. (1982) Cannabis and cancer chemotherapy: a comparison of oral delta-9-THC and prochlorperazine. *Cancer* **50**, 636–645.
129. Vachon, L., Fitzgerald, M. X., Solliday, N. H., Gould, I. A. and Gaensler, E. A. (1973) Single-dose effect of marihuana effect: bronchial dynamics and respiratory-center sensitivity in normal subjects. *N. Engl. J. Med.* **288**, 985–989.
130. Vaysse, P. J., Gardner, E. L. and Zukin, R. S. (1987) Modulation of rat brain opioid receptors by cannabinoids. *J. Pharmacol. Exp. Ther.*, **241**, 534–539.
131. Venance, L., Piomelli, D., Glowinski, J. and Giaume, C. (1995) Inhibition by anandamide of gap junctions and intercellular calcium signalling in striatal astrocytes. *Nature* **376**, 590–594.
132. Vitez, T. S., Way, W. L., Miller, R. D. and Eger, E. I. D. (1973) Effects of delta-9-tetrahydrocannabinol on cyclopropane MAC in the rat. *Anesthesiology* **38**, 525–527.
133. Weinberg, D., Lande, A., Hilton, N. and Kerns, D. L. (1983) Intoxication from accidental marijuana ingestion. *Pediatrics* **71**, 848–849.
134. Weiss, J. L., Watanabe, A. M., Lemberger, L., Tamarkin, N. R. and Cardon, P. V. (1972) Cardiovascular effects of delta-9-tetrahydrocannabinol in man. *Clin. Pharmacol. Ther.* **13**, 671–684.
135. Wiesbeck, G. A., Schuckit, M. A., Kalmijn, J. A., Tipp. J. E., Bucholz, K. K. and Smith, T. L. (1996) An evaluation of the history of a marijuana withdrawal syndrome in a large population. *Addiccation* **91**, 1469–1478.
135a.Wilens, T. E., Biederman, J., and Spencer, T. J. (1997) Case study: adverse effects of smoking marijuana while receiving tricyclic antidepressants. *J. Am. Acad. Child Adolesc. Psychiatry.* **36**, 45–48.
136. Williams, S. J., Hartley, J. P. R. and Graham, J. D. P. (1976) Bronchodilator effect of delta-1-THC administered by aerosol to asthmatic patients. *Thorax* **31**, 720.
137. Wu, H. D., Wright, R. S., Sassoon, C. S. and Tashkin, D. P. (1992) Effects of smoked marijuana of varying potency on ventilatory drive and metabolic rate. *Am. Rev. Respir. Dis.* **146**, 716–721.
138. Wu, T. C., Tashkin, D. P., Djahed, B. and Rose, J. E. (1988) Pulmonary hazards of smoking marijuana as compared with tobacco. *N. Engl. J. Med.*, **318**, 347–351.
139. Zalcman, S., Liskow, B., Cadoret, R. and Goodwin, D. (1973) Marijuana and amphetamine: the question of interaction. *Am. J. Psychaitry* **130**, 707–708.
140. Zurier, R. B., Rossetti, R. G., Lane, J. H., Goldberg, J. M., Hunter, S. A. and Burstein, S. H. (1998) Dimethylheptyl-THC-11 oic acid: a nonpsychoactive antinflammatory agent with a cannabinoid template structure. *Arthritis Rheum.* **41**, 163–170.
141. Zwillich, C. W., Doekel, R., Hammill, S. and Weil, J. V. (1978) The effects of smoked marijuana on metabolism and respiratory control. *Am. Rev. Respir. Dis.* **118**, 885–891.

19

Interactions of Marihuana and THC with Other Drugs
What We Don't, But Should, Know

Leo E. Hollister

Abstract

Marihuana use involves more than one substance. Not only is tetrahydrocannabinol (THC), the active psychoactive component, present, but also one or both other major cannabinoids, cannabidiol (CBD) and cannabinol (CBN).At present, evidence indicates that neither of these other two cannabinoids affects the action of THC. For practical purposes, THC alone is a model for the psychoactive action of marihuana. Alcohol is the social drug most used with marihuana, such use often being deliberate. Both have similar intoxicating effects, but these additive effects have not led to serious interactions. Stimulants often reverse some of the effects of THC, but the "high" from cocaine may be additive to that from THC. The interaction is so mild that no pattern of combined use has appeared. The same is true of the hallucinogen phencyclidine. So far as therapeutic drugs are concerned, few data are available. Although medical marihuana is not officially approved, marihuana has been tried empirically for treating a variety of medical disorders, such as nausea and vomiting associated with cancer chemotherapy, wasting syndrome associated with AIDS, and spasticity from neurological diseases. In each instance, other drugs are also present. So far, no adverse interactions from such use have been reported. However, this might not reflect the true prevalence. Unless one looks for something, one is not likely to find it.

1. INTRODUCTION

I last reviewed this subject at a New York Academy of Sciences meeting in 1976 *(1)*. In preparing this review some 22 years later, I was struck by the fact that so little had really changed. The published literature, at least in regard to studies in humans, has been rather silent. Usually, such silence indicates that no meaningful interactions have been observed in the real life use of marihuana as compared with experimental studies. A review of interactions of marihuana an Δ^9-tetrahydrocannabinol (THC), mainly covering experimental animal

From: *Marihuana and Medicine*
Edited by: G. G. Nahas et al.   © Humana Press Inc., Totowa, NJ

literature with some clinical studies published before 1984, appeared in that year *(2)*. No other reviews have appeared that had any bearing on clinical aspects of marihuana use.

Study of interactions of marihuana and other drugs are of interest from several points of view. Almost all social drugs are used in combination with others, not always concurrently. Presumably, such interactions might pose some danger of obtaining greater effects from marihuana than anticipated; these would hardly be serious, as no deaths have ever been ascribed to use of marihuana. On the other hand concurrent use of marihuana might increase or decrease the effects of therapeutic drugs, which might be more serious. Another use of the study of interactions is to obtain clues to the mechanism of actions of the drug, in this case THC. However, the discovery during the past decade of specific cannabinoid receptors as well as endocannabinoids, has apparently solved this problem *(3–5)*.

The purpose of this review will be to review the literature of the past decade or two, emphasizing possible interactions in humans and their occurrence in the real world of drug use rather than under experimental conditions. This goal will not always be possible, because of the relative dearth of studies bearing on the last situation.

2. INTERACTIONS BETWEEN Δ^9-THC and Other Cannabinoids

The biosynthetic pathway of THC begins with cannabidiol (CBN), proceeds to THC, and ends with the formation of cannabinol (CBN). As plant material from which marihuana is obtained varies greatly in the time it is harvested, varying relative concentrations of these three cannabinoids occur. A sample containing relatively large amounts of CBD compared to CBN was probably taken while the plant was still young, whereas the reverse would indicate that the plant was rather farther along in THC production. It is virtually impossible that THC could exist alone in marihuana without one or both of the other cannabinoids. Thus, the combination of drugs most often taken in marihuana use is one containing combinations of THC with CBD and CBN.

For many years it was thought that the clinical effects of marihuana were accounted for by all the cannabinoids. With the availability of pure materials it became possible to test each alone. A pharmacokinetic interaction between CBD and THC and its metabolites was reported in mice. Pretreatment with CBD increased brain levels of THC threefold, as well as increasing other THC metabolites *(6)*. However, in clinical use, CBD and THC become available simultaneously.

On the other hand two separate pharmacokinetic studies in humans failed to show any significant interaction between THC and CBD or CBN *(7, 8)*. Furthermore, clinical tests in humans of both CBD and CBN showed both to be essentially devoid of clinical activity *(9)*. Even when each was studied in combination with THC in measured amounts, it was impossible to show any significant interaction *(10)*. Thus, one can confidently conclude, that in humans, any interactions between the cannabinoids and THC are of little significance and that the psychoactivity of marihuana rests solely in its content of THC.

3. INTERACTIONS WITH OTHER SOCIALLY ABUSED DRUGS

The social drug most commonly taken with marihuana is alcohol. Such combinations are used deliberately to enhance the effects of marihuana. This folk practice is well-substantiated by a number of studies showing enhanced clinical effects of THC by alcohol *(2,11,12)*. Both drugs have similar effects and time-courses of action: Initial euphoria followed by sedative effects later. There have been no reports of serious interactions from this deliberately sought additive effect.

A similar situation might be expected to prevail with concurrently used sedatives, based on literature from animal studies. In mice, the catalepsy and loss of righting influence induced by THC was enhanced by pretreatment with benzodiazepines (13). It is difficult to bring to mind any two drugs more innocuous in terms of lethality than THC and benzodiazepines. Despite the possible allure of such combinations, their combined use has not become a social practice. The same kinds of additive effects are seen in animals treated with THC and barbiturates, a potentially more dangerous combination. Fortunately such use must be rare.

In general, animal studies indicate that many of the effects of THC are reversed by stimulants (2,10). THC decreased the increased locomotor activity induced in mice by stimulants and decreased lethality of cocaine (10). Similar findings were reported from pretreatment with THC on methamphetamine-induced locomotor activity and lethality (14). In one clinical study, seven subjects were given an intranasal dose of cocaine 30 minutes following a marihuana cigarette. Plasma cocaine concentrations were almost twice those following a placebo marihuana cigarette. The only change noted was that the latency of cocaine effects was reduced, probably because marihuana caused some vasodilation of the nasal mucosa (15). In another study of this interaction, seven subjects smoked a marihuana cigarette followed in 13 minutes by intravenous doses of cocaine. This combination produced larger and more prolonged ratings of "stimulated and "high." This result suggests an additive effect between the two drugs (14). Because the interactions were so mild, combined use has not been reported in humans; fortunately, the THC equivalent of the "speedball" (combined use of cocaine and heroin) has not become the fashion.

A couple of studies of interactions between phencyclidine (PCP) and THC have been reported in animals. Both THC and PCP decreased the rate of response to a fixed schedule reinforcement for food. When administered together, the effects were increased further (11). A pharmacokinetic interaction between THC and PCP was studied in dogs. When both drugs were administered together, PCP metabolism was inhibited with resultant higher serum PCP levels (17). Once again, there is little indication that these two mind-altering drugs are used together, which is probably fortunate.

4. INTERACTIONS BETWEEN THC AND OTHER THERAPEUTIC AGENTS

Therapeutic claims for THC have increased rapidly during the past decade, but little is known of interactions of marihuana when used therapeutically with other drugs. One of the most reasonable therapeutic uses of marihuana or THC has been to ameliorate the nausea and vomiting associated with cancer chemotherapy. Thus, cannabinoids will be used simultaneously with many highly toxic cancer drugs, such as cisplatin, doxorubicin, and others. Already, the literature supports the use of orally administered THC in such cases (18,19). An in vitro study has been reported that CBD inhibits metabolism of cyclosporine with the potential to increase levels in humans and produce toxic effects. However, in none of the reports of use of THC or marihuana in patients simultaneously undergoing cancer chemotherapy has there been any mention of increased toxicity of anticancer drugs (20). Nonetheless, the absence of such reports may signify that no attempt was made to look for them. This avenue of research should be encouraged.

A somewhat similar situation applies to the therapeutic use of orally administered THC in treating the wasting syndrome associated with AIDS. Modest weight gains have been produced by orally administered THC with continued weight loss among comparison patients who received placebo (20,21). In this case, THC would be used concurrently with various drugs (nucleoside homologs and protease inhibitors) that have high levels of intrinsic toxicity. Once again, the reported studies have not mentioned any interactions of consequence when THC was added to the existing drug treatments of AIDS and its complications. Here, too, we lack knowledge.

THC or marihuana has been used for treating spasticity associated with neurologic disorders, such as multiple sclerosis and spinal cord injury (22,23). Since THC may be added to ongoing regimens of muscle relaxants, it would be of some interest to know whether such combined uses might be harmful. In one animal study in which THC was given with muscle relaxants, it was found to increase the desired effect of the latter drugs (12). In this case, the interaction might be advantageous.

Two cases reports of hypomania or manic reactions followed the use of fluoxetine and disulfiram concurrently with marihuana (24,25). As both the interacting drugs have well-known effects on inhibiting drug metabolism, it is possible that this was the mechanism in these two isolated cases.

5. CONCLUSIONS

The expanding social and now possible therapeutic use of marihuana and THC contrasts to the relative lack of information about drug interactions between cannibinoids and other drugs. The recent literature, such as it is, focuses mainly on animal studies with few being pertinent to the way cannabinoids are used in the real world. Whether the recent silence about interactions indicates that all is well or whether it indicates that no one is looking is a question that needs answering.

REFERENCES

1. Hollister, L. E. (1976) Interactions of delta-9-tetrahydrocannabinol with other drugs. *Ann. NY Acad. Sci.* **281**,212–218.
2. Nahas, G. C. (1984) *Marihuana in Science and Medicine* Raven, New York, pp.189–197.
3. Herkenham, M., Lynn, A. B., Little, M. D., Johnson, M., Melvin, B., De Costa, B. R. and Rice, K. C. (1960) Cannabinoid receptor localization in brain. *Proc. Natl. Acad. Sci. USA* **87**,1931–1936.
4. Holleltt, A. C., Bidaut-Russell, M., Devane, W. A., Melvin, L. S., Johnson, M. R., and Herkenham, M. (1960) The cannabinoid receptor, biochemical, anatomical and behavioral characterization. *Trends Neurosci.* **13**,420–423.
5. Devane, W. A. (1994) New dawn of cannabinoid pharmacology. *Trends Pharmacol. Sci.* **15**,40–41.
6. Bornheim, L. M., Kim, K. Y., Perottti, B. Y. T., and Benet, L. Z. (1994) Effect of cannabidiol (CBD) pretreatment on the kinetics of tetrahydrocannabinol (THC) metabolites in brain. *Can. J. Physiol. Pharmacol.* **72 (suppl 1)** 292.
7. Agurell, S., Carlsson, S., Lindgren, J. E., Ohlssson, A., Gillespie, H., and Hollister, L. E. (1981) Interactions of delta-1-tetrahydrocannabinol cannabinol and cannabinol following oral administration in man. Assay of cannabinol and cannabidiol by mass fragmentography. *Experientia* **37**,1090–1091.
8. Hunt, R. A., Jones, R. T., Herning, R. I., and Bachman, J. (1981) Evidence that cannabidiol does not significantly alter the pharmacokinetics of tetrahydrocannabinol in man. *J. Pharmacokinetics Biopharmaceutics* **9**,245–260.
9. Hollister, L. E. (1973) Cannabidiol and cannabinol in man. *Experientia* **29**,825–826.
10. Hollister, L. E. and Gillespie, H. K. (1975) Interactions in man of delta-9-tetrahydrocannabinol. II. Cannabidiol and cannabinol. *Clin Pharmacol. Ther.* **18**, 80–82.
11. Doty, P., Dykstra, L. A., and Picker, M. J. (1992) Delta-9-tetrahydrocannabinol interactions with phencyclidine and ethanol. Effects on accuracy and rate of responding. Pharmacol. *Biochem. Behav.* **43**,61–70.
12. Nishikami, J., Hamajima, K., Watanabe, K., Yamamoto, I., and Yoshimura, H. (1987) The interaction of cannabinoids with various drugs. *J. Pharm. Sci.* **76, S43.**
13. Pertwee, R. G. and Greentree, R. G. (1988) Delta-9-tetrahydrocannabinol-induced caltalepsy in mice enhanced by pretreatment with flurazepam or chlordiazepoxide. *Neuropharmacology* **27**.486–491.
14. Lukas, S., Sholar, M., Kouri, E., and Mendelson, J. H. (1992) Marihuana smoking increases plasma cocaine levels and subjective reports of euphoria in male volunteers. *Pharmacologist,* **34**, abstract 386.

15. Foltin, R. W., Fischman, M. W., and Kelly, T. H. (1992) Behavior effects of ethanol and marihuana, alone and in combination with cocaine in humans. Proc. Committee on Problems of Drug Dependence. NIDA Res. Monograph **109,** 218.

16. Yamamoto, I, Umebayashi, E., Watanebe, E., and Yoshimura, R. (1988) Interactions of cannabis extract, delta-9-tetrahydrocannabinol and 11-hydroxy-delta-8-tetrahydrocannabinol with methamphetamine in mice. *Commun. Subst. Abuse* **9,**107–116.

17. Godley, P. J., Moore, E. S., Wooworth, J. R., and Fineg, J. (1991) Effects of ethanol and delta-9-tetrahydro-cannabinol on phencyclidine disposition in dogs. *Biopharm. Drug Dispos.* **12,**189–199.

18. Lane, M., Vogal, C. L., Ferguson, J., Dransow, S., Saiers, J. L., Hamm, J., Salva, K., Wiernik, P. H., Holroyde, C. P., Hammill, S., Shepherd, K., and Plasse, T. (1990) Dronabinol and prochlorperazine in combination for treatment of cancer. *J. Pain Symptom Manage* **6,**352–359.

19. Vinciguerra, V., Moore, T., and Brennan, E. (1988) Inhalation marihuana as an antiemetic for cancer chemotherapy. *NY State J. Med.* **88,**525–528.

20. Gorter, R. (1991) Management of anorexia-cachexia associated with cancer and HIV infection. *Oncology* **5(suppl 9),** 13–16.

21, Mattes, R. D., Engelmann, K., Shaw, L. M., and Elsoholy, M. A. (1994) Cannabinoids and appetite stimulation. *Pharmacol. Biochem. Behav.* **49,**187–195.

22. Ungerleider, J. T., Andyrsiak, T., Fairbanks, L., Ellison, G. W. and, Myers, L. W. (1987) Delta-9-THC in the treatment of spasticity associated with multiple sclerosis. *Adv. Alcohol Substance Abuse* **7(1),**39–50.

23. Meinck, H., Schonle, P. W., and Conrad, B. (1989) Effect of cannabis of spasticity and ataxia in multiple sclerosis. *J. Neurol.* **239,**120–122.

24. Jaeger, W., Benet, L. Z., and Bornheim, L. M. (1996) Inhibition of cyclosporine and tetrahydrocannabinol metabolism by cannabidiol in mouse and human microsomes. *Xenobiotica* **26,**275–284.

25. Lacoursiere, R. B. and Swatek, R. (1983) Adverse interaction between disulfiram and marihuana: a case report. *Am. J. Psychiatry* **140,**243–244.

26. Stoll, A. L., Cole, J. O., and Lukas, S. L. (1991) Letter. A case of mania as a result of fluoxetine-marihuana interaction. *J. Clin Psychiatr.* **52,** 280–281.

20

Marihuana and the Lung

Donald P. Tashkin

Abstract

Habitual marijuna use may lead to the following effects on the lung: acute and chronic bronchitis; extensive microscopic abnormalities in the cells lining the bronchial passages, some of which may be premalignant; overexpression of molecular markers of progression to lung cancer in bronchial tissue; abnormally increased accumulation of inflammatory cells (alveolar macrophages) in the lung; and impairment in the function of these immune-effector cells (reduced ability to kill microorganisms and tumor cells) and in their ability to produce protective inflammatory cytokines. Clinically, the major pulmonary consequences that may ensue from regular marijuana use are pulmonary infections and respiratory cancer. Infections of the lung are more likely in marijuana users because of a combination of smoking-related damage to the ciliated cells in the bronchial passages (the lung's first line of defense against inhaled microorganisms) and marijuana-related impairment in the function of alveolar macrophages (the principal immune cells in the lung responsible for defending it against infection). Patients with pre-existing immune deficits caused by AIDS or cancer chemotherapy might be expected to be particularly vulnerable to marijuana-related pulmonary infections. Furthermore, biochemical, cellular, genetic, animal, and human studies all suggest that marijuana is an important risk factor for the development of respiratory cancer. However, proof that habitual use of marijuana does in fact lead to respiratory cancer must await the results of well-designed case-control epidemiologic studies that should now be feasible after the passage of 30 years since the inititation of widespread marijuana use among young individuals in our society in the mid-1960s.

1. INTRODUCTION

Since tobacco is known to be the most important cause of chronic obstructive pulmonary disease (COPD) and lung cancer and to predispose to respiratory tract infection (because of smoking-related damage to the lung's defenses against infection, e.g., the mucociliary apparatus of the tracheobronchial tree), it is reasonable to be concerned about a possible relation between habitual use of the second most widely smoked substance in the United States, namely

From: *Marihuana and Medicine*
Edited by: G. G. Nahas et al.   © Humana Press Inc., Totowa, NJ

marijuana, and similar pulmonary consequences. This chapter will review the evidence that addresses this question.

2. COMPARISON OF THE SMOKE CONTENTS OF MARIJUANA AND TOBACCO

The smoke contents of marijuana and tobacco reveal many of the same gas phase constituents, including chemicals known to be toxic to respiratory tissue, such as hydrocyanic acid, acetaldehyde, and acrolein, (1,2), which are present in somewhat similar concentrations in the smoke from the same quantity of marijuana and tobacco. The particulate phase (tar) constituents of marijuana and tobacco smoke are also generally similar, with the major exception that marijuana contains Δ^9-THC and other cannabinoid compounds not found in tobacco, whereas tobacco tar contains nicotine not found in marijuana. It is particularly noteworthy that the tar phase of marijuana smoke contains many of the same carcinogenic compounds contained in tobacco smoke, including nitrosamines, reactive aldehydes and up to a 50% higher concentration of polycyclic aromatic hydrocarbons (PAHs), such as benz[α]anthracene and benz[α]pyrene. Benz[α]pyrene was recently identified as a key factor promoting human lung cancer (3).

3. ANIMAL STUDIES

Studies in animals exposed to varying doses of marijuana smoke for from 12–30 months have shown extensive damage in dogs (4) and monkeys (5) to the smaller airways, which are the major site of injury caused by tobacco-related COPD, as well as acute and chronic pneumonia in rats (6,7) and monkeys (5). On the other hand, rats exposed for 1 year to increasing doses of marijuana smoke failed to demonstrate any anatomic or functional evidence of emphysema, whereas such evidence was apparent in tobacco-exposed rats (8).

4. HUMAN STUDIES

Human studies conducted in the 1970s yielded mixed results: some reported an association between regular marijuana use and chronic bronchitis and emphysema (9,10), whereas others failed to find such a relationship (11,12). These studies may be criticized because of deficiencies in experimental design, including failure to control adequately for the important confounding variable of tobacco, only small numbers of participants, lack of follow-up evaluation, and probable selection biases. More recent studies in humans have systematically evaluated the effects of habitual use of marijuana on respiratory symptoms, lung function, airway pathology, and the structure and function of alveolar macrophages, which are the lung's key immune-effector cells.

4.1 Symptoms of Chronic Bronchitis

Tashkin et al. (13) studied a large sample of volunteers recruited from the Los Angeles area, including 144 heavy, habitual smokers of marijuana only (MS) and 135 smokers of marijuana plus tobacco (MTS), as well as 70 smokers of tobacco only (TS) and 97 nonsmokers (NS). Compared to NS, a significantly higher proportion of MS (15–20%) acknowledged symptoms of chronic bronchitis (chronic cough and phlegm production). Whereas 20–25% of TS also reported symptoms of chronic bronchitis, the proportion of symptomatic TS did not differ significantly from that of symptomatic MS (despite a marked disparity in the amount of each substance smoked per day: 3–4 joints of marijuana versus >20 cigarettes of tobacco), and no additive effects of marijuana and tobacco were noted. Similar findings were reported by Bloom et al. *(14)* in a randomly stratified sample of young individuals (15–40 years of age) residing in the Tucson area, with the exception that these investigators noted an additive effect of marijuana and tobacco that was not observed in the Los Angeles study.

4.2. Lung function

In the Tucson study *(14)*, regular marijuana use (approximately 1 joint per day on the average) by young persons was associated with significant impairment in measurements that reflect the function of the small airways (the major site of COPD); these changes were even greater than those noted in young regular tobacco smokers, and the effects of both marijuana and tobacco appeared to be additive. The authors concluded that regular marijuana smoking was a risk factor for the development of COPD, which, in its advanced stages, is characterized by disabling shortness of breath. In contrast, the Los Angeles study *(13)* failed to find any impairment in small-airway function in association with even heavier regular use of marijuana (3–4 joints per day), although mild, statistically significant narrowing of large, central airways was noted in the marijuana users. Recently, a longitudinal analysis of the lung function results obtained in Los Angeles *(15)* revealed an accelerated rate of decline in lung function with age in the tobacco-smoking participants (consistent with an increased risk for developing symptomatic COPD later in life), but failed to find such an effect in the marijuana smokers. The mixed findings from these two studies leave open the question as to whether habitual smoking of marijuana, in the absence of tobacco, can lead to COPD.

4.3. Airway Pathology

4.3.1. VISUAL AND MICROSCOPIC EVIDENCE OF AIRWAY INJURY

Bronchoscopy was performed in 53 NS, 40 MS, 31 TS, and 44 MTS who participated in the Los Angeles study *(16,17)* to ascertain whether regular smoking of marijuana with or without tobacco might cause damage to the airways and lung that might not be reflected by abnormalities in lung function. Visual inspection of the appearance of the large, central airways showed that a large proportion of smokers of marijuana or tobacco alone (but rarely nonsmokers) showed evidence of increased redness (erythema) and swelling (edema) of the airway tissues and increased mucous secretions. Moreover, the findings in the combined smokers of both marijuana and tobacco appeared additive *(18)*. These visual findings were correlated with microscopic evidence of increased numbers and size of small blood vessels in the bronchial wall, tissue edema, and replacement of the normal ciliated columnar epithelial cells lining the inner surface of the bronchial wall by mucus-secreting goblet cells.

Microscopic findings in biopsies of the bronchial mucosa revealed that a much higher proportion of MS than NS (and a proportion comparable to, if not greater than, that of TS) exhibited a variety of cellular abnormalities. The latter included abnormal proliferation of cells (reserve cells, goblet cells), transformation of normal ciliated cells into abnormal cells resembling skin (squamous metaplasia), accumulation of inflammatory cells, and abnormalities in the cell nuclei *(16,17)*. Some of these changes (e.g., nuclear alterations and squamous metaplasia) have been described as precursors to the subsequent development of lung cancer in tobacco smokers *(19)* and thus may be considered to be premalignant. Smokers of both marijuana and tobacco exhibited these microscopic cellular abnormalities to the greatest extent, suggesting an additive injurious effect of marijuana and tobacco on airway tissue. These findings in healthy, largely nonsymptomatic young marijuana smokers confirm and extend previous bronchoscopic observations of Tennant *(20)* in symptomatic United States servicemen who smoked cannabis (in the form of hashish) heavily. In addition, these microscopic findings may explain the relatively high proportion of marijuana smokers who complain of chronic cough and phlegm, because overproduction of mucus by the increased numbers of mucus-secreting cells in the face of diminished numbers of ciliated cells whose function is to transport mucus toward the mouth by rapid ciliary motion might leave cough as the only mechanism to remove mucus from the airways. Furthermore, since normal mucociliary function serves to cleanse the lung of inhaled particles, including bacteria, that deposit on the mucus lining of the airways, marijuana-related airway damage, by interfering with this important function, impairs the lung's first line of defense against infection.

4.3.2. MOLECULAR MARKERS OF PRECANCER PROGRESSION

A specific combination of genes (oncogenes, tumor suppressor genes) that are responsible for regulating cell growth must be activated and/or mutated for lung cells to transform into cancerous cells. Bronchoscopic biopsies from 63 participants in the Los Angeles study (12 MS, 9 MTS, 14 TS, and 28 NS) were examined for alterations in some of the genes known to be involved in the development of lung cancer (21). These included epidermal-growth-factor receptor (EGFR), Ki-67 (a nuclear proliferation protein responsible for cell division), and the p53 tumor-suppressor gene (whose mutant protein product has lost the ability normally to suppress cell growth). Immunohistology was used to detect the overexpression of the protein products of these genes by epithelial cells in the bronchial biopsies (21). EGFR and Ki-67 were markedly overexpressed in the biopsies from MS compared to NS (and even to a greater extent than in the biopsies from TS), and effects of marijuana and tobacco were additive. Expression of the p53 oncogene (which may play a role in as many as 75% of all lung cancers) was found only in a smoker of marijuana plus tobacco, as well as a combined smoker of marijuana, cocaine, and tobacco. These results reflect molecular evidence of extensive growth dysregulation in these relatively young smokers of marijuana alone and, particularly, in the combined smokers of marijuana and tobacco, implying an important role of marijuana use in progression to lung cancer.

4.4 Alveolar Macrophages

Alveolar macrophages are the principal immune-effector cells in the lung and are primarily responsible for protecting the lung against infectious microorganisms. A saline rinse (bronchoalveolar lavage, or BAL) was used in participants in the Los Angeles study at the time of bronchoscopy to harvest cells from the air spaces in the lung; over 90% of these cells were alveolar macrophages. Approximately two or three times as many alveolar macrophages were obtained from the lungs of marijuana or tobacco smokers, respectively, as from nonsmokers, and the effects of smoking both substances were additive (22). These observations indicate that regular marijuana smoking produces an inflammatory response, i.e., an accumulation of increased numbers of alveolar macrophages, in the lung. Under the electron microscope, alveolar macrophages from marijuana or tobacco smokers showed a striking increase in size and complexity of inclusion bodies in their cytoplasm (probably caused by ingestion by these cells of particulate material in the smoke), and macrophages from combined smokers of marijuana and tobacco were nearly completed filled by these inclusions (23). It might be expected that the packing of these important cells with large inclusion bodies would interfere with their function. To evaluate this possibility, investigators in the Los Angeles study examined the following aspects of alveolar macrophage function.

4.4.1. ABILITY TO INGEST AND KILL FUNGAL ORGANISMS

Alveolar macrophages from MS showed an approximately 30% reduced ability to kill *Candida albicans* compared to NS. This reduction in normal fungal killing function was statistically significant and comparable to the impairment in killing activity of macrophages from TS. No marijuana- or tobacco-related defect in ingestion (phagocytosis) of the fungus was noted (24).

4.4.2. Ability to Ingest and Kill Pathogenic Bacteria

Macrophages from MS, but not from TS, showed a significant (average of 25%) impairment in their ability to ingest *Staphylococcus aureus*. Moreover, macrophages from MS, but not from TS, were significantly impaired (by close to 60% on the average) in their ability to kill these bacteria, compared with the killing activity of NS *(25)*.

4.4.3. Ability to Produce Reactive Oxygen Intermediates

Assays of superoxide production by alveolar macrophages showed a trend toward reduced basal (unstimulated) production by cells from MS compared to NS and a striking inability of macrophages from MS to increase production of superoxide to the same extent as that exhibited by TS when stimulated *(24)*. Moreover, both resting and stimulated superoxide production by macrophages from combined smokers of marijuana and tobacco was reduced in comparison with that from the cells of smokers of tobacco alone. These findings suggest a marijuana-related impairment in the ability of alveolar macrophages to produce reactive oxygen compounds that are needed to combat infection.

4.4.4. Ability to Kill Tumor Cell Targets

As part of their overall function in the lung's immune defense system, alveolar macrophages play an important role in restricting the growth of and killing tumor cells. In a cytotoxicity assay, macrophages from MS, but not from TS, showed a significant impairment in their ability to kill tumor target cells (either small-cell carcinoma cells or erythroleukemia cells), compared to macrophages from NS *(25)*.

4.4.5. Ability to Produce Cytokines

Alveolar macrophages from marijuana smokers, when stimulated with bacterial endotoxin, were depressed in their ability to produce a variety of proinflammatory cytokines (including TNF-α, IL-6 and GM-CSF), but not immunosuppressive cytokines *(25)*. Since cytokines are important regulators of macrophage function, this marijuana-related decrease in inflammatory cytokine production by cells from MS could provide a mechanism for the depression in the immune-effector function (fungal, bacterial, and tumor-cell killing) of the macrophages from MS.

5. EFEECTS OF MARIJUANA ON THE IMMUNE SYSTEM: IMPLICATIONS FOR RESPIRATORY TRACT INFECTION

5.1. In Vitro and Animal Studes

Cannabinoid receptors have been identified on leukocytes *(26)*. The presence of THC-receptors on immune cells is consistent with observations that THC is capable of modulating immune responses. In vitro and animal studies suggest that THC has a general immunosuppressive effect on a variety of immune cells, including macrophages, natural killer cells, and T cells *(27–31)*. Mice pretreated with Δ^9-THC prior to infection with a sublethal dose of *Legionella pneumophila*, a cause of community-acquired and opportunistic bacterial pneumonia, failed to develop cell-mediated protective immunity and died when rechallenged with the organism; on the other hand, control mice not pretreated with Δ^9-THC became immune to repeated infection and survived *(32)*.

5.2. Immune Deficits in Marijuana Smokers

As noted previously, alveolar macrophages from the lungs of healthy, habitual marijuana smokers were suppressed in their ability to kill fungal and bacterial organisms, as well as tumor cells. Moreover, the same cells were suppressed in their ability to release proinflammatory cytokines. These findings suggest that marijuana may be an immunosuppressant with clinically significant effects on host defense, which could have potentially serious health consequences in patients with pre-existing immune deficits caused by AIDS, organ transplantation (receiving immunosuppressive therapy to prevent rejection of the transplant), or cancer (receiving immunosuppressive chemotherapy). The latter possibility is supported by reports of fungal and bacterial pneumonias in patients with AIDS or organ transplantation who used marijuana *(33,34)*. Moreover, among HIV-positive individuals, active marijuana use has been found to be a significant risk factor for rapid progression from HIV infection to AIDS and acquisition of opportunistic infections and/or Kaposi's sarcoma *(35,36)*.

6. ROLE OF MARIJUANA IN RESPIRATORY CANCER

Several lines of evidence suggest that marijuana may play an important role in the development of respiratory cancer, as described below.

The tar phase of marijuana smoke contains many of the same carcinogenic compounds contained in tobacco smoke, including nitrosamines, reactive aldehydes and up to a 50% higher concentration of carcinogenic polycyclic hydrocarbons (PAHs), including benz[α]pyrene *(1)* Benz[α]pyrene, which has recently been shown to promote mutations in the p53 oncogene *(3)*, is believed to play an important role in human cancer.

One marijuana cigarette was shown by Wu and colleagues *(37)* to deposit four times as much tar in the lung as that deposited by a single filtered tobacco cigarette of approximately the same weight. The higher content of carcinogenic PAHs in marijuana tar and the greater deposition of marijuana tar in the lung act together to amplify exposure of the marijuana smoker to the carcinogens in the tar phase. It is noteworthy, however, that marijuana cigarettes that are smoked recreationally contain approximately one-half the quantity of marijuana compared to the amount of tobacco contained in an average tobacco cigarette.

Preliminary findings suggest that marijuana smoke activates cytochrome P-450 1A1 (CYP1A1), the enzyme primarily responsble for converting PAHs, such as benz[α]pyrene, into active carcinogens *(38)*. PAHs in tar are known to be themselves capable of inducing the CYP1A1 enzyme through a pathway that involves binding to a receptor (AHR) in the cell which then becomes complexed to a nuclear transporter protein (ARNT). This complex is translocated into the cell nucleus where promoter sequences on DNA are activated and the gene that codes for the CYP1A1 enzyme is transcribed. Recent studies have shown that bronchial epithelial cells in biopsies from marijuana smokers stain strongly for the antibody to the CYP1A1 enzyme, whereas staining is absent or only weak in biopsies from nonsmokers, implying that regular exposure to marijuana smoke induces the CYP1A1 enzyme in vivo *(38)*. Incubation of liver cells in vitro with tar from marijuana smoke is also capable of activating the CYP1A1 enzyme *(38)*. Marijuana tar induced comparable numbers of mutations to those produced by tar from the same quantity of tobacco in a common bacterial assay for mutagenicity *(39)*. Painting tar from marijuana smoke on the skin of mice produced lesions correlated with malignancy *(40)*.

Exposure of hamster lung cell cultures to marijuana or tobacco smoke over a period of two years led to accelerated malignant transformation within 3–6 months of marijuana exposure compared to control (unexposed) cell cultures; moreover, the changes in the cells exposed to marijuana smoke were more impressive than those in the tobacco-exposed cells *(41)*.

Biopsies of bronchial lining tissue of habitual marijuana smokers demonstrated extensive cellular alterations, some of which may be considered premalignant; effects of smoking both marijuana and tobacco on these cellular changes were additive *(17)*. Bronchial immunohistology revealed overexpression of molecular markers of lung-tumor progression in smokers of marijuana *(21)*.

Alveolar macrophages from marijuana-only smokers have reduced ability to kill tumor-cell targets *(25)*.

THC inhibits the development of antitumor immunity both in vitro and in vivo. Antitumor immunity depends on the ability of antigen-presenting dendritic cells to stimulate the proliferation of T lymphocytes that selectively recognize and destroy tumor cells, but not normal cells. In in vitro studies in which dendritic cells and T cells were incubated in the presence or absence of THC, THC suppressed T cell proliferation in a dose-dependent manner *(42)*. At the same time, THC inhibited the release of protective proinflammatory cytokines (interferon-γ) that may help mediate the T-cell proliferative response.

Pretreatment of mice with THC for 2 weeks prior to implanting Lewis lung-cancer cells (a nonsmall-cell immunogenic carcinoma) into the animals caused larger, faster-growing tumors. THC-stimulated enhanced growth of these tumors was correlated with the production by cells associated with the tumor of decreased amounts of proinflammatory cytokines (e.g., interferon-γ) and increased amounts of immunosuppressive cytokines (e.g., transforming growth factor-β and interleukin-10) *(43)*. These results suggest that THC impairs the development of anti-tumor immunity in vivo and parallels the findings of THC-related inhibition of anti-tumor immunity in the in vitro studies cited above.

Several case-series reports indicate an unexpectedly large proportion of marijuana users among cases of lung cancer *(44,45)* and upper aerodigestive tract cancers (cancers of the oral cavity, pharynx, and larynx) *(44,46,47)* that occurred before age 45 years. These case-series reports suggest that marijuana may play a role in the development of human respiratory cancer. Without a control group, however, the effect of marijuana use on cancer risk cannot be estimated, nor can the potentially confounding effect of tobacco and other risk factors be controlled.

The only epidemiologic study that examined an association between marijuana and cancer was recently published by Sidney and colleagues *(48)*. These investigators at Kaiser Permanente in Northern California followed a cohort of 65,000 health plan members 15–49 years of age in 1979–1985, at which time they completed self-administered questionnaires about marijuana use and other health-related factors. This cohort was followed for detection of the development of new cancers until 1993. Over this period of time 182 tobacco-related cancers were detected, of which 97 were lung malignancies. No effects of lifetime or current marijuana use on the risk of these cancers was found. The major limitation of this study is that those subjects who are likely to have been heavy or long-term users of marijuana were probably not followed long enough to detect an effect on cancer risk since the peak incidence or respiratory cancer occurs in later life. Moreover, despite the large cohort size, there may not have been a sufficient number of heavy and/or long-term marijuana smokers to observe an effect. Well-designed case-control studies are required to address the question more conclusively as to whether regular use of marijuana is a significant risk factor for the development of respiratory cancer.

REFERENCES

1. Hoffmann, D., Brunneman, D. K., Gori, G. B., and Wynder, E. L. (1975) On the carcinogenicity of marijuana smoke. *Recent. Adv. Phytochem.* **9,** 63–81.
2. Novotny, M., Lee, M. L., and Bartle, K. D. (1976) A possible chemical basis for the higher mutagenicity of marijuana smoke as compared to tobacco smoke. *Experientia.* **32,** 280–282.
3. Dinissenko, M. F., Pao, A., Tang, M-S, and Pfeifer, G. P. (1996) Preferential formation of benz[α]pyrene adducts at lung cancer mutational hotspots in p53. *Science* **274,** 430–32.
4. Roy, P. E., Magnan-Lapointe, F., Huy, N. D., and Boutet, M. (1976) Chronic inhalation of marijuana and tobacco in drugs: pulmonary pathology. *Research Communications in Chemical Pathology and Phamacology.* **14:** 305–307.

5. Fligiel, S. E. G., Beals, T. F., Tashkin, D. P., Paule, M. G., Scallet, A. C., Ali SF, Bailey JR, and Slikker W Jr. (1991) Marijuana exposure and pulmonary alterations in primates. *Pharmacol. Biochem. Behav.* **40,** 637–642.

6. Fleischman, R. W., Baker, J. R., and Rosenkrantz, H. (1979) Pulmonary pathologic changes in rats exposed to marijuana smoke for one year. *Toxicol. Appl. Pharmacol.* **47,** 557–566.

7. Rosenkrantz, H. and Fleischman, R. W. (1979) Effects of cannabis on lung. In: Nahas, G. and Payton, W. D. H. (eds.) *Marijuana: Biological Effects.* Oxford, England, Pergamon Press, pp. 279–299.

8. Huber, G. L., Mahajan, V. K. (1988) The comparative response of the lung to marihuana or tobacco smoke inhalation. In: *Marijuana: An International Research Report. Proceedings of Melbourne Symposium on Cannabis 2-4 September, 1987.* (Cheser G, Consroe P, Musty R., eds.) National Campaign Against Drug Abuse. Monograph Series No. 7, Australian Government Publishing Service, Canberra, pp. 19–24.

9. Chopra, G. S. (1973) Studies on psycho-clinical aspects of long-term marihuana use in 124 cases. *Int. J. Addict.* **8,** 1015–1026.

10. Hall, J. A. S. (1975) Testimony in marijuana-hashish epidemic and its impact on United States security, In: *Hearings of the Committee on the Judiciary, United States Senate.* Government Printing Office, pp. 147–154.

11. Rubin, V. and Comitas, L. (1975) Respiratory function and hematology. In: *Ganja in Jamaica: A Medical Anthropological Study of Chronic Marihuana Use.* The Hague, Mouton, pp. 87–102.

12. Boulougouris, J. C., Panayiotopoulos, C. P., Antypas, E, Liakos, A., and Stefanis, C. (1976) Effects of chronic hashish use on medical status in 44 users compared with 38 controls. *Ann. NY Acad. Sci.* **282,**168–172.

13. Tashkin, D. P., Coulson, A. H., Clark, V. A., Simmons, M., Bourque, L. B., Duann, S., Spivey, G. H., and Gong, H: Respiratory symptoms and lung function in habitual, heavy smokers of marijuana alone, smokers of marijuana and tobacco, smokers of tobacco alone, and nonsmokers. *Am. Rev. Respir. Dis.* **135,** 209–216.

14. Bloom, J. W., Kaltenborn, W. T., Paoletti, P., Camilli, A., and Lebowitz, M. S. (1987) Respiratory effects of non-tobacco cigarettes. *Br. Med. J.* **295,** 516–518.

15. Tashkin, D. P., Simmons, M. S., Sherrill, D., and Coulson, A. H. Heavy habitual marijuana smoking does not cause an accelerated decline in FEV_1 with age: a longitudinal study. *Am. J. Respir. Crit. Care Med.* **155,** 141–148.

16. Gong, H. Jr, Fligiel, S., Tashkin, D. P., and Barbers, R. G. (1987) Tracheobronchial changes in habitual, heavy smokers of marijuana with and without tobacco. *Am. Rev. Respir. Dis.* **136,** 142–149.

17. Fligiel, S. E. G, Roth, M. D., Kleerup, E. C., Barsky, S. H., Simmons, M. S., and Tashkin, D. P. (1997) Tracheobronchial histopathology in habitual smokers of cocaine, marijuana and/or tobacco. *Chest.* **112,** 319–326.

18. Roth, M. D., Kleerup, E. C., Arora, A., Barsky, S., and Tashkin, D. P. (1998) Airway inflammation in young marijuana and tobacco smokers. *Am. Rev. Respir. Crit. Care Med.* **157,** 928–937.

19. Auerbach, O., Stout, A. P.,. Hammond, E. D.,and Garfinkel, L. (1961) Changes in bronchial epithleium in relation to cigarette smoking and its relation to lung cancer. *N. Engl. J. Med.* **265,** 253–267.

20. Tennant, F. S. Jr. (1980) Histopathologic and clinical abnormalities of the respiratory system in chronic hashish smokers. *Subst. Alcohol. Actions Misuse* **1,** 93–100.

21. Barsky, S. H., Roth, M. D., Kleerup, E. C., Simmon, M., and Tashkin, D. P. (1998) Molecular alterations in bronchial epithelium of habitual smokers of marijuana, cocaine and/or tobacco. *J. Natl. Cancer Inst.* (in press).

22. Barbers, R. G., Gong, H. Jr, Tashkin, D. P., Oishi, J., and Wallace, J. M. (1987) Differential examination of bronchoalveolar lavage cells in tobacco cigarette and marijuana smokers. *Am. Rev. Respir. Dis.* **135,** 1271–1275.

23. Beals, T. F., Fligiel, S. E. G., Stuth, S., and Tashkin, D. P. (1989) Morphological alterations of alveolar macrophages from marijuana smokers. *Am. Rev. Respir. Dis.* **139 (Part 2),** A336.

24. Sherman, M. P., Campbell, L. A., Gong, H. Jr, Roth, M. D., and Tashkin, D. P. (1991) Respiratory burst and microbicidal characteristics of pulmonary alveolar macrophages recovered from smokers of marijuana alone, smokers of tobacco alone, smokers of marijuana and tobacco and nonsmokers. *Am. Rev. Respir. Dis.* **144,** 1351–1356.

25. Baldwin, G. C., Tashkin, D. P., Buckley, D. M., Park, A. N., Dubinett, S. M., and Roth, M. D. (1997)Habitual smoking of marijuana and cocaine impairs alveolar macrophage function and cytokine production. *Am. J. Respir. Crit. Care. Med.* **156,**1606–1613.

26. Bouaboula, M., Rinaldi, M., Carayon, P., Carillon, C., Delpech, B., Shire, D., LeFur, G., and Casellas, P. (1993) Cannabinoid-receptor expression in human leukocytes. *Eur. J. Biochem.* **214,** 173–80.

27. Huber, G. L., Simmons, G. A., McCarthy, C. R.,Cutting, M. B., Laguarda, R., and Pereira, W. (1975) Depressant effect of marihuana smoke on antibactericidal activity of pulmonary alveolar macrophages. *Chest.* **68,** 769–773.

28. Huber, G. L., Pochay, V. E., Pereira, W., Shea, J. W., Hinds, W. C., First, M. W., and Sornberger, G. C. (1980) Marijuana, tetrahydrocannabinol, and pulmonary antibacterial defenses. *Chest* **77,** 403–410.

29. Klein, T. S., Kawakami, Y., Newton, C., and Friedman, H. (1991) Marijuana components suppress induction and cytolytic function of murine cytotoxic T cells *in vitro* and *in vivo. J. Toxicol. Environ. Health.* **32,** 465–77.

30. Kusher, D. I., Dawson, L. O., Taylor, A. C., and Djeu, J. Y. (1994) Effect of the psychoactive metabolite of marijuana, delta-9-tetrahydrocannabinol (THC), on synthesis of tumor necrosis factor by human large granular lymphocytes. *Cellular Immunol.* **154,** 99–108.

31. Tindall, B. Philipot, C. R., Cooper, D. A., Gold, J., Donovan, B., Penny, R., and Barnes, T. (1988) The Sydney AIDS project: Development of acquired immune deficiency syndrome in a group of HIV seropositive homosexual men. *Aust. NZ J. Med.*

32. Newton, C. A., Klein, T. W., and Friedman, H. (1994) Secondary immunity to Legionella pneumophilia and Th1 activity are suppressed by Δ^9-tetrahydrocannabinol injection. *Infection and Immun.* **62,** 4015–20.

33. Denning, D. W., Follansbee, S. E., Scolaro, M., Norris, S., Edelstein, H., and Stevens, D. A. (1991) Pulmonary aspergillosis in the acquired immunodeficiency syndrome. *N. Engl. J. Med.* **324,** 654–662.

34. Caiaffa, W. T., Vlahov, D., Graham, N. M., Astemborski, J., Solomon, L., Nelson, K. E., and Muñoz, A. (1994) Drug smoking, *Pneumocystis carinii* pneumonia, and immunosuppresion increase risk of bacterial pneumonia in human immunodeficiency virus-seropositive infection drug users. *Am. Rev. Respir. Dis.* **150,** 1493–1498.

35. Newell, G. R., Mansell, P. W., Wilson, M. B., Lynch, H. K., Spitz, M. R., and Hersh, E. M. (1985) Risk factor analysis among men referred for possible acquired immune deficiency syndrome. *Preventive Medicine* **14,** 81–91.

36. Tindall, B., Philipot, C. R., Cooper, D. A., gold, J., Donuvan, B., Penny, R., and Barnes, T. (1988) The Sydney AIDS project: Development of acquired immune deficiency syndrome in a group of HIV seropositive homosexual men. *Aust. NZ J. Med.*

37. Wu, T-C, Tashkin, D. P., Djahed, B., and Rose, J. E. (1988) Pulmonary hazards of smoking marijuana as compared with tobacco. *N. Engl. J. Med.* **318,** 347–351.

38. Marques-Magallanes, J. A., Tashkin, D. P., Serafian, T., Stegeman, J., and Roth, M. D. (1997) *In vivo* and *in vitro* activation of cytochrome P4501A1 by marijuana smoke. Presented by DP Tashkin at the 1997 Symposium on the Cannabinoids of the International Cannabinoid Research Society, Stone Mountain, GA, June, 1997, International Cannabinoid Research Society Program and Abstracts, ISBN# 09658053-0-1, p.78.

39. Wehner, F. C., Van Rensburg, S. J., and Theil, P. F. (1980) Mutagenicity of marijuana and Transkei tobacco smoke condensates in the Salmonella/microsome assay. *Mutat. Res.* **77,** 135–142.

40. Cottrell (1973)

41. Leuchtenberger, C., and Leuchtenberger, R. (1976) Cytological and cytochemical studies of the effects of fresh marihuana cigarette smoke on growth and DNA metabolism of animal and human lung cultures. In: *The Pharmacology of Marijuana* (Braude MC, Szara S eds.). Raven, New York, p. 595–612.

42. Roth, M. D., Zhu, L., Sharma, S., Stolina, M., Park, A. N., Chen, K., Tashkin, D. P., and Dubinett, S. M. (1997) Δ^9-tetrahydrocannabinol inhibits antigen-presentation *in vitro* and anti-tumor immunity *in vivo.* Presented at the 1997 Symposium on the Cannabinoids of the International Cannabinoid Research Society, Stone Mountain, GA, June, 1997, International Cannabinoid Research Society Program and Abstracts, ISBN# 09658053-0-1, p. 79.

43. Zhu, L., Sharma, S., Stolina, M., Chen, K., Park, A., Roth, M., Tashkin, D. P., and Dubinett, S. M. (1997) THC-mediated inhibition of the antitumor immune response. Presented at the 19th Southern California Pulmonary Research Conference, Palm Springs, CA, January.

44. Taylor, F. M. III. (1988) Marijuana as a potential respiratory tract carcinogen: A retrospective analysis of a community hospital population. *South. Med. J.* **81,** 1213–1216.

45. Sridhar, K. S., Raub, W. A., Weatherby, N. L., Metsch, L. R., Surratt, H. L., Inciardi, J. A., Duncan, R. C., Anwyl, R. S., and McCoy, C. B. (1994) Possible role of marijuana smoking as a carcinogen in the development of lung cancer at a young age. *J. Psychoactive Drugs* **26,** 285–88.

46. Donald, P. J. (1991) Advanced malignancy in the young marijuana smoker. *Adv. Exp. Med. Biol.* **288,** 33–46.

46. USDHEW. (1979)*Smoking and Health. A Report of the Surgeon General.* DHEW Publication No.(PHS) 79-50066. Washington, DC:USGPO.

47. Endicott, J. N., Skipper, P., and Hernandez, L. (1993) Marijuana and head and neck cancer. *Adv. Exp. Med. Biol.* **335,** 107–113.

48. Sidney, S., Beck, J. E., Tekawa, I. S., and Quesenberry, C. P., Jr. (1997) Marijuana use and cancer incidence. *Am. J. Public Health* 585–590.

21 Marihuana Smoking, a Possible Carcinogen or Cocarcinogen

George Hyman

Abstract

Marihuana smoking may act as a carcinogen or co-carcinogen. It contains several proven carcinogens such as nitrosoamine and benzene, and is known to damage the respiratory epithelium, including the nasopharynx. There is also a proven decrease in cellular and humoral immunity. These facts, coupled with reports in the literature of multiple cases of cancer of the respiratory tract in the young with the average age at onset of 26 years, highlight this hazard. The AIDS population (whose life-span is now being prolonged) are the most susceptible to this potential effect of marihuana smoking.

None of the claims for the benefits of marihuana inhalation for protection against the side-effects of chemotherapy, or for relief of a variety of symptoms in the AIDS patient, stand up against more effective and wiser alternatives. Thus, a 2-mg tablet of granisetron taken one hour before chemotherapy affords a 24-hour protection from nausea and vomiting, and megestrol taken orally will relieve the anorexia and weight loss.

What is more important to the marihuana smoker is the damage to cells of the respiratory tract and its possible role as a carcinogen or cocarcinogen *(1,2)*. Marihuana smoke contains 50% more carcinogen than a tobacco cigarette of the same weight. When added to tobacco cigarette smoking and frequent use of alcohol, the potential of increased risk of cancer of the respiratory tract becomes even greater. The literature of carcinoma of the respiratory tract includes a striking number of young patients under the age of 40 (almost always of the squamous-cell variety). This increase in the number of cases requires careful evaluation. Several of the reports *(4–7)* decribed cases of lung cancer in a series of patients of an average age of onset at 26 years; and many of the tumors were at an advanced stage.

The damaging effects of marihuana smoking on the lungs and respiratory tract mucosa have been reported and studied for many years following the report from the American Thoracic Society in 1975 *(8)*. Tissue culture of lungs exposed to marihuana smoke display anomalies in mitosis and DNA complement and cellular proliferation *(9)*.

From: *Marihuana and Medicine*
Edited by: G. G. Nahas et al.   © Humana Press Inc., Totowa, NJ

Even more serious may be the reported decrease in cellular and humoral immunity *(10,11)*. This is particularly ominous in those infected by HIV, in whom impaired immunity may be compounded by marihuana smoke.

In the past, early death from AIDS was anticipated and, therefore, a potential carcinogenic effect of marihuana was not problematic. With the antiretroviral triple therapy for AIDs, life can be extended for years. Any carcinogen introduced in a immunodepleted patient may produce a carcinoma of the lung in a group of individuals already susceptible to other neoplasms such as lymphoma and Kaposi's sarcoma.

What an irony to control AIDS in years ahead while increasing the risk of a marihuana-induced lung cancer epidemic. In view of medicinal marihuana's risks, even as additional research continues; cessation of medical use of marihuana smoking is mandatory in AIDS patients.

REFERENCES

1. Hoffman, D., Brunnemann, K. D., Gori, G. S., and Wynder, E. L. (1975) On the carcinogenicity of marihuana smoke. *Recent Adv. Phytochem.* **9,** 63–81.
2. Wehner, F. C., Van Rensurg, S. J., and Theil, P. F. (1980) Mutagenicity of marihuana and Transkei tobacco smokes condensates in the *Salmonella*/microsome assay. *Muta. Res.* **77,** 135–142.
3. Donald, P. J. (1986) Marihuana smoking—possible cause of head and neck carcinoma in young patient. *Otlaryngol. Head Neck Surg.* **94,** 517–521.
4. Tashkin, D. O., Coulson, A. H., Clark, V. A., Simmons, M., Bourque, L. B., Duann, S., Spivey, G. H., and Gong, H. (1987) Respiratory symptoms and lung function in habitual, heavy smokers of tobacco alone, and nonsmokers. *Am. Rev. Respir. Dsi.* **135** 209–216.
5. Taskin, D. P. (1997) Potential respiratory and infectious comlications of medical marihuana: suggested monitoring procedures. Presented by D. P. Tashkin at the 1997 Symposium on the Cannabinoids of the International Cannabinoid Research Society, Stone Mountain, GA, June, 1997, International Cannabinoid Research Society Program and Abstracts, p.89.
6. Taylor, F. M., III. (1988) Marihuana as a potential respiratory tract carcinogen. A retrospective analysis of a community hospital population. *S. Med. J.* **81,** 1213–1216.
7. Sridhar, K: S., Raub, W. A., and Weatherby, N. L., et al. (1994) Possiblerole of marihuana smoking as a carcinogen in the development of lung cancer at a young age. *J. Psychoactive Drugs* **26** 285–288.
8. American Thoracic Society. (1975) Position paper: marihuana and the lungs. *Am. Thoracic. Soc. News* Spring, 7.
9. Leuchtenberger, C., Leuchtenberger. R., and Ritter, U. (1973) Effects f marihuana and tobacco smoke on DNA and chromosomal compliment in human lung expants. *Nature* **242,** 403–404.
10. Peterson, B. H., Lemberger, L. Graham, J., and Dalton, B. (1975) Alternations in the cellular-mediated immune responsiveness of chronic marihuana smokers. *Psychopharmacol. Commun.* **1,** , 67–74.
11. Nahas, G. G., Desoize, B., Armand, J. P., Hsu., J., and Morishima, A. (1975) Natural canabinoids: apparent depression of nucleic acids and protein synthesis and cultures of human lymphocytes. *In*: (Szara, S. and Braude, X, eds.) Raven, New York, pp. 177–188.

22 Cardiovascular Effects of Marihuana and Cannabinoids

Renaud Trouve and Gabriel Nahas

Abstract

In the isolated heart THC produces a biphasic effect on heart rate with an initial increase followed by a decrease. THC also decreases coronary flow and cardiac contractile force. The depressant effect of THC on cardiac contraction and coronary flow is antagonized by CBD and by Ca^{2+} antagonists. In humans, THC and marihuana induce increases in heart rate and blood pressure. In the supine position, postural hypotension is observed because of the peripheral vasodilation produced by the drug. THC produces a deregulation of the baroreflex. In dogs, cats, and rats, THC produces hypotension and bradycardia, indicating a predominance of the interaction of the parasympathetic outflow by THC in these animals. Marihuana smoking increases coronary insufficiency in patients with ischemic cardiac disease. Self-administration of cocaine before exercise will result in an increase in the tachycardia and a decreased efficiency. Marihuana smoking and THC have no therapeutic cardiac properties and are contraindicated in patients with coronary problems.

1. INTRODUCTION

The cardiovascular effects of marihuana have been extensively studied in experimental preparations and in humans. They have been attributed to its main psychoactive ingredient, THC. Its mechanism of action on the heart, which includes interaction of the drug with the central and autonomic nervous systems, is not entirely clarified. Other cannabinoids such as CBD and CBN have limited cardiovascular properties, but may interact with THC and modify its effect.

2. STUDIES IN VITRO AND ON THE ISOLATED HEART

Bose[1] reported that *Cannabis* extracts have a relaxing effect in vitro in smooth muscle of rabbit intestine and uterus, and antagonize the spasmogenic effect of carbachol and histamine. Gill and Paton[2] also reported that Δ^9-THC inhibited the contracture of ileum and aortic

From: *Marihuana and Medicine*
Edited by: G. G. Nahas et al.   © Humana Press Inc., Totowa, NJ

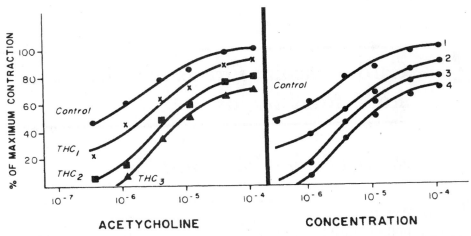

Fig. 1. Inhibition by delta-9-THC of acetylcholine-induced contraction of uterine muscle strip in two preparations of rate uterine muscle. From Schwartz and Nahas (3).

strip. Schwartz and Nahas (3) observed that Δ^9-THC 10^{-5} to $10^{-4}\,M$ in vitro inhibits the acetylcholine-induce contraction of uterine muscle strip in the rat (Fig. 1).

Manno and Manno[4] reported that Δ^9-THC in doses of 0.1–0.4 mg reduces the force of contraction of the isolated heart with little or no effect on heart rate. Other authors using the rat heart or guinea pig heart-lung preparations reached similar conclusions (5–7). Smiley et al.[8] reported that in the isolated perfused rat heart, THC and CBN decrease contractile force while increasing the rate; whereas CBD produced bradycardia arrhythmias and asystole. However, the experimental design used by the authors resulted in accumulation of cannabinoids in the heart and prevented the study of dose-response effects and of the cardiac interaction of these different cannabinoids.

Trouve and Nahas (9) investigated the effect of THC, CBD, and CBN administered separately or in combination to a heart preparation specially designed to avoid cumulative effects of the drug and to obtain dose-response effects (10). These studies will be described as originally published.

2.1 Methods

Wistar rats weighing 200–300 g and maintained on a standard laboratory diet were anesthetized with ether. The heart is excised and placed in a saline-buffered heparinized solution at 4°C. The aorta is cannulated and attached to the base of the retrograde perfusion column of a modified Langendorff preparation which has been described in a separate publication. This system allows for continuous storage, analysis, and display of coronary flow, heart rate, and differential pressure (ΔP) between minimal diastolic and peak systolic supra-aortic pressures. This latter measurement may be considered an index of cardiac performance.

The Langendorff perfused heart is studied in a closed system with automatic regulations to maintain constancy of the perfusion column (Krebs-Henseleit + 0.5% albumin or 25–30% washed erythrocyte suspension); and continuous recording of rate, coronary flow, and supravalvular aortic pressure. A microcomputer with software interface is used for storage treatment and on line analysis of the recorded variables. In 38 preparations perfused with Krebs-Henseleit, minimal diastolic (61.2 ± 2.8 mmHg) is significantly below and peak systolic (98.7 ± 3.6 mmHg) significantly above perfusion pressure (80 mmHg). Pressure difference between minimal diastolic and peak systolic (ΔP) is 37.5 ± 1.8 mmHg. Increases in perfusion pressure will be associated with increases of coronary flow and ΔP, which are also increased by isoprenaline administration. Oxygen consumption decreased by 76% when perfusion pressure was lowered from 80 to 60 mmHg in hearts perfused with a 30% suspension of washed erythrocytes. All of these experimental results were interpreted as indicating that ΔP measured in this system resulted from an ejected volume (x acceleration) from the heart. The ejected volume corresponds to a valvular leak caused by the rigid nature of the system which is devoid of aortic compliance. ΔP may be considered an index of left ventricular performance, an indication that the Langendorff preparation studied under the present conditions is a working heart. A 100-μL volume constant-infusion syringe for time administration of cardioactive drugs may be inserted at the base of the perfusion column to obtain dose-response effects.

The cannabinoids supplied by NIDA (National Institute of Drug Abuse) with chromatographic analysis indicating 99.5% purity are stored in the dark at 4°C. Before use, these samples were reanalyzed by mass spectrometry liquid-gas chromatography and similar results were obtained. Δ^9-THC was supplied diluted in ethanol, whereas CBD and CBN supplied in crystalline form were resuspended in ethanol. All drugs were diluted in a solution containing 10% Tween-80 in buffered saline and 2.5% ethanol, a solution in which the fat-soluble cannabinoids are well-solubilized (11). The test substance is administered during 1 minute by means of an electrically powered syringe containing 100 μL as described (10), to obtain dose–response effects. Dose–response effects of each cannabinoid were studied on four to seven hearts.

The pharmacokinetic profile of Δ^9-THC in this system was determined by administering the tritiated compound in a single bolus and recovering coronary output every 30 seconds for the next 10 minutes. Retention and elimination time of the drug was then calculated so as to perform subsequent dose–response curves of the drug at proper intervals and avoid its accumulation in the heart. It was observed that after administration of a single bolus of tritiated THC in the system, 98% of the radioactivity had been eliminated after 10 minutes. Cannabinoids were therefore administered at intervals of 10 minutes or more, after all variables had been restored to their initial control values, and the measurement performed during the period just preceding drug administration was considered to be a control measurement.

2.2 Analysis of Data

The analog-to-digital conversion of the physiological markers recorded by this system will give a greater precision than that of conventional recording methods. Under controlled, stable conditions, the reproducibility of coronary outflow, pressure, and rate measurements are better than ± 1%. Therefore a variation in these measurements performed on the same preparation during its 1-hr period of stability and exceeding ± 3% is significant ($P < 0.01$). Effects produced by the different compounds administered are processed by the computer and expressed as a fraction of the preceding control measurement which has been previously recorded and stored. A change greater than 2% (0.02) from control is significant ($P < 0.05$), and for a change greater than 3% (0.03), $\Delta P < 0.01$.

2.3. Results

Administration of the vehicle (10% Tween, 80% isotonic saline, 2.5% ethanol) did not alter any of these recorded markers. THC administered to five preparations (Fig. 2) produced a biphasic effect on cardiac frequency, first an increase with THC concentrations of 2.05 to 7.75×10^{-6} M. Maximum recorded increase was 24% above control with 7.75×10^{-6} M. With

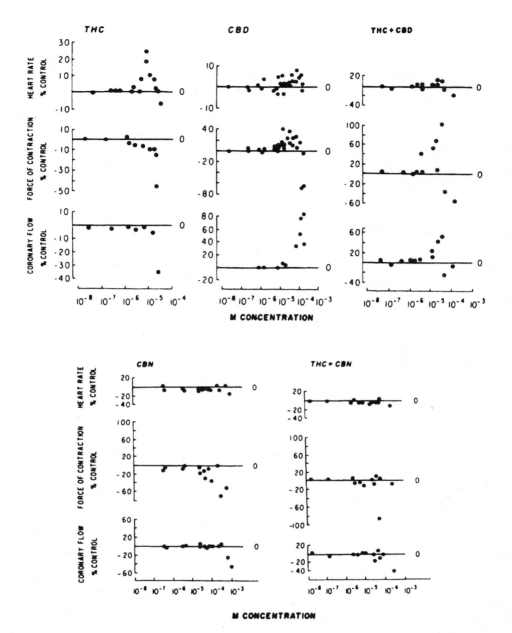

Fig. 2.

higher dosage there was a progressive decrease in frequency toward and below control. With similar doses of THC, ΔP and coronary flow decreased progressively. ΔP was 50% below control when THC concentration was 3×10^{-5} M. All cardiac activity stopped with THC 3.4×10^{-5} M. Similar results are observed with 11 OH Δ^9-THC, the hydroxylated active metabolite of THC.

CBD administered to seven preparations produced small increments in frequency limited to 8% above control, and a dose-related increase of pulse pressure (4–42%) and coronary flow (7–55%). Cardiac arrest occurred with 2.66 to 3.4×10^{-4} M, a dose nine times higher than that occurring with THC (Fig. 2).

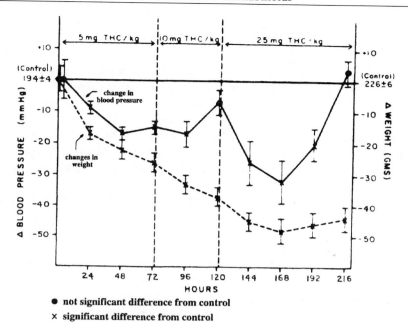

Fig. 3.

Cannabinol (CBN) 10^{-6} *M* to 10^{-4} *M* tends to decrease rate and pulse pressure in the presence of a stable coronary flow. When administered in equivalent amounts with THC, heart rate increases caused by THC were no longer present. Cannibycyclol and cannibachromene had significant effects up to a dose of 10^{-5} *M*, which decreased contractile force.

When THC and CBD are administered simultaneously to five preparations in equimolar concentrations, 10^{-7} to 10^{-4} *M*, the effects of CBD predominate. There is a limited change in rate, whereas contractile force and coronary flow increase with THC concentrations of 1.23×10^{-6} *M* to 5.6×10^{-5} *M*. Cocaine in the range of 10^{-7} *M* to 10^{-4} *M* concentration produces a transient small increase in heart rate and pulse pressure. Cocaine administered in equimolar concentration of THC mitigated the depressant effect of this drug on pulse and heart rate.

2.4. Discussion

The cardiac chronotropic effects of THC in vitro are observed within a very narrow range of concentrations: 4.2×10^{-6} *M* to $2.0 \times 10\ 10^{-5}$ *M*. Higher concentrations are toxic: 3.3×10^{5} *M* THC produces asystole. Other in vitro effects of THC on lymphocytes or nerve cells are observed within a similar narrow range of concentrations: 10^{-6} *M* to 10^{-5} *M*. The concentrations of THC used in this study were calculated from amount administered and coronary flow; they are 10–50 times higher than plasma concentrations associated with cardiac effects. However, THC and cannabinoids tend to adhere to glass and other surfaces, and tissue concentrations of these drugs, following their in vitro administration, are consequently reduced by these amounts and may be lower by a factor of 10 than the concentrations administered (*11*).

CBD will induce asystole with concentrations of 2.3×10^{-4} *M*, nine times the concentration of THC that stops cardiac activity. CBN appears to have a cardiac activity different from that of THC and CBD: decreasing rate and pulse pressure in the presence of a constant coronary flow.

The cellular mechanisms that mediate the cardiac effects of these cannabinoids are not clear. The tachycardia induced by THC in the isolated heart could be caused in part to by its action on catecholaminergic receptors that the drug has been reported to potentiate (*12*). The brief duration of the tachycardia induced by THC and its "biphasic" effect might be caused by the release and depletion by THC of catecholamine stores from the isolated rat heart. These stores are limited; THC might in addition interfere with uptake mechanisms. The mechanisms of the depressing effect of THC on contractile force and coronary flow cannot be presently ascertained. There is some limited evidence in humans of a weakening of cardiac contractility by THC (*13*): In a study of marihuana and placebo cigarette smokers with coronary heart disease, THC *per se* contributed to the observed reduction of stroke index, cardiac index, and ejection fraction.

The mechanisms of the cardiac effect of CBD are unclear. CBD 10^{-6} *M* decreases by 50% calcium ATPase activity(*14*), a property that might account in part for its effects on coronary flow and ΔP.

2.5. Animal Preparations.

The antagonistic effects of THC and CBD have also been reported in animal preparations since the first observation of Carlini et al. (*15*): CBD blocks THC-induced catatonia in mice, corneal areflexia in rabbits, aggressiveness in REM sleep-deprived rats, and minimizes in unanesthetized rabbits the depressant effect of THC on heart rate, respiration, and rectal temperature (*16,17*).

CBD antagonizes the effect of THC on operant behavior of rodents and Rhesus monkeys (*18,19*). It has also been reported that CBD inhibits the epileptic seizures induced by THC in the genetically epileptic rabbit. According to some authors (*20,21*), CBD blocks the increase in heart rate of THC when simultaneously administered with this drug; others (*22,23*) failed to observe such antagonistic effects of CBD. Therefore, it is not clear to what extent the direct cardiac effects of THC could be antagonized in human by CBD.

The major cardiovascular effects of a single dose of Δ^9-THC in most animal species studied are bradycardia, decreased cardiac reflexes, and hypotension. As a result, cardiac output and cerebral blood flow are usually decreased. These tests were carried out in anesthetized cats (*24–26*) anesthetized dogs (*27,28*), unanesthetized dogs (Nahas and Hardy, unpublished observation), and anesthetized rat (*24,29*). This bradycardia seems to be of central origin and caused by an increased vagal outflow and in the rat is inhibited by atropine (*24*). Borgen and Davis (*30*) reported that CBD (25 mg/kg, i.v.) causes a significant attenuation of the depressant effect of THC (3 mg/kg, i.v.) on heart rate and rectal temperature of unanesthetized rabbits. Tolerance to THC-induced bradycardia in rodents was reported after 10 days of treatment by Ford and McMillan (*31*).

Dewey (*32*) reported that in anesthetized dogs a dose of 1–10 mg/kg of THC intravenously produced a drop in arterial pressures (systolic, diastolic, and mean), in heart rate, in systemic vascular resistance, and cardiac output (*33*). This drop in arterial pressure, which lasted two to three hours, was not suppressed by vagotomy or the use of β-adrenergic agents, suggesting a complicated interactive mechanism of blood-pressure deregulation.

In rats, following THC administration, the observed effects depend on the route of administration. Intragastric administration of 10–20 mg/kg of THC did not change arterial pressure but induced a decrease in heart rate. When administered intraperitoneally, 0.4–4 mg/kg of THC induces a mild-to severe drop in mean blood pressure that lasted for several hours after a 4 mg/kg dose of marihuana. Dewey reported a similar transient pressure response followed by hypotension and bradycardia in the rat (*34*).

Doherty et al. reported dose-related hypotension and bradycardia in vivo in anesthetized cats (35). These effects were limited in contrast to the recorded progressive respiratory depression leading to respiratory failure.

Some of the factors that account for the THC-induced bradycardia observed in animal preparations might include a central reduction of sympathetic tone, which slows the heart by increasing vagal tone a central stimulation of vagal activity and an activation of peripheral chemoreceptors that elicits a reflex bradycardia (36). In the spontaneously hypertensive rat (SHR) 10–20 mg/kg of THC administered intragastrically will also lower blood pressure. Tolerance to this effect develops within a week (37) (Fig. 3).

In contrast with other animal species, sympathetic outflow stimulation by THC dominates in humans, leading to tachycardia, which can be controlled in part by β-blockers. THC has a dual effect on the autonomic system by interacting with sympathetic and parasympathetic outflow. The physiologic balance of both systems is impaired by THC.

2.6. Developmental Effects

Effects of THC on chicken embryonic heart cells in culture include changes in enzymatic activity (GOT, LDH, HBD), decrease of glucose consumption, lactate production, and contraction rate after 6–18 hours of exposure (38). After 72 hours of exposure, all these factors were decreased, suggesting an inhibition of short half-life proteases.

Sassenrath et al. reported one case of myocardial alteration in the offspring of a rhesus monkey treated with THC daily (39). Scherwitz et al. examined potential paternal risk factors in the etiology of isolated ventricular septal defects in infants (40). A significant association was found between paternal marihuana use and the defect. Other compounding variables include race and patterns of cocaine abuse.

3. STUDIES IN HUMANS

The most striking effect of THC-containing *Cannabis* in human observed by all routes of administration is a dose-related tachycardia which may increase by 30–60% over control rate. This consistently observed physical manifestation of *Cannabis* intoxication was first reported in 1940 by the authors of the La Guardia Report. Previous studies of *Cannabis* intoxication, such as the Indian Hemp Drug Commission Report of 1894 or subsequent ones from India or the Middle East failed to mention this basic physiological change.

In one study on marihuana smokers, 65% of the increase in heart rate observed could be associated with the concentration of Δ^9-THC in the cigarette (41). Dose–response increases in heart rate of subjects inhaling from a spirometer uniform amounts of *Cannabis* smoke were reported by Renault et al. (42) (Fig. 4). A reproducible dose effect was observed in individual subjects, whereas variance between subjects in their heart–rate response to marihuana inhalation was great. No difference was found between experienced and inexperienced smokers. Marihuana smoking suppressed the normal sinus arrhythmia as well as the bradycardia associated with the Valsalva maneuver. With the highest Δ^9-THC concentration (6.5 mg), maximum heart rates were in the range of 140–160/min. The increase in pulse parallels the intensity of the brain functional effects. If the drug induces euphoria (or anxiety) a marked increase in heart rate occurs-whereas if it induces somnolence or sedation, a moderate rise is observed. The maximum increase in rate is observed within 15–30 minutes after smoke inhalation, lasts for 30–40 minutes, and is followed by a slow decline over a period of four to five hours.

Maximal tachycardia and psychoactive effects occur concurrently 10–15 minutes after the peak of plasma THC concentration (43).

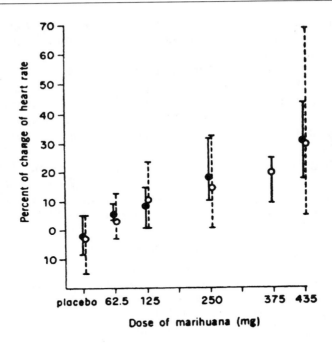

Fig. 4.

Equal amounts of THC administered intravenously or ingested produces similar increases in heart rate (*44–46*).

Tolerance may develop to this THC effect of *Cannabis* (*47*). After 18–20 days of 210 mg a day of THC administration, the same test marihuana cigarette produced a 7% increase in heart rate instead of a 45% increase in the control period. In this tolerant state, increasing the dose of THC reinstates the tachycardia along with the euphoric effect. The Δ^9-hydroxy THC and the analog dimethylheptyl pyran (DMHP) show a similar action.

Karniol et al. (*20*) reported that CBD administration blocks the increase in heart rate of THC when simultaneously administrated with this drug. Hollister and Gillespie (*22*) and Dalton et al. (21) failed to observe such antagonistic effects of CBD. The latter authors noted however an antagonistic action of CBD on the psychoactive effects of THC.

Propranolol, in doses sufficient to block the beta-adrenergic receptors of the heart, in association with atropine, prevents the increase in heart rate induced by THC (*48,49*). With lower doses of propranolol such blockage is not observed. R. H. Miller et al. (*50*) studied the effect of THC on the conducting system, showing an acceleration of sinus cycle and recovery time, no action on atrial refractory periods, and facilitation of measures of sinoatrial and AN nodal conduction; and they point out the similarity of these effects to those of isoprenaline and atropine.

This effect of THC on the autonomic nervous system has been dissociated from the psychoactive effects of the drug: In subjects administered 30–45 μg/kg intravenously, treatment with atropine and propranolol abolished any effect of THC on heart rate, but the subjective and EEG effects remained as intensive (*51*).

The occurrence of acute ECG anomalies and arrhythmias in marihuana smokers have been reported by a number of investigators. Thus, Johnson and Domino (*41*) noted premature ventricular contractions (PVCs) in 2 of 15 subjects; they also noted T-wave flattening, commonly of a degree less than that produced by moderate exercise. Kochar and Hosko (52) noted in seven subjects a gross flattening of T wave in one, some flattening in another, and PVCs at five per minute in a third. R. H. Miller et al. (50) reported frequent multifocal PVCs in one subject of six in their study of conduction mechanisms. On the other hand, there are a considerable number of studies that report no abnormalities (44,53). It would appear that ECG abnormalities occur no more frequently than would be expected from the degree of sympathetic cardioacceleration observed.

There is some limited evidence on weakening of cardiac contractility by THC. Prakash et al. (13) reported in a study of marihuana and placebo cigarette smokers with coronary heart disease, that THC *per se* contributed to the observed reduction of stroke index, cardiac index, and ejection fraction.

3.1. Hemodynamic and Peripheral Effects

These effects are a function of the nature of exposure (acute or chronic) of the dose and of the body position. Acute exposure in humans lying supine usually causes a modest increase in blood pressure (which is not always apparent) (48,54–56). On assuming upright position, orthostatic hypotension of significant magnitude may occur (57,58).

Cardiac output in the supine position is increased by as much as 30% after an injection of THC (59,60). This increase can be attributed to the increase in heart rate (61) with changes in the ventricular contraction periods (increase in ejection time and shortening of the preinjection period) (62).

Increase in cardiac output in the presence of little or no increase in blood pressure indicates that a substantial decrease in peripheral resistance is taking place under the influence of THC. The change in resistance varies among different vascular beds, being greatest in the vessels of the skeletal muscles and minimal in those of the skin.

Chronic exposure to large doses of Δ^9-THC or of marihuana cigarettes exerts different effects (57,63). Systolic and diastolic pressure tend to fall as the heart rate slows from the high levels caused by initial *Cannabis* administration. Postural hypotension is also accentuated. With oral administration, the extent of postural hypotension is increasingly related to the amount of plasma volume increase (57,63).

The above-mentioned studies lead to the following analysis: THC produces a reduction of sympathetic tone to the blood vessels and vasodilation, insufficient to produce a fall in blood pressure in the presence of postural stress. The same factor will account for the attenuation of reflex vasomotor responses such as the cold pressor test or vasoconstriction of the fingers in response to deep inhalation. Associated with this THC-induced peripheral vasodilation may be feelings of warmth and small falls of body temperature, subsequent feelings of chill, and an occasional headache. However, the mechanisms by which THC interacts with the autonomic nervous system (sympathetic and parasympathetic) are unclear. The data are insufficient to determine to what extent the respective contributions are mediated through central nervous receptors, and by peripheral ones. Both appear to be operative. The most striking peripheral vasodilator response to THC in humans, that of the conjunctiva, seems to be related to a peripheral effect of THC. Conjunctival blood vessel congestion is one of the most constant signs following marihuana smoking, but its cause remains unknown. It is dose-related and relatively slow in onset, peaking at about one hour, and persists for hours. Its time course is more prolonged than the effects on heart-rate. The reddening is accentuated by alcohol. Because the vasodilation is not accompanied by any sensation or inflammatory response, it is hardly likely to be mediated by histamine or related peptides, or by an axon reflex.

3.2. Exercise

Smoking marihuana (2% THC) decreased duration of exercise and caused tachycardia, additive to that of exercise (*64*). Arakian et al. (*65*) studied the effect of marihuana on cardiorespiratory responses to submaximal exercise (15 min at 750 kg/m/min). Cigarettes containing 7.5 mg THC or placebo were smoked by six subjects 20 minutes before the test. Oxygen consumption rose with placebo, heart rate rose from 65 to a peak of 130/per minute with exercise, and had returned to normal in 25–30 minutes thereafter, whereas with marihuana, the heart rate rose from 85 to a peak of 150 per min. and returned to 85 per minute after exercise. The increase in O_2 consumption observed after marihuana smoking could be accounted for by the increase in heart rate caused by the drug, which is added to the physiological tachychardia of exercise. During exercise, deregulation of the baroreflex by marihuana will result in a decrease in the efficiency of the cardiac pump.

3.3. Plasma Volume, Sodium Retention

Although acute administration of THC has little effect, chronic ingestion of large doses of THC causes a gain in body weight and plasma volume caused by sodium retention (*44*). The change in plasma volume seems to be causally related to orthostatic hypotension. Mechanisms responsible for this retention might be a direct effect of THC on kidney, with an inhibition of sodium excretion (*66*).

3.4. Marihuana Smoking and Coronary Insufficiency

Aronow and Cassidy reported that in human subjects with documented coronary impairment, the smoking of one calibrated marihuana cigarette decreased the duration of exercise before onset of angina by 50%, as compared to the same control group without smoking a placebo (*67*). This result was mainly attributed to the increase in heart rate and its effects on cardiac load and oxygen consumption. In a subsequent study, marihuana smoking was compared with the effects of a nicotine-containing cigarette in a group of coronary-impaired patients (*68*). After smoking the nicotine-containing cigarette, time to angina during exercise was reduced by 23% compared to a reduction of 50% after marihuana. Marihuana smoking is contraindicated in patients prone to coronary insufficiency.

4. MECHANISMS OF ACTION

The exact mechanism responsible for the direct effects of cannabinoids on the isolated heart are not clear. Present studies indicate that THC interacts with the catecholamine and their receptors in the heart. Catecholamine stores in the rat heart are limited and could help account for the brief stimulating effect of THC on the rate of the isolated heart. Administration of norepinephrine will reverse the depressant effect of THC on cardiac contraction. The negative effects of THC on pulse pressure (muscular contraction), and coronary flow might be accounted for by its interaction. It has been reported that THC might interfere with Ca^{2+} ATPase. Receptors to THC have only been recently reported in the heart (probably on the cardiac vessels) and the cannabinoid CB_1 receptor is coupled to the G protein that inhibits adenylcyclase and voltage gated Ca^{2+} current (*69*).

Cardiac effects of CBD might be accounted by its calcium antagonist activity. It has been reported that CBD 10^{-6} M decreases by 50% calcium channel ATPase activity in the isolated heart. The increase in pulse pressure (proportional to the force of contraction and the ejected volume of fluid) is compatible with this property. One would expect a decrease in muscular strength of contraction depending on which stage of the cellular calcium pathways the effect occurs; it is possible to observe a biphasic effect in vivo with some calcium-channel blockers.

This effect is based on a better segregation of Ca^{2+} and relaxation of the ventricular wall during diastole, which further results into better compliance of the ventricle and diastolic filling. On the following ejection, cardiac contractile force increases due to Starling's law (greater cardiac fiber distension). Cardiac distension will have a positive influence as long as the filling volume is limited (and the ventricle has not become too compliant).

The antagonism between CBD and THC and between CBD and cocaine observed in other experiments might be explained by a similar mechanism. These results are similar to those obtained with THC and nitrendipine or cocaine and nitrendipine. This observation would corroborate the marked increase in coronary flow seen with CBD, much greater than an increase needed for metabolic adjustment caused by increased cardiac performance.

THC and some other cannabinoids might produce their biological effects by interacting with CB_1 and CB_2 receptors and their natural ligands, inducing a basic deregulation of homeostatic functions at the cellular and organ levels.

Anandamide also has an hypotensive action, mediated by CB_1 receptors as reported by Varga (70). This depressor response is inhibited upon administration of SR 141176A, a cannabinoid receptor antagonist or attenuated by spinal cord section or alpha-receptor blockade. This suggests that the depressor effect of anandamide occurs through a basic receptor mechanism that regulates vascular tone by modulating the activities of cholinergic and catecholeminergic outflow.

REFERENCES

1. Bose, B. C., Saifi, A. Q., and Bhagwat, A. W. (1963) Effect of *Cannabis indica* on hexobarbital sleeping time and tissue respirationof rat brain. *Arch. Int. Pharmacodyn. Ther.* **141**, 520–524.
2. Gill, E. W. and Paton, W. D. M. (1970) Pharmacological experiments *in vitro* on the active principles of cannabis, in *The Botany and Chemistry of Cannabis* (Joyce, C. R. B. and Curry, S. H., eds.), Churchill, London, UK, pp. 165–173.
3. Schwartz, I. W. and Nahas, G. G. (1984) Inhibition of smooth muscle contraction by THC, in *Marihuana in Science and Medicine* (Nahas, G. G., ed.), Raven, New York, pp. 160.
4. Manno, B. R. and Manno, J. E. (1973) Some cardiovascular actions of delta-9-tetrahydrocannabinol in the rat. *Toxicol. Appl. Pharmacol.* **25**, 451.
5. Beaconsfield, P., Oakley, C., Carpi, A., Rainsbury, R., and Del Basso, P. (1974) Cardiac effect of delta-9-tetrahydrocannabinol on a heart-lung preparation and on the intact animal. *Eur. J. Cardiol.* **2**, 167–173.
6. Benmoyal, E., Cote, G., and Morin, Y. (1971) A direct action of delta-9-tetrahydrocannabinol ingestion on myocardial contractility. *Clin. Res.* **19**, 758.
7. Huy, N. D., McNicholl, J., and Roy, P. E. (1972) The acute effects delta-9-tetrahydrocannabinol (THC) on the left ventricular function of isolated hearts. *Clin. Res.* **20**, 910.
8. Smiley, K. A., Karler, R., and Turkanis, S. A. (1976) Effects of canabinoids on the perfused rat heart. *Res. Commun. Chem. Pathol. Pharmacol.* **14**, 659–675.
9. Nahas, G., Trouve, R. (1985) Effects and interactions of cannabinoids on the isolated heart. *Proc. Soc. Exp. Biol.* **180**, 312–316.
10. Trouve, R. and Nahas, G. (1985) Cardiac dynamics of the Langerdorff perfused heart. *Proc. Soc. Exp. Biol. Med.* **180**, 303–311.
11. Rosenkrantz, H., Thompson, G. R., and C, B. M. (1972) Oral and parentenal formulations of marihuana constituents. *J. Pharm. Sci.* **61**, 1106–1112.
12. Bloom, A. S. (1982) Cannabinoids and neurotransmitter receptors. *Brain Res.* **235**, 370–375.
13. Prakash, R., Aronow, W. S., Warren, W. M., Laverty, W., and Gottschalk, L. A. (1975) Effects of marihuana and placebo marihuana smoking on hemodynamics in coronary disease. *Clin. Pharmacol. Ther.* **18**, 90–95.
14. Collins, F. G. and Haavik, C. O. (1979) Effects of cannabinoids on cardiac microsomal ca++ATPase activity and calcium uptake. *Biochem. Pharmacol.* **28**, 2303–2306.
15. Carlini, E. A., Santos, M., V, C., D., and B., F, K. (1970) Structure activity relationship of four tetrahydrocannibinols and the pharmacological activity of five semi-purified extracts of Cannabis sativa. *Psychopharmagologia* **18**, 82–85.
16. Karniol, I. G. and Carlini, E. A. (1973) Pharmacological interaction between cannabidiol and delta-9-tetrahydrocannabinol. *Psychopharmacologia* **33**, 53–61.

17. Borgen, L. A. and Davis, W. M. (1977) Cannabidiol interaction with delta-9-tetrahydrocannabinol. *Commun. Chem. Pathol. Pharmacol.* **16**, 1–8.
18. Zuardi, A. W., Finkelfarb, E., A, B. O. F., E, M. R., and Karniol, I. G. (1981) Characteristics of the stimulus produced by the mixture of cannabidiol with delta-9-tetrahydrocannabinol. *Arch. Int. Pharmacodyn.* **249**, 137–146.
19. Brady, K. T. and L, B. R. (1980) The effect of delta-9-tetrahydrocannabinol alone and in combination with cannabidiol on fixed-interval performance in rhesus monkeys. *Psychopharmacology* **72**, 21–26.
20. Karniol, I. G., Shirakawa, I., Kasiniski, N., Pfeferman, A., and Carlini, E. A. (1974) Cannabidiol interferes with the effect of delta-9-tetrahydrocannabinol in the rat. *Eur. J. Pharmacol.* **28**, 172–177.
21. Dalton, W. S., Martz, R., Lemberger, L., Rodda, B. E. and Forney, R. B. (1976) Influence of cannabidiol on delta-9-tetrahydrocannabinol effects. *Clin. Pharm. and Ther.* **19**, 300–309.
22. Hollister, L. E. and Gillespie, L. E. (1975) Interactions of delta-9-THC and CBD. *Clin. Pharmacol. Ther.* **18**, 80–84.
23. Benowitz, N. L., Nguyen, I., and Jones, R. T. (1980) Cardiovascular effect of cannabinoids. *Clin. Pharmacol. Ther.* **28**, 115–123.
24. Graham, J. D. P. and Li, D. M. F. (1973) Cardiovascular and respiratory effects of cannabis in cat and rat. *Br. J. Pharmacol.* **49**, 1–10.
25. Hardman, H. F., Domino, E. F. and Seevers, M. H. (1971) General pharmacological actions of some synthetic tetrahydrocannabinol derivatives. *Pharmacol. Rev.* **23**, 295–315.
26. Vollmer, R. R., Cavero, I., Ertel, R. J., Solomon, T. A. and Buckley, J. P. (1974) Role of the central autonomic nervous system in the hypotension and bradycardia induced by (–)-delta-9-transtetrahydrocannabinol. *J. Pharm. Pharmacol.* **26**, 186–192.
27. Dagirmanjian, R. and Boyd, E. S. (1962) Some pharmacological effects of two tetrahydrocannabinol. *J. Pharmacol. Exp. Ther.* **135**, 25–33.
28. Dewey, W., Yonle, L., Harris, L., Reavis, W. M., Griffin, E. D. J. and Newby, E. V. (1970) Some cardiovascular effects of trans-delta-9-THC. *Pharmacologist* **12**, 259.
29. Milzoff, J. R., Forney, R. B., Stone, C. J. and Allen, D. O. (1971) The cardiovascular effects of delta-9-THC in vagotomized rats. *Pharmacologist* **13**, 247.
30. Borgen, L. A. and Davis, W. M. (1974) Cannabidiol interaction with delta-9-tetrahydrocannabinol. *Res. Commun. Chem. Pathol. Pharmacol.* **7**, 633–670.
31. Ford, R. D. and McMillan, D. E. (1971) Behavioral tolerance and cross tolerance to 1-delta-9-tetrahydrocannabinol and 1-delta-8-tetrahydrocannabinol in pigeons and rats. *Fed. Proc.* **30**, 279.
32. Dewey, W. L. (1986) Cannabinoid pharmacology. *Pharmacol. Rev.* **38**, 151–178.
33. Mechoulam, R., Devane, W. L., and Glasser, R. (1992) Cannabinoid geometry and Biological activity in marijuana/cannabinoids Neurobiology and neurophysiology (Laura Murphy and Andrzej Bartke eds) C.R.C Press, Boca Baton.
34. Dewey, W., Harris, L., Howes, J., Granchelli, F., Pars, H., and Razdan, R. (1970) Pharmacology of some marihuana constituents and two heterocyclic analogues. *Nature* **226**, 1265–1267.
35. Doherty, P. A., McCarthy, L. E., and Borison, H. L. (1983) Respiratory and cardiovascular depressant effects of nabilone, N-methyllevonantradol and delta 9-tetrahydrocannabinol in anesthetized cats. *J. Pharmacol. Exp. Ther.* **227**, 508–516.
36. Paton, W. (1982) Cannabis and the cardiovascular system, in *Report of the Expert Group on the Effects of Cannabis Use* The Advisory Council on the Misuse of Drugs (Members Letter to the Home Secretatry), London, p. 9.
37. Nahas, G. G., Schwartz, I. W., and Adamec, J. (1973) Tolerance to delta-9-THC in the spontaneously hypertensive rat. *Proc. Soc. Exp. Biol. Med.* **142**, 58–60.
38. Choisy, H., Choisy, G., Millart, H., and Legris, H. (1979) Influence of delta-9-tetrahydrocannabinol on contraction rate and enzymatic activity of embryonic heart cells, in *Marihuana, Biological Effects, Advances in the Biosciences* vol. 22,23. (Nahas, G., and Paton, W., eds.), Pergamon Press, New York pp. X–X.
39. Sassenrath, E., Chapman, L., and Goo, G. (1979) Reproduction in rhesus monkeys chronically exposed to delta-9-tetrahydrocannabinol, in *Advances in the Biosciences* vol. 22,23 (Nahas, G., and Paton, W., eds.), Pergamon Press, New York pp. 501–512.
40. Scherwitz, L., Perkins, L., Chesney, M., Hughes, G., Sidney, S., and Manolio, T. (1992) Hostility and health behaviors in young adults: the CARDIA study. *Am. J. Epidemiol.* **136**, 136–145.
41. Johnson, S. and Domino, E. F. (1971) Some cardiovascular effects of marijuana smoking in normal volunteers. *Clin. Pharmacol. Ther.* **12**, 762–768.

42. Renault, P. F., Schuster, C. R., Heinrich, R., and Freeman, D. (1971) Marijuana: standardized smoke adminis- tration and dose effect curves on heart rate in humans. *Science* **174**, 589–591.

43. Ohlsson, A., Lindgren, J. E., Wahlen, A., Agurell, S., Hollister, L. E., and Gillespie, H. K. (1980) Plasma delta-9-tertrahydrocannabinol concentration and clinical effects after oral and intravenous administration and smoking. *Clin. Pharmacol. Ther.* **28**, 409–416.

44. Benowitz, N. L. and Jones, R. T. (1975) Cardiovascular effects of prolonged delta-9-tetrahydrocannabinol ingestion. *Clin. Pharmacol. Ther.* **18**, 287–297.

45. Perez-Reyes, M., DiGuiseppi, S., Davis, K. H., Shindler, V. H., and Cook, C. E. (1982) Comparison of effects of marihuana cigarettes of 3 different potencies. *Clin. Pharmacol. Ther.* **31**, 617–624.

46. Agurell, S., Carlsson, S., Lindgren, J. E., Ohlsson, A., Widman, M., Gillespie, H., and Hollister, L. (1986) Pharmacokinetic and metabolism of delta-1-tetrahydrocannabinol. *Pharmacol. Rev.* **38**, 21.

47. Benowitz, N. L. and Jones, R. T. (1977) Prolonged delta-9-tetrahydrocannabinol ingestion: effects of sympa- thomimetic amines and autonomic blockades. *Clin. Pharmacol. Ther.* **21**, 336–342.

48. Beaconsfield, P., Ginsburg, J., and Rainsbury, R. (1972) Marijuana smoking: cardiovascular effects in man and possible mechanisms. *N. Engl. J. Med.* **287**, 209–212.

49. Perez-Reyes, M., Lipton, M. A., Timmons, M. C. et al. (1973) Pharmacology of orally-administered delta-9- tetrahydrocannabinol. *Clin. Pharmacol. Ther.* **14**, 48–55.

50. Miller, R. H., Dhingra, R. C., Kanakis, C., Amatry-Leon, F., and Rosen, K. M. (1977) The electrophysiologi- cal effects of delta-9-tetrahydrocannabinol (cannabis) on cardiac conduction in man. *Am. Heart J.* **94**, 740–747.

51. Bachman, J. A., Benowitz, N. L., Herning, R. I., and Jones, R. T. (1979) Dissociation of autonomic and cog- nitive effectsof THC in man. *Psychopharmacology* **61**, 171–175.

52. Kochar, M. S. and Hosko, M. J. (1973) Electrocardiographic effects of marihuana. *JAMA* **225**, 25–27.

53. Hollister, L. E. (1974) Structure-activity relationships in man of cannabis constituents and homologs, and metabolism of delta-9-tetrahydrocannabinol. *Pharmacology* **11**, 3–11.

54. Allentuck, S. (1941) Medical aspects of the marijuana problem in the City of New York, in *The Marijuana Papers* (Soloman, D. A., ed.), Bobbs-Merrill, Indianapolis in, pp. 269–284.

55. Hollister, L. E. (1971) Actions of various marihuana derivatives. *Pharmacol. Rev.* **23**, 349–358.

56. Isbell, H., Gorodetsky, G. W., Jasinski, D., Claussen, U., Spulak, F., and Korte, F. (1967) Effect of (–) delta-9- *trans*tetrahydrocannabinol in man. *Psychopharmacologia* **11**, 184–188.

57. Benowitz, N. L., Rosenberg, J., Rogers, W., Bachman, J., and Jones, R. T. (1979) Cardiovascular effects of intravenous delta-9-tetrahydrocannabinol: autonomic nervous mechanisms. *Clin. Pharmacol. Ther.* **25**, 440–446.

58. Kanakis, C. J., Pouget, J. M., and Rosen, K. M. (1976) The effects of delta-9-tetrahydrocannabinol (cannabis) on cardiac performance with and without beta blockage. *Circulation* **53**, 703–707.

59. Malit, L. A., Johnstone, R. E., Bourke, D. I., Kulp, R. A., Klein, V., and Smith, T. C. (1975) Intravenous delta- 9-tetrahydrocannabinol: effects of ventilatory control and cardiovascular dynamics. *Anesthesiology* **42**, 666–673.

60. Tashkin, D. P., Levisman, J. A., and Abbasi, A. S. (1977) Short-term effects of smoked marihuana on left ven- tricular function in man. *Chest* **72**, 20–26.

61. Gash, A., Karliner, J. S., Janowsky, D., and Lake, C. R. (1978) Effects of smoking marihuana on left ventrical performance and plasma norepinephrine: studies in normal men. *Ann. Intern. Med.* **89**, 448–452.

62. Weiss, J. L., Watanabe, A. M., Lemberger, L., Tamarkin, N. R., and Cardon, P. V. (1972) Cardiovascular effects of delta-9-tetrahydrocannabinol in man. *Clin. Pharmacol. Ther.* **13**, 671–684.

63. Bernstein, J. G., Becker, D., Babor, T. F., and Mendelson, J. H. (1974) Physiological assessments: cardiopul- monary function, in *The Use of Marijuana: A Psychological and Physiological Inquiry* (Mendelson, J. H., Rossi, A. M., and Meyers, R. E., eds.), Plenum Press, New York, pp. 147–160.

64. Shapiro, B. J., Reiss, S., Sullivan, S. F., Tashkin, D. P., Simmons, M. S., and Smith, R. T. (1976) Cardiopul- monary effects of marijuana smoking during exercise. *Chest* **70**, 441.

65. Arakian, E. V., Horwath, S. M., Michael, E. D., and Jacobs, S. (1979) Effect of marihuana on cardiorespira- tory responses to submaximal exercise. *Clin. Pharmacol. Ther.* **26**, 777–781.

66. Santos-Martinez, J., Gonzales-Castillo, M. A., Toro-Goyco, E. (1984) Effect of (–)-delta-9-tetrahydrocannibinol on fractional sodium and potassium excretion in the dog, in *The Cannabinoids: Chemical, Pharmacologic and Therapeutic Aspects* (Agurell, S., Dewey, W. L., and Willete, R. E., eds.), Academic Press, New York.

67. Aronow, W. S. and Cassidy, J. (1974) Effect of marihuana and placebo-marihuana smoking on angina pec- toris. *N. Engl. J. Med.* **291**, 65–67.

68. Aronow, W. S. and Cassidy, J. (1975) Effect of smoking marihuana and of a high-nicotine cigarette on angina pectoris. *Clin. Pharmacol. Ther.* **17**, 549–554.
69. Howlett, A. C. (1995) Cannabinoid compounds and signal transduction mechanisms, in (Pertwee, R. G., ed.), Academic, London, pp. 167–204.
70. Varga, K., Lake, K., Martin, B. R., and Kunos, G. (1995) Novel antagonist implicates the CB1 cannabinoid receptor in the hypotensive action of anandamide. *Eur. J. Pharmacol.* **278**, 279–283.

23 The Immune Response and Marihuana

Harris Rosenkrantz

Abstract

THC significantly inhibits the humoral and cellular mediated immune responses of rats in a dose-related fashion. A similar immunosuppressive effect is produced by marihuana smoke delivered by an automatic inhaler (equivalent inhibition is not produced by marihuana smoke from which THC has been removed). Doses of THC administered were calculated so as to correspond to the doses used in human consumption.

1. INTRODUCTION

The fermenting fervor of dispute related to contrary marihuana findings continues to diminish the credibility of research efforts in this field. No doubt scientific and public communities desire a rapid resolution of discrepancies in order to assume rational positions on legal aspects of marihuana use. Unfortunately, the pendulum of evidence swings erratically through an arc of harmful to not harmful in critical areas of cannabinoid research. The questions of mental performance, teratogenicity, endocrine dysfunction, and immunological impairment potentially induced by marihuana have at the moment not yielded uniformly conclusive answers. The issues remain of paramount importance since the number of users steadily increases, and the quality of illicit cannabinoid agents is constantly being improved *(21)*.

The contrary results reported for the effects of marihuana and pure cannabinoids on immunological defense mechanisms are being examined. Even before the announcements of an apparent marihuana suppression of the cell-mediated immune response *(22,23)*, several ancillary factors suggested that marihuana might interfere with immunological mechanisms: tobacco smoking was an immunosuppressant of both humoral *(6,24,34)* and cellular *(33,35)* immune pathways; marihuana, like tobacco, stimulated the pituitary-adrenal axis *(3,21)*, which could initiate involution of the thymus *(3,28)*, a primary organ of the immune system; cannabinoids have a remarkable affinity for lung tissue *(7,28)*, a major organ of phagocytosis, providing prolonged exposure of drug to macrophages regardless of route of administration of cannabinoids *(7,28)*; marihuana has influenced alveolar macrophage structure, function, and mobilization *(7,20)*; *Cannabis* use has evoked allergic reactions *(18,30)*; cannabinoids

From: *Marihuana and Medicine*
Edited by: G. G. Nahas et al.   © Humana Press Inc., Totowa, NJ

might perform as haptenes because of their nearly complete binding to plasma proteins *(3,21)*; and cannabinoids have repressed bone marrow leukopoiesis *(3,13)*. Perhaps other indirect evidence exists that has escaped attention.

Of course, despite possible prediction of a physiological or biochemical effect of a drug that has not been tested in a specific cellular process, a direct demonstration of cause and effect is mandatory. However, when direct evidence is obtained and then is unconfirmed or refuted, the resolution of the discrepancy is often difficult. This is the present situation for proof of the interaction of cannabinoids and the immune mechanisms as documented in Table 1. Using blood lymphocytes from marihuana users and two types of in vitro tests–T-cell rosette formation or incorporation of tritiated thymidine in the presence of a mitogen or particulate antigen–some investigators *(4,22)* found inhibition of cell-mediated immunity, but others did not *(14,36)*. A skin test was also negative *(32)*. On the other hand, mouse skin allografts survived longer *(17)* and splenic lymphocytes were inhibited by Δ^9-tetrahydro-cannabinol (Δ^9-THC) *(17)*. When the in vitro influence of cannabinoids on cell-mediated immunity was tested, thymidine incorporation into lymphocytes and T-cell rosette formation were suppressed *(1,4,5)*. The humoral immune response of the blood lymphocytes of marihuana users was not affected *(4,36)*. In contrast, splenic lymphocytes from rodents given Δ^9-THC were impaired as determined by three different methods *(16,17,27)*.

The review of the above investigations disclosed a distinction between human and animal studies in that the findings on rodents were consistent. Although immunosuppression of the humoral response was observed after oral administration of Δ^9-THC, it was important to substantiate this finding for marihuana smoke. The present investigation evaluated this potential interaction of marihuana with the humoral immune pathway under conditions simulating marihuana smoking in humans through use of an automatic inhalator. The immunosuppression obtained by the inhalation route was similar to that obtained by corresponding oral doses of Δ^9-THC in the same strain of rat.

2. METHODS AND MATERIALS

The inhalation and oral studies were independently conducted at different times but employing the same personnel and environmental factors. Fischer rats weighing approximately 110–140 g were housed in pairs of the same sex in wire suspension cages $7 \times 9.5 \times 7$ inches. Both sexes were used in the inhalation study, but only females were tested in the oral trial. All animals were fed commercial rat chow and water ad libitum and were in a room regulated for a 12-hour dark/light circadian cycle and maintained at $23 \pm 2°C$.

2.1. Cannabinoid Materials And Doses

Marihuana cigarettes contained approximately 2.1% Δ^9-THC, 0.17% cannabidiol, and 0.15% cannabinol; corresponding maximum values for marihuana placebo cigarettes were 0.05%, 0.01%, and 0.01%, respectively. Oral preparations were solutions of 96% pure synthetic (–)-trans-Δ^9-THC in USP grade sesame oil; the latter served as vehicle control. All cannabinoids were supplied by the National Institute on Drug Abuse, (NIDA) and were stored at 5°C. Before use, cigarettes were maintained at 60% humidity and 23°C for 24–48 hours.

The Δ^9-THC doses for both routes of administration were selected to be relative to those consumed by humans. This was determined, as outlined in Table 2, by expressing doses on the basis of body surface area and encompassing the Δ^9-THC dose range for an average quality of marihuana (1% THC) and of hashish (5% THC) *(26,28)*. An average human body weight of 50 kg has been assumed to represent the spectrum of weights of young to older

Table 1
Cannabinoid Effects on the Cell-Mediated and Humoral Immune Responses

Cannabinoid	Dose (mg/kg)	Route	Species	Cell type and source	Mitogen or antigen		Methodology	Finding	Reference
					Route	Type			
Cell-mediated immune response									
Marihuana	4 ×/wk[a]	Lungs	Human	Lymphocyte, blood	In vitro	SRBC[b]	T-cell rosette	Inhibition	4
	4 ×/wk	Lungs	Human	Lymphocyte, blood	In vitro	PHA; MLC[b]	^{3}H-thymidine incorp.	Inhibition	22
	3 ×/wk	Lungs	Human	Lymphocyte, blood	In vitro	PHA	^{3}H-thymidine incorp.	No change	36
	3 ×/wk	Lungs	Human	Lymphocyte, blood	intraderm.	2,4-DNCB[b]	Skin test	No change	32
	1 ×/wk	Lungs	Human	Macrophage, alevoli	none	None	Morphology	Change	20
Marihuana ext.	2 µg/ml	In vitro	Human	Leukocyte, blood	none	None	Migration	Inhibition[e]	31
Δ^9-THC	2–22 µM	In vitro	Human	Lymphocyte, blood	In vitro	PHA	^{3}H-thymidine incorp.	Inhibition	1
		In vitro	Rat	Lymphocyte, spleen	In vitro	PHA	^{3}H-thymidine incorp.	Inhibition	1
	$9 \times 10^{-7}M$	In vitro	Human	Lymphocyte, blood	In vitro	SR BC	T-cell rosette	Inhibition[d]	4
	$2 \times 10^{-4}M$	In vitro	Human	Lymphocyte, blood	In vitro	PHA; MLC	^{3}H-thymidine incorp.	Inhibition[f]	5
	210 × 14 days	Oral	Human	Lymphocyte, blood	In vitro	PHA	^{3}H-thymidine incorp.[e]	No change	14
	$1.6 \times 10^{-5}M$	In vitro	Mouse[g]	Lymphocyte, spleen	In vitro	Δ^9-THC	^{3}H-thymidine incorp.	Stimulation	23
	50–200	Oral	Mouse	Lymphocyte, spleen	In vitro	PHA	^{3}H-thymidine incorp.	Inhibition	17
	50–200	Oral	Mouse	Lymphocyte, spleen	Skin	Allograft	Graft survival	Increased	17
	0.3–1.3	IP	Rat	Macrophage, perit.	intraderm.	Adjuvant	Migrat. inhib. factor	Suppressed	8
Humoral immune response									
Marihuana	4 ×/wk	Lungs	Human	Lymphocyte, blood	In vitro	SR BC-hemolysin[h]	B-cell rosette	No change	4
	3 ×/wk	Lungs	Human	Lymphocyte, blood	In vitro	Pokeweed	^{3}H-thymidine incorp.	No change	36
Δ^9-THC	140	IP	Mouse	Lymphocyte, spleen	IP	SR BC	Plaque formation	Inhibition	16
	25–200	Oral	Mouse	Lymphocyte, spleen	In vitro	Lipopoly. B[i]	^{3}H-thymidine incorp.}	Inhibition	17
	1–10	Oral	Rat	Lymphocyte, spleen	IP	SR BC	Serum antibodies	Inhibition	27

[a]Time since last use of marihuana variable.
[b]SR BC = sheep red blood cells; PHA = phytohemagglutinin; MLC = mixed lymphocyte culture (allogeneic cells); 2,4-DNCB = 2,4-dinitrochlorobenzene.
[c]Leukocytes from both marihuana smokers and nonsmokers responded similarly.
[d]Inhibition also induced by cannabinol and cannabidiol.
[e]A decreased incorporation of ^{3}H-leucine and ^{3}H-uridine was also seen.
[f]Inhibition also obtained with various cannabinoids and 11-OH metabolites.
[g]Sensitized to Δ^9-THC.
[h]Trypsinized sheep red blood cells coated with antisheep hemolysin for detection of B-cell C_3 receptor.
[i]E. coli lipopolysaccharide B.

Table 2
Relevancy of Δ^9-Tetrahydrocannabinol Doses and Routes of Administration Used in Animals as
Compared to Humans

	mg/kg Δ^9-THC (marihuana, 1% THC; hashish, 5% THC)		
Route[a]	Human[b]	Rat[c]	Mouse[c]
Inhalation, 1 cig/day	0.1–0.5	0.7–3.5	1–6
3 cigs/day	0.3–1.5	2–10	4–18
6 cigs/day	0.6–3.0	4–20	7–36
Approx. LD$_{50}$	[d]	36–42	40–60[e]
Oral	0.3–1.5	2–10	4–18
	0.9–4.5	6–30	10–54
	1.8–9.0	12–63	20–100
Approx. LD$_{50}$	[d]	800–1200	1400–2200

[a]In humans, oral route requires three times the inhalation dose.
[b]Assumes 50 kg mean body weight and 50% loss of THC during smoking.
[c]Dose based on body surface area; conversion factor of 7 and 12 for rat and mouse, respectively.
[d]As a guide, intravenous LD$_{50}$ in monkey was about 100 mg/kg and orally it was estimated to be approximately 15,000 mg/kg.
[e]n value; however, intravenous and inhalation values in rat shown to be nearly identical.

marihuana users. Several investigators have shown that 50% of the Δ^9-THC in marihuana is destroyed and/or entrapped in the residual butt during smoking *(3,26)*. Therefore, 1% Δ^9-THC (10 mg/g) marihuana and 5% Δ^9-THC (50 mg/g) hashish would provide 5 and 25 mg THC, respectively, or 0.1–0.5 mg/kg body weight for each gram of *Cannabis* preparation smoked.

The oral dose in humans is approximately three times the inhalation dose. Body surface area conversion factors from humans to rat and mouse are seven and 12, respectively. Data are given for these two rodents because they, in addition to man, have been used for immunological studies with marihuana and Δ^9-THC. The relationship of LD$_{50}$ values to these calculated Δ^9-THC doses in human and actual Δ^9-THC doses used in rodents arc included as reference points of efficacy and safety *(26)*. On the basis of the above considerations, it was decided to use Δ^9-THC inhalation doses of 0.7,2, and 4 mg/kg and intragastric doses of 1,5, and 10 mg/kg.

2.2. Treatment Protocols

The three prerequisites for obtaining meaningful data on the potential interaction of Δ^9-THC and the humoral immune response were: approximation of the type of human smoking conditions; administration of known doses of the drug; and maintenance in the animal model of identical environmental surroundings for the two routes of administration used by humans. To achieve these objectives, we compared smoking conditions in the automatic inhalator with smoking procedures used by humans, as outlined in Table 3. Tobacco users (United States brands) generally inhale a 30 to 40 mL puff volume of two-second duration and retain smoke in their lungs for approximately 15 seconds before expelling it. A fresh puff is consumed each minute. Tobacco investigators have used the tobacco reference cigarette (University of Kentucky) to calibrate their smoking machines accordingly *(26)*. The naive marihuana smoker inhales and expires the marihuana smoke similarly to the tobacco smoker. However,

Table 3
Simulation of Human Marihuana Use in Rats Exposed to Marihuana Smoke
in an Automatic Smoking Machine

Parameter	Marihuana (NIDA)	Placebo (NIDA)	Tobacco (Ky ref.)	Tobacco (U.S. brands)
Cigarette weight (gm)	1011 ± 19	861 ± 17	1114 ± 13	1100 ± 15
Total particulates (mg/8 puffs)	24 ± 3	18 ± 3	26 ± 3	2–31
Butt length (mm)	33 ± 4	31 ± 2	35 ± 2	35 ± 3
Puff volume (mL/cig)	35–200[a]	50 ± 2[b]	35 ± 2	30–40
Puff duration (seconds)	2–15[a]	2 ± 0.1[b]	2 ± 0.1	2 ± 0.1
Exposure interval (seconds)	15–45[a]	30 ± 0.2[b]	15 ± 0.1	10–20
Purge period (seconds)	15–30[a]	30 ± 0.2[b]	43 ± 0.1	40–50

[a]Naive marihuana smoker at lower end and experienced smoker at higher end.
[b]Conditions selected for the rat were a 50-ml puff simultaneously from each of three marihuana or placebo cigarettes over a two-seconds puff duration for a 30-seconds exposure interval, followed by 30 seconds of fresh air each min *(7,26)*.

the experienced *Cannabis* consumer deviates from these conditions by inspiring approximately a 50 to 200-mL puff for 8–10 seconds and retaining the smoke for 30–60 seconds before exhaling *(26)*. For the present rat inhalation study, a 150-mL puff volume (50 mL from each of three cigarettes) was automatically delivered to a constant-volume smoke chamber by simultaneously smoking three marihuana (or placebo) cigarettes. Each minute the cigarettes were puffed for two seconds, the smoked retained in the inhalator for 30 seconds, followed by displacement of the smoke with fresh air for 30 seconds. The cycle of events was repeated each minute. The smoking apparatus permitted simultaneous exposure of 8–10 rats *(26)*.

The estimation of Δ^9-THC doses relied on direct and indirect (recovery of Δ^9-THC from total particulates trapped on filter pads inserted between smoked cigarettes and the entrance to animal holders) gas chromatographic analyses of marihuana smoke. Several such determinations on different lots of marihuana cigarettes yielded Δ^9-THC concentrations in smoke of 0.6–0.9 µg/mL after four puffs, and 1.8–2.5 µg/mL after eight puffs by both analytical approaches. No cigarettes were used for more than eight puffs. When more than eight puffs were used, additional fresh cigarettes were ignited to replaced expended ones without interrupting the automatically controlled smoking sequence. Since the concentration of Δ^9-THC in smoke was known for four and eight puffs, summation of values afforded estimates of smoke Δ^9-THC concentrations in those instances in which 12 or 16 puffs were employed. Variation of the puff number permitted variation of Δ^9-THC dose during inhalation.

The Δ^9-THC concentration in smoke was converted to the usual expression of dose (mg/kg) by consideration of the following facts: the rat tidal volume was approximately 0.8 ml; the rat respiration rate was 40–80/30 seconds (lower level adjusts for Δ^9-THC-induced hypopnea) *(26)*; each exposure period lasted 30 seconds there were 4, 8, or 16 exposure periods (4, 8, or 16 puffs); and the mean Δ^9-THC smoke concentration was 0.7, 2, and 4 µg/mL for 4, 8, and 16 puffs, respectively. Since the tidal volume was taken as 0.8 ml, the concentration of inspired Δ^9-THC was 0.6, 1.6, and 3.2 µg/ml for 4, 8, and 16 puffs, respectively. Therefore, the concentration of Δ^9-THC in tidal air times the mean respiration rate per exposure times the number of exposures equals the quantity of Δ^9-THC entering the rodent nasal passages. For example, in the instance of eight puffs, the equation would be 1.6 µg/mL × 60 respirations × eight exposures = 768 μg Δ^9-THC/rat. However, rodents are obligatory nasal breathers, and it has been shown that 50% of smoke particulates are filtered out in the rodent nasal turbinates *(26)*. Of the quantity (50%) that reaches the lungs, 80% is absorbed into the pulmonary circulation *(26)*. Therefore, the 768 μg Δ^9-THC/rat is reduced to 307 μg/rat or 0.3 mg/150 g body weight. This value is converted to 2 mg/kg. Similar calculations for 4 and 16 puffs yield Δ^9-THC inhalation doses of 0.7 and 4 mg/kg, respectively.

The mechanical smoking sequence and doses outlined above were incorporated into the inhalation treatment protocol. Five rats of each sex, after conditioning to the inhalator, were simultaneously exposed once daily during the morning for 5 days to 4, 8, or 16 puffs of marihuana. Control rats were exposed to placebo smoke, whereas others were sham-treated (placed in the smoking machine but not given smoke). On the first day of exposure, each rat received a single intraperitoneal injection of 0.5 mL of a 50% suspension of washed sheep red blood cells (SRBC) in isotonic saline.

Orally treated female rats (eight per group) received a daily Δ^9-THC dose of 1,5, or 10 mg/kg, and control animals were given sesame oil (0.5/100 g body weight) for five days. All rats were injected with SRBC in an identical manner to those used in the inhalation study. Δ^9-THC or vehicle was withheld from other control rats in the presence and absence of SRBC in order to estimate efficacy of antigenic stimulation and to determine background levels of functional splenic antibody cells, respectively. Five days after SRBC injection, the animals were decapitated and blood specimens were collected.

2.3. Preparation of Cells

SRBC were obtained in Alsever's fluid from the same donor sheep for both studies. When used for immunization, SRBC were washed three times in isotonic saline. For serological use, SRBC were rinsed three times and diluted to a 1% suspension in 0.01 M phosphate-buffered saline (PBS) at pH 7.3. In the plaque formation test, a 20% suspension of washed SRBC in medium 199 provided SRBC as indicator cells.

Splenic cells were obtained by fragmentation of each teased spleen, suspended in medium 199, through a mesh-60 grid. Viable splenic lymphocytes were determined by dye exclusion of 0.2% trypan blue, and suspensions of 2×10^7/mL viable cells in medium 199 were used for counting antibody-forming cells (AFC) in the localized hemolysis in gel (LHG) plaque-formation test.

2.4. Hemochemical and Physiological Parameters

Medium 199 was used both as a diluent of cells and in the preparation of gels because it improved sensitivity of the LHG method *(27)*. Gel plates (100 × 15 mm) consisted of 7.5 ml of 1.2% agarose for the lower layer, and after this layer was solidified, the upper layer containing 0.1 mL of 20% SRBC and 0.1 ml of 2×10^7/mL viable splenic cells in 0.6% agarose was deposited on the lower layer. Gelation proceeded initially for 20 minutes at 23°C and then for two hours at 37°C. When gelation was completed, the surface of the gel was coated with 1 mL of 20% guinea pig complement, which had been absorbed with an equal volume of packed SRBC for 60 minutes at 4°C. After the complement was added, the gel plates were incubated for 50 minutes at 37°C, and excess complement solution was then decanted. The specificity of AFC and the extent of background interference were estimated by preparing gel plates with SRBC or viable splenic cells alone and in the presence or absence of complement. Hemolytic plaques on experimental gel plates were corrected for those counted on control gel plates.

Serum antibody titers (expressed as the reciprocal) to SRBC were measured by a standard hemagglutination (HT) procedure using a microtiter apparatus (27). Heat-inactivated (30 minutes at 56°C) sera were serially diluted in PBS, and each dilution received an equal volume of 1% SRBC in PBS. After gentle agitation for 50 seconds, the reaction plates were incubated for two hours at 23°C and the highest dilution having definitive hemagglutination was noted.

A preliminary attempt was made to detect circulating antibodies with a rabbit antiserum to rat IgG in the sera of rats exposed to marihuana smoke. Standard double-diffusion commercial gel plates were used.

In addition to the hemochemical procedures, we observed some behavioral and physiological changes. Animals were observed for signs of CNS inhibition or stimulation, and exploratory activity, rectal temperature, and respiration rate were measured. At the beginning of treatment and at autopsy, we recorded body weights and calculated the growth rate from the ratio of final body weight to initial body weight. During necropsy, animals were inspected for gross pathology and wet weights of spleen, thymus, and adrenals were measured.

3. RESULTS

The experimental design permitted evaluation of the inductive phase of the primary immune response in coincidence with that period of time during which drug tolerance did not develop fully. The credibility of findings relies strongly on concomitant measurements of the number of AFC, HT, and splenic weights by the two routes of cannabinoid administration and at doses used by humans. The behavioral and physiologic manifestations substantiated drug expression. The students t-test was applied for each parameter.

3.1. Behavioral and Physiological Findings

Generally, Δ^9-THC activity occurred sooner and with more intensity via the inhalation route than the oral route (Table 4). In addition, recovery from daily aberrations induced by drug took place more quickly by the inhalation route. After inhalation of marihuana smoke, both sexes displayed a dose-related CNS inhibition and reductions in exploratory activity and respiration rate. Ataxia and incoordination were commonly seen soon after removal from the smoking apparatus. A borderline hypothermia and decrease in growth rate were associated with the high dose. Daily changes were essentially reversed in four to six hours. No gross pathology was seen in any animals. A non-dose-related decrease (18–35%) in absolute and relative thymus weights occurred for both sexes. There was a 15% increase in female adrenal weights at the high dose. Also at the high dose, absolute and relative spleen weights diminished approximately 18%.

Intragastric administration of Δ^9-THC initiated behavioral changes three to four hours after treatment. The more intense CNS inhibition was expressed as ataxia and incoordination. Only at 10 mg/kg was there a fall in exploratory activity and respiration rate (Table 4). A slight increase in rectal temperature and a borderline decrease in growth rate occurred at the high dose. Abnormal signs disappeared six to eight hours after gavage. No gross pathological changes were found. Thymic and adrenal weights were unchanged. Absolute and relative splenic weights were reduced 11–15% at both 5 and 10 mg/kg (Table 5).

3.2. Hemochemical Findings

By and large, the results obtained with each sex exposed to marihuana smoke were similar; therefore, their respective hemochemical data have been combined for presentation in

Table 4
Behavioral and Physiological Changes in Rats Exposed to Marihuana Smoke or Treated Orally with Δ⁹-THC for 5 days[a]

Δ⁹-THC (mg/kg)	CNS inhibition		Exploratory activity		Rectal temperature		Respiration rate		Growth Rate	
	Day in study (left)	Change (%) (right)	Day in study (left)	Change (%) (right)	Day in study (left)	Change (%) (right)	Day in study (left)	Change (%) (right)	Day in study (left)	Change (%) (right)
Marihuana smoke inhalation										
Placebo	3	+10%	5	−31%[b]	5	±0%	5	−15%	6	−3%
0.7	3	+5	5	−16	5	+4	5	−12	6	+4
2	2	+33[b]	3	−48[b]	3	+4	3	−25[b]	6	−3
4	1	+72[b]	1	−60[b]	3	−3[b]	1	−28[b]	6	−9[b]
Oral Δ⁹-THC										
Vehicle										
1	5	+5	5	±0	5	±0	5	±0	6	+4
5	3	+20[b]	4	−10	5	+1	4	−10	6	+14
10	2	+50[b]	3	−25[b]	3	+5[b]	3	−25[b]	6	−10[b]

[a] Inhalation values were derived from a comparison of values during treatment with those measured before treatment on the same animals; in the oral study, treated values are compared to those of vehicle control.
[b] p < 0.01–0.05.

Table 5+Marihuana Smoke Inhalation and oral Δ⁹-THC Suppression of the Humoral Immune Response in Rats

Δ⁹-THC (mg/kg)		Antibody-forming cells (×10⁶) (mean ± SD)		Hemagglutination titer (recip. of dil.) (mean ± SD)		Spleen weight (mg/100 gm FBW) (mean ± SD)	
Inhalation	Oral	Inhalation	Oral	Inhalation	Oral	Inhalation	Oral
plac.	veh.	145 ± 41	189 ± 27	209 ± 52	185 ± 21	276 ± 29	297 ± 12
0	0	155 ± 23	165 ± 17	204 ± 49	184 ± 17	236 ± 23	303 ± 16
0.7	1	69 ± 35	57 ± 7[a]	147 ± 65	69 ± 9[a]	252 ± 25	311 ± 7
2	5	60 ± 40[a]	84 ± 12[a]	131 ± 52[a]	98 ± 11[a]	264 ± 28	266 ± 5[a]
4	10	34 ± 24[a]	43 ± 9[a]	123 ± 49[a]	63 ± 9[a]	227 ± 23[a]	255 ± 9[a]

[a] p < 0.05–0.01 as compared to controls; there were 8–10 rats per group (equal numbers of both sexes in the inhalation study).

Table 5. However, female controls (placebo and sham-treated) tended to have a larger number of AFC than male control rats. In any case, for both sexes, there was a dose-related decline in AFC. The decrease was 61–74% in females and 24–75% in males as compared to the mean AFC values of placebo and sham-treated groups. The HT values for all control animals (placebo and sham-treated) of both sexes were in close agreement. A dose-related decrease of 22–44% was observed for males, but a similar decrement for females was independent of dose. An attempt to identify and quantitate the presence of serum IgG in treated rats using a rabbit antiserum to rat IgG was unsuccessful. In a group of untreated rats (neither sham treated nor exposed to marihuana or placebo smoke), the IgG precipitin reaction was clearly detectable up to serum dilutions of 1:32.

In the oral study, AFC was reduced 56–78% and HT was decreased 48–66% at all doses (Table 5).

4. DISCUSSION

Despite the discrepancy of findings on marihuana's influence on the immune processes in humans, it has been demonstrated in this study by parallel changes in three parameters that relevant doses of marihuana and Δ^9-THC in the rat are immunosuppressant. By both preferred routes of administration used by human cannabinoid consumers, the primary immune response to SRBC was inhibited. As many precautions as possible were taken to obtain reliable results. The inbred Fischer rat strain meets the National Institutes of Health (NIH) standards of immunogenetic homogeneity (monitored at Charles River Breeding Laboratories by riciprocal skin homografting) and has a remarkably low incidence of pulmonary disease (essential for inhalation studies). The drug doses used were not lethal or intoxicating to the point of irreversible debilitation. The inhalation exposure conditions were reliably reproducible. The contribution of carbon monoxide toxicity was virtually eliminated by using a single daily exposure, by providing fresh air for one-half of each exposure cycle, and by restricting the number of marihuana puffs to a quantity that did not cause death when the tobacco reference cigarette was used. The immunity investigation was confined to five days, a time for optimal expression of AFC and HT responses to SRBC in the Fischer rat (27). Finally, any criticism as to the use of SRBC as a suitable antigenic stimulant for B-cell proliferation and maturation may be countered by the recent report of similar findings of Δ^9-THC inhibition of the humoral response to E. coli lipopolysaccharide B (17).

Although the present study evaluated the inductive phase of the primary immune response, it has been demonstrated that the productive phase is also impaired by oral Δ^9-THC (27). To interpret the suppression of both the inductive and productive phases of the humoral pathway, it would seem reasonable to infer that the early processing of antigenic information is implicated. At least in part, the initial step of phagocytizing particulate antigen by lung, liver, and splenic macrophages may be involved. The macrophage processing of antigen is a prerequisite for stimulation of immunocyte maturation and proliferation. Cannabinoids could interfere with macrophage function by causing structural alterations, inhibiting biochemical pathways, or altering transport mechanisms. Others have reported structural and functional changes in alveolar macrophages in marihuana smokers and in rodents and lung-explant cultures treated with cannabinoids (3,7,8,20,28). It has been postulated that altered lysosomal integrity could explain reduced cellular immunity (12). Cannabinoids have been shown to affect cell membranes and transport in erythrocytes, bull spermatozoa, iris cells, and ileal cells (9,10,15,25). Mitochondrial energy metabolism during antigenic processing must be sustained. Although there is no direct evidence for changes in macrophage mitochondria, Δ^9-THC has impaired mitochondrial function in hepatocytes (2,19).

Whereas the administration of Δ^9-THC orally established a definitive situation of cause and effect, the inhalation of marihuana smoke presented a more complex situation. One must contend with both the cannabinoid content and the physicochemical properties of the pyrolytic products. Research findings on tobacco smoke have shown that the immune system is affected by noncannabinoid smoke ingredients. Cigarette smoke suppressed the cellular immune pathway and the primary and secondary immune humoral responses, depressed the number and function of splenic plaque-forming cells, and inhibited macrophage protein synthesis *(6,11,24,29,33–35)*.

In many instances, chronic exposures were performed in the evaluation of both arms of the immune mechanism. However, in the present study, subacute exposure to placebo smoke did not inhibit the humoral response, implicating cannabinoids more strongly as immunosuppressants.

Perhaps it is appropriate to comment on the unresolved disagreement on a potential cannabinoid effect on human immune systems. Clinical investigators have tried to establish the general health, use of noncannabinoid drugs, and frequency of marihuana consumption. On the other hand, the environmental setting, the Δ^9-THC content of *Cannabis* (a variation from a trace quantity to 3% depending upon country of origin), and actual previous use of marihuana remain questionable variables.

It seems reasonable to conclude that pure Δ^9-THC, at reasonable doses, is immunosuppressive in rodents and that cannabinoids in marihuana smoke have a similar effect since placebo marihuana smoke did not elicit an equivalent inhibition. The inability to detect a reduction in the release of IgG during the primary immune response may have been caused, in part, by the fact that IgM is the first immunoglobulin to be released in the primary immune response. Documentation is sufficient to encourage continued investigation of *Cannabis* constituents in the area of immunobiology and immunochemistry. The important consideration of the role of immunosuppression in relationship to tolerance and other adaptive processes seen for other physiological parameters during prolonged treatment with Δ^9-THC or marihuana smoke must be entertained.

ACKNOWLEDGMENTS

The author expresses his appreciation to Henry J. Esher, Miasnig Hagopian, Andrew J. Miller, Rosa A. Sprague, and Jeffrey Grant for collaborative efforts. Special thanks are extended to Monique C. Braude and the National Institute on Drug Abuse for supplies of cannabinoids and financial support under NIH Grant No. DA 00932–01.

Reprinted with permission from Marihuana: Chemistry, Biochemistry and Cellular Effects (Nahas, G.; Paton, W. D. and Idanpaan-Heikkila, J., eds.), Springer-Verlag, New York, 1976, pp. 441–456.

REFERENCES

1. Armand, J. -P., Hsu, J. T. and Nahas, G. G. (1974) inhibition of blastogenesis of T lymphocytes by Δ^9-THC. *Fed. Proc.* **33**, 539.
2. Bino, T. A., Chari-Bitron, and Shahar, A. (1972) Biochemical effects and morphological changes in rat liver mitochondria exposed to Dl-tetrahydrocannabinol. *Biochim. Biophys. Acta* **288**, 195–202.
3. Braude, M. C. and Szara, S. (eds.) (1975) *The Pharmacology of Marihuana.* Raven, Press. New York.
4. Cushman, P. and Khurana, R. (1975) Effects of marihuana smoking and tetrahydrocannabinol on T-cell rosettes. *Fed. Proc.* **34**, 783.
5. DeSoize, B., Hsu, J., Nahas, G. G. and Morishima, A. (1975) Inhibition of human lymphocyte transformation *in vitro* by natural cannabinoids and olivetol. *Fed. Proc.* **34**, 783.

6. Esher, H. J., Menninger, F. F., Jr., Bogden, A. E. and Mason, M. M. (1973) Immunological deficiency associated with cigarette smoke inhalation by mice: primary and secondary hemagglutinin response. *Arch. Environ. Health* **27**, 99–104.

7. Fleischman, R. W., Sprague, R. A., Hayden, D. W., Braude, M. C. and Rosenkrantz H. (1975) Chronic marihuana inhalation toxicity in rats. *Toxicol. Appl. Pharmacol.* **34**, 467–478.

8. Gaul, C. C. and Mellors, A. (1975) Δ^9-tetrahydrocannabinol and decreased macrophage migration inhibition activity. *Res. Commun. Chem. Pathol. Pharmacol.* **10**, 559–564.

9. Gibermann, E. S., Gothilf, A., Shahar, and Bino, T. (1975) Effects of Δ^9-tetrahydrocannabinol on the membrane permeability of bull spermatozoa to potassium. *J. Reprod. Fertil.* **42**, 389–390.

10. Green, K. and Pederson, J. E. (1973) Effect of Δ^9-tetrahydrocannabinol on aqueous dynamics and ciliary body permeability in the rabbit. *Exp. Eye Res.* **15**, 499–507.

11. Holt, P. G. and Keast, D. (1973) Cigarette smoke inhalation: effects on cells of the immune series in the murine lung. *Life Sci.* **12**, 377–383.

12. Irvin, J. E. and Mellors, A. (1975) Δ^9-tetrahydrocannabinol-uptake by rat liver lysosomes. *Biochem. Pharmacol.* **24**, 305–306.

13. Johnson, R. J. and Wiersema, V. (1974) Effects of a Δ^9-tetrahydrocannabinol (Δ^9-THC) metabolite on bone marrow myelopoiesis. *Res. Commun. Chem. Pathol. Pharmacol.* **8**, 393–396.

14. Lau, R. J., Lerner, C. B., Tubergen, D. G., Benowitz, N., Domino, E. F. and Jones, R. T. (1975) Non-inhibition of phytohemagglutinin (PHA) induced lymphocyte transformation in humans by Δ^9-tetrahydrocannabinol (Δ^9-THC). *Fed. Proc.* **34**, 783.

15. Laurent, B., Roy, P. E. and Gailis, L. (1974) Inhibition by Δ^9-tetrahydrocannabinol of a sodium-potassium ion transport ATPase from rat ileum. *Can. J. Physiol. Pharmacol.* **52**, 1110–1113.

16. Lefkowitz, S. S. and Yang, C. (1975) Drug induced immunosuppression of the plaque forming cell response. 75th Meeting, *Am. Soc. Microbiol.* p. 81.

17. Levy, J. A., Munson, A. E., Harris, L. S. and Dewey, W. L. (1975) Effects of Δ^9-THC on the immune response of mice. *Fed. Proc.* **34**, 782.

18. Liskow, B., Liss, J. L. and Parker, C. W. (1971) Allergy to marihuana. *Ann. Intern. Med.* **75**, 571–573.

19. Mahoney, J. M. and Harris, R. A. (1972) Effect of Δ^9-tetrahydrocannabinol on mitochondrial processes. *Biochem. Pharmacol.* **21**, 1217–1226.

20. Mann, P. E. G., Cohen, A. B., Finley, T. N. and Ladman, A. J. (1971) Alveolar macrophages. Structural and functional differences between non-smokers and smokers of marijuana and tobacco. *Lab. Invest.* **25**, 111–120.

21. *Marihuana and Health*. (1974) Fourth Report to the U.S. Congress, Department of Health, Education and Welfare Publ. No. (ADM) 75–181, pp. 1–152.

22. Nahas, G. G., Sucia-Foca, N., Armand, J. -P. and Morishima, A. (1974) Inhibition of cellular mediated immunity in marihuana smokers. *Science* **183**, 419–420.

23. Nahas, G. G., Zagury, D., Schwartz, I. W. and Nagel M. -D. (1973) Evidence for the possible immunogenicity of Δ^9-tetrahydrocannabinol (THC) in rodents). *Nature* **243**, 407–408.

24. Nulsen, A., Holt, P. G. and Keast, D. (1974) Cigarette smoking, air pollution, and immunity. Model system. *Infect. Immun.* **10**, 1226–1229.

25. Raz, A., Schurr, A. and Livne, A. (1972) The interaction of hashish components with human erythrocytes. *Biochim. Biophys. Acta* **274**, 269–272.

26. Rosenkrantz, H. and Braude, M. C. (1974) Acute, subacute and 23-day chronic marihuana inhalation toxicities in the rat. *Toxicol. Appl. Pharmacol.* **28**, 428–441.

27. Rosenkranz, H., Miller, A. J. and Esber, H. J. (1976) Δ^9-Tetrahydrocannabinol suppression of the primary immune response in rats. *J. Toxicol. Environ. Health* **1**, 119–125.

28. Rosenkranz, H., Sprague, R. A., Fleischman, R. W. and Braude, M. C. (1975) Oral Δ^9-tetrahydrocannabinol toxicity in rats treated for periods up to six months. *Toxicol. Appl. Pharmacol.* **32**, 399–417.

29. Roszman, T. L., Elliott, L. H. and Rogers A. S. (1975) Suppression of lymphocyte function by products derived from cigarette smoke. *Am. Rev. Respir. Dis.* **111**, 453–456.

30. Schapiro, C. M., Orlina, A. R., Unger, P. and Billings, A. A. (1974) Antibody response to cannabis. *J.A.M.A.* **230**, 81–82.

31. Schwartzfarb, L., Needle, M. and Chavez-Chase, M. (1974) Dose-related inhibition of leukocyte migration by marihuana and Δ^9-tetrahydrocannabinol (THC) in vitro. *J. Clin. Pharmacol.* **14**, 35–41.

32. Silverstein, M. J. and Lessin P. J. (1974) Normal skin test responses in chronic marijuana users. *Science* **186**, 740–741.

33. Thomas, W. R., Holt, P. G. and Keast D. (1973) Cellular immunity in mice chronically exposed to fresh cigarette smoke. *Arch. Environ. Health* **27**, 372–375.

34. Thomas, W. R., Holt, P. G. and Keast, D. (1973) Effect of cigarette smoking on primary and secondary humoral responses in mice. *Nature* **243**, 240.

35. Thomas, W. R., Holt, P. G. and Keast, D. (1974) Recovery of immune system after cigarette smoking. *Nature* **248**, 358–359.
36. White, S. C., Brin, S. C. and Janicki, B. W. (1975) Mitogen-induced blastogenic responses of lymphocytes from marihuana smokers. *Science* **188**, 71–72.

24 Marihuana and the Immune System

Guy A. Cabral

Abstract

Marihuana has been shown to decrease host resistance to bacterial, protozoan, and viral infections in experimental animal models and in vitro systems. Recent immuno epidemiological studies suggest that marihuana may also influence the outcome of viral infections in humans. The main substance in marihuana that exerts these immuno depressive effects is its major psychoactive constituent Δ^9-tetrahydrocannabinol (THC). This cannabinoid alters the function of an array of immune cells including lymphocytes, natural killer cells, and macrophages, thereby affecting their capacity to exert anti microbial activities. Two modes of action by which THC affects immune responsiveness have been proposed. At sites such as the lung that are subject to exposure to high concentrations of THC and other cannabinoids contained in marihuana smoke, THC may alter cellular membranes because of its highly lipophilic nature. In contrast, at sites distal to the lung, THC at relatively low concentrations may exert its suppressive effects on immune cells by interacting with cannabinoid receptors CB_1 and CB_2. No controlled longitudinal epidemiological studies have yet correlated the immunosuppressive effects of *Cannabis* smoke on the incidence of infections or viral disease in different segments of the population.

1. INTRODUCTION

Δ^9-tetrahydrocannabinol (THC) is the major psychoactive component in marihuana and can produce a variety of effects in humans including alterations in mood, perception, cognition and memory, psychomotor activity, and consciousness (*1*). THC also has been reported to account for the majority of the immunosuppressive properties attributed to marihuana. In vivo and in vitro studies have indicated that THC impairs cell-mediated immunity (*2–4*), humoral immunity (*5,6*), and cellular defenses against a variety of infectious agents (*7–10*). Although the immunosuppressive effects of THC have been well-documented in experimental studies, no clinical epidemiological studies have been performed yet to relate marihuana consumption with an increased incidence of infectious disease. Gross et al. (*11*) reported that marihuana consumption altered responsiveness of human papillomavirus to α-2a treatment and suggested that THC could be a cofactor that influences the outcome of viral infection. In

From: *Marihuana and Medicine*
Edited by: G. G. Nahas et al.   © Humana Press Inc., Totowa, NJ

addition, immunoepidemiological studies using univariant and multivariant analyses have implied an association between marihuana use and the progression of human immunodeficiency virus (HIV) (12). However, longitudinal epidemiological studies in humans using biological or clinical approaches have not been undertaken or completed. Most of the completed studies to define the effects of marihuana on the immune system have been conducted using animal models and in vitro systems.

2. IN VIVO STUDIES

The classical experiments with guinea pigs and mice that have been used for nearly a century have documented the effects of cannabinoids on host infection. These experimental animals have well-defined immune systems that have been extensively investigated in virology and bacteriology. They allow for definition of the factors of host resistance that are targeted by drugs and permit the conduct of experiments under stringent controlled conditions. As a result, acquisition of statistically significant data with minimal confounding variables present in human populations such as environmental toxic exposures and multiple drug use is possible. Morahan et al. (13) demonstrated that mice exposed to THC were compromised in their ability to resist infection to viral and bacterial agents. In these experiments, BALB/C mice administered 200 mg THC/kg intraperitoneally on two consecutive days exhibited decreased resistance to infection with either *Listeria monocytogenes* or herpes simplex virus type 2 (HSV2). These relatively high doses of THC were administered parenterally rather than through inhalation of marihuana smoke, and a linkage between the immunosuppressive properties of THC in vitro was obtained. Mishkin and Cabral (14) and Cabral et al. (15) confirmed that THC increased in a dose-related fashion the susceptibility to herpes virus infection in guinea pigs and mice. The THC dose-dependent relationship to the decreased resistance to HSV2 infection not only implicated cellular elements of the immune system as targets of THC, but also implied a role for a cannabinoid receptor in this process. Mishkin and Cabral (14) demonstrated that decreased antiviral responsiveness involved elements of both cellular and humoral immunity. THC delayed the onset, and inhibited the magnitude, of the delayed hypersensitivity response (DHR) to HSV2 when administered intravaginally to mice. Administration of THC resulted also in significant reductions in antibody production in response to HSV2. A reduction of T-lymphocyte-dependent cell-mediated immunity also has been found to be associated with THC administration (16,17). Similar inhibitory effects of THC on HSV2 were demonstrated in a guinea-pig model, for which the clinical manifestations and sequelae associated with herpes genitalis closely mimic the human disease (15). Animals treated with THC and infected intravaginally with HSV2 experienced a rapid onset of primary disease marked by greater severity of frank lesions and amounts of virus shed from the vagina when compared with similarly infected vehicle control animals. In addition, THC-treated guinea pigs experienced a higher frequency of recurrent HSV2 infection.

THC alters host resistance to infectious agents other than the herpes virus. Specter et al. (18) reported that THC augments murine retroviral-induced immuno suppression and infection. These results suggested that marihuana could serve as a cofactor, in conjunction with opportunistic pathogens, in the progression of infection with retroviruses, including HIV. In addition, THC has been shown to induce cytokine-mediated mortality of mice infected with *Legionella pneumophila (19)*. Mice administered two injections of THC (8 mg/kg), before and after a sublethal dose of *Legionella* experienced acute collapse and death. The THC-induced mortality resembled cytokine-mediated shock. Acute-phase serum from these animals contained significantly elevated levels of tumor necrosis factor (TNF) and interleukin 6 (IL-6).

Some have claimed that the doses (0.2–100 mg/kg) of THC administered by different routes to guinea pigs and mice, the standard animals for studies in infectious agents, are beyond those used by marijuana smokers. Rosenkrantz (20) has determined the relevance of THC doses and routes of administration used in rats and mice as compared to those absorbed by humans. By taking levels and body surface area as markers, it was established that a dose of 10–12 times greater was required in mice than in humans for similar effects. A similar scale is used by Martin. One hundred ng/kg in mice would correspond to 8 ng/kg in man, a dose consumed by heavy marihuana smokers (21).

3. IN VITRO STUDIES

Many in vitro studies performed in several laboratories have complemented those on animals, and have allowed identification of specific cellular and subcellular elements of the immune system targeted by THC. These experiments required primary cell populations such as murine splenocytes, purified macrophages, and lymphocytes from various rodents and humans, and immortalized cell types that exhibit macrophage-like or T-lymphocyte-like properties. The effect of THC on macrophage function is a major focus of research since these cells play a pivotal role in host resistance to viruses and bacteria. Macrophages are chemotactically attracted to sites of initial microbial invasion; they engulf and degrade infectious particles, and present engulfed antigens as processed peptides in the context of their major histocompatibility complex (MHC) class II molecules to T-helper lymphocytes to initiate a cascade of immune responsiveness. Macrophages also secrete effector molecules that exhibit potent immunomodulatory and antimicrobial activities, and restrict in an interferon-independent fashion the replication of viruses within the macrophage and the cells to which they attach. These latter properties are referred to as intrinsic (22,23) and extrinsic antiviral activities (24), respectively. Such antiviral activities play an important role in limiting the spread and dissemination of virus from the primary site of infection to distal sites. THC has no effect on macrophage *intrinsic* antiviral activity (25), but exerts a dose-dependent inhibition on macrophage *extrinsic* antiviral activity (9).

THC has also enhanced in vitro the growth of *Legionella pneumophila*, an opportunistic pathogen that infects macrophages in vivo and in vitro. Arata et al. (26) reported that treatment of macrophages from permissive A/J mice with THC (8–10 p*M*) enhanced the growth of *Legionella* within these cells. THC exposure will also overcome macrophage restriction of the growth of *Legionella*, normally induced by lipopolysaccharide activation. Burnette-Curley et al. (10) examined the effects of THC on the capacity of *Bacillus Calmétte-Guérin* (BCG)-activated macrophages to exert amoebicidal activity against *Naegleria fowleri*, free-living amebae that can cause a fatal disease in humans know as primary amebic meningoencephalitis (PAME) (27). Peritoneal macrophages from mice receiving BCG in concert with THC (25 and 50 mg/kg) exhibited in vitro a drug-dose–related inhibition in their ability to lyse *Naegleria*.

4. MECHANISM OF ACTION

4.1. Effects Mediated Through Membrane Perturbation

The manner in which THC exerts its immuno suppressive activities has not been determined. It has been suggested that, since THC is a highly lipophilic molecule, it interacts with cellular membranes and affects membrane fluidity, thereby altering selective permeability (28). Surface-membrane selective permeability, with attendant increases in intracellular sodium, have been proposed as the mode by which certain viruses shutdown host-cell macro-

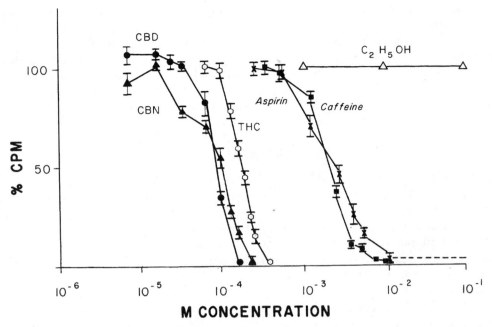

Fig. 1. Inhibitory effects of different cannabinoids (THC, CBD, CBN) on PHA-induced human lympho-cyte transformation as measured by ³H thymidine incorporation (20% pooled serum in the medium). CBD and CBN are more cytotoxic than THC (from ref. *33*).

molecular synthesis (*29,30*). THC may have a similar effect on cells; such alterations in membranes may also account for the inhibition of macromolecular precursor transport pro-duced by THC (*31*). Alternatively, THC could effect a morphological disruption of cellular membranes (*32*). Such disruption could alter compartments of protein synthesis and/or post translational events, affect intercellular communication and suppress secretion of immunoregulatory molecules. Other cannabinoids, such as CBD and CBN, also inhibit macromolecular synthesis (Fig. 1) in cultured lymphocytes to a greater extent than THC (*33*). The membrane effect of cannabinoids may be especially marked on the immune cells of the lung, which are directly exposed to the elevated concentrations of THC and other cannabi-noids contained in marihuana smoke.

4.2. Effects Mediated Through Cannabinoid Receptors

A second mode of action by which THC and other cannabinoids alter the function of the immune system has been proposed. Cannabinoid receptors have been located within the brain and the immune system. The first of these receptors, CB_1, is found primarily in brain and neural tissues. It has been cloned from rat (*34*), mouse (*35*), and human (*36*) tissues and exhibits greater than 97% amino acid sequence identity across species. The CB_2 receptor was originally identified in a human leukemia HL60 library as a cDNA fragment that displayed 68% homology with the CB_1 receptor. The CB_1 and CB_2 receptors have seven transmem-brane loci and are negatively coupled to adenylyl cyclase through a G-inhibitory protein and elicit signal-transductional activities through a cAMP second-messenger cascade (*37–40*). Cannabinoid receptors have been identified within cells of the immune system through detec-tion of their messenger RNAs using reverse transcription polymerase chain reaction (RT-PCR) and Northern blot analysis (*41–43*). However, a major difference in the tissue

Table 1
Cannabinoid Receptor Distribution in Immune Cells and Tissues

Cell Type/Tissue	Species	Receptor Subtype	Reference
B lymphocytes	human	CB2	44
Lymph Nodes	rat	CB[a]	45
Macrophages	human	CB2	44
Mast Cells	rat	CB2	57
Natural Killer Cells	human	CB2	44
Peripheral Mononuclear Cells	human	CB2	44,57
	rat		
Peyer's Patches	rat	CB[a]	45
Spleen	rat	CB2	41, 43–45, 57
	human	CB[a]	
	mouse	CB1	
	rat	CB[a]	
T4 Lymphocytes	human	CB2	44
T8 Lymphocytes	human	CB2	44
Tonsils	human	CB2	44
Thymus	human	CB2	44

[a]Detection method did not allow for discrimination of receptor subtype.

distribution and levels of expression of these receptors has been recognized. Transcripts for the CB_1 receptor are found primarily in neural tissue and, to a smaller extent, in peripheral tissues including the adrenal gland, bone marrow, heart, lung, prostate, testis, thymus, tonsils, and spleen (41,42,44). In contrast, transcripts for the CB_2 have been identified only in immune tissues (43,44). The relative levels of CB_2 mRNA vary in human blood-cell populations. B lymphocytes express the highest levels of CB_2 mRNA, followed in order by natural killer cells, monocytes, polymorphonuclear neutrophils, T8 lymphocytes, and T4 lymphocytes (44). Transcripts for CB_1 and CB_2 have been found also in transformed immune cell types. A rank order of CB_2 transcript expression similar to that in primary human cell types has been found for human cell lines belonging to the myeloid, monocytic, and lymphoid lineages (44). In addition, transcripts of the CB_1 have been identified in immune cells and tissues (41,42). Thus, immune regulation effected by cannabinoid receptors may involve both the CB_1 and CB_2 subtypes. Cannabioid-receptor protein has been detected in rat lymph nodes, Peyer's patches, and spleen (45), and on membranes of myelomonocytic U937 cells using ³HCP55940 as ligand (42). Immunohistochemical analysis using anti receptor antibodies has confirmed that the CB_2 receptor subtype as a protein entity is expressed in immune cells and tissues. Expression of CB_2 has been detected in rat spleen (45), and in association with B-lymphocyte–enriched areas of the mantle of secondary lymphoid follicles in human tonsil sections (44). Table 1 lists the currently known distribution of cannabinoid receptors in immune cells and tissues.

The sequestration of the CB_2-receptor subtype to immune cells and tissues implicates this receptor as having a role in immune-function modulation and regulation. A direct linkage between the presence of cannabinoid receptors and immune-function activities has still to be investigated. Kaminski et al. (47) demonstrated that suppression of the humoral immune response by cannabinoids was partially mediated through inhibition of adenylate cyclase by a pertussis-toxin-sensitive G-protein–coupled mechanism. THC and the synthetic bicyclic cannabinoid CP55940 inhibited the lymphocyte proliferative response and the sheep erythrocyte IgM antibody-forming cell response of murine splenocyte to phorbol-1 2 myristate-1 3-acetate (PMA) plus the calcium ionophore ionomycin. THC also modulated differentially the capacity of macrophages to process antigens which is a requisite for the activation of CD4+T lymphocytes (48). The alterations in processing were elicited in a drug-dose–dependent fashion and at concentrations extending to the nanomolar range consistent with a receptor-mediated mode of action. THC has been reported to suppress a fixation-resistant costimulatory signal to helper T cells in part by diminishing expression of macrophage heat-stable antigen (49).

5. DISCUSSION

Cumulative data from in vivo and in vitro studies indicate that THC has immunosuppressive properties and that it can compromise host resistance to a variety of infectious agents in experimental animals. However to date, epidemiological control studies similar to those performed with tobacco or alcohol have not been carried out in human populations in order to assess a decreased resistance to infections or other pathology related to immune dysfunction. And yet multiple epidemiological studies have been carried out to determine the incidence of marihuana use among different human populations, especially among the young. But they have not reported any physiological or medical markers. Similar longitudinal studies to evaluate the effects of marihuana smoking on these markers are urgently needed. The use of animal models, in which infectious disease processes mimic closely those in humans, affords a unique opportunity to examine the potential of drugs of abuse to alter immune function and host resistance. These animal models permit the conduct of experiments under controlled conditions, and may be replicated in different laboratories. The cumulative data on the effects of THC that have been obtained with these models strongly suggest that the deleterious effects of THC as they relate to host resistance to infections should be applicable to humans.

In vivo and in vitro data indicate that macrophages are a major target of THC. Studies employing murine and guinea pig animal models indicate that this cannabinoid decreases host resistance to herpesvirus genital infection and to infection by bacteria and protozoa. In this context, THC exposure has been shown to alter extrinsic antiviral activity, but does not appear to alter intrinsic antiviral activity (9,25). Whereas the cellular events for the THC-induced suppression of macrophage function remains to be defined, it is apparent that they do not involve dysfunction of effector cell-target cell contact (10). Furthermore, since THC exerted similar suppression of antiviral activities in different mammalian species, the inhibitory effects of this drug on host resistance may represent a general biological phenomenon.

The mechanism by which THC alters function of macrophages, T-lymphocytes, and NK cells in response to infection remains to be defined. It has been reported that two mechanisms may be responsible for the immunosuppressive activity of THC (50). The first, caused by the lipophilicity of THC (28), is a nonspecific interaction of the drug with the cell membrane components that may result in cellular dysfunction. This property of THC may account, in part, for its immunosuppressive effects at high concentrations on immune cells (31,33). These high concentrations target lung alveolar macrophages, which are exposed to persistent elevated concentrations of marihuana smoke. Perturbation of membranes could result in the disruption of intracellular compartments that are involved in the synthesis, posttranslational modification, and/or secretion of effector molecules which exhibit antiviral and antibacterial activities (15,51–54). Second, specific signal-transduction pathways are coupled with a cannabinoid receptor. Matsuda et al. (34) were the first to clone a neural cannabinoid receptor (CB$_1$). This receptor is coupled to a G protein (55) so that binding of cannabinoids results in inhibition of adenylate cyclase, a decrease in levels of CAMP (50,56), and inhibition of N-type calcium channels (38). The identification of a second peripherally localized cannabinoid receptor (CB_2) (43), which is expressed on macrophages and lymphocytes, suggests that a receptor-mediated mechanism is also operative in the immune system and may account for the dysregulation caused by the attachment of THC to this receptor. Such a receptor-mediated mode of action for THC is consistent with relatively low concentrations of the drug, which would be present in sites distal from the lung.

6. CONCLUSION

THC alters host defenses to bacterial, protozoan, and viral infection in experimental animals. This decrease in host resistance results from the immunosuppressive action of this cannabinoid on the function of macrophages, T lymphocytes, and natural killer cells. Little is known concerning the potential of cannabinoids other than THC to alter immune function, except for the properties of cannabidiol and cannabinol to inhibit the macromolecular synthesis of cultured lymphocytes in a concentration similar to that of THC (33). THC alters antimicrobial activity in vivo and in vitro, indicating that marihuana use does carry the risk of decreased resistance to infections in humans. A quantitative clinical determination of the extent, time, or duration of the immunosuppression induced by marihuana will require controlled epidemiological studies similar to those performed with tobacco. Marihuana is a cofactor that can increase the severity of infection by microbial agents by altering host resistance. Epidemiological data suggest that HIV-positive marihuana smokers progress to symptomatic AIDS more rapidly than those who do not smoke marihuana. Epidemiological surveys recording frequency of marihuana use and incidence of physiopathological and infectious markers should be undertaken.

REFERENCES

1. Dewey, W. L. (1986) Cannabinoid pharmacology. *Parmcol. Rev.* **38**, 151–178.
2. Nahas, G. G., Suciu-Foca, N., Armand, J. P., and Morishima, A. (1974) Inhibition of cellular mediated immunity in marihuana smokers. *Science* **183**, 419–420.
3. Cushman, P. and Khurana, R. (1976) Marihuana and T lymphocyte rosettes. *Clin. Pharmacol. Ther.* **19**, 310–317.
4. Klein, T. W., Newton, C., Widen, R., and Friedman, H. (1985) The effect of delta-9-tetrahydrocannabinol and 11-hydroxy-delta-9-tetrahydrocannabinol on T-lymphocyte and B-lymphocyte mitogen responses. *J. Immunopharmacol.* **7**, 451–466.
5. Munson, A. E., Levy, J. A., Harris, L. S., and Dewey, W. L. (1976) Effects of delta-9-tetrahydrocannabinol on the immune system, in *The Pharmacology of Marijuana* (Braude, M. C., and Szara, S., eds.) Raven, New York, pp. 187–197.
6. Baczynsky, W. O. T. and Zimmerman, A. M. (1983) Enhanced growth of *Legionella pneumophila* tetrahydrocannabinol-treated macrophages. *Proc. Soc. Exp. Biol. Med.* **199(1)**, 65–67.
7. Klein, T. W., Newton, C., and Friedman, H. (1987) Inhibition of natural killer cell function by marijuana components. *J. Toxicol. Environ. Health* **20**, 321–332.
8. Lopez-Cepero, M., Friedman, M., Klein, T., and Friedman, H. (1986) Tetrahydrocannabinol-induced suppression of macrophage spreading and phagocyte activity in vitro. *J. leuk. Biol.* **39**, 679–686.
9. Cabral, G. A. and Vásquez, R. (1991) Marijuana decrease macrophage antiviral and antitumor activities. *Adv. Biosci.* **80**, 93–105.
10. Burnette-Curley, d., Marciano-Cabral, F., Fischer-Stenger, K., and Cabral, G. A. (1993) Δ-9-tetrahydrocannabinol inhibits cell contact-dependent cytotoxicity of bacillus Calmétte-Guérin-activated macrophages. *Int. J. Immunopharmacol.* **15**, 371–382.
11. Gross, G., Roussaki, A., Ikenberg, H., and Dress, N. (1991) Genital warts do not respond to systemic recombinant interferon alpha-2a treatment during cannabis consumption. *Dermatol.* **183**, 203–207.
12. Tindall, B., Cooper, D. A., Donovan, B., Barnes, T., Philpot, C. R., Gold, J., and Penny, R. (1988) The Sydney AIDS Project: development of acquired immnodeficiency syndrome in a group of HIV seropositive homosexual men. *Aust. N.Z. J. Med.* **18(1)**, 8–15.

13. Morahan, P. S., Klykken, P. C., Smith, S. H., Harris, L. S., and Munson, A. E. (1979) Effects of cannabinoids on host resistance to Listeria monocytogenes and herpes simplex virus. *Infect. Immun.* **23**, 670–674.
14. Mishkin, E. M. and Cabral, G. A. (1985) Delta-9-tetrahydrocannabinol decreases host resistance to herpes simplex virus type 2 vaginal infection in $B_6C_3F_1$ mice. *J. Gen. Virol.* **66**, 2539–2549.
15. Cabral, G. A., Mishkin, E. M., Marciano-Cabral, F., Coleman, P., Harris, L., and Munson, A. E. (1986) Effect of delta-9-tetrahydrocannabinol on herpes simplex virus type 2 vaginal infection in the guinea pig. *Proc. Soc. Exp. Biol.* **182**, 181–186.
16. Klykken, P. C., Smith, S. H., Ley, J. A., Razdan, R., and Munson, A. E. (1977) Immuno suppressive effects of 8.9-eposyhexahdrocannabinol (EHHC). *J. Pharmacol. Exp. Ter.* **201**, 573–579.
17. Smith, S. H., Harris, L. S., Uwaydah, L. M., and Munson, A. E. (1978) Structure-activity relationships of natural and synthetic cannabinoids in suppression of humoral and cell-mediated immunity. *J. Pharmacol. Exp. Ther.* **207**, 165–170.
18. Specter, S. C., Lancz, G., Westrich, G., and Friedman, H. (1991) Delta-9-tetrahydrocannabinol augments murine retroviral induced immunosuppression and infection. *Int. J. Immunopharmacology* **13(4)**, 411–417.
19. Klein, T. W., Newton, C., Widen, R., and Friedman, H. (1993) Delta-9-tetrahydrocannabinol injection induces cytokine-mediated mortality of mice infected with *Legionella pneumophila. J. Pharmacol. Exp. Ther.* **267(2)**, 635–640.
20. Rosenkrantz H. (1976) The immune response and marihuana, in *Marihuana: Chemistry, Biochemistry & Cellular Effects.* (Nahas G. G., Paton W. D. M., and Idanpaan-Heikkila J., eds.) Springer-Verlag, New York, p. 441.
21. Hembree, W. C., Nahas G., Zeidenberg, P. and Huang, H. F. S. (1979) Changes in human spermatozoa associated with high dose marihuana smoking, in *Marihuana: Biological Effects, Analysis, Cellular Responses, Reproduction and Brain.* (Nahas G. G. and Paton W. D. M., eds.) Pergamon, New York, pp. 429–439.
22. Stevens, J. G. and Cook, M. L. (1971) Restriction of herpes simplex virus by macrophages. N analysis of the cell-virus integration. *J. Exp. Med.* **133**, 19–38.
23. Selgrade, M. K. and Osborne, J. E. (1974) Role of macrophages in resistance to murine cytomegalovirus. *Infect. Immun.* **10**, 1381–1390.
24. Morahan, P. S., Glasgow, L. A., Crane, J. L., Jr., and Kern, E. R. (1977) Comparison of antiviral and antitumor activity of activated macrophages. *Cell Immunol.* **28**, 404–415.
25. Cabral, G. A. and Vásquez, R. (1992) Delta-9-tetrahydrocannabinol suppresses macrophage extrinsic antiherpesvirus activity, in *Cannabis: Physiopathology, Epidemiology, Detection* (Nahas, G. G. and Latour, C., eds.) CRC Press, Boca Raton, FL, pp. 137–153.
26. Arata, S., Klein, T. W., Newton, C., and Friedman, H. (1991) Tetrahydrocannabinol treatment suppresses growth restriction of Legionella pneumophila in murine macrophage cultures. *Life Sci.* **49**, 473–479.
27. Marciano-Cabral, F. (1988) Biology of *Naegleria* spp. *Microbiol. Revs.* **52**, 114–133.
28. Wing, D. R., Leuschner, J. T. A., Brent, G. A., Harvey, D. J., and Paton, W. D. M. (1985) Quantification of in vivo membrane associated delta-9-tetrahydrocannabinol and its effects on membrane fluidity, in *Proceedings of the 9th International Congress of Pharmacology 3rd Satellite Symposium on Cannabis* (Harvey, D. J., ed.) IRL Press, Oxford, UK pp. 411–418.
29. Carrasco, L. and Smith, A. E. (1976) Sodium ions and the shut-off of host cell protein synthesis by piconviruses. *Nature (London)* **264**, 807–809.
30. Garry, R. F., Bishop, J. M., Parker, S., Westbrook, K, Lewis, G., and Waite, M. R. F. (1979) Na+ and K+ concentrations and the regulation of protein synthesis in sindbis virus-infected chick cells. *Virology* **96**, 108–120.
31. Desoize, B., Leger C., and Nahas, G. G. (1979) Plasma membrane inhibition of macromolecular precursor transport by THC. *Biochemical Pharmacology*, **28**, 1113–1118.
32. Poddar, M. K., Mitra, G., and Ghosh, J. J. (1978) Delta-9-tetrahydrocannabinol-induced changes in brain ribosomes. *Toxicol. Appl. Pharmacol.* **46**, 737–757.
33. Nahas, G. G., Morishima, A., and Desoize, B. (1977) Effects of cannabinoids on macromolecular synthesis and replication of cultured lymphocytes. *Fed. Proc.* **36**, 1748–1752.
34. Matsuda, L. A., Lolait, S. J1, Brownstein, M. J., Young, A. C., and Bonner, T. I. (1990) Structure of a cannabinoid receptor and functional expression of the cloned cDNA. *Nature* **346**, 561–556.
35. Chakrabarti, A., Onaivi, E. S., and Chaudhuri, G. (1995) cloning and sequencing of a cDNA encoding the mouse brain-type cannabinoid receptor protein. *DNA Seq.-J. Seq. Map* **5**, 385–388.
36. Gérard, C., Mollereau, C., Vassart, G., and Parmentier, M. (1990) Nucleotide sequence of a human cannabinoid receptor cDNA. *Nucleic Acids Res.* **18**, 7142.
37. Howlett, A. C., Qualy, J. M., and Khachchatrian, L. L. (1986) Involvement of Gi in the inhibition of adenylate cyclase by cannabimimetic drugs. *Mol. Pharmacol.* **29**, 307–313.
38. Mackie, K. and Hille, B. (1992) Cannabinoids inhibit N-type calcium channels in neuroblastoma-glioma cells. *Proc. Natl. Acad. Sci. USA* **89**, 3825–3829.

39. Selley, D. E., Stark, S., and Childers, S. R. (1996) Cannabinoid receptor stimulation of [^{35}S]GTPγ S binding in rat brain membranes. *Life Sci.* **59**, 659–668.

40. Childers, S. R. and Deadwyler, S. A. (1996) Role of cyclic AMP in the actions of cannabinoid receptors. *Biochem. Pharmacol.* **52**, 819–827.

41. Kaminski, N. E., Abood, M. E., Kessler, F. K., Martin, B. R., and Schatz, A. R. (1992) Identification of a functionally relevant cannabinoid receptor on mouse spleen cells that is involved in cannabinoid-mediated immune modulation. *Mol. Pharmacol.* **42**, 736–742.

42. Bouaboula, M., Rinaldi, M., Carayon, P., Carillon, C., Delpech, B., Shire, D. Le Fur, G., and Casellas, P. (1993) Cannabinoid-receptor expression in human leukocytes. *Eur. J. Biochem.* **214**, 173–180.

43. Munro, S., Thomas, K. L., and Abu-Shaar, M. (1993) Molecular characterization of a peripheral receptor for cannabinoids. *Nature* **365**, 61–65.

44. Galiègue, S., Mary, S., Marchand, J., Dussossoy, D., Carrière, D., Carayon, P., Bouaboula, M., Shire, D., Le Fur, G., and Casellas, P. (1995) Expression of central and peripheral cannabinoid receptors in human immune tissues and leukocyte subpopulations. *Eur. J. Biochem.* **232**, 54–61.

45. Lynn, A. B. and Herkenham, M (1994) Localization of cannabinoid receptors and nonsaturable high-density cannabinoid binding sites in peripheral tissues of the rat: implications for receptor-mediated immune modulation by cannabinoids. *J. Pharmacol. Exp. Ther.* **268**, 1612–1623.

46. Dove-Pettit, D. A., Anders, M. P., and Cabral, G. A. (1996) Cannabinoid receptor expression in immune cells. *Adv. Exp. Med. Biol.* **402**, 119–129.

47. Kaminski, N. E., Koh, W. S., Yang, K. H., Lee, M., and Kessler, F. K. (1994) Suppression of the humoral immune response by cannabinoids is partially mediated through inhibition of adenylate cyclase by a pertussis toxin-sensitive G-protein coupled mechanism. *Biochem. Pharmacol.* **48**, 1899–1908.

48. McCoy, K. L., Gainey, D., and Cabral, G. A. (1995) Δ^9-Tetrahydrocannabinol modulates antigen processing by macrophages. *J. Pharmacol. Exp. Ther.* **273**, 1216–1223.

49. Clements, D., Cabral, G. A., and McCoy, K. L. (1996) Delta-9-tetrahydrocannabinol selctively inhibits macrophage co-stimulatory activity and down-regulates heat-stable antigen expression. *J. Pharmacol. Exp. Ther.* **277**, 1315–1321.

50. Felder, C. C., Joyce, K. E., Briley, E. M., Mansouri, J., Mackie, K., Blond, O., Lai, Y., Ma, A. L., and Mitchell, R. L. (1995) Comparison of the pharmacology and signal transduction of the human cannabinoid CB$_1$ and CB$_2$ receptors. *Mol. Parmcol.* **48**, 443–450.

51. Watzl, B., Scuderi, P., and Watson, R. R. (1991) Marijuana components stimulate human peripheral blood mononuclear cell secretion of interferon-gamma and suppress interleukin-1-alpha *in vitro*. *Int. J. Immunopharmacol.* **13**, 1091–1097.

52. Nakano, Y., Pross, S. H., and Friedman, H. (1992) Modulation of interleukin 2 activity by delta-9-tetrahydrocannabinol and stimulation with concanavalin A, phytohemagglutinin, or anti-CD3 antibody. *Proc. Soc. Exp. Biol. Med.* **20**, 165–168.

53. Zheng, Z. M., Specter, S., and Friedman, H. (1992) Inhibition by delta-9-tetrahydrocannabinol of tumor necrosis factor alpha production by mouse and human macrophages. *Int. J. Immunopharmacology* **14**, 1445–1452.

54. Fisher-Stenger, K., Dove Pettit, D. A., and Cabral, G. A. (1993) Δ^{9}Tetrahydrocannabinol inhibition of tumor necrosis factor-alpha: suppression of post-translational events. *J. Pharmacol. Exp. Ther.* **267**, 1558–1565.

55. Houston, D. B. and Howlett, A. C. (1993) Solubilization of the cannabinoid receptor from rat brain and its functional interaction with guanine nucleotide-binding proteins. *Mol. Pharmacol.* **43**, 17–22.

56. Howlett, A. C., Champion, T. M., Wilken, G. H., and Mechoulam, R. (1990) Stereochemical effects of 11-OH-^{8}-tetrahydrocannabinol-dimethylheptyl to inhibit adenylate cyclase and bind to the cannabinoid receptor. *Neuropharmacology* **29**, 161–165.

57. Facci, L., Dal Toso, R., Romanello, S., Buriani, A., Skaper, S. D., and Leon, A. (1995) Mast cells express a peripheral receptor with differential sensitivity to anandamide and palmitoylethanolamide. *Proc. Natl. Acad. Sci. USA* **92**, 3376–3380.

25

How to Design the Ideal Drug of the Future

Paul Janssen

The ideal drugs of the future, theoretically at least, are drugs that are 100% effective all the time. Theoretically, this is something that is highly desirable, but in practice of course, impossible. That does not mean that we shouldn't try to move in that direction. A second property of an ideal drug of the future is that it should have no, absolutely no, undesirable side effects—zero. Now again, such a drug does not exist, and it is very unlikely that we will find such a drug in the years to come. But we should try to get as close to it as possible. A third property of an ideal drug is optimal compliance. In other words, a drug that is so easy to administer that patients or doctors, or whoever is involved, will never forget to administer or to take it. In this respect, of course, progress has been made. There are such practically ideal drugs like vaccines, but they are still the exception and not the rule. And then finally, an ideal drug should be a drug with as low a production cost as possible, because everybody constantly complains about drugs being too expensive. In order to lower the cost of drugs, they have to be inexpensive to manufacture. We must not forget that.

Now research, in my vocabulary, is simply defined as mainly those things we do in the laboratory, in our office, or elsewhere, to satisfy our own curiosity. In other words, research has certain topics that are of interest to a scientist, and he or she thinks about them, as do the teams surrounding them. Together, they carry out the necessary experiments to answer the problem. And as soon as one's curiosity is satisfied, that, as far as my definition is concerned, is the end of research. But it is only then that development starts because development, in my vocabulary again, is unfortunately those things we have to do to convince the rest of the world, which is very different and, in my opinion, very much more difficult than research. The rest of the world meaning, in practical terms, the so-called authorities to start with, and then later on the user and the professions, such as the medical profession, the veterinary profession, agricultural profession, and so on.

During the 1930s, my father was a general practitioner, and there were four other general practitioners in the town where I was born. He and four other MDs were serving 60,000 patients. There were no specialties, and there was no hospital. And I remember that my father was a great skeptic. He didn't really believe in the usefulness of drugs in general because this

From: *Marihuana and Medicine*
Edited by: G. G. Nahas et al.   © Humana Press Inc., Totowa, NJ

was before the sulfonamides, and there was very little one could do, of course with morphine, being on the one hand of course effective but dangerous, with digitoxin, or with mercurial diuretics. It was quiet obvious that the unwanted effects were more obvious than the desirable effects. And except for some vaccines, he was very skeptical, except for one drug, and that drug happened to be marihuana. That is why I am trying to explain it a little bit.

In the town where I was brought up in, there were maybe 10 or 20 cases of trigeminal neuralgia. And for many years, the five doctors in town tried to alleviate the incredible pain of these patients without any success. As you all know, even morphine has practically no effect. These patients certainly do not respond to placebos, that's for sure. And I remember, as a boy, these women mostly entering the office with their face in their hands and being miserable, as miserable as one could be. Now in the same street there was a pharmacist by the name of Edouard Cornil who was interested in plants in general, and in marihuana in particular. He made extracts of plants that he imported from all over the world. I remember my father using alcoholic extracts of marihuana that Edouard Cornil imported from India, or from an area that was then called India. In these days it is probably Pakistan. Each time he made such a concoction, or extract, my father would try it on these 10 or 20 patients suffering from very severe trigeminal neuralgia, involving 1,2, or 3 parts of the nerve. When the batch was really effective, then he could literally make these patients pain-free with orally given drops. Unfortunately, many batches, particularly those that came from Saudi Arabia, somehow did not contain the active ingredient. The difficulty was to find an active batch, and of course in those days, nobody had the slightest idea what the active ingredient could be.

When I started doing research in the early 1950s, one of the ideas that stuck in my mind was to try to find out what this was all about. But the chemistry, unfortunately, was completely unknown, as we have heard this morning, and I decided against trying to do that simply because I thought that, chemically speaking, it was too difficult for me. I believe that this decision was not wrong because the answer to that simple question was only given in the 1960s, as we have also heard this morning. So with that brief introduction let me stop and wait for your questions. At my age I have very few, or no secrets, so ask me whatever you want.

Q: (Dr. Nahas) Would you comment on your methods, using computers to screen and select active molecules?

A: The discovery of drugs traditionally, has been a question of serendipity as you know. Practically all active drugs that are known today have been discovered by coincidence, or by somebody with an open mind. As you know, the human mind is like a parachute: it works better when it is open. In modern times at least, new drugs have been the result of working on chemical leads, and trying to refine these chemical leads, to improve upon them, and eventually get a drug which is closer to the ideal drug than the chemical lead itself, and good enough to be marketed. That's what modern drugs are all about. The challenge that I am involved with recently is the question of whether or not it is possible to discover new drugs with no chemical leads.

Is it possible to use a computer for discovering new chemical leads? This is what we do at the Center for Molecular Design where I work these days. One of the things we are doing is to try to select a few so-called molecular targets. These are, in all instances, proteins that have been crystallized and have been studied very carefully by crystallographers so that we know their three-dimensional structure in great detail. Most of these so-called targets have something to do with virology; there are quite a number of targets that are known, and they have something to do with the AIDS virus; for instance, reverse transcriptase and proteases that are with the influenza virus. So, it is possible to display the structure of these target molecules on a computer screen, and to have all the coordinates in the computer memory using a program that we are working on. Employing genetic algorithm methods, this program combines chemical fragments in thousands of ways per day. Each time the computer makes a new artificial chemical molecule on the screen, the program then determines, with sufficient precision, whether or not the new molecule has high docking energy or low docking energy.

In other words, whether the new chemical molecule has high binding affinity or low binding affinity to the target. This program we have at the moment can handle the problem with approximately 10,000–20,000 molecules per day. By the end of the day, we can actually print out, or look at the screen, and pick out those molecules that were made by the computer and have, according to the computer, a surprisingly high affinity to the target. Then we can use those molecules that are on the first screen sufficiently active in theory at least, and use much slower but much more refined program to find out what the probable confirmation of the molecule is and how it actually interacts with the target molecule in molecular detail.

This type of approach was thought to be impossible until very recently. At least I certainly thought it would be completely impossible to find molecules this way, but I have to contradict myself now, because as I told Dr. Nahas, in recent months it is becoming obvious that the computer can indeed find at least interesting new lead compounds at the rate, for some target molecules, that is surprisingly high. The problem is that at the moment, our programs are still too slow. In other words, the number of possibilities, when we present these fragments to the computer, are so huge that we would have to examine millions of possible combinations. But the computer is too slow. We can only look at 10,000–20,000 molecules per day, which on the one hand is a lot of molecules, but in relative terms, is not enough.

A second shortcoming of the program as it exists, is that we don't know yet how to write software that allows the computer to carry out a certain number of very important chemical modifications. For instance, we insert two rings, and would like the computer to fuse these rings. This is something that the program cannot yet do. We are working on it.

In a couple of months, I am almost certain the program will probably have reached a stage where even that is possible. As a result, the number of possibilities will then increase. It is also predictable that the speed of the computers will increase year after year. Even today, there are computers much faster than ours that are available. However, these faster computers are so expensive that it is out of the question to use them on a routine basis.

Q: (Dr. Nahas) What you really need, is some method, or mechanism, for the very accurate measurement of the microdimension of your receptors, and which you want to bind with your ligands ... is that right?

A: Yes, a deviation of one angstrom is too much. The required precision is very high. That, of course, limits the number of available possibilities, of available targets. For instance, when a crystallographer looks at a protein, with a resolution of, let us say, two angstroms: he or she finds in most proteins what we call 'water threads.' In other words, no longer is water present in some proteins, but apparently in most of them. These 'water threads' are literally threads that play a structural function that in some target molecules is not to be neglected. Now this was not known until about one year ago. And therefore, we need target molecules that are crystallized, and that have been studied by several crystallographers with a resolution of much less than three angstroms. Three angstroms is not good enough. Now that limits the number of known targets to about five.

Q: (unidentified questioner) Couldn't you use it to try to get some new anticoagulants? because the existing ones have such horrible side effects.

A: We could, for instance, use very well-known enzymes like trypsin or chymotrypsin or thrombin or other enzymes; actually, not thrombin, because its molecular structure is not known in sufficient detail. We might look for inhibitors for trypsin or chymotrypsin, but *a priori* this is unlikely to be useful in medical practice.

Unfortunately, in the field of anticoagulants, most of the target molecules that we can think of are not proteins, but glycoproteins or lipoproteins. The disadvantage of these lipoproteins is that they can not be crystallized. So, one of the problems that we are facing is to try to undo lipoproteins from their lipids, and try to find out what happens when the resulting protein is uncrystallized, whether or not it maintains its properties. It is protein that goes through a lipid bilayer once. As such, native neuraminidase of the influenza virus can not be crystallized because of the fact that it goes through a lipid bilayer. But fortunately, with a few small tricks, it is possible to clip off the carboxyl terminus, which is relatively small, and the remaining molecule retains all of its catalytic activities, and can be crystallized. It is with this compound that we are actually working. We are trying to do the same thing with P-450 s. As you know, all P-450 s of the human body are proteins that go through a lipid bilayer at least once or twice. At the moment, we are trying, together with investigators in Germany and in Russia, to clip this small part of the P-450, mono-oxygenase usually, to try to find out whether we can crystallize lipid-bound P-450 and actually investigate it using our new methods.

The same is true for receptors in general. As you know, the more classical receptors go through membranes seven times. Certainly the G-protein-coupled receptors do and these receptors of course can not be crystallized. We have to get rid of the lipids first, and this also is something we are working toward, but it is going to be very difficult. Michel in Germany, who won a Nobel prize for having done that for the Light Center, is trying to do it. He hopes and believes that it can be done. So let us hope for the best, because if this could be done, and if G-protein-coupled receptors could be freed from their lipids, and could be crystallized, and would theoretically at least still be active as the receptors, then we could apply our approach to the most classical receptors, maybe the G-coupled receptors. All other receptors are also bound to lipids and are therefore not fit to this particular way of studying proteins to which we are engaged at the moment. So, thus far the number of possibilities are limited and one should not exaggerate their importance.

Q: There is increased interest on the part of some people in developing drugs that can be delivered by inhaled route for systemic effects, not for effects of the lung. Until now, most inhaled drugs have been used to treat pulmonary problems, such as asthma, broncho-obstruction, or bronchitis. But if you could deliver a drug-like insulin in a very fine particle size so that it reaches the alveolar level and gets absorbed, than you could abrogate problems associated with intramuscular injection. But, in regard to THC, we are all aware that one of the limitations is the acceptability or tolerability of oral THC for the treatment of nausea and vomiting is that when given by the oral route, it may be poorly absorbed, or erratically absorbed. Do you have any interest, experience, or knowledge of what needs to be done to develop a drug like a cannabinol that could be effectively administered by inhalation as a very fine particle, and thereby be systemically absorbed?

A: I could only offer a few suggestions and the suggestion that crosses my mind is the trick that works for vitamin A and vitamin D. As you know, highly lipid-soluble vitamins when given orally in oily solution are not absorbed at all. But if you make a suspension, or a colloidal suspension with Tween for instance, then the oral absorption of vitamins A and D can be increased to 100% simply because these Tween particles, with an average size of 1 micrometer, are taken up, not by the blood stream, but by the lymphatic system.

This was something that was described in 1950 by a pediatrician named Popper here in New York. Practically all of the vitamin A and D used in Europe, at least, is no longer dissolved in oil as it used to be, but in a colloidal solution. This might work for a very potent lipophilic compound chemically related to tetrahydrocannabinol

Q: Oral delivery, then, as a suspension?

A: By oral route.

Q: By orally, you mean primarily by suspension?

A: By suspension the problem is even more formidable because a very long time ago, like many other people, we had studied what the properties of something that reaches the small alveoli should be like. And one of the requirements is that the small droplets, which are supposed to reach the small alveoli, that are important for instance in asthma, cannot have a diameter of more than I micrometer, 1 micron that is. And that is technically very difficult, because before they get there they tend to coagulate. To prevent this tendency of these molecules to interact with themselves, rather than to penetrate the bronchial tree, is notoriously difficult. It has been tried, by many people for insulin, but it never worked. The reason probably is that the small particles prefer to interact with themselves, rather than go unaltered through this very long bronchial tree.

People have tried as you know intranasal administration too. The intranasal route, theoretically at least, should be easier than the bronchial route, but again I do not know anybody, or any article in the literature, claiming success with insulin via the nasal route.

IV MARIHUANA AND REPRODUCTIVE FUNCTION

26

Cannabinoid Receptors in Sperm

Herbert Schuel, Michael C. Chang, Lani J. Burkman, Robert P. Picone, Alexandros Makriyannis, Arthur M. Zimmerman, and Selma Zimmerman

Abstract

Mammalian and invertebrate sperm contain receptors for a wide variety of neurotransmitters that regulate sperm functions required for fertilization such as motility and the initiation of the acrosome reaction. The acrosome reaction is a ligand-stimulated secretory event in sperm that enables the sperm to penetrate the egg's investments and to fuse with the egg's plasma membrane. Previous studies in our laboratory using [3H]CP-55,940 showed that sea urchin sperm contain cannabinoid receptors that are remarkably similar to cannabinoid receptors found in mammalian brain and peripheral organs. Cannabinoid agonists and anandamide (an endogenous ligand for cannabinoid receptors in mammalian tissues) inhibit fertilization in sea urchins by blocking the acrosome reaction. These findings, taken together with other studies showing that the gene for the human brain cannabinoid receptor also is expressed in the human testis and that anandamide is synthesized in the female reproductive tract in mammals, suggested to us that human sperm may contain cannabinoid receptors. We have obtained preliminary evidence that [3H]CP-55,940 binds to putative cannabinoid receptors in live human sperm in a saturable manner, and that cannabinoid ligands affect in vitro capacitation of human sperm. These findings show that functional cannabinoid receptors are present in sperm, suggest that sperm cannabinoid receptors and their endogenous ligands may regulate normal sperm functions required for fertilization within the female reproductive tract in humans, and also imply that smoking marijuana may affect these processes in vivo.

From: *Marihuana and Medicine*
Edited by: G. G. Nahas et al.   © Humana Press Inc., Totowa, NJ

1. INTRODUCTION

Historically, we first become aware of the the existence of a specific receptor and its endogenous ligand(s) indirectly by virture of the pharmacological effects produced by plant products that are used as drugs in medicine and/or for illicit purpuses. This situation also applies to cannabinoids that are the pharmacologically active substances found in *Cannabis*. Marijuana has been used for millenia because of its medicinal and psychoactive properties *(1)*. The primary psychoactive cannabinoid in marijuana is $(-)\Delta^9$-tetrahydrocannabinol [$(-)\Delta^9$-THC] *(2)*. It is now clear that $(-)\Delta^9$-THC and other cannabinoids affect a wide variety of physiologic processes in organs outside the central nervous system by acting directly on non-neural cells in the reproductive *(3–10)*, immune *(11–13)*, and urinary *(14)* systems. However, despite extensive studies, the mechanism(s) by which cannabinoids produce their biological effects is poorly understood. Cannabinoids are extremely hydrophobic compounds and tend to partition into biological membranes *(15)*. The recent discovery of cannabinoid receptors in brain (CB_1) and in peripheral tissues (CB_2) may provide the basis for understanding the physiological actions of cannabinoids *(16,17)*. Cannabinoid receptors are G-protein regulated and affect signal transduction mechanisms in mammalian somatic cells. Several endogenous ligands for central and peripheral cannabinoid receptors have been identified, including arachidonylethanolamide (anandamide) and related fatty acid derivatives *(18,19)*.

The use of marijuana is on the rise among young adults in America *(102)*. This situation may have significant clinical ramifications for human fertility. Cannabinoids are known to affect all reproductive functions studied thus far in humans and/or laboratory animals by: inhibiting secretion of gonadotrophic hormones by the pituitary gland and affecting secretion of steroids by the gonads *(20–27)*; inhibiting ovulation *(28,29)*; inhibiting sperm production and increasing the incidence of sperm with abnormal nuclei and acrosomes *(30–39)*; inhibiting the motility of ejaculated sperm *(40–42)*; affecting early embryonic development, hatching of the blastocyst from the zona pellucida, and implantation the blastocyst into the uterine endometrium *(3,10,43–45,101)*; and reducing the number of pregnancies carried to term *(29,46,47)*.

The gene for the human brain cannabinoid receptor (CB_1) also is expressed in the human testis *(48,49)*. Anandamide is synthesized in the testis and in the female reproductive tract of mammals *(44,45,50)*. These observations are suggestive of possible roles for sperm cannabinoid receptors and their endogenous ligands in regulating sperm functions required for fertilization. However, in studies on human populations of marijuana users or in experiments on laboratory mammals, it is not possible to discriminate between reduced fertility resulting from a direct effect on fertilization and indirect effects on other reproductive functions or behaviors. Whereas large quantities of human sperm can be obtained from volunteers, eggs are not readily available since human females normally produce only one egg each month and a surgical procedure is required to collect it. Furthermore, there are significant ethical concerns to the use of live human eggs for research purposes.

2. CANNABINOID RECEPTORS IN SEA URCHIN SPERM

Sea urchin gametes have been extensively used as an in vitro model system to study fertilization and early embryonic development for over a century because: these processes normally take place externally in sea water; large quantites of mature gametes can be easily collected from adult animals; and eggs undergo synchronous fertilization and development following insemination in vitro *(51)*. These features make it possible to directly treat eggs and sperm with a drug to assess its effects on fertilization processes under carefully controlled laboratory conditions.

The fertilizing capacity of sperm depends upon their ability to swim to the egg's surface and then to undergo the acrosome reaction. The acrosome reaction is a ligand-stimulated secretory event in sperm that enables the sperm to penetrate the egg's investments and fuse with the egg's plasma membrane. Unfertilized eggs are surrounded by extracellular investments that must be penetrated by the fertilizing sperm before it can activate the egg: vitelline layer and jelly coat in sea urchins, zona pellucida and cumulus oophorus in mammals (52,53). In sea urchins the acrosome reaction in the fertilizing sperm is stimulated by a glycoprotein ligand located the egg's jelly coat, and in humans and other mammals it is stimulated by a glycoprotein (ZP3) located in the egg's zona pellucida (52,54–56). Physiological acrosome reactions in mammalian sperm also can be stimulated by progesterone that is secreted by follicular cells in the matrix of the cumulus oophorus surrounding the unfertilized egg (57). The sperm receptor for ZP3 is regulated by a pertussis toxin sensitive G-protein, whereas the progesterone receptor is not (58,59). The biological significance of these dual physiological triggers for the acrosome reaction in the immediate vicinity of the unfertilized human egg is poorly understood. However, redundant mechanisms for stimulating physiological acrosome reactions at the egg surface may enhance the probability of successful fertilization.

Studies with sea urchin gametes provided the first evidence that cannabinoids can **directly** inhibit the process of fertilization by reducing the fertilizing capacity of sperm (4). However, cannabinoids enhanced sperm motility under these conditions, which suggested to us that they may inhibit fertilization by affecting the acrosome reaction. Subsequent studies showed that anandamide and (-)Δ^9-THC reduce sperm fertility in sea urchins by inhibiting the egg jelly-stimulated acrosome reaction in a dose-dependent manner (5–7,60). The inhibitory effects of anandamide and (-)Δ^9-THC on sea urchin sperm are completely reversible. Sperm regain their ability to undergo the acrosome reaction and to fertilize eggs upon removal of cannabinoid agonists. Anandamide and (-)Δ^9-THC do not block the acrosome reaction in sea urchin sperm that is triggered by ionophores such as ionomycin which promotes Ca^{2+} influx and nigericin which activates K^+ channels in sperm and somatic cells (5–7). These findings suggest that cannabinoids and anandamide affect events in the stimulation-secretion coupling mechanism of sperm prior to the opening of ion channels. The opening of Ca^{2+} and K^+ channels are essential signal transduction events in the egg jelly-stimulated acrosome reaction in sea urchin sperm (61,62), and similar events are associated with the zona pellucida- and progesterone-stimulated acrosome reactions in mammalian sperm (57,58,63). Our findings on sea urchin sperm are consistent with observations showing that cannabinoid receptors modulate signal-transduction systems in a wide variety of mammalian cells (reviewed in ref. 17), and are suggestive of a general role for cannabinoid receptors and their ligands in regulating signal-transduction processes in cells (5,7).

Ultrastructural observations on sea urchin sperm showed that the membrane fusion step in exocytosis of the acrosomal granule is blocked by cannabinoids (60). This finding is consistent with observations that cannabinoid agonists and anandamides inhibit secretion of neurotransmitters by peripheral nerve, of hormones by the pituitary gland, and of inflammatory mediators such as serotonin by mast cells (25,64,65,103), and is suggestive of a general role of cannabinoid receptors in regulating stimulation-secretion coupling mechanisms by cells (5,7). Our ultrastructural observations also revealed that cannabinoids cause the formation of lipid deposits in the subacrosomal fossa and in the centriolar fossa of treated sperm. The nuclear envelope is fragmented in close proximity to these lipid deposits (60). The lipid deposits disappear from treated sperm after the cannabinoids are removed by washing and the sperm regain their capacity to undergo egg jelly-stimulated acrosome reactions and to fertilize eggs. This shows that cannabinoids do not damage the sperm since the cells are struc-

Table 1
Binding Properties of Cannabinoid Receptors in Sea Urchin Sperm and Mammalian Tissues

Binding properties	Sea urchin sperm[a]	Rat brain (minced)[b]	Cloned human brain CB1[c]	Rat cerebellum mem.[c]	Rat Cerebral Cortex Mem.[d]	Mouse Spleen Cells[e]
K_D (nM)	5.16 ± 1.02	15.0 ± 3.0	3.3 ± 0.7	2.3 ± 0.4	0.133 ± 0.011	0.91
Hill Coef.	0.98 ± 0.004	NR	NR	NR	0.88 ± 0.08	~1
K_i CP55,940 (nM)	2.18 ± 0.5	15.0 ± 3.0	3.7 ± 0.1	NR	0.068 ± 0.006	NR
K_i (-)D^{9}THC (nM)	830.0 ± 180	420.0 ± 51	53.0 ± 0.1	NR	1.6 ± 0.56	NR
K_i (+)D^{9}THC(nM)	3700.0 ± 520	7700.0 ± 2100	>900	NR	NR	NR
B_{max} (pM/mg prot.)	2.44 ± 0.42	0.9	7.0 ± 0.5	2.5 ± 0.3	1.85 ± 0.26	NR
Receptors/cell	710.0 ± 122	NR	NR	NR	NR	~1000

NR, not Reported.
[a]ref. 71.
[b]ref. 94.
[c]ref. 95.
[d]ref. 16.
[e]ref. 11.
From: ref. 71.

trually and functionally intact after the ligand is washed away. These unexpected findings suggested that the lipid deposits in sea urchin sperm may represent hydrolysis product(s) derived from the fragmented nuclear envelope, possibly reflecting cannabinoid-induced activation of phospholipase(s) within the sperm. Subsequent studies showed that cannabinoids activate calcium-dependent phospholipase A_2 (PLA$_2$) activity in homogenates of sea urchin sperm (66). Arachidonic acid that is released from membrane phospholipids by the actions of PLA$_2$ and/or its metabolites may act as second messengers within sperm to block signal transduction events associated with the acrosome reaction (67). Furthermore, (-)Δ^9-THC is significantly more potent than (+)Δ^9-THC in activating PLA$_2$ in sperm homogenates (68). Stereoselectivity is a characteristic feature of receptor-mediated reactions. Cannabinoids are known to activate PLA$_2$ in mammalian somatic cells by receptor-mediated reactions (69, 70), which suggested to us that sea urchin sperm may contain functional cannabinoid receptors that regulate the acrosome reaction.

Using the highly potent synthetic cannabinoid agonist [^{3}H]CP,55940 (Table 1), we showed that sea urchin sperm contain a high-affinity cannabinoid receptor that is remarkably similar to cannabinoid receptors in mammalian brain and nonneural tissues. (71). These data suggest that live sea urchin sperm contain a single class of cannabinoid binding sites and the absence of significant cooperative interactions The rank order of potency to inhibit specific binding of [^{3}H]CP,55940 to live sea urchin sperm **and** to inhibit the egg-jelly stimulated acrosome reaction is: CP-55,940 > (-)Δ^9-THC > (+)Δ^9-THC. These results support our hypothesis that the sperm cannabinoid receptor modulates the acrosome reaction.

We believe that sperm cannabinoid receptors and endogenous anandamides may have normal functional roles during fertilization in sea urchins. The prevention of polyspermy is a critical event in normal fertilzation (reviewed in ref. 51). Many sperm are likely to be in the vicinity of an unfertilized egg during the process of fertilization. As soon as the first sperm activates the egg, other sperm in the vicinity of the egg represent a potential hazard to normal development. Penetration of the egg by more than one sperm (polyspermy) results in abnormal cleavage and death of the embryo. We postulated that anandamides may be produced by the egg after it is activated by the fertilizing sperm to prevent other sperm in the vicinity from undergoing the acrosome reaction, and thereby help to prevent polyspermic fertilization (7,71). This hypothesis is supported by recent observations that ovarian sea urchin eggs contain the enzymatic apparatus to produce anandamide and related acyl-ethanolamides *(72)*.

3. CANNABINOID RECEPTORS IN HUMAN SPERM

The gene for the human brain cannabinoid receptor (CB$_1$) also is expressed in the human testis *(49)*. This finding taken together with our observations on sea urchin sperm led us to postulate that human sperm would contain similar cannabinoid receptors *(71)*. This hypothesis is also supported by observations that anandamide can be synthesized within the testis and the female reproductive tract of mammals *(43–45,50)*.

We have obtained preliminary evidence for the presence of cannabinoid receptors in ejaculated human sperm *(7,8,73)*. Specific binding of [³H]CP-55,940 to live human sperm is saturable, and comparable to that previously obtained with sea urchin sperm. These findings raise the possibility that endogenous anandamides and cannabinoids may have functional roles in the process of fertilization in humans similar to those that we have seen in sea urchin gametes.

In addition to affecting the acrosome reaction during fertilization, anandamides and cannabinoid agonists may influence the process of sperm capacitation within the female reproductive tract in humans. Unlike sea urchin sperm, which can fertilize eggs immediately upon release into sea water, ejaculated human sperm require several hours of exposure to secretions of the female reproductive tract before they acquire the capacity to fertilize eggs in vivo *(53)*. Capacitated sperm exhibit hyperactivated motility and can undergo the acrosome reaction when they contact an unfertilized egg. Sperm can be capacitated in vitro by incubation in culture media supplemented with serum albumins *(74)*. Whereas a significant portion of viable sperm undergo premature acrosome reactions during in vitro capacitation, the great majority of motile sperm free in the oviductal lumen retain their acrosomes until they arrive at the surface of an unfertilized egg *(53,75)*. These findings suggest that unknown factors present within the female reproductive tract prevent premature acrosome reactions during capacitation *in vivo*. Do endogenous anandamides produced within the uterus and oviduct in mammals *(43–45)* have functional roles in modulating sperm motility and premature acrosome reactions during capacitation in vivo? Experiments are now being conducted in our laboratory to answer this question using (-)Δ^9-THC and R-methanandamide (AM-356), a potent anandamide analog that is resistant to hydrolysis by cellular amidases *(93)*. Preliminary observations indicate that both AM-356 and (-)Δ^9-THC affect the induction of premature acrosome reactions and hyperactivated motility in human sperm during in vitro capacitation *(8,9,73)*.

4. DISCUSSION

The observations described above show that functional cannabinoid receptors are present in both sea urchin and human sperm, and suggest that endogenous anandamides may regulate sperm functions required for fertilization. Mature invertebrate and mammalian sperm cells contain a wide variety of receptors for neurotransmitters (acetylcholine, adenosine, biogenic amines, progesterone, amino acids, nuropeptides, natriuretic-like peptides, and eicosanoids) and pyschoactive drugs such as cocaine, nicotine, and opioids *(8,9,54,57,71–74,76–87)*. These receptors modulate normal sperm functions that are essential for fertilization such as respiration, capacitation, motility, chemotaxis, and the acrosome reaction. Cannabinoid receptors in human and sea urchin sperm are another example of what appears to be a general biological phenomenon.

There may be significant medical ramifications to the presence of cannabinoid receptors in human sperm. Our findings raise the possibility that sperm cannabinoid receptors and endogenous anandamides may regulate normal sperm functions within the female reproductive tract required for capacitation and fertilization (8,9,73). Anandamide is known to be produced within the female reproductive tract (43–45). It is possible that certain currently unexplained types of human infertility may be caused by aberrant cannabinoid receptors in mature sperm, and/or abnormal synthesis of anandamides within the female reproductive tract. The smoking of marijuana by women also could affect normal sperm functions required for fertilization within the female reproductive tract. Furthermore, the gene for human CB_1 is also expressed in the human testis (49), and anandamide is known to be synthesized within the mammalian testis (50). Whereas the cells within the testis that produce these signal molecules have yet to be identified, the detection of cannabinoid receptors in mature sperm indicate that spermatogenic cells within the testis probably synthesize cannabinoid receptors. These findings suggest that cannabinoid receptors in spermatogenic cells and endogenous anandamides may regulate sperm production within the testis. This possibility also may account for previous observations that marijuana smoke and cannabinoids adversely affect sperm production in humans and laboratory animals (30–39). Marijuana and cannabinoids are also known to affect the functions of Sertoli cells (88,89) and Leydig cells (21,22) within the testis. This could contribute to the adverse effects of cannabinoids on sperm production. Whereas additional research is required to resolve these issues, it appears that endogenous anandamides and exogenous cannabinoids can affect multiple sperm functions within the male and female reproductive tracts.

Cannabinoid receptors and their endogenous ligands have beeen found in somatic and reproductive cells of invertebrates and mammals (3,5–9,12,17,44,71,72,86,105). Furthermore, cannabinoids are known to affect cyclic nucleotide metabolism in protozoa (90), whereas anandamides and related substances have been found in modern plants (91,92). Taken together these findings suggest that cannabinoid receptors and their endogenous ligands have an ancient origin in evolutionary history that may predate the origin of multicellular animals and plants. Within this context, the psychoactive effects induced by *Cannabis* should be viewed as but one aspect of a signal system that has existed for over 600 million years and that has a general role in modulating the functions of cells both within and outside of the central nervous system. What we refer to as "cannabinoid receptors" are actually receptors for endogenous ligands such as the anandamides. It is a quirk of evolution that certain cannabinoids produced by the *Cannabis* plant happen to bind to these receptor sites.

NOTE ADDED IN PROOF

The attention of many investigators remains focused upon the psychoactive properties of cannabinoids and their effects on brain functions (96). However, it is now clear that functional cannabinoid receptors also are located in non-neural cells outside of the nervous system, including phagocytic cells and lymphocytes in the immune system (11–13,48); type-II alveolar cells in the lung (97); smooth muscle and endothelial cells in the vascular system (98–99,106); human breast cancer cells (100); renal endothelial cells and mesangial cells in the kidney (14); mature sperm cells (8–9,71,73); early mouse embryos (3,10,101); as well as epithelial cells and stromal cells of the mouse uterus (43–45). Non-neural cannabinoid receptors, which normally react with endogenous ligands to modulate physiological functions within the body, may account, at least in part, for the pharmacological effects produced by marijuana outside of the central nervous system. These processes may be potential targets for novel therapeutic agents. This would require the development of suitable high affinity and selective ligands to avoid problems associated with smoking of marijuana, e.g., psychoactive effects, abuse potential, controlled dosing, immunosuppression, and the potential carcinogenic hazard of marijuana smoke, etc. (96).

Previous studies showed that anandamide and cannabinoid agonists reduce the fertilizing capacity of sea urchin sperm (4–7,71). We have begun to search for similar effects in humans using the hemizona assay which was originally developed to evaluate the fertilizing potential of sperm collected from men presenting to infertility clinics *(104)*. Our preliminary observations suggest that AM-356 significantly inhibits tight binding of capacitated sperm to the human zona pellucida in the hemizona assay *(73)*. The finding is predictive of failed fertilization in human IVF clinics *(104)*, and represents the first evidence for a possible role for sperm cannabinoid receptors and endogenous anandamides in regulating fertilization processes in humans.

ACKNOWLEDGMENTS

Supported in part by a Multidisciplinary Research Pilot Project grant from the University at Buffalo, SUNY to H.S. and L.J.B., and by NIDA grants DA-03801 and DA-09158 to A.M. We also thank Raphael Mechoulam for providing us with samples of anandamide for use in our studies on sea urchin sperm, for reading this manuscript, and for providing us with his critical comments.

REFERENCES

1. Mechoulam, R (1986) The pharmacohistory of Cannabis satavia. In: *Cannabinoids as Therapeutic Agents* (Mechoulam, R., ed.) CRC Press, Boca Raton, FL pp 1–19.
2. Mechoulam R, Devane A, Breuer A, Zahalka J (1991): A random walk through a cannabis field. *Pharmacol. Biochem. Behav.* **40,** 461–464.
3. Paria BC, Das KS, and Dey KS (1995): The preimplantation mouse embryo is a target for cannabinoid ligand-receptor signaling. *Proc. Natl. Acad. Sci.* **92,** 9460–9464.
4. Schuel H, Schuel R, Zimmerman AM, and Zimmerman S (1987) Cannabinoids reduce fertility of sea urchin sperm. *Biochem. Cell. Biol.* **65,** 130–136.
5. Schuel H, Berkery D, Schuel R, Chang MC, Zimmerman AM, and Zimmerman S (1991) Reduction of the fertilizing capacity of sea urchin sperm by cannabinoids derived from marihuana. I. Inhibition of the acrosome reaction induced by egg jelly. *Mol. Reprod. Devel. 29,* 51–59.
6. Schuel H, Chang MC, Berkery D, Schuel R, Zimmerman AM, and Zimmerman S. (1991) Cannabinoids inhibit fertilization in sea urchins by reducing the fertilizing capacity of sperm. *Pharmacol. Biochem. Behav.* **40,** 609–615.
7. Schuel H, Goldstein E, Mechoulam R, Zimmerman AM, and Zimmerman S (1994) Anandamide (arachidonylethanolamide), a brain cannabinoid receptor agonist, reduces fertilizing capacity in sea urchins by inhibiting the acrosome reaction. *Proc. Natl. Acad. Sci. USA* **91,** 7678–7682.
8. Schuel H, Burkman LJ, Picone RP, Bo T, and Makriyannis A (1997): Cannabinoid receptors in human sperm. *Mol. Biol. Cell.* **8,** 325A.
9. Schuel H, Burkman LJ, Hill WA, Picone RP, and Makriyannis A (1997) Evidence for cannabinoid receptors in human sperm. *1997 Symposium on Cannabinoids.* International Cannabinoid Research Society, Burlington VT. p 70.
10. Yang ZM, Paria BC, and Dey SK (1996) Activation of brain-type cannabinoid receptors interferes with preimplantation mouse embryo development. *Biol. Reprod.* **55,** 756–761.
11. Kaminski NE, Abood ME, Kessler FK, Martin BR, and Schatz AR (1992) Identification of a functionally relevant cannabinoid receptor in mouse spleen cells that is involved in cannabinoid-mediated immune modulation. *Mol. Pharmacol.* **42,** 736–742.
12. Stefano GB, Liu Y, and Goligorsky MS (1996) Cannabinoid receptors are coupled to nitric oxide release in invertebrate immunocytes, microglia, and human monocytes. *J. Biol. Chem.* **271,** 19238–19242
13. Zimmerman AM, Titishov N, Mechoulam R, and Zimmerman S (1991) Effects of stereospecific cannabinoids on the immune system. *Adv. Exp. Med. Biol.* **288,** 71–80.
14. Deutsch DG, Goligorsky MS, Schmid PC, Krebsbach RJ, Das SK, Dey SK, Arreaza G, Thorup C, Stefano G, and Moore LC (1997) Production and physiological actions of anandamide in the vasculature of the rat kidney. *J. Clin. Invest.* **100,** 1538–1546.
15. Makriyannis A, and Rapaka RS (1990) The molecular basis of cannabinoid activity. *Life Sci.* **47,** 2173–2184.
16. Devane WA, Dysarz FA, Johnson MR, Melvin LS, and Howlett AC (1988) Determination and characterization of a cannabinoid receptor in rat brain. *Mol. Pharmacol.* **34,** 605–613.
17. Matsuda LA (1997) Molecular aspects of cannabinoid receptors. *Critical Rev. Neurobiol.* **11,** 143–166.

18. Devane WA, Hanus L, Breuer A, Partwee, RG, Stevenson LA, Griffin G, Gibson D, Mandelbaum A, Etinger A, and Mechoulam R (1992) Isolation and structure of a brain constituent that binds to the cannaboid receptor. *Science.* **258,** 1946–1949.
19. Mechoulam R, Hanus L, and and Martin BR (1994) Search for endogenous ligands of the cannabinoid receptor. *Biochem. Pharmacol.* **48,** 1537–1544.
20. Bloch E, Thysen B, Morrill GA, Gardner E, and Fujimoto G. (1978): Effects of cannabinoids on reproduction and development. *Vitamines and Hormones* **36,** 203–258.
21. Burstein S, Hunter SA, Shoupe TS, and Taylor P (1978) Cannabinoid inhibition of testosterone synthesis by mouse Leydig cells. *Res. Commun. Chem. Pathol. and Pharmacol.* **19,** 557–560.
22. Dalterio S, Bartke A, and Mayfield D (1981) Δ^9-tetrahydrocannabinol increases plasma testosterone concentrations in mice. *Science.* **213,** 581–583.
23. Harclerode, J (1984) Endocrine effects of marijuana in the male: preclinical studies. *NIDA Res. Monogr.* **44,** 46–64.
24. Kolodny RC, Masters WH, Kolodner RM, and Toro G (1974) Depression of plasma testosterone levels after chronic intensive marihuana use. *N. Engl. J. Med.* **290,** 872–874.
25. Murphy LL, Newton SC, Dhali J, and Chavez D (1991) Evidence for a direct anterior pituitary site of delta-9-tetrahydrocannabinol action. *Pharmacol. Biochem. Behav.* **40,** 603–607.
26. Murphy LL, Cher J, Steger RW, and Bartke A (1994) Effects of Δ^9-tetrahydrocannabinol on copulatory behavior and neuroendocrine responses of male rats to female conspecifics. *Pharm. Biochem. Behav.* **48,** 1011–1017.
27. Smith CG, Smith MT, Besch NF, Smith RG, and Asch RH (1978) Effect of delta-9-tetrahydrocannabinol (THC) on female reproductive function. In: *Marihuana: Biological Effects* (Nahas GG and Paton WDM, eds.) Pergamon Press, Oxford, pp. 449–468.
28. Field E, and Tyre L (1986) Blockade of first ovulation in pubertal rats by delta-9-tetrahydrocannabinol: requirement for advanced treatment due to early initiation of the critical period. *Biol. Reprod.* **34,** 512–516.
29. Powell DJ, and Fuller RW (1983) Marihuana and sex: strange bedpartners. *J. Psychoactive Drugs* **15,** 269–280.
30. Dalterio S, Badr F, Bartke A, and Mayfield D (1982) Cannabinoids in male mice: effects on fertility and spermatogenesis. *Science.* **216,** 315–316.
31. Hembree WC, Nahas GG, Zeidenberg P, and Huang HFS (1979) Changes in human spermatozoa associated with high dose marihuana smoking. In: *Marihuana: Biological Effects* (Nahas, GG and Paton WDM, eds.) Pergamon Press, Oxford, pp. 429–439.
32. Huang HFS, Nahas GG, and Hembree WC (1978) Effects of marihuana inhalation on spermatogenesis of the rat. In: *Marihuana: Biological Effects* (Nahas GG and Paton WDM, eds.) Pergamon Press, Oxford, pp. 419–427.
33. Issidorides MR (1978) Observations in chronic hashish users: nuclear abberations in blood and sperm and abnormal acrosomes in spermatozoa. In: *Marihuana: Biological Effects* (Nahas GG and Paton WDM, eds.) Pergamon Press, Oxford, pp. 377–388.
34. Morrill GA, Kostellow AB, Ziegler DH, and Fujimoto GI (1983) Effects of cannabinoids on function of testis and secondary sex organs in the Fischer Rat. *Pharmacol.* **26,** 20–28.
35. Thompson GR, Mason MM, Rosenkrantz H, and Braude MC (1973) Chronic oral toxicity of cannabinoids in rats. *Toxicol. Applied. Pharmacol.* **25,** 373–390.
36. Tilak SK, and Zimmerman AM (1984) Effects of cannabinoids on macromolecular synthesis in isolated spermatogenic cells. *Pharmacol.* **29,** 343–350.
37. Zimmerman AM, Zimmerman S, and Raj AY (1978) Effects of cannabinoids on spermatogenesis in mice. In: *Marihuana: Biological Effects* (Nahas GG and Paton WDM, eds.) Pergamon Press, Oxford, pp. 407–418.
38. Zimmerman AM, Bruce WR, and Zimmerman S (1979) Effects of cannabinoids on sperm morphology. *Pharmacol.* **18,** 143–147.
39. Zimmerman AM, Murer-Orlando ML, and Richer (1986) Effects of cannabinoids on spermatogenesis *in vivo*: a cytological study. *Cytobios* **45,** 7–15.
40. Hong CY, Chaput de Saintogne DM, and Turner P (1981) Δ^9-tetrahydrocannabinol inhibits human sperm motility. *J. Pharm. Pharmacol.* **33,** 746–747.
41. Perez LE, Smith CG, and Asch RH (1981) Δ^9-tetrahydrocannabinol inhibits fructose utilization and motility in human, rhesus monkey, and rabbit sperm in vitro. *Fertil. Steril.* **35,** 703–705.
42. Shahar A, and Bino T (1974) *In vitro* effects of Δ^9tetrahydrocannabinol (THC) on bull sperm. *Biochem. Pharmacol.* **23,** 1341–1342.
43. Das SK, Paria BC, Chakraborty I, and Dey SK (1995) Cannabinoid ligand-receptor signaling in the mouse uterus. *Proc. Natl. Acad. Sci. USA* **92,** 4332–4336.
44. Paria BC, Deutsch DD, and Dey SK (1996): The uterus is a potential site for anandamide synthesis and hydrolysis: differential profiles of anandamide synthase and hydrolase activities in the mouse uterus during the periimplantation period. *Mol. Reprod. Devel.* **45,**183–192.

45. Schmid PC, Paria BC, Krebsbach RJ, Schmid HHO, and Dey SK (1997) Changes in anandamide levels in mouse uterus are associated with uterine receptivity for embryo implantation. *Proc. Natl. Acad. Sci.* **94**, 4188–4192.

46. Abel, E. L. (1984) Effects of Δ^9-THC on pregnancy and offspring in rats. *Neurobehav. Toxicol. Teratol.* **6**, 29–32.

47. Rosenkrantz H (1978) Effects of cannabinoids on fetal development of rodents. In: *Marihuana: Biological Effects* (Nahas GG and Paton WDM, eds.) Pergamon Press, Oxford, pp. 479–500.

48. Galiegue S, Mary S, Marchand J, Dussossoy D, Carriere D,Carayon P, Bouaboula M, Shire D, Le Fur G, and Casellas P (1995) Expression of central and peripheral cannabinoid receptors in human immune tissues and leukocyte populations. *Eur. J. Biochem.* **232**, 54–61.

49. Gerard CM, Mollereau C, Vassart G, and Parmentier M (1991) Molecular cloning of a human cannabinoid receptor which is also expressed in testis. *Biochem. J.* **279**, 129–134.

50. Sugiura T, Kondo S, Sukagawa A, Tonegawa T, Nakane S, Yamashita A, and Waku K (1996) Enzymatic synthesis of anandamide, an endogenous cannabinoid receptor ligand, through N-acylphosphatidylethanolamine pathway in testis: involvement of Ca^{2+}-dependent transacylase and phosphodiesterase activities. *Biochem. Biophys. Res. Comm.* **218**, 113–117.

51. Schuel H (1984) The prevention of polyspermic fertilization in sea urchins. *Biol. Bull.* **167**, 271–309

52. Wassarman PM (1987) The biology and chemistry of fertilization. *Science.* **235**, 553–560.

53. Yanagimachi R (1994) Mammalian fertilization. In: The Physiology of Reproduction, Second Edition, vol. 1 (Knobil E and Neil JD eds.) Raven, New York, pp. 189–317.

54. Garbers DL (1989) Molecular basis of fertilization. *Annu. Rev. Biochem.* **58**, 719–742.

55. Keller SH, and Vacquier VD (1994) The isolation of acrosome-reaction-inducing glycoproteins from sea urchin egg jelly. *Devel. Biol.* **162**, 304–312.

56. Van Duin VM, Polman JEM, De Breet ITM, Van Ginneken K, Bunschoten H, Grootenhuis A, Brindle J, and Aitken RJ (1994) Recombinant human zona pellucida protein ZP3 produced by chinese hamster ovary cells induces the human sperm acrosome reaction and promotes sperm-egg fusion. *Biol. Reprod.* **51**, 607–617.

57. Meizel S (1997) Amino acid neurotransmitter receptor/chloride channels of mammalian sperm and the acrosome reaction. *Biol. Reprod.* **56**, 569–574.

58. Bailey JL, and Storey BT (1994) Calcium influx into mouse spermatozoa activated by solubilized mouse zona pellucida, monitored with the calcium fluorescent indicator, Fluo-3. Inhibition of the influx by three inhibitors of the zona pellucida induced acrosome reaction: tyrphostin A28, pertussis toxin, and 3-quinclidinyl benzilate. *Mol. Reprod. Devel.* **39**, 297–308.

59. Tesarik J, Carreras A, and Mendoza C (1993) Differential sensitivity of progesterone- and zona pellucida-induced acrosome reactions to pertussis toxin. *Mol. Reprod. Devel.* **34**, 183–189.

60. Chang MC, and Schuel H (1991) Reduction of the fertilizing capacity of sea urchin sperm by cannabinoids derived from marihuana. II. Ultrastructural changes associated with inhibition of the acrosome reaction. *Mol. Reprod. Devel.* **29**, 60–71.

61. Beltran C, Zapata O, and Darszon A (1996) Membrane potential regulates sea urchin sperm adenylylcyclase. *Biochemistry.* **35**, 7591–7598.

62. Guerrero A, and Darszon A (1989) Evidence for the activaiton of two different Ca^{2+} channels during the egg jelly-induced acrosome reaction of sea urchin sperm. *J. Biol. Chem.* **264**, 19593–19599.

63. Ward CR, and Kopf GS (1993) Molecular events mediating sperm activation. *Devel. Biol.* **158**, 9–34

64. Facci L, Toso RD, Romanello S, Buriani A, Skaper SD, and Leon A (1995) Mast cells express a peripheral cannabinoid receptor with differential sensitivity to anandamide and palmitoylethanolamide. *Proc. Natl. Acad. Sci. USA* **92**, 3376–3380.

64. Roth SH (1978) Stereospecific presynaptic inhibitory effect of Δ^9-tetrahydrocannabinol on cholinergic transmission in the myenteric plexus of the guinea pig. *Can. J. Physiol. Pharmacol.* **56**, 968–975.

66. Chang MC, Berkery D, Laychock SG, and Schuel H (1991) Reduction of the fertilizing capacity of sea urchin sperm by cannabinoids derived from marihuana. III. Activation of phospholipase A_2 in sperm homogenate by Δ^9-tetrahydrocannabinol. *Biochem. Pharmacol.* **42**, 899–904.

67. Axelrod J, Burch RM, and Jelsema CL. (1988) Receptor-mediated activation of phospholipase A_2 via GTP-binding proteins: arachidonic acid and its metabolites as second messengers. *Trends Neurosci.* **11**, 117–123.

68. Chang MC, Laychock SG, Berkery D, Schuel R, Zimmerman AM, and Zimmerman S (1991) Effects of (-) and (+) enantiomers of delta-9-tetrahydrocannabinol on sea urchin sperm function. *J. Cell. Biol.* **115**, 320A.

69. Burstein S (1992): Eicosanoids as mediators of cannabinoid action, In: *Marijuana/Cannabinoids: Neurobiology and Neurophysiology,* (Murphy, L. and Bartke, A. eds.) CRC Press, Boca Raton, FL, pp. 73–91.

70. Burstein S, Budrow J, Debatis M, Hunter SA, and Subramanian A (1994) Phospholipase participation in cannabinoid-induced release of free arachidonic acid. *Biochem. Pharmacol.* **48**, 1253–1264.

71. Chang MC, Berkery D, Schuel R, Laychock SG, Zimmerman AM, Zimmerman S, and Schuel H (1993) Evidence for a cannabinoid receptor in sea urchin sperm and its role in blockade of the acrosome reaction. *Mol. Reprod. Devel.* **36,** 507–516.

72. Bisogno T, Ventriglia M, Milone A, Mosca M, Cimino G, and Di Marzo V (1997) Occurrence and metabolism of anandamide and related acyl-ethanolamides in ovaries of the sea urchin *Paracentrotus lividus. Biochim. Biophys. Acta.* **1345,** 338–348.

73. Burkman LJ, Schuel H, Shasanya S, Bruno J, Azarias A, Makriyannis A, and Crickard K (1997) Cannabinoids can alter human sperm acrosome reactions. Annual Meeting of the American Soc. for Reprod. Medicine, abstract.

74. Meizel S (1985) Molecules that initiate or help stimulate the acrosome reaction by their reaction with the mammalian sperm surface. *Am. J. Anat.* **174,** 285–302.

75. Burkman LJ (1990) Hyperactivated motility of human spermatozoa during in vitro capacitation. In: *Controls of Sperm Motility,* (Gagnon, E., ed.) CRC Press, Boca Raton, FL, pp. 304–329.

76. Anderson, R. A., Feathergill, K. A., Rawlins, R. G., Mack, S. R., Zaneveld L.J.D. (1995) Atrial natriuretic peptide: a chemoattractant of human spermatozoa by a guanylate cyclase-dependent pathway. *Mol. Reprod. Devel.* **40,** 371–378.

77. Bandivdekar AH, Segal SJ, and Koide, SS (1991) Binding of 5-hydroxytryptamine analogs by isolated *Spisula* sperm membrane. *Invert. Reprod. Devel.* **21,** 43–46.

78. Basuray R, De Jong C, and Zaneveld LJD (1990) Evidence for a role for cysteinyl leukotrienes in mouse and human sperm function. *J. Androl.* **11,** 47–51.

79. Blackmore PF, Neulen J, Lattanzio F, and Beebe SJ (1991) Cell surface-binding sites for progesterone mediate calcium uptake in human sperm. *J. Biol. Chem.* **266,** 18655–18659.

80. Cariello L, Zanetti L, Spagnuolo A, and Nelson L (1986) Effects of opoids and antagonists on the rate of sea urchin sperm progressive motility. *Biol. Bull.* **171,** 208–216.

81. Florman HM, and Storey BT (1981) Inhibition of in vitro fertilization of mouse eggs: 3-quinuclidinyl benzilate specifically blocks penetration of zonae pellucidae by mouse spermatozoa. *J. Exp. Zool.* **216,** 159–167.

82. Nelson L (1978) Chemistry and neurochemistry of sperm motility control. *Fed. Proc.* **37,** 2543–2547.

83. Sastry RBV, Janson VE, and Owens LK (1991) Significance of substance P-and enkephalin-peptide systems in the male genital tract. *Ann. NY Acad. Sci.* **632,** 339–353.

84. Shen MR, Linden J, Chen SS, and Wu SN (1993) Identification of adenosine receptors in human spermatozoa. *Clin. Exp. Pharmacol. Physiol.* **20,** 527–534.

85. Ward CR, Kopf GS, and Storey BT (1994) Solubilization and partial purification from mouse sperm membranes of the specific binding activity for 3-quinuclidinyl benzilate, a potent inhibitor of the zona pellucida-induced acrosome reaction. *Mol. Reprod. Devel.* **39,** 423–432.

86. Yazigi RA, Odem RR, and Polakowski KL (1991) Demonstration of specific binding of cocaine to human spermatozoa. *J. Am. Med. Assoc.* **266,** 1956–1959.

87. Wenger T, Fragakis G, Probonas K, Toth BE, and Yiannakakis N (1994) Anandamide (endogenous cannabinoid) affects anterior pituitary hormone secretion in the adult male rat. *Neuroendocrinol Letters* **16,** 297–303.

87. Young RJ, and Laing JC (1991) The binding characteristics of cholinergic sites in rabbit spermatozoa. *Mol. Reprod. Devel.* **28,** 55–61.

88. Heindel JJ, and Keith WB (1989) Specific inhibition of FSH-stimulated cAMP accumulation by Δ^9-tetrahydrocannabinol in cultures of rat Sertoli cells. *Toxicol. Applied. Pharmacol.* **101,** 124–134.

89. Holmes SD, Lipschultz LI, and Smith RG (1983) Effect of cannabinoids on human Sertoli cell function in vitro. *Archiv. Androl.* **11,** 245–251.

90. Zimmerman S, Zimmerman AM, and Laurence H (1981) Effect of Δ^9-tetrahydrocannabinol on cyclic nucleotides in synchronously dividing Tetrahymena. *Can. J. Biochem.* **59,** 489–493.

91. Kuehl FA, Jacob TA, Ganley OH, Ormond RE, and Meisinger MAP (1957) The identification of N-(2-hydroxyethyl)-palmitamide as a naturally occurring anti-inflammatory agent. *J. Am. Chem. Soc.* **79,** 5577–5578.

92. Tomaso E, Beltramo M, and Piomelli D (1996) Brain cannabinoids in chocolate. *Nature.* **382,** 677–678.

93. Abadji, V., Lin, S., Taha, G., Griffin, G., Stevenson, L. A., Pertwee, R. G., and Makriyannis, A. (1994) (R)-methanandamide: a chiral novel anandamide possessing high potency and metabolic stability. *J. Med. Chem.* **37,** 1889–1893.

94. Herkenham M, Lynn AB, Little MD, Johnson MR, Melvin LS, de Costa BR, and Rice KC (1990) Cannabinoid receptor localization in brain. *Proc. Natl. Acad. Sci. USA* **87,** 1932–1936.

95. Felder CC, Veluz JS, Williams HL, Briley EM, and Matsuda LA (1992) Cannabinoid agonists stimulate both receptor-and non-receptor mediated signal transduction pathways in cells transfected with and expressing cannabinoid receptor genes. *Mol. Pharmacol.* **42,** 838–845.

96. Felder CC, and Glass M (1998) Cannabinoid receptors and their endogenous agonists. *Ann. Rev. Pharmacol. Toxicol.* **38,** 179–200.

97. Rice W, Shannon JM, Burton R, and Fieldeldey D (1997) Expression of brain type cannabinoid receptor (CB1) in alveolar type-II cells in the lung—regulation by hydrocortisone. *Eur. J. Pharmacol.* **327,** 227–232.

98. Hillard CJ, Gebremedhin D. Lange AR, Campbell WB, Harder DR, and Hudetz AG (1997) Cannabinoid receptors (CB1) of cerebral arterial muscle cells inhibit L-type calcium current: does the CB1 receptor play a role in the regulation of cerebral blood flow? *1997 Symposium on Cannabinoids.* International Cannabinoid Research Society, Burlington, VT, p. 73.

99. Sugiura T, Kodaka T, Nakane S, Kishimoto S, Kondo S, and Waku K (1998) Detection of an endogenous cannabinimetic molecule, 2-arachidonoylglycerol, and cannabinoid CB1 receptor mRNA in human vascular cells: is 2-arachidonoylglycerol a possible vasomodulator? *Biochem. Biophys. Res. Comm.* **243,** 838–843.

100. Di Marzo V, Melck D, Bisogno T, and De Petrocellis L (1998) Anandamide potently and selectively inhibits human breast cancer cell proliferation through interference with endogenous prolactin action. *1998 Symposium on Cannabinoids.* International Cannabinoid Research Society, Burlington, VT, in press.

101. Paria BC, Ma W, Andrenyak DM, Schmid PC, Schmid HHO, Moody DE, Deng H, et al. (1998) Effects of cannabinoids on preimplantation mouse embryo development and implantation are mediated by brain-type cannabinoid receptors. *Biol. Reprod.* **58,** 1490–1495.

102. Turner CF, Ku L, Rogers SM, Lindberg LD, Pleck JH, and Sonenstein FL (1998) Adolescent sexual behavior, drug use, and violence: increased reporting with computer survey technology. *Science* **280,** 867-873.

103. Ishac EJN, Jiang L, Lake KD, Varga K, Abood ME, and Kunos G (1996) Inhibition of exocytotic noradrenaline release by presynaptic cannabinoid receptors on peripheral sympathetic nerves. *Br. J. Pharmacol.* **118,** 2023–2028.

104. Burkman LJ, Coddington CC, Franken DR, Oehninger SC, and Hodgen GD (1990) The Hemizona Assay (HZA): Assessment of fertilizing potential by means of human sperm binding to the human zona pellucida. In: *Laboratory Diagnosis and Treatment of Infertility.* (BA Keel and B Webster, eds.). CRC Press, Boca Raton, FL, pp. 213–228.

105. Stefano GB, Salzet B, and Salzet M (1997) Identification and characterization of the leech CNS cannabinoid receptor: coupling to nitric oxide release. *Brain Res.* **753,** 219–224.

106. Stefano GB, Salzet M, and Bilfinger TV (1998) Long-term exposure of human blood vessels to HIV gp120, morphine, and anandamide increases endothelial adhesion of monocytes: uncoupling of nitric oxide release. *J. Cardiovasc. Pharmacol.* **3,** 862–868.

107. Sepe N, De Petrocellis L, Montanaro F, Cimino G, and Di Marzo V (1998) Bioactive long chain N-acylethanolamines in five species of edible bivalve molluscs. Possible implications for mollusc physiology and sea food industry. *Biochim. Biophys. Acta.* **1389,** 101–111.

27

Effects of Cannabinoids on Spermatogenesis in Mice

Arthur M. Zimmerman, Selma Zimmerman and A. Yesoda Raj

Abstract

Sperm morphology was investigated in hybrid mice of genotype (C57BL × C3H)F_1 following treatment with Δ^9-tetrahydrocannabinol (Δ^9-THC), cannabinol (CBN) and cannabidiol (CBD). Mice were treated for five consecutive days and 35 days after the last intraperitoneal injection the epididymal sperm were scored in the light microscope and assessed in the scanning electron microscope. The Δ^9-THC (5 and 10 mg/kg) and CBN (10 and 25 mg/kg)-treated mice had a statistically higher incidence of abnormal sperm than the vehicle (dimethylsulfoxide)-treated controls. Normal sperm have a smooth kidney-shaped head with a prominent hook; abnormal sperm displayed heads without hooks, banana-shaped heads, amorphous heads, and folded heads.

Cytogenetic assessment of primary spermatocytes obtained from mice treated with CBN (10 mg/kg), CBD (10 mg/kg) and Δ^9-THC (10 mg/kg) for five days showed an increase in the number of ring and chain translocations when cells were assessed 16 days after the last dose. The incidence of translocations in the cannabinoid-treated animals was three to five fold greater than the vehicle controls (DMSO). The significance of the results is discussed in terms of the potential genetic effects of the cannabinoids.

1. INTRODUCTION

The action of marihuana has been more clearly defined since 1970, when purified Δ^9-tetrahydrocannabinol (Δ^9-THC, also designated Δ^1-THC) became available for investigation (*see* refs. 2.27 for reviews). Various reports in the literature suggest that marihuana and Δ^9-THC affect growth, development, and reproduction. Our laboratory is interested in determining the influence of marihuana on spermatogenesis. In such an analysis, it is fruitful to use various cannabinoids to determine whether they differ from one another in their effect on spermatogenesis.

From: *Marihuana and Medicine*
Edited by: G. G. Nahas et al.   © Humana Press Inc., Totowa, NJ

Spermatogenesis is a complicated process in which the differentiation of sperm is controlled by an intricate neurohormonal mechanism. Thus in analyzing marihuana's action on sperm differentiation, it is important to consider whether marihuana acts directly on the sperm-forming cells via interference with genetic and/or cellular mechanisms or indirectly by affecting the neuroendocrine functions that regulate spermatogenesis. In view of the complex interaction between spermatogenesis and testosterone levels as well as the contribution of the sperm cell to fetal development, it is pertinent to briefly review the literature with respect to the effects of marihuana on testosterone levels, fetal development and spermatogenesis.

1.1 Influence of Cannabinoids on Testosterone

Conflicting reports in the literature make it difficult to ascertain whether cannabinoids affect plasma testosterone levels in humans. Kolodny and coworkers report a depression of plasma testosterone after chronic (20) or acute (21) marihuana use. In contrast to these reports, Mendelson et al. (26) and Schaefer et al. (32) were unable to demonstrate a depression of plasma testosterone. It is possible, however, as Kolodny and coworkers (21) have pointed out, that the discrepancies may be explained by methodological differences in the investigations. Recent studies by Hembree et al. (16) show that in a hospital setting, daily heavy use of marihuana is not associated with a decrease in serum testosterone levels.

Reports of testosterone levels in rodents suggest that Δ^9-THC depresses testosterone levels (9,34). In vitro studies also show an inhibitory effect of cannabinoids on testosterone (4). In addition, cannabinoids decrease the weight of accessory sex glands in mice and rats (5,6,7,29).

1.2 Teratogenic Effects of THC

Teratogenic effects of Δ^9-THC are also difficult to evaluate since various routes of administration, varying times of treatment during gestation, and different dosages have been used. In rabbits, Δ^9-THC treatment induced eventrations and hairlip (11). In mice, high dosages of Δ^9-THC caused exencephaly and cleft palate (18). Using more moderate dosages of Δ^9-THC, Mantilla-Plata and coworkers reported induction of cleft palate in Swiss Webster mice (24,25). Moreover, teratogenic effects induced by Δ^9-THC were potentiated by treatment with phenobarbita (13). Teratogenic effects of tetrahydrocannabinol were also demonstrated in Zebrafish (35). However, other investigators did not observe teratogenic effects in hamsters, rabbits, mice, and rats following treatment with marihuana or specific cannabinoid extracts (10,12,19,30,31).

1.3 Effects of Marihuana on Spermatogenesis

Cannabinoids induced disruption of spermatogenesis in mice that was accompanied by Leydig cell degeneration (7). In humans, marihuana induced a reduction of sperm concentration and total sperm count, however, there was no indication of abnormal sperm morphology (16).

It is difficult to ascertain the mechanism of the effect of marihuana, however, it should be emphasized that a simple dose-response relationship between sperm reduction and sperm production has not been established and is unlikely in view of the multifactorial nature of the system (16).

2. SPERM MORPHOLOGY AND MUTAGENICITY

Spermatogenesis is a complex process involving germ-cell differentiation, the result of which is a highly structured, species-specific cell, called a spermatozoon. Early investigations showed that the incidence of abnormal sperm morphology increases following ionizing radiation (23,28). Recently, quantitative measurements of radiation dosage revealed that the incidence of abnormalities is radiation dose-dependent and the frequency of abnormal sperm morphology is a function of the specific strain of mice irradiated (3).

Sperm morphology appears to be under genetic control, however, the mechanism by, which abnormal sperm are produced has not been elucidated. It is interesting to note that F_1 and F_2 progeny of irradiated male mice have an elevated incidence of abnormal sperm and, in specific individuals the high proportion of abnormal sperm are found for several generations (17). One possible explanation for induction of abnormal sperm is directly induced genetic damage to spermatogenic cells (37,39).

Wyrobek et al. (39) investigated the possibility that abnormal sperm morphology resulted from chromosomal abnormalities, i.e., whether chromosomal translocation in the diploid germ cell, or chromosomal imbalance (aneuploidy) within the haploid cell (spermatid) caused sperm-head abnormalities. The investigators measured the incidence of abnormal sperm in mice, heterozygous and homozygous for 24 various reciprocal and Robertsonian translocations. Diploid cells of these mice contain translocated chromosomes, and a predictable proportion of the gametes carry translocated chromosomes. The investigators report that the levels of sperm-head shape abnormalities were not related to the presence of translocated chromosomes in the germ cells or chromosome aneuploidy in the spermatid cells.

During the last several years more than 60 chemicals have been tested on mice, and sperm morphology has been assessed (15,37,38). The sperm of hybrid male mice of genotype (C57BL × C3H)F_1 were examined at 1, 4, and 10 weeks after the mice received five consecutive daily intraperitoneal injections of various chemical agents. The fraction of sperm with abnormal shape in the treated mice was compared to that of nontreated controls. Among the agents investigated, approximately 45 of them were considered mutagenic in mammalian cells in vivo, that is, agents known to cause heritable mutations, dominant lethal mutations, somatic mutations, and chromosomal aberrations. The sperm assay method gave a success rate of 67% for the known mutagens as compared with a 64% success rate seen with the Ames *Salmonella* assay for the same panel of agents. It must be emphasized that depending upon the choice of agents tested, the success rate may vary.

It is evident that no single test will identify all potential mutagenic agents, however, by using a battery of tests, such as the *Salmonella* test, micronuclei assay, and sperm abnormality assay, it is possible to increase the successful identification of potentially deleterious agents. Employing both the sperm abnormality assay and the *Salmonella* assay, Heddle and Bruce[15] report a success rate of 89% for the panel of 61 compounds they investigated.

3. INFLUENCE OF CANNABINOIDS: SPERM MORPHOLOGY AND CYTOGENETICS

In view of the reports that suggest that cannabinoids affect spermatogenesis and cause teratogenic effects we initiated a program to investigate the effects of specific cannabinoids on sperm differentiation. We wish to report on two aspects of this study, namely: the consequences on sperm morphology when germinal cells in the primary spermatocyte stage were exposed to cannabinoids (40) and a cytogenetic study of primary spermatocytes that were exposed to cannabinoids during the spermatogonium stage.

3.1 General Methodology

3.1.1. SPERM CELL PREPARATION

The procedure for evaluation of sperm morphology was essentially that of Wyrobek and Bruce (37,38). Young hybrid male mice genotype (C57BL × C3H)F_1 from Bio Breeding

Laboratories (Canada) were obtained at 11–14 weeks of age. The animals received five daily intraperitoneal injections of a specific cannabinoid, mitomycin C, or vehicle. Thirty-five days after the last treatment, the cauda epididymis was removed from the test animal and a sperm suspension was prepared. The epididymal sperm were assayed for sperm abnormality. Sperm scored at this time were assumed to have been in the early primary spermatocyte stage at the time of drug treatment. Cells were prepared for light microscopy or scanning-electron microscopy. For light microscopy, the sperm suspension was stained with 1% eosin Y in aqueous solution. The smears were prepared and 800 sperm from each animal were scored under × 400 magnification. The slides were scored using a double-blind procedure. For scanning-electron microscopy, epididymal sperm were fixed in 2.5% glutaraldehyde in phosphate-buffered saline (PBS)- at pH 7.3 for a minimum of 30 minutes. Following fixation, the cells were washed by centrifugation three times with PBS and three times with glass-distilled water. The cells were frozen with liquid nitrogen, dehydrated in a Speedivac-Pearse tissue drier Model I (Edwards High Vacuum, Sussex, UK), and coated with a thin layer of gold. The specimens were viewed in the Cambridge S180 Scanning Electron Microscope at an accelerating voltage of 30 KV.

3.1.2. Cannabinoids

The cannabinoids investigated were Δ^9-tetrahydrocannabinol (5 and 10 mg/kg), cannabinol (10 and 25 mg/kg), and cannabidiol (10 and 25 mg/kg). Mitomycin C (0.6 mg/kg) was used as a positive control. Since all agents were dissolved in dimethylsulfoxide, a vehicle control group was established in which the animals received 0.1 mL dimethylsulphoxide. Higher concentrations of THC, CBN, and CBD were also tested. However, because of the toxicity of the cannabinoids there was a high mortality and no animals survived the 35-day recovery period (Table 1). In general, Δ^9- and Δ^8-THC were the most toxic of the cannabinoids investigated and none of the animals survived a dosage of 25 mg/kg. CBD was the least toxic, as 60% of the animals survived at 25 mg/kg. The order of toxicity in the cannabinoid series was Δ^9- and Δ^8-THC > CBN > CBD.

3.1.3. Cytogenetic evaluation

Cannabinoids were administered to mice as previously described for five days. The testes were excised from the test animal 16 days after the last treatment, at which time primary spermatocytes were evaluated for aberrations. Testes were rinsed in 2.2% sodium citrate and the tunica was removed. The tubules were gently squeezed on a glass plate in a drop of 2.2% sodium citrate solution. The cells were washed by centrifugation and placed into 1% sodium citrate. Methanol/acetic acid (3:1 v/v) was used as a fixative. The fixative solution was replaced two times; cells were placed on slides, air dried, and stained with aceto-orcein *(1)*.

3.2. Sperm Morphology Assay

The percentage of abnormal sperm in the (C57BL × C3H)F$_1$ strain of mice is consistently low and the mean frequency of abnormalities as reported by Wyrobek and Bruce *(17)* is 1.8% with 9% interval for the population extending from 1.2–3.4. Zimmerman et al. *(40)*, report non-treated control values (*n* = 14) of 1.54 ± 0.11 SE for the average incidence of abnormal sperm. Individual values are considered positive when the treated group exceeds the control group by 1% *(38)*. The individual values for sperm abnormality are summarized in Table 1 and each value is compared statistically to the DMSO series where the average value was 1.86. Thus an agent is considered to display a positive response in the sperm assay when the sperm abnormalities exceed 3% (a guideline).

Table 1
Percent of Abnormal Sperm Following Treatment

| Treatment | Number of animals | | % survived | Averages | ±SE | P Value[a] |
	Initial	Survivors				
Control	15	14	93	1.54	0.11	.095
DMSO 0.1 mL/animal	15	15	100	1.86	0.17	–
Mit. C 0.6 mg/kg	20	9	45	9.22	1.08	.000[b]
Δ⁹-THC						
10 mg/kg	24	11	46	5.26	1.58	.003[b]
5 mg/kg	30	24	80	3.82	0.81	.003[b]
CBN						
25 mg/kg	31	4	13	8.63	3.40	.049[b]
10 mg/kg	27	15	56	3.26	0.69	.045[b]
CBD						
25 mg/kg	23	14	64	2.51	0.37	.057
10 mg/kg	21	12	57	2.40	0.62	.334
Mit. C 2.4 mg/kg	6	0				
Δ⁹-THC 300 mg/kg	4	0				
100 mg/kg	4	0				
75 mg/kg	10	0				
50 mg/kg	10	0				
25 mg/kg	10	0				
CBN 300 mg/kg	4	0				
100 mg/kg	4	0				
50 mg/kg	7	0				
CBD 300 mg/kg	4	0				
100 mg/kg	4	0				
50 mg/kg	7	0				
Δ⁹-THC 300 mg/kg	4	0				
100 mg/kg	4	0				
25 mg/kg	4	0				

[a]Derived from t-test comparison to DMSO.
[b]Significant at the 5% level.

Mitomycin C, the positive control, elicited a sperm abnormality of over 9%. Δ⁹-THC at 5 and 10 mg/kg gave values of 3.82 and 5.26%, respectively. These values were statistically significant at the 5% level when compared to the DMSO controls. CBN at 10 and 25 mg/kg produced values of 3.26 and 8.63% respectively; these were also significantly different from the DMSO values at the 5% level. In the CBD series, however, the frequency of abnormally shaped sperm was not significantly different from the DMSO controls, at either the low (10 mg/kg) or high (25 mg/kg). dose.

The data is plotted in Fig. 1, where it can be seen that the results of THC and CBN at both low and high dosages are considered positive according to the criteria proposed by Wyrobek and Bruce (38). CBD values, although slightly higher than the DMSO controls, do not exceed the 3% guideline, and statistically are not different from the DMSO controls.

The strong positive effect recorded with 25 mg/kg CBN may result from the fact that only four of the 31 mice treated survived the 35-day recovery period. This factor probably contributed to the strong positive response. However, this is not the only explanation since more

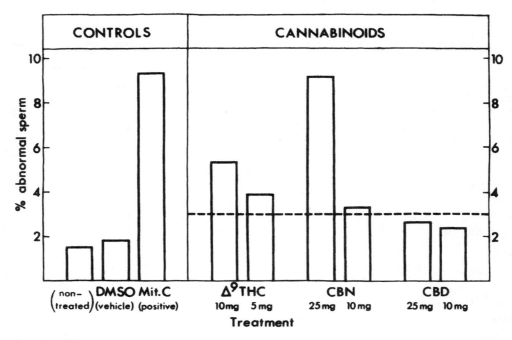

Fig. 1. The effects of cannabinoids on sperm morphology. The mice in each series were treated for 5 days with one of the cannabinoids, vehicle (DMSO) or mitomycin C. The dosage shown below each cannabinoid is expressed in mg/kg. Each value represents the percent of abnormal sperm observed 35 days after the last treatment. The dashed line at the 3% level represents the demarcation line above which induced abnormalities are considered to be deleterious. (From the work of Zimmerman et al.[40].)

than 50% of the animals survived at the lower dose of CBN (10 mg/kg), yet the incidence of abnormal sperm is statistically greater than the DMSO controls.

3.3. Sperm Morphology as Visualized in the Scanning-Electron Microscope

The shape of murine sperm from nontreated normal and drug-treated animals was evaluated in the scanning-electron microscope *(40)*. Representative normal sperm are illustrated in Fig. 2A,B. The normal sperm has a kidney-shaped head with a prominent curved hook on the top. Several different abnormal sperm were identified; they included heads without hooks, banana-shaped heads, amorphous heads, and folded heads. In Fig. 2C–F, representative sperm from animals receiving 10 mg/kg of Δ^9-THC are shown.

3.4. Cytogenetics

In order to further ascertain the effects of cannabinoids on spermatogenesis, a cytogenetic evaluation was initiated. Mice were trearted for five consecutive days with a specific cannabinoid and 16 days after the last treatment the primary spermatocytes were prepared for cytological evaluation. The prophase meiotic cells (at diakinesis) were scored for ring and chain translocations, chromosome breaks, deletions, and aneuploidy. Cells evaluated at this time were assumed to have been in the spermatogonium state (2–3 weeks earlier) when the cannabinoids were administered to the animals (cf. ref. *8*).

The average number of ring and chain translocations in non-treated and DMSO controls were 0.87 and 1.22 per 100 cells analyzed, respectively. In the mitomycin C-treated mice the value was 6.73; the percentage of *translocations* in the Δ^9-THC, CBN, and CBD cells were

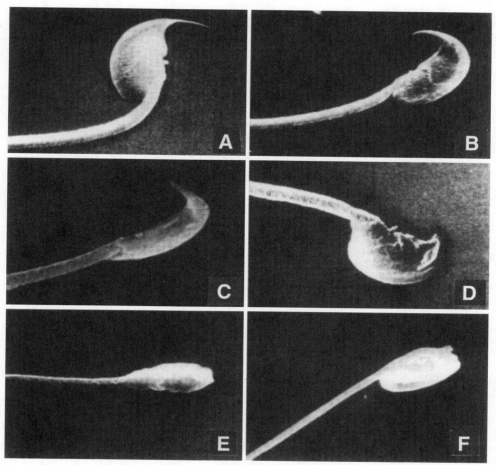

Fig. 2.   Scanning-electron micrographs of epididymal sperm obtained from control and Δ^9-THC-treated mice. In the normal sperm (**A** and **B**) the most characteristic feature is the hook that protrudes from the head. Abnormal sperm comprised between 3.8 and 5.2% of population from THC-treated mice. The abnormal-shaped sperm head included (**C**) banana-shaped heads, (**D**) sperm heads without hooks, and (**E**) amorphous heads. Folded heads (**F**) were occasionally observed, but were not included in the scoring for abnormal sperm since it is possible that these shapes may be fixation artifacts. (From the work of Zimmerman et al.[40].)

5.74, 4.95, and 6.48%, respectively. In general, the incidence of translocations in the cannabinoid treated animals was three-to five fold greater than the DMSO controls. The total number of abnormalities in the cannabinoid-treated animals was approximately twice as great as in the control animals (Table 2, Fig. 3); there was no appreciable difference in the observed number of chromosome breaks, deletions, and aneuploidy between the different treatments. In summary, the major aberrations induced by the cannabinoids were ring and chain translocations.

4. CONCLUDING REMARKS

In general, these experiments demonstrate an increased incidence of abnormally shaped sperm heads in Δ^9-THC- and CBN-treated hybrid mice (C57BL × C3H)F$_1$. However, the

Table 2
Cytogenetic Analysis of Primary Spermatocytes[a]

Drug	Animal	Total cells analyzed	Translocations ring and chain	Chromosome breaks	Aneuploidy	Percentages Translocation	Total abnormalities
Control	1	164	2	3	3	1.20	4.87
	2	152	1	4	4	0.65	5.92
	3	130	1	4	4	0.76	6.92
						0.87	5.90 avg.
DMSO	1	156	3	6	4	1.92	8.33
	2	187	1	4	3	0.53	4.27
						1.22	6.30 avg.
Mit. C	1	127	6	2	–	4.72	6.29
(0.6 mg/kg)	2	183	16	6	5	8.74	14.75
						6.73	11.74 avg.
CBN	1	226	10	12	8	4.42	13.27
(10 mg/kg)	2	146	8	2	2	5.47	8.21
						4.95	10.72 avg.
THC	1	199	17	6[b]		8.54	11.55
(10 mg/kg)	2	122	7	5	5	5.73	13.93
	3	135	3	4	5	2.96	8.88
						5.74	11.45 avg.
CBD	1	121	11	7	–	9.09	14.8
(10 mg/kg)	2	198	7	6	4	3.53	8.58
	3	161	11	5	3	6.83	11.80
						6.48	11.72 avg.

[a]5 days[1] treatment; analyses 16 days after last dose.
[b]Chromosome deletions.

exact mechanism for induction of the abnormal sperm has not been established. In the present experiments, the cytogenetic evidence indicates that cells exposed to cannabinoids in the spermatogonia stage show an increase in the number of ring and chain translocations when observed in the primary spermatocyte stage. The relationship of these translocations to sperm morphology remains unclear. Further evidence of chromosome breakage following cannabinoid treatment may be seen from the work of Zimmerman and Raj (unpublished) in our laboratory, who found that Δ^9-THC, CBN, and CBD gave a positive response in the micronucleus test system (cf. refs. *14,36*). The Wyrobek et al. *(39)* study refutes a direct relationship between the presence of a translocation and/or aneuploidy condition in cells undergoing spermatogenesis and the formation of an abnormally shaped sperm head. Nevertheless, their experiments do not rule out the possibility that translocations involving chromosomal segments other than those observed may be more directly involved in the development of sperm with normal head shape. It is of interest to note that, in our studies, CBD treatment (10 mg/kg) resulted in the highest percentage of translocations but was least effective in inducing sperm-head abnormalities.

Alternative hypotheses that may be proposed for the induction of abnormal sperm are point mutation or modified gene function, which may affect protein structure or cell metabolism. The current investigation does not allow us to conclude that these cannabinoids are

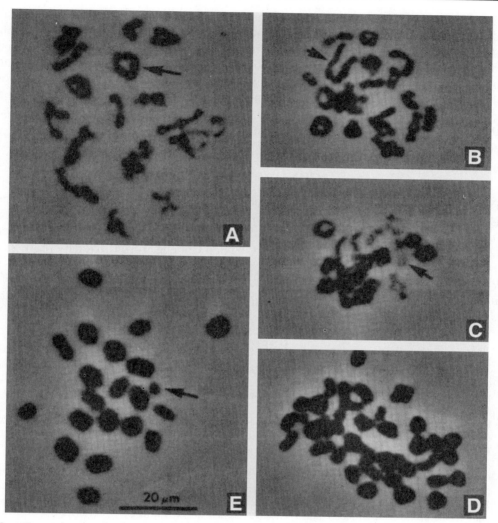

Fig. 3. Photomicrographs of primary spermatocyte at diakinesis illustrating ring and chain translocations and early metaphase chromosomes showing aneuploidy and broken segments induced by Δ⁹-THC.
Mice were treated for 5 days with 10 mg/kg of Δ⁹-THC and the primary spermatocytes were assessed 16
days after the last treatment. (**A**) Translocation ring of four chromosomes and 18 bivalents. (**B**) Translocation chain of four chromosomes. (**C**) Translocation chain of three chromosomes. (**D**) Aneuploid cell showing 30 bivalents. (**E**) Broken chromosome segment and 20 bivalents.

mutagenic. Reports from our laboratory *(41)* and those of Legator and coworkers *(22,33)*
suggest that Δ⁹-THC is not mutagenic. We reported negative findings using a battery of tests,
including the Ames *Salmonella* assay and tests with fibroblasts from normal and *Xeroderma*
patients in which chromosome aberrations, sister chromatid exchanges, and unscheduled
DNA synthesis were assessed. Legator and coworkers *(22,23)* and I also reported a failure to
detect mutagenic effects of Δ⁹-tetrahydrocannabinol using the Ames *Salmonella* test,
micronucleus assay, dominant lethal test, and host-mediated assay.

The apparent contradictory reports from our own laboratory and other laboratories
requires us to be cautious in the interpretation of our results. It may be that the specific strain

of mice (C57BL × C3H)F$_1$ used in these experiments metabolize cannabinoids to intermediary compounds and that these metabolites interfere directly with the germ cells, resulting in identifiable meiotic aberrations (translocations) and sperm-head aberrations. It is also possible that the cannabinoids and/or their metabolites induce sperm-head abnormalities by interfering with spermiogenesis. In conclusion, we wish to emphasize the need for additional information concerning the effect of cannabinoids and their metabolities on cytogenetic structure and sperm morphology. We also propose that the effect of these drugs on protein synthesis and cell metabolism be studied in cells involved in spermatogenesis in order to ascertain biochemical alterations that may play a role in sperm formation.

ACKNOWLEDGMENTS

The authors wish to express their gratitude to Helen Laurence for her expert technical assistance and their thanks to Eric Y. C. Lin for his assistance with the scanning-electron microscope. This investigation was supported by a grant from National Research Council (to A. M. Z.) and a Minor Research Grant from Glendon College, York University (to S. Z.).

Reprinted with permission from Marihuana: Biological Effects, Analysis, Metabolism, Cellular Responses, Reproduction, and Brain, (G. G. Nahas, W. D. M. Paton, eds.) Pergamon Press, New York, 1979. pp. 407–418.

REFERENCE

1. Adler, I. D. (1974) Comparative cytogenetic study after H treatment of mice spermatogonia with Mitomycin C. *Mutat. Res.* **23**, 369–371.
2. Braude, M. C. and Szara, S., (eds.) (1976) *Pharmacology of Marihuana.* vol. 1 and 2. Raven, New York. 1976.
3. Bruce, W. R., Furrer, R., and Wyrobek, A. J. (1974) Abnormalities in the shape of murine sperm after acute testicular X irradiation. *Mutat. Res.* **23**, 381–386.
4. Dalterio, S., Bartke, A., and Burstein, S. (1977) Cannabinoids inhibit testosterone secretion by mouse testes in vitro. *Science* **196**, 1472–1473.
5. Collu, R., Letarte, J., Leboeuf, G., and Ducharme, J. R. (1975) Endocrine effects of chronic administration of psychoactive drugs to prepubertal male rats. 1.⁹-tetrahydrocannabinol. *Life Sci.*, **16**, 533–542.
6. Dixit., V. P. and Lohiya, N. K. (1975) Effects of cannabis extract in the response of accessory sex organs of adult male mice to testosterone. *Indian J. Physiol. Pharmacol.* **19**, 98–100.
7. Dixit, V. P., Sharma, V. N., and Lohiya, N. K. (1974) The effect of chronically administered cannabis extract on the testicular function of mice. *Eur. J. Pharmacol.* **26**, 111–114.
8. Ehling, U. H. (1974) Differential spermatogenic response of mice to the induction of mutations by antineoplastic drugs. *Mutat. Res.* **26**, 285–295.
9. Esber, H. J., Rosenkrantz, H., and Bogden, A. E. (1976) Assessment of the effect of Δ⁹ tetrahydrocannabinol on testicular and thyroid hormone levels in rats. *Fed. Proc.* **35**, 727.
10. Fleischman, R. W., Hayden, D. W., Rosenkrantz, H., and Braude, M. C. (1975) Teratologic evaluation of ⁹-tetrahydrocannabinol in mice, including a review of the literature. *Teratology* **12**, 47–50.
11. Fournier, E., Rosenberg, E., Hardy, N., and Nahas, G. G. (1976) Teratologic effects of cannabis extracts in rabbits: a preliminary study. In: *Marihuana Chemistry, Biochemistry and Cellular Effects* Nahas, G. G. ed.). Springer-Verlag, New York, pp. 457–468.
12. Haley, S. L., Wright, P. L., Plank, J. B., Keplinger, M. L., Braude, M. C., and Calandra, J. C., (1973) The effect of natural and synthetic ⁹-tetrahydrocannabinol on fetal development. *Toxicol. Appl. Pharmacol.* **25**, 450. (abstract).
13. Harbison, R. D., Mantilla-Plata, B., and Lubin, S. J. (1977) Alteration of Δ⁹-tetrahydrocannabinol induced teratogenicity by stimulation and inhibition of its metabolism. *J. Pharmacol. Exp. Ther.* **202**, 455–465.
14. Heddle, J. A. (1973) A rapid in vivo test for chromosomal damage. *Mutat. Res.* **18**, 187–190.
15. Heddle, J. A. and Bruce, W. R. (1977) On the use of multiple assays for mutagenicity, especially the micronucleus, Salmonella, and sperm abnormality assays. In: *Progress in Genetic Toxicology.* Scott, D. Bridges B. A. and Sobels, F. H. eds.). Elsevier/North-Holland Biomedical Press, Amskradam, pp. 265–274.

16. Hembree, W. C., Zeidenberg, P., and Nahas, G. G. (1976) Marihuana's effects on human gonadal function. In: *Marihuana, Chemistry, Biochemistry and Cellular Effects* (Nahas, G. G., ed.). Springer-Verlag, New York, pp. 521–532.

17. Hugenholtz, A. P. and Bruce, W. R. year? Induction and transmission of elevated levels of abnormality shaped murine sperm. *Can. J. Genet. Cytol.*, in press.

18. Joneja, M. G. (1976) A study of teratological effects of intravenous, subcutaneous and intragastric administration of ^{9}-tetrahydrocannabinol in mice. *Toxicol. Appl. Pharmacol.* **36**, 151–162.

19. Joneja, M. G. (1977) Effects of ^{9}-tetrahydrocannabinol on hamster fetuses. *J. Toxicol. and Environ. Health* **2**, 1031–1040.

20. Kolodny, R. C. Masters, W. H., Kolodner, R. M., and Toro, G. (1974) Depression of plasma testosterone levels after chronic intensive marihuana use. *N. Engl. J. Med.* **290**, 872–874.

21. Kolodny, R. C., Lessin, P., Toro, G., Masters, W. H., and Cohen, S. (1976) Depression of plasma testosterone with acute marihuana administration. In: *Pharmacology of Marihuana* (Braude, M. C. and Szara, S, eds.). Raven, New York, pp. 217–225.

22. Legator, M. S., Weber, E., Connor, T., and Stoeckel, M. (1976). Failure to detect mutagenic effects of Δ^9-tetrahydrocannabinol in the dominant lethal test host-mediated assay, blood- urine studies and cytogenetic evaluation with mice. In: *Pharmacology of Marihuana* (Braude, M. C. and Szara, S., eds.). Raven, New York, pp. 699–709.

23. Macleod, J., Hotchkiss, R. S., and Sitterson, B. W. (1964) Recovery of male fertility after sterilization by nuclear radiation. *J. Am. Ass.* **187**, 637–641.

24. Mantilla-Plata, B. and Harbison, R. (1976) Alteration of Δ^9-tetrahydrocannabinol induced prenatal toxicity by phenobarbital and SKF-525A. In: *Marihuana, Chemistry, Biochemistry and Cellular Effects* (Nahas, G. G. ed.). Springer-Verlag, New York, pp. 469–480.

25. Mantilla-Plata, B. Clewe, G. L., and Harbison, R. D. (1975) ^{9}-tetrahydrocannabinol-induced changes in prenatal growth and development of mice. *Toxicol. Appl. Pharmacol.* **33**, 333–340.

26. Mendelson, J. H., Kuehnle, J., Ellingboe, J., and Babor, T. F. (1974) Plasma testosterone levels before, during and after chronic marihuana smoking. *N. Engl. J. Med.* **291**, 1051–1055.

27. Nahas, G. G., (ed.) (1976) *Marihuana Chemistry, Biochemistry and Cellular Effects.* Springer-Verlag, New York.

28. Oakberg, E. F. and Diminno, R. L. (1960) X-ray sensitivity of primary spermatocytes of the mouse. *Intern. J. Radiation. Biol.* **2**, 196–209.

29. Okey, A. B. and Truant, G. S. (1975) Cannabis demasculinizes but is not estrogenic. *Life Sci.* **17**, 1113–1118

30. Pace, H. B., Davis, W. M., and Borgen, L. A. (1971) Teratogenesis and marihuana. *Ann. N.Y. Acad. Sci.* **191**, 123–131

31. Rosenkrantz, H. and Braude, M. C. (1976) Comparative chronic toxicities of ^{9}-THC administered by inhalation or orally in rats. In *Pharmacology of Marihuana* (Braude, M. C. and Szara S., eds.). Raven, New York, pp. 571–584.

32. Schaefer, C. F., Gunn, C. G., and Dubowski, K. M. (1975) Normal plasma testosterone concentrations after marihuana smoking. *N. Engl. J. Med.* **292**, 867–868.

33. Stoeckel, M., Weber, E., Connor, T., and Legator, M. S. (1975) Failure to detect mutagenic effects of ^{9}-tetrahydrocannabinol in *in vitro* and *in vivo* studies with mice. *Murat. Res.* **31**, 313–314.

34. Symons, A. M., Teale, J. D., and Marks, V. (1976) Effect of ^{9}-tetrahydrocannabinol on the hypothalamicpituitary-gonadal system in the maturing male rat. *J. Endocrinol.* **68**, 43P–44P (abstract)

35. Thomas, R. J. (1975) The toxicologic and teratologic effects of $^9\Delta$-tetrahydrocannabinol in the Zebrafish embryo. *Toxicol. Appl. Pharmacol.* **32**, 184–190.

36. Von Ledebur, M., and Schmid, W. (1973) The micronucleus test. Methodological aspects. *Mutat. Res.* **19**, 109–117.

37. Wyrobek, A. J. and Bruce, W. R. (1975) Chemical induction of sperm abnormalities in mice. *Proc. Nat. Acad. Sci. U.S.A.* **72(11)**, 4425–4429.

38. Wyrobek, A. J. and Bruce, W. R. The induction of sperm shape abnormalities in mice and humans. In *Chemical Mutagens* Hollaender, A. and de Serres, eds.). Plenum, New York, in press.

39. Wyrobek, A. J., Heddle, J. A., and Bruce, W. R. (1975) Chromosomal abnormalities and the morphology of mouse sperm heads. *Can. J. Genet. Cytol.* **17**, 675–681.

40. Zimmerman, A. M., Bruce, W. R., and Zimmerman, S. (1979) Effects of cannabinoids on sperm morphology. *Pharmacol.* in press.

41. Zimmerman, A. M., Stich, H., and San, R. (1978) Non-mutagenic action of cannabinoids in vitro. *Pharmacol.* **16**, 333–343.

28

Effects of Marihuana Inhalation on Spermatogenesis of the Rat

Hosea F. S. Huang, Gabriel G. Nahas, and Wylie C. Hembree III

Abstract

The effect of marihuana smoking on spermatogenesis was studied in normal mature rats and in post-vitamin-A-treated, vitamin-A-deficient rats. A specific decrease in epididymal sperm was noted only after inhalation of marihuana smoke for a period of 75 days at 16 puffs/day. In the absence of tissue and urine cannabinoid levels, no direct comparison to human use can be made, although the amount of THC, as calculated by Rosenkrantz, is comparable to that used in humans. Spermatogenesis may be specifically affected by marihuana smoking as indicated by increased dissociation of sperm head and tail and by the histological changes observed in seminiferous tubule. Marihuana exposure had little effect on DNA-specific activity after H^3-thymidine administration, although a modest decrease in DNA synthesis, accompanied by a total decrease in germ-cell number, cannot be excluded by this experimental design. Elevations in serum FSH levels following marihuana exposure may indicate a specific and sensitive effect upon Sertoli cell function.

1. INTRODUCTION

The effect of cannabinoids on male gonadal function has been reported frequently. We have found that marihuana smoking in human volunteers resulted in a reduction in sperm count[1] and an increase of abnormal sperm morphology. Although other labs have reported that marihuana smoking caused reduction of serum testosterone. (3), we found no significant change of serum testosterone in our patients (1). The time course of the decline in sperm count suggests that spermatogenesis might be a target for marihuana effects. In rodents, treatment with *cannabis* extracts has been reported to cause spermatogenic arrest, abnormal spermatogenic cell association, and reduction in sperm production (4,5). However, the specificity and mechanism of cannabinoid action upon male gonadal function has not been clarified. In an attempt to investigate the specific effects of marihuana smoking on spermatogenesis of the

From: *Marihuana and Medicine*
Edited by: G. G. Nahas et al. © Humana Press Inc., Totowa, NJ

rat, a series of experiments was undertaken using a special device, a Walton smoke exposure machine, to deliver marihuana smoke to animals in amounts approximating those in human consumption.

2. MATERIALS AND METHODS

Normal mature male Sprague-Dawley rats (250 g) were caged in an air-conditioned, light-controlled animal room, given *ad lib* water and commercial rat pellet. Vitamin-A-deficient (VAD), rats were prepared by raising 21-day-old weanling male Sprague Dawley rats on a vitamin-A-deficient diet *(6)*. Spermatogenesis of vitamin-A-deficient rats was reinitiated by oral feeding of 1 mg vitamin A and maintained by a return to a normal diet.

Marihuana cigarettes, containing approximately 1.75%Δ^9-THC and 0.027% cannabinol, and marihuana placebo cigarettes were supplied by the National Institute on Drug Abuse. All cannabinoid material was stored at 5°C and was maintained at 60% humidity and 22–23% for 48 hours before being used.

2.1 Inhalation Procedure

A Walton smoke exposure machine (Process Instruments, Brooklyn, N Y) with a three-cigarette capacity was used throughout the experiments. Using this machine, rats in each treatment protocol were exposed each morning either to marihuana placebo smoke or to marihuana smoke. Inhalation dosages of marihuana smoke are expressed as number of puffs per exposure. Rats exposed to four and 16 puffs of marihuana smoke inhale approximately 0.4 and 3 mg of Δ^9-THC per kg of body weight according to the calculation method of Rosenkrantz *(7)*.

2.2 Treatment Protocol

Normal mature male rats were assigned to one of the following five groups. Group 1, the laboratory control group, received no treatment throughout the experimental period. Group 2, the machine control group, was allowed to go through the machine for one cycle daily but received no smoke. Group 3, the placebo control group, was exposed to 16 puffs of marihuana placebo cigarette smoke daily. Group 4, the low-inhalation-dosage group, was exposed to four-puffs of marihuana smoke daily. Group 5, the high-inhalation-dosage group, was exposed to 16 puffs of marihuana smoke daily. Two sets of studies were undertaken in which rats received 30 exposures in 30 days and 75 exposures in 90 days.

Animals in experiments using post – vitamin-A-treated, vitamin-A-deficient (PVA-VAD) rats were assigned to one of the following groups. Group 1, machine control group, exposed to machine for one cycle daily for five days before and 10 days after vitamin A feeding. Group 2, placebo control group, exposed to 16 puffs of marihuana placebo cigarette smoke five days before 10 days after vitamin A feeding. Group 3, exposed to 16 puffs of placebo smoke for five days before and to 16 puffs of marihuana smoke for 10-days after vitamin A feeding. Group 4, exposed to 16 puffs of marihuana smoke 10 days before and 10 days after vitamin A feeding.

3. RESULTS

Weight gain was slightly retarded ($p <0.10$) by 30 high-dose marihuana smoke exposures. Although 75 daily exposures to the machine also resulted in reduced growth rate as compared to laboratory control animals, the machine control animals and low-dose-inhalation animals gained significantly more weight than either the placebo control animals or the high-dose-inhalation animals ($p < 0.05$).

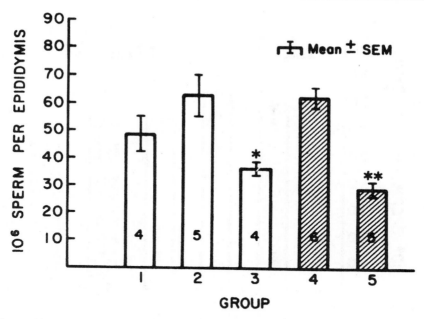

Fig. 1. Effects of 30 daily exposures of marihuana smoke on rat epididymal sperm count, expressed as mean ± SEM × 10⁶. Number inside each bar represents the number of animals used. Group 1, laboratory control. Group 2, machine control. Group 3, placebo control. Group 4, four-puff marihuana. Group 5, 16-puff marihuana.* Significantly different from group 2 ($p < 0.01$);** significantly different from group 1 ($p < 0.05$), groups 2 and 4 ($p < 0.01$) and group 3 ($p < 0.10$)

The testis and seminal vesicle of rats in the high-inhalation group were significantly smaller ($p < 0.05$) when compared to that of laboratory control, machine control, and low-inhalation groups.

Animals in groups 2–5 had a significantly higher adrenal gland weight ($p < 0.05$) than the laboratory control group only after 75 exposures.

The effect of long-term exposure to marihuana smoke on testicular function caused a significantly reduced epididymal sperm count. Although exposure to placebo smoke for 30 days also caused a reduction in total epididymal sperm (Fig. 1), the sperm count in the 16-puff marihuana exposure rats was significantly lower ($p < 0.10$) than that of the placebo-smoking rats. After 75 exposures of 16 puffs of marihuana smoke, sperm production was significantly affected as shown in Fig. 2. Rats that received either placebo smoke or four puffs of marihuana smoke also had lower epididymal sperm count as compared to lab control and machine control groups, although the differences were not statistically significant.

A qualitative change in rat sperm was noted in addition to the quantitative change in sperm number. Sperm taken from the cauda epididymidis of rats exposed to 30 daily 16-puff marihuana smoking tended to have a higher incidence of dissociated head and tail (Fig. 3) as compared to sperm taken from rats of other groups. Quantitation of this observation is currently being undertaken.

Histological observation of testicular sections reveals that there were observable changes after 30 daily exposures to 16-puff marihuana smoke. Dramatic changes were noted after 75 daily exposures to marihuana smoke, however. These abnormalities include early release of spermatocytes and spermatids as well as disorganized or incomplete cellular association, shown in Fig. 4. Note the presence of sperm in most of the tubules of the four-puff mari-

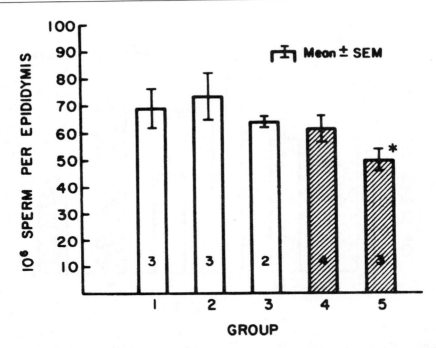

Fig. 2. Effects of 75 daily exposures of marihuana smoke on rat epididymal sperm count, expressed as mean ± SEM × 10⁶. Number inside each bar represents the number of animals used. Experimental design as described in Fig. 1. *Significantly different from groups 1 and 3 ($p < 0.05$) and 2 and 4 ($p < 0.025$).

huana-smoking rats in spite of tubular disorganization and in contrast to the tubules of the 16-puff marihuana-smoking rat.

Twenty-four hours after intratesticular injection of 10 μCi ³H-thymidine, there was no significant change in DNA-specific activity of collagenase, DNAase, trypsin-treated testicular cells[8] in association with high-dose placebo and marihuana smoking. After 75 daily exposures to four-puff marihuana smoke, however, testicular DNA-specific activity increased as compared to machine controls and to laboratory animals.

When PVA-VAD rat model was used, acute marihuana smoking produced a more pronounced effect. Under normal conditions, supermatogenesis of PVA-VAD rats is reinitiated after vitamin A feeding. Pachytene spermatocytes can be seen 10–14 days after vitamin A administration (6). When VAD rats were exposed to 16-puff marihuana smoke for 10 days before vitamin A administration, and then 10 days after vitamin A treatment, regeneration of spermatogenesis was markedly impaired in two of three animals. Both degeneration of pachytene spermatocytes and a decreased proliferation of germ cells were observed.

4. DISCUSSION

Both endocrine and cellular biochemical functions of the testis are directed toward the production of functionally normal male gametes, spermatozoa. Any factor that might alter hormone production or responsiveness, or interfere with cell division or differentiation will be reflected in a decreased efficiency of sperm production. In the rat, in which estimation of sperm production by repeated ejaculation is technically difficult, total epididymal sperm count provides a more accurate index of sperm production. The significant reduction in epi-

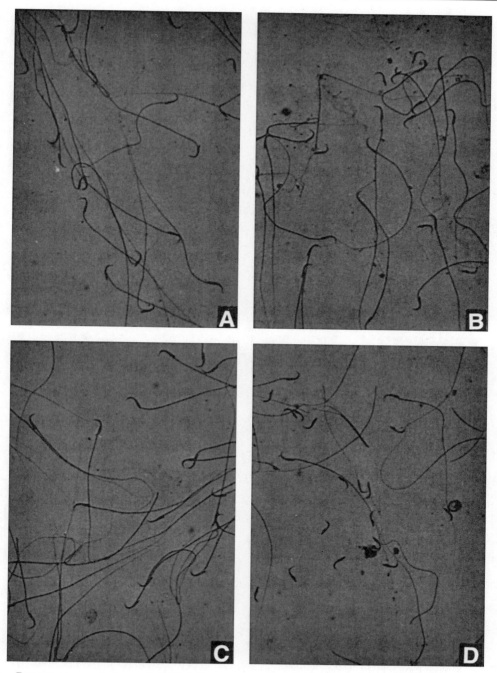

Fig. 3.   Rat sperm morphology after 30 daily exposures to (**A**) machine, (**B**) 16 puffs of placebo mari-huana smoke, (**C**) four puffs of marihuana-smoke, (**D**) 16 puffs of puffs of marihuana smoke.

didymal sperm count after chronic exposure to a high dose of marihuana smoke suggests a specific effect of cannabinoids upon spermatogenesis. After 30 daily exposures of 16 puffs/per day, inhalation of smoke from both placebo and marihuana cigarettes was associated with a significant decrease in sperm count. Smaller amounts of marihuana smoking did not alter sperm count. However, after 75 exposures, epididymal count was normal in placebo-

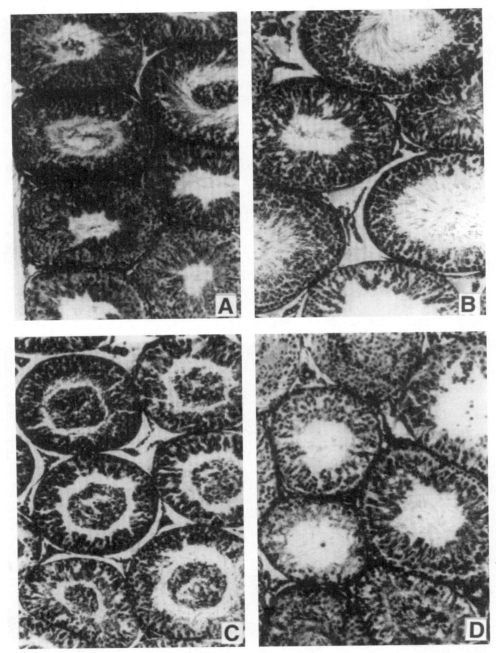

Fig. 4. Photomicrograph of testicular histology from rat after 75 exposures to (**A**) machine, (**B**) 16 puffs of placebo marihuana smoke, (**C**) four puffs of marihuana smoke, (**D**) 16 puffs of marihuana smoke.

smoking rats, whereas reduced sperm number was sustained in the 16-puff marihuana-smoking animals. These data suggest that spermatogenesis may be adversely affected by components of the marihuana placebo, as well as by marihuana. Further, a specific marihuana effect may become apparent only after prolonged exposure. This finding is supported by abnormal cellular association of seminiferous tubules seen after 75 exposures. A similar reduction in sperm count has been reported in mice (4) and rats (5) treated with marihuana extract.

Germ-cell DNA-specific activity following ³H-thymidine injection was used as an index of spermatogonial proliferation. In spite of a significant reduction in epididymal sperm count after 30 daily exposures to large amounts of marihuana smoke, there was no significant change in ³H-thymidine incorporation into testicular DNA. This suggests that inhibition of germ-cell division is not the dominant action of marihuana in the rat. The significance of the increased DNA-specific activity after 75 exposures in the four-puff marihuana group is not certain and requires further study. On the other hand, in the vitamin-A-deficient rat, marihuana smoke does appear to inhibit early spermatogonial proliferation in response to vitamin A. Inhibition of spermatogenic regeneration and depressed testicular incorporation of ³H-thymidine was noted in marihuana-smoking PVA-VAD rats if the VAD rats were exposed to marihuana smoke prior to vitamin A feeding. Studies that define the relationship between spermatogonial proliferation in the VAD and PVA-VAD rat model and that in the normal rat are in progress.

It has been suggested that spermatogenesis may be adversely affected by marihuana smoking in humans (1,9). The higher incidence of dissociated sperm heads and tails, incomplete cellular association, and release of spermatocytes and early spermatids suggest that marihuana smoking may also interfere with spermatogenesis in rats.

Sertoli cells play a central role in the regulation of spermatogenesis. They form the blood–testis barrier regulating the entry of circulating substances into germ cells; each germ cell maintains direct cellular contact with Sertoli cells throughout spermatogenesis and they control the final release of sperm into seminiferous tubules (10). Serum follicle stimulant harm (FSH) is frequently used as an indicator of spermatogenic function, and the FSH-inhibiting factor, inhibin (11,12), may be associated with Sertoli cells (13), the Sertoli cell-spermatogonial unit (14), or with a certain stage of spermiogenesis (2). In humans, an elevated serum FSH is frequently associated with a severe reduction of sperm production or with degenerating seminiferous tubules (15). In preliminary studies, we have found that serum FSH was significantly higher than that of the machine and laboratory control groups in rats exposed to the 16-puff marihuana dose for 30 days and to the four-puff and 16-puff dose for 75 exposures. Placebo exposure did not alter FSH levels. If confirmed, these results indicate that marihuana may alter Sertoli cell or spermatogonial function, prior to or separate from the effect upon sperm production. This effect upon FSH secretion may be more sensitive and specific than other effects previously described.

ACKNOWLEDGMENT

The authors wish to thank Lorraine Billig and Diane T. W. Wang for their technical assistance. This study was supported by NIDA grant 5 ROIDA00894.

Reprinted with permission from Marihuana: Biological Effects, Analysis, Metabolism, Cellular Responses, Reproduction and Brain (G. G. Nahas and W. D. M. Paton, eds.) Pergamon Press, New York, 1979, pp. 419–427.

REFERENCES

1. Hembree, W. C., Zeidenberg, P., and Nahas, G. G. (1976) Marihuana effects upon human gonadal function. In: *Marihuana Chemistry, Biochemistry and Cellular Effects* (Nahas G. G., Paton, W. D. M, and J. Idanpaan Heikkila, eds. Springer-Verlag, New York, pp. 521–532.
2. Huang, H. F. S., Dyrenfurth, I., and Hembree, W. C. (1978) Incomplete feedback regulation of FSH in the vitamin A deficient rat. Annual Meeting of the Endocrine Society, 60th, p. 79.

3. Kolodny, R. C., Masters, W. H., Kolodner, R. M., and Toro, G. (1974) Depression of plasma testosterone levels after chronic intensive marihuana use. *N. Engl. J. Med.* **290**, 872–847.
4. Dixit, V. P., Sharma, V. N., and Lohiya, N. Y. (1974) The effect of chronically administered cannabis extract on the testicular function of mice. *Eur. J. Pharmacol.* **26**, 111–114.
5. Fujimoto, G. 1., Rosenbaum, R. M., Ziegler, D., Rettura, G., and Morrill, G. A. (1978) Effects of marihuana extract given orally on male rat reproduction and gonads. Annual Meeting of the Endocrine Society, p. 373.
6. Huang, H. F. S. and Hembree, W. C. (1978) Hormonal histological and biochemical characteristics of spermatogenesis (SG) in vitamin A deficient (VAD) and in post-vitamin A treated rats. Annual Meeting of the American Society of Andrology, 3rd, p. 39.
7. Rosenkrantz, H. The immune response and marihuana. In: *Marihuana, Chemistry, Biochemistry and Cellular Effects* Nahas, G. G., Paton, W. D. M., and Idänpään-Heikkilä, X. X. eds) Springer-Verlag, N.Y. pp. 441–456, 1976.
8. Bellve, A. R., Cavicchia, J. C., Michelle, C. F., O'brien, D. A., Bhatnagar, Y. M., and Dym, M. (1977) Spermatogenic cells of the prepuberal mouse. Isolation and morphological characterization. *J. Cell. Biol.* **74**, 68–85.
9. Huang, H. F. S., Nahas, G. G., and Hembree, W. C. (1978) Morphological changes of spermatozoa during marihuana induced depression of human spermatogenesis. *Fed. Proc.* **37(3)**, 739.
10. Fawcett, D. W. (1975) Ultrastructure and function of Sertoli cell. In: *Handbook of Physiology* (Hamilton, D. W., and Greep, R. O., eds.) American Physiology Society, Washington, DC pp. 21–55.
11. Mccullagh, D. R. (1932) Dual endocrine activity of the testis. *Science, N.Y.* **76**, 19–20.
12. Setchell, B. P., Davies, R. V., and Main, S. J. (1977) Inhibin. In: The Testis Johnson, A. D. and Gomes, W. R. eds.) Academic, New York pp. 190–227.
13. Steinberger, A. and Steinberger, E. (1976) Secretion of an FSH-inhibiting factor by cultured Sertoli cells. *Endocrinology* **99**, 918–921.
14. Krueger, P. M., Hodgen, G. D., and Sherins, R. J. (1974) New evidence for the role of the Sertoli cell and spermatogonia in feedback control of FSH secretion in male rats.
15. Franchimont, P., Millet, D., Vendesely, E., Letawe, J., Legros, J. J., and Netter, A. (1972) Relationship between spermatogenesis and serum gonadotropin levels in azoospermia and oligospermia. *J. Clinc. Endocr. Metab.* **34**, 1003–1008.

29 Changes in Human Spermatozoa Associated with High-Dose Marihuana Smoking

Wylie C. Hembree III, Gabriel G. Nahas,
P. Zeidenberg, and Hosea F. S. Huang

Abstract

We have shown that 4 wk of high-dose marihuana use (8–20 cigarettes/d) in 16 healthy, chronic marihuana smokers was associated with a significant decline in sperm concentration and total sperm count during the fifth and sixth weeks after the first exposure. This was preceded by a decrease in sperm motility and accompanied by a reduction in the number of sperm with normal morphology. In 12 of 16 subjects, a highly significant decrease was noted, which was sustained until the end of the study in 11 subjects.

No evidence was obtained suggesting a hormonal mechanism for observed effects. The most likely explanation is a direct cannabinoid effect on the germinal epithelium during spermiogenesis. Loss of motility response to cyclic AMP and a phosphodiesterase inhibitor, theophylline, in two subjects indicates that the sperm produced following cannabinoid exposure may also have structural or biochemical defects in sperm function. The improvement in sperm motility following cessation of chronic smoking raises some optimism concerning the reversibility of the abnormalities and, if confirmed in additional subjects, gives further credence to the causal relationship between acute marihuana exposure and the abnormalities subsequently observed. No conclusion can be reached regarding the possibility of adverse effects of acute or chronic marihuana use upon human reproduction. On the other hand, it is essential that further studies be undertaken that will examine this possibility.

Marihuana smoking in men has been reported to reduce testosterone *(13)* and pituitary hormone levels *(14)* and to be associated with gynecomastia *(7)*. We previously reported that 4 wk of inhalation of large quantities of marihuana in a controlled hospital environment was associated with a highly significant decrease in the concentration of ejaculated sperm and in

From: *Marihuana and Medicine*
Edited by: G. G. Nahas et al.   © Humana Press Inc., Totowa, NJ

the total sperm count in three of the four chronic marihuana smokers studied *(8)*. Because the fall in sperm count was neither preceded by nor associated with a significant fall in serum testosterone, luteinizing hormone (LH), and follicle-stimulating hormone (FSH) concentrations in these initial studies, it was proposed that cannabinoids may exert a direct effect on the germinal epithelium, thereby suppressing total sperm production.

Numerous agents are known to exert direct testicular effects. In animals, testosterone alone can maintain normal spermatogenesis *(27)*. By contrast, X-irradiation *(16)*, antimetabolites *(29)*, perhaps estrogens *(1)*, viruses, and the humoral factors associated with an anaphylactic reaction *(18)* are known to reduce the number of ejaculated sperm by direct action on the testis. In addition, genitourinary tract infections can reversibly depress sperm number, motility, and morphology *(3)*. Hypogonadotropism will also result in varying degrees of oligozoospermia. Although "stress" is popularly believed and has been reported to be associated with depression of sperm counts *(15)*, the studies are limited and poorly controlled. Approximately 10% of otherwise normal adult males have idiopathic oligospermia. Most agents known to alter the number of ejaculated sperm also reduce the extent and quality of sperm motility and the fraction of sperm with normal morphology.

The worldwide prevalence of cannabinoid use and proposed clinical applications make it necessary to determine whether cannabinoids exert any effect(s) on the male reproductive system and, if so, whether such effect(s) are harmful and/or reversible. The complexity of the male reproductive system requires that animal model systems be developed to study both the morphological and the biochemical details of the consequences of treatment with cannabinoids. Studies from this and other laboratories are reported elsewhere in this volume *(11)*.

Studies to determine the effects of marihuana smoking on human spermatogenesis have been continued in an effort to investigate the consistency of our initial observations and to determine the specificity of the results. Herein, we report data from 12 additional subjects in whom changes in the number of ejaculated sperm were associated with 1 mo of high-dose cannabinoid exposure; we describe a simple in vitro assay of sperm function and the changes in response to the assay associated with marihuana smoking; and we describe the results using a protocol for examining the *reversibility* of abnormal spermatogenesis in chronic marihuana users.

CLINICAL PROTOCOL

Regular marihuana users, age 18–29, were admitted to the New York State Psychiatric Institute Clinical Research Center for 9–12 wk's, during which time all activities inside and outside the hospital were under 24-hr surveillance. Subjects were selected who had no acute or chronic illnesses known to affect reproductive function. Each had a normal physical examination, including normal testicular size and the absence of a varicocele. Because of the observations made in the initial four subjects, only men with total sperm counts greater than 100 million, normal motility, and normal morphology were selected.

Semen specimens were obtained twice weekly by masturbation and analyzed for routine clinical parameters: volume, concentration, percent motility, progression of motility, and morphology. The period of prior sexual continence was noted. Once weekly, blood was obtained for testosterone, LH, and FSH; a total of five samples drawn at 15-min intervals. This procedure was utilized to ascertain a range of hormone levels, mindful that sampling could occur during the onset or following one of the frequent episodic secretory bursts of LH or FSH release *(23)*. After a 3–4-wk control period during which there was no smoking, each subject was allowed to smoke *ad libitum* marihuana cigarettes prepared by the National Institute of Drug Abuse and standardized to contain 2% Δ^9-tetrahydrocannabinol. The number of cigarettes varied daily between 6 and 20, averaging 8/d throughout the 4-wk smoking period. Subsequently, measurement of each parameter continued during an additional 3–4 wk non-smoking period.

A similar protocol is being utilized in a group of chronic marihuana smokers to study the effect of cannabinoid withdrawal on the characteristics of ejaculated sperm. Subjects are examined by one of us (W.H.) and are screened for multidrug use. Selection is based on the consistent observation of one or more abnormalities of the semen analysis in chronic smokers who have no apparent cause, e.g., a varicocele, genitourinary tract infection, hormone deficiency or excess, or testicular atrophy. Each subject is first studied for 2–3 mo as an outpatient. Although each person who volunteers for the study is motivated in part by his desire to stop using marihuana, only those individuals are selected who indicate that they would continue to smoke if they did not participate. Should anyone desire to stop before completion of the 3-mo outpatient protocol, they are urged to do so; they may continue to participate as nonsmoking outpatients or are admitted if adequate outpatient control data have been obtained.

During the outpatient phase of the study, semen specimens are submitted every 2 wk, five blood samples are drawn for hormone levels and the first-voided morning urine is obtained for total cannabinoids (by radioimmunoassay) and creatinine. Volunteers are then admitted to the General Clinical Research Center of the Presbyterian Hospital for 90 d during which time sperm production is assessed using the same protocol as that employed for the studies of high-dose smoking effects.

Adrenal function is monitored by weekly 24-hr urine samples for 17-ketosteroids and 17-ketogenic steroids, as well as cortisol levels in those samples obtained in weekly blood tests. Subjects may leave the hospital on occasion for less than 8 hr and, upon return, blood alcohol levels are measured and urine is obtained for cannabinoids and a drug screen.

Total urinary cannabinoids are measured by radioimmunoassay, utilizing a modification of the method described by Collaborative Research, Inc. (2) and by Dr. Vincent Marks (28). ^{3}H-Δ^9-tetrahydrocannabinol (11.7 Ci/mmol) was obtained from Collaborative Research, Inc. and purity confirmed by thin layer chromatography (17), [^{14}C] tetrahydrocannabinol (101 μCi/mg, NIDA) was utilized as a standard to ascertain precise standard solubility, and antisera were furnished by Dr. Marks and purchased from Collaborative Research, Inc. Unbound ^{3}H-Δ^9-THC was precipitated by dextran-coated charcoal and log-linear standard curves were obtained over a range from 0.3 to 5.0 ng/tube. Twenty microliter aliquots of diluted urine were assayed in duplicate at four dilutions. For each urine sample assayed, the cannabinoid concentration was calculated using only the data from aliquots containing THC-equivalent amounts of cannabinoids within the standard range. If nonparallelism was demonstrated, the urine was reassayed.

The response of sperm motility to cyclic nucleotides and to phosphodiesterase inhibitors has been reported (24). In known fertile donors, we have shown that the increment in motility produced by addition of theophylline is inversely proportional to the initial motility (9).

In these experiments, semen was diluted in Bavister's solution, control and treatment samples were brought to the concentration of cyclic AMP (10 mM) and theophylline (10 mM), which produces maximal stimulation of motility, each tube was incubated at 37°C in 95% O_2; 5% CO_2, and the percent progressive motility was determined at hourly intervals for four to five hours. A typical response is shown in Fig. 1, the rate of decay of motility in the control samples being approximately the same as that of the treated samples after the initial period of stimulation. Cyclic AMP is often associated with an initial fall in motility below control levels (shown here) or with late stimulation. Thus, percent stimulation is calculated from both 1-hr and 4-hr data. Data are calculated as the fractional motility of the treated sample as

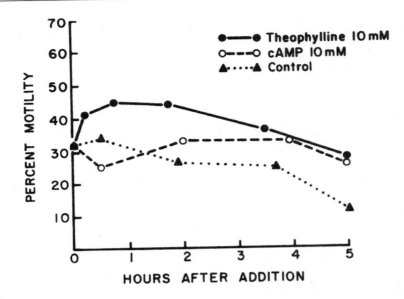

Fig. 1. Response of sperm motility to theophylline and cyclic AMP. Semen was diluted in Bavister's solution and incubated at 37°C in 95% O_2 and 5% CO_2. Percent motility was determined at hourly intervals. Theophylline final concentration (10 mM) and cAMP final concentration (10 mM) are those yielding maximum stimulation in donors.

compared to that of the control and reported as percents: % motility$_{theo}$/% motility$_{control}$ × 100 = percent motility response.

RESULTS

Sperm Concentration

Data from 16 subjects are shown in Fig. 2. Details of semen characteristics from each subject are reported elsewhere *(10)*. The average sperm concentration during the 4-wk presmoking control period was used to normalize individual data during subsequent weeks in each subject so that direct comparisons could be made between subjects and group statistics could be calculated. For the group, a significant reduction in sperm concentration occurred during the first ($p < 0.001$) and second weeks ($p < 0.01$) of the postsmoking period. No significant change in semen volume occurred in any subject. In 12/16 subjects, a sustained decrease in sperm concentration, below the 95% confidence limits calculated for the control period, was observed after 3 wk (five subjects) or 4 wk (two subjects) of smoking, or during the first (three subjects) or second week (two subjects) postsmoking. These decreases were sustained for at least 2 wk and remained low until the end of the study in 11 subjects. There was a trend toward normal in the group as a whole during the third and fourth week postsmoking (Fig. 2). There was also a significant decrease in percent mobility and the percent of sperm with normal morphology, which occurred during the fourth week of smoking and during the first nonsmoking week, respectively.

Motility Response

Response of sperm motility to theophylline and AMP was studied in two subjects, TP and RS. TP had no significant change in sperm concentration, although sperm motility and mor-

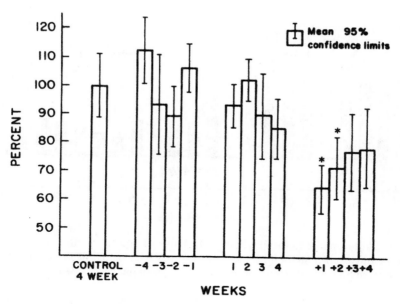

Fig. 2. Marihuana effect upon sperm concentration—grouped data. Sperm concentration for each subject is compared by normalizing each value to the sperm concentration during the control period, using the average from the 4-wk control period as 100%. Brackets represent 95% confidence limits. Numbers on the abscissa represent weeks of study during the presmoking (−4 to − 1), smoking (1 to 4), and post-smoking (+1 to +4) periods. Changes were statistically significant (*) at + 1 wk ($p < 0.001$) and + 2 wk ($p < 0.01$) postsmoking.

phology decreased during the postsmoking period. Although there was no significant decrease in motility, responsiveness to theophylline at 1 h and 4 h began to decrease by the second week of smoking (Fig. 3), with a highly significant loss of responsiveness during the smoking ($p < 0.001$) and postsmoking ($p < 0.001$) periods (Fig. 4). Response to cAMP was also markedly diminished during the postsmoking period. Subject RS, who had smoked large quantities of marihuana in the 2 wk prior to admission, had a significant and sustained fall in sperm count 2 wk after admission. Thus, he was not given additional marihuana, and he agreed to remain in the hospital for the 90-d study period. These data are not included in the 16 subjects. During the first 30 d (presmoking), sperm motility remained normal and motility stimulation was similar to that observed in TP. Marked variations in motility were observed during the designated smoking and postsmoking periods. During the final 30-d, postsmoking period, motility response both to theophylline and to cyclic AMP was virtually absent (Fig. 5).

Marihuana Withdrawal

Complete data on semen characteristics and urinary cannabinoid levels are available in only one subject. JP, a 24-y-old student who used a Bong to smoke 1–2 marihuana cigarettes/d, had urinary cannabinoid levels comparable to subjects smoking 5–10 cigarettes/d. Although sperm concentration and total sperm counts were normal (Fig. 6), percent motility was abnormal (Fig. 7). After admission, urinary cannabinoid levels declined to the limit of assay detection within 5 d and remained low, except for four admitted indiscretions of a single cigarette (days 109, 114, 120, and 152). Only one semen specimen, which was obtained after 10 d of sexual continence and following an 8-d emergency pass for personal business, contained a significantly increased sperm density (day 108). Otherwise, there was no other

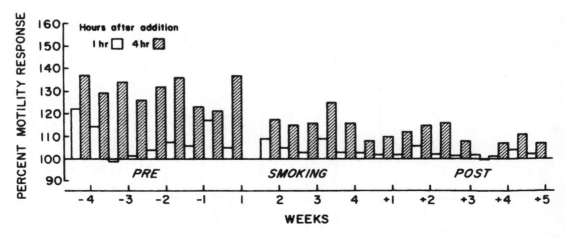

Fig. 3. Sperm motility response to theophylline. Calculation of percent motility response is based upon control percent motility at 1 h and 4 h as 100%. (See text.) Bars represent the responses in individual semen specimens from Subject TP. Weeks of the study are shown on the abscissa.

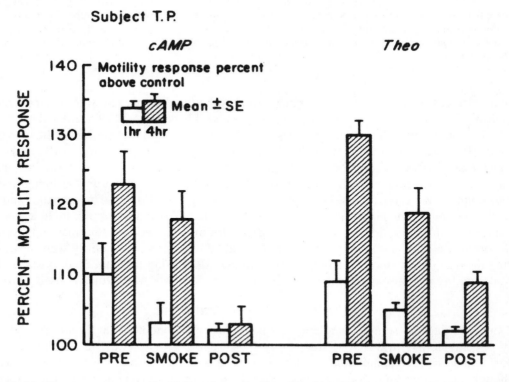

Fig. 4. Motility response to cyclic AMP and theophylline. In subject TP, the average motility response to cAMP (left) and to theophylline (right) during the presmoking control period (PRE), smoking period (SMOKE), and postsmoking period (POST) are shown 1 h (open bar) and 4 h (hatched bar). Brackets represented two standard errors; 1 h responses to cAMP are decreased during the smoking and postsmoking periods ($p < 0.001$). Responses to theophylline are also decreased at both 1 h ($p < 0.01$) and 4 h ($p < 0.001$).

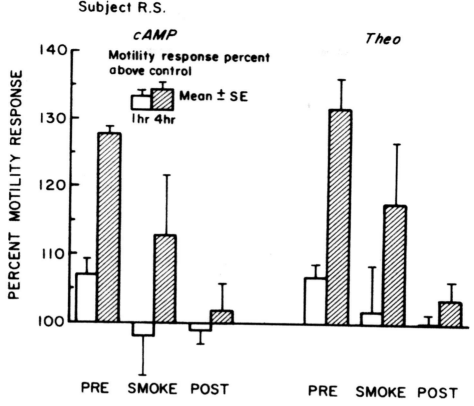

Fig. 5. Motility response to cyclic AMP and theophylline. Subject RS, as in Fig. 4. No marihuana was smoked during the 12-wk study. (See text.) Responses to cAMP and theophylline are reduced at 1 h and 4 h only during the postsmoking period ($p < 0.001$) (week, 9–12).

significant increase in sperm density, total sperm count, or semen volume (Fig. 7). However, sperm motility rose to normal levels within 40 d of hospitalization ($p < 0.01$) and remained increased throughout ($p < 0.05$). Analyses of sperm morphology, though incomplete, indicate an increase in abnormal, nonovoid forms of sperm, with a marked alteration of the acrosome (Fig. 8).

DISCUSSION

Sperm production is a complex process requiring 74 d within the testicular tubule with an average of 11 d transit time, thereafter, required for sperm to appear in the ejaculate. The variability in the number of sperm per ejaculate in serial specimens has been well documented *(6,25)*, with the coefficients of variation ranging between 10 and 40%. In serial specimens, only sperm morphology remains constant *(19)*, in the absence of major perturbing events. Thus, in this experimental design in which sperm number is compared before and after marihuana exposure, there must be an average change of 20–80% (depending on the variance in each sample) if the change is to attain statistical significance. The optimal control period for assessing sperm production and sperm quality is 6 mos, or two spermatogenic cycles, with semen specimens obtained at regular intervals of no less than every 2 wk *(25)*. In this manner, a realistic determination can be made of individual variability while spontaneous trends in

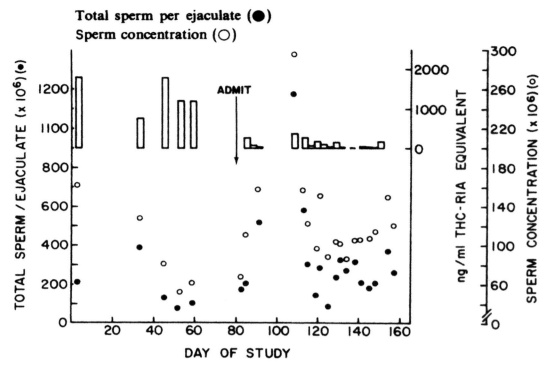

Fig. 6. Sperm production following marihuana withdrawal. Subject JP. Total sperm per ejaculate (*) is shown on the left and sperm concentration (○) on the far right. Urinary cannabinoids at ng/mL of THC radioimmunoassay equivalent are shown by open bars on the near right. Hospitalization and cessation of marihuana began d 80 of the study.

data tend to exclude gonadotropin inhibition, with secondary Leydig cell suppression, as a likely mechanism.

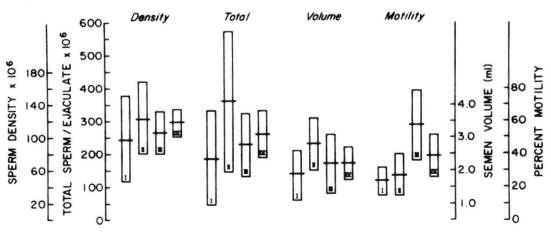

Fig. 7. Changes in semen characteristics following marihuana withdrawal. Subject JP. Open bars represent the 95% confidence limits and horizontal lines the mean sperm density, total sperm per ejaculate, semen volume, and percent sperm motility in semen specimens obtained during d 1–60 (I), d 80–115 (II), d 116–140 (III), and d 140–160 (IV) of the study. Sperm motility was significantly greater than control (I) during periods III ($p < 0.01$) and IV ($p < 0.05$). No other significant changes were noted.

sperm production can be excluded. Attempts to ensure that the period of sexual continence prior to ejaculation is approximately the same for each analysis will reduce the intrinsic experimental variability. This is especially true if sperm number is low. In our experiments, a period of 36–60 h of prior sexual continence was requested. Compliance was not always observed, perhaps accounting for the broad fluctuations observed in some subjects.

In the data reported herein, four to eight specimens were examined during the 4-wk control period; the coefficients of variation were in the predictable range. Data from 2-wk periods were grouped for comparison to the control period and an average decrease in sperm density of 35% was required to achieve statistical significance. The probability that four successive samples would fall below the 95% confidence limits is less than 1%. Thus, the significance of the changes observed in the grouped data was confirmed by linear analyses in 12/16 of the individual subjects.

A limitation in the interpretation of quantitative studies of human spermatogenesis is the fact that sperm number per ejaculate may not directly correlate with sperm production. Rather, sperm count is also a function of smooth muscle contraction of the ductus deferens, ampulla of the vas, and seminal vesicle (through the thoracic–lumbar–sympathetic outflow) (12), closure of the posterior bladder neck (sympathetic and parasympathetic) and of clonic contraction of pelvic striated muscle (parasympathetic sacral outflow). In our studies, we cannot exclude the possibility that marihuana smoking results in deficient ampullary and ductus deferens contraction; there would be no alteration in seminal fluid volume. However, if bladder neck closure was incomplete, causing partial retrograde ejaculation, or if prostatic and/or seminal vesicle fluid emission was reduced, there would have been a decrease in semen volume. This was observed in only one subject, although change in seminal fluid volume preceded that in the total sperm count.

Acute and chronic prostatitis or seminal vesiculitis may result in abnormalities of sperm number, motility, and morphology (3). Similarly, acute viral infection can totally abolish sperm count, presumably because of a transient orchitis (18). None of our subjects had evidence of male reproductive tract infection and each denied a history of recent illness. It is unlikely that a randomly acquired infectious process could have been responsible for the decline in sperm number, which bore a synchronous relationship to the protocol. Only four subjects were hospitalized at a time and the study of the 16 subjects took place over a 2-y period.

It must be emphasized that our data do not establish that the observed changes in semen characteristics were caused by effects of inhaled cannabinoids upon the testis. Yet, alternative explanations are either highly unlikely or untestable in the human. Thus, if the data are a reflection of changes in sperm production, it is appropriate to consider possible mechanisms. First, an indirect effect of THC on spermatogenesis could result from hormone suppression, either at the hypothalamic–pituitary level or at the Leydig cell level. Although no sustained reduction in LH, FSH, or testosterone could be demonstrated, this experimental design could not exclude the possibility that intermittent acute suppression is associated with smoking. Whether intermittent gonadotropin suppression causes a reduction in sperm number is not known. However, induction of temporary azoospermia by exogenous testosterone has been utilized as a therapeutic measure in oligospermic individuals (22), the mechanism of suppression being pharmacologic hypogonadotropism. In our experience, administration of 200 mg testosterone enanthate every 2 wk causes a sustained suppression of both LH and FSH within 1 wk after the first injection. Reduction of sperm number below the 95% confidence limits was observed in a few patients by 6 wk, although the average time required was 8 wk. This is in contrast to the 4-wk average onset of statistically significant changes following high-dose marihuana smoking. Another difference is that hormonally induced azoospermia is associated with either improvement or lack of change in sperm motility and morphology. Thus, our

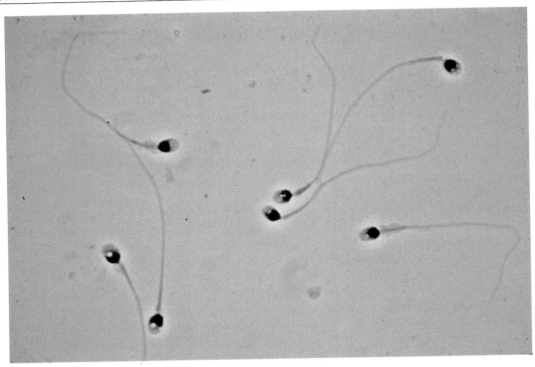

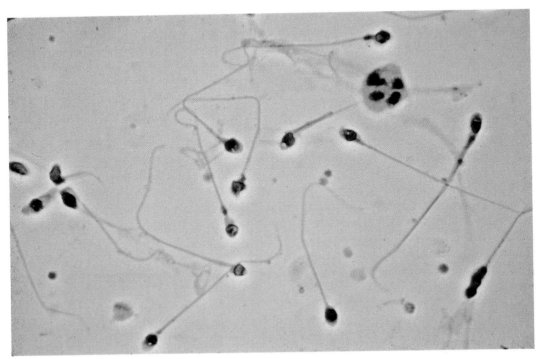

Fig. 8. *Top:* Normal ovoid shape human spermatazoa sampled from tobacco smoker and moderate alcohol drinker. *Bottom:* Nonovoid and immature form present among ovoid shape human spermatazoa sampled from daily marihuana smoker.

Marihuana has been reported to exert estrogenic effects in rodents and in men (7,26). Both THC and marihuana extracts are found to be active agonists in in vitro assays of estrogenic activity (21). Estrogen is known to induce azoospermia via gonadotropin suppression and direct testicular effects, although evidence of neither was noted. Therefore, unless there is selective testicular uptake of marihuana products, direct action on the germinal epithelium via an estrogen (or antiandrogen) mechanism is unlikely.

Δ^9-THC has been reported to alter membrane stability and to interfere with cell division and metabolism by a nonspecific change in membrane permeability (4). The time of maximum effect noted in these studies, 4–5 wk after initiation of marihuana smoking, is consistent with an action upon spermiogenesis. This phase of spermatogenesis, which is primarily morphogenetic, is coordinated through the Sertoli cell, which maintains membrane contact with all germ cells. Sertoli cells contain highly complex, membranous subcellular organelles that are contiguous to developing spermatids (5). Functional or anatomic disruption of Sertoli cell function could reduce sperm number, as well as result in the production of abnormally shaped sperm and/or sperm in which the biochemical and structural machinery for motility is altered. It should be pointed out that the total 8-wk study period in this protocol is not sufficient time to observe any changes that might have occurred as a result of decreased spermatogonial division, increased spermatogonial degeneration, or inhibition of meiosis. Such effects would have been manifested between 40 and 80 d following marihuana exposure.

Few methods are available to assess the fertilizing capacity of human sperm in vitro. Specific anatomical defects in sperm are associated with absence of biochemical properties, e.g., ATPase phosphohydrolase deficiency and absence of sperm tail dynein arms in situs inversus (20). Recently, we have attempted to develop assay systems the responses to which correlate with the fertilizing capacity of sperm. Abnormal responses of sperm motility to the phosphodiesterase inhibitors, theophylline and caffeine, have been reported (21). In this study, we showed progressive loss of responsiveness to both theophylline and to cyclic AMP in two marihuana subjects. It remains to be determined whether this abnormality is characteristic of sperm in chronic marihuana smokers (Fig. 8). Although there are no data in humans which suggest that marihuana adversely affects reproduction, it is essential that efforts be made to characterize the abnormalities noted and to assess their potential consequences upon reproductive capacity and fetal development. It is hoped that studies of this type will shed some light on this possibility.

We have begun studies to determine the extent to which abnormalities in ejaculated sperm found in chronic marihuana smokers are reversible. The results of the study reported herein indicate that an improvement in sperm motility occurred 35 d after hospital admission and cessation of marihuana smoking. Sperm morphology and hormone data are not yet complete. Although we can conclude nothing from this single study, it does indicate that an improvement in semen characteristics can occur during hospitalization, unlike the previous studies in which sperm motility either declined or remained unchanged. Such observations, if confirmed, speak against the results as being nonspecific effects of hospitalization and further validate the claim of a specific marihuana effect.

ACKNOWLEDGMENT

This study was supported by NIDA grant 5ROIDA 00894. The collaboration of Drs. Sidney Malitz, Jerome Jaffe, and Donald Klein of the New York State Psychiatric Institute is gratefully acknowledged.

Reprinted with permission from Marihuana: Biological Effects, Analysis, Metabolism, Cellular Responses, Reproduction and Brain (G. G. Nahas and W. D. M. Paton, eds.), Pergamon, Press, New York, 1979, pp. 429–439.

REFERENCES

1. Adler, A., Burger, H., Davis, J., Dalmonis, A., Hudson, B., Sarfaty, G. and Stratton, M. (1968) Carcinoma of prostate: Response of luteinizing hormone and testosterone to oestrogen therapy. *Br. Med. J.* 1–28.
2. Chase, A. R., Kelley, P. R., Taunton-Rigby, A., Jones, R. T. and Harwood, T. (1976) Quantitation of Cannabinoids in Biological Fluids by Radioimmunoassay. Research Monograph Series #7, Cannabinoid Assays in Humans, US HEW Alcohol, Drug Abuse and Mental Health Administration.
3. Derrick, F. C. and Dahlberg, B. (1976) Male genital tract infections and sperm viability, in *Human Semen and Fertility Regulation in Men* (E. S. E. Hafez, eds.), Mosby, St. Louis, MO, p. 389.
4. Desoize, B., Leger, C., Banchereau, J. and Nahas, G. G. (1978) Inhibitory effects of diazepam and other psychotropic drugs on blastogenesis of cultured T lymphocytes. *Fed. Proc.* **37**, 739.
5. Dym, M. and Cavicchia, J. C. (1978) Functional morphology of the testis. *Biol. Reprod.* **18**, 1–15.
6. Freund, M. (1963) Effect of frequency of emission on semen output and on estimate of daily sperm production in man. *J. Reprod. Fertil.* **6**, 269.
7. Harmon, J. and Aliapoulios, M. A. (1972) Gynecomastia in marihuana users. *N. Engl. J. Med.* **287**, 936.
8. Hembree, W. C., Zeidenberg, P. and Nahas, G. G. (1976) Marihuana's effects on human gonadal function, in *Marihuana: Chemistry, Biochemistry, and Cellular Effects*, (Nahas, G. G., ed.), Springer-Verlag, New York.
9. Hembree, W. and Overstreet, J. (1977) Defects in human sperm function in clinical infertility. reduced zona pellucida penetration in vitro, in *The Testis in Normal and Infertile Men* (P. Troen and H. R. Nankin, eds.), Raven Press, New York, p. 513.
10. Hembree, W. C., Zeidenberg, P., Nahas, G. G., Dyrenfurth, I. and Linkie, D. Evidence for a direct effect of marihuana smoking upon the characteristics of ejaculated human spermatozoa, in preparation.
11. Huang, H. F. S., Nahas, G. G. and Hembree, W. C. Effects of Marihuana Inhalation on Spermatogenesis of the Rat, this volume, Chapter 27.
12. Kedia, K. and Markland, C. (1975) *Effect of Sympathectomy and Drugs on Ejaculation in Control of Male Fertility* (Q. J. Sciarra, C. Markland, and J. J. Speidel, eds.), Harper and Row, New York. p. 240.
13. Kolodny, R. C., Masters, W. H., Kolodner, R. M. and Toro, G. (1974) Depression of plasma testosterone levels after chronic intensive marihuana use. *N. Engl. J. Med.* **290**, 872.
14. Kolodny, R. C. (1975) Paper Presented at First Meeting of the International Academy of Sex Research, State University of New York at Stony Brook, 13 September.
15. Kreuz, L. E., Rose, R. M. and Jennings, J. R. (1972) Suppression of plasma testosterone levels and psychological stress. *Arch. Gen. Psychiat.* **26**, 479.
16. Lacy, D. (1963) Comparison of effects produced by high doses of ionizing radiation and oestrogenic hormone on the seminiferous tubules of rat testes, in *Effects of Ionizing Radiation on the Reproductive System* (W. D. Carlson and F. X. Gassner, eds.), Pergamon Press, Oxford, England, p. 103.
17. Leighty, E. G. (1973) Metabolism and distribution of cannabinoids in rats after different methods of administration. *Biochem. Pharmacol.* **22**, 1613.
18. Macleod, J. (1967) A testicular response during and following a severe allergic reaction. *Fertil. Steril.* **13**, 531.
19. Macleod, J. and Gold, R. Z. (1951) The male factor in fertility and infertility. II. Spermatozoon counts in 1000 men of known fertility and in 1000 cases of infertile marriage. *J. Urol.* **66**, 436.
20. Peterson, H. and Rebbe, H. (1975) Absence of arms in the axoneme of immobile human. Spermatozoa. *Biol. Reprod.* **12**, 541.
21. Rifka, S. M., Sauer, M., Hawks, R. L., Cutler, G. B. and Loriaux, D. L. (1978) Marihuana as an estrogen. Ann. Meeting, The Endocrine Soc., 60th, p. 200.
22. Rowley, M. J. and Heller, C. G. (1972) The testosterone rebound phenomenon in the treatment of male infertility. *Fertil. Steril.* **23**, 498.
23. Santen, R. J. and Bardin, C. W. (1973) Episodic luteinizing hormone secretion in man. Pulse analysis, clinical interpretation, physiologic mechanisms. *J. Clin. Invest.* **52**, 2617.
24. Schoenfeld, C., Amelar, R. D. and Dubin, L. (1975) Stimulation of ejaculated human spermatozoa by caffeine. *Fertil. Steril.* **26**(2), 158.
25. Sherins, R. J., Brightwell, D. and Sternthal, P. M. (1977) Longitudinal analysis of semen of fertile and infertile men, in *The Testis in Normal and Infertile Men* (P. Troen and H. R. Nankin, eds.), Raven Press, New York, p. 473.
26. Solomon, J., Cocchia, M. A., Gray, R., Shattuck, D. and Vossmer, A. (1976) Uterotropic effects of delta-9-tetrahydrocannabinol in ovariectomized rats. *Science* **192**, 559.
27. Steinberger, E., Swerdloff, R. S. and Horton, R. (1977) The control of testicular function, in *Frontier in Reproduction and Fertility Control. A Review of the Reproductive Sciences and Contraceptive Development* (R. O. Greep and M. A. Koblinsky, eds.), The MIT Press, Cambridge, MA. p. 264.
28. Teale, J. D., Forman, E. J., King, L. J., Piall, E. M. and Marks, V. (1975) The development of a radioimmunoassay for cannabinoids in blood and urine. *J. Pharm. Pharmacol.* **27**, 465.
29. Van Thiel, D. H., Sherins, R. J., Myers, G. H., JR. and Devita, V. T., Jr. (1972) Evidence for a specific seminiferous tubular factor affecting follicle stimulating hormone secretion in man. *J. Clin. Invest.* **51**, 1009.

30

Tolerance to the Reproductive Effects of Δ⁹-Tetrahydrocannabinol

Comparison of the Acute, Short-Term, and Chronic Drug Effects on Menstrual Cycle Hormones

Carol Grace Smith, Ramona G. Almirez, Pamela M. Scher and Riccardo H. Asch

1. INTRODUCTION

The reproductive effects of marihuana and Δ⁹-tetrahydrocannabinol (THC) have received much attention from the scientific community for the past several years. Early clinical reports indicated that chronic marihuana use may be associated with decreased hormone levels and infertility. Later studies failed to confirm these findings. Studies in laboratory animals clearly demonstrate that THC has pronounced effects on reproductive hormones and on ovulation and spermatogenesis, and have provided much information on how these effects are produced. These studies have not, however, provided much insight into the apparent discrepancy in the pronounced drug effects reported in laboratory animal studies and the less impressive effects of absence of disruptive effects reported in clinical studies. Since much of our knowledge of human reproductive physiology has been obtained from studies in laboratory animals, it is difficult to ascribe these differences to species variations. It is more likely that the discrepancies in laboratory animal studies and the clinical studies are based on differences in experimental designs and failure to consider the role of the development of drug tolerance in the conclusions of these studies.

The sexually mature rhesus monkey is one of the best experimental animal models for extrapolating to the human reproductive system. The female commonly has a 28-day menstrual cycle that is controlled by negative and positive feedback mechanisms between gonadal steroids and pituitary gonadotropins similar to those found in the human menstrual cycle. Specific amounts of marihuana can be administered to these animals and reproductive parameters can be examined directly. The purpose of this review is to summarize the effects of acute, short-term (less than 30 days), and chronic treatment with THC on the primate men-

From: *Marihuana and Medicine*
Edited by: G. G. Nahas et al.   © Humana Press Inc., Totowa, NJ

strual cycle. Particular emphasis will be place on the studies that examine the development of tolerance to the reproductive effects of THC.

2. RESULTS

2.1. Acute Effects of THC on Menstrual Cycle Hormones

It is now well established that THC decreases the circulating levels of follicle-stimulating hormone (FSH) and luteinizing hormone (LH) in various species (1–4) including primates of both sexes (5). This inhibition in ovariectomized rhesus monkeys ranges from 50 to 80% of basal levels and lasts for up to 24 hours after a single dose (dose dependent). This inhibitory effect can be reversed by the administration of the hypothalamic gonadotropin releasing hormone (GnRH), indicating a hypothalamic site of action for the THC (6,7).

Acute administration of THC also causes a decrease in the circulating levels of prolactin for up to 180 minutes in both male and female rhesus monkeys (8) and in other species (9). This effect on prolactin again indicates a hypothalamic site of action for THC.

The acute effects of THC on menstrual cycle hormones have been studied in the rhesus monkey using both in vivo and in vitro techniques (10). In the in vivo studies, THC (2.5 mg/kg) or vehicle (3% Tween-80 in saline) was administered by an intramuscular injection to rhesus monkeys on day 20, 21, or 22 of the menstrual cycle. Progesterone levels were measured at six-hour intervals for the first 24 hours after treatment. THC caused a significant decrease in progesterone levels during this 24-hour period. This decrease was reversed by the administration of human chorionic gonadotropin (HCG) at six hours after THC administration. This stimulatory effect on HCG could be observed as early as 30 minutes after injection, and normal progesterone levels were observed from 180 minutes to 48 hours after the HCG injection. These results indicate that the acute effect of THC on progesterone levels is mediated by an indirect effect on pituitary gonadotropins rather than direct effects on the ovarian synthesis and secretion of progesterone.

This conclusion is supported by in vitro studies of basal progesterone production by dispersed cells from the rhesus monkey corpus luteum. The corpora lutea were surgically removed from the ovaries six to eight days after ovulation. These dispersed cells will continue to produce progesterone for several hours without adding gonadotropin to the medium. THC or marihuana extract was added to the cell suspension to a final concentration of up to 50 mcM. Neither THC nor marihuana extract had any effect on progesterone production at any concentration up to 50 mcM (limit of drug solubility). However, a number of other in vitro studies with cannabinoids have shown that these drugs disrupt gonadal steroidogenesis, protein and nucleic acid synthesis, glucose utilization, prostaglandin synthesis, and cyclic AMP concentrations in various species including mice, rats, and pigs and in various tissues including Leydig cells, granulosa cells, and luteal cells (11–15). Clearly, the weight of evidence points to a pronounced in vitro effect of THC on gonadal function.

This generates a conflict between the in vivo studies that show no direct effect on gonadal steroid production with these in vitro results; therefore, special attention to the details of the in vitro methods is warranted. All of the cannabinoids studied in these in vitro systems are poorly water soluble. If the solubility of the compound is exceeded, the actual tissue level may be greater than the concentration added to the medium. Unlike the studies with dispersed luteal cells from rhesus monkeys, most of the other in vitro systems use tissues that require the addition of a gonadotropin to the incubation medium to stimulate steroid production. The integrity of the in vitro environment and the function of the poly peptide hormones added to the incubations may be compromised in the presence of these drugs. Until adequate information is available on the actual levels of these drugs in the media and in the tissues and on the chemical identity of the drugs throughout the incubation period, the conclusions drawn from all in vitro studies will remain tentative.

2.2. Short-Term Effects of THC on Menstrual Cycle Hormones

The effects of short-term administration of THC on the menstrual cycle in the rhesus monkey has been studied in our laboratories. One such study examined the effect of THC administration on follicular development and ovulation (16). The rhesus monkeys used in these studies had normal menstrual cycles. The first day of menses was designated as day I of the cycle, and ovulation normally occurs on about day 15 (average day 15 ± 1 day SD). To determine whether THC administration would affect ovulation in these monkeys, THC (2.5 mg/kg) or vehicle (3% Tween-80 in saline) was injected daily from day 1 to day 18 of the cycle. Blood was drawn daily from days 8 to 18 of the cycle and then every other day until the occurrence of menses. The hormones that were measured included total estrogens, LH, and progesterone. Serial laparoscopies were done twice weekly to observe follicular maturation, ovulation, and corpus luteum formation. None of the five THC-treated monkeys exhibited estrogen rises of LH surges, and none of the THC-treated monkeys ovulated before the next menses. The period of disruption that followed the short-term THC treatment ranged from 55 to 145 days. After this period, normal hormone levels and ovulation were observed in all monkeys. This study shows that the inhibitory effect of THC on gonadotropin secretion is sufficient to disrupt ovulation and that the subsequent disruption of the menstrual cycle may last as long as several months. When exogenous gonadotropins were administered to monkeys treated with THC during the first 18 days of the cycle, ovulation was restored and normal luteal function followed. The successful induction of ovulation and normal luteal function in this study using exogenous gonadotropins in the presence of antiovulatory doses of THC clearly supports the hypothesis of a central action of the drug rather than an action directly at the gonad. These results are consistent with studies from other laboratories that show that THC treatment causes an inhibition of ovulation in rats (7) and rabbits (3) by a reversible inhibition of gonadotropin secretion.

Similar results were obtained in studies in which THC was administered to rhesus monkeys during the luteal phase of normal ovulatory cycles (17). The daily administration of THC (2.5 mg/kg) had no effect on serum progesterone levels or on the length of the luteal phase. Again, the posttreatment period was marked by an absence of normal levels of estrogens, gonadotropins, and progesterone. The prolactin levels recorded during the posttreatment period were four to five times greater than prolactin levels in normal ovulatory cycles. A separate study was done in which increasing doses of HCG were administered from days 6 to 10 after ovulation (day 6, 30 IU; day 7, 60 IU; day 8, 90 IU; day 9, 180 IU; day 30, 360 IU). This treatment with HCG during the luteal phase in control animals resulted in augmentation of the progesterone levels to four to five times greater than those of control cycles. The daily injections of THC (2.5 mg/kg) had no effect on the HCG-induced progesterone rise when compared to either vehicle treatment or control responses. These results show that THC has no direct effect on luteal function during normal cycles. Further, THC has no direct effect on corpus luteum function stimulated by HCG administration. The lack of an effect of THC on HCG-stimulated corpus luteum function is particularly important, since this experimental condition mimics progesterone secretion in early pregnancy.

2.3. Chronic Effects of THC on the Primate Menstrual Cycle

Drug tolerance can be defined as a decrease in pharmacologic response that results from prior exposure to the drug. This phenomenon has been reported with repeated administration of THC in humans and laboratory animals to the behavioral and cardiac effects of THC administration. Tolerance can develop by several mechanisms including metabolic tolerance or an increased metabolic clearance of the drug from the body. Cellular or adaptive tolerance occurs when the organ system through homeostatic mechanisms loses its sensitivity to the drug's actions. Either of these mechanisms could be involved in the development of tolerance to the reproductive effects of THC. The chronic studies described here were designed to study the effects of chronic THC on the primate menstrual cycle and to examine the mechanisms involved in the development of tolerance. The study was designed to continue drug treatment for at least one year or until tolerance developed and normal cycles were restored.

Five female rhesus monkeys with normal menstrual cycles were used in this study. Ovulation was detected by monitoring plasma estrogen, LH, and progesterone levels and by laparoscopic examination. Daily vaginal swabbings were utilized to detect the onset of vaginal bleeding and duration of menses. Each monkey was followed for one control cycle and one vehicle treatment cycle before the THC treatment began. On day 1 of the third cycle the monkeys began receiving thrice weekly injections of 2.5 mg/kg THC or 1.25 mg/kg THC. The injections were given on a Monday-Wednesday-Friday schedule (at noon), and blood sampled on each treatment day immediately before injection. THC was obtained from the National Institute on Drug Abuse in solution in absolute ethanol. The ethanol was evaporated under a constant stream of nitrogen gas, and the residue was homogenized in Emulphor (polyethoxylated vegetable oil and ethanol) in saline. The drug or vehicle was administered by an intramuscular injection. The blood level of THC obtained with the 2.5 mg/kg dose of THC given three times per week in monkeys is equivalent to moderate-to-heavy use of marihuana (five to six joints per day; three times per week). Blood levels of THC were measured by RIA where adequate serum was available after hormone measurements (19). The maximum blood level of THC was an average of 300 ng/mL at 60 minutes after injection. The blood level had decreased to an average of 20 ng/mL by 12 hours, and this trough level was maintained until the next dose at 48 hours. These parameters did not change significantly throughout the studies.

All monkeys exhibited normal hormone levels and ovulation during the control and vehicle cycles. Cycle lengths were within normal limits for the colony. After the drug injections began, none of the monkeys ovulated or showed normal hormone levels. After the tolerance to the drug effects developed, normal cycles were reestablished. Ovulation was again detected by laparoscopy and normal hormone levels were observed.

Vehicle administration produced no significant change in prolactin levels. The comparisons were made between pretreatment prolactin values from control and vehicle cycles (sample size about 24 values/monkey); treatment prolactin values during the period of disruption (sample size about 48 values/monkey); and prolactin values during the two cycles after tolerance (sample size 24 values/monkey). There appears to be some decrease in the average prolactin levels during the period of disruption produced by the chronic drug treatment for the three monkeys treated with the 2.5 mg/kg dose of THC (19C; 103C; 237C). Whether this is caused by direct drug effects or is secondary to disrupted menstrual cycles cannot be determined. It is clear, however, that the previously observed elevations in prolactin levels following discontinuation of short-term drug treatment are not observed with chronic drug treatment. Some recovery in the average prolactin level was observed after tolerance developed and normal menstrual cycles were restored in these three monkeys.

3. DISCUSSION

This chronic study demonstrates the disruptive effects of chronic THC administration on the primate menstrual cycle. Since both gonadotropins and sex steroids are at basal levels during the period of disruption, it is likely that there is a direct suppression of hypothalamic/pituitary activity. This study also demonstrates that with chronic drug treatment tolerance develops to the inhibitory effect of THC and normal cycles are re-established.

The mechanism for the tolerance to the effect of THC is not known. Tolerance develops to other pharmacologic effects of THC including euphoria and tachycardia. Behavioral tolerance has been reported in rhesus monkeys and was observed in the present study. Preliminary data from this study and complete pharmacokinetic studies in humans and laboratory animals indicate that increased drug metabolism or clearance is not a major factor in the development of tolerance (19). It is likely that the tolerance that develops to the reproductive effects of THC is caused by adaption of neural mechanisms in the hypothalamus rather than to increased metabolism of the drug.

The results of the present study are consistent with the one clinical study of young women who used marihuana regularly (20). These women experienced changes in menstrual cycles associated with decreased prolactin levels. However, the development of tolerance and return to apparently normal menstrual cycles may mean that normally fertile young women who use marihuana regularly may not notice much change in their menstrual cycles. Drug effects may be more obvious during adolescence, in young women who have some other menstrual irregularities, or if pregnancy occurs. The present studies also demonstrate that the development of tolerance must be considered as a variable in reproductive studies in young men and women who use marihuana and may help to explain some of the conflicting data in human and laboratory animal studies.

Reprinted with permission from The Cannabinoids: Chemical, Pharmacologic, and Therapeutic Aspects (Agurell, S.; Dewey, W. and Willette, R., eds.), Academic Press, New York, 1984, pp. 471–485.

REFERENCES

1. Marks, B. H. (1973) Delta-l-tetrahydrocannabinol and luteinizing hormone secretion. *Prog. Brain Res.* **39**, 331.
2. Dalterio, S., Bartke, A., Roberson, C., Watson, D. and Burstein, S. (1978) Direct and pituitary-mediated effects of THC and cannabinol on the testis. *Pharmacol. Biochem. Behav.* **8**, 673.
3. Besch, N. R., Smith, C. G., Besch, P. K. and Kaufman, R. H. (1977) The effect of marihuana (delta-9-tetrahydrocannabinol) on the secretion of luteinizing hormone in the ovariectomized rhesus monkey. *Am. J. Obstet. Gynecol.* **128**, 635.
4. Asch, R. H., Fernandez, E. O., Smith, C. G. and Pauerstein, C. J. (1979) Precoital single doses of delta-9-tetrahydrocannabinol block ovulation in the rabbit, *Fertil. Steril.* **31**, 331.
5. Smith, C. G., Besch, N. F. and Asch, R. H. (1980) Effects of marihuana on the reproductive system. In: *Advances in Sex Hormone Research* (Thomas, J. A. and Singhal, R., eds.) Urban and Schwartzenberg, Baltimore, M D, p. 273.
6. Smith, C. G., Besch, N. F., Smith, R. G. and Besch, P. K. (1979) Effect of tetrahydrocannabinol on the hypothalamic-pituitary axis in the ovariectomized rhesus monkey. *Fertil. Steril.* **31**, 331.
7. Nir, I., Ayalon, D., Tsafriri, A., Cordova, T. and Lindner, H. R. (1973) Suppression of the cyclic surge of luteinizing hormone secretion and of ovulation in the rat by delta-1-tetrahydrocannabinol. *Nature* **243**, 470.
8. Asch, R. H., Smith, C. G., Siler-Knodr, T. M. and Pauerstein, C. J. (1979) Acute decreases in serum prolactin concentrations caused by delta-9-tetrahydrocannabinol in nonhuman primates. *Fertil. Steril.* **32**, 571.
9. Kramer, J. and Ben-David, M. (1978) Prolactin suppression by (–)-delta-9-tetrahydrocannabinol (THC): involvement of serotonergic and dopaminergic pathways. *Endocrinology* **102**, 452.
10. Almirez, R. G., Smith, C. G. and Asch, R. H. (1982) The effects of marihuana extract and delta-9-tetrahydrocannabinol on luteal function in the rhesus monkey. *Fertil. Steril.* **37**, 306.
11. Ayalon, D., Nir, I.,. Cordova, T., Bauminger, S., Puder, M., Naor, Z., Kashi, R., Zor, U., Harell, A. and Lindner H. R. (1977) Acute effect of delta-1-tetrahydrocannabinol on the hypothalamo-pituitary ovarian axis in the rat. *Neuroendocrinology* **23**, 31.

12. Burstein, S., Hunter, S. and Shoupe, T. S. (1979) Cannabinoid inhibition of rat luteal cell progesterone synthesis. *Res. Commun. Chem. Pathol. Pharmacol.* **24**, 413.

13. Dalterio, S., Bartke, A. and Burstein, S. (1976) Cannabinoids inhibit testosterone secretion by mouse testes in vitro. *Science* **196**, 1472.

14. Reich, R., Laufer, N., Lewysohn, O., Cordova, T., Ayalon, D. and Tsafriri, A. (1982) In vitro effects of cannabinoids on follicular function in the rat. *Biol. Reprod.* **27**, 223.

15. Jakubovic, A. and McGreer, P. L. (1976) In vitro inhibition of protein and nucleic acid synthesis in rat testicular tissue by cannabinoids. In: *Marihuana: Chemistry, Biochemistry, and Cellular Effects* Nahas, G. G., Paton, W. D. M., and Idanpaan-Heikkila, J., eds.), Springer-Verlag, New York, p. 223.

16. Asch, R. H., Smith, C. G., Siler-Knodr, T. M. and Pauersteinr C. J. (1981) Effects of delta-9-tetrahydrocannabinol during the follicular phase of the rhesus monkey (macaca mulatta). *J. Clin. Endocrinol. Metab.* **52**, 50.

17. Asch, R. H., Smith, C. G., Siler-Knodr, T. M. and Pauerstein, C. J. (1979) Effects of delta-9-tetrahydrocannabinol administration on gonadal steroidogenic activity in vivo. *Fertil. Steril.* **32**, 576.

18. Lemberger, L. and Rubin, A. (1978) Cannabis: role of metabolism in the development of tolerance. *Drug Metab. Rev.* **8**, 59.

19. Cook, C. E., Seltzman, H. H., Schindler, V. H., Tallent, C. R. and Chin, M. M. (1982) The analysis of cannabinoids in biological fluids. In: *Cannabinoid Assays in Body Fluids* (Hawks, R. L. ed.). NIDA Research Monograph, No. 42, U. S. Government Printing Office, Washington, DC.

20. Bauman, J. E. (1980) Marihuana and the female reproductive system. Testimony before the Subcommittee on Criminal Justice of the Committee on the Judiciary, U. S. Senate. In: *Health Consequences of Marihuana Use*, U. S. Government Printing Office, Washington, DC, p. 85.

31 Marihuana Effects on Pituitary and Gonadal Hormones in Women

Jack H. Mendelson and Nancy K. Mello

Abstract

A series of studies were carried out to assess the acute and chronic effects of marihuana smoking on pituitary and gonadal hormone levels in women. Plasma samples for analysis of luteinizing hormone (LH), estradiol, progesterone, and prolactin were obtained from 16 women prior to and following smoking one marihuana cigarette that contained 1.8% THC or a 1-g placebo cigarette. A small but statistically significant decrement ($p < 0.02$) in LH levels was observed following marihuana smoking in contrast to placebo smoking during the luteal phase of the menstrual cycle. However, the decrease in LH probably was not biologically significant since all LH levels were within the normal range for healthy adult women. Marihuana smoking was also followed by a small but statistically significant decrease in prolactin levels during the luteal phase of the menstrual cycle, but this probably was not biologically significant. The hormonal effects of daily marihuana smoking over 21 days were studied in 21 women who lived on a clinical research ward for 33 days. Women worked at a simple operant task to acquire marihuana cigarettes. Each marihuana cigarette contained 1.8% Δ^9-THC. Blood samples for analysis of LH, estradiol, and progesterone were collected on alternate days before, during, and after marihuana smoking. Normal ovulatory menstrual cycles were observed, and there was no evidence of a marihuana dose-related suppression of ovulation or disruption of luteal phase function in women classified as heavy (6.1 ± 1.45 cigarettes per day), moderate (2.72 ± 0.16 cigarettes per day) or occasional (0.90 ± 0.22 cigarettes per day) marihuana smokers. These data indicate that smoking marihuana at the dose levels observed for 21 days did not disrupt the menstrual cycle in healthy adult women.

1. INTRODUCTION

In the early 1980s, the United States Institute of Medicine and the Addiction Research Foundation of Canada issued committee reports that emphasized the need for more informa-

From: *Marihuana and Medicine*
Edited by: G. G. Nahas et al.   © Humana Press Inc., Totowa, NJ

tion about the effects of marihuana upon reproductive function in women (*1,2*). Preclinical studies published in 1979 indicated that D9-tetrahydrocannabinol (THC) suppressed luteinizing hormone (LH) levels in female rabbits and rhesus monkeys (*3–5*). One study of marihuana use by women reported that marihuana smokers had shorter menstrual cycles, but no significant abnormalities in LH and estradiol were detected (*6*). Our group examined the acute effects of marihuana on LH, estradiol and progesterone in women during the follicular and luteal phases of the menstrual cycle. This study was originally published in the *Journal of Pharmacology and Experimental Therapeutics* in 1986 (*7*), and the methods and major findings are summarized below.

1.1 Acute Effects of Marihuana on Luteinizing Hormone (LH), Estradiol, and Progesterone During the Follicular and Luteal Phases of the Menstrual Cycle

"Sixteen healthy adult females provided informed consent for participation in this study. All had normal physical examinations, medical, and mental history evaluations and normal laboratory (biochemistry and hemogram) studies. No subject had any past or current history of alcohol or drug abuse, and urine screens for drugs (opiates, barbiturates, tranquilizers, stimulants and depressants) were negative upon admission to the ward. All women reported normal menstrual cycles and none used birth control medication or intrauterine devices. No women had received any form of prescription medication for at least one year before the study, and none had ever received gonadotropins or steroids. No subjects were pregnant as determined by the human chorionic gonadotropin β-subunit test. Before the study, subjects completed daily diaries reporting morning basal body temperature and menstrual function for three consecutive menstrual cycles. Subjects were also interviewed during the luteal and follicular phases of each cycle, and phase status was confirmed by plasma estradiol and progesterone levels."

"Eight women were studied during the follicular phase of the menstrual cycle. These women were between 21 and 33 years of age (mean = 25), and their mean frequency of marihuana use was 14.4 times/month. Eight women were studied during the luteal phase of the menstrual cycle. They were between 21 and 30 years of age (mean = 24.6), and mean frequency of marihuana use was 14.3 times per month."

"Subjects were admitted to a residential research facility for five consecutive days, which involved one day of acclimation, a second day for marihuana or placebo administration, a drug-free day, a fourth day for marihuana or placebo administration, and a final drug-free day. Marihuana or placebo was administered on day two or four in a randomized counterbalanced design to control for sequence effects. Subjects consumed a balanced diet and had access to nonalcoholic beverages and snacks. No drug use occurred other than placebo or marihuana cigarette administration."

"Marihuana or placebo cigarette administration and plasma sampling procedures for pituitary gonadal hormones were identical for all subjects. Subjects did not consume food for 12 hours before the initiation of each study, which was begun at approximately 9 AM. An indwelling intravenous cannula with a heparin lock was connected to a slow infusion of 5% dextrose in saline. Baseline blood specimens were collected at 30-minute intervals for 120 consecutive minutes before administration of marihuana or placebo."

"After baseline samples were collected, each woman smoked either a 1-g marihuana cigarette containing 1.8% THC or a 1-g marihuana placebo cigarette (standardized cigarettes were provided by the National Institute on Drug Abuse). Subjects were instructed to take a

deep inhalation of the marihuana or placebo cigarette once every 30 seconds and retain the inhaled smoke for 2–4 seconds. Under these conditions, subjects smoked a 1-g marihuana or placebo cigarette within 10 to 12 minutes."

"Blood samples were collected at 15, 20, 25, 30, 45, 60, 90, 120, 150, and 180 minutes after initiation of marihuana or placebo. Blood samples were centrifuged immediately after collection, and aliquots of plasma were stored at –70°C for subsequent analysis of LH, estradiol, and progesterone."

"LH was assayed as described previously (8). Results are expressed as nanograms of LER-907 standard per milliliter of plasma. Mean intra- and interassay C.V.s were 7 and 11%. Progesterone was assayed without solvent extraction using kits purchased from Radioassay Systems Laboratories (Carson, CA). The mean intra-assay C.V. was 8.%. Interassay C.V.s were 7.0 and 13.6% for controls that averaged 27.6 and 1.12 ng/mL. 17β Estradiol was assayed without solvent extraction using kits purchased from Serono Laboratories (Boston, MA). Intra- and interassay C.V.s were 6.0 and 7.3 %."

"ANOVA was carried out to ascertain whether significant changes in plasma hormone levels occurred after marihuana or placebo smoking at zero time. Stability of baseline hormone values before marihuana or placebo smoking (–120 min to zero time) was also determined by ANOVA. If ANOVA revealed a significant main (placebo or marihuana) effect, paired comparison tests were used to determine at which time points significant effects occurred."

"No statistically significant changes in plasma estradiol and progesterone levels were found following marihuana in contrast to placebo cigarette smoking. Figure 1 shows mean LH levels prior to marihuana or placebo smoking and at 60, 90, and 120 minutes following marihuana or placebo smoking. A significant decrease in LH levels were observed following marihuana in contract to placebo smoking during the luteal phase of the menstrual cycle (p < 0.02). However, no significant differences in LH levels were observed following marihuana in contrast to placebo smoking during the follicular phase of the menstrual cycle."

The acute effects of marihuana smoking on prolactin levels in women were reported in the *Journal of Pharmacology and Experimental Therapeutics* in 1985 (9). Although we detected a statistically significant difference between marihuana and placebo effects during the luteal phase of the menstrual cycle, the decrement in plasma prolactin levels observed following marihuana smoking was relatively small (2–6 ng/mL) and probably was not biologically significant. Normal prolactin levels range between 3 and 18 ng/mL in healthy adult females.

1.2. Assessment of chronic effects of marihuana use on pituitary and gonadal hormones in women.

In 1985 we reported studies of operant acquisition of marihuana by women in the *Journal of Pharmacology and Experimental Therapeutics (10)*, and our methods and major findings are summarized below.

Marihuana acquisition and use patterns were studied in 21 women on a clinical research ward. Women could earn one-gram marihuana cigarette or 50 cents in 30 minutes of performance on a second-order Fixed-Ratio 300 (Fixed-Interval 1 sec:S) schedule of reinforcement. A 7-day drug-free baseline was followed by 21 days of marihuana availability and a postmarihuana drug-free period of 5 days. Five heavy marihuana users smoked an average of 6.1 (± 1.45) marihuana cigarettes per day and increased marihuana use significantly through time

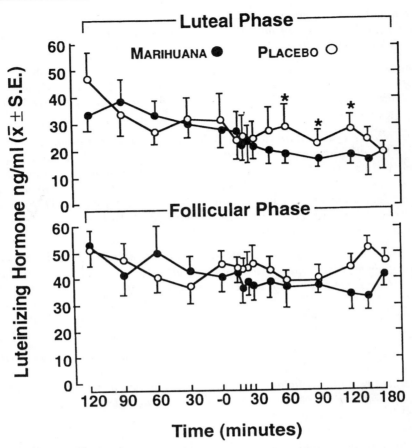

Fig 1. LH levels (mean ± SE) before and after (zero time) marihuana (●) or placebo (○) cigarette smoking during the luteal and follicular phases of the menstrual cycle. Placebo vs marihuana, $p < 0.02$. (Adapted from ref. 7 with permission.)

($p < 0.001$). Seven moderate marihuana users smoked an average of 2.72 (± 0.16) marihuana cigarettes per day and used significantly less marihuana through time ($p < 0.01$). Nine occasional marihuana users smoked less than one cigarette per day (0.90 ± 0.22) and maintained stable patterns of marihuana use. Women who increased marihuana use during the premenstruum reported significantly greater premenstrual dysphoria on the Premenstrual Assessment Form than women whose marihuana use decreased or remained the same ($p < 0.05$ to 0.01). There were no marihuana dose-related effects on operant performance. The heavy, moderate, and occasional marihuana smokers did not differ in operant purchase points earned, hours worked, or money earned. Each marihuana dose-group earned an equivalent number of purchase points during the drug-free periods and the period of marihuana availability. Some subjects continued to work for money when smoking 15–20 marihuana cigarettes per day and periods of maximal operant work coincided with periods of maximal marihuana smoking (noon–midnight). There was an inverse relationship between reported duration of unemployment and amount of marihuana used. Marihuana smoking did not change the amount and temporal distribution of tobacco smoking in 16 women who also used tobacco cigarettes. One woman had signs and symptoms of withdrawal after smoking an average of 11.62 (±1.47) marihuana cigarettes per day for 21 days (*10*).

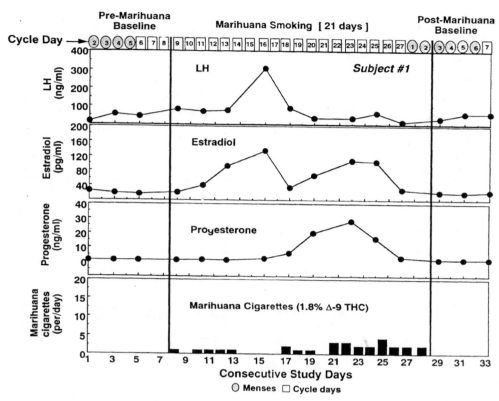

Fig. 2. The effects of occasional marihuana smoking on LH, estradiol, and progesterone levels across the menstrual cycle in a woman. Days of the menstrual cycle before, during, and after 21 days of marihuana smoking are shown at the top of the figure. Menstruation is indicated by shaded circles and cycle days after menstruation are shown as squares. Consecutive days of the study are shown on the abscissa. Plasma levels of LH (ng/mL, estradiol (pg/mL) and progesterone (ng/mL) are shown in rows 1–3 as indicated on the left ordinate. The number of marihuana cigarettes (1.8% Δ^9-THC) smoked each day during the 21 days of marihuana availability are shown in row 4.

Blood samples for analysis of LH, estradiol, and progesterone were collected on alternate days before, during, and after the 21-day period of marihuana smoking. Data for three illustrative subjects who were occasional, moderate, or heavy marihuana smokers are shown in Figs. 2–4. Each figure shows the day of the menstrual cycle, plasma levels of LH, estradiol, and progesterone and the number of marihuana cigarettes smoked each day. This 33-day inpatient study spanned one complete menstrual cycle in two of the three subjects.

Figure 2 shows one woman who was an occasional marihuana smoker (1.4 ± 0.2/day). Her menstrual cycle began on the day of admission and a periovulatory LH surge (308 ng/mL) was detected on cycle day 16, followed by increases in progesterone to levels of 28.2 ng/mL on cycle day 23. Figure 3 shows data for a moderate marihuana smoker ($\bar{x}$) = 4.3 ± 0.4 cigarettes per day) whose menstrual cycle began on study day 2. A periovulatory LH surge of 131 ng/mL was detected on cycle day 16 and progesterone levels peaked at 24.7 ng/mL on cycle day 25. Figure 4 shows data for a heavy marihuana smoker ($\bar{x}$) = 11.6 ± 1.5 cigarettes per day). A periovulatory LH surge of 160 ng/mL was detected on day 11 of the menstrual cycle that began on the second day of marihuana smoking. This woman smoked an average of 6.5 ± 0.6 marihuana cigarettes during the 11 days before ovulation, then increased marihuana

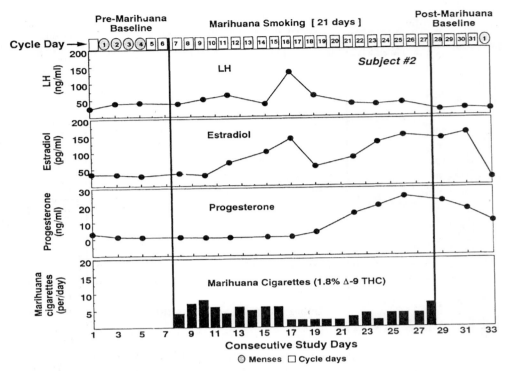

Fig. 3. The effects of moderate marihuana smoking on LH, estradiol, and progesterone levels across the menstrual cycle in a woman. Days of the menstrual cycle before, during and after 21 days of marihuana smoking are shown at the top of the figure. Menstruation is indicated by shaded circles and cycle days after menstruation are shown as squares. Consecutive days of the study are shown on the abscissa. Plasma levels of LH (ng/mL), estradiol (pg/mL) and progesterone (ng/mL are shown in rows 1–3 as indicated on the left ordinate. The number of marihuana cigarettes (1.8% Δ^9-THC) smoked each day during the 21 days of marihuana availability are shown in row 4.

smoking to average 17.2 ± 1.7 during the final 9 days of marihuana availability. Peak post-ovulatory progesterone levels of 27.6 ng/mL were detected immediately after the marihuana smoking period.

It is apparent that these three women had normal ovulatory menstrual cycles during the period of marihuana smoking. Hormonal levels during the periovulatory surge were normal and the postovulatory elevation in progesterone indicated that luteal phases were adequate. Normal hormonal profiles were also observed in 20 women in whom LH, E2, and progesterone data were evaluated. Of the nine women classified as occasional marihuana smokers, eight had mid-cycle LH surge and luteal phase elevation in progesterone. Of the seven women classified as moderate marihuana smokers, 7 had a mid-cycle LH surge and luteal phase elevation in progesterone. Of the five women classified as heavy marihuana smokers, 5 had a mid-cycle LH surge and a luteal phase elevation in progesterone. No woman was amenorrheic during the period of observation.

In summary, data obtained in this study did not reveal any marihuana-induced derangements in regulation of anterior pituitary or ovarian hormones across the menstrual cycle. Although this study was carried out under controlled research ward conditions for a period of 33 consecutive days, it is possible that frequent high-dose marihuana smoking over many

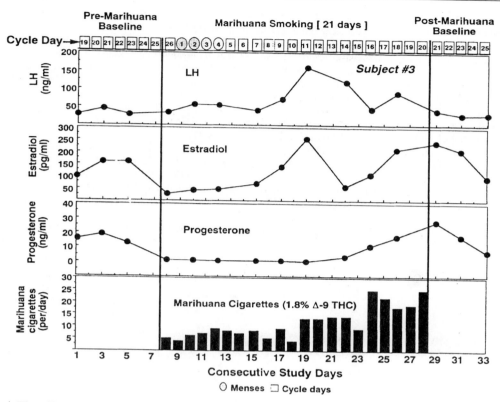

Fig. 4. The effects of heavy marihuana smoking on LH, estradiol, and progesterone levels across the menstrual cycle in a woman. Days of the menstrual cycle before, during, and after 21 days of marihuana smoking are shown at the top of the figure. Menstruation is indicated by shaded circles and cycle days after menstruation are shown as squares. Consecutive days of the study are shown on the abscissa. Plasma levels of LH (ng/mL), estradiol (pg/mL) and progesterone (ng/mL), are shown in rows 1–3 as indicated on the left ordinate. The number of marihuana cigarettes (1.8% Δ^9-THC) smoked each day during the 21 days of marihuana availability are shown in row 4.

months or years could compromise reproductive hormone function in women. However, these data suggest that the medical use of marihuana over relatively short periods should not disrupt the menstrual cycle.

ACKNOWLEDGMENTS

The American Society for Pharmacology and Experimental Therapeutics has provided permission to reproduce materials originally published in the *Journal of Pharmacology and Experimental Therapeutics (refs. 7,10)*. This research was supported in part by grants K05-DA00064, K05-DA00101, R01-DA02905, and P50-DA04059 from the National Institute on Drug Abuse, National Institutes of Health.

REFERENCES

1. Fehr, K. O. and Kalant, H.: eds. (1983) *Cannabis and Health Hazards*. Addiction Research Foundation, Toronto.
2. *Marihuana and Health* (1981) Report of a Study by a Committee of the Institute of Medicine, Division of Health Sciences Policy, National Academy Press, Washington, DC.

3. Asch, R. H., Fernandez, E. O., Smith, C. G. and Pauerstein, C. J. (1979) Blockage of the ovulatory reflex in the rabbit with delta-9-tetrahydrocannabinol. *Fertil. Steril.* **31,** 331–334.

4. Smith, C. G., Besch, R. G., Smith, R. G. and Besch, P. K. (1979) Effects of tetrahydrocannabinol on the hypothalamic-pituitary axis in the ovariectomized rhesus monkey. *Fertil. Steril.* **31,** 335–339.

5. Smith, C. G., Smith, M. T., Besch, N. F., Smith, R. G., and Asch, R. H. (1979) The effects of Δ^9-tetrahydrocannabinol (THC) on female reproductive function, In: *Marihuana: Biological Effects* (Nahas, C.G. and Paton, W.D.M. eds.) Pergamon, Oxford, pp. 449–467.

6. Bauman, J. E., Kolodny, R. C., Dornbush, R. L., and Webster, S. K. (1979) Effectos endocrinos del uso cronico de la mariguana en mujeres, In: *Cauadernos Cientificos CEMESAM (Centro Mexicano de Estudios en Salud Mental,* (Julio, D.F., ed.) CEMESAM, Mexico, pp. 85–97.

7. Mendelson, J. H., Mello, N. K., Ellingboe, J., Skupny, A. S. T., Lex, B. W., and Griffin, M. (1986) Marihuana smoking suppresses luteinizing hormone in women. *J. Pharmacol. Exp. Ther.* **237,** 862–866.

8. Mendelson, J. H., Ellingboe, J., Kuehnle, J. C. and Mello, N. K. (1978) Effects of chronic marihuana use on integrated plasma testosterone and luteinizing hormone levels. *J. Pharmacol. Exper. Ther.* **207,** 611–617.

9. Mendelson, J. H., Mello, N. K. and Ellingboe, J. (1985) Acute effects of marihuana smoking on prolactin levels in human females. *J. Pharmacol. Exp. Ther.* **232,** 220–222.

10. Mello, N. K. and Mendelson, J. H. (1985) Operant acquisition of marihuana by women. *J. Pharmacol. Exp. Ther.* **235,** 162–171.

32

Cannabinoid Ligand–Receptor Signaling During Early Pregnancy in the Mouse

*Bibhash C. Paria, Sanjoy K. Das,
and Sudhansu K. Dey*

Abstract

The recent identification and cloning of brain-type and spleen-type cannabinoid receptors (CB-1R and CB2-R, respectively) provide evidence that many of the effect of cannabinoids are mediated via these receptors. Using multiple appoaches (RT-PCR, Scatchard analysis, autoradiographic binding, cAMP assay, Western blotting, and immunocytochemistry), we demonstrated that functional CB1-R receptors are present in the preimplantation embryo and uterus. The levels of CB1-R in the embryo are much higher than those in the brain. Furthermore, the mouse uterus has the anandamide synthesizing and hydrolyzing capacities that are differentially regulated during the peri-implantation period. The uterus contains the highest levels of anandamide yet discovered in a mammalian tissue. These results suggest that preimplantation mouse embryos are possible targets for cannabinoid ligand-receptor signaling. Indeed, activation of embryonic cannabinoid receptors by natural and synthetic cannabinoid ligands interferes with preimplantaion embryo development, and this effect is completely reversed by a specific CB1-R antagonist. These results suggest that cannabinoid effects on embryo develpment are mediated by CB1-R We also observed that Δ^9-tetrahydrocannabinol [(-)THC] infused in the presence of cytochrome P450 inhibitors interfered with blastocyst implantation. This adverse effect was reversed by coinfusion of CB1-R antagonist. Collectively, these results demonstrated that cannabinoid effects on embryo development and implantation are mediated by embryonic and/or uterine CB1-R.

1. INTRODUCTION

Marijuana has been used for centuries as a psychoactive drug. Δ^9-tetrahydrocannabinol [(-)THC], an active component of marijuana, primarily contributes to the psychoactive effects. Marijuana and its cannabinoid derivatives induce a wide spectrum of effects including analgesia, antiemetic, anticonvulsion, attenuation of intraocular pressure in glaucoma, anti-

From: *Marihuana and Medicine*
Edited by: G. G. Nahas et al. © Humana Press Inc., Totowa, NJ

inflammation and immunosuppression *(1,2)*. One of the major concerns among many central and peripheral effects of habitual marijuana smoking, or exposure to cannabinoid derivatives is their reported adverse effects on reproductive functions, including fetal loss, pregnancy failure, retarded embryonic development and reduced fertilizing capacity of sperm (reviewed in ref. *2–6*). The mechanisms by which these effects of cannabinoids are mediated remained poorly defined for many years. The identification and cloning of G-protein-coupled cannabinoid receptors in the brain (CB1-R) and spleen (CB2-R) *(7–9)* have begun to provide evidence that many of the central and peripheral effects of cannabinoids are mediated via these receptors. Furthermore, isolation of two endogenous cannabinomimetic lipid derivatives, anandamide (*N*-arachidonoylethanolamide) and 2-AG (*sn*-2-arachidonoylglycerol) from brain and other tissues *(10–15)* suggests that cannabinoid ligand–receptor signaling may be normally operative in the central nervous system *(10,11)*, although the physiological significance of this signaling pathway is yet to be defined.

The CB1-R and CB2-R genes were previously shown to be primarily expressed in the brain and spleen *(8,9)*. However, there is evidence now that other tissues also express these receptors, such as the testis, spleen, and peripheral blood leukocytes *(16–18)*. The expression of cannabinoid receptors in the spleen and leukocyte has been associated with the anti-inflammatory and immunosuppressive roles of cannabinoids *(17,18)*. The observation of reduced fertilizing capacity of sperm exposed to cannabinoid ligands is consistent with the detection of CB1-R mRNA in the testis and cannabinoid binding sites in the sperm *(5,6,16)*. However, the effects and mode of action of cannabinoids in embryo and uterus remained largely undefined and controversial in spite of the numerous reports published in this field during the last two decades *(3,4)*. Sporadic reports of adverse effects of cannabinoid exposure on embryonic growth and development in several species including the rodent *(19–21)* prompted us to examine whether the preimplantation mouse embryo can express functional cannabinoid receptors and whether cannabinoid agonists can influence their development in vitro. We also examined whether uterus could be a major source of anandamide that could interact with embryo.

2. EXPRESSION OF CANNABINOID RECEPTORS IN THE PREIMPLANTATION MOUSE UTERUS AND EMBRYO

To examine whether CB1-R mRNA is expressed in the mouse uterus, Northern blot hybridization and RT-PCR were employed. As previously reported *(11)*, Northern blot analysis detected a 6.0 kb transcript in total brain RNA or pregnant uterine poly (A)$^+$ RNA samples (Fig. 1A). The abundance of CB1-R mRNA was markedly lower in the uterus. However, a predominant 1.2-kb transcript was detected in the uterus, and showed higher accumulation on days 4 and 7 of pregnancy as compared to that on day 1. Whether this smaller transcript is the result of alternate splicing or represents a truncated form of the receptor is not known. RT-PCR also detected CB1-R mRNA in the uterus (Fig. 1B), confirming the results of Northern blot hybridization *(22)*. In contrast, RT-PCR could not detect CB2-R mRNA in the uterus, although this mRNA was detected in the rat or mouse spleen (Fig. 1C). In the preimplantation mouse embryo *(23)*, CB1-R mRNA was primarily detected from the four-cell through the blastocyst stages (Fig. 2A), whereas CB2-R mRNA was present from the one-cell through the blastocyst stages (Fig. 2B).

3. ANANDAMIDE BINDING SITES IN THE BLASTOCYST

Anandamide binding to the preimplantation embryos was examined by autoradiography. Numerous binding sites for ^{3}H-anandamide were evident within a short period of autoradiographic exposure. Unlabeled cannabinoid ligands competed for this binding. The binding

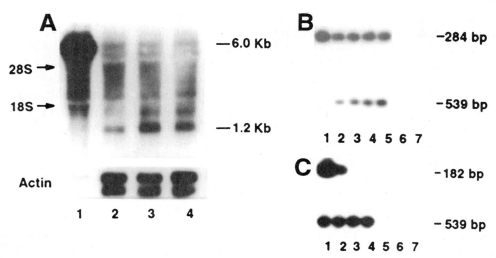

Fig. 1. Analysis of cannabinoid receptor transcripts in the uterus. **(A)** Northern blot analysis of CB1-R. Lane 1: Total RNA (6.0 μg) from the whole brain; poly(A)+ uterine RNA (10 μg) from days 1, 4, and 7 of pregnancy, respectively. The blot was reprobed with β-actin. **(B)** Southern analysis of RT-PCR-amplified products of CB1-R (284 bp) and -actin (539 bp). Lanes: 1, brain; 2, day 1 pregnant uterus; 3, day 4 pregnant uterus; 4, ovariectomized uterus; 5, THC-treated ovariectomized uterus; 6, brain RNA without the RT reaction, and 7, primer control. After 2 weeks of rest, adult ovariectomized mice were given a subcutaneous injection of sesame oil (0.1 mL) or (-)THC (2.5 mg/kg body weight in oil) and killed 6 hours later. **(C)** Southern analysis of RT-PCR-amplified products of CB2-R (182 bp) and β-actin (539 bp). Lanes: 1, rat spleen; 2, mouse spleen; 3, day 1 pregnant uterus; 4, day 4 pregnant uterus; 5 and 6, rat and spleen RNA without the RT reaction, respectively; 7, primer control. Reprinted with permission from ref. *22*.

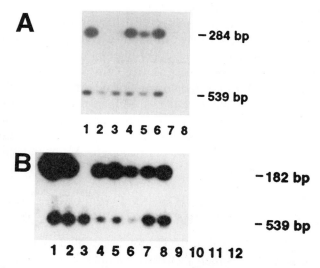

Fig. 2. Analysis of CB1-R and CB2-R transcripts in the preimplantation mouse embryo. **(A)** Southern blot analysis of RT-PCR-amplified products of CB1-R (284 bp) or β-actin (539 bp). Lanes: 1, mouse brain; 2–6, embryos at one-cell, two-cell, four-cell, eight-cell/morula, and blastocyst stages, respectively; 7, mouse brain RNA without RT reaction; 8, primer control. **(B)** Southern blot analysis of RT-PCR-amplified products of CB2-R (182 bp) or -actin (539 bp). Lanes: 1, rat spleen; 2, mouse spleen; 3, day 1 pregnant uterus; 4–8, embryos at one-cell, two-cell, four-cell, eight-cell/morula, and blastocyst stages, respectively; 9–11, rat spleen, mouse spleen, and mouse blastocyst RNA without RT reaction, respectively; 12, primer control. These experiments were performed twice with similar results. Reprinted with permission from ref. *23*.

sites were primarily localized in the trophectoderm, but not in the inner cell mass (23). Scatchard analysis showed that anandamide binds to a single class of high-affinity sites in day 4 blastocysts with an apparent K_d of 1.0 nM and B_{max} of 0.09 fmol/blastocyst (Fig. 3A). In contrast, the apparent K_d and B_{max} for day 4 pregnant mouse brain membranes were 1.8 nM and 18.8 pmol/mg protein, respectively (data not shown). Cannabinoid agonists, Win 55212-2 (K_i 2.1 nM), CP 55,940 (K_i 1.8 nM), (-)THC (K_i: 1.8 nM) and the CB1-R antagonist, SR141716A (K_i 1.4 nM), but not the inactive (+)THC (cannabidiol) (K_i 4.8 μM), competed for the ^{3}H-anandamide binding in day 4 blastocysts (Fig. 3B). The apparent K_d (1.2 nM) and B_{max} (0.09 fmol/blastocyst) for WIN 55212-2 binding to blastocysts were also comparable to those of anandamide binding (24).

4. IMMUNOREACTIVE CB1-R PROTEIN IN PREIMPLANTATION EMBRYOS

Whether the CB1-R mRNA is translated in preimplantation mouse embryos was examined by Western blotting and immunohistochemistry using antipeptide antibodies to CB1-R. To determine that the antibodies were specific to CB1-R, Western blotting was first performed (24). The population of CB1-R is thought to be in higher abundance in the mammalian brain. Two major bands of 59 kDa and 54 kDa were detected in rat brain membranes, whereas a predominant band of 54 kDa was observed in mouse brain membranes (Fig. 4). In blastocyst preparations, a major band of 59 kDa and a minor band of 54 kDa were detected. The 54 kDa band is consistent with the predicted size of the CB1-R (8). The 59-kDa band in the rat brain or mouse blastocyst suggests possible glycosylation of the receptor protein (25). These bands were not detected when preneutralized antibodies with an excess of the antigenic peptide were used. Three bands of 64, 59, and 53 kDa proteins were reported previously in the rat brain (25). In addition, a 55-kDa protein was detected in Sf9 cells expressing the rat CB1-R cDNA from a baculovirus expression vector (26).

Immunohistochemistry was used to detect distribution of CB1-R protein in preimplantation mouse embryos (24). Little or no immunoreactive CB1-R was detected in one-cell embryos, whereas distinct signals were evident in embryos from two-cell through blastocyst stages. In the morula, immunoreactive CB1-R were detected primarily in outside cells, whereas it was predominantly detected in trophectoderm cells of blastocysts. Little or no reactivity was detected in the inner cell mass (Fig. 5). Preneutralized antibodies with an excess of the antigenic peptide failed to show any positive immunostaining in preimplantation embryos (data not shown). The patterns of immunostaining are consistent with our previous observation of autoradiographic distribution of anandamide binding sites in preimplantation mouse embryos (23).

5. EFFECTS OF CANNABINOIDS ON THE FORSKOLIN-STIMULATED CAMP ACCUMULATION IN THE BLASTOCYST

In the brain, CB1-R is a member of the G protein-coupled superfamily and inhibits adenylyl cyclase and N-type Ca^{++} channels (8,9). To examine whether the embryonic cannabinoid receptors were coupled to G proteins (G_i), the effects of (-)THC (10 μM) or (+)THC (10 μM) on forskolin (5 μM)-stimulated cAMP accumulation in blastocyst homogenates were measured with or without pertussis toxin (5 μM) pretreatment (23). (-)THC, but not (+)THC, inhibited forskolin-stimulated cAMP accumulation and this inhibition was prevented by pertussis toxin pretreatment (Fig. 6). This suggests that cannabinoid receptors in the blastocyst are coupled to G_i and the response is specific to the active cannabinoid.

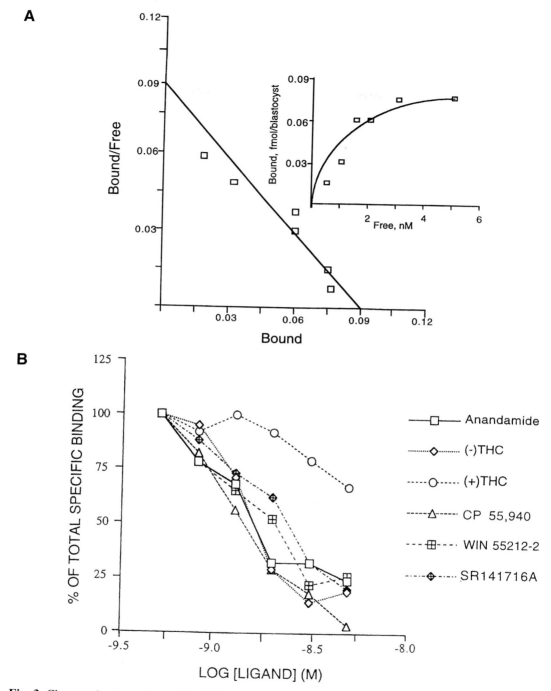

Fig. 3. Characterization of cannabinoid binding in day 4 blastocysts. **(A)** Scatchard analysis of ^{3}H-anandamide binding in day 4 mouse blastocysts. (Inset) Equilibrium binding kinetics. The apparent K_d and B_{max} of anandamide binding in the embryo were 1.0 nM and 0.09 fmol/blastocyst, respectively, while those in the brain were 1.8 nM and 18.8 pmol/mg membrane protein, respectively (data not shown). **(B)** Competition by cannabinoid agonists, CP 55,940, WIN 55212-2, (-)THC (active cannabinoid), (+)THC (inactive cannabinoid), or SR141716A (CB1-R antagonist) for anandamide binding in day-4 blastocysts. Whereas CP 55,940 (K_i 1.8 nM), WIN 55212-2 (K_i 2.1 nM), (-)THC (K_i: 1.8 nM) or SR141716A (K_i 1.4 nM) efficiently displaced anandamide binding, (+)THC (K_i 4.8 μM) was a poor competitor. Reprinted with permission from ref. *24*.

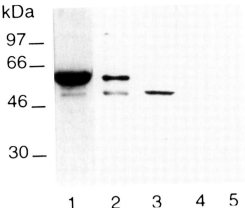

Fig. 4. Western blot analysis of CB1-R of mouse blastocysts or brain membranes. Day-4 blastocyst preparation and brain membranes were immunoblotted using rabbit antipeptide antibodies to CB1-R. Lane 1, day 4 mouse blastocysts (approximately 59 and 54 kDa bands); lane 2, rat brain membranes (approximately 59 and 54 kDa bands); lane 3, mouse brain membranes (approximately 54 kDa band), lanes 4 and 5, rat or mouse brain membranes immunoblotted with antibodies preneutralized with excess of antigenic peptide, respectively. Two hundred day 4 blastocysts were used in this experiment. Molecular size markers are indicated. Reprinted with permission from ref. 24.

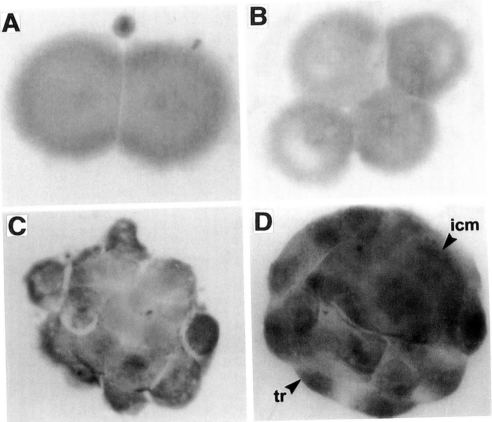

Fig. 5. Immunohistochemistry of CB1-R in preimplantation mouse embryos. Brightfield microphotographs (X 400) of representative two-cell (A), four-cell (B), morula (C) and blastocyst (D) are shown. Red deposits indicate positive immunostaining. Incubation of embryos in antibodies preneutralized with excess of antigenic peptide showed no positive staining (data not shown); tr, trophectoderm; icm, inner cell mass. Reprinted with permission from ref. 24.

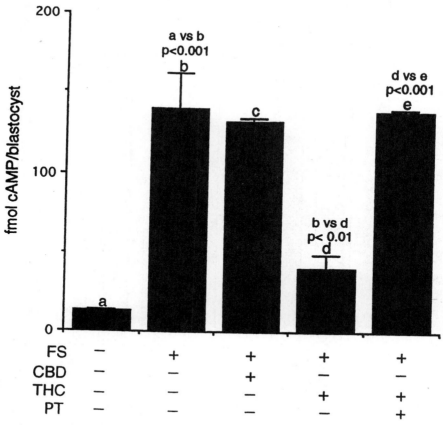

Fig. 6. Effects of cannabinoid agonists on forskolin-stimulated cAMP accumulation in the preimplantation embryo. . Results are the mean ± SD of triplicate experiments. Statistical comparisons (t test) are shown: FS, forskolin; PT, pertussis toxin. Reprinted with permission from ref. 23.

6. EFFECTS OF CANNABINOID AGONISTS ON PREIMPLANTATION EMBRYO DEVELOPMENT:

To examine whether cannabinoid ligands influence preimplantation embryo development, two-cell embryos were cultured in the presence or absence of various synthetic or natural cannabinoid agonists (23,24). All of the agonists [(-)THC, CP 55,940, Win 55212-2, and anandamide] exhibited inhibition of embryonic development to blastocysts (23,24). As shown in other systems (8,9), THC was relatively less potent than the other cannabinoid agonists in this response. The developmental arrest primarily occurred between the four-cell and eight-cell stages. The failure of (+)THC and arachidonic acid to interfere with embryonic development suggests that the effects of cannabinoid agonists on embryo development was not caused by nonspecific toxic effects. The adverse effects of cannabinoids on embryo development were reversed when two-cell embryos were cultured in the presence of a CB1-R specific antagonist SR141716A (8 nM) plus the same concentrations of anandamide, WIN 55212-2 or CP 55,940; 87.5, 87.1, or 96.5% of two-cell embryos developed into blastocysts, respectively. SR141716A (8 nM) alone had no deleterious effects on embryonic development; more than 90% of two-cell embryos developed into blastocysts (Fig. 7). Embryos that developed into blastocysts in the presence of an agonist plus SR141716A or SR141716A

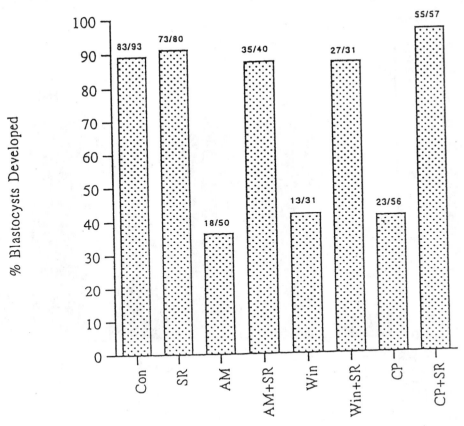

Fig. 7. Effects of cannabinoid agonists and/or the CB1-R antagonists on preimplantation embryo development. Two-cell embryos were cultured in Whitten's medium in the absence or presence of anandamide (AM, 7 nM), Win 55212-2 (WIN, 7 nM), or CP 55,940 (CP, 4 nM) with or without SR141716A (SR, 8 nM) for 72 hours. After termination of culture, the number of embryos that developed to blastocysts was scored. The numbers at the top of each bar indicate the number of blastocysts that developed/total number of two-cell embryos cultured. Each experiments were repeated 3–6 times with controls run simultaneously. Statistical analysis was performed using X^2 and Fisher exact tests. The number of 2-cell embryos developing into blastocysts decreased significantly ($p < 0.05$) when they were cultured in the presence of cannabinoid agonists alone as compared with two-cell embryos cultured in the absence of the agonists, agonists plus SR 141716A or SR141716A alone. The control culture medium contained the same concentration of the vehicle (<0.1% ethanol) used to dissolve the test agents. Reprinted with permission from ref. *24*.

alone were viable, since about 50% of these blastocysts implanted when transferred into uteri of synchronized day 4 pseudopregnant mice (data not shown).

The adverse effects of cannabinoid agonists were also noted in trophoectoderm cell number of blastocysts that escaped the developmental arrest *(24)*. The CB1-R antagonist, SR141716A, was also effective in reversing this adverse effect of cannabinoids (Table 1). Blastocysts developed from the two-cell stage in culture in the absence of any cannabinoids or in the presence of SR141716A alone had an average of 40 trophoectoderm cells. In contrast, the trophoectoderm cell number reduced to about 30 cells/blastocyst when embryos were grown in the presence of a cannabinoid agonist. This reduction in trophoectoderm cell number was completely reversed when embryos were cultured in the presence of

Table 1
Effects of Cannabinoid Agonists and/or CB1-R Antagonist on Trophoectoderm (Tr) and Inner
Cell Mass Cell (ICM) Number of blastocysts (mean ± SEM)

Treatment	No. of Tr cells[a]	No. of ICM cells[a]
Control (<0.1% ethanol)	44.2 ± 1.2 (27)	10.3 ± 0.3 (25)
SR141716A	44.7 ± 1.1 (19)	10.7 ± 0.3 (17)
Anandamide	28.4 ± 1.6 (5)	8.0 ± 1.0 (5)
SR141716A + anandamide	45.6 ± 1.0 (5)	10.0 ± 0.4 (6)
WIN 55212-2	35.8 ± 1.7 (6)	9.5 ± 0.2 (6)
SR141716A + Win 55212-2	45.4 ± 1.4 (11)	11.1 ± 0.4 (11)
CP 55,940	34.3 ± 1.3 (14)	10.2 ± 0.4 (14)

Two-cell embryos were cultured in the presence or absence of anandamide (7 nM), Win 55212-2 (7 nM), CP-55,940 (4 nM), and/or SR141716A (8 nM) for 72 hours.
[a]The numbers in parentheses indicate the number of blastocysts analyzed in each group.
Reprinted with permission from ref. 24.

Table 2
Effects of Anandamide on Blastocyst Hatching in Vitro

Treatment	No. of embryos cultured	No. of Embryos developed to Blastocysts	Hatched blastocysts	
			No.	%
Anandamide, nM				
0	42	41	24	58.5
10	42	41	22	53.7
20	45	43	14	32.68[a]
Anandamide (20 nM) plus SR (10 nM)	43	43	29	67.4
SR, 10 nM	31	31	21	67.7

Eight-cell embryos (10–12 embryos per group) were cultured in the presence or absence of anandamide and/or SR141716A (SR) for 48 hours. Each experiment was repeated 3–4 times.
[a]$p < 0.05$ (χ^2test) compared with other groups. Reprinted with permission from ref. 12.

an agonist with SR141716A. The number of inner cell mass cells was not significantly altered under any of these experimental conditions. Collectively, the results suggest that cannabinoid effects on preimplantation embryo development are mediated primarily via embryonic CB1-R.

7. BLASTOCYST GROWTH AND HATCHING IN VITRO

To study effects of anandamide on blastocyst growth and hatching in vitro, eight-cell embryos recovered on day 3 (1000–1030) were cultured in groups (10–12 embryos/group) for 84 hours in 25 µL of Whitten's medium in the absence or presence of anandamide and/or SR141716A (12). Anandamide inhibited zona-hatching of blastocysts in vitro, and these detrimental effects of anandamide are reversed by SR141716A (Table 2).

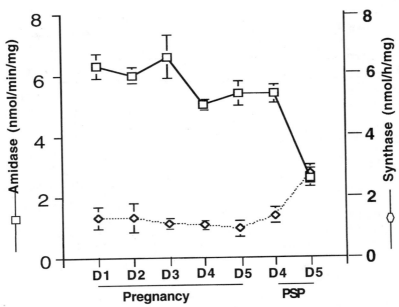

Fig. 8. Uterine anandamide synthase and amidase activity on different days of pregnancy or pseudopregnancy. Whole-uterine microsomes (100 µg) from days 1–5 (D1–D5) of pregnancy or days 4 and 5 of pseudopregnancy (PSP) were incubated under standard optimal conditions as based on initial enzyme kinetics to measure the synthase and amidase activities. Amidase activity on day 4 of pregnancy was significantly lower ($p < 0.05$) than those on days 1–3. Similarly, the amidase activity on day 5 of pseudopregnancy was significantly lower ($p < 0.01$) than that on day 4. The synthase activity on day 5 of pseudopregnancy was higher 9 ($p < 0.05$) than those of days 1–5 of pregnancy or day 4 of pseudopregnancy. Values are mean ± SD and analyzed by student's *t*-test. Reprinted with permission from ref. *33*.

8. ANANDAMIDE SYNTHASE AND AMIDASE ACTIVITIES IN THE PERIIMPLANTATION MOUSE UTERUS

The mechanism of anandamide synthesis remains an open question. There is evidence for the synthesis of anandamide via enzymatic condensation of free arachidonic acid and ethanolamine *(27–30)*, and this synthesis was reported to be independent of ATP and coenzyme A. Very recent evidence suggests that anandamide is synthesized in rat brain by the transacylation-phosphodiesterase pathway rather than by N-acylation of ethanolamine *(31,32)*. Our findings of relatively low substrate requirement (K_m of 3.8 µ*M* and 1.2 m*M* for arachidonic acid and ethanolamine, respectively) for uterine anandamide synthase activity suggests direct N-acylation of ethanolamine as a possible pathway for anandamide synthesis in the uterus *(33)*.

We obtained differential patterns of uterine anandamide synthase and amidase activities during early pregnancy and pseudopregnancy (Fig. 8). The levels of the synthase activity remained virtually unchanged, whereas those of the amidase activity exhibited modest fluctuations on days 1–5 of pregnancy. In contrast, significant increases in uterine-synthase activity with concomitant decreases in amidase activity were observed on day 5 (nonreceptive phase) of pseudopregnancy as compared to that observed on day 4 (receptive phase) of pregnancy or pseudopregnancy *(33)*. When these enzyme activities were examined in separated implantation versus interimplantation sites on days 5-7, an inverse relationship was noted between the two enzyme activities. Whereas levels of the synthase activity were lower at the sites of embryo implantation, the levels were higher at the interimplantation sites (Fig. 9A). In contrast, the reverse was true for the amidase activity (Fig. 9B). In average, the levels of anandamide synthase activity were fourfold and those of amidase activity were threefold higher in the day 4 pregnant mouse brain that those in the pregnant uterus. It is interesting to note that the changing uterine levels of anandamide with pregnancy are reflected in changing pattern of uterine anandamide synthase and amidohydrolase activity *(12)*. Mouse uterus contains the highest levels of anandamide ever found in any mammalian tissues. The levels reach 1345 pmol/μmol lipid P (20 nmol/g tissue) in day 7 interimplantation sites, whereas the brains of the same mice contained only 10–14 pmol/g tissue (data not shown).

9. EFFECT OF THC ON IMPLANTATION

We previously observed that single or repeated injections of (-THC) failed to affect implantation in the mouse *(34)*. We surmised that (-THC) was rapidly metabolized to inactive forms in vivo and did not reach a critical level in the uterus to affect embryo development and implantation. As shown in Table 3, infusion of (-)THC (20 μg/h) alone again failed to prevent implantation, whereas (-)THC plus combined treatment of metyrapone and clotrimazol (50 mg/kg), known inhibitors of cytochrome P450 enzyme system *(35)*, inhibited implantation in 12 of 13 (92%) mice. Miniosmotic pumps containing the drugs were placed in mice on day 2 of pregnancy and continued through day 5. Metyrapone and clotrimazole were first injected 2 h before the installation of pumps and injected twice daily until day 4 of pregnancy. On day 5 of pregnancy, implantation sites were determined by an intravenous injection of 0.1 ml of 1% Chicago blue B in saline 5 minutes before killing. However, coadministration of SR141716A (5 μg/h) with (-)THC completely reversed the implantation-inhibitory effects of (-)THC plus the cytochrome P-450 inhibitors. In contrast, infusion of (+)THC with clotrimazole and metyrapone was not effective in inhibiting implantation *(36)*. A large number of blastocysts (68%) recovered on day 5 from mice treated with (-)THC plus the combination of metyrapone and clotrimazole was zona encased.

10. DISCUSSION

The cannabinoid receptors expressed in the brain are thought to be the mediators of many of the central effects exerted by cannabinoids, whereas the receptors expressed in the spleen and leukocytes are associated with the anti-inflammatory and immunosuppressive effects of these agonists *(17,18)*. The expression of cannabinoid receptors in the testis *(16)* and the presence of cannabinoid binding sites in sperm correlates with their reduced fertilizing capacity after exposure to cannabinoid ligands *(5,6)*. These observations suggest that the activation of G_i-protein-coupled cannabinoid receptors is capable of evoking a wide spectrum of responses depending on the cell types involved. This is further documented by the expression of cannabinoid receptors in the mouse uterus and modulation of uterine gene expression by THC *(22)*.

The results of our investigation establish that preimplantation mouse embryos also express functional cannabinoid receptors and respond to cannabinoid ligands in vitro. The differential temporal expression of the CB1-R and CB2-R mRNAs in the embryo during the preimplantation period is an interesting observation, the significance of which is not yet clear. The CB2-R mRNA could be of maternal origin which persisted through the blastocyst stage, whereas the accumulation of CB1-R mRNA appears to be associated with the activation of the embryonic genome. The overlapping expression of these two embryonic receptors throughout the preimplantation period suggests that the embryo could be a target for the cannabinoid ligands at any stage during this period. However, it is not known whether these

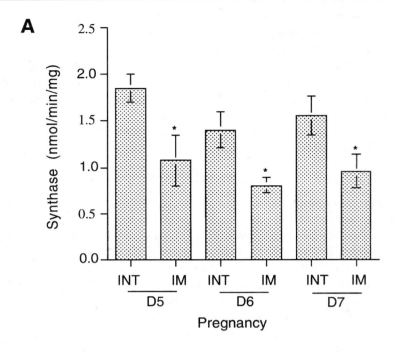

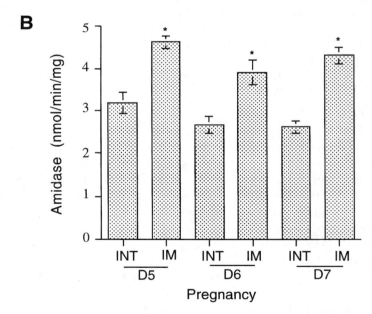

Fig. 9. The anandamide synthase and amidase activities in uterine implantation and interimplantation sites on days 5–7 (D5–D7 of pregnancy. Microsomal proteins (100 μg/point) from surgically separated implantation (IM) and interimplantation (INT) sites were incubated under standard optimal conditions as based on initial enzyme kinetics to measure the **(A)** synthase and **(B)** amidase activity. The synthase activities in the interimplantation sites were always higher (*$p < 0.05$) than those in the implantation sites. In contrast, the amidase activities in the interimplantation sites were higher (*$p < 0.05$) than those in the interimplantation sites. Values are mean ± SD and analyzed by student t-test. Reprinted with permission from ref. *33*.

Table 3
Effects of Infusion of (-)THC or (+)THC on Implantation

Treatments	No. of mice	No. of mice with IS	No. of mice without IS	No. of IS	No. of blastocysts recovered
(-)THC	4	4	0	11.5 ± 2.0	0
(-)THC+Met+Clot	13	1	12	3	91(62)
(+)THC+Met+Clot	6	5	1	10.3 ± 1.7	5
(-)THC+Met+Clot+SR	10	10	0	13.2 ± 1.3	0
Met+Clot	5	4	1	8.3 ± 2.0	8
Met+Clot+SR	4	4	0	9.5 ± 3.3	0
(-)THC+Clot	7	1	6	10	43(26)
(-)THC+Met	7	7	0	11.0 ± 1.4	0
(+)THC+Clot	4	4	0	11.0 ± 2.1	0
Clot	4	4	0	11.3 ± 1.6	0

Miniosmotic pumps containing (-)THC (active), (+)THC (less active), (-)THC + SR141716A (SR) or (+)THC + SR were placed subcutaneously under the back skin from days 2–5 of pregnancy. The release rate of (-)THC or (+)THC was 20 µg/h, whereas that of SR was 5 µg/h. The cytochrom P450 inhibitors metyrapone (Met) plus clotrimazole (Clot) (50 mg/kg each), or Met and Clot each (100 mg/kg) alone were injected twice daily intraperitoneally from days 2–4 of pregnancy. Implantation sites were examined by intravenous injections of 0.1 mL of 1% Chicago blue dye on day 5. Blue bands along uterine horns indicated implantation sites(IS). Uteri without IS were flushed with Whitten's medium to recover blastocysts. Mice without IS or blastocysts were excluded from the experiments. (-)THC, but not (+)THC, inhibited implantation in the presence of cytochrome P450 inhibitors and this inhibition was reversed by a CB1-R antagonist, SR141716A. Numbers within paranthe-ses indicate the number of zona-encased blastocysts.

two receptors behave differently in response to ligand activation during development. Identi-fication of anandamide binding sites by autoradiography and Scatchard analysis of ^{3}H-anan-damide suggests a high-affinity single class of cannabinoid binding sites in the blastocyst, and considering the total cell number (about 50) and protein content (approximately 20 ng) of day 4 mouse blastocysts (37), it is apparent that mouse blastocysts have many more high affinity cannabinoid receptors than in the mouse brain. This is perhaps the first report of any Scatchard analysis in the preimplantation mouse embryo. The inhibitory effects of cannabi-noid agonists on preimplantation embryo development at low nanomolar concentrations are consistent with the presence of a large population of high-affinity receptors in the embryo. The results of Western blotting also suggest that the CB1-R protein is in higher abundance than that in the brain. Rat brain CB1-R has consensus sequence for three potential sites of N-linked glycosylation on the extracellular N-terminus of the receptor (8) and Western blot analysis has confirmed N-linked glycosylation of the rat brain CB1-R (25). Our results sug-gest that the mouse blastocyst CB1-R, like the rat brain, is primarily glycosylated as opposed to the mouse brain CB1-R.

The reversal of the cannabinoid-induced inhibition of embryonic development by a CB1-R antagonist (SR141716A) at a low nanomolar concentration strongly suggests that the brain-type receptors are primarily responsible for the observed effects of cannabinoids. The primary effects of cannabinoids appear to be targeted at the outer cells of embryos that constitute the trophectoderm. This is consistent with the patterns of cannabinoid binding (23) and immunos-taining, and reduction of trophoectoderm cells in blastocysts. Although the CB2-R mRNA is expressed, it is not yet known whether this receptor mRNA is efficiently translated in the preimplantation mouse embryo, or whether this receptor subtype has any functions in the preimplantation embryo. SR141716A is considered to be a preferred antagonist to CB1-R. This compound displays 1000-fold higher affinity for the central receptors (CB1-R) than for peripheral receptors (CB2-R) *(38,39)*. The successful competition of anandamide binding by SR141716A with a K_i of 1.4 nM suggests that cannabinoid-binding sites are primarily of brain-type. CP 55,940, (-)THC or anandamide have been observed to be essentially equipotent in interacting with CB1-R or CB2-R, although WIN 55212-2 or cannabinol was found to bind to CB2-R with higher affinity than to the CB1-R *(11)*. The availability of specific antibodies, or a specific antagonist or agonist to CB2-R will be required to explore the interactions of cannabinoid agonists with this receptor subtype and its roles in preimplantation embryos. In this respect, our recent studies showed that a selective CB2-R agonist, AM 663 even at 20 nM showed no deleterious effects on embryo development (data not shown). The effects of 2-AG or anandamide on embryo development were not reversed by SR144528, a CB2-R antagonist (data not shown).

Inhibition of forskolin-stimulated cAMP accumulation in the blastocyst by THC and its prevention by pertussis toxin pretreatment suggest that embryonic cannabinoid receptors are coupled to G_i proteins. However, the physiological significance of cannabinoid receptors in the preimplantation embryo is not yet clearly understood. In this respect, it should be noted that G_i-like proteins are present in the preimplantation mouse embryo *(40)*. If cannabinoid ligands are available to the embryo during its normal development, it may modulate the intracellular concentration of cAMP and/or Ca^{++} in the embryo. These two second messengers, involved in important signal-transduction pathways, are implicated in cell proliferation, differentiation, and gene expression. In this respect, cAMP has been implicated in zygotic gene activation and blastocyst expansion *(41,42)*, whereas intracellular Ca^{++} plays an important role in cell polarity and embryonic compaction necessary for morula to blastocyst transformation *(43,44)*. The failure of embryos to proceed beyond the eight-cell stage after exposure to cannabinoid ligands in culture could be because of the inhibition of Ca^{++} channels resulting from the activation of the cannabinoid receptors. Therefore, tight regulation of the levels of cAMP and Ca^{++} is likely to be critical for normal embryonic development and growth. Although embryonic arrest after exposure to cannabinoids in vitro is consistent with in vivo findings of retarded embryonic development and pregnancy failure following chronic exposure to exogenous cannabinoids *(19–21)*, it still cannot be ascertained whether the in vivo effects of cannabinoids are mediated directly via these embryonic receptors or by some other mechanism.

Although mouse uterus contains high levels of anandamide *(12)* and has the capacity to synthesize anandamide *(33)*, whether this tissue contains and/or synthesizes 2-AG is not known. We have demonstrated that although lower levels of anandamide are associated with uterine receptivity for implantation, higher levels are correlated with uterine refractoriness to implantation. These results suggested that increased levels of a cannabinoid agonist in the target tissues would interfere with blastocyst implantation. Indeed, infusion of CP 55,940 (a synthetic cannabinoid) via miniosmotic pumps during the preimplantation period, prevented implantation and this inhibition was reversed by coadministration of CP 55,940 with SR141716A *(12)*. In contrast, a single or repeated injections of (-)THC *(34)* or continuous infusion of (-)THC during the preimplantation period failed to affect the implantation process, suggesting either this process is unresponsive to (-)THC or this cannabinoid was rapidly metabolized to its inactive forms and/or cleared from the system. The rapid metabolism and/or clearance appear to be the most reasonable explanation, because infusion of (-)THC interfered with implantation only in the presence of cytochrome P450 inhibitors. Therefore, inhibition of implantation by (-)THC only in presence of P450 inhibitors suggests that under normal conditions females can protect against the adverse effect of cannabinoid on early pregnancy by the P450-linked enzyme system present in the uterus and possibly in the embryo. Because CB1-R is present in both the preimplantation embryo and uterus, it is possible that the adverse effects of (-)THC on implantation were mediated via the uterus and/or embryo. The observed inhibition of implantation by (-)THC could be caused by failure of the uterus to achieve the receptive state. On the other hand, the recovery of large number of zona encased blastocysts on day 5 of pregnancy suggests that (-)THC interfered with blastocyst growth and functions. Thus, cannabinoids may affect both the embryo and the uterus, and disturb the synchronous development of the blastocyst and uterus for successful implantation. Finally, the reversal of (-)THC-induced inhibition of implantation by SR141716A strongly suggests that these effects were mediated via CB1-R. In conclusion, these results place the uterus and embryo as important and physiologically relevant target for cannabinoid ligand-receptor signaling.

ACKNOWLEDGMENT

This work was supported by grants from National Institute of Drug Abuse (DA06665). The center grants (HD 0252 and HD 33994) provided access to core facilities.

REFERENCES

1. Dewey, W. L. (1986) Cannabinoid pharmacology. *Pharmacol. Rev.* **38**, 151–178.
2. Martin, B. R, Compton, D. R., Prescott, W. R., Barrett, R. L., and Razdan, R. K. (1995) Pharmacological evaluation of dimethylheptyl analogs of delta 9-THC: reassessment of the putative three-point cannabinoid-receptor interaction. *Drug Alcohol Depend.* **37**, 231–240.
3. Bloch, E., Thysen, B., Morrill, G. A., Gardner, E., and Fujimoto, G. (1978) Effects of cannabinoids on reproduction and development. *Vitam. Horm.* **36**, 203–258.
4. Smith, C. G. and Asch, R. H. (1987) Drug abuse and reproduction. *Fertil. Steril.* **48**, 355–373.
5. Chang, M. C., Berkery, D., Schuel, R., Laychock, S. G., Zimmerman, A. M., Zimmerman, S., and Schuel, H. (1993) Evidence for a cannabinoid receptor in sea urchin sperm and its role in blockade of the acrosome reaction. *Mol. Reprod. Dev.* **36**, 507–516.
6. Schuel, H., Goldstein, E., Mechoulam, R., Zimmerman, A.M., and Zimmerman, S. (1994) Anandamide (arachidonoylethanolamide), a brain cannabinoid receptor agonist, reduces sperm fertilizing capacity in sea urchins by inhibiting the acrosome reaction. *Proc. Natl. Acad. Sci. USA* **91**, 7678–7682.
7. Howlett, A. C. (1995) Pharmacology of cannabinoid receptors. *Annu. Rev. Pharmacol. Toxicol.* **35**, 607–634.
8. Matsuda, L. A., Lolait, S. J, Brownstein, M. J, Young, A. C., and Bonner, T. I. (1990) Structure of a cannabinoid receptor and functional expression of the cloned cDNA. *Nature* **346**, 561–564.
9. Munro, S., Thomas, K. L., and Abu-Shaar, M. (1993) Molecular characterization of a peripheral receptor for cannabinoids. *Nature* **365**, 61–65.
10. Devane, W. A., Hanus, L., Breuer, A., Pertwee, R. G., Stevenson, L. A., Griffin, G., Gibson, D., Mandelbaum, A., Etinger, A., and Mechoulam, M. (1992) Isolation and structure of a brain constituent that binds to the cannabinoid receptor. *Science* **258**, 1946–1949.
11. Felder, C. C., Veluz, J. S., Williams, H. L., Briley, E. M., and Matsuda, L. A. (1992) Cannabinoid agonists stimulate both receptor- and non-receptor-mediated signal transduction pathways in cells transfected with and expressing cannabinoid receptor clones. *Mol. Pharmacol.* **42**, 838–845.
12. Schmid, P. C., Paria, B. C., Krebsbach, R. J., Schmid, H. H., and Dey, S. K. (1997) Changes in anandamide levels in mouse uterus are associated with uterine receptivity for embryo implantation. *Proc. Natl. Acad. Sci. USA* **94**, 4188–4192.
13. Mechhoulam, R., Ben Shabat, S., Hanus, L., Ligumsky, M., Kaminski, N. E., Schatz, A. R., Gopher, A., Almog, S., Martin, B. R., Compton, D. R., Pertwee, R. G., Griffin, G., Bayewitch, M., Barg, J., and Vogel, Z. (1995) Identification of an endogenous 2-monoglyceride, present in canine gut, that binds to cannabinoid receptors. *Biochem. Pharmacol.* **50**, 83–90.
14. Sugiura, T., Kondo, S., Sukagawa, A., Nakane, S., Shinoda, A., Itoh, K., Yamashita, A., and Waku, K. (1995) 2-arachidonoylglycerol: a possible endogenous cannabinoid receptor ligand in brain. *Biochem. Biophys. Res. Commun.* **215**, 89–97.
15. Stella, N., Schweitzer, P., and Piomelli, D. (1997) A second endogenous cannabinoid that modulates long-term potentiation. *Nature* **388**, 773–777.

16. Gerard, C. M., Mollereau, C., Vassart, G., and Parmentier, M. (1991) Molecular cloning of a human cannabinoid receptor which is also expressed in testis. *Biochem. J.* **279,** 129–134.

17. Kaminski, N. E., Abood, M. E., Kessler, F. K., Martin, B. R., and Schatz, A. R. (1992) Identification of a functionally relevant cannabinoid receptor on mouse spleen cells that is involved in cannabinoid-mediated immune modulation. *Mol. Pharmacol.* **42,** 736–742.

18. Bouaboula, M., Rinaldi, M., Carayon, P., Carillon, C., Delpech, B., Shire, D., LeFur, G. , and Gasellas, P. (1993) Cannabinoid-receptor expression in human leukocytes. *Eur. J. Biochem.* **214,** 173–180.

19. Nahas, G. and Latour, C. (1992) The human toxicity of marijuana. *Med. J. Aust.* **156,** 495–497.

20. Rosenkrantz, H. (1979) Effects of cannabis on fetal development of rodents. In: *Marihuana: Biological Effects* (Nahas, G. G. and Paton, W. D. M. eds.), Pergamon, Oxford, pp. 479-499.

21. Dalterio, S., and Bartke, A. (1981) Fetal testosterone in mice:effect of gestational age and cannabinoid exposure. *J. Endocrinol.* **91,** 509–514.

22. Das, S. K., Paria, B. C., Chakraborty, I., and Dey, S. K. (1995) Cannabinoid ligand-receptor signaling in the mouse uterus. *Proc. Natl. Acad. Sci. USA* **92,** 4332–4336.

23. Paria, B. C., Das, S. K., and Dey, S. K. (1995) The preimplantation mouse embryo is a target for cannabinoid ligand-receptor signaling. *Proc. Natl. Acad. Sci. USA* **92,** 9460–9464.

24. Yang, Z-M., Paria, B. C., and Dey, S. K. (1996) Activation of brain-type cannabinoid receptors interfere with preimplantation mouse embryo development. *Biol. Reprod.* **55,** 756–761.

25. Song, C. and Howlett, A. C. (1995) Rat brain cannabinoid receptors are N-linked glycosylated proteins. *Life Sci.* **56,** 1983–1989.

26. Pettit, D. A., Showwalter, V. M., Abood, M. E., and Carbal, G. A. (1994) Expression of a cannabinoid receptor in baculovirus-infected insect cells. *Biochem. Pharmacol.* **48,** 1231–1243.

27. Deutsch, D. D. and Chin, S. A. (1993) Enzymatic synthesis and degradation of anandamide, a cannabinoid receptor agonist. *Biochem. Pharmacol.* **46,** 791–796.

28. Kruszka, K. K. and Gross, R. W. (1994) The ATP-and CoA-independent synthesis of arachidonoylethanolamide. *J. Biol. Chem.* **269,** 14,345–14,348.

29. Devane, W. A. and Axelrod, J. (1994) Enzymatic synthesis of anandamide, the endogenous ligand for the cannabinoid receptor, by brain membrane. *Proc. Natl. Acad. Sci. USA* **91,** 6698–6701.

30. Ueda, N., Kurahashi, Y., Yamamoto, S., and Tokunaga, T. (1995) Partial purification and characterization of the porcine brain enzyme hydrolyzing and synthesizing anandamide. *J. Biol. Chem.* **270,** 23823–23,827

31. Di Marzo, V., Fontana, A., Cadas, H., Schinelli, S., Cimino, G., Schwartz, J. C., and Piomelli, D. (1994) Formation and inactivation of endogenous cannabinoid anandamide in central neurons. *Nature* **372,** 686–691

32. Sugiura, T., Konda, S., Sukagawa, A., Tonegawa, A., Nakane, S., Yamashita, A., and Waku, K. (1996). Enzymatic synthesis of anandamide, an endogenous cannabinoid receptor ligand, through N-acylphosphatidylethanolamine pathway in testis: involvement of Ca^{++} dependent transacylase and phosphodiesterase activities. *Biochem. Biophys. Res. Commun.* **218,** 113–117.

33. Paria, B. C., Deutsch, D. D., and Dey, S. K. (1996) The uterus is a potential site for anandamide synthesis and hydrolysis: Differential profiles of anandamide synthase and hydrolase activities in the mouse uterus during the periimplantation period. *Mol. Reprod. Dev.* **45,** 183–192.

34. Paria, B. C., Kapur, S., and Dey, S. K. (1992) Effects of 9-ene-tetrahydrocannabinol on uterine estrogenicity in the mouse. *J. Steroid Biochem. Mol. Biol.* **42,** 713–719.

35. Bonin, A., Miguel, R. D., Fernandez-Ruiz, J. J., Cebeira, M., and Ramos, J.A. (1994) Possible role of the cytochrome P-450-linked monooxygenase system in preventing delta-tetrahydrocannabinol-induced stimulation of tuberoinfundibular dopaminergic activity in female rats. *Biochem. Pharmacol.* **48,** 1387–1392.

36. Paria, B. C., Ma, W., Andrenyak, D. M., Schmid, P. C., Schmid, H. H. O., Moody, D. E., Deng, H., Makriyannis, A., and Dey, S. K. (1998) Effects on preimplantation mouse embryo development and implantation are mediated by brain-type cannabinoid receptors. *Biol. Reprod.* **58** (in press)

37. Brinster, R. L. (1973) Nutrition and metabolism of the ovum, zygote, and blastocyst, In: *Handbook of Physiology* (Greep, R. O. and Astwood, E. B., eds.), Am. Physiol. Soc., Bethesda, MD, section 7, vol. 2, pp. E165–E185.

38. Rinaldi-Carmona, M., Barth, F., Heaulme, M., Alonso, R., Shire, D., Congy, C., Soubrie, P., Breliere, J-C., and Le Fur, G. (1995) Biochemical and pharmacological characterization of SR141716A, the first potent and selective brain cannabinoid receptor antagonist. *Life Sci.* **56,** 1941–1947.

39. Rinaldi-Carmona, M., Barth, F., Heaulme, M., Shire, D., Calandra, B., Congy, C., Martinez, S., Maruani, J., Neliat, G., Caput. D., Ferrara, P., Soubrie, P., Breliere, J. C., and Le Fur, G. SR141716A, a potent and selective antagonist of the brain cannabinoid receptor. *FEBS Let.* **350,** 240–244.

40. Jones, J. and Schultz, R. M. (1990) Pertussis toxin-catalyzed ADP-ribosylation of a G protein in mouse oocytes, eggs and preimplantation embryos: developmental changes and possible functional roles. *Dev. Biol.* **139,** 250–262.

41. Manejwala, F., Kaji, E., and Schultz, R. M. (1989) Development of activatable adenylate cyclase in the preimplantation mouse embryo and role for cyclic AMP in blastocoel formation. *Cell* **46,** 95–103.
42. Poueymirou, W. T. and Schultz, R. M. (1989) Regulation of mouse preimplantation embryo development: inhibition of synthesis of proteins in the two-cell embryos that require transcription by inhibitors of cAMP-dependent protein kinase. *Dev. Biol.* **133,** 588–599.
43. Pakrasi, P.L. and Dey, S.K. (1984) Role of calmodulin in blastocyst formation in the mouse. *J. Reprod. Fertil.* **71,** 513–517.
44. Ducibella, T., and Anderson, E. (1975) Cell shape and membrane change in the eight-cell mouse embryo: prerequisites for morphogenesis of the blastocyst. *Dev. Biol.* **47,** 45–48.

33

Effects of Cannabis on Fetal Development of Rodents

Harris Rosenkrantz

Abstract

The majority of teratologic studies on marihuana and Δ^9-THC in rodents have been negative but serious observations of cleft palate in mice and eventrations in rabbits remain unexplained. There has been agreement on the increased incidence of *in utero* deaths. To clarify the potential effects of cannabinoids on fetal development, studies were performed in rodents using the inhalation and oral routes. The Δ^9-THC doses in marihuana smoke were 0.8–3.8 mg/kg, which correlated with plasma Δ^9-THC levels of 73–297 ng/mL and carboxyhemoglobin levels between 21 and 60%. Oral Δ^9-THC doses were 5–600 mg/kg for mice and 12–50 mg/kg for rats. An automatic inhalator provided a 50-mL puff from each of three NIDA cigarettes in a two-second puff, retention of smoke for a 30-second exposure interval followed by a 30-second fresh air purge each min. Exposure to smoke was performed during days 6–15 of gestation. Oral studies included a similar treatment protocol but in addition the number of treatments and days of treatment were varied to establish the time of greatest effect on fetal development. The embryocidal effect of marihuana and Δ^9-THC was demonstrated by two routes and in two rodent species. In fact, whole litter resorption was encountered and two to five treatments around days 7 to 9 of gestation were sufficient to induce embryotoxicity. At least in mice, the fetocidal effect appeared to be related to vaginal bleeding, possibly a consequence of interrupted development of fetoplacental circulation and deranged hormone balance. No drug-related teratogenic effects were found.

1. INTRODUCTION

Over the past 10 years, *Cannabis* and a few cannabinoid constituents have been investigated for potential effects on the reproductive process and fetal development in animals. Despite assessment of the complete spectrum of reproductive function from coital performance in parents to postnatal behavior of progeny, controversial conclusions remain *(54)*. The disparity in teratogenic findings, including chromosomal aberrations, could not always be attributed to vari-

From: *Marihuana and Medicine*
Edited by: G. G. Nahas et al.   © Humana Press Inc., Totowa, NJ

ation in species, dose or route of administration. No argument exists as to the need to resolve any discrepancies in reproductive findings. It is essential that some estimate of physiologic risk of marihuana use be obtained as a guideline for human females in the gravid state.

In the evaluation of *Cannabis* for potential influence on fetal development, it is necessary to consider three possibilities of pharmacologic action of cannabinoids: individual cannabinoid effects; changes related to pure cannabinoid interaction; and alterations initiated by interaction of cannabinoid and noncannabinoid components present during pyrolysis of marihuana. Whereas the teratogenic assessment of pure cannabinoids, individually or in combination, may be achieved in a straightforward fashion, the evaluation of the contribution of pyrolytic products, like carbon monoxide, in marihuana smoke is subject to greater complexity. It cannot be overemphasized that reproductive risk in humans must be related to use of *Cannabis* in the usual manner of smoking marihuana.

In the instance of pure cannabinoids, the oral or intraperitoneal (ip) routes of administration have been favored, but both routes are unnatural and require large quantities of drug *(23)*. It would have been more reasonable to utilize the intravenous (iv) route since acute LD_{50} values of Δ^9-tetrahydrocannabinol (Δ^9-THC) are similar for intravenous and inhalation routes *(79)*. A second advantage is that much smaller doses of pure cannabinoids are needed as compared with other routes and suitable intravenous drug formulations are available *(80)*. In addition, the onset and duration of behavioral effects are similar by intravenous and inhalation routes. However, it should be mentioned that in great part Δ^9-THC oral effects have adequately compared with those by inhalation *(73,76)*.

The use of marihuana smoke in contrast to pure cannabinoids affords the advantage of similarity to use of *Cannabis* in humans. However, simulation of human marihuana smoking can be compromised by variation in marihuana potency based on Δ^9-THC content and by variability in the ratios of cannabinoid constituents depending on the source of *Cannabis*. For example, the Mexican variety contains much more Δ^9-THC than cannabidiol (CBD) or cannabichromene (CBCH), whereas in Turkish marihuana, the latter two predominate *(56,75,78)*.

Other factors beside cannabinoid content exert influences that must be considered in order to mimic human marihuana smoking. Among the chemical factors to be considered are transformations of cannabinoid structure during pyrolysis, cannabinoid destruction during the burning process, generation of carbon monoxide (CO), and the chemical profile of noncannabinoid pyrolytic products. The influence of the latter can be evaluated by comparison with a suitable placebo marihuana (which at the moment is not available) and the others are amenable to direct measurement *(74)*.

Biological factors that must be standardized in order to reliably reproduce conditions for the inhalation of marihuana smoke include puff volume, puff duration, puff frequency, duration of exposure, and appearance and clearance of carboxyhemoglobin (COHb). In animal paradigms, cannabinoid doses relevant to man should be documented by determination of plasma cannabinoid levels. In general, the biological factors may be controlled through the use of automatic smoking machines. The measurement of cannabinoid and CO in the smoke chamber in conjunction with analyses of COHb and plasma cannabinoid in the animals can establish greater credibility of marihuana inhalation studies *(73,77)*.

In relationship to studies of *Cannabis'* effects on fetal development, additional factors of animal species, strain, and source provide problems of standardization. Particularly in the mouse, the incidences of reported cleft palate evoked by Δ^9-THC varied from 0 to 70% *(23)*. The mouse appears to have a greater susceptibility to cleft palate than other species *(5,6)*. It is difficult to estimate genetic drift of a mouse strain from breeder to breeder. It would appear that knowledge of circulating cannabinoid would aid in resolving differences in incidences of cleft palate when disagreement exists (Table 1).

Table 1
Fetal development After Administration of Cannabinoids During Organogenesis

Cannabinol preparation	Dose, mg/kg	Species	route	Teratogenicity (type)	No teratogenicity
				Literature references	
Cannabis, resin or extract	16	Mouse	IP	Persaud & Ellington, 1967 (stunting)	
	4	Rat	IP	Persaud & Ellington, 1968 (syndactyl, encephalocele)	
	0.5–15	Rat	PO		Miras,1965; Haley *et al.* 1973; Keplinger *et al.*, 1973; Wright *et al.*, 1976
	23–300	Hamster	SC	Geber &Schramm, 1969 (runting)	Pace *et al.*, 1971
	15–500	Rabbit	SC, PO	Fournier *et al.*, 1976 (eventration, hairlip)	Geber & Schramm, 1969; Wright *et al.*, 1976
THC	50–300	Mouse	IP	Mantilla-Plata *et al.*, 1975, 1976; Harbison *et al.*, 1977 (cleft palate)	Philips *et al.*, 1971; Fleischman et al, 1975
	3–300	Mouse	IV, SC		Joneja, 1976; Maker et al., 1974
	400	Mouse	PO	Joneja, 1976 (exencephaly, cleft palate)	
	1–250	Rat	PO, SC		Borgen et al., 1971, 1973; Pace et al., 1971; Uyeno, 1973; Banerjee et al., 1975~ Vardaris et al., 1976; Wright et al., 1976
	25–500	Hamster	po		Joneja, 1977
	1–15	Rabbit	po		Haley *et al.*, 1973; Wright *et al.*, 1976
	2.4	Monkey	po		Sassenrath & Chapman, 1975
	10 ppm	Zebra fish	iv, po	Thomas, 1975 (curved spine, bulb tail)	
	1–2	Chick	ip		Jakubovic *et al.*, 1976
Marihuana (1.1% Δ^9-THC)	1–3	Rat	Lung		Fried ,1976
(2.6% Δ^9-THC)	1–4	Rat	Lung		Rosenkrantz *et al.*,1978
	1–4	Mouse	Lung		Rosenkrantz et al., 1978

At the moment, in the absence of plasma Δ^9-THC analyses, only the disparities and not the reasons for the discrepancies can be reviewed. When cannabis resin or extract was tested, runting was observed in mice treated intraperitoneally (67) and in hamsters treated subcutaneously (sc) (29). However, the results in hamster could not be confirmed (66). In the rat treated ip, syndactyl and encephalocoele were seen (68) but oral treatment with a similar dose was negative (34,45,59). Low doses of oral crude marihuana extract or Δ^9-THC given to albino rats were also not teratogenic (99). Eventrations and hairlip were reported for rabbits given cannabis extract subcutaneously or orally (24), but earlier and recent studies in this species failed to implicate *Cannabis* as a teratogen (29,99).

Equally confusing but serious reports of teratogenicity induced by pure Δ^9-THC have been published. High doses of Δ^9-THC (50-400 mg/kg) administered to mice intraperitoneally (52,53) or orally (42) have evoked a 30–70% incidence of cleft palate. However, recently the group that consistently found a high incidence of cleft palate in mice have reported other findings on the Harlan Swiss mouse (36). Δ^9-THC doses of 200 mg/kg only on days 12 and 13 or 50 mg/kg on days 10 and 11 initiated a 9–10% incidence of cleft palate. No cleft palate occurred when 50 mg/kg was given on days 8, 9, 12, and 13 or when 200 mg/kg was administered on days 8, 9, 10, and 11. The absence of cleft palate induction by Δ^9-THC in mice was also noted by others using various routes of administration (23,51,69). Joneja (42), who did observe cleft palate formation after oral Δ^9-THC, could not substantiate this in mice treated intravenously or subcutaneously

Administration of Δ^9-THC (25–500 mg/kg) orally to hamsters was also essentially devoid of teratogenic activity (43). Δ^9-THC given to rats orally or subcutaneously (4,8,9,66,92,94), to rabbits orally (34), to monkeys orally (82), and to chickens intraperitoneally (41) was not teratogenic. Zebrafish placed in a medium containing 10 ppm of Δ^9-THC produced offspring with curved spines and bulbous tails (91).

Despite the disparity in the findings of *Cannabis*-evoked teratogenic effects, a common observation has been an increased incidence of *in utero* deaths (22,23,26,42,53,54,77,93). Although cannabinoid-induced embryotoxicity is of paramount importance as a risk factor in the use of marihuana, the observations of cleft palate formation in mice and eventrations in rabbits cannot simply be dismissed.

Because of the controversial findings of cannabinoid-induced abnormalities in rodent progeny, the present studies were performed. Both the route of inhalation and oral treatment were utilized to permit comparison of crucial findings in two rodent species by two routes of administration. No teratogenic effects were observed in rodents after exposure to marihuana smoke (26,27,77) but embryotoxicity was prevalent in mice (77).

2. METHODS AND MATERIALS

The inhalation investigation was conducted to establish whether marihuana smoke itself containing doses of Δ^9-THC relevant to humans could elicit embryotoxicity. Other studies with larger oral doses of pure Δ^9-THC were performed to delineate the time of greatest fetal sensitivity to cannabinoid-induced fetal resorption. In addition, experiments were designed to clarify the finding of cannabinoid-evoked whole-litter resorption, which compromised confirmation of pregnancy of rodent dams (22).

The inhalation and oral studies were performed at different times but, where possible, the same personnel were used and environmental factors were kept similar.

2.1. Animal Housing, Care, and Mating

All animals were procured from the same source (Charles River Breeding Laboratories, Wilmington, MA). Two strains of mice, CD-1 and Swiss-Webster, and Fischer 344 rats were studied. Female mice weighing 30–40 g were housed five per cage and female rats weighing 135–150 g were housed three per cage. The dimensions of the wire-mesh suspension cages were 24 × 18 × 17 cm. Individual sexually mature males of either species were kept in similarly constructed but larger breeding cages. Mice in advanced pregnancy were transferred to plastic cages to prevent loss of pups if early parturition occurred.

Commercial rodent chow pellets and water were freely available. Each animal room had a 12-hour light/dark circadian cycle to minimize the effects of hormonal surges. Ambient room temperature was 23 ± 2°C and there were six to eight air changes per hour.

Mating of rodents for the inhalation studies were performed inhouse. One shipment of each species was used. The estrus cycle was determined in rats by vaginal smear and two females at proestrus were transferred to the breeding cage of one fertile male. Positive mating was confirmed by the presence of sperm in the vaginal tract and the day of this occurrence was considered day 0 of gestation. As pregnant rats were obtained, they were arbitrarily randomized into control and treated groups till there were approximately 30 pregnant rats per group. The estrus cycles of mice were too variable to depend on mating during proestrus; two females were permitted to remain with one male for one to three days until sperm was found in the vagina. Randomization was like that for the rat.

In the oral studies, rodents were obtained three-days pregnant from the breeder, whose larger breeding colony could provide more accurate conception rates and adequate numbers of rodents as needed. As above, day 0 of gestation was the day the presence of a vaginal plug and/or sperm was found the morning after mating.

2.2 Cannabinoid Materials and Doses

Marihuana cigarettes contained approximately 2.8% Δ^9-THC and less than 0.2% of each of the major cannabinoids. Cannabinoid-extracted marihuana served as placebo cigarettes. Oral preparations were sesame oil solutions of 96% pure synthetic (-)-*trans* Δ^9-THC; drug formulations of 3.75–15 mg/mL were used for rats and 15–60 mg/mL for mice. All cannabinoids were supplied by the National Institute on Drug Abuse: marihuana cigarettes were lot RTI 2055-53; placebo cigarettes were lot RTI 205534; and pure Δ^9-THC was lot QCD-84924. Cannabinoid materials were stored at 5°C but before use, cigarettes were placed at 60% humidity and 23°C for 24–48 hours.

The doses selected for inhalation studies were estimated on the basis of rodent tidal volumes, respiration rates, duration and number of exposure periods (puffs), and concentration of Δ^9-THC in the smoke as previously described (73). These calculated values were corrected for pyrolytic losses and for losses caused by entrapment in nasal passages. For example in the rat: 3.3 µg/mL (Δ^9-THC concentration in smoke) x 0.8 mL (tidal volume) x 60 (respiration rate) x 12 puffs = 1.9 mg/200 g rat or 9.5 mg/kg; 50% loss in rat nasal turbinates and 20% loss in lungs yield a dose of approximately 3.8 mg/kg. In the mouse: 3.3 µg/mL x 0.16 mL x 60 x 12 puffs = 0.38mg/40 g mouse or 9.5 mg/kg; losses similar to those in rat yield a dose of approximately 3.8 mg/kg.

The rodent inhalation doses were relevant to marihuana use in man. Assuming a 50-kg body weight and correcting for Δ^9-THC losses during smoking, it has been estimated that Δ^9-THC doses of marihuana with 2.6% Δ^9-THC would be approximately between 0.3–1.8 mg/kg in humans depending on consumption of one to six marihuana cigarettes per day (73). On the basis of body surface area, these human doses would be similar to 2–20 mg/kg in rats and mice. Because oral doses in humans needed to elicit similar effects to those by inhalation are known to be three to six times larger, relevant oral doses in rodents would be approximately 6–70 mg/kg in rat and 12–200 mg/kg in mice corrected for body surface areas (73) The acute inhalation LD$_{50}$ in these rodent species was approximately 40–50 mg/kg and the acute oral LD_{50} was approximately 1000–2000 mg/kg, the mouse being less sensitive than rat to Δ^9-THC given by the oral route *(73)*. Furthermore, female rodents were more sensitive to oral Δ^9-THC than males.

Dosimetry in the present inhalation studies was directly monitored (suborbital blood specimens) by determination of COHb by the Dubowski spectrophotometric method *(17)* and plasma Δ^9-THC levels were measured by a gas chromatographic procedure through the courtesy of Battelle Columbus Laboratories.

2.3. Treatment Protocols

Of considerable importance in the inhalation studies was to simulate smoking conditions in rodents that closely mimic those in humans. In addition, it was anticipated to obtain plasma Δ^9-THC levels and relate these to reported circulating levels in humans. *Cannabis* consumers inspire a puff volume of 50–200 mL during a 2- to 10-second period and retain the smoke in their lungs for 15–60 seconds *(73)*. In the rodent teratology studies, an automatic smoking machine was used which delivered a 150-mL puff volume (50 mL from each of three cigarettes) over a two-second period and the smoke was retained in a 400-mL constant volume smoke chamber for 30 seconds. The smoke was displaced with a fresh air purge for 30 seconds. The complete cycle was repeated each min and was equivalent to one puff/minute.

Multiple rodents were exposed simultaneously by attachment of a circular array of four to nine cone-shaped lucite holders to each side of the smoke chamber. The Swiss-Webster mouse strain and the Fischer 344 rat strain were used in inhalation studies. The former was selected because of the report of others of a high incidence of Δ^9-THC-evoked cleft palate *(53)*. The rat strain was chosen because of a considerable archive of marihuana data on the Fischer rat *(76)*. Groups of successfully mated rodents were exposed during days 6 to 15 of gestation to four puffs (0.8 mg/kg), eight puffs (2.6 mg/kg) or 12 puffs (3.8 mg/kg). Two control groups were used, one being exposed to eight puffs of placebo smoke and the second group was placed in the inhalator in the absence of smoke (sham treated). A reduced number of placebo puffs, compared with the marihuana high dose, were used because cannabinoid-extracted marihuana has been found to generate approximately 30% more carbon monoxide and induce mortality.

The oral treatment protocols were varied in accordance with exploration of the mechanism of embryotoxicity: effect of number of Δ^9-THC treatments on fetal viability in rats and mice; determination of gestational days of greatest susceptibility to embryotoxicity in rats; and confirmation of complete fetal resorption in rats whose pregnancies were unequivocally established by laparotomy. The rats were of the Fischer 344 strain and the mice were the CD-1 strain. The gavage volume of drug formulation administered to rats was 0.5 mL/150 g body weight and that for mice was 0.2 mL/20 g body weight.

In the first oral study, weekly shipments of three-day pregnant rats were randomized to achieve approximately 50 rats/group, who received Δ^9-THC doses of 12.5, 25, or 50 mg/kg. One control group received the sesame oil vehicle and a second control group were sham treated. Weekly shipments of three-day pregnant mice were also randomly assigned to two treatment protocols: approximately 75 mice per group were orally administered Δ^9-THC doses of 5, 15, or 50 mg/kg or were treated with vehicle; and approximately 90 mice per group received oral Δ^9-THC doses of 150, 300, or 600 mg/kg and control groups were given vehicle or were sham treated. Rats and mice were treated either for 2, 5, 8, or 10 days commencing on day 6 of gestation, the longest duration of treatment terminating on day 15 of gestation. Rodents on the shorter treatment schedules were sacrificed the day after the last treatment.

In the second oral study approximately 200 rat dams were distributed among 10 groups. One-half the groups received an oral Δ^9-THC dose of 50 mg/kg and the others were given vehicle, matched treated and control groups being treated on days 5 to 7, 6 to 8, 7 to 9, 8 to 10, or 9 to 11 of gestation and all were sacrificed on day 14.

In the third oral study, pregnancy was confirmed by laparotomy, an exact count of embryos was recorded and approximately 20 dams per group were orally administered Δ^9-THC at 50 mg/kg or vehicle or were sham treated on days 6–9 of gestation. Approximately one-half the rats in each group were sacrificed on day 12 and the other half on day 16 of gestation.

2.4. Teratology Procedures

Except for the early sacrifices in the variable treatment schedules of oral studies 1 and 2 and on laparotomized dams in study 3, all other animals underwent caesarian delivery on days 18 to 20. Euthanasia was by carbon dioxide inhalation and standard observations were made for the classical teratology experiments and abbreviated ones for the studies on the mechanism of embryotoxicity. Briefly, the abdominal wall of each dam was incised and reflected to expose the uterine horns; fetal swellings and metrial glands were counted under a magnifier illuminator; the uterine horns were opened from apex to cervix and the numbers of live, dead, and resorbed fetuses were determined; each fetus was individually weighed and placed upon a sponge relative to its position in the uterine horns; and, each fetus was sexed and examined for external defects.

Approximately equal numbers of male and female pups were randomly transferred into labeled vials containing 95% ethanol for bone clearing or Bouin's solution for fetal slicing. As a general procedure, the first and second fetuses were placed in alcohol and the third in Bouin's solution. When gross skeletal defects were evident, the fetus went into alcohol; fetuses with external indication of soft-tissue injury were immersed in Bouin's solution. Approximately one-third of the fetuses were preserved for evaluation of soft tissue changes and two-thirds were prepared for the evaluation of skeletal anomalies.

Examination of fetuses for soft-tissue anomalies was performed according to the Wilson technique (98). Bouin's solution (8 days) was replaced by 80% ethanol (5–6 days), which in turn was replaced by distilled water prior to cutting the fetus. Legs and tail were clipped from their trunk junctures and the head severed at the level above the ears by slicing through the mouth. Five to six slices were made between front of eyes to ears. Transverse slices (0.5–2 mm) were made of the trunk from the regions of the shoulders to a caudal area beyond the kidneys. Included were the heart, liver, kidney, and genitourinary regions. A dissecting microscope was used for closer viewing of slices and the sections were stained with 0.1% aqueous cresyl violet mixed 1:20 with 2% acetic acid. Differential coloration yielded a purple stain for bone, red for cartilage, dark blue for glands, blue-green for other tissue (background color was yellow). The coloration lasted approximately 4 hours in water and stained sections were returned to 80% ethanol.

Bone clearing was accomplished by fixing fetuses in 95% ethanol for 48–96 hours after which they were transferred to 1% potassium hydroxide until the skeleton was clearly visible (24–72 hours). A subsequent transfer into alkaline alizarin R (1:100; 1% aqueous alizarian R in 1 percent potassium hydroxide) for two days provided a violet-red staining of the skeletal tissue. The stained fetuses were immersed in Mall's solution (20% glycerol in 1% potassium hydroxide) for one to two days to remove excess stain and were placed into a 35% glycerol solution for inspection. Storage of specimens was in 50% glycerin.

Statistical analysis of the significance of change of the usual teratologic parameters were based on the Student's t test. Chi-square analysis was performed using the numbers of embryos before and after treatment with experimental N unit (5). Whole-litter resorption was subjected to Fisher's exact probability using dams as the experimental unit. Percent whole-litter resorption and fetal mortality were based on embryo counts made at laparotomy.

3. RESULTS

It is of some importance to mention behavioral changes observed in the rodent species at the cannabis doses used since prolonged gross intoxication can compromise the teratological findings. Approximately 30% of the Swiss-Webster mice exposed to marihuana smoke exhibited a dose-related CNS-inhibition manifested by ataxia, dyspnea, and inactivity at the high dose in the first two hours from which the animals rapidly recovered by the third hour. This temporal pattern of events occurred for four to five days of postexposure, but tolerance to CNS-inhibition developed thereafter. The majority of placebo-exposed mice displayed similar, but more intense, behavioral changes which included instances of tremors, convulsions, and lethality. The observation of cyanosis in many placebo mice suggested their behavioral changes were related to CO intoxication. There were minor incidences of CNS stimulation at all doses of marihuana before and after development of tolerance to CNS inhibition. Sham-treated mice behaved normally.

Approximately 20% of rats at the mid-dose and 50% at the high dose of marihuana responded only with a depression of activity and all animals behaved normally by the end of the day. About 10% of the low-dosed rats exhibited hyperactivity. As in the instance of mice, many placebo rats were depressed and some were cyanotic. In general, tolerance developed to the CNS inhibition in marihuana-exposed groups between days 3 and 5 and the usual second phase of CNS stimulation was a minor occurrence. Sham-treated rats behaved normally.

In the oral studies with pure Δ^9-THC, mice predominantly exhibited a dose-related decrease in voluntary activity to which tolerance developed in three to four days. Hypersensitivity was noted in approximately 25% of high-dosed mice during days 5 to 7 of treatment. Control mice behaved normally. Less than 20% of the high-dosed rats vocalized and were sedated or depressed after the first treatment. Thereafter, approximately 75% of high-dosed rats were depressed during two subsequent treatments but all groups of Δ^9-THC-treated rats behaved normally during continued treatment. One-half of the mid-dosed animals and approximately 30% of the low-dosed rats were depressed during the first three oral treatments, whereas an equal number displayed hyperactivity. Some vocalization occurred at the lower doses and approximately 35% of the rats in these groups behaved aggressively after five treatments. Δ^9-THC groups were normal during continued treatment, whereas control rats behaved normally throughout treatment with sesame oil vehicle.

A pilot study in rats using oral Δ^9-THC doses of 75–300 mg/kg revealed considerable *Cannabis* intoxication and mortality. Therefore, none of these doses were considered realistic or relevant in the rat teratology investigations and were abandoned.

3.1. Reproductive Findings

Because most of the teratology data have or will soon appear in other publications, such data will not be presented in detail here *(22, 77)*. Instead, simplified tables referring to the significance of changes observed in dams and fetuses in all studies have been provided herein. More stress has been placed on the embryotoxicity observations and appropriate data have been supplied on this aspect of fetal development.

3.1.1. Dam Changes

In the inhalation studies on both rodent species, there were no significant adverse effects on conception rate, dam growth rate, total number of implants, and number of implants per dam (Table 2). On the other hand, the number of dams with early fetal resorptions was signif-

Table 2

Teratology Parameters Evaluated on CD-1 Mice, Swiss-Webster Mice, and Fischer Rats Orally Treated or Exposed to Inhalation of D9-Tetrahydrocannabinol During gestation Days 6–15 and Sacrificed Near Term[a].

	CD-1 mice		Swiss-Webster mice	Fischer 344 rats	
Parameters evaluated	Oral Δ^9-THC 5–50 (mg/kg)	Oral Δ^9-THC 150–600 (mg/kg)	Inhalation Δ^9-THC 0.8–3.8 (mg/kg)	Oral Δ^9-THC 12.5–50 (mg/kg)	Inhalation 0.8–3.8 (mg/kg)
Dams ($n = 30$–50):					
Effect on pregnancy[b]	$p < 0.01$	$p < 0.01$	NS	$p < 0.1$	NS
Premature delivery	NS	NS	NS	NS	NS
Growth rate	NS	$p < 0.01$	NS	$p < 0.1$	NS
Number implants/dam	NS	NS	NS	NS	NS
Number with					
(a) Early resorption	$p < 0.05$'	$p < 0.01$	$p < 0.01$	$p < 0.05$[c]	NS
(b) Late resorption	NS	NS	NS	NS	NS
(c) Dead fetuses	NS	NS	NS	NS	NS
Fetuses (n = 350–550):					
Litter weight	NS	$p < 0.01$	NS	$p < 0.01$	NS
Mean fetal weight	NS	$p < 0.05$	NS	$p < 0.05$	NS
Sex ratio	NS	NS	NS	NS	NS
Early resorptions	$p < 0.05$'	$p < 0.05$	$p < 0.01$	$p < 0.05$	NS
Late resorptions	NS	NS	NS	NS	NS
Dead non-resorbed	NS	NS	NS	NS	NS
Total fetal mortality	$p < 0.05$	$p < 0.01$	$p < ODI$	$p < 0.01$	NS

[a]NS, nonsignificant compared with sham and/or sesame oil controls in oral studies or with sham and placebo marihuana (free of cannabinoids) controls in inhalation studies.

[b]This parameter relates to pregnancy interruption in oral studies and to inhibition of conception rate in inhalation studies.

[c]Only at higher doses.

icantly increased in a dose-related fashion among marihuana-exposed Swiss-Webster mice. In contrast, marihuana inhalation did not evoke a similar significant change of this parameter in rats. There was no significant difference between treated and control groups of either species in regard to the numbers of dams with late fetal resorptions or dead fetuses.

In the oral studies on CD-1 mice, who were procured three-days pregnant, a dose-related interruption of pregnancy occurred (Table 2). At the larger doses (150–600 mg/kg), dam growth rate was significantly inhibited but loss in dam weight was related to resorption of fetuses and not dam intoxication. Total number of implants and number of implants per dam were unchanged at all Δ^9-THC doses. The number of dams with early fetal resorptions, but not with late resorptions or dead fetuses, was significantly increased at doses greater than 25 mg/kg in a non–dose related manner.

Orally treated rat dams exhibited pregnancy interruption but the finding was of borderline significance (Table 2). This was also true for dam growth rate. As in the instance of mice, a non–dose-related increase in the number of dams with early fetal resorptions occurred at higher doses in rat dams.

Table 3.
Summary of Fetal Anomalies in CD-1 Mice, Swiss-Webster Mice, and Fischer 344 Rats Orally Treated or Exposed to Inhalation of D9-Tetrahydrocannabinol During Gestation Days 6–15 and Sacrificed Near Term

Species	Route of administration	Δ^9-THC dose (mg/kg)	Number of fetuses	Percent anomalies (all types)					
				External	Types	Soft-tissue	Types	Skeletal	Types
CD-1 mice	Oral	Sham	755	2.2	2[a]	0.5	5[b]	7.5	3[c]
		Vehicle	1265	2.1	2[a]	13.2	7[b]	7.9	3[c]
		5–50	1310	2.5	2[a]	18.7	7[b]	16.2	3[c]
		150-600	795	2.3	2[a]	13.3	5[b]	14.5	3[c]
Swiss-Webster mice	Inhalation	Sham	263	0		1.1	2[d]	0	
		Placebo	202	0		1.0	2[d]	0	
		0.8–3.8	853	0		0.6	2[d]	0	
Fischer rats	Oral	Sham	677	0					
		Vehicle	563	0					
		12.5–50	1472	0					
	Inhalation	Sham	287	0		1.0	2[d]	0	
		Placebo	230	0		0.4	2[d]	0	
		0.8–3.8	799	0		0.4	2[d]	0	

[a]Major findings were skin hemorrhages and backwardly curved hindlimbs.
[b]Major anomalies were hydronephrosis, hemorrhages, hydrocephalus, cleft palate, hemothorax, hemoperitoneum, and hepatic focal pale areas.
[c]Major abnormalities were missing 5th sternebrae, hole in 6th sternebrae, and extra right or left ribs.
[d]Major anomalies were hydronephrosis and hydrocephalus; one low-dosed female rat had cleft palate.

3.1.2. FETAL CHANGES

In the inhalation studies on rodents, total litter weight, mean fetal weight, and sex ratio were unaltered for both species (Table 2). In contrast, there was a dose-related elevation in early resorption of mouse fetuses but not rat fetuses. The increase in total fetal mortality was attributable to early fetal resorption alone since there were no significant changes in late fetal resorption or fetal deaths.

Fetal changes among mice treated orally with pure Δ^9-THC substantiated the findings obtained after marihuana inhalation (Table 2). In addition to the increase in early fetal resorption, and thus fetal mortality, the larger doses of Δ^9-THC (150–600 mg/kg) induced a significant decrease in total litter weight and mean fetal weight. These changes originated in the excessive loss of fetuses caused by early resorptions. Similarly, rats treated orally with Δ^9-THC had a significant increase in early resorptions concomitant with decrements in total litter weight and mean fetal weight.

A summary of the rodent fetal abnormalities encountered is outlined in Table 3. There were no significant differences in the numbers of incidences or types of external defects, soft-tissue anomalies, or skeletal abnormalities for either species exposed to marihuana smoke or treated orally with pure Δ^9-THC. Among the orally treated CD-1 mice, the major external findings in both treated and control fetal groups were skin hemorrhages and backwardly curved hindlimbs. Soft-tissue anomalies in all groups included hydronephrosis, hydrocephalus, a rare observation of cleft palate, hemothorax, hemoperitoneum, and occasional hepatic focal pale areas. Skeletal aberrations encompassed missing 5th sternebrae, a hole in the 6th sternebrae and an extra right or left rib. Orally treated rats had fetuses virtually free of teratological signs.

Table 4
Pregnancy Rates and Number of Mouse Dams Exhibiting Fetal Resorption After Treatment with Δ⁹-Tetrahydrocannabinol During Gestation Days 6–15 and Sacrificed Near Term

Mouse strain	Route of adminis- tration	Δ⁹-THC dose (mg/kg)		Number of expected pregnancies				Percent with early resorptions	
				Theoret- ical (N)	Found (N)	In doubt (N)	Pregnancy rate[a] (%)	One or more resorption	All resorbed
CD-1 mice	Oral	Sham	(3)[b]	71	65	6	67	47	4
		Veh.	(4)	114	107	7	60	40	9
		5	(1)	40	40	0	71	50	0
		10	(1)	40	40	0	68	65[c]	0
		50	(1)	40	38	2	56	66[c]	5
		150	(4)	111	64	47	26[d]	82[d]	65[d]
		300	(3)	67	20	47	20[d]	96[d]	76[d]
		600	(3)	68	7	61	3[d]	100[d]	95[d]
Swiss-Webster mice	Inhalation	Sham	(1)	23	23	0	62	52	0
		Placebo	(1)	19	19	0	63	63	0
		0.8	(1)	29	29	0	62	66	0
		2.6	(1)	27	27	0	70	70	0
		3.8	(1)	30	30	0	70	73'	0

[a]Based on actual numbers of mice mated and unequivocally established pregnant by presence of at least one fetus.
[b]Values in parenthesis indicate number of studies performed.
[c]$p < 0.05$.
[d]$p < 0.01$.

Swiss-Webster mice exposed to marihuana smoke did not have fetuses with external or skeletal defects, but there were a few incidences of soft-tissue anomalies of hydronephrosis and hydrocephalus in both treated and control groups. The fetuses of rats exposed to marihuana smoke had similar insignificant changes to those observed for mice.

3.2. Mechanism of Embryotoxicity

The prevalent observation of embryotoxicity in both inhalation and oral teratology studies stimulated closer examination of this adverse effect of *Cannabis*. Based on a sufficient number of studies, it was apparent that the pregnant state of some animals was always in doubt. There was a lack of sufficient residual embryonic tissue for identification. This was a crucial circumstance since it compromised the significance of *Cannabis*-related pregnancy interruption or inhibition of conception rate. In order to understand the reason for the doubtful pregnancies and to relate them to the process of embryotoxicity, all reproductive data were pooled from similar studies and were organized on the basis of known pregnancy rates for each rodent species (Table 4 and 5). The theoretical pregnancy rates were 55–70% for mice and 80–95% for rats. These pregnancy rates were equally applied to treated and control groups.

In the oral studies on mice, there were approximately 1–8% pregnancies in doubt in control groups. On the contrary, treated groups had a nearly dose-related 42–90% doubtful pregnancies at doses above 10 mg/kg. These doubtful pregnancies resulted in pregnancy rates not being in agreement with the theoretical one for dams treated with Δ⁹-THC doses of 150–600 mg/kg. The percentage of doubtful pregnancies correlated with the percentage of dams having fetal resorptions. Moreover, there was a close correlation between the incidence of doubt-

Table 5
Pregnancy Rates and Number of Rat Dams Exhibiting Fetal Resorption After Treatment with Δ^9-Tetrahydrocannabinol During Gestation Days 6–15 and Sacrificed Near Term[a]

Rat strain	Route of administration	Δ^9-THC dose (mg/kg)	Theoret-ical (N)	Found (N)	In doubt (N)	Pregnancy rate[b] (%)	One or more resorption	All resorbed
			Number of expected pregnancies				Percent with early resorptions	
Fischer 344	Oral	Sham	70	70	0	94	21	0
		Vehicle	65	65	0	94	32	0
		12.5	63	55	8	79	45	12[d]
		25.0	64	55	9	77	50[c]	18[d]
		50.0	61	51	10	69[c]	74[d]	25[d]
Fischer 344	Inhalation	Sham	31	31	0	91	13	0
		Placebo	30	30	0	85	30	0
		0.8	30	30	0	86	27	0
		2.6	30	30	0	77	23	0
		3.8	33	33	0	92	21	0

[a]Oral results are the mean of three studies and there was one inhalation study.
[b]Based on actual numbers of rats mated and unequivocially established pregnant by presence of at least one fetus.
[c]$p < 0.05$.
[d]$p < 0.01$.

ful pregnancies and the percentage of dams with whole-litter resorptions. There were no doubtful pregnancies in the inhalation study with mice (Table 4). There also were no incidences of whole litter resorption but there was a significant increase in the percentage of dams with fetal resorptions.

A similar assessment of reproductive data was performed for the rat studies (Table 5). There were no doubtful pregnancies in oral vehicle control groups. On the other hand, approximately 13–16% of doubtful pregnancies was possible among orally treated rat dams. However, only the high-dosed group had a pregnancy rate significantly different from that of control groups. Of more certainty was a dose-related increase in the percentage of dams with fetal resorptions and whole litter resorptions.

The doses of Δ^9-THC used in the rat marihuana inhalation studies were insufficient to initiate significant changes in fetal resorption. There were no pregnancies in doubt (Table 5).

3.2.1. TEMPORAL PATTERN OF EMBRYOTOXICITY

The effect of the number of treatments on fetal viability was established by administration of two to 10 oral treatments during the critical phase of organogenesis (Table 6). Since the embryotoxicity response was not dose related, the data on Δ^9-THC groups were pooled for simplicity. After two treatments on days 6 and 7 of gestation in mice, there were no dams with resorptions in vehicle or sham-treated controls. In contrast, 74% of treated dams had fetal resorptions. Treatment for five days in mice elicited fetal resorptions in 50–64% of controls and 100% in Δ^9-THC groups. A total of eight oral treatments resulted in 60–67% control dams having fetal resorptions. Ten consecutive treatments during gestation days 6 to 15 evoked fetal resorptions in approximately 42% control dams and 100% in Δ^9-THC groups.

Table 6
Temporal Patterns of Embryotoxicity in CD-1 Mice and Fischer Rats Given Oral Δ^9-Tetrahydrocannabinol

Treatment on gestation days	Sacrifice on gestation day	CD-1 mice[a]			Fischer 344 rats[a]		
		Sham	Vehicle	> 100 mg/kg	Sham	Vehicle	> 12 mg/kg
0–7	8	0/12	0/13	20/27	0/8	0/8	0/23
6–10	11	7/14	7/11	15/15	0/10	0/10	13/28
6–13	14	8/12	9/15	16/18	2/10	2/9	10/22
6–15	17–19	7/16	6/15	17/17	5/21	7/19	27/44

Number of dams with resorptions/total dams

[a]Results on Δ^9-THC groups, 150, 300, and 600 mg/kg, for mice and 12.5, 25, and 50 mg/kg for rats, were pooled for a simpler presentation.

A similar temporal pattern of dams with fetal resorptions was observed in rats receiving more than two treatments with Δ^9-THC (Table 6). After two treatments, no control or treated dams had fetal resorptions. Continued treatment for five days instituted no resorptions in control rats but 46% of Δ^9-THC dams had resorptions. When eight consecutive treatments were administered, approximately 16% control dams had resorptions, whereas 45% of treated dams were involved. Ten treatments produced fetal resorptions in 24–37% control dams and 61% in Δ^9-THC dams.

When whole-litter resorptions were related to the number of treatments, there was a significant dose-related increase in whole-litter resorption among mice (53–100%) after two to five dosages of oral Δ^9-THC (22). Vehicle and sham-treated control mice had approximately a 6% incidence of whole litter resorptions. In the instance of rats, the response was not strictly dose related and the incidences of whole-litter resorption was 18–32% after five treatments. Both control groups had a 0–2% incidence of whole-litter resorption.

In a study in which rats were orally treated with 50 mg/kg on days 5–7, 6–8, 7–9, 8–10, or 9–11 and sacrificed on day 14 of gestation, optimal susceptibility to embryotoxicity occurred between days 7 and 9 of gestation (22). At this time interval, 36% of Δ^9-THC-treated dams had whole-litter resorptions and none of the vehicle controls did.

In the investigation on rats in which pregnancy was unequivocally confirmed by laparotomy, 50 mg/kg given orally on days 6 to 9 of gestation induced whole litter resorption in 27 percent of dams sacrificed on day 12 and in 42 percent of dams sacrificed on day 16. Neither vehicle control or sham-treated dams exhibited whole litter resorption at either sacrifice interval (22).

3.2.2. EMBRYOTOXICITY AND VAGINAL BLEEDING

Vaginal bleeding at midgestation has been considered a sign of pregnancy in rodents (95) but in the present investigation, vaginal bleeding correlated with decreases in uterine weights and fetal resorption in mice (Table 7). An oral Δ^9-THC dose of 150 mg/kg induced approximately a 21% incidence of fetal resorptions in conjunction with a 94% reduction in dam uterine weights and a 9% incidence in dam vaginal bleeding. At 300 mg/kg 68% fetal resorptions occurred concomitantly with a 93% decline in uterine weights and a 33% incidence of vaginal bleeding in dams. The highest Δ^9-THC dose of 600 mg/kg had corresponding values of 100% fetal resorptions, a 97% reduction in uterine weights and 36% of dams exhibited vaginal bleeding. There was approximately 8% fetal resorptions, normal uterine weights, and

Table 7
Interrelationship of Mouse Embryotoxicity, Dam Uterine Weights and Dam Vaginal Bleeding
Evoked by Δ^9-Tetrahydrocannabinol Administered During Organogenesis

Mouse strain	Route of administration	Δ^9-THC dose, mg/kg	Early fetal resorptions		Uterine weights mean ± SD	Dam vaginal bleeding	
			Resorption/ total	Fetuses, %		Bled/ total;	Dams, %
CD-1 mice[a]	Oral	Sham	77/755	10.2	5.8 ± 6.3	0/71	0
		Vehicle	83/1343	6.2	7.6 ± 7.8	1/114	1
		150	120/565	21.2[b]	0.4 ± 0.6[b]	10/111	9[b]
		300	123/181	68.0[b]	0.5 ± 0.8[b]	22/67	33[b]
		600	87/87	100.0[b]	0.2 ± 0.1[b]	24/68	36[b]
Swiss-Webster mice	Inhalation	Sham	17/284	6.0		0/31	0
						0/45	0
		Placebo	18/229	7.9		0/33	0
		0.8	46/331	13.9[b]		0/33	0
		2.6	37/352	10.5[b]		0/33	0
		3.8	46/332	13.9[b]		0/39	0

[a]Mean results of three studies.
[b]Results significant at $p < 0.05$–0.01.

only 1 of 185 dams displayed vaginal bleeding in combined control groups. Of the 56 treated mice exhibiting vaginal bleeding, 18 had one or two resorptions, eight had multiple resorptions, and 30 had whole-litter resorptions.

Among the Swiss-Webster mice exposed to marihuana smoke during days 6–15 of gestation, none were observed to have vaginal bleeding. Similarly none of the control dams, placebo-exposed or sham-treated dams had signs of vaginal bleeding.

3.3. Dosimetry

It was not feasible to estimate plasma Δ^9-THC levels during treatment. However, for the sake of monitoring equivalence of smoke exposure of treated and control dams, COHb concentrations were determined (Table 8). It should be pointed out that the COHb analytical procedure used tended to have an approximately 10% error on the high side. Furthermore, animals exposed to smoke develop some tolerance to smoke intoxication during continued treatment and symptoms of smoke toxicity diminished with time. In effect, COHb levels are tolerated that initially are debilitating. For example, a single continuous exposure of rodents, particularly mice, to marihuana or tobacco smoke for a period of time necessary to induce COHb levels of 35–45% evoked lethality. With prolonged treatment, these and higher levels of COHb did not induce mortality. It has been demonstrated that CO is cleared from the blood within 2 hours after each exposure.

The COHb concentrations attained in the present study were dose related and COHb levels of treated and placebo groups were similar (Table 8). In rats, mice, hamsters, and guinea pigs exposed to single or multiple doses of tobacco smoke, nonlethal mean COHb values between 25 and 60% have been reported (7,61,71).

Upon completion of the marihuana inhalation studies, it was found that plasma Δ^9-THC levels were dose related (Table 8). Moreover, the range of plasma Δ^9-THC concentrations in the rodents approximated those reported for humans (2,28,33,50,72,86,90).

Table 8
Correlation of Estimated Δ^9-THC Dose, Plasma Δ^9-THC Levels and Carboxyhemoglobin Concentrations[a]

Dosimetry		Levels of plasma D9-THC and carboxyhemoglobin						
		Pregnant mouse		Pregnant rat		Non-pregnant rat[b]		Human male
Estimated Δ^9-THC, mg/kg	Puffs (3 cigs.)	THC, ng/mL	COHb, %	THC, ng/mL	COHb, %	THC, (ng/ml)	COHb, %	THC, ng/mL
Placebo	6	0	33 ± 15	0	54 ± 4			
0.8	4	73 ± 15	29 ± 11	81 ± 60	21 ± 12			
2.6	8	123 ± 21	43 ±13	183 ± 54	45 ± 9			
3.8	12	200 ± 34	60 ±16	297 ± 75	54 ± 10			
Placebo	12					0	49 ± 9	
0.4	4					76 ± 27	15 ± 4	40–80[c]
1.1	8					179 ± 81	25 ± 10	
2.2	16					319 ± 135	42 ± 9	200–500[d]

[a]Marihuana (2–2.8% Δ^9-THC) inhalation between days 6 and 15 of gestation for pregnant animals and 20 consecutive days for nonpregnant rats. Males used for mating were not exposed to marihuana.

[b]Male and female rats not used in reproductive studies; literature values after single inhalation or intravenously radiolabeled dose (5 mg/kg) were 68–270 ng/mL for mouse and rat (Gill et al., 1974; Leighty, 1973; Willinsky et al., 1974).

[c]Acute study using one radiotracer labeled marihuana cigarette (Skinner, 1972; Galanter et al., 1972; Agurell et al., 1973; Lemberger, 1973; Rosenfeld et al., 1974).

[d]Chronic marihuana users consuming unknown number of cigarettes (Gross et al., 1974; Teale et al., 1974).

For the sake of comparison, plasma Δ^9-THC findings from a chronic inhalation study in nonpregnant rats are included in Table 8 *(22)*. Others have reported a range of 68–270 ng/mL for mice and rats after a single exposure to marihuana smoke or a Δ^9-THC intravenous dose of 5 mg/kg *(30,49,97)*.

3.4. Postnatal Development

In a separate pilot experiment in which dams were treated with an oral Δ^9-THC dose of 1, 5, or 10 mg/kg or sesame oil vehicle during 21 days of gestation, they were permitted to deliver their offspring. The pups remained with their natural mothers until they achieved a body weight of 30–40 g. At this time one-half the offspring of each treated and control group was given a single oral dose of Δ^9-THC of 10 mg/kg. The other one-half of pups received sesame oil. Nearly all pups from Δ^9-THC-treated mothers exhibited a dose-related hypersensitivity and approximately 10–25% of them responded with involuntary vertical jumping ("popcorn" response). The half receiving vehicle behaved normally. None of the offspring from vehicle control dams responded to sesame oil in an abnormal fashion. Administration of Δ^9-THC evoked CNS inhibition.

4. DISCUSSION

The unequivocal embryocidal effect of marihuana and its major psychoactive agent, Δ^9-THC, has been demonstrated in rodents. The ability of *Cannabis* products to elicit whole-litter resorptions in which no vestigial embryonic tissue could be discerned was also established. Although the embryocidal effect was not always dose related, it occurred at Δ^9-THC doses that were relevant to heavy, chronic marihuana use in humans.

It was determined that two oral treatments of Δ^9-THC in mice or five in rats commencing on day 6 of gestation were adequate to induce embryotoxicity. The period of greatest susceptibility to fetal resorption was between days 7 and 9 of gestation, which was in agreement with the findings of other investigators (42,53).

The mechanism of embryotoxicity was not identified but there was a correlation between midgestation vaginal bleeding and excessive fetal resorption. This observation suggested that there may have been a direct effect of *Cannabis* on the endometrium and associated development of the fetoplacental circulatory tree. On the other hand, a similar result could have been accomplished indirectly by a deficiency of hormones necessary to maintain normal pregnancy. In regard to a potential direct effect by *Cannabis*, it is known that Δ^9-THC traverses the placental barrier of mice (25,35,44,81), rats (94), hamsters (39), and dogs (55), and deposits in yolk sac, fetal tissues, and amniotic fluid.

In the instance of a potential indirect effect through alteration of hormone secretion, both tracer disposition studies and hormone measurements have associated marihuana components with endocrine glands. Δ^9-THC doses penetrate the blood–brain barrier (1,83) and reach the critical areas of the pituitary gland (48,55,58,81) and hypothalamus (18,37,84) of a variety of species including monkey. An antigonadotrophic effect of Δ^9-THC was not mediated through the pituitary (87) but there is ample evidence that growth hormone levels (15,46), LH levels (88,89), FSH levels (19), and prolactin levels (11,13,47) are suppressed in rats. Adrenal steroidogenesis is inhibited by cannabinoids (96) as well as steroid metabolism (57).

A number of effects have been elicited by *Cannabis* products directly on the rodent uterus. Ovulation has been inhibited (63), uterine weights depressed (16,65), and water and glycogen content were deranged (12). The earlier confusion revolving around the uterotropic effect of Δ^9-THC has been partially resolved by the demonstration of different binding sites for estrogens and cannabinoids(64). Although not investigated directly on the uterus, Δ^9-THC has been shown to influence nucleic acid and protein synthesis and the activity of lysosomes (10,60).

One additional point must be addressed and that is the contribution of CO on fetal development in inhalation studies with marihuana. In the present studies there was a significant difference between the number of fetal resorptions in treated groups compared with placebo groups. However, it can be reasoned that CO may have contributed to the extent of embryotoxicity because of diminution in the available oxygen to fetuses. Other investigators have reported toxic changes in fetal rats and pups at COHb concentrations less than 20%. Persistent neurotoxic effects (20), cardiac hypertrophy (70), and reduced birth rates(21) have been seen. Slight numbers of fetal mortality were observed in rats exposed to carbon monoxide (32), but virtually none after exposure to tobacco (71). Neonatal mortality was significantly increased (35% versus 1% in controls) among rabbits at COHb levels of 18% (3). Fetal brain injury occurred, but there was no embryotoxocity in monkeys exposed to carbon monoxide intoxication (31). There is a paucity of data on the mouse in part because of their greater sensitivity to carbon monoxide (38). Minimal effects on pregnant rats and their fetuses were observed after exposure to tobacco smoke (62).

Despite the discrepancies in *Cannabis*-evoked teratological signs, the conclusion that cannabinoids are embryotoxic cannot be avoided. Furthermore the deposition of cannabinoids in fetal tissue for periods long enough to affect postnatal development must be reckoned with since fetal cannabinoid levels may be augmented during lactation (14,25,40). The residual sensitivity of offspring to Δ^9-THC has been demonstrated in the present studies on rats and EEG changes in fetal guinea pigs have extended into the postnatal period (85).

ACKNOWLEDGMENT

The author recognizes the extensive contributions of both professional and technical staff members to these studies: Robert W. Fleischman, John R. Baker, Jean Fredette, R. Jeffrey Grant, Phyllis Hughes, Rachel Haskell, Jack Metterville, and Forrest Tibbetts. Supported in part by NIDA contracts HSM 42-71-79 and 271-76-3320.

Reprinted with permission from Marihuana: Biological Effects, Analysis, Metabolism, Cellular Responses, Reproduction and Brain (G. G. Nahas and W. D. M. Paton, eds.) Pergamon, Press, New York, 1979, pp. 479–499.

REFERENCES

1. Agnew, W. F., Rumbaugh, C. L., and Cheng, J. T.(1976), The uptake of Δ^9-tetrahydrocannabinol in choroid plexus and brain cortex *in vitro* and *in vivo*. *Brain Res.* **109,** 335–366.
2. Agurell, S., Gustafsson, B., and Holstedt, B. (1973), Quantitation of Δ1-tetrahydrocannabinol in plasma from cannabis smokers. *J. Pharm. Pharmacol.* **25,** 554–558.
3. Astrup, P., Olsen, H. M., Trolle, D., and Kjeldsen, K., (1972) Effect of moderate carbon-monoxide exposure on fetal development. *Lancet*, 1220–1222.
4. Banerjee, B. M., Galbreath, C., and Sofia, R. D. (1975), Teratologic evaluation of synthetic Δ^9-tetrahydro-cannabinol in rats. *Teratology* **11,** 99–102.
5. Becker, B. A., (1975) in *Toxicology*, (Casarett, L. J. and Doull, J. eds.) Macmillan, New York, pp. 313–332.
6. Biddle, F. G. (1977) 6-Aminonicotinamide-induced cleft palate in the mouse: the nature of the difference between the A/J and C57BL/6J strains in frequency of response and its genetic basis. *Teratology* **16,** 301–312.
7. Binns, R., Beven, J. L., Wilton, L. V., and Lugton, W. G. D. (1976) Inhalation toxicity studies on cigarette smoke. 11. Tobacco smoke inhalation dosimetry studies on small laboratory animals. *Toxicology* **6,** 197–206.
8. Borgen, L. A., Davis, W. M., and Pace, H. B. (1971) Effects of synthetic Δ^9-tetrahydrocannabinol on pregnancy and offspring in the rat. *Toxicol. Appl. Pharmacol.* **20,** 480–486.
9. Borgen, L. A., Davis, W. M., and Pace, H. B. (1973) Effects of prenatal Δ^9-tetrahydrocannabinol on the development of rat offspring. *Pharmacol. Biochem. Behav.* **1,** 203–206.
10. Braude, M. C. and Szara, S. (1976) *Pharmacology of Marihuana*, vol. 2, Raven Press, New York, 461–492.
11. Bromley, B. and Zimmerman, E. (1976) Divergent release of prolactin and corticosterone following Δ^9-tetrahydrocannabinol injection in male rats. *Fed. Proc.* **35,** 220.
12. Chakravarty, I. and Ghosh, J. J. (1977) Effect of cannabis extract on uterine glycogen metabolism in prepubertal rats under normal and estradiol-treated conditions. *Biochem. Pharmacol.* **26,** 859–863.
13. Chakravarty, I., Sheth, A. R., and Ghosh, J. J. (1975) Effect of acute Δ^9-tetrahydrocannabinol treatment on serum luteinizing hormone and prolactin levels in adult female rats. *Fertil. Steril.* **26,** 947–948.
14. Chao, F.-C., Green, D. E., Forrest, I. S., Kaplan, J. N., Winship-Ball, A., and Braude, M. C. (1976) The passage of 14C-Δ^9-tetrahydrocannabinol into the milk of lactating squirrel monkeys. *Res. Comm. Chem. Pathol. Pharmacol.* **15,** 303–317.
15. Collu, R., Letarte, J., Leboeuf, G., and Ducharme, J. R. (1975) Endocrine effects of chronic administration of psychoactive drugs to prepubertal male rats. I. Δ^9-Tetrahydrocannabinol. *Life Sci.* **16,** 533–542.
16. Dixit, V. P., Arya, M., and Lohiya, N. K. (1975) The effect of chronically administered cannabis extract on the female genital tract of mice and rats. *Endokrinologie* **66,** 365–368.
17. Dubowski, K. M. (1964) Measurement of hemoglobin derivatives, in (Sunderman, F. W. and Sunderman, F. W., Jr, eds.), *Haemoglobin: Its Precursors and Metabolites*, Lippincott, Philadelphia, pp. 49–60.
18. Erdmann, G., Just, W. W., Thel, S., Werner, G., and Wiechmann, M., (1976) Comparative autoradiographic and metabolic study of Δ^8 and Δ^9-tetrahydrocannabinol in the brain of the marmoset callithrix jacchus. *Psychopharmacol.* **47,** 53–58.
19. Esber, H. J., Rosenkrantz, H., Kuo, E. H., and Braude, M. C. (1975) Serum hormone levels in non-pregnant rats after chronic oral treatment with Δ^9-tetrahydrocannabinol. *Fed. Proc.* **34,** 783.
20. Fechter, L. D. (1978) Persistent neurotoxic effects of mild prenatal carbon monoxide exposure. 17th Ann. Meet. *Soc. Toxicol.*105.
21. Fechter, L. D. and Annau, Z. (1977) Toxicity of mild prenatal carbon monoxide exposure. *Science* **197,** 680–682.
22. Fleischman, R. W., Hayden, D. W., Naqvi, R. H., Rosenkrantz, H., and Braude, M. C., The embryotoxic effects of cannabinoids in rats and mice. *J. Environ. Pathol. Toxicol.* (being reviewed).

23. Fleischman, R. W., Hayden, D. W., Rosenkrantz, H., and Braude, M. C. (1975) Prenatal effects of Δ^9-tetrahydrocannabinol in mice including a review of the literature. *Teratology* **12**, 47–50.

24. Fournier, E., Rosenberg, M., Hardy, N., and Nahas, G. G. (1976) Teratologic effects of cannabis extracts in rabbits, in *Marihuana: Chemistry, Biochemistry and Cellular Effects,* (Nahas, G. G., ed.) Springer-Verlag, New York, pp. 457–468.

25. Freudenthal, R. I., Martin, J., and Wall, M. E. (1972) Distribution of Δ^9-tetrahydrocannabinol in the mouse. *Brit. J. Pharmacol.* **44**, 244–249.

26. Fried, P. A. (1976) Short and long-term effects of prenatal cannabis inhalation upon rat offspring. *Psychopharmacology* **50**, 285–291.

27. Fried, P. A. and Nieman, G. W. (1973) Inhalation of cannabis smoke in rats. *Pharmacol. Biochem. Behav.* **1**, 371–378.

28. Galanter, M., Wyatt, R. J., Lemberger, L., Weingartner, H., Vaughan, T. B., and Roth, W. T. (1972) Effects on humans of delta-9-tetrahydrocannabinol administered by smoking. *Science* **176**, 934–936.

29. Geber, W. F. and Schramm, L. C. (1969) Effect of marihuana extract on fetal hamsters and rabbits. *Toxicol. Appl. Pharmacol.* **14**, 276–282.

30. Gill, E. W. and Lawrence, D. K. (1974) Blood and brain levels of Δ^1-tetrahydrocannabinol in mice. The effect of 7-hydroxy-Δ^1-tetrahydrocannabinol. *Biochem. Pharmacol.* **23**, 1140–1143.

31. Ginsberg, M. D. and Myers, R. E. (1976) Fetal brain injury after maternal carbon monoxide intoxication. *Neurology* **26**, 15–23.

32. Grabowski, C. T. (1976) Postnatal effects on rats of prenatal exposure to carbon monoxide. *Teratology* **13**, 23a.

33. Gross, S. J., Soares, J. R., Wong, S. L. R., and Schuster, R. E. (1974) Marijuana metabolites measured by a radioimmune technique. *Nature* **252**, 581–582.

34. Haley, S. L., Wright, P. L., Plank, J. B., Keplinger, M. L., Braude, M. C., and Calendra, J. C. (1973) The effect of natural and synthetic Δ^9-tetrahydrocannabinol on fetal development. *Toxicol. Appl. Pharmacol.* **25**, 450.

35. Harbison, R. D. and Manttlla-Plata, B. (1972) Prenatal toxicity, maternal distribution and placental transfer of tetrahydrocannabinol. *J. Pharmacol. Exp. Ther.* **180**, 446–453.

36. Harbison, R. D., Mantilla-Plata, B., and Lubin, D. J. (1977) Alternation of Δ^9-tetrahydrocannabinol-induced teratogenicity of stimulation and inhibition of its metabolism. *J. Pharmacol. Exp. Ther.* **202**, 455–465.

37. Hattori, T. and Mcgeer, P. L. (1977) Electron microscopic autoradiography and Δ^8-(^{3}H)-tetrahydrocannabinol localization in brain tissue. *Toxicol. Appl. Pharmacol.* **39**, 307–311.

38. Hilado, C. J. and Cumming, H. J. (1977) Effect of carbon monoxide on Swiss albino mice. *J. Combust. Toxicol.* **4**, 216–230.

39. Idanpaan-Heikkila, J. E., Fritchie, G. E., Englert, L. F., Ho, B. T. and McIsaac, W. M. (1969) Placental transfer of tritiated-1-Δ^9-tetrahydrocannabinol. *N. Engl. J. Med.* **281**, 330–332.

40. Jakubovic, A., Hattori, T., and Mcgeer, P. L. (1973) Radioactivity in suckled rats after giving carbon-14-labeled tetrahydrocannabinol to the mother. *Eur. J. Pharmacol.* **22**, 221–223.

41. Jakubovic, A., McGeer, P. L., and Fitzsimmons, R. C. (1976) Effects of Δ^9-tetrahydrocannabinol and ethanol on body weight protein and nucleic acid synthesis in chick embryos. *J. Toxicol. Environ. Health* **1**, 441–447.

42. Jonfja, M. G. (1976) A study of teratologic effects of intravenous, subcutaneous and intragastric administration of Δ^9-tetrahydrocannabinol in mice. *Toxicol. Appl. Pharmacol.* **36**, 151–162.

43. Joneja, M. G. (1977) Effects of Δ^9-tetrahydrocannabinol on hamster fetuses. *J. Toxicol. Environ. Health* **2**, 1031–1040.

44. Kennedy, J. S. and Waddell, W. J. (1972) Whole-body autoradiography of the pregnant mouse after administration of ^{14}C-Δ^9-THC. *Toxicol. Appl. Pharmacol.* **22**, 252–258.

45. Keplinger, M. L., Wright, P. L., Haley, S. L., Plank, J. B., Braude, M, C. and Calandra, J. C. (1973) The effect of natural and synthetic delta-9-tetrahydrocannabinol on reproductive and lactation performance in albino rats. *Toxicol. Appl. Pharmacol.* **25**, 449.

46. Kokka, N. and Garcia, J. F. (1974) Effects of Δ^9-THC (tetrahydrocannabinol) on growth hormone and ACTH secretion in rats. *Life Sci.* **15**, 329–338.

47. Kramer, J. and Ben-David, M. (1974) Suppression of prolactin secretion by acute administration of Δ^9-THC in rats. *Proc. Soc. Exp. Biol. Med.* **17**, 482–484.

48. Layman, J. M. and Milton, A. S. (1971) Distribution of tritium labelled Δ^1-tetrahydrocannabinol in the rat brain following intraperitoneal administration. *Br. J. Pharmacol.* **42**, 308–310.

49. Leighty, E. G. (1973) Metabolism and distribution of cannabinoids in rats after different methods of administration. *Biochem. Pharmacol.* **22**, 1613–1621.

50. Lemberger, L. (1973) Tetrahydrocannabinol metabolism in man. *Drug Metab. Dispos.* **1**, 461–468.

51. Maker, B. S., Khan, M. A., and Lehrer, G. M. (1974) The effect of self regulated Δ^9-tetrahydrocannabinol consumption of pregnant mice and offspring. *Fed. Proc.* **33**, 540.

52. Mantilla-Plata, B., Clewe, G. L., and Harbison, R. D. (1975) Δ^9-Tetrahydrocannabinol-induced changes in prenatal growth and development of mice. *Toxicol. Appl. Pharmacol.* **33,** 333–340.

53. Mantilla-Plata and Harbison, R. D. (1976) Influence of alteration of tetrahydrocannabinol metabolism on tetrahydrocannabinol-induced teratogenesis, in *Pharmacology of Marihuana*, vol. 2, (Braude, M. C. and Szara, S. eds.) Raven, New York, pp. 733–746.

54. *Marihuana and Health* (1977) Sixth Annual Report to Congress, Department of Health, Education and Welfare, Publ. No. (ADM) 77–443.

55. Martin, B. R., Dewey, W. L., Harris, L. S., and Bechner, J. S. (1976) ^{3}H-Δ^9-tetrahydrocannabinol distribution in pregnant dogs and their fetuses. *Res. Comm. Chem. Pathol. Pharmacol.* **17,** 457–470.

56. Martin, B. R., Harvey, D. J., and Paton, W. D. M. (1977) Biotransformation of cannabidiol in mice: identification of new acid metabolites. *Drug. Metab. Disp.* **5,** 259–267.

57. Maskarinec, M. P., Shipley, G., Novotny, M., Brown, D. J., and Forney, R. B. (1978) Different effects of synthetic delta-9-tetrahydrocannabinol and cannabis extract on steroid metabolism in male rats. *Experientia* **34,** 88–89.

58. Mcisaac, W. M., Fritchie, G. E., Idanpaan-Heikkila, J. E., Ho, B. T., and Englert, L. F. (1971) Distribution of marihuana in monkey brain and concomitant behavioral effects. *Nature* **230,** 593–594.

59. Miras, C. J. (1965) Some aspects of cannabis action. in *Hashish: Its Chemistry and Pharmacology* (Wolstenholme, G. E. W. and Knight, J. eds.) Little, Brown, Boston, MA, pp. 37–52.

60. Nahas, G. G., Paton, W. D. M., and Idanpaan-Heikkila, J. E. (1976) *Marihuana, Chemistry, Biochemistry and Cellular Effects*. Springer-Verlag, New York, pp. 3–556.

61. Nettesheim, P., Guerin, M. R., Kendrick, J., Rubin, I., Stokely, J., Creasia, D., Maddox, W., and Caton, J. E. (1975) Control and maximization of tobacco smoke dose in chronic animal studies, in *Proceedings of the Tobacco Smoke Inhalation Workshop on Experimental Methods in Smoking and Health Research*. DHEW Publ. No. (NIH) 75-906. (Gori, G. B., ed.) pp. 17–26.

62. Nikitovitch-Winer, M. B., and Ferry, J. D. (1973) Influence of smoking on reproductive process in the rat. *Proc. Un. Kent. Tobacco & Health Res. Inst. Rep.* **4,** 337–359.

63. Nir, I., Ayalon, D., Tsafrirl A., Cordova, T., and Lindner, H. R. (1973) Δ^1-Tetrahydrocannabinol: suppression of the cyclic surge of LH secretion and of ovulation in the rat. *Nature* **243,** 470.

64. Okey, A. B. and Bondy, G. P. (1978) Δ^9-Tetrahydrocannabinol and 17-ß-estradiol bind to different macromolecules in estrogen target tissue. *Science* **200,** 312–314.

65. Okey, A. B. and Truant, G. S. (1975) Cannabis-demasculinizes rats but is not estrogenic. *Life Sci.* **17,** 1113–1118.

66. Pace, H. B., Davis, W. M., and Borgen, L. A. (1971) Teratogenesis and marihuana. *Ann. NY Acad. Sci.* **191,** 123–131.

67. Persaud, T. V. N. and Ellington, A. C. (1967) Cannabis in early pregnancy. *Lancet* **2,** 1306.

68. Persaud, T. V. N. and Ellington, A. C. (1968) Teratogenic activity of cannabis resin. *Lancet* **2,** 406–407.

69. Phillips, R. N., Turk, R. F., and Forney, R. B. (1971) Acute toxicity of Δ^9-tetrahydrocannabinol in rats and mice. *Proc. Soc. Exp. Biol. Med.* **136,** 260–263.

70. Prigge, E. and Hochrainer, D. (1977) Effects of carbon monoxide inhalation on erythropoiesis and cardiac hypertrophy in fetal rats. *Toxicol. Appl. Pharmacol.* **42,** 225–228.

71. Reckzeh, G., Donten Will, W., and Leuschner, F. (1975) Testing of cigarette smoke inhalation for teratogenicity in rats. *Toxicology* **4,** 289–295.

72. Rosenfeld, J. J., Bowins, B., Roberts, J., Perkins, J., and Macpherson, A. S. (1974) Mass fragmentographic assay for Δ^9-tetrahydrocannabinol in plasma. *Anal. Chem.* **46,** 2232–2234.

73. Rosenkrantz, H. (1976) The immune response and marihuana, in *Marihuana: Chemistry, Biochemistry and Cellular Effects*. (Nahas, G. G., ed.) Springer-Verlag, New York, pp. 441–456.

74. Rosenkrantz, H. and Braude, M. C. (1974) Acute, subacute and 23-day chronic marihuana inhalation toxicities in the rat. *Toxicol. Appl. Pharmacol.* **28,** 428–441.

75. Rosenkrantz, H. and Braude, M. C. (1975) Rat inhalation toxicity of Turkish marihuana. *Pharmacologist* **17,** 181.

76. Rosenkrantz, H. and Braude, M. C. Comparative chronic toxicities of Δ9-tetrahydrocannabinol administered by inhalation or orally in rat, in *The Pharmacology of Marihuana*. (Braude, M. C. and Szara, S. eds.) Raven, New York, pp. 571–584, 1976. 1

77. Rosenkrantz, H., Fleischman, R. W., and Baker, J. R. (1978) Embryotoxicity of marihuana by inhalation. *Fed. Proc.* **37,** 737.

78. Rosenkrantz, H., Hayden, D. W., and Braude, M. C. (1976) Inhalation toxicity of Turkish marihuana, cannabichromene and cannabidiol. *Fed. Proc.* **35,** 643.

79. Rosenkrantz, H., Heyman, I. A., and Braude, M. C. (1974) Inhalation, parenteral and oral LD 50 values of Δ^9-tetrahydrocannabinol in Fischer rats. *Toxicol. Appl. Pharmacol.* **28,** 18–27.

80. Rosenkrantz, H., Thompson, G. R., and Braude, M. C. (1972) Oral and parenteral formulations of marihuana constituents. *J. Pharm. Sci.* **61,** 1106–1112.

81. Ryrfeldt, A., Ramsay, C. H., Nilsson, I. M., Widman, M., and Agurell, S. (1973) Whole-body autoradiography of Δ^1-tetrahydrocannabinol in the rat. *Psychopharmacol.* **27,** 141–156.

82. Sassenrath, E. N. and Chapman, L. F. (1975) Tetrahydrocannabinol-induced manifestations of the "marihuana syndrome" in group-living macaques. *Fed. Proc.* **34,** 1666–1670.

83. Schou, J., Prockop, L. D., Dahlstrom, G., and Rohde, C. (1977) Penetration of delta-9-tetrahydrocannabinol and 11-hydroxy-delta-9-tetrahydrocannabinol through the blood-brain barrier. *Acta Pharmacol. Toxicol.* **41,** 33–38.

84. Shannon, M. E. and Fried, P. A. (1972) The macro- and microdistribution and polymorphic electroencephalographic effects of Δ^9-tetrahydrocannabinol in the rat. *Psychopharmacol.* **27,** 141–156.

85. Singer, P. R., Seibetta, J. J., and Rosen, M. G. (1973) Simulated marihuana smoke in the maternal and fetal guinea pig. *Am. J. Obs. Gyn.* **117,** 331–340.

86. Skinner, R. F. (1972) Determination of submicrogram amounts of Δ^9-THC (tetrahydrocannabinol) and its metabolites. *Proc. West. Pharmacol. Soc.* **15,** 136–138.

87. Smith, C. G., Besch, N. F., Smith, R. G., and Besch, P. K. (1978) Mechanism for the anti-gonadotrophic action of tetrahydrocannabinol (THC). *Fed. Proc.* **37,** 724.

88. Smith, C. G. and Moore, C. E. (1976) Effect of delta-9-tetrahydrocannabinol (THC) on the secretion of male sex hormone in the rhesus monkey. *The Pharmacologist* **18,** 248.

89. Symons, A. M., Teale, J. D., and Marks, V. (1976) Effect of Δ^9-tetrahydrocannabinol on the hypothalamicpituitary-gonadal system in the maturing male. *J. Endocrin.* **68,** 43P–44P.

90. Teale, J. D., Forman, E. J., King, L. J., and Marks, V. (1974) Radioimmunoassay of cannabinoids in blood and urine. *Lancet* **2,** 533–555.

91. Thomas, R. J. (1975) Toxicologic and teratologic effects of Δ^9-tetrahydrocannabinol in the zebrafish embryo. *Toxicol. Appl. Pharmacol.* **32,** 184–190.

92. Uyeno, E. T. (1973) Δ^9-Tetrahydrocannabinol administration during pregnancy of the rat. *Proc. West. Pharmacol. Soc.* **16,** 64–67.

93. Uyeno, E. T. (1975) Δ^9-Tetrahydrocannabinol administered to pregnant rats. *Pharmacologist* **17,** 181.

94. Vardaris, R. M., Weisz, D. J., Fazel, A., and Rawitch, A. B. (1976) Chronic administration of delta-9-tetrahydrocannabinol to pregnant rats: studies of pup behavior and placental transfer. *Pharmacol. Biochern. Behav.* **4,** 249–254.

95. Venable, J. W. (1939) Intrauterine bleeding in the pregnant albino rat. The " placental sign ". *Anat. Rec.* **74,** 273–293.

96. Warner, W. and Harris, L. S. (1978) Inhibition of corticosteroidogenesis by delta-9-tetrahydrocannabinol. *Endocrinology* **101,** 1815–1820.

97. Willinsky, M. D., Kalant, H., Meresz, O., Endrenyi L., and Woo, N. (1974) Distribution and metabolism *in vivo* of carbon 14-labeled tetrahydrocannabinol in the rat. *Eur. J. Pharmacol.* **27,** 106–119.

98. Wilson, J. C. and Warkry, J. (1964) Methods of administering agents and detecting malformations in experimental animals, in *Teratology, Principles and Techniques,* University of Chicago Press, Chicago, IL, pp. X–X.

99. Wright, P. L., Smith, S. H., Keplinger, M. L., Calandra, J. C., and Braude, M. C. (1976) Reproductive and teratologic studies with Δ^9-tetrahydrocannabinol and crude marihuana extract. *Toxicol. Appl. Pharmacol.* **38,** 223–235.

34

Prenatal Exposure to Cannabis and Fetal Development

David D. Cozens, Gabriel G. Nahas, and David Harvey

Abstract

The purpose of these experiments was to determine the effects of *Cannabis* extracts on fetal development when administered to pregnant rabbits in doses calculated to approximate those that may be reached in human consumption. Two series of experiments were conducted using 84 New Zealand rabbits. They were treated with *Cannabis* extracts administered by gastric intubation or by subcutaneous administration from days 6–18 of gestation. The animals were sacrificed on day 29. During pregnancy, treated rabbits showed a lower mean gain in body weight than did the control animals.

The mean weights of the fetuses treated with *Cannabis* extracts were lower than those of fetuses from control animals. The differences were statistically significant for rabbits receiving the equivalent of 3 and 5 mg/kg THC per day via the oral route ($p < 0.01$ and 0.05) and for rabbits receiving 5 mg/kg THC per day by the subcutaneous route ($p < 0.001$). The mean weights of the placentae of the treated animals were lower than those of the control animals (following oral administration, $p < 0.05$, and following subcutaneous administration, $p < 0.01$). Whereas these studies demonstrate that *Cannabis* extracts are fetotoxic in the rabbit, there was no indication that treatment had increased the incidence of major malformation. However, the fetuses of the animals treated with cannabis extract showed an increased incidence of minor skeletal and visceral anomalies.

1. INTRODUCTION

The smoking of the flowering tops of *Cannabis sativa*, either in its natural form (marihuana) or after extraction (hashish), has become after tobacco the most frequently and voluntarily inhaled xenobiotic in American society. In 1980, 42 million Americans were estimated to have used the drug, and three million, most below the age of 40 consumed it daily. Surveys also indicate that 10% of high school seniors smoke marihuana every day (*1*). On the basis of

From: *Marihuana and Medicine*
Edited by: G. G. Nahas et al.   © Humana Press Inc., Totowa, NJ

these figures, it may be estimated that close to one million women of childbearing age are current users.

The effects of *Cannabis* extracts and of its major psychoactive constituents, Δ^9-tetrahydro-cannabinol (THC) on fetal development has been extensively studied in animals. Although the production of major malformations by xenobiotics which are usually designated as teratologic may be the most obvious demonstration of their damaging effect on fetal development and maturation, it is only an extreme manifestation of their fetotoxic potential. Less apparent and more subtle manifestations of this fetotoxicity are: lower birth weight, retarded growth, and neurological and behavioral anomalies (designated behavioral teratology).

Although reports of the teratogenicity of cannabis extracts and THC are conflicting *(2–18)*, fetotoxicity of these xenobiotics has been clearly documented in four mammalian species *(14,15,17,19)*. And yet, there are only a few fragmentary reports linking the use of marihuana alone during pregnancy to impaired fetal development.

In this paper, we report our studies of the fetotoxic effects of *Cannabis* extracts in the rabbit. Next we review the few reports in the clinical literature linking marihuana use during pregnancy to impaired fetal development.

2. EXPERIMENTAL STUDIES

The purpose of the experiments described here was to determine the effect on fetal development of *Cannabis* extracts administered to pregnant rabbits in doses calculated to approximate those which may be reached in human consumption. Such doses have been empirically established *(20)* by comparing blood levels reached in rodents following exposures to different dose schedules of THC to those measured in humans. Furthermore, the doses were selected to produce minimal measurable effects on the maternal organism: They amounted to: 0.6–5.0 mg/kg of THC equivalent per day, administered intragastrically or subcutaneously. They correspond to approximately one-fiftieth of the LD_{50} in rats.

3. METHODS

Two series of experiments were conducted using 84 New Zealand white rabbits allocated to two control groups and four experimental groups. The protocol adopted was that used by the Huntingdon Research Centre over the last 17 years for the assessment of the effect of more than 350 chemical compounds on the fetal development of this animal *(21)*. The females were treated from the 6th through the 18th day of gestation.

The alcohol extract of *Cannabis* was supplied by Monique Braude of the National Institute on Drug Abuse (NIDA), Rockville, Maryland. Two batches were used, one containing 3% THC, 5% cannabidiol (CBD) plus cannabichromene (CBC), and 15% cannabinol (CBN). The second contained 13% of THC, 1.7% of CBD plus CBC, and 1.2% of CBN. Analysis was performed using the mass spectrometer-GLC technique *(26)*.

In the first series of studies, *Cannabis* extract batch 1 was used. The extract was prepared as an emulsion in sesame oil at 1:10 dilution and was administered to the rabbits by gastric intubation. The doses were 1 mL/kg, equivalent to 3 mg/THC, 5 mg CBD plus CBC, and 15 mg CBN/kg, and 0.2 mL/kg, equivalent to 0.6 mg THC, 1 mg CBD plus CBC, and 3 mg CBN/kg. The control group received sesame oil *(19)*.

In the second series of experiments, the cannabis extract batch 2 was administered subcutaneously in an isotonic saline solution containing 1% Tween-80 or orally as an emulsion in sesame oil.

A 1-mL/kg dose was equivalent to 5 mg THC, 0.65 mg CBD plus CBC, and 0.45 mg CBN/kg. The control group was treated subcutaneously with the saline–Tween-80 vehicle.

The animals were sacrificed on day 29. The ovaries and uteri were examined to determine the number of corpora lutea, the number and distribution of live fetuses, and the number of resorptions. The fetuses were weighed and evident abnormalities noted. They were then dissected to determine visceral abnormalities. The skeletons were then stained and examined (22). The analysis of the results considered the whole litter as the experimental unit (23). All values expressed as percentages were first calculated for each litter and the group values calculated as means of the individual percentages. Statistical analyses using the litter as the basic sample were performed by the nonparametric method described by Kruskal and Wallis (24) and Luthra (25).

In a third experiment, 0.5 or 1 mL of *Cannabis* extract (containing 3 mg THC, 5 mg CBD and CBC, and 15 mg CBN/mL) was administered to five pregnant rabbits via the oral route from days 15–18 of gestation. Blood samples were withdrawn from 30 minutes to 1 hour after the last dose, and the animals were then sacrificed. After extraction, the cannabinoids were measured in the plasma and in the whole fetus from each litter, using the method described by Harvey (26).

4. RESULTS

During pregnancy, treated rabbits showed a lower mean gain in body weight than did the control animals (Fig. 1). Some animals given 3 or 5 mg THC equivalent showed a loss in weight during the course of treatment, but regained it when administration of the *Cannabis* extract ceased after day 18. No other specific signs were observed in the pregnant females, apart from local tissue reaction around the injection sites of those given the extract subcutaneously.

The effects on the progeny are described in Tables 1 and 2. The mean weights of the fetuses treated with cannabis extract were lower than those of fetuses from control animals. The differences were statistically significant for rabbits receiving the equivalent of 3 and 5 mg/kg THC per day via the oral route ($p < 0.01$ and 0.05) and for rabbits receiving 5 mg/kg THC per day by the subcutaneous route ($p < 0.001$). Also, in the second series of experiments, the mean weights of the placentae of the treated animals were lower than those of the control animals (following oral administration, $p < 0.05$, and following subcutaneous administration, $p < 0.01$).

There was no indication that treatment had increased the incidence of major malformation (21,22). However, the fetuses of the animals treated with *Cannabis* extract showed an increased incidence of minor skeletal and visceral anomalies, which probably reflects the reduced fetal weights.

The plasma concentrations of THC, CBD, and CBN following three consecutive doses were of the order of 2.5–13 ng/mL for THC and for CBN and could not be detected for CBD (Table 3). No cannabinoids were detected in the fetal tissues.

5. DISCUSSION

Maternal treatment of New Zealand white rabbits with *Cannabis* was not associated with an increased incidence of grossly malformed young. Our results are thus in general agreement with those of Wright et al. (14) and Sofia et al. (18). Similar results have been obtained following the administration of cannabis or THC to other species, e.g., to the rat and the mouse by Rosenkrantz (16) and to the rhesus monkey by Sassenrath (17). However, in common with many other studies in which *Cannabis* or THC was administered orally (12–14,16), parenterally (3,4,10,13,18), or by inhalation (11), there were signs of impaired fetal growth. The mechanisms of these adverse effects on maternal and fetal growth as well as upon the placenta have not been fully established. Cannabinoids are known to reduce

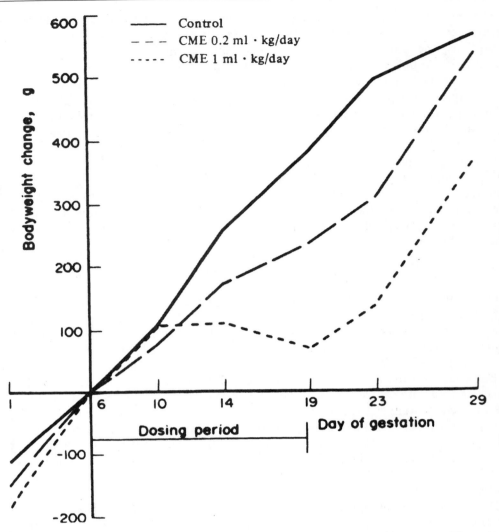

Fig. 1. Effects of THC on weight gain of gestating rabbits treated with cannabis extracts, The animals were treated with crude marihuana extracts (CME) administered orally in sesame oil. These extracts contained 3% THC, 5% CBD + CBC, and 15% CBN. (———) Control; (———) CME 0.2 mL/kg/day; (———) CME 1 mL/kg/day.

maternal food consumption *(18)* and to impair protein, RNA, and DNA biosynthesis required for cell proliferation *(27,28)*. *Cannabis* is also reported to inhibit human placental cytochrome P-450, which plays a significant role in the synthesis of placental estrogen *(29)*; together with progesterone, placental estrogen is involved in the regulation of the fetal placental circulation. The production of LH, FSH, and prolactin may also be impaired by cannabinoids at nanomolar concentrations acting on the hypothalamo-pituitary axis *(30–32)*.

The maternal plasma cannabinoid concentrations, found in five assays in rabbits, were very low compared with those reported in animals and in humans receiving similar intake *(4,10,16,33,34)*. This may be due to the difference in gastric absorption via intragastric intubation, from absorption via parenteral administration, or exposure by inhalation. The low concentrations may also reflect more rapid excretion of cannabinoids in the rabbit, which

Table 1

Effects of Intragastric Administration of Cannabis Extract on Fetal Development of the New Zealand Rabbit (mean litter data)

Grp	Number of animals	Number viable fetuses			Number of resorptions			Implants	Corpora lutea	%Loss pre-implantation	% Fetal loss	Litter weight (g)	Weight of fetus (g)
		male	female	total	early	late	total						
1[a]	12	3.9	4.3	8.2	1.0	0.3	1.3	9.4	10.8	11.8	9.6	334.3	42.0
2[b]	16	4.6	4.0	8.6	0.6	0.7	1.3	9.9	11.3	12.8	12.0	334.8	39.7
3[c]	14	4.6	4.1	8.7	0.6	0.7	1.3	10.0	11.1	9.4	12.7	229.5[d]	34.7[**e]

[a] Control treated with sesame oil.
[b] Treated with 0.2 ml/kg of sesame oil emulsion containing 0.6 mg of THC, 1 mg of CBD + CBC, and 3 mg of CBN.
[c] Treated with 1ml/kg of sesame oil emulsion containing 3 mg of THC, 5 mg of CBD +CBC, and 15 mg of CBN.
[d*] $p < 0.05$ (Kruskal-Wallis test).
[e**] $p < 0.01$ (Kruskal-Wallis test).

Table 2

Effects of Cannabis Extract on Fetal Development in the New Zealand Rabbit (mean litter data)

Group	Number of animals	Number viable fetuses			Number of resorptions			Im-plants	Corpora lutea	%Loss preim-plantation	% Fetal loss	Litter weight (g)	Weight of fetus (g)	Total placental weight (g)	Placer weight (g)
		Male	Female	total	early	late	total								
4[a]	14	3.8	4.6	8.4	0.5	0.5	1.0	9.4	11.2	16.5	10.9	363.4	45.26	47.7	5.94
5[b]	14	4.2	5.2	9.4	0.9	1.0	1.9	11.3	11.9	5.1	19.3	330.7	370.2[***f]	43.2	4.91[**e]
6[c]	14	3.8	5.2	9.0	0.5	0.3	0.8	9.8	11.2	12.7	8.0	351.6	39.90[*d]	43.4	4.98[*]

[a] Control treated by subcutaneous injection of 1 ml/kg of isotonic solution containing 1% Tween 80.
[b] Treated by subcutaneous injection of 1ml/kg of cannabis extract dissolved in the preceding solution and containing 5 mg of THC, 0.65 mg of CBD + CBC, and 0.45 mg of CBN.
[c] Treated by intragastric administration of 1 ml/kg of cannabis extract in sesame oil and cotnaining 5 mg THC, 0.65 mg of CBC and CBC, and 0.45 mg of CBN.
[d*] $p < 0.05$ (Kruskal-Wallis test).
[e**] $p < 0.01$ (Kruskal-Wallis test).
[f***] $p < 0.001$ (Kruskal-Wallis test).

Table 3
Plasma Concentrations of Cannabinoids in Pregnant Females Receiving Cannabis Extracts

Number of rabbit	Dose (ml · kg/d) from 15th to 18th day	Time of sampling (after the last dose) (h)	Concentrations (ng/mL)		
			CBN	THC	CBD
51	0.5	0.5	0[b]	T[a]	0[b]
52	0.5	1.0	13.0	4.0	T
53	0.5	0.5	2.5	3.0	0
55	1.0	0.5	3.0	4.5	0
56	1.0	1.0	4.3	4.5	0

Doses were 0.5–1 ml/kg. Each mL contained 3 mg of THC, 5 mg of CBD + CBC, and 15 mg of CBN.
[a] T, traces (limit of detection = 0.5 ng/ml).
[b] O, No cannabinoids were detected in fetal tissues.

takes place mainly via the renal route *(35)*. It should also be recalled that in other species, THC has been recovered from the fetus following administration to the dam *(36–39)*. In the present studies, it may be possible that concentrations of cannabinoids lower than 0.5 ng/g, which could not be detected by the method used, might have reached the fetus. It would seem that the fetotoxicity observed in these studies might be caused in great part by the effect of the drug on the maternal organism in the brain and placenta, which are affected by nanomolar concentrations of the drug (Fig. 2) *(16,17)*.

It is not always appreciated that although the production of gross malformation by a substance may be the most obvious demonstration of its embryofetal toxicity, this is only part of the spectrum of possible signs of such toxicity. At one extreme may lie lethality, followed by teratogenicity, then by fetal growth retardation, whereas at the other extreme may lie more subtle events, such as changes in the behavior of the offspring. Thus, our observation of reduced maternal body weight gain and of impaired placental and fetal growth at low doses and low plasma levels corresponding to those used in moderate human consumption *(20)* should not be dismissed. Reduced fetal weight has been a consistent finding in animals born from *Cannabis*-treated females.

At the more subtle level, there have been reports that maternal administration of *Cannabis* is associated with reduced concentrations of neonatal rat brain macromolecules *(25)*, with possible learning deficits in rats *(40,41)*, and also with subtle behavioral changes in the offspring of chronically exposed monkeys *(17)*. Effects produced *in utero*, such as altered fetal brain biochemistry *(25)* or those leading to altered male reproductive performance *(42)* may be exacerbated in the early neonatal period by cannabinoids ingested with the maternal milk *(43)*.

6. REVIEW OF CLINICAL REPORTS

The use of *Cannabis* has been mentioned in six clinical reports describing congenital malformations in offspring of mothers who had consumed the drug during pregnancy *(44–48;* H.Q. Quazi et al., personal communication). In the first five, the use of *Cannabis* was associated with that of other psychoactive drugs (LSD, amphetamines, barbiturates) and major malformations were reported. In Qazi et al., *(49)*, the mothers admitted smoking marihuana daily during pregnancy, yet categorically denied use of alcohol and other psychoactive substances. The two resulting infants displayed symptoms of intrauterine growth retardation—lower birth weight, shorter height, smaller head circumference, abnormal neurological manifestations, and facial anomalies. The fathers of these two infants drank alcohol, but were not alco-

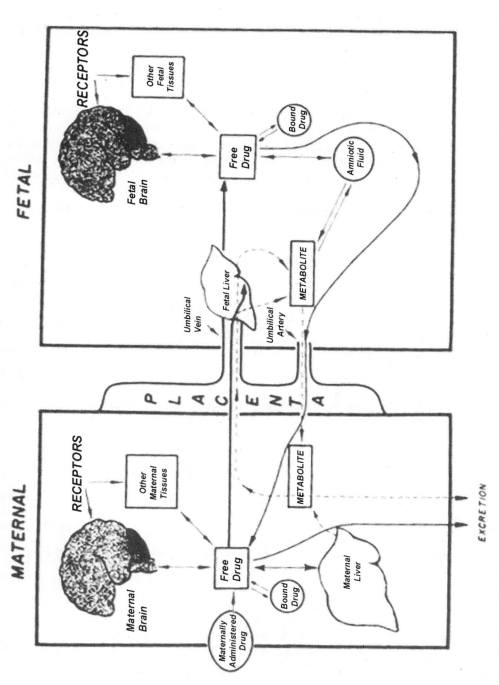

Fig. 2. Distribution and biotransformation of drugs in a maternal-placental-fetal unit. THC, or its metabolites, may affect directly fetal development by crossing the placenta, or indirectly by acting on the maternal organism: the brain (hypothalamus) that regulates gonadotropin secretion and the placenta that regulates fetal circulation and nutrition.

holics, and smoked marihuana. The relationship of paternal drinking to abnormal fetal development remains to be explored. The contribution of paternal *Cannabis* smoking to offspring anomalies should also be examined, since chronic marihuana smokers present an increased incidence of abnormal, nonovoïd forms of sperm *(50)*. The anomalies observed on the two infants born to marihuana-smoking mothers were similar to those described in the fetal alcohol syndrome, which was first scientifically documented in 1968 *(51)*, confirming observations made since recorded history.

7. CONCLUSION

Experimental studies and preliminary clinical observations indicate that *Cannabis* use during pregnancy is fetotoxic. In view of the widespread usage of marihuana among young women of childbearing age and among prospective fathers, systematic epidemiological studies should be undertaken to determine the extent of incidence of neonatal and postnatal morphological, neurological, and behavioral anomalies associated with prenatal marihuana exposure.

Reprinted with permission from: Banbury Report 11, Cold Spring Harbor Laboratory, New York, 1982, pp. 473–484.

REFERENCES

1. Johnston, L.D., J.G. Bachman, and P.M. O'Malley. (1981). Student drug use in America. 1975–1980. National Institute on Drug Abuse, Rockville, MD.
2. Persaud, T.V. and A.C. Ellington. (1968). Teratogenic activity of cannabis resin. *Lancet* **ii,** 406.
3. Geber, W.F. and L.C. Schramm. (1969). Effect of marihuana extract on fetal hamsters and rabbits. *Toxicol. Appl. Pharmacol.* **14,** 276.
4. Harbison, R.D. and B. Mantilla-Plata. (1972). Prenatal toxicity, maternal distribution and placental transfer of THC. *J. Pharmacol. Exp. Ther.* **180,** 446.
5. Borgen, L.A., W.M. Davis, and H.B. Pace. (1971). Effects of synthetic delta-9-THC on pregnancy and offspring in the rat. *Toxicol. Appl. Pharmacol.* **20,** 480.
6. Haley, S.L., P.L. Wright, J.B. Plank, M.L. Keplinger, M.C. Braude, and J.C. Calendra. (1973). The effect of natural and synthetic delta-9-THC on fetal development. *Toxicol. App. Pharmacol.* **25,** 450.
7. Keplinger, M.L., P.L. Wright, S.L. Haley, J.B. Plank, M.C. Braude, and J.C. Calandra. (1973). The effect of natural and synthetic delta-9-THC on reproductive and lactation performance in albino rats. *Toxicol. Appl. Pharmacol.* **25,** 449.
8. Banerjee, B. M., Galbreath, C., and Sovia, R. D. (1975). Teratologic evaluation of synthetic delta-9-THC in rats. *Teratology* **11,** 99.
9. Fleischman, R.W., D.W. Hayden, H. Rosenkrantz, and M.C. Braude. (1975). Prenatal effects of delta-9-THC in mice including a review of the literature. *Teratology* **12,** 47.
10. Mantilla-Plata, B., G.L. Cleve, and R.D. Harbison. (1975). Delta-9-THC induced changes in prenatal growth and development of mice. *Toxicol. Appl. Pharmacol.* **33,** 333.
11. Fried, P.A. (1976). Short and long term effects of prenatal cannabis inhalation upon rat offspring. *Psychopharmacology* **50,** 285.
12. Fournier, E., E. Rosenberg, N. Hardy, and G.G. Nahas. (1976). Teratologic effects of cannabis extracts in rabbits, in *Marihuana—Chemistry, Biochemistry and Cellular Effects* (Nahas, G.G. and Paton, W.D.M.) eds, Springer-Verlag, New York, p. 457.
13. Joneja, M.G. (1976). A study of teratological effects of intravenous, subcutaneous and intragastric administration of delta-9-THC in mice. *Toxicol. Appl. Pharmacol.* **36,** 151.
14. Wright, P.L., S.H. Smith, M.L. Keplinger, J.C. Calandra, and M.C. Braude. (1976). Reproductive and teratologic studies with delta-9-THC and crude marihuana extract. *Toxicol. Appl. Pharmacol.* **38,** 223.
15. Rosenkrantz, H., R.W. Fleischmann, and J.R. Baker. (1978). Embryotoxicity of marihuana by inhalation. *Fed. Proc.* **37,** 737.
16. Rosenkrantz, H. (1979). Effects of cannabis on fetal development of rodents, in *Marihuana: Biological Effects* (Nahas, G.G. and Paton, W.D.M., eds.), Pergamon, Oxford, UK, p. 479.

17. Sassenrath, E.N., L.F. Chapman, and G.P. Goo. (1979). Reproduction in rhesus monkeys chronically exposed to delta-9-THC, in *Marihuana: Biological Effects* (Nahas, G.G. and Paton, W.D.M., eds.), Pergamon, Oxford, UK,.p. 501.

18. Sofia, R.D., J.E. Strasbaugh, and B.N. Banerjee. (1979). Teratologic evaluation of synthetic delta-9-THC in rabbits. *Teratology* **19**, 361.

19. Cozens, D.D., R. Clark, A.K. Palmer, N. Hardy, G.G. Nahas, and D.J. Harvey. 1979. The effect of crude marihuana extract on embryonic and fetal development of the rabbit, in *Marihuana: Biological Effects* (Nahas, G.G. and Paton, W.D.M. eds.), Pergamon, Oxford, UK, p. 469.

20. Rosenkrantz, H. (1976). The immune response and marihuana, in *Marihuana: Chemistry, Biochemistry and Cellular Effects* (Nahas, G.G. and Paton, W.D.M.) eds., Springer-Verlag, New York, p. 441.

21. Palmer, A.K. (1968). Spontaneous malformations of the New Zealand white rabbit: the background to safety evaluation tests. *Lab. Anim.* **2**, 195.

22. Cozens, D.D. (1965). Abnormalities of the external form and of the skeleton in the New Zealand white rabbit. *Food Cosmet. Toxicol.* **3**, 695.

23. Weil, C.S. (1970). Selection of the valid number of sampling units and a consideration of their combination in toxicological studies involving reproduction, teratogenesis or carcinogenesis. *Food Cosmet. Toxicol.* **8**, 177.

24. Kruskal, W.H. and W.A. Wallis. (1952). Use of ranks in one criterion variance analysis. *J. Amer. Stat. Assoc.* **47**, 582.

25. Luthra, Y.K. (1979). Brain biochemical alterations in neonates of dams treated orally with delta-9-THC during gestation and lactation, in *Marihuana: Biological Effects* (Nahas, G.G. and Paton, W.D.M.) eds., Pergamon, Oxford, UK, p. 531..

26. Harvey, D.J. (1978). Comparison of fourteen substituted silyl derivatives for the characterization of alcohols, steroids and cannabinoids by combined gas-liquid chromatography and mass spectrometry. *J. Chromatogr.* **147**, 291.

27. Nahas, G.G., A. Morishima, and B. Desoize. (1977). Effects of cannabinoids on macromolecular synthesis and replication of cultured lymphocytes. *Fed. Proc.* **36**, 17 48.

28. Stein, G.S., M.J. Mon, A.E. Haas, R.L. Jansing, and J.L. Stein. (1979). Cannabinoids: the influence on cell proliferation and macro molecular biosynthesis, in *Marihuana: Biological Effects* (Nahas, G.G. and Paton, W.D.M., eds.), Pergamon, Oxford, UK, p. 171.

29. Stanley, R.L., P.K. Besch, and N.F. Besch. (1979). The effect of THC on the cytosol and microsomal fractions of the human term placenta. *Pharmacologist* **21**, 204.

30. Kramer, J. and M. Ben-David. (1974). Suppression of prolactin secretion by acute administration of delta-9-THC in rats. *Proc. Soc. Exp. Biol. Med.* **17**, 482.

31. Chakravarty, I., P.G. Shah, A.R. Sheth, and J.J. Ghosh. (1979). Mode of action of delta-9-tetrahydrocannabinol on hypothalamo-pituitary function in adult female rats. *J. Reprod. Fert.* **57**, 113.

32. Smith, C.G., M.T. Smith, N.F. Besch, R.G. Smith, and R.H. Asch. (1979). Effect of delta-9-tetrahydrocannabinol on female reproductive function, in *Marihuana: Biological Effects* (Nahas, G.G. and Paton, W.D.M., eds.), Pergamon, Oxford, UK, p. 449.

33. Agurell, S., Gustafsson, B., and Holmstedt, B. (1973). Quantitation of Δ^1-THC in plasma from cannabis smokers. *J. Pharm. Pharmacol.* **25**, 554.

34. Garrett, E.R. (1979). Pharmacokinetics and disposition of delta-9-tetrahydrocannabinol and its metabolites, in *Marihuana: Biological Effects* (Nahas, G.G. and Paton, W.D.M. eds.), Pergamon, Oxford, UK, p. 105.

35. Agurell, S., Nilsson, I. M., Ohlsson, A., and Sandberg, F. (1970). On metabolism of tritium labelled Tetrahydrocannabinol in the rabbit. *Biochem. Pharmacol.* **19**, 1333.

36. Pace, H.B., W.M. Davis, and L.A. Borgen. (1971). Teratogenesis and marihuana. *Ann. NY Acad. Sci.* **191**, 123.

37. Harbison, R.D., B. Mantilla-Plata, and D.J. Lubin. (1977). Alteration of delta-9-THC: induced teratogenicity of stimulation and inhibition of its metabolism. *J. Pharmacol. Exp. Ther.* **202**, 455.

38. Kennedy, J.S. and W.J. Waddell. (1972). Whole-body autoradiography of the pregnant mouse after administration of ^{14}C-delta-9-THC. *Toxicol. Appl. Pharmacol.* **22**, 252.

39. Martin, B.R., W.L. Dewey, L.S. Harris, and J.S. Bechner. (1976) 3 3H-delta-9-THC distribution in pregnant dogs and their fetuses. *Res. Comm. Chem. Pathol. Pharmacol.* **17**, 457.

40. Gianutsos, G. and E.R. Abbatiello. (1972). The effect of prenatal cannabis sativa on maze learning ability in the rat. *Psychopharmacologia* **27**, 117.

41. Vardaris, R.M., D.J. Weisz, A. Fazel, and A.B. Rawitch. (1976). Chronic administration of delta-9-THC to pregnant rats: studies of pup behavior and placental transfer. *Pharmacol. Biochem. Behav.* **4**, 249.

42. Dalterio, S. and A. Bartke. (1979). Prenatal exposure to cannabinoids alters male reproductive function in mice. *Science* **205**, 1420.

43. Chao, F.C., D.E. Green, I.S. Forrest, J.N. Kaplan, A. Winship-Ball, and M.C. Braude. (1976) The passage of 14C-delta-9-THC into the milk of lactating squirrel monkeys. *Res. Comm. Chem. Pathol. Pharmacol.* **15**, 303.

44. Hecht, F., R. Beals, M. Lees, H. Jolly, and P. Roberts. (1968). Lysergic-acid diethylamide and cannabis as possible teratogens in man. *Lancet* **ii**, 1087.

45. Carakushansky, G., R.L. Neu, and L.T. Gardner. 1969. Lysergide and cannabis as possible teratogens in man. *Lancet* **i**, 150.

46. Geleherter, D. (1970). Lysergic acid diethylamide (LSD) and exstrophy of the bladder. *J. Pediatr.* **77**, 1065.

47. Bogdanoff, B., L.B. Rorke, M. Yanoff, and W.S. Warren. (1972). Brain and eye abnormalities: possible sequelae to prenatal use of multiple drugs including LSD. *Am. J. Dis. Child.* **123**, 145.

48. Jacobson, C.B. and C.M. Berlin. (1972). Possible reproductive detriments in L.S.D. users. *JAMA* **222**, 1367.

49. Qazi, Q.H., Mariano E., Milman D.H., Beller E., and Crombleholme W. (1985) Abnormalities in offspring associated with prenatal marihuana exposure. *Dev. Pharmacol. Ther.* **8**, 141–148.

50. Hembree, W., H. Huang, and G.G. Nahas. (1979). Effects of marihuana smoke on spermatogenesis in rats, in *Marihuana: Biological Effects* (Nahas, G.G. and Paton, W.D.M. eds.), Pergamon, Oxford, UK, p. 429.

51. Lemoine, P., H. Harousseau, J.P. Borteyru, and J.C. Menuet. (1968). Les enfants du parents alcooliques: Anomalies observees, a propos de 127 cas. *Quest. Med.* **25**, 477.

35

Maternal or Paternal Exposure to Cannabinoids Affects Central Neurotransmitter Levels and Reproductive Function in Male Offspring

Susan L. Dalterio, Richard W. Steger, and Andrzej Bartke

Abstract

A single prenatal exposure to cannabinol or cannabidiol reduced brain norepinephrine and dopamine and hypothalamic NE concentrations, but increased brain levels of serotonin and its metabolite, 5-hydroxyindoleacetic acid. In addition, testicular testosterone concentrations and seminal vesicles weights were reduced in animals exposed to CBN. In contrast, seminal vesicles weights were increased in CBD-exposed males. Prenatal exposure to the major psychoactive component of marihuana, δ^9-tetrahydrocannabinol on one of the last four days of gestation did not affect these parameters.

The F_1 male offspring of male mice treated with CBN, CBD, or THC presented evidence of reduced fertility and testicular chromosomal abnormalities. In addition, two of the F_1 male offspring of the THC-treated mice sired litters containing pups with severe congenital malformations.

These findings indicate that maternal or paternal exposure to cannabinoids can influence developmental and reproductive functions in offspring. Thus, cannabinoids appear to be both mutagenic and teratogenic in mice.

1. INTRODUCTION

Marihuana, and its main psychoactive component Δ^9-tetrahydrocannabinol (THC), have been reported to exert a wide range of effects on reproductive performance [1]. Association of chronic marihuana use by men with decreased plasma testosterone levels, reduced sperm counts, and impotence has been reported [2,3]. In adult male mice acutely exposure to THC

From: *Marihuana and Medicine*
Edited by: G. G. Nahas et al. © Humana Press Inc., Totowa, NJ

or chronic treatment with CBN, a relatively nonpsychoactive cannabinoid, can decrease plasma testosterone, prolactin, and gonadotropin levels. Whereas the suppression of prolactin secretion may involve alterations in serotonergic and dopaminergic activity (7), the central mechanisms by which THC alters gonadotropin release are not clear, although direct effects of THC on the hypothalamic-pituitary axis have been suggested (8,9).

In general, the reports of the effects of THC on central nervous system (CNS) neurotransmitters are conflicting, with investigators presenting evidence of increased or decreased levels of norepinephrine (NE) and serotonin (5-HT) after THC treatment (10–13). Recently, low concentrations of THC have been shown to stimulate dopamine (DA) and NE uptake by hypothalamic and striatal synaptosomes whereas higher concentrations inhibited DA and NE uptake (13). In the mouse, THC has been shown to increase synaptosomal DA synthesis in striatum at low doses, but decreases DA synthesis at higher doses (14). In addition to these effects of cannabinoids on the CNS it is apparent that these compounds can directly affect the steroidogenic and spermatogenic functions of the testes in several species of laboratory animals (1,4,15). Although the mechanisms responsible for cannabinoid-induced alterations in testicular function remain to be elucidated, available evidence suggests that interference with gonadotropic stimulation (15), reduction in testicular synthesis of proteins, lipids, and nucleic acids (17), and prostaglandins (18,19), glucose utilization (20), or activity of cholesterol esterase (21,22) may be involved in the reduction of testicular steroidogenesis.

The testicular hormonal milieu is critical for normal spermatogenesis and at present it cannot be determined whether cannabinoid-induced suppression of spermatogenesis in mice (23), or in humans (24) is secondary to a reduction in testosterone production or caused by a direct action on the germinal epithelium. Cannabinoids have been reported to influence acrosomal morphogenesis and condensation of chromatin in sperm heads as well as inhibit sperm maturation (25).

On the basis of these findings it can be concluded that cannabinoids affect adult male reproductive functions. However, the possible implications for male fetal development have been given less attention. We have previously reported that exposure of female mice to either THC or CBN on the last day of gestation and for the first six days postpartum resulted in long-term alterations in body-weight regulation and reproductive functions in their male offspring (5,6). Effects of perinatal exposure to cannabinoids on the male reproductive system did not become evident until after weaning (21 days of age). During and after sexual maturation, male mice exposed to THC had reduced testes weights and elevated levels of plasma luteinizing hormone (LH). In contrast, CBN-exposed males had reduced concentrations of these hormones after sexual maturation. Copulatory behavior was also reduced in adult males exposed to either THC or cannabinol (CBN) during the perinatal period of sexual differentiation (5,6). Biochemical changes, including alterations in brain RNA synthesis, in neonatal rats have been induced by THC administration during pregnancy (26) and effects of prenatal cannabinoid exposure on development and learning have been reported (27,28).

The present experiments were designed to further characterize the consequences of perinatal exposure of male mice to THC or CBN, or to the nonpsychoactive component cannabidiol (CBD). In particular, we have examined the concentrations of brain amines in adult male mice prenatally exposed to these compounds.

We have previously reported that treatment of adult male mice with THC, CBN, or CBD reduced fertility and resulted in chromosomal abnormalities (15). In the present study we have examined the consequences of paternal exposure to cannabinoids on the subsequent fertility of their male offspring.

2. METHODS

Primiparous female mice obtained from our colony of radomly bred animals received a single oral administration of THC, CBN, or CBD at a dose of 50 mg per kg on one of the last four days of gestation. On the first day postpartum, litters were culled to five or six male pups; the offspring were weaned at 21 days of age and housed in groups of three until adulthood (60–80 days).

Half of the animals in each treatment group were castrated in connection with ongoing studies on the effects of prenatal cannabinoid exposure on androgen receptor levels in seminal vesicles. Castrations were performed under ether anesthesia and the testes were removed, weighed, homogenized in distilled water (9:1 w/v) and stored frozen for the radioimmunoassay determination of testosterone as described previously (29,30). Two days postcastration the males were sacrificed by cervical dislocation and the brain was quickly removed and stored frozen for measurement of amine concentrations.

Prior to the amine assay, the brains were partially thawed and the hypothalamus was dissected free. The hypothalamus consisted of a tissue block 2.0-mm deep extending from the rostral margin of the mammillary body to the rostral border of the optic chiasm and laterally to the hypothalamic sulci. The hypothalamic block and the remaining brain tissue were weighed and sonicated in 0.1 N $HClO_4$ containing 3-methoxy-4-hydroxy-phenethanol (MOPET) as a standard for the indole amine assay, dihydroxybenzylamine (DHBA) as an internal standard for the catecholamine assay and 1.0 mM sodium metabisulfate.

Indolamines were separated by high-performance liquid chromotography (HPLC) and quantitated by electrochemistry (29). Standards were run concurrently, and 5-HT and 5-hydroxyindoleaceticacid (5-HIAA) were calculated by comparison of peak heights with those of the standards. Values were corrected for recovery of the internal standard which averaged 97.3 ± 1.2%. The intra-assay coefficient of variation was 5.6% for 5-HT, and 7.2% for 5-HIAA.

Catecholamines were prepared for chromatography as previously described (29,30). Norepinephrine, DA and DHBA were separated by HPLC and quantitated by electrochemistry. The recovery of DHBA averaged 82.3 ± 1.1% and the intra-assay coefficient of variation was 6.1% for NE and 6.7% for DA.

For groups and parameters in which no significant differences were found caused by the time of prenatal treatment, results from animals exposed to cannabinoids on the different days of gestation were combined for further statistical analysis and presentation. In studies concerning the effects of paternal exposure to cannabinoids on the subsequent fertility of their male offspring, adult male mice were treated with THC, CBN, or CBD (50 mg/kg) three times a week for five weeks, using 18 males per group as described previously (15). The males were individually housed with a different adult female each during the third, fourth, and fifth week of treatment and during the first and fourth posttreatment weeks. In each treatment group, half of the pregnant females were allowed to deliver and raise their pups. The surviving F_1 male offspring were weaned at 21 days of age, and housed in groups of four until adulthood (60–80 days). Each F_1 male was given the opportunity (during a one-week cohabitation period) to mate with at least three different females. Females were sacrificed between days 15 and 19 of gestation for determination of the number of corpora lutea, resorptions, dead fetuses, live and still births, and postnatal deaths. The overall percentage of females impregnated was also recorded. Female mice who failed to become pregnant were remated to known fertile males to verify their fertility.

3. RESULTS

3.1. Maternal Exposure

At two days postcastration the concentrations of NE in hypothalamus and NE and DA in the remaining brain were slightly reduced in CBN- and CBD-exposed animals in comparison to castrated controls. In contrast, levels of 5-HT and 5-HIAA were significantly elevated in both the hypothalamus and the remaining brain in these mice. Exposure to THC during the latter part of gestation did not significantly affect brain amine concentrations. There were no significant differences in the weights of the brain or hypothalamic tissue blocks or in body weight among the animals in the different treatment groups.

Testicular testosterone concentrations were reduced in adult male mice exposed to CBN, although testes weights were not affected. The weights of the seminal vesicles were increased by CBD exposure, but were significantly reduced by CBN exposure. Exposure to THC did not influence these parameters.

3.2. Paternal Exposure

The F_1 male offspring of the CBD-treated male mice successfully impregnated all the females with whom they were paired, as did the offspring of the oil-treated control mice. However, the F_1 male offspring of the THC and CBN-treated animals had significantly reduced reproductive performance.

For the analysis of results on F_1 male fertility, offspring from each treatment group were classified into three categories. The first included the males that had successfully impregnated all the females with whom they were paired, with all the resulting litters being normal by the standards of our breeding colony, that is litter size of at least 10 pups and less than 10% pre- or postnatal mortality. The second category consisted of those males in which one out of three matings deviated from these criteria. Finally, the third category consisted of those males whom did not produce a single pregnancy that met our criterion of normalcy.

Among the THC and CBN-exposed offspring, a significant percentage, 36% of the THC and 21% of the CBN-F_1 males, fell into the third category. In addition, in two litters sired by F_1 males from THC-treated fathers, one contained an exencephalic fetus, whereas another pup (delivered alive at autopsy on day 19) exhibited exencephaly, spina bifida, and exteriorized intestines. Testes from the most severely affected group of males were examined cytogenetically and, in testes obtained from two out of eight animals, chromosomal abnormalities in the form of ring and chain translocations, nondisjunction, and aneuploidy were observed, as was a reduction in testicular weights.

4. DISCUSSION

The present findings indicate that alterations in brain amine levels in adulthood may result from prenatal exposure to cannabinoids. The relatively nonpsychoactive CBN and CBD altered brain and hypothalamic concentrations of NE, DA, 5-HT, and 5-HIAA as well as testicular testosterone concentrations and seminal vesicles weights, whereas prenatal THC exposure during late gestation did not appear to influence these parameters. However, we have recently observed that exposure to THC during the mid-portion of gestation did result in altered brain amine levels in adult mice (Dalterio and Steger, unpublished observation). In view of our earlier findings of long-term alterations in other parameters of endocrine and behavioral function in male mice exposed to THC during the perinatal period (5,6), it is possible that critical time periods exist for cannabinoid-induced alterations in developmental processes. We are currently investigating this issue as well as planning experiments to determine effects of perinatal cannabinoid exposure on amine uptake and turnover.

Although we do not know the precise mechanism by which castration differentially affected cannabinoid-exposed animals, it is known that castration stimulates amine turnover in normal animals (31). It is possible that cannabinoid exposure resulted in a differential responsiveness to the surgical stress associated with castration. We have previously reported that adult male mice treated with cannabinoids exhibit a differential hormonal response to stressful stimuli (32). However, we have also reported that the release of pituitary gonadotropin three weeks postcastration is altered in animals perinatally exposed to THC (33) and it is doubtful that surgical stress could be a factor in these observations. It is possible that alterations in catecholamines, which are known to have a role in the regulation of gonadotropin release (34), may be involved. We have also reported that perinatal, but not pre-pubertal, exposure to THC reduces responsiveness of the vas deferens in vitro to NE and D-Ala^2-Met-enkephalin (35).

It is conceivable that the reported effects of prenatal cannabinoid exposure on development and learning are also related to cannabinoid-induced changes in concentrations of these neurotransmitters (27,28). We have previously reported that adult copulatory behavior was reduced differentially by THC or CBN (5,6). Although the influence of neurotransmitters on sexual behavior are not clear (36), it is conceivable that changes in behavioral responsivity to stimuli from conspecifics may result from cannabinoid-induced alterations in brain catecholamines during critical periods of sexual differentiation.

Another factor that may be related to the observation that castration brought out an effect of prenatal cannabinoid exposure that was not otherwise observed concerns the presence of gonadal steroids, which can modulate amine levels (37). We have shown that the gonadal steroids modulate the acute hormonal responses to THC administration in adult mice (38). In addition to the possible influences of surgical stress or the presence of gonadal steroids we have also demonstrated that environmental factors such as the presence of female con-specifics can interact with effects of perinatal cannabinoid exposure. In an earlier study we noted that prepubertal cannabinoid-exposed males responded to housing with an immature female as a stressful situation, as suggested by increased adrenal weights and reductions in the weights of the testes and seminal vesicles (5). Thus, the precise mechanism by which castration appears to reveal the effects of prenatal cannabinoid exposure on CNS neurotransmitter levels is at present unclear. However, based on our earlier studies these findings appear to be consistent with cannabinoid-induced alterations in physiological responsivity to events which disturb homeostatic conditions.

In mice, maternal exposure to cannabinoids appears capable of inducing teratogenesis in male offspring. These effects are observed after a single prenatal exposure or repeated exposure during the perinatal periods of development (5,6). In addition, the effects on the male offspring, including alterations in body weight regulation, pituitary-gonadal function, sexual behavior, and central neurotransmitter concentrations, are not inconsistent with results of cannabinoid administration to immature or adult males (1).

Evidence from studies of paternal exposure to cannabinoids indicates that these compounds, in addition to their reported embryocidal or teratogenic potential (1) also may be mutagenic. We have shown that brief or repeated exposure in adulthood to psychoactive or nonpsychoactive components of *Cannabis* affects the endocrine system and fertility and that these effects were not rapidly reversible, were associated with chromosomal abnormalities, and in some cases, with reductions in testicular weights and alterations in plasma hormone concentrations (15). Although the mechanisms by which cannabinoids influence the genetic apparatus are unclear, we observed that the F_1 male offspring of cannabinoid-treated male mice exhibited reductions in reproductive performance, as well as cytogenetic abnormalities similar in type and frequency to those observed in their treated sires (15). This strongly suggests that cannabinoid effects on fertility can be transmitted from one generation to the next. In addition, it must be stressed that these F_1 males were survivors of matings in which indications of subfertility and perinatal loss had been observed, and therefore these animals do not represent the most seriously affected offspring of the cannabinoid-treated males. The observation of severe congenital defects in F_2 offspring of THC-treated males suggests that cannabinoids may affect polygenetic systems involved, not only in reproductive functions, but with a wide range of developmental processes as well.

It is evident that either maternal or paternal exposure to cannabinoids, whether psychoactive or nonpsychoactive, are capable of producing long-term alterations in reproductive functions in their male offspring. Furthermore, it is evident that in either situation, that is, pregestational or gestational exposure, the effects of cannabinoids may not become apparent until maturational or environmental factors require physiological responses, particularly those involving the endocrine system.

Reprinted with permission from The Cannabinoids: Chemical, Pharmacologic, and Therapeutic Aspects (S. Agurell, W. Dewey, R. Willette, eds.) Academic Press, Orlando, 1984, pp. 411–425.

REFERENCES

1. Bloch, E., Thysen, B., Morrill, G. A., Gardner, E. and Fujimoto, G. (1978) Effects of cannabinoids on reproduction and development. *Vitam. Horm.* **36**, 203–258.
2. Kolodny, R. C., Lessin, P., Toro, G., Masters, W. H. and Cohen, S. (1976) Depression of plasma testosterone with acute marihuana administration, in *The Pharmacology of Marihuana* (Braude, M. C. and Szara, S., eds.), Raven, Press, New York, pp. 217–225.
3. Kolodny, R. C., Masters, W. H., Kolodner, R. M. and Toro, G. (1974) depression of plasma testosterone levels after chronic intensive marihuana use. *N. Engl. J. Med.* **290**, 872–874.
4. Dalterio, S., Bartke, A., Roberson, C., Watson D. and Burstein, S. (1978) Direct and pituitary-mediated effects of Δ^9-THC and cannabinol on the testis. *Pharmacol. Biochem. Behav.* **8**, 673–678.
5. Dalterio, S. (1980) Perinatal or adult exposure to cannabinoids alters male reproductive functions in mice. *Pharmacol. Biochem. Behav.* **12**, 143–153.
6. Dalterio, S. and Bartke, A. (1979) Perinatal exposure to cannabinoids alters male reproductive function in mice. *Science* **205**, 1420–1422.
7. Kramer, J. and Ben-David, M. (1978) Prolactin suppression by (–)-Δ^9-tetrahydrocannabinol (THC): involvement of serotonergic and dopaminergic pathways. *Endocrinology* **103**, 452–457.
8. Smith, C. G., Besch, N. F., Smith, R. G. and Besch, P. K. (1979) Effects of tetrahydrocannabinol on the hypothalamic-pituitary axis in the ovariectomized Rhesus monkey. *Fertil. Steril.* **31**, 335–339.
9. Asch, R. H., Smith, C. G., Siler-Knodr, T. M. and Pauerstein, C. J. (1979) Effects of Δ^9- tetrahydrocannabinol on gonadal steroidogenic activity in vivo. *Fertil. Steril.* **32**, 576–582.
10. Fuxe, K. and Johnson, G. (1971) The effect of tetrahydrocannabinol on central monoamine neurons. *Acta Pharm. Suec.* **8**, 695–701.
11. Ho, B. T., Taylor, D. V., Fritchie, G. E., Englert, G. E. and McIsaac, W. M. (1973) Neuropharmacological study of Δ^9-tetrahydrocannabinol in monkeys and mice. *Brain Res.* **38**, 163–170.
12. Harris, L. S., Dewey, W. L. and Razdan, R. (1972) Cannabis: it's chemistry, pharmacology, and toxicology, in *Drug Addiction II* (Martin, W. R., ed.) Handbook of Experimental Pharmacology, **45**, 371–429.
13. Dewey, W. L., Poddar, M. K. and Johnson, K. M. (1979) The effects of cannabinoids on rat brain synaptosomes, in *Marihuana, Biologic Effects* (Nahas, G. G. and Paton, W. D. M. eds.) Pergamon, Oxford, UK p. 343.
14. Bloom, A. S. (1982) Effect of Δ^9-tetrahydrocannabinol on the synthesis of dopamine and norepinephrine in mouse brain synaptosomes. *J. Pharmacol. Exp. Ther.* **221**, 97–103.
15. Dalterio, S., Badr, F., Bartke, A. and Mayfield, D. (1982) Cannabinoids in male mice: effects on fertility and spermatogenesis. *Science* **216**, 315–316.
16. Tyrey, L. (1980) Δ^9-tetrahydrocannabinol: a potent inhibitor of episodic luteinizing hormone secretion. *J. Pharmacol. Exp. Ther.* **213**, 300–308.
17. Jakubovic, A., McGeer, E. G. and McGeer, P. L. (1979) Effects of cannabinoids on testosterone and protein synthesis in rat testis Leydig cells in vitro. *Molec. Cell. Endocrinol.* **15**, 41–50.
18. Burstein, S., Levin, E. and Varanelli, C. (1973) Prostaglandins and cannabis II: inhibition of biosynthesis by the naturally occurring cannabinoids. *Biochem. Pharmacol.* **22**, 2905–2910.
19. Dalterio, S., Bartke, A., Harper, M. J. K., Huffman, R. and Sweeney, C. (1981) Effects of cannabinoids and female exposure on the pituitary-testicular axis in mice: possible involvement of prostaglandins. *Biol. Reprod.* **24**, 315–322.

20. Husain, S. and Lame, M. W. (1981) Inhibitory effects of Δ^9-tetrahydrocannabinol on glycolytic substrates in the rat testis. *Pharmacology* **23**, 102–112.

21. Shoupe, T. S., Hunter, S. A., Burstein, S. H. and Hubbard, C. D. (1980) Nature of the inhibition of cholesterol esterase by Δ^1-tetrahydrocannabinol. *Enzyme* **25**, 87–91.

22. Burstein, S., Hunter, S. A. and Shoupe, T. S. (1979) Site of inhibition of Leydig cell testosterone by Δ^1-tetrahydrocannabinol. *Molec. Pharmacol.* **15**, 663–640.

23. Dixit, V. P., Sharma, V. N. and Lohiya, N. K. (1974) The effect of chronically administered cannabis extract on the testicular function in mice. *Eur. J. Pharmacol.* **26**, 111–114.

24. Hembree, W. C., Nahas, G. G., Zeidenberg, P. and Dyrenfurth, I. (1976) Marihuana effects of the human testis. *Clin. Res.* **24**, 272A.

25. Issidorides, M. R. (1979) Observations in chronic marihuana users: nuclear aberrations in blood and sperm and abnormal acrosomes in spermatozoa, in *Marihuana, Biological Effects* (Nahas, G. G. and Paton, W. D. M. eds.) Pergamon, Oxford, UK, p 377.

26. Luthra, Y. K. (1979) Brain biochemical alterations in neonates of dams treated orally with Δ^9-tetrahydrocannabinol during gestation lactation, in *Marihuana, Biological Effects* (Nahas, G. G. and Paton, W. D. M., eds.) Pergamon, Press, Oxford, UK, p. 531.

27. Fried, P. A. (1976) Short and long term effects of prenatal cannabis inhalation upon rat offspring. *Psychopharmacology* **50**, 285–291.

28. Raduoco-Thomas, S., Magnan, F., Grove, R. N., Singh, P., Garcon, F. and Raduoco-Thomas, C. (1976) Effect of chronic administration of Δ^9-THC on learning and memory in developing mice, in *The Pharmacology of Marihuana* (Braude, M. C. and Szara, S, eds.) Raven, New York, p. 487.

29. Steger, R. W., DePaolo, L., Asch, R. H., and Silverman, A. V. (1982) Interactions of Δ^9-tetrahydrocannabinol (THC) with hypothalamic neurotransmitters controlling luteinizing hormone and prolactin release. *Neuroendocrinology* (submitted).

30. Steger, R. W., Bartke, A. and Goldman, B. D. (1982) Alterations in neuroendocrine function during photoperiod-induced testicular atrophy and recrudiscence in the golden hamster. *Biol. Reprod.* **26**, 437–444.

31. Bapna, J., Neff, N. H. and Costa, E. (1971) A method for studying norepinephrine and serotonin metabolism in small regions of the brain: effect of ovariectomy on amine metabolism in anterior and posterior hypothalamus. *Endocrinology* **89**, 1345–1349.

32. Dalterio, S., Michael, S. D., Macmillan, B. T. and Bartke, A. (1981) Differential effects cannabinoid exposure and stress have on plasma prolactin, growth hormone and corticosterone levels in male mice. *Life Sci.* **28**, 761–766.

33. Dalterio, S., Bartke, A. and Sweeney, C. (1981) Interactive effects of ethanol and Δ^9-tetrahydrocannabinolon endocrine functions in male mice. *J. Androl.* **2**, 87–93.

34. Barraclough, C. A. and Wise, P. M. (1982) The role of catecholamines in the regulation of pituitary luteinizing hormone and follicle-stimulating hormone secretion. *Endocrinol. Rev.* **3**, 91–119.

35. Dalterio, S., Blum, K., Dellalo, L., Sweeney, C., Briggs, A. and Bartke, A. (1980) Perinatal exposure to Δ^9-THC in mice: altered enkephalin and norepinephrine sensitivity in vas deferens. *Subs. Alcohol Actions/Misuse* **1**, 467–478.

36. Gessa, G. L. and Tagliamonte, A. (1975) Role of brain serotonin and dopamine in male sexual behavior, in *Sexual Behavior: Pharmacology and Biochemistry* Raven, New York, p. 117.

37. Wise, P. M., Rance, N. and Barraclough, C. A. (1981) Effects of estradiol and progesterone on catecholamine turnover in discrete hypothalamic regions on ovariectomized rats. *Endocrinology* **108**, 2186–2193.

38. Dalterio, S., Bartke, A., Michael, S. and Macmillan, B. (1980) Gonadal steroids influence the effects of Δ^9-tetrahydrocannabinol in male mice. *Biol. Reprod.* **22**, 117A.

36 Reproduction in Rhesus Monkeys Chronically Exposed to Δ^9-Tetrahydrocannabinol

E. N. Sassenrath, L. F. Chapman, and G. P. Goo

Abstract

Data is reported from 46 matings between 11 undrugged adult rhesus monkey breeders and eight comparable breeders that had received daily oral doses of Δ^9-THC at 2.4 mg per kg for a 5-yr period. Matings of drugged breeders showed no decrease in conceptions, but a 42% reproductive loss for matings of THC-treated females compared to an 8–11% loss for matings of undrugged females. The observed losses were not related to parity of mother or duration of drug intake and were nonspecific relative to stage of pregnancy; i.e., they occurred as resorptions, abortions, fetal deaths, stillbirths, and neonatal deaths. Nonviable term offspring appeared grossly normal, but exhibited a variety of nonspecific abnormalities on histopathological evaluation.

Viable offspring of drugged mothers also appeared grossly normal. However, male infants had significantly lower birth rates. In general, offspring of THC-treated mothers tended to show subtle behavioral differences from control offspring in both responsivity to environmental stimuli and adaptability in peer social environments.

The nonspecific and variable nature of these effects in a controlled primate test system suggests that such effects would be difficult to document in relation to marihuana use in the human population.

1. INTRODUCTION

During the last decade a number of studies have focused on the question of the possibility that marihuana use may present a significant risk for the offspring of exposed parents. Only a few, inconclusive, observations have been reported on humans (4,15). Almost all of these studies have utilized rodents, in part because of their obvious practical advantages in

From: *Marihuana for Medicine*
Edited by: G. G. Nahas et al.   © Humana Press Inc., Totowa, NJ

terms of low cost, large number of animals per litter, and relatively brief gestation period. In general, these studies have utilized an experimental model in which marihuana extracts or synthetic THC has been administered to pregnant females for a relatively brief time (assumed to be a critical period). The results of such studies have recently been summarized in a number of articles, including Fleishman et al. (7), Braude (3), Fournier et al. (8), and Harbison et al. (14), among others. In brief, reported abnormalities and other did not. Differences in species and strains, routes of administration, dosage, stage of gestation, and duration of exposure during pregnancy, as well as environmental conditions, details of experimental design, and other factors have been suggested as possible explanations of the divergence in the implications of specific studies for evaluation of potential hazards to human reproduction.

Several early studies (9,10,18,19) reported embryotoxicity, fetal toxicity, and specific teratological malformations in rats, guinea pigs, hamsters, and rabbits associated with exposure to natural Cannabis extracts during pregnancy. In general, the amounts of the agents reported to result in frank teratology were well beyond the range used by humans. A number of later studies with synthetic THC failed to produce specific congenital malformations (12,17), even with relatively large amounts of the agent. However, some (but not all) investigators have continued to report an increase in embryotoxicity and fetal toxicity (5,7,8,13,14,20,26); the amounts used have often been large, but the observation of dose-dependent increases in fetal and embryonic deaths emphasizes the importance of assessing the possibility that lower levels of exposure might result in significant human risk.

Whereas the method of administering suspected teratogenic agents only during presumed critical periods is an important and valid component of the assessment of reproductive hazards associated with a given pharmacologically active agent, in some instances it may not result in complete assessment. For example, the usual pattern of marihuana exposure is not duplicated by heavy dosage limited to brief periods during pregnancy: a much more common pattern is chronic exposure beginning months and years before pregnancy. In addition to the possibility of direct damage to male or female gametes, the capacity of the mother to develop adequate fetal life-support following conception could be adversely affected by changes in any of the variety of systems that contribute (endocrine, hematological, vascular, and so on). The perinatal period is also pertinent; exposure to THC interferes with maternal milk production (17).

Laboratory primates offer obvious advantages as animal models for assessment of human reproductive hazards. The principal disadvantages of using laboratory primates for this purpose lie in the slow rate of reproduction and high costs associated with controlled studies on sufficient numbers of animals. To our knowledge, only a single study with laboratory primates has been reported. Grilly, Ferraro, and Braude (11) examined the reproductive histories of eight chimpanzees that had been exposed to various amounts of Cannabis or THC from 5 to over 150 times during a period which ended 1.5 months to 1.5 years before conception. One of the mothers experienced a miscarriage at three months. The remaining infants appeared normal at birth.

In 1973 we began a series of observations on possible social behavior changes associated with chronic long-term exposure to THC (23,24). These behavioral studies generated an opportunity to observe certain aspects of reproductive capacity under the condition of long-term chronic exposure in laboratory primates. The program has also permitted exploration of possible behavioral and developmental abnormalities in the live-birth offspring of THC-treated parents.

There is evidence from rodent studies to indicate that exposure of the pregnant rat to THC (10 mg/kg) on days 10–12 of gestation results in behavioral and developmental changes in the offspring. Cross fostering did not reduce these adverse effects, indicating a direct action on the developing fetus.

Although studies with nonhuman species inevitably must be evaluated with caution in terms of their relevance to humans, the rhesus monkey is a particularly attractive animal model for exploration of potential human reproductive risks from exposure to THC. For example, in addition to the obvious similarities common to other simian species, it is known that the metabolism of THC in the rhesus follows pathways more closely related to those of humans than those utilized by certain other simians (27).

We report here a summary of current data from ongoing studies. At this time, several major conclusions are apparently well established, with adequate numbers of animals for statistical evaluation. For other questions, the number of animals studied is still too small to permit firm conclusions, and other components (notably observations of the offspring of THC-treated parents) remain incomplete; nevertheless, in view of the paucity of information regarding reproductive function in primates treated with *Cannabis*, we have included brief descriptions of these incomplete studies as a preliminary report.

2. METHODS

2.1. Subjects

Breeders were 19 sexually mature colony-born rhesus monkeys, progressing from an age range of 3–4 years to 8–9 years during the 5-year study.

All females were mated in three to five sequential years during the study; all were primiparous at first conception. The males also were inexperienced breeders on first matings. In all matings, breeding behavior appeared normal. After timed matings, sperm plugs were observed and/or sperm recovered by vaginal swabbing of the female.

2.2. Drug Administration

Δ^9-THC was given orally daily on preferred food to 5 of 12 female breeders and to 3 of the 7 male breeders, starting 3–18 months prior to first mating. During four of the five breeding seasons, THC was given at 2.4 mg per kg per day. To clarify the reproductive effect of dosage, the level was raised to 4.8 mg per kg for both males and females prior to the third breeding season (October, 1975) and maintained at that level for females until weaning or loss of infant, after which the 2.4 mg per kg dose level was reinstituted.

2.3. Breeding

During the first three breeding seasons, all conceptions occurred in group settings of 4–6 monkeys per cage. Breeding groups were left intact through births and weaning until second season conceptions were confirmed. Thereafter, all group-bred females were removed to individual cages after conception to assure standardization of prenatal and postnatal mother-infant environments.

During the fourth and fifth breeding seasons, additional timed matings were instituted for indoorcaged breeders. Females were caged in the same room as the male, and moved to his cage for 2–4 hours daily for 5–7 days mid-menses. This interval was calculated to cover estrus for each female on the basis of daily records of vaginal bleeding to define menses.

Pregnancies were initially confirmed by cessation of regular menses together with the appearance of "placental sign" vaginal discharge. After 30 days, pregnancies were evaluated periodically by bimanual palpation (for size) and by detection of fetal heart-beat (for viability).

There were a total of 46 matings for five breeding seasons: i.e., 19 each for THC-treated and control females; and 27 each for THC-treated and control males.

Table 1
Comparison of Reproductive Loss for 46 Pregnancies from Matings Between THC-Treated and Undrugged (Control) Males and Females

Matings			Births			Group difference	
Mother x father	n	Lost	Viable	Percent loss	Comparison matings	c^2	
THC x cont	14	6	8	42%	Cont-Cont	$p < .05$	
THC x all	19	8	11	42%	Cont-All	$p < .005$	
Cont x THC	14	2	12	14%	Cont-Cont	NS	
All x THC	19	4	15	21%	All-Cont	NS	
Cont x Cont	13	1	12	8%			
Cont x All	27	3	24	11%			
All x Cont	27	7	20	26%			

THC = THC-treated parent.
Cont = undrugged parent.
All = drugged + undrugged parent.
p = Significance from contingency tables for Chi-square test(6).

3. RESULTS

3.1. Reproductive Potential of THC-Treated Breeders

No differences in sexual function were observed between breeders under long-term daily treatment with THC at 2.4 mg per kg per day, compared to the undrugged controls with respect to cyclic endocrine changes or observable responses to sexual stimuli. The regularity and duration of menses were similar for drugged and undrugged females, as were the behavioral sexual receptivity and the regularity of conceptions in a group-breeding environment or in timed matings of breeder pairs. Cyclic changes in plasma levels of progesterone and estrogen in the females were also within the normal range. Similarly, outdoor-caged THC-treated males were comparable to undrugged controls, both in mean elevation of plasma testosterone levels during the breeding season and in the annual rhythm of this hormone. For both males and females, if THC-related effects on these measures were present during long-term chronic drug exposure, they were overshadowed by inter-individual variability in these measures.

3.2. Reproductive Deficit for THC-treated Breeders

As shown in Table 1, based on 46 matings among 8 THC-treated and 11 nondrugged control breeders, the percent of pregnancies which did *not* result in viable offspring surviving to six months of age was higher for THC-treated mothers mated with undrugged fathers (42% loss) than for undrugged females mated with undrugged males (8%). This deficit did not change when matings with drugged fathers was included for both THC-treated and undrugged females. The Chi-square test for significance of group differences confirms that reproductive deficit differs from control levels only when considering matings with THC-treated mothers and regardless of the drug status of the father. In this study, matings between drugged females and drugged males have been too few to permit evaluation of possible interaction effects.

The distribution of reproductive loss occurred throughout the course of pregnancy and parturition as shown in Table 2. Losses occurred at a variety of stages in development: including

Table 2
Distribution of Reproductive Loss for Different Stages of Pregnancy Relative to Drug Status of Parent

Parents			Offspring mortality					
Drug status			In utero			Perinatal		Postnatal
Mother Father		Number matings	RE	AB	ED	SB	ND	ID
THC or THC × Cont		19	2(1)	1^T	2(2)		I^T	2(1)
Cont × THC		14		1			1	
Cont × Cont		13					1	

RE = resorption, SB = stillbirth,
AB = Abortion, ND = Neonatal death,
FD = Fetal death, ID = infant death.
T = Mating with THC-treated father.
() = Number of females contributing to deficit.

in utero, as abortions and fetal deaths; at term, as stillbirths and neonatal deaths; and as postnatal infant deaths. Although the number of animals studied is small, the data indicate a nonspecific distribution of conceptus losses during gestation and shortly after birth for pregnancies of THC-treated females.

If reproductive loss is viewed relative to parity of mother, as in Table 3, the distribution again appears random. There is no evidence of greater loss during first pregnancies than during subsequent pregnancies. Neither is there evidence of increasing or decreasing risk with successive pregnancies.

To evaluate effects of environmental differences during successive birthing seasons, the success of individual matings in shown in Table 4 as they occurred for each female in each breeding season. Again, losses appear to be distributed randomly. It is of interest, however, that, in the year of higher THC dosage (1976) pregnancy losses occurred earlier in pregnancy as abortions and resorptions rather than later fetal, neonatal, or infant deaths.

The higher dose of THC does not appear to increase the contribution of drugged males (noted by T superscript) to reproductive loss. Further, no effect related to drugged fathers appeared during the last two seasons when THC-treated males were bred only to undrugged control females.

One major difference between THC-treated and undrugged control female breeders was apparent in assessment of body-weight changes during the course of the study. The mean body weight gain of THC-treated females during all pregnancies which came to full term was significantly less than that of undrugged control females: i.e., the percent body weight gain for 12 term pregnancies in THC-treated females was 10 ± 5 compared to 20 ± 9 for 21 term pregnancies in undrugged controls ($t = 3.11$; $p = 0.005$). In contrast, the average nonpregnant body weight gain per year was comparable between THC-treated and control females when individuals were equated for age and weight data were taken only during months when females were neither pregnant or lactating. The annual whole body-weight gains for all females on this study also fell in the range of the norms established for colony-born rhesus monkeys by other workers (2).

Table 3
Reproductive Deficit for Successive Pregnancies of Individual Female Breeders Relative
to Parity of Mother

Females		Number of pregnancies				
Drug	I.D.	1	2	3	4	5
THC	6586	+[T]	(F)	+		
	6604	(A)[T]	+	(F)		
	6627	+	(I)	(I)	+	+
	6668	(N)[T]	+[T]	+[T]	+	
	6840	+	(R)	+	(R)	
		2/5	3/5	2/5	1/3	0/1
		40%	60%	40%	33%	
None	6666	(A)	+	+	(F)[T]	+[T]
	6737	+	+	+	+	+[T]
	6756	+[T]	(N)[T]	+[T]	+	+
	6989	+	+	+[T]		
	7024	+	+[T]	+[T]		
	7054	+	+	+[T]	+[T]	
	6962	+[T]	+			
		1/7	1/6	0/6	1/4	0/3
		14%	16%	0%	25%	0%

A = abortus, N = neonatal death;
F = fetal death, R = resorption;
I = infant death,
T = mating with THC-treated male.

3.3. Pathological Observations

Histopathological evaluation of all offspring in this study has not been completed: many offspring are still under observation for behavioral evaluation. However, observations on a limited number of offspring are completed and of interest here.

Of seven early fetal and neonatal deaths prior to 1978, three were partially autolysed and one was a mummified fetus from an *in utero* death. Lesions observed in two offspring of THC-treated mothers and one offspring of a control mother mated with a THC-treated father are shown in Table 5. These included hydrocephalus, inguinal hernia, ectopic pancreas, and umbilical and myocardial degeneration. Two infants showing hydrocephalus were offspring of a THC and a control mother mated with the same drug-treated male in different birth years.

Since monkey births occur primarily at night and females normally eat the placental tissue after birth, fresh placentas were not usually available for examination. However, it has been possible to obtain one fresh placenta by caesarian section within 24 hours after death of a late third trimester fetus (140 days) of a THC-treated mother. This had gross morphological and vascular abnormalities of both lobes and was massively infarcted. Placentas from caesarian section deliveries of viable term infants of two undrugged control mothers (with vaginal prolapses) showed no comparable abnormality. This pathology has not been observed in placentas obtained from caesarian-section delivery of term pregnancies in the rhesus colony.

Table 4
Reproductive Deficit in Successive Breeding Seasons for Individual Female Breeders

Females		Breeding season (year of birth)				
Drug	I.D.	1974	1975	1976	1977	1978
THC	6586			$+^T$	(F)	+
	6604			$(A)^T$	+	(F)
	6627	+	(I)	(I)	+	+
	6668	$(N)^T$	$+^T$	$+^T$		+
	6840		+	(R)	+	(R)
		1/2	1/3	3/5	1/4	2/5
		50%	33%	60%	25%	40%
Control	6666	(N)	+	+	$(F)^T$	$+^T$
	6737	+	+	+	$+^T$	$+^T$
	6756	$+^T$	$(N)^T$	$+^T$	+	+
	6989			+	$+^T$	$+^T$
	7024			+	$+^T$	$+^T$
	7054	+	+		$+^T$	$+^T$
	6962				$+^T$	+
		1/4	1/4	0/5	1/7	0/7
		25%	25%	0%	14%	0%

A = abortus, N = neonatal death;
F = fetal death; R = resorption;
I = infant death;
T = mating with THC-treated male.
THC dosage was doubled (to 4.8 mg per kg) during pregnancy and lactation in the 1976 birthing season only.

Table 5
Pathological Changes Noted in Three of the Early Neonatal and Infant Deaths in this Study

Offspring No.	Mother	Father	Pathological changes
7932	THC	THC	Stillbirth with hydrocephalus. umbilical artery degeneration; myocardial degeneration; renal cortical necrosis.
16088	THC	Cont	Infant, 2.5 months with inguinal hernia (resulting in intestinal obstruction); ectopic pancreas within the intestinal wall and pancreatic atrophy.
8239	Cont	THC	Neonatal death with hydrocephalus and inguinal hernia.

3.4 Infants of THC-Treated Parents

Surviving infants of THC-treated parents appeared grossly normal. However, birth weights of male offspring of THC-treated mothers were significantly smaller than offspring of control mothers. They were also significantly smaller than a larger reference sample of colony male offspring with comparable pre- and postnatal environments, as shown in Table 6. All birth weights of male offspring of THC-treated females fell below the mean and

Table 6
Comparison of Mean Birth Weights of Infants Born to THC-Treated and Undrugged Parents

Experimental group		N	Birth weight (g)		Comparison group	Significance	
Offspring	Parents		(mean)	(SD)		t	p
Males	THC-mothers	7	430.6	52.1	Control mothers	2.59	0.025
					Experimental controls	2.83	0.01
					Colony controls	3.07	0.005
	THC-fathers	3	483.3	123.3	Experimental controls	0.61	NS
					Colony controls	0.80	NS
	Control mothers	7	527.8	84.4	Colony controls	0.27	NS
	Experimental controls[a]	2	540.0	7.1	Colony controls	0.38	NS
	Colony controls	54	519.6	74.1			
Females	THC-mothers	6	471.7	48.8	Control mothers	0.77	NS
					Experimental controls	0.36	NS
					Colony controls	0.56	NS
	THC-fathers	6	510.8	72.1	Experimental controls	0.62	NS
	Control mothers	15	496.3	72.0	Colony controls	0.50	NS
	Experimental controls	8	485.0	79.6	Colony controls	0.06	NS
	Colony controls	48	486.7	63.3			

[a]Experimental controls: Offspring of undrugged parents.

median of the reference sample. Birth weights of male offspring of THC-treated fathers (with control mothers) or nondrugged parents (experimental controls), however, were distributed throughout the range of birth weights of the reference sample, as were the weights of female offspring of THC-treated mothers.

Surviving offspring from this study have also been subjected to a series of behavioral characterizations during their first year of life. The behavior of the first season's offspring of THC-treated mothers was suggestive of hyperactivity and overresponsiveness to environmental stimuli, together with a lack of appropriate cautious or avoidance behaviors in novel environments. In order to study this further, the gestation, parturition, and preweaning environments have been carefully standardized for subsequent mother-infant pairs to minimize the contribution of early environmental differences to subsequent observed behavioral differences in offspring.

To date, we have characterized nine infants from one week to one year of age and are studying an additional eight newborns. The data suggest that offspring of THC-treated mothers show enhanced responsivity—both autonomic and behavioral—to visual and auditory stimuli; less fear and avoidance behavior in a novel environment; and overstimulation and assertiveness in response to peer socialization. Sex differences in these infant responses are apparent as well as differences in maternal behavior between THC-treated and undrugged mothers; data on a larger number of mother-infant pairs is essential to assess adequately these drug-related effects on offspring behavior.

4. DISCUSSION

This study has examined the reproductive outcome of five breeding seasons in rhesus monkeys exposed to THC at a level equivalent to moderately heavy marihuana usage in the

United States. The number of animals treated was necessarily small in comparison to rodent studies, and the data are insufficient to answer a number of important questions. However, in terms of statistical significance, several findings can be expressed with confidence.

First, it was established clearly that daily maternal oral intake of THC in the range of 2.4–4.8 mg/kg resulted in significant reproductive casualties. The rate of reproductive loss in the treated animals was approximately 40%; reproductive loss in specific control animals and in a large breeding program at the same center approximated 10%. There was some evidence that the higher dosage (4.8 mg/kg) resulted in a greater and earlier loss. Reproductive losses occurred from the first trimester to early infant death. The pattern of reproductive deficit indicated embryonic and fetal toxicity and was not characterized by specific consistent congenital anomalies. Survivors appeared morphologically normal. Exposure of the father (but not the mother) to chronic THC in the same dose range did not result in significant reproductive loss beyond control levels.

Secondly, a sufficient number of animals were studied to permit the conclusion, with a high level of statistical confidence, that the birth weight of male infants born to THC-treated mothers is less than comparable control weights. The birth weights of all male infants born to THC-treated mothers were all less than the mean or median birth weights of control animals. The mean birth weight of female offspring of THC-treated mothers was not significantly less than mean control birth rate. This finding is in keeping with the greater vulnerability of male conceptions to adverse prenatal, perinatal, and neonatal influences in macaques monkeys and in humans(22). The probable pathological basis for the observed increase in reproductive loss remains a matter of speculation. A nonspecific, variable drug action on gametes of long-term THC-treated parents might be relevant; however, the evidence from these studies is not supportive of such a hypothesis. There was no evidence of a deficit related to drug exposure of the sperm of THC-treated fathers. Also, evidence for a contribution of direct damage to the ova is lacking. Our studies revealed no evidence for a cumulative effect over sequential pregnancies in individual drugged females.

The absence of frank teratology and the nonspecific nature of pregnancy interruption and morphological changes suggest that a proximal cause of drug-related decrements may be impairment of the maternal support for the fetus, possibly caused by alternations of the complex mechanisms involved in establishing an optimally functioning placental circulation and other aspects of the overall fetal support system. The observations of placental infarction and umbilical degeneration in pathological evaluation of a few late-pregnancy deaths support this possibility, as does the lower body-weight gain during pregnancy of THC-treated mothers.

In broad terms, the present study indicates that in the rhesus monkey, chronic exposure to moderately large amounts of THC results in embryotoxicity and fetotoxicity. There was no evidence of specific teratology in the sense of a specific reproducible pattern of congenital malformation. Surviving infants were grossly normal in appearance. This overall pattern of findings is similar to that recently observed by Rosenkrantz et al.(21) in rodents. They found that exposure to relatively small (0.9–3.5 mg/kg) amounts of THC inhaled in smoke on days 5 and 6 of gestation resulted in significant embryotoxicity in mice, but not in specific teratological patterns.

Although behavioral characterization of viable offspring from this study is still in progress, current data suggest that the offspring of THC-treated mothers show altered autonomic and behavioral responsiveness to visual, auditory, and social environmental stimuli.

The limitations and qualifications that must be applied in extrapolating findings based on animal models in evaluating potential human health hazards are well known. However, the results of the present study with laboratory primates, and those of a number of investigators who have observed increased embryotoxicity and fetotoxicity with moderate levels of THC exposure, raise the possibility that exposure of the human female to marihuana in amounts in relatively common use may be associated with an increased risk of reproductive loss. There is also evidence suggesting that surviving infants may also be at increased risk for subsequent behavioral and developmental abnormalities, although there is no evidence of increased risk of physical abnormality in these offspring.

If, indeed, marihuana use in the moderately heavy range is associated in humans with increased reproductive hazard, a question arises as to why the increased risk has not been readily recognized in clinical practice, since marihuana use during childbearing age is widespread. Clues to the answers may lie in the observations with animal models that viable offspring do not appear physically unusual, the embryotoxic and fetotoxic actions are variable in this dosage range; one pregnancy may terminate early, but the next may result in a live birth, and finally, animals that die *in utero* do not exhibit a consistent teratological pattern.

These factors combine in such a manner that the type of increased reproductive risk suggested by the studies with animal models would be unusually difficult to recognize in the human population. A number of associated problems concerned with identifying the amount of marihuana exposure as well as problems of multiple drug exposure add to the difficulties of designing and conducting studies to assess potential reproductive risks in humans.

The delayed definition of the fetal alcohol syndrome may also be instructive. Despite a long history of recognition that heavy alcohol consumption might be related to increased reproductive risks, a specific syndrome was not defined until a decade ago; it is now recognized that this syndrome is not rare.

Although there are many difficult problems in conducting human clinical studies on this question, these considerations underscore the need for additional information regarding the possibility that increases in reproductive hazards may be associated with human exposure to marihuana.

ACKNOWLEDGMENT

We wish to acknowledge the continuing cooperation and support of the administration and staff of the California Primate Research Center, especially members of Pathology Services of the Primate Medicine Unit, which performed all autopsy and histopathology evaluations of subjects in this study.

Δ^9THC has been supplied by the National Institute on Drug Abuse.

This investigation was supported by USPHS grant DA-00135. Additional partial support has been provided by USPHS grants RR-00169 to the California Primate Research Center and RR-05684 to the School of Medicine, University of California, Davis.

Reprinted with permission from Marihuana: Biological Effects, Analysis, Metabolism, Cellular Responses, Reproduction and Brain (G. G. Nahas and W. D. M. Paton, eds.) Pergamon, Press, New York, 1979, pp. 501–512.

REFERENCES

1. Borgen, L. A., Davis, W. M. and Pace, H. B. (1973) Effects of prenatal delta-nine-tetrahydrocannabinol on the development of rat offspring. *Pharmacol. Biochem. Behav.* **1**, 203.
2. Bourne, G. H. (1975) Collected anatomical and physiological data from the rhesus monkey in *The Rhesus Monkey*, vol. 1, (Bourne, G. H., ed.). Academic, New York.
3. Braude, M. C. (1976) Genetics and reproduction, introduction in *Pharmacology of Marihuana*, vol. 2, (Braude M. C. and Szara, S., eds) Raven, New York.
4. Carakushansky, G., Neu, R. L. and Gardner, L. I. (1969) Lysergide and cannabis as possible teratogens in man. *Lancet* **1**, 150.

5. Clarren, S. K. and Smith, D. W. (1978) The fetal alcohol syndrome. *New Eng. J. Med.* **298**, 1063.
6. Finney, D. J., Latscha, R., Bennett, B. M. and Hsu, P. (1963) *Tables for testing Significance in a 2 × 2 Contingency Table.* University Press, Cambridge.
7. Fleischman, R. W., Hayden, D. W., Rosenkrantz, H. and Braude, M. C. (1975) Teratologic evaluation of Δ^9-tetrahydrocannabinol in mice, including a review of the literature. *Teratology.* **12**, 47.
8. Fournier, E., Rosenberg, E., Hardy, N. and Nahas, G. (1976) Teratologic effects of cannabis extracts in rabbits: a preliminary study in *Marihuana: Chemistry, Biochemistry, and Cellular Effects* (Nahas, G. G., ed.) Springer-Verlag, New York, pp. 457–468.
9. Geber, W. F. and Schramm, L. C. (1969) Effects of marihuana extract on fetal hamsters and rabbits. *Toxic. Appl. Pharmacol.* **14**, 276.
10. Geber, W. F. and Schramm, L. C. (1969) Teratogenicity of marihuana extract as influenced by plant origin and seasonal variation. *Arch. Int. Pharmacol. Ther.* **177**, 224.
11. Grilly, D. M., Ferraro, D. P. and Braude, M. C. (1974) Observations on the reproductive activity of chimpanzees following long-term exposure to marihuana. *Pharmacology* **11**, 304.
12. Haley, S. L., Wright, P. L., Plank, J. B., Keplinger, M. L., Braude, M. C. and Calandra, J. C. (1972) The effect of natural and synthetic delta-9-tetrahydrocannabinol on fetal development. *Toxicol. Appl. Pharmacol.* **25**, 450.
13. Harbison, R. D. and Mantilla-Plata, B. (1972) Prenatal toxicity, maternal distribution and placental transfer of tetrahydrocannabinol. *J. Pharmacol. Exp. Ther.* **180**, 446.
14. Harbison, R. D., Mantilla-Plata, B. and Lubin, D. J. (1977) Alternation of ^{9}-tetrahydrocannabinol-induced tetratogenicity by stimulation and inhibition of its metabolism. *Jour. Pharm. Exp. Ther.* **202**, 455.
15. Hecht, F., Beals, R. K., Lees, M. H., Jolly, H. and Roberts, P. (1968) Lysergic acid diethylamide and cannabis as possible teratogens in man. *Lancet* **2**, 1087.
16. Joneja, M. G. (1977) Effects of Δ^9-tetrahydrocannabinol on hamster fetuses. *J. Tox. Envir. Health.* **2**, 1031.
17. Pace, H. B., Davis, W. M. and Borgen, L. A. (1971) Teratogenesis; and marijuana. *Ann. N. Y. Acad. Sci.* **191**, 123.
18. Persaud, T. V. N. and Ellington, A. C. (1967) Cannabis in early pregnancy. *Lancet* **2**, 1306.
19. Persaud, T. V. N. and Ellington, A. C. (1968) Teratogenic activity of canabis resin. *Lancet* **2**, 406
20. Phillips, R. N., Turk, R. F. and Forney, R. B. (1971) Acute toxicity of delta-nine tetrahydrocannabinol in rats and mice. *Proc. Scott. Exp. Biol. Med.* **136**, 260.
21. Rosenkrantz, H., Fleishman, R. W. and Baker, J. R. (1978) Embryotoxicity of marihuana by inhalation. *Fed. Proc.* **37(3)**, 737 (Abstract).
22. Sackett, G., Holm, R. and Landesman-Dwyer, S. (1975) Vulnerability for abnormal development: pregnancy outcomes and sex differences in macaque monkeys in *Aberrant Development in Infancy: Human and Animal Studies* (Ellis N. R., ed.) Wiley New York.
23. Sassenrath, E. N. and Chapman, L. F. (1975) Tetrahydrocannabinol-induced manifestations of the 'marihuana syndrome' in group-living macaques. *Fed. Proc.* **34**, 1666 (1975).
24. Sassenrath, E. N. and Chapman, L. F. (1976) primate social behavior as a method of analysis of drug action: studies with THC in monkeys. *Fed. Proc.* **35**, 2238
25. Sassenrath, E. N., Goo, G. P. and Chapman, L. F. Behavioral effects of acute and long-term chronic exposure to Δ^9-THC in group-living rhesus monkeys. pp. 693–712).
26. Uyeno, E. T. (1973) Delta-nine tetrahydrocannabinol administration during pregnancy of the rat. *Proc. West. Pharmacol. Soc.* **16**, 64.
27. Wursch, M. S., Otis, L., Green, D. E. and Forrest, I. S. (1972) ^{3}H-^{9}-tetrahydrocannabinol metabolism in rhesus and squirrel monkeys. *Proc. West. Pharmacol. Soc.* **15**, 68.

37 The Effects of Maternal Marihuana Use During Pregnancy on Fetal Growth

Steven J. Parker and Barry S. Zuckerman

Abstract

This paper reviews the literature and presents findings from an epidemiologic study conducted in Boston, MA concerning the effects of maternal marihuana use during pregnancy on fetal growth. After controlling for potentially confounding variables, a positive maternal urine assay for marihuana during pregnancy and/or in the immediate postpartum period was associated with a 79 g decrease in birthweight ($p = 0.04$) and a 0.5-cm decrement in length ($p = 0.02$), compared to nonusers. No association between prenatal marihuana use and congenital anomalies, shortened gestation, or decreased head circumference was found. The effects of marihuana on neonatal body composition suggest that impaired fetal growth may have been caused by fetal hypoxia. Implications for future research and interventions are discussed.

1. INTRODUCTION

Fetal growth is an important and easily quantified outcome of pregnancy. Low birthweight is often associated with later adverse health and developmental outcomes for children. As a result of current research on the effects of maternal health behaviors during pregnancy, many factors have been shown to have a deleterious effect on fetal growth. These include poor maternal nutrition before and during pregnancy, chronic medical conditions, and the use of substances such as cigarettes, excessive alcohol and, most recently, cocaine. This chapter will summarize our investigations *(1,2)* of the effects on fetal growth of a commonly used, but little studied, psychoactive drug: marihuana. We shall also discuss the important methodological issues that must be addressed in any such future research.

2. PHARMACOLOGY

The principle psychoactive chemical of marihuana is 1-Δ^9-tetrahydrocannabinol (THC). Whereas most research focuses on Δ^9-THC, over 400 different chemicals have been identi-

From: *Marihuana for Medicine*
Edited by: G. G. Nahas et al. © Humana Press Inc., Totowa, NJ

fied in marihuana smoke (3). After inhalation, more than one-half of the Δ^9-THC is absorbed into the bloodstream (4). It is primarily bound to serum lipoproteins and other plasma proteins (5). Following hydroxylation in the liver, most metaboliltes of Δ^9-THC are eliminated in feces and urine (5). Because it has a strong affinity for lipids, Δ^9-THC is stored and accumulates in fatty tissues of the body (6). A single dose of Cannabis in humans has a tissue half-life of seven days and may take up to 30 days to be completely excreted (7). For this reason marihuana has been shown to accumulate in the body following chronic use (8).

Like all psychoactive drugs, marihuana is capable of crossing the placenta. There is evidence in animals that Δ^9-THC may concentrate in the placenta following administration (9). Placental transfer is highest early in gestation and diminishes as pregnancy progresses (10). Most animal studies demonstrate higher maternal than fetal serum Δ^9-THC levels following administration (5). p.4).

The inhalation of marihuana smoke in animals produces maternal ventilation/perfusion abnormalities, with subsequent fetal hypoxia lasting about 60 minutes (11). Smoking marihuana is also associated with higher blood carbon monoxide lasting about 60 minutes (17). Thus, marihuana may pose a hazard to fetal growth through its indirect effect of decreasing fetal oxygenation as well as through a potential direct drug effect.

3. STUDIES IN HUMANS

The prevalence of marihuana use during pregnancy has been estimated as between 5 and 34%, depending on the population studied (1). Epidemiologic studies are utilized to study the effects of maternal drug use during pregnancy on the human fetus. Such studies, however, contain inherent methodological difficulties that often make interpretation of their results problematic. These include difficulty in the accurate assessment of the amount, timing, and duration of maternal drug use and the coexistence of multiple confounding variables (e.g., cigarettes, alcohol and other illicit drugs, malnutrition, inadequate prenatal care, medical illness) with maternal drug use. Additionally, there are a paucity of outcome variables in the neonatal period that can detect subtle consequences of maternal drug use. Finally, studies of maternal drug use during pregnancy tend to focus on neonatal effects. Long-term follow-up studies are far more difficult to conduct because of high attrition rates and the increasing importance of confounding environmental, social, and health variables in the child's life.

Only six studies with large enough sample sizes to control for confounding variables have addressed the effects of Cannabis on human fetal growth. These investigations have reported conflicting results. Some have shown a deleterious effect of Cannabis on fetal growth (13–15), whereas others have not (16,17). A potential link between maternal marihuana use and major malformations has been suggested by one large study (20), but most have not found such an association (16,18,19). Finally, the reported effects of maternal Cannabis use on the duration of gestation have ranged from an increased length of gestation (13), to no effect (14,20), to a decreased length of gestation (15,16,19).

One explanation for the conflicting reports may have been the reliance of these studies on maternal self-report to ascertain marihuana use. Without urine testing, some marihuana users may have been misclassified as non-users, thereby obscuring the association between marihuana use and fetal growth. We therefore undertook an investigation of the effects of maternal marihuana smoking during pregnancy that identified use through urine testing and maternal self-report.

4. METHODS

Pregnant women were recruited from the general prenatal clinic at Boston City Hospital. The only requirements for participation were the ability to speak English or Spanish and willingness to give informed consent. Recruitment occurred from July, 1984 through June, 1987.

A total of 1664 women initially agreed to participate in the study. Of this sample, 1226 mother/infant pairs (74%) completed the study. The demographics of study participants were representative of the women in our inner-city urban hospital: young (73% were less than 29 years), poor (54% earned less than $12,000/yr), non-white (47% were United States-born black, 19% were foreign-born black, and 18% were Hispanic), and poorly educated (41% did not graduate high school).

Women were assessed once prenatally and once in the immediate postpartum period. They were interviewed to elicit the timing, frequency, and quantities of use of marihuana, cigarettes, alcohol, cocaine and other drugs before and during pregnancy. Health and nutritional information was gathered, as well as maternal demographic and psychosocial characteristics. After the prenatal and postpartum interviews, participants were asked for a urine sample to assay for illicit drugs. Cannabinoid metabolites were detected by enzyme-mediated immunoassay technique (EMIT). A sample was defined as positive if the level of cannabinoid metabolites was greater than 0.02 mg/L. Positive samples were then confirmed by high-pressure liquid chromatography (HPLC).

The infants of study participants were assessed between 8 and 72 hours after delivery by a pediatrician who was blind to maternal status. The infants were weighed on a Detecto scale, their length was measured on a Holtain Infantometer, and head circumference determined with a cloth tape. A general pediatric and neurological examination was then conducted, followed by a careful search for major and minor congenital morphologic anomalies. Following this examination, information was abstracted from the infant's medical record.

5. RESULTS

A total of 278 women reported using marihuana during pregnancy (Table 1). An additional 53 women denied use of marihuana during pregnancy but had a positive urine assay in the prenatal and/or perinatal period. Thus, 331 of 1,226 (27%) women in our study used marihuana during pregnancy.

Table 2 reports the frequency of self-reported marihuana use during pregnancy of women who had at least one positive urine assay and those who did not. Women with a positive urine assay for marihuana reported much more frequent use than did those women who reported marihuana use but had negative urine assays. This finding underscores the significance of the 16% (53/331) of marihuana users who would not have been identified as users had urine assays not been performed. Since these women were likely to have been relatively heavy marihuana users, their misclassification as nonusers would have diminished any subsequently measured marihuana effects.

Prenatal maternal marihuana use was highly intercorrelated with other drug use. For example, of the women who were marihuana users, 80% smoked cigarettes (vs 30% of nonusers, $p < 0.0001$), 76% drank some alcohol (vs 51% of nonusers, $p < 0.0001$), 46% used cocaine (vs 7% of nonusers, $p < 0.0001$), and 8% used opiates (vs 3% of nonusers, $p < .01$). Additionally, women with positive urine assays for marihuana had fewer prenatal visits than did nonusers (7.9 vs 9.2, $p < 0.001$) and gained less weight during pregnancy than did non users (28 vs 31 pounds, $p < 0.05$).

Table
Marijuana Use During Pregnancy

	Urine Assay		
	Positive	Negative	Total
Self-report positive	149	129	278
Self-report negative	53	895	948
TOTAL	202	1024	1226

Table 2
Frequency of Reported Marijuana Use During Pregnancy by Positive or Negative Urine Assay for Marihuana[a]

Frequency	Positive Assay (n = 149)	Negative Assay (n = 129)
3 or more times per week	42%	19%
1–2 times per week	30%	26%
1–3 times per month	19%	24%
Less than 1 time per month	9%	31%

[a] Chi square 29.4 df 3; $p < 0.0001$.

Table 3
Univariate Analysis: Positive Urine Assay and Neonatal Growth, Gestational Age, and Anomalies

	Nonuse	Positive Assay	Significance
Birthweight (g)	3260	2980	< 0.001
Length (cm)	49.8	48.3	< 0.001
Head circumference (cm)	34.3	33.4	< 0.001
Gestational age (wk)	39.2	38.9	N.S.
Congenital anomalies			
≥ 3 minor or 1 major	9%	9%	N.S.
≥ 1 minor	38%	45%	N.S.

Table 3 displays the univariate relationship between the use of marihuana during pregnancy and the infants' growth, gestational age, and presence of anomalies. Marihuana use was significantly correlated with a diminished birthweight, a smaller length, and a smaller head circumference. Marihuana use was *not* associated with shorter duration of pregnancy or to an increase in minor or major congenital anomalies.

Since prenatal marihuana use was associated with other drug use and risk factors that have an adverse impact on fetal growth, a multiple aggression analysis was performed. After controlling for these and other potentially confounding variables, a positive maternal assay for marihuana metabolites was still associated with a significant diminution in mean newborn weight (79 g), length (0.52 cm), but not head circumference (Table 4). Infants of women with a positive urine assay for marihuana had a 50% higher risk of being low birthweight (less than 2500 g) than infants whose mothers did not use drugs. In order to assess the importance of urine assays in ascertaining marihuana use, these analyses were repeated using maternal self-report (rather than a positive urine assay) of marihuana use as the independent variable, a methodology comparable to previous studies in which urine assays were not used. These analyses revealed that maternal self-report alone was *not* significantly correlated with impaired fetal growth.

We further assessed the effects of prenatal maternal marihuana use on neonatal fat and lean body mass *(2)*. Marihuana exposure was associated with decreased arm muscle mass and decreased body nonfat mass, but with normal fat stores. These findings remained after controlling for maternal cigarette use and nutritional status during pregnancy. This pattern of decreased lean body mass and normal fat stores in infants exposed to marihuana is consistent with a hypoxic or other nonnutritional mechanism *(21)* and is similar to that seen in babies exposed to maternal tobacco-cigarette smoking. Because marihuana smoking increases carbon monoxide levels and diminishes oxygenation, we speculate that the effects of marihuana on fetal growth may be mediated by these factors, rather than caused by a primary drug effect.

6. CONCLUSION

The results of our investigation demonstrate that maternal marihuana use during pregnancy is associated with impaired fetal growth. The data on neonatal body composition suggests that the mechanism of this effect may be through impaired fetal oxygenation. Whether there is also a direct drug effect on the fetus remains unclear. Our study does not support an association of marihuana use with a shortened duration of pregnancy or with neonatal congenital anomalies.

This study demonstrates the critical need for biological markers in the study of maternal marihuana use. Had urine tests for marihuana not been performed, we would have not identified 16% of the marihuana users during pregnancy. Such misclassification of the most frequent marihuana users as nonusers would have obscured the significant association between prenatal marihuana use and decreased fetal growth. Urine testing or some other biological marker of use must now be seen as a necessity for any subsequent research in this area.

Finally, our research has led us to the conclusion that the impact of any single drug or risk factor on the fetus is rarely as significant as the *cumulative* effects of a maternal lifestyle that involves multiple risk factors. Adverse health behaviors can have an additive or synergistic detrimental effect on the fetus. For example, in our study if a woman used marihuana alone her infant's mean weight was 79 g less than if she engaged in no behaviors that posed a risk for her infant. However, if the mother had a positive urine assay for marihuana and cocaine and smoked cigarettes and had a poor weight gain during pregnancy, her infant weighed 416 g less than did a mother without these factors. Interventions targeting pregnant women who use psychoactive drugs may need to focus on multiple aspects of their unhealthy lifestyle, rather than any individual drug in order to be effective.

Reprinted with permission from Advances in the Biosciences, Vol. 80, Pergamon Press, Great Britain, 1991, pp. 55–63.

REFERENCES

1. Zuckerman, B., Frank., Hingson R., Amaro H., Levenson S., Kayne H., Parker S., Vinci R., Aboagye K., Fried L., Cabral H., Timperi R. and Bauchner H. (1989) Effects of maternal marijuana and cocaine use on fetal growth. *New Engl. J. Med.* **320**, 762–766.

2. Frank, D., Bauchner, H., Parker, S., Huber, A., Kyei-Aboagye, K., Cabral, H and Zuckerman, B.(1990) Neonatal body proportionality and body composition following in utero exposure to cocaine and marijuana. *J. Peds.*
3. Turner C. (1980) Marijuana research and problems: an overview. *Phar. Int.* **1**, 93.
4. Renault P., Shuster C., Heinrich R. and Freeman D. (1971) Marijuana: standardized smoke administration and dose-effect curves on heart rate in humans. *Science* **174**, 589.
5. Abel, E. (1983) *Marihuana, Tobacco, Alcohol and Reproduction.* CRC Press, Boca Raton, FL.
6. Kruez D. and Axelrod J. (1973) Delta-9-tetrahydrocannabinol: localization in body fat. *Science* **179**, 391.
7. Nahas G. (1976) *Marihuana: Chemistry, Biochemistry and Cellular effects.* Springer-Verlag, New York.
8. Lemberger L., Tamarkin N., Axelrod J. and Kopin I. (1971) Delta-9-tetrahydrocannabinol: metabolism and disposition in long-term marijuana smokers. *Science* **173**, 72.
9. Harbison R. and Mantilla-Plata B. (1972) Prenatal toxicity, maternal distribution and placental transfer of tetrahydrocannabinol. *J. Pharmacol. Exp. Ther.* **180**, 446.
10. Indanpaan-Heikkila J., Fritchie G., Englert L., Ho B. and McIsaac W. (1969) Placental transfer of tritiated tetrahydrocannabinol. *N. Engl. J. Med.* **281**, 330.
11. Clapp, J., Wesley, M., Cooke, R., Pekals, R. and Holstein, C. (1986) The effects of marihuana smoke on gas exchange in ovine pregnancy. *Alcohol Drug Res.* **7**, 85.
12. Wu T., Tashkin D., Djahed B. and Rose J. (1988) Pulmonary hazards of smoking marijuana as compared to tobacco. *N. Engl. J. Med.* **318**, 347.
13. Tennes M., Avitable N., Blackard C., Boyles C., Hassoin B., Holmes L. and Kreye M. (1985) Marijuana: prenatal and postnatal exposure in the human, In: *Current Research on the Consequences of Maternal Drug Abuse* (Pinkert T., ed.) NIDA Research Monograph 59, Washington, D.C.: Government Printing Office (DHHS Publication no. (ADM) 85: 1400), p. 48.
14. Hingson R., Alpert J., Day N., Dooling E., Kayne H., Morelock S., Oppenheimer E., Rosett H., Weiner L. and Zuckerman B. (1982) Effects of maternal drinking and marihuana use on fetal growth and development. *Pediatrics* **70**, 539.
15. Hatch E. and Bracken M. (1986). Effect of marijuana use in pregnancy on fetal growth. *Am. J. Epidemiol.* **124**, 986.
16. Fried, P., Watkinson, B. and Willan, A. (1984) Marijuana use during pregnancy and decreased length of gestation. *Am. J. Obstet. Gynecol.* **150**, 23.
17. Kline J., Stein Z. and Hutzler M. (1987) Cigarettes, alcohol and marijuana: varying association with birthweight. *Int. J. Epidemiol.* **16**, 44.
18. Tennes M. and Blackard C. (1980) Maternal alcohol consumption, birthweight and minor physical anomalies. *Am. J. Obstet. Gynecol.* **138**, 774.
19. Gibson G., Bayhurst P. and Colley D. (1983) Maternal alcohol, alcohol, and cannabis consumption and the outcome of pregnancy. *Aust. N. Z. Obstet. Gynecol.* **23**, 16.
20. Linn S., Schoenbaum S., Monson R., Stubblefield P. and Ryan K. (1984) The association of marijuana use with outcome of pregnancy. *Am. J. Public Health* **73**, 1161.
21. Frisancho, A., Klayman, J. and Matos, J. (1977) Newborn baby composition and its relationship to linear growth. *Am. J. Clin. Nutr.* **30**, 704.

V CANNABINOIDS IN THE TREATMENT OF PAIN

38

Central Mechanisms of Pain and Analgesia

Lars Terenius

Pain remains the major complaint and symptom. Despite recent advances in the understanding of the neurobiology of pain, the pharmacologic targets and tools remain the same: the antipyretic antiinflammatory analgesics, which block the generation of noxious eicosanoids from the arachidonic acid cascade, and opiates, which act on the endogenous opioid systems. As pointed out by Brune in 1998, the conventional distinction of peripherally acting analgesics ("antipyretics") versus centrally acting ("opiates") does not represent the proper profile of the respective group of agents. In this chapter, I will mainly discuss the opioid systems, since no other central endogenous system has yet been found therapeutically useful. It should be remembered that existing therapies are not adequate, or they are not properly utilized, since a great number of patients do not obtain adequate pain relief. Chronic pain, which by definition represents a therapeutic failure, is a common and severely dehabilitating condition.

The term pain describes both a sensation (like vision, hearing, etc.) and a subjective experience that is coupled to anxiety and suffering. Clinical pain always has an affective component and involves the spinal cord and higher CNS mechanisms. Severe pain has a global influence on the brain's metabolic activity, as indicated by studies using in vivo imaging techniques. Thus, besides activation of specific pathways, generalized brain activation is observed. The affective component of pain is often the most disturbing. Injection of an opiate at low doses can reduce suffering to an acceptable level and will not affect the sensory aspects. "It still hurts but it does not matter."

INTERINDIVIDUAL DIFFERENCES IN THE SENSITIVITY TO PAIN

Animal experiments indicate that there are genetic differences in the sensitivity to pain. For instance, the hypertensive SHR line of Wistar rats is less sensitive to pain than normoten-

From: *Marihuana and Medicine*
Edited by: G. G. Nahas et al.   © Humana Press Inc., Totowa, NJ

sive animals *(1)*. The hyposensitivity is reduced by naloxone, suggesting that the difference is due to release of opioid peptides in the CNS *(2)*.

Also patients with hypertension are less pain sensitive. Recently it was observed that normotensives with risk of developing hypertension are hyposensitive *(3)*. Dyck *(4)* observed that neuropathic pain occurs more frequently in patients with a genetic predisposition.

We have addressed interindividual differences in the sensitivity to clinical pain using an experimental paradigm. Patient-controlled self-medication with opiates is a valuable asset in the treatment of postoperative pain. Each patient uses a motor-controlled pump that delivers opiate intravenously and injects the opiate on demand. It appears that injections occur with a regular frequency, which keeps the plasma level of the injected opiate at a pseudo-steady-state level for several hours *(5)*. This steady-state level may be used as an objective measure of the pain experience ("suffering"). Interestingly, individual patients titrate to different plasma levels (differing by a factor of 3–5). We were also able to perform lumbar punctures of each individual and measure levels of opioid peptides by a receptor assay. Relating the level of opioid peptide in the cerebrospinal fluid (CSF) to the pseudo-steady-state level of meperidine, an inverse relationship was observed. Thus, the patient with low endogenous opioid activity requires more opiate to feel comfortable and vice versa *(5)*.

In another study, a group of primigravidae volunteered to donate a lumbar CSF sample in early labor. The women were offered epidural analgesia. Those who chose an epidural had lower levels of the opioid peptide, dynorphin A *(6)*. This peptide occurs in spinal interneurons, which form contacts with primary afferents from the viscera. Another opioid peptide, β-endorphin, of higher central origin showed no difference between those who chose or did not choose the epidural. Experiments in rats have indicated that dynorphin peptides play an important role in labor analgesia. Blocking dynorphin with antagonists or with antibody causes strong irritation and lowers surviving pup numbers. Taken together these studies point to a role of opioid peptides in the control of acute pain.

Indirect evidence exists that the placebo effect, which is always relevant in the treatment of pain, is mediated by opioid peptides. Naloxone has been reported to at least partially inhibit the placebo response *(7)*. Probably a much greater source of individual variation is the influence of sex hormones. It is well known that, in general, women have lower pain thresholds. However, these differences are small. More important, there are large sex differences in the incidence of certain pains. For instance, fibromyalgia is almost uniquely diagnosed in females whereas postherpetic neuralgia has high prevalence in men. A recent review article emphasizes the need for future studies into mechanisms underlying these sex differences. This much neglected field deserves indepth study.

CHRONIC PAIN

Pain may be chronic (persists for more than 6 mo) because of a chronic painful condition. Chronic inflammatory conditions can be treated with the antipyretic/antiinflammatory agents. Chronic pain due to malignancy is always emotionally laden and responds to opiates. Chronic use of opiates is not without complications and side-effects such as constipation may limit compliance. Optimally used, opiates remain the drugs of choice.

A large group of patients suffers from chronic pain without any diagnosable pathology in tissues and organs except primary afferent neurons and the CNS. This kind of pain may be called "neurogenic" and seems to arise from distorted activity in CNS pathways, in the spinal cord, or in the brain. A frequent cause is deafferentation or other types of communicative dysfunction. We have asked whether patients in such pain conditions for more than 6 mo (i.e., with a chronic ailment) have normal or altered opioid peptide activity.

OPIOID PEPTIDES IN CHRONIC NEUROGENIC PAIN

Opioid peptides have been analyzed in lumbar CSF from a series of patients with pain of at least 6 mo duration. Quite surprisingly, it was observed that patients with neurogenic pain tended to have lower opioid peptide levels than a group of healthy volunteers. Patients with chronic afferent pain due to rheumatoid arthritis or malignancy showed values close to those in the comparison group. A third group of patients with idiopathic pain that had no obvious somatic origin and where a psychogenic component was indicated, showed values higher than those in the comparison group *(8)*. Patients with neurogenic pain are generally refractory to opiate treatment. Partial relief can often be obtained with transcutaneous electric stimulation (TENS) or acupuncture. It has been observed that pain relief induced by acupuncture–like TENS or classic acupuncture–is partially reversed by naloxone. We have shown that this kind of stimulation increases the CSF levels of enkephalin peptides, which have substantial affinity for the naloxone-sensitive mu-opioid receptors. High-frequency TENS, which, on the other hand, reportedly induces nonopioid analgesia, releases dynorphin peptides into the CSF *(9)*. The dynorphin peptides mainly act on kappa-receptors, which have low naloxone sensitivity.

Patients with fibromyalgia have also been subjected to neurochemical analysis. These patients do not appear to have deviant CSF levels of opioid peptides. However, substance P levels are markedly elevated and particularly in those who smoke *(10)*. Substance P is a major peptide in the C-fiber afferents which are relevant for clinical pain. Opiates are known to inhibit the release of substance P from C-fibers but do not offer relief in this condition. The significance of the observation is therefore not clear.

OTHER CENTRAL ACTING PAIN-MODULATING SUBSTANCES

It is surprising that there are really no alternatives to opiates in severe "afferent" pain with an emotional overload. Experimental screening in animals has identified nonopioid compounds that act as analgesics, but they have not yet reached the clinic. Opiate-refractory pain represents a particular challenge. Animal models have been developed to investigate these painful disorders. Section of a peripheral nerve in a rat limb (axotomy) may cause paresthesias and abnormal self-mutilating behavior, which indicates that the animal experiences strong irritation or pain. The behavioral changes are accompanied by extensive changes in neurotransmitters/neuropeptides of the primary afferent neuron *(11)*. Such changes may give leads to new therapeutic agents.

Cannabinoids are well-known in medicine by themselves, or in combination with other centrally acting substances. The most active principles, Δ^9-THC, act through the so-called CB-1 receptor, which is widespread in the CNS. As reviewed elsewhere, there is evidence that the active principles also release endogenous opioids and certain central actions of Δ^9-THC are blocked by naloxone. It is also interesting that chronic use of cannabinoids upregulates the expression of the proenkephalin gene *(12)*. Apparently, the cannabinoids are intimately linked to opioid systems.

CONCLUSIONS

The urge to relieve pain must have developed as human beings acquired conscious knowledge during evolution. The two major classes of presently used analgesics are derived from herbal medicines (opium poppy and coca leaves) and have been in use for several thousand years. Cannabis has also been attributed analgesic properties as confirmed in present-day pharmacologic studies of its active principles. As discussed elsewhere, these principles, notably Δ^9-THC, to some extent probably act through the release of opioid peptides. It is interesting that knock-out manipulation of mice that lack a functional pro-enkephalin gene, one of the three opioid peptide precursor genes, leads to lower nociceptive thresholds, higher irritability, and aggressiveness *(13)*. Thousands of years of folk medicine and industrial drug development have so far failed to identify alternative centrally acting analgesics of similar potency and utility as the opioids. Thus, the opioid system remains the main target for centrally induced analgesia.

REFERENCES

1. Maixner, W., Touw, K. B., Brody, M. J., Gebhart, G. F. and Long, J. P. (1982) Factors influencing the altered pain perception in the spontaneously hypertensive rat. *Brain Res* **237**, 137–145.
2. Saavedra, M. M. (1981) Naloxone reversible decrease in pain sensitivity in young and adult spontaneously hypertensive rats. *Brain Res* **209**, 245–249.
3. Page, G. D. and France, C. R. (1997) Objective evidence of decreased pain perception in normotensives at risk for hypertension. *Pain* **73**, 173–180.
4. Dyck, P. J. (1994) Inherited neuronal atrophy and degeneration of peripheral sensory neurons. In Dyck, P. J., Thomas, P. K., Lambert, L. A. and Bunge, R. (Eds.). *Peripheral Neuropathy, 2nd ed.*, Saunders, Philadelphia.
5. Tamsen, A., Hartvig, P., Dahlström, B., Wahlström, A. and Terenius, L. (1980) Endophins and on-demand pain relief (letter). *Lancet* **1**, 769–770.
6. Lyrenäs, S., Nyberg, F., Willdeck-Lund, G., Lindström, L., Lindberg, B. and Terenius. L. (1987) Endorphin activity in cerebospinal fluid prior to elective cesarean section and in early puerperium. *Ups J Med Sci* **92**, 37–45.
7. Benedetti, F. (1996) The opposite effects of the opiate antagonist naloxone and the cholecystokinin antagonist proglumide on placebo analgesia. *Pain* **64**: 535–543.
8. Almay, B. G., Johansson, F., von Knorring, L., Terenius, L. and Wahlström, A. (1978) Endorphins in chronic pain. I. Differences in CSF endorphin levels between organic and psychogenic pain syndromes. *Pain* **5**, 153–162.
9. Han, J. S., Chen, X. H., Sun, S. L., Xu, X. J., Yuan, Y., Yan, S. C., Hao, J. X. and Terenius, L. (1991) Effect of low- and high-frequency TENS on Met-enkephalin-Arg-Phe and dynorphin A immunoreactivity in human lumbar CSF. *Pain* **47**, 295–298.
10. Vaerøy, H., Helle, R., Førre, Ø., Kåss, E. and Terenius, L. (1988) Elevated CSF levels of substance P and high incidence of Raynaud phenomenon in patients with fibromyalgia: new features for diagnosis. *Pain* **32**, 21–26.
11. Hökfelt, T., Zhang, X. and Wiesenfeld-Hallin, Z. (1994) Messenger plasticity in rimary sensory neurons following axotomy and its functional implications. *Trends Neurosci* **17**, 22–30.
12. Manzanares, J., Corchero, J., Romero, J., Fernandez-Ruiz, J. J., Ramos, J. A. and Fuentes, J. A. (1998) Chronic administration of cannabinoids regulates proenkephalin mRNA levels in selected regions of the rat brain. *Mol Brain Res* **55**, 126–132.
13. Konig, M., Zimmer, A. M., Steiner, H., Holmes, P. V., Crawley, J. N., Brownstein, M. J. and Zimmer, A. (1996) Pain responses, anxiety and aggression in mice deficient in pre-proenkephalin. *Nature* **383**, 535–538.

39 Pharmacology of Chronic Pain

Andy Dray, Laszlo Urban,
and Anthony Dickenson

Abstract

Chronic pain, which is associated with prolonged tissue damage or injuries to the peripheral or central nervous system, results from a number of complex changes in nociceptive pathways. These include alterations of cell phenotype and changes in the expression of proteins such as receptors, transmitters, and ion channels, as well as modifications of neural structure, for example, cell loss, nerve regeneration, and synaptic reorganizations. The resultant increase in neural excitability can be reduced with receptor-selective drugs that block peripheral or central chemical mediators or that control ectopic activity or cellular phenotype changes. In this article, Andy Dray, Laszlo Urban, and Anthony Dickenson focus on some current mechanistic aspects of chronic pain imposed by inflammation and peripheral neuropathy, and review, in particular, the molecular changes involving the pharmacology of nociceptive pathways, since these have important implications for the management of pain.

Definitions of pain states can be rather subjective and imprecise. On the one hand, acute transient pain is associated with negligible tissue damage and is thought to serve as a physiological warning to guard the integrity of the organism. On the other hand, chronic pain is associated with tissue damage, inflammation, or neuropathologies and the pain sensations outlast their biological usefulness. Moreover, in chronic pain states there is a superimposition of many other processes onto the basic events of nociception, which alters the relationship between stimulus and the response and affects the ability to modulate the resultant pain states. Indeed, it is likely that some of the specific changes that relate to the type of injury and accompanying inflammation or neuropathology affect the qualities of pain sensation and reaction to it.

From: *Marihuana and Medicine*
Edited by: G. G. Nahas et al.   © Humana Press Inc., Totowa, NJ

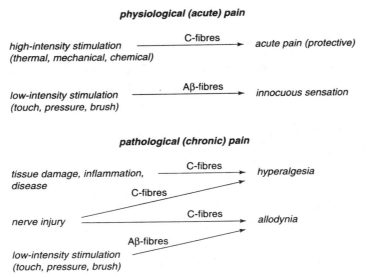

Fig. 1. Under normal physiological conditions, nociceptive signals generated by C-fibers initiate acute pain and a protective reflex. Activation of low-threshold Aβ-fibers by innocuous stimuli does not induce pain. In pathological pain following various types of injury or nerve damage. C-fibers become hypersensitive and induce hypersensitivity in sensory pathways, resulting in an enhanced and persistent response following sensory nerve stimulation. Under these conditions, low-intensity Aβ-fiber stimulation induces pain (allodynia).

In chronic pain, a rudimentary understanding is beginning to emerge of the complexity of events that occur in nociceptive pathways. Some of these events occur in precise time windows during the development and consolidation of the pain state, and can range from changes in the excitability of fine afferent nerves to drastic alterations in their cellular phenotype with the expression of new molecules, including neurotransmitters, enzymes, and chemical receptors (1–4). In addition, chronic central alterations in the neurochemistry of pain signaling produce hypersensitivity, which enhances and prolongs relatively low levels of afferent input and allows normally innocuous stimuli to be perceived as painful (Fig. 1). Structural changes, particularly following peripheral nerve injury, include loss of spinal interneurones, inappropriate rearrangements of afferent nerve processes in the spinal cord (5–6) and proliferation of sympathetic fibres into sensory ganglia, which are not normally innervated to any significant degree (6). The occurrence of the changes outlined above and their particular features are by no means uniform and depend on the type of tissue injury, the involvement of specific types of afferent fibre and the participation of the immune system. In addition, chronic pain conditions do not always result from peripheral injuries but can result from organic or affective disorders of the CNS. These latter processes are poorly understood. Furthermore, chronic pain behavior has added complexities, since human reactions can be modified by the environmental or sociological setting.

PERIPHERAL PHARMACOLOGY OF PAIN

Inflammation

Fine afferent C and Aβ nociceptive nerves are activated by a number of potentially harmful stimuli, but their sensitivity to the chemicals generated by tissue damage and inflammation is particularly notable (Fig. 1). The activation of afferent nerves induces an axon reflex and the

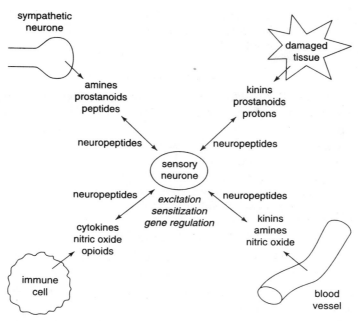

Fig. 2. A variety of chemical factors released from blood vessels, damaged tissues, sympathetic neurons, and immune cells activate or sensitize primary sensory neurones or alter their cellular phenotype. There is a dynamic interaction between these tissues and the effects of neuropeptides released by sensory nerves. These produce changes in blood flow and blood vessel permeability, stimulate immune cells, and activate sympathetic nerves.

release of sensory neuropeptides, particularly substance P, neurokinin A (NKA), and calcitonin gene-related peptide (CGRP). These peptides also change the excitability of sensory nerves and nearby postganglionic sympathetic fibres. They also activate immune cells, alter local blood flow, and induce the release of other active substances by plasma extravasation (Fig. 2). Finally, a number of other peptides such as nerve growth factor (NGF), which are normally secreted by target tissues to regulate growth and to maintain cellular phenotype of sensory and sympathetic neurones, may be increased by inflammation and nerve damage *(7)*.

Chemical pain transduction involves interactions with membrane receptors that are coupled to ion channels and second messenger systems, resulting in changes in membrane excitability and cell phenotype. In this environment, many chemical stimuli are available to initiate cascades of signals. Hence, there is enormous potential for signal amplification and modulation, as well as an opportunity for synergisms between neural and nonneural tissues. Such interactions are important in producing hyperalgesia, but must also be viewed as important mechanisms contributing to tissue regeneration and repair following injury.

Bradykinin

Bradykinin is a potent algogen produced during injury and inflammation. The pain and inflammation mediated by kinins involve effects on the more commonly observed bradykinin B_2 receptor. However, B_1 receptors are expressed during prolonged inflammation and make a significant contribution to the hyperalgesia*(8)*. Other inflammatory products, including cytokines such as interleukin (IL)-1, -6, and -8 and tumour necrosis factor-α (TNF-α), also induce hyperalgesia by facilitating induction of B_1 receptors, by stimulation of prostanoid production and by activation of sympathetic neurons. In keeping with this, hyperalgesia can be reversed by indomethacin, by a novel IL-1 antagonist Lys-D-Pro-Thr, or by sympathectomy and antagonists of adrenoceptors *(9)*.

Prostanoids

A variety of prostanoids (PGE$_2$, PGI$_2$, and LTB$_4$) that are produced during inflammation are known either to excite nociceptors or, more usually, to sensitize them to other stimuli and, thus, contribute to peripheral hyperalgesia. Indeed, inhibition of the synthetic and constitute enzyme, cyclooxygenase-1, is believed to be the basis for the analgesic and anti inflammatory actions of nonsteroidal anti inflammatory drugs (NSAIDs). More recently, another form of cyclooxygenase, cyclooxygenase-2, has been shown to be induced by inflammation. Cyclooxygenase-2 is also susceptible to NSAIDs *(10)*, but some NSAIDs are more potent against one form of the enzyme than the other.

5-Hydroxytryptamine

5-Hydroxytryptamine (5-HT) is released from platelets and mast cells, and produces mild and transient pain by direct activation of sensory neurons via 5-HT$_3$ receptors. 5-HT also induces a direct sensitization of nociceptors via 5-HT$_1$ and 5-HT$_2$ receptors*(11)*. A possible basis for sensitization by 5-HT, as well as by bradykinin and prostanoids, is a reduction of the slow, inhibitory afterpotential that follows the action potential in some sensory neurones. The inhibition is due to cAMP generation and a reduction of the inhibitory K$^+$ current. The overall effect is to increase the likelihood that the neurone will respond to a relatively weak stimulus with a train of action potentials rather than with a single spike.

Histamine

Histamine, one of the best known inflammatory mediators, evokes the sensations of itch at low concentrations and pain at higher concentrations *(12)*. There is surprisingly little information on how these effects are produced, but activation of histamine H$_1$ receptors may increase membrane Ca^{2+} permeability *(13)* and the release of tachykinins and CGRP *(13)*, resulting in further complex interactions including vascular changes and mast-cell degranulation.

Nitric Oxide

Several inflammatory mediators, including substance P and bradykinin, stimulate vascular endothelial cells to release the vasodilator nitric oxide (NO). NO is important for intercellular communication in peripheral tissue and in the CNS, including nociceptive pathways. This is usually achieved via the activation of guanylate cyclase and the production of cGMP *(14)*. Sensory neurons synthesize NO and increase cGMP concentrations in satellite cells in sensory ganglia following stimulation with an NO donor such as sodium nitroprusside. NO does not directly alter sensory neuron excitability, but acts indirectly in the antinociceptive effects of acetylcholine and morphine and promotes tachyphylaxis to bradykinin *(15)*. Paradoxically, inhibitors of nitric oxide synthase (NOS), such as L-NAME, are also antinociceptive in neuropathic and chemically induced pain *(14)*. This effect may be partly exerted in the spinal cord and will be discussed later. However, peripheral NO mechanisms may be involved in neuropathic pain since NOS is induced in sensory ganglia following peripheral axotomy. Furthermore, both the pain and ectopic discharges that occur in peripheral fibers are reduced by NOS inhibition *(16)*. How NOS inhibition alters nerve excitability is unclear, but changes in peripheral blood flow may contribute to this effect.

Opioids

Recent evidence indicates a novel role of endogenous opioids in peripheral inflammation (17). This involves the unmasking of opioid receptors together with the arrival of immunocompetent cells at the site of damage. These cells possess both opioid receptors and the capacity to synthesize opioid peptides (17). Because of the rapidity with which sensitivity to opioids is seen in the periphery, synthesis of new receptors is unlikely. However, it is well established that opioid receptors are synthesized in the sensory neuron cell body and are transported in both central and peripheral directions. The centrally directed receptors become the presynaptic receptors on the spinal terminals of the C-fibers and the peripheral receptors become active only after local tissue damage. All three opioid receptors (μ, δ, and K) are likely to be present in the periphery, since their respective agonists produce a receptor-selective reduction in the excitability of afferent fibres as well as of sympathetic fibers (18).

Nerve Growth Factor

Inflammation stimulates increased synthesis of NGF in fibroblasts, keratinocytes, and Schwann cells. NGF induces prolonged changes in sensory neuron excitability and alterations of cell phenotype that are associated with the development of hyperalgesia (7). High concentrations of NGF act on tyrosine-kinase-linked receptors to regulate cellular transcription factors (such as the octomer Oct-2) and thereby specific gene expression (19). Importantly, NGF increases the synthesis, axoplasmic transport, and neuronal content of substance P and CGRP, thereby making greater amounts available for release from central and peripheral terminals of sensory neurons. It also regulates at least two types of ion channel in sensory neurons: the capsaicin receptotion channel complex and the tetrodotoxin-resistant Na^+ channel (1). Sensory neuronal connectivity and function may also be modified by the promotion of axonal sprouting at central and peripheral terminals of nociceptive neurones (7). In addition, there is likely to be a subtle interplay between nerves, invasive inflammatory cells, and resident cells at sites of tissue damage, since NGF stimulates the release of histamine as well as lipid mediators (for example, LTC_4) from these cells. The synthesis of NGF is also stimulated by cytokines such as IL-β and TNF-α. To complete this positive feedback loop, cytokine production is, in turn, upregulated by substance P released from the sensory nerves. These effects make it highly likely that a selective NGF antagonist would be an effective analgesic and antiinflammatory agent.

Cytokines

A variety of cytokines are released by phagocytotic and antigen-presenting cells of the immune system during inflammation. Neurokinins also stimulate cytokine release from macrophages. As mentioned earlier, cytokines stimulate a number of other systems, and, importantly, can induce phenotypic changes in neurons. For example, IL-1, through the production of leukemia inhibitory factor (LIF), stimulates the expression of substance P in sympathetic neurons (20) and it is possible that release of this neuropeptide stimulates afferent fibers and contributes further to neurogenic inflammation.

Sympathetic Fibers

Some of the postulated interactions of sympathetic fibers are shown in Fig. 3. Other direct interactions of sympathetic nerves or sympathetic transmitters with afferent fibers have not been easy to demonstrate (21). During inflammation, afferent fibers may be sensitized by prostanoids released from sympathetic fibers (22), and following peripheral nerve injury,

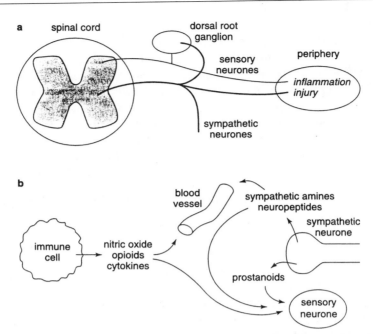

Fig. 3.(a) Peripheral nerve injury induces sprouting of sympathetic fibers that innervate dorsal root ganglia and affect the activity of C-fibers and A-fibers through α-adrenoceptors. **(b)** During inflammation, postganglionic sympathetic nerve fibers also sensitize sensory neurons (via prostanoid release) and contribute to plasma extravasation by changing blood flow in microvessels and by neuropeptide release. Immune cells release cytokines, nitric oxide, and opioid peptides to affect the vasculature and nerve activity.

sympathetic nerve stimulation or the administration of noradrenaline can excite some Aβ- and C-fiber afferents via α-adrenoceptors *(6,22)* These findings may partially explain causalgia and sympathetically mediated pain, since these conditions may be ameliorated by sympathectomy or by treatment with the α_2-adrenoceptor agonist, clonidine. Sympathetic fibers also contribute to the production of plasma extravasation by affecting vascular caliber and vascular permeability, as well as by affecting neuropeptide release from fine afferents.

Neuropathic Pain

A number of diverse substances have been used with varying degrees of success in the treatment of neuropathic pain and trigeminal neuralgia. These include the antidepressant drug amitriptiline, the anticonvulsants carbarnazepine and phenytoin, the antiarrythmic drug mexiletine, and the local anaesthetic agents lidocaine and tocainide *(23)*. Several of these compounds reduce ectopic activity, induced by peripheral axotomy or nerve lesions, in neuroma tissue and sensory ganglia, at concentrations that do not block nerve conduction *(24)*. The mechanism underlying this effect is the block of activated Na^+ channels *(23)*, suggesting that abnormal ion channel activity is associated with the nerve damage and related pain (Fig. 4). Indeed, Na^+ channels accumulate in large diameter peripheral nerves at the sites of nerve injury *(25)* and these channels may have unusual properties. On the other hand, some of these drugs may be active in the CNS. Amitriptyline and carbanazepine block NMDA receptors *(26)*, which are important in producing central hyperexcitability in chronic pain, and lidocaine also blocks hyperexcitability in the spinal cord *(21)*. Further studies on the actions of

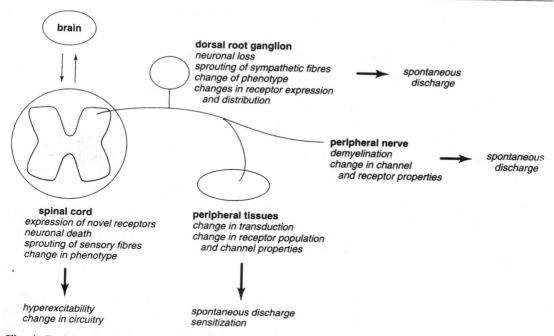

Fig. 4. Peripheral nerve damage induces ectopic activity in peripheral nerve fibers (neuroma) and in sensory ganglion cells. Fibers degenerate due to damage and loss of neurotrophic support. Structural and neurochemical reorganization occurs in the spinal cord. This contributes to an enhancement of excitability and produces exaggerated responses to C-fiber stimulation, and it also allows normally innocuous Aβ-fiber-mediated stimuli to induce pain.

these drugs are required, since inhibition of abnormal neuronal discharge is seen as an important target for treating spontaneous and evoked pain.

Disturbances of peripheral nerve excitability in neuropathic pain may also occur through alterations in K^+ or Ca^{2+} ion function as well as by altered local blood flow. Since inhibition of K^+ conduction increases nerve excitability, it may be worth evaluating K^+ channel activators in suppressing ectopic nerve activity. Furthermore, Ca^{2+} channel blockers such as nimodipine improve experimental diabetes- and cisplatin-induced neuropathy *(28)*, possibly by improving local blood flow or by altering the excitability of peripheral afferent and sympathetic nerves. These findings should be used in the development of new therapies.

CENTRAL PHARMACOLOGY OF CHRONIC PAIN

Glutamate Receptors

Glutamate-mediated transmission is of fundamental importance in the hyperexcitability that is induced in the spinal cord and other central pathways in chronic pain. Indeed, NMDA receptor antagonists are powerful inhibitors of the maintained increase of excitability in dorsal horn cells *(3)*, and both competitive antagonists (D-AP5 and CPP) as well as non competitive antagonists (dizocilpine) potently inhibit the pain of inflammation as well as that of ischemic and neuropathic injuries *(29,30)*. In addition, metabotropic glutamate receptor antagonists (e.g., L-AP3) may reduce the spinal hyperexcitability that occurs during inflammation.

NMDA Receptors

Spinal NMDA receptors are critical for producing "wind-up" in the spinal cord. This is characterized by an increase in the excitability and discharge frequency of neurons in the dorsal horn. It is produced uniquely by repetitive stimulation of C-fiber afferents and requires sensory neuropeptides (Fig. 4). Wind-up is not normally seen following stimulation of large Aβ-fibers (3,31) but this may also occur following a peripheral injury (31).

The prevention of these central hyperexcitability changes by the preemptive blockade of nociceptive input has been proposed as a means of increasing the efficacy of postoperative analgesia. However, the outcomes of several studies that used local anesthetics to block peripheral input and other analgesics to block central nociception have been controversial. It is possible that the substances used did not block nociceptive input effectively, or that the block could not be maintained for long enough. A small degree of breakthrough activity might readily induce wind-up and other hyperexcitability phenomena. Perhaps a combination of a long-acting local anesthetic with the selective inactivation of C-fibers with capsaicin may provide an alternative way of inhibiting C-fiber discharges for prolonged periods. A comparison of preemptive and post operative treatments with morphine have shown analgetic benefits of the former strategy (32). Indeed, giving morphine after central hyperexcitability was established would predictably produce less analgesia, since NMDA-dependent wind-up would break through. This can be overcome, however, by the administration of greater amounts of opioid. In addition, combinations of agents with complementary mechanisms of action, such as local anesthetics or NMDA antagonists, administered together with an opioid may potentiate each others effects and provide improved analgesia (33).

Tachykinin Receptors

Although A- and C-fibers release excitatory amino acids, it is the corelease of neuropeptides, particularly substance P and neurokinin A, that enables wind up to occur. Substance P activates postsynaptic tachykinin NK_1 receptors and neurokinin A has selectivity for NK_2 receptors. NK_1 receptor antagonists, such as CP96345 and RP67580, are not particularly effective against acute C-fiber-evoked activity in the spinal cord, whereas the NK_2 receptor antagonists MEN10376 and L659874 are effective to some extent (34). However, NK_1 antagonists attenuate both wind-up and the increase in spinal excitability produced by repetitive C-fiber stimulation or peripheral inflammation suggesting that the availability of substance P and the presence of NK_1 receptors enable the prolonged NMDA receptor-induced excitability changes to occur.

Inflammation

During inflammation, there is increased glutamate and aspartate release in the spinal dorsal horn and increased synthesis of neurokinins in sensory ganglion cells as well as an increase in their transport and release in the spinal cord (37,38). Similar changes occur with CGRP, but the importance of this abundant sensory peptide in spinal excitability is unclear, since it does not support the excitability changes induced by NMDA. However, it may increase the activity of substance P. The increased synthesis of sensory neuropeptides can be powerfully stimulated by NGF, which is produced in excess in inflamed tissues.

There is also a time-dependent increase in binding of substance P in the dorsal horn, and particularly an upregulation and expression of postsynaptic NK_1 receptors. In keeping with

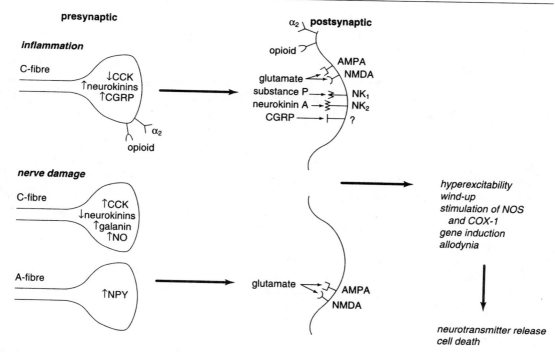

Fig. 5. Dynamic alterations in C- and A-fibers during inflammation and injury. Inflammation induc upregulation of neurokinins but a downregulation of cholecystokinin (CCK) in C-fibers. The excitability of these fibers is reduced by presynaptic oplo Spinal excitability is increased by the interplay between synaptic and nonsynaptic release of glutamate and a number of neuropeptides. These act via specific receptors to induce secondary changes including stimulation of nitric oxide synthase (NOS) and cyclooxygenase as well as wind-up and gene expression. Damage to peripheral fibers also induces changes in peptide expression in C-fibers and hyperexcltability in the spinal cord. Large A-fibers may also change their phenotype and activate nociceptive pathways.

this, CP96345 and RP67580 potently block C-fiber-evoked activation of the spinal neuron. An important role for NK_1 receptors in hyperalgesia is further indicated, since NK_1 receptor antagonists or antibodies against substance P attenuate or block hyperalgesic behavior.

The opioid peptide dynorphin is also significantly increased in the spinal cord. Its time-course outlasts that of substance P and follows the time-course of hyperalgesia more closely *(2)*. However, it is unclear whether in these circumstances dynorphin is involved in maintaining or compensating for spinal hyperexcitability.

The increased availability and release of sensory neuropeptides result in other trophic effects that may also indirectly affect spinal excitability. These include an increased blood flow *(41)*, and an activation of neuroglia to release neuroactive substances, including prostanoids and amino acids *(41)*.

Neuropathic Hyperalgesia

By contrast, the hyperalgesia associated with peripheral neuropathy appears to be mediated by different mechanisms than those involved in inflammation (Fig. 5). For example, the neuropeptide content of sensory ganglia undergoes prolonged depletion following axotomy or may be decreased temporarily (for 45 d) following nerve crush or partial axotomy and then return to normal levels *(42)*. Neurokinin and CGRP losses result, in part, from the absence of target-derived NGF, while some sensory neuropeptides are upregulated, including neuropeptide Y in large myelinated neurons *(4)* and vasoactive intestinal peptide and galanin in small sensory neurons *(4)*.

NMDA and peptide-receptor mechanisms *(3)* may also account for the spinal hyperexcitability following peripheral nerve injury, during which normally innocuous mechanical stimuli, such as light touch, may evoke a feeling of intense pain (allodynia). However, in neuropathic pain, further contribution to central hyperexcitability may occur through loss of inhibitory interneurons by the excitotoxicity mediated by excessive glutarnate release *(43)* (Fig. 5). Another important consequence of this is an upregulation of $GABA_B$ receptors, possibly on presynaptic afferent nerve terminals, and is reflected in the increased analgesic effectiveness of the $GABA_B$ receptor agonist, L-baclofen. In addition, the regeneration of damaged AB-fibers induces axonal sprouting into dorsal horn regions, which are normally innervated by nociceptive C-fiber afferents. Thus, stimulation of AB-fibres, which normally give rise to innocuous signals, may then inappropriately activate spinal nociceptive pathways *(5)* (Fig. 4). The increased excitability changes may be counterbalanced by the inhibitory influences of GABA, as mentioned above, and by the enhanced release of galanin from spinal neurons and from fine afferent nerve fibres *(4)*.

It is significant that neuropathic hyperalgesia appears insensitive to acute intrathecal treatment with capsaicin, which selectively inactivates C-fibers. It is also unaffected by NK_1 receptor antagonists, suggesting that neuropeptide-releasing fibers are not significantly involved in maintaining hyperalgesia *(40,44)*. However, it has also been suggested that activity of fine afferent fibers is necessary to maintain spinal hyperexcitability in neuropathic pain *(45)*. Neuropathic pain can be consistently ameliorated by NMDA receptor antagonists and may also be relieved by sympathectomy and by adrenoceptor antagonists *(21)*. It is not clear how the sympathetic nervous system supports the hyperalgesic state, but several mechanisms are postulated. Vascular supersensitivity and proliferation of postganglionic sympathetic fibers occurs after peripheral axotomy with increased innervation of neurons and blood vessels in sensory ganglia. In keeping with this, sympathectomy and sympatholytic drugs produce a profound reduction of neuropathic pain.

Nitric Oxide

Although NO has also been implicated in the induction and maintenance of chronic pain states *(14)*, it does not appear to be important in acute nociception *(46)*. Whereas NO is produced in sensory ganglia or in dorsal horn neurons, few NOS-positive primary afferent terminals are found in the spinal dorsal horn*(47)*. However, NOS expression is upregulated in both small and large sensory neurons following peripheral axotomy *(16)* and after carrageenan-induced inflammation. This may be a nonspecific response to injury, affecting the excitability of many spinal structures as well as afferent fibers. However, NOS is also colocalized in large preganglionic cells of the intermediolateral nucleus and in periaqueductal cells in the intermediate lamina *(47)*, structures associated with central control of sympathetic activity that may contribute to sympathetically maintained pain. In keeping with a role for NO mechanisms in chronic pain, the NOS inhibitors L-NAME and 7-nitroindazole block thermal hyperalgesia and aversive pain behavior evoked by intrathecal NMDA, as well as the pain of neuropathy and inflammatory hyperalgesia *(14,16)*.

Central Pain

In most cases of central changes in nociceptive pathways, there is clear evidence that the hypersensitivity results from peripheral nerve activity. Indeed, disordered central processing can be interrupted by the administration of local anesthetics in the periphery *(44)*. However, there are other pathological circumstances (e.g., head trauma and stroke) where a central lesion may be the cause of pain. A number of antidepressant and anticonvulsant drugs, including amitriptyline and carbamazepine, have been useful in treating central pain. These drugs block Na^+ channels and are likely to block pain-generating ectopic activity in the brain. Clearly, further studies of centrally generated pain and its therapeutic management are necessary.

Opioids

There is abundant clinical evidence that opioids are efficacious in chronic pain. However, when the pain is associated with inflammation or neuropathy, opioid sensitivity can be significantly changed *(48)*. For example, the enhanced central actions of opioids after inflammation are unlikely to result from direct receptor changes, since binding studies reveal no marked differences. Changes in opioid peptide synthesis may contribute as mentioned earlier, but altered spinal transmission involving cholecystokinin (CCK) has also been proposed. This peptide, which is found predominantly in intrinsic dorsal horn neurons, interferes with morphine analgesia in normal animals via actions at the CCK_B receptor *(49)*. In inflammation, the levels and/or release of CCK are reduced (Fig. 5), thus removing an endogenous negative influence on morphine analgesia *(50)*.

Reduced sensitivity to opioids also occurs in some neuropathic pain conditions, but the reasons for this remain to be elucidated. After nerve section, reduced morphine sensitivity is accompanied by an induction of CCK in afferent fibers, which may be responsible for the reduced opioid actions. Opioid sensitivity is restored by CCK receptor antagonists*(48)*. There are several other explanations for reduced opioid sensitivity in neuropathic pain. These include: (1) degeneration of the C-fiber afferents and loss of the presynaptic μ- and δ-opioid receptors; (2) the inability of opioids to overcome the increased activity in second-order spinal neurons because of the expression of new mechanisms such as wind-up; (3) pathological transmission of pain evoked by large diameter A-fibers, which are poorly responsive to opioids since these fibers do not possess opioid receptors; and (4) the formation of morphine metabolites with agonistic (morphine-6-glucuronide) or potential antagonistic (morphine-3-glucuronide) properties that may contribute to unpredictable analgesia, especially after long-term therapy. Although at present the relative contribution of these factors is unclear, in all cases, with the exception of CCK in which environmental factors are important, these negative influences can be overcome by opioid dose-escalation.

$α_2$-Adrenoceptors

Increased activation of noradrenaline-mediated pathways has been proposed as a mechanism to explain the increased sensitivity to opioids in inflammatory hyperalgesia. Activation of the $α_2$-adrenoceptor, which is located postsynaptically to noradrenergic terminals originating from the brain stem and midbrain, produces not only an inhibition of nociception but will synergize with the effect of μ-opioid agonists*(51)*. Whether $α_2$-adrenoceptor agonists alone will be useful analgesics depends on the incidence of side-effects such as sedation, hypotension, and motor effects. However, probes for the mRNA for $α_2$-adrenoceptor subtypes reveal a differential location in sensory, autonomic, and motor areas in the spinal cord, and hence selective agents might circumvent some of these problems*(52)*. The degree of synergy between $α_2$-adrenoceptor and μ-opioid receptor agonists, particularly with the newer potent agonists such as dexmedetomidine, is so powerful that combinations of threshold doses are effective and would be expected to produce fewer side-effects.

NSAIDs

As mentioned earlier, multiple forms of cyclooxygenase have been identified in peripheral tissues and an important central role for NSAIDs in analgesia has been proposed. Indeed, there is good evidence for the release of prostanoids in the spinal cord following depolarization and C-fiber stimulation*(53)*. Moreover, NSAIDs reduced the hyperalgesia induced by NMDA and substance P, indicating that receptor actions of these substances can trigger prostanoid release. Most convincing, however, is that spinal administration of NSAIDs reduced the prolonged pain response produced by peripheral administrations of formalin with the order of potency reflecting their ability to inhibit cyclooxygenase activity.

CONCLUSION

A diversity of changes in the peripheral and central processing of pain signals occurs during chronic pain, in which there is an apparent loss of the biological significance of pain signaling as an organic protective measure. Chronic pain, therefore, is a sign of major distress in the functioning of the nervous system, and is comparable to other chronic disorders of brain and behavior that have potentially fatal consequences. The manifold changes that occur include neurochemistry alterations in many different types of cell, changes in cellular phenotype and morphological rearrangements in the nervous system. Among these processes, there are abundant targets through which pain therapy can be addressed, including a range of molecular targets in peripheral sensory and sympathetic nerve fibers, in the spinal cord and in higher centers. Increased information on these targets allows a more constructive attitude to the disastrous implications of chronic pain. In addition, thoughtful treatment can begin with the acknowledgment that chronic pain is mechanistically diverse and is the outcome of multisystem dysfunction.

Reprinted with permission from Trends in Pharmacological Sciences, 15: 190–197.

REFERENCES

1. Rang, H. P., Bevan, S. J. and Dray, A. (1994) *Br. Med. Bull.* **47**, 543–548.
2. Dubner, R. and Ruda, M. A. (1992) *Trends Neurosci.* **15**, 96–103.
3. McMahon, S. B., Lewin, G. R. and Wall, P. D. (1993) *Curr. Biol.* **3**, 602–610.
4. Hokfelt, T., Zhang, X. and Wiesenfelt-Hallin, Z. (1994) *Trends Neurosci.* **17**, 22–30.
5. Woolf, C. J., Shortland, P. and Coggeshall, R. E. (1993) *Nature* **355**, 75–78.
6. McLachlan, E. M., Janig, W., Devor, M. and Michaellis, M. (1993) *Nature* **363**, 543–546.
7. Lewin, G. and Mendell, L. M. (1993) *Trends Neurosci.* **16**, 353–359.
8. Dray, A. and Perkins, M. (1993) *Trends Neurosci.* **16**, 99–104.
9. Ferriera, S. H., Lorenzetti, B. B. and Poole, S. (1993) *Br. J. Pharmacol.* **110**, 1227–1231.
10. Mitchell, J. A., Akarasereenont, P., Thiernermann, C., Flower, R. J. and Vane, J. R. (1993) *Proc. Natl. Acad. Sci. USA* **90**, 11693–11697.
11. Rueff, A. and Dray, A. (1992) *Neuroscience* **50**, 899–905.
12. Kolzenburg, M. and McMahon, S. (1993) *Trends Neurosci.* **15**, 497–501.
13. Tani, E., Shiosaka, S., Sato, M., Ishikawa, T. and Tohyama, M. (1990) *Neurosci. Lett.* **115**, 171–176.
14. Meller, S. T. and Gebhart, G. F. (1993) *Pain* **52**, 127–136.
15. McGhee, D. S., Goy, M. F. and Oxford, G. S. (1992) *Neuron* **9**, 315–324.
16. Wiesenfelt-Hallin, Z., Hao, J-X, Xu, X-J. and Hokfelt, T. (1993) *J. Neurophysiol.* **70**, 2350–2353.
17. Stein, C. (1992) *Anesth. Analg.* **76**, 182–191.
18. Andreev, N., Urban, L. and Dray, A. (1994) *Neurosci.* **58**, 793–798.
19. Wood, J. N. et al. (1992) *J. Biol. Chem.* **267**, 17787–17791.
20. Jonakait, G. M. (1993) *Trends Neurosci.* **10**, 419–423.
21. McMahon, S. B. (1991) *Br. Med. Bull.* **47**, 584–600.
22. Levine, J. O., Fields, H. L. and Basbaum, A. J. (1993) *J. Neurosci.* **13**, 2273–2286.

23. Tanelian, D. L. and Brose, W. G. (1991) *Anesthesiology* **74**, 949–951.
24. Devor, M., Wall, P. D. and Catalan, N. (1992) *Pain* **48**, 261–268.
25. Devor, M., Govrin-Lippman, R. and Agelides, K. (1993) *J. Neurosci.* **13**, 1976–1992.
26. Watanebe, Y., Saito, H. and Abe, K. (1993) *Neuropharmacology* **32**, 479–486.
27. Fraser, H., Chapman, V. and Dickenson, A. H. (1992) *Pain* **49**, 33–41.
28. Kappelle, A. C. et al. (1993) *Eur. J. Pharmacol.* **250**, 43–49.
29. Schaible, H-G. and Grubb, B. D. (1993) *Pain* **55**, 5–54.
30. Coderre, T. J. and Melzack, R. (1992) *J. Neurosci.* **12**, 3665–3670.
31. Thompson, S. W. N., Dray, A. and Urban, L. *J. Neurosci.* (in press)
32. Richmond, C. E., Bromley, L. M. and Woolf, C. J. (1993) *Lancet* **342**, 73–75.
33. Chapman, V. and Dickenson, A. H. (1992) *Brain Res.* **573**, 321–323.
34. Munro, F. E., Fleetwood-Walker, S. H., Parker, R. M. C. and Mitchell, R. (1993) *Neuropeptides* **25**, 299–305.
35. Laird, J. M. A., Hargreaves, R. J. and Hill, R. G. (1993) *Br. J. Pharmacol.* **109**, 713–718.
36. Thompson, S. W. N., Urban, L. and Dray, A. (1993) *Brain Res.* **625**, 100–108.
37. Donnerer, J., Schuligoi, R. and Stein, C. (1992) *Neuroscience* **49**, 693–698.
38. Valtschanoff, J. G., Weinberg, R. J. and Rustioni, A. (1992) *Neuroscience* **50**, 685–696.
39. McCarson, K. E. and Krause, J. E. (1994) *J. Neurosci.* **14**, 712–720.
40. Birch, P. J., Harrison, S. M., Hayes, A. G., Rogers, H. and Tyers, M. B. (1992) *Br. J. Pharmacol.* **105**, 508–510.
41. Freedman, J., et al. (1988) *Neuroscience* **27**, 267–278.
42. Villar, M. J., et al. (1989) *Neuroscience* **33**, 587–604.
43. Sugimoto, T., Bennetr, G. J. and Kajander, K. C. (1990) *Pain* **42**, 205–213.
44. Yamamoto, T. and Yaksh, T. L. (1992) *Pain* **51**, 329–334.
45. Gracely, R., Lynch, S. A. and Bennett, G. J. (1993) *Pain* **52**, 251–253.
46. Malmberg, A. B. and Yaksh, T. L. (1993) *Pain* **54**, 291–301.
47. Valtschanoff, J. G., Weinberg, R. J. and Rustioni, A. (1992) *J. Comp. Neurol.* **320**, 1–14.
48. Stanfa, L. C., Dickenson, A. H., Xu, X-L. and Wiesenfeld-Hallin, Z. (1994) *Trends Pharmacol. Sci.* **15**, 65–66.
49. Stanfa, L. C. and Dickenson, A. H. (1993) *Br. J. Pharmacol.* **108**, 967–973.
50. Wiertelak, E. P., Maier, S. F. and Watkins, L. R. (1992) *Science* **256**, 830–833.
51. Hylden, J. L. K., Thomas, D. A., Iadorola, M. J., Nahin, R. L. and Dubner, R. (1991) *Eur. J. Pharmacol.* **194**, 135–143.
52. Nicholas, A. P., Pierbone, V. and Hokfelt, T. (1993) *J. Comp. Neurol.* **328**, 575–594.
53. Malmberg, A. B. and Yaksh, T. L. (1992) *Science* **257**, 1276–1279.

40   Antipyretic Analgesic Drugs

Kay Brune

1. INTRODUCTION

Pain is the most impressive symptom of a disturbed homeostasis in a segment of the body or an organ. It originates (with few exceptions) from stimulation of the so-called tissue nociceptors. Their stimulation results in depolarisation of C-fibers. The stimulus will be transferred to the dorsal horn of the spinal cord, and may then, depending on facilitating or inhibiting modulation, be conducted through the spinothalamic tract to the medulla oblongata *(1,2)*. Here, in the hypothalamus and the thalamus, additional processing takes place before the information is translated into the sensation of "pain." The subjective feeling of pain may be influenced by further factors such as distraction. In principle, the production of pain can be modulated, either amplified or reduced, at all of the aforementioned levels.

To date there have been no anatomical or functionally distinct nociceptors clearly defined. The term "nociceptor" thus refers to the existing fine nerve terminations in the tissue, which are responding with different sensitivities (over a wide dynamic range) to a great number of (polymodal) stimuli *(1)*. If the tissue is injured, the sensitivity of the majority of these sensors increases under the influence of the disturbed homeostasis *(1)*. An increased concentration of protons and potassium ions, but also bradykinin, histamine, and serotonin are able to activate these receptors (Fig. 1). According to our present understanding two groups of mediators are particularly able to modulate their sensitivity over a considerable range, prostaglandins (PGs) and opioid peptides. Whereas presumably the prostaglandins released from constitutively present cyclooxygenase 1 or induced cyclooxygenase 2 of invading leukocytes in traumatized (inflamed) tissue *(3)* lead to a sensitization or activation of the nociceptors, the opioid peptides induce a deactivation, probably at the same level. It is obvious that regulation of nociceptor sensitivity comprises a first means for analgesic action *(1)*.

In the spinal cord these relationships are less clear. We presently believe that it is at this level that the second and possibly even more important step of pain modulation occurs *(1,2,4)*. In the spinal cord, the transmitter of the information originating from the nociceptors is (stimulatory) glutamate. This substance is not alone in this processing, because substance P (SP) acts as a cotransmitter *(1)*. This transmission is modulated by means of other mediators *(1,4,5)*. The aminergic mediators, noradrenaline (NA) and serotonin, primarily mediate

From: *Marihuana and Medicine*
Edited by: G. G. Nahas et al.   © Humana Press Inc., Totowa, NJ

Activators and Modulators
of Polymodal (wide dynamic range)
Nociceptors

C-Fiber Terminal

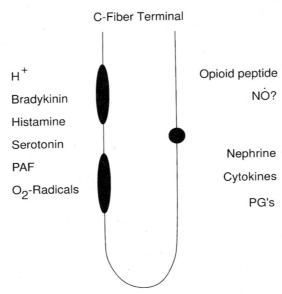

H$^+$ Opioid peptide

Bradykinin   NO?

Histamine

Serotonin

PAF   Nephrine

O$_2$-Radicals   Cytokines

                             PG's

Fig. 1. Activators and modulators of polymodal (wide dynamic range) receptors (nociceptors). Noxious tissue injury leads, in addition to other effects, to a release of potassium ions, protons, and bradykinin and to the synthesis of prostaglandins (PGs). These ions and mediators, e.g., bradykinin, stimulate the nociceptors. Histamine and serotonin released from mast cells, thrombocytes and other cells, facilitate vasodilatation and extravasation of plasma (inflammation). Prostaglandins increase the sensitivity of the nociceptors and enhance the inflammatory effect of other mediators. Opioid peptides should have an inhibitory influence on the nociceptors. The role of nitric oxide (NO), cytokines, and noradrenaline (NA) in the genesis of pain are issues of present research.

the so called descending inhibition. Certainly, of importance are the opioid peptides, glycine and gamma-aminobutyric acid (GABA) released from the interneurons, the D$_2$, and E$_2$-PGs and thromboxane (TX) released from the nerve cells themselves or from the glial cells by both cyclooxygenase 1 and 2 (6). Finally, an important role is probably played by nitric oxide (NO) released from specific interneurons (5). The possible effect of prostaglandin inhibition by a metabolite of THC, like 11 THC oic acid, in the dorsal horn of the spinal cord, has not been demonstrated (see Chapter 44). As summarized (Fig. 2), nociceptive (painful) stimuli cause nociceptor-depolarization that is transmitted to the spinal cord and the CNS finally leading to pain. This process is mediated and/or amplified by the activity of PGs, glycine, and SP. The opioid peptides, serotonin and NA, but probably also GABA, NO, and anandamide reduce the transmission and by this means serve as analgesics.

It is suggested that similar modulatory mechanisms also take place in the medulla oblongata, hypothalamus, thalamus, and other centers. Our knowledge concerning the significance of these structures and the crucial mediators is not yet sufficiently consolidated for presentation in an overview. However, it does appear that the PGs amplify the impulses related to pain in these higher centers as well as some aminergic mediators, but certainly the opioid peptides reduce them.

Modulation of Synaptic Transmission
of Nociceptive Information in Spinal Cord

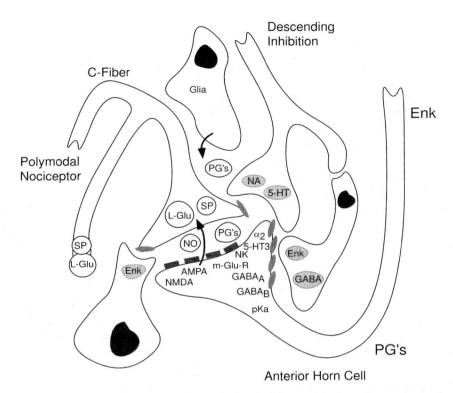

Fig. 2. The modulation of synaptic transmission at the level of the nociceptive afferents in the dorsal horn of the spinal cord (modified from Yaksh, T.L. Refresher course at the "7th World Congress on Pain", August, 1993, Paris, France) Glutamate (Glu) and substance P (SP), which are the neurotransmitters of the nociceptive afferents (C-fibers), transmit the nociceptive information via the synapses inside the "substantia gelatinosa" of the dorsal horn of the spinal cord to neurones projecting via the anterior cord (Tr. spinothalamicus) to the thalamus. Prostaglandins (PGs), released from the nerve terminations and the surrounding glial cells, facilitate synaptic transmission. Serotonin, noradrenaline (NA), and opioid peptides may inhibit the nociceptive transmisssion by effects on action on pre- and postsynaptic receptors. Aminergic transmitters ("antinociceptive") are released from the neurons of the descending endogene that stems from the area of the periaqueductal gray matter, the nuc. raphe magnus and locus coeruleus. The opioid peptides are probably released from inteneurons.

On the basis of the above information, it can be suggested that pain relief can be obtained on three levels:

1. Blocking or reducing the sensitivity of the nociceptors by local anesthetics and inhibitors of PG synthesis (possibly also opioids and proinflammatory cytocines).
2. Reducing spinal transmission by inhibiting PG synthesis or by activation of the opioid receptors (possibly amplified by adrenergic, serotonergic, and GABA-ergic drugs or even cannabinoids).
3. Activation of the opioid receptors in the medulla oblongata, hypothalamus, and thalamus.

Besides these means of achieving analgesia, there is the possibility of reducing the gluta-minergic transmission (by e.g., ketamine) or, at least theoretically, of decreasing (increasing?) NO synthesis in the spinal cord. These possibilities are either special situations (ketamine in intensive care) or yet not clinically realizable (inhibition of NO synthesis).

2. ANTIPYRETIC ANALGESIC DRUGS

The aim of this contribution is to discuss a group of substances that, according to present knowledge, influence the hyperalgesia mediated by PGs (increased nociceptor sensitivity, intensified transmission of pain-related impulses in the spinal cord). Because PGs are not only mediators within the framework of developing and processing pain but also contribute to the regulation of temperature homeostasis (in the hypothalamus) all substances that are analgesic through complete or partial inhibition of PG synthesis are also antipyretic agents.

It is reasonable, therefore, to describe this group of agents as antipyretic analgesics (ASA) and to differentiate them from opiates and opioids which, beside their analgesic actions, also produce sedative and euphoric effects. They may hence be termed "narcotic analgesics." The terms used in the literature instead of antipyretic analgesics such as "nonopioid (weak) analgesics" and such, appear to be lacking in sense because the supposedly "weak" analgesic, acetylsalicylic acid, often has a more potent effect, e.g., in rheumatic or posttraumatic injury, than the opioids.

2.1. Classification

The group of antipyretic analgesics can be divided into three subgroups. On one hand there are a series of acidic agents that pharmacologically derive from salicylic and acetylsalicylic acid. They possess in common, some presumably essential physicochemical properties, including lipophilic-hydrophilic polarity, a pKa between 3 and 5, and a very high protein binding in human and animal organisms (Table 1). To this group belong from the chemical point of view, also arylacetic acids, arylpropionic acids, fenamates, and different keto-enolic acids as oxicams and phenylbutazone.

The second group consists of nonacidic derivatives of phenazone including prodrugs such as metamizol (dipyrone). This group has different physicochemical characteristics, e.g., its representatives are neutral or moderately alkaline, bind only in limited proportion to plasma proteins, and do not have hydrophilic-lypophilic polarity (Table 2). Finally, the third group consists to date of only one drug, paracetamol (acetaminophen), an almost neutral substance with limited polarity and protein binding (Table 2).

Important for the therapy of pain is the classification into acids on the one hand and nonacidic compounds on the other. The reason for this lies in the fact that the acidic antipyretic analgesics show clear anti-inflammatory effects at therapeutic doses, whereas the nonacidic agents exert only analgesic effects at normally nontoxic doses. A possible explanation for these differences is presented in the following section.

2.2. Effects and Mechanisms of Action of the Antipyretic Analgesics (ASA)

Systematic experiments showed that the antipyretic analgesics produced measurable antinociceptive reactions in animal models (6,7). Phenazone and its derivates were most effective in spastic pain, whereas paracetamol demonstrated analgesic effects in animal experiments, only in large doses. Recent research in humans (8) illustrates a comparable spectrum of action of these drugs and confirms the clinical experience of rheumatologists who consider the anti-inflammatory acids as antirheumatics and phenazone and paracetamol as pure analgesics. For a long time it remained unclear why such differences in action exist.

Table 1

Acidic Antipyretic Analgesics (Anti-Inflammatory Antipyretic Analgesics, NSAIDS): Chemical Classes, Structures, Physicochemical and Pharmacological Data, Therapeutic Dosage

Chemical class Monosubstance (subclass)	Structure	pKa	Plasma protein binding	$t_{1/2}{}^a$	$t_{max}{}^b$	Oral bioavailability	Daily dosage in adults
Salicylates Acetylsalicylic acid (active metabolite)		3.5 2.9	50–70% 80–95% dose dependent	~0.25 h 2.5–4.5 h dose dependent	~0.25 h 0.5–2 h	50–70% 80–100%	1–4 g
Arylacetic acids Diclofenac (Fenac-class)		3.9	99.7%	1–2 h	1–12 h very variable	30–80% first pass	50–150 mg
Arylpropionic acids (Profen-class) Ibuprofen		4.6	99.5%	1.5–2.5 h	0.5–2 h	80–100%	0.6–2.4 g

(Table 1 continues)

Table 1 (continued)

Chemical class Monosubstance (subclass)	Structure	pKa	Plasma protein binding	$t_{1/2}^a$	t_{max}^b	Oral bioavailability	Daily dosage in adults
Ketoprofen		5.3	99.2%	1.5–2.5 h (~8 h)	1–2 h	~100%	150–200 mg
Naproxen		4.1	99.7%	13–15 h	2–4 h	90–100%	0.5–1 g
Keto-enol acids Piroxicam (Oxicam)		5.9	99.3%	14–160 h (~50 h) very variable EHC[c]	~2 h 2. Peak: 4–8 h	~100%	20 mg initially: 40 mg

[a]Terminal half-life of elimination.

[b]Time to reach maximum plasma concentration after oral administration.

[c]EHC, enterohepatic circulation.

Table 2
Nonacidic Analgesics: Chemical Classes, Structures, Pharmacokinetic Data, Therapeutic Dosage

Chemical class Monosubstance	Structure	Plasma protein binding	$t_{1/2}{}^{a}$	$t_{max}{}^{b}$	Oral bioavailability	Daily dosage in adults
Aniline derivates Paracetamol (acetaminophen)		5–50% dose dependent	1.5–2.5 h	0.5 h–1.52 h	70–100% dose dependent	1–4 g —
Pyrazolinones[c] Phenazone (antipyrine)		<10%	11–12 h	0.5–2 h	~100% dose dependent	1–4 g

[a]Terminal half-life of elimination.
[b]Time to reach maximum plasma concentration after oral administration.
[c]Terms like pyrazole and, incorrectly, pyrazolone are also in use.

A first answer was given by the research of the pharmacologist Lim. He demonstrated that ASAs had above all, an analgesic effect when administered directly into the traumatized painful tissue of an experimental animal. By contrast, opiates and opioids show distinct effects especially after they reach the central nervous system, the spinal cord and brain *(9)*. Phenazone derivates are qualitatively as effective as salicylates, though only in very high doses. On the basis of these experimets the different analgesic drugs were categorized until recently as peripherally and centrally active agents. This classification no longer appears to be appropriate, as the following comments will show.

At the end of the 1960s Vane and coworkers (London) demonstrated that ASA and other analgesic acids (not salicylic acid) act as potent inhibitors of PG synthesis *(3,10)*. At similar dosage phenazone and paracetamol had only very weak (phenazone), or no activity (antaminophen) *(10,11)*. Vane concluded that inhibition of PG synthesis in inflamed tissue reduced the production of pain and inflammation. Recent physiological studies have demonstrated that, as previously mentioned, the release of PGs, occurs in inflamed tissue, leads to an increase in nociceptor sensitivity (Fig. 1). My coworkers and I showed that the anti-inflammatory acids, on the basis of their high protein binding and their acidic character, readily leave the blood in inflamed tissue and are sequestered therein (Fig. 3) *(12)*. Consequently they inhibit PG synthesis first of all in inflamed tissue, and thereby reduce pain and other PG-mediated symptoms of inflammation. On the basis of their local high concentrations in inflamed tissue, they are also able to curb numerous other processes, e.g., complement activation, histamine release, leukocyte invasion, and so on, thus exhibiting a broad, though reversible action. On the basis of these data, it is clear why anti-inflammatory analgesic acids are active especially in inflammatoy pain: they prevent the release of inflammation and lead to a normalization of nociceptor sensitivity *(7)*. Therefore, in a strict sense, they are "antihyperalgesic." The nonacidic antipyretic analgesics hardly inhibit PG synthesis in inflamed tissues and, probably, this is the reason why they do not exhibit an anti-inflammatory effect. How they mediate their analgesic effects remained somewhat hypothetical until recently.

We now have evidence that a reduction of nociceptor activation-dependent prostaglandin release in the spinal cord is the mechanism of action of these drugs *(7)*. Recent experiments performed by different research groups confirm that nonacidic antipyretic analgesics readily cross into the central nervous system (CNS; Fig. 3) and reduce PG synthesis there even at relatively low concentrations *(12)* and presumably in this way produce an analgesic effect. Since the acidic anti-inflammatory analgesics also pass into the central nervous system (although more slowly), it is understandable why these agents mediate some analgesic effects in the spinal cord and clear antipyretic action in the hypothalamus in addition to their peripheral effects *(6,7)*. It appears, however, that the concentrations achieved in the CNS are not sufficient to curb PG production to the same extent as in inflamed tissue. Why a reduction of PG synthesis in the central nervous system is sufficient for mediating these central analgesic effects is the topic of ongoing research. Also the question of what the contribution of additional mediators such as NO and opioid peptides (Fig. 2) is another topic of intensive investigation at the present time.

2.3. The Use of Antipyretic Analgesics

On the basis of the spectrum of actions and of the side effects, it is obvious that in inflammatory (rheumatic) pain, anti-inflammatory acids should be administered, whereas in complaints with temporary and limited inflammatory symptoms, e.g., colic pain, phenazone (propyphenazone or metamizol where available) is indicated (Table 3). In influenza-like (common cold) infections accompanied by pain and fever, paracetamol may be used. Naturally, this approach is indicated only after cautious consideration of the existing contraindica-

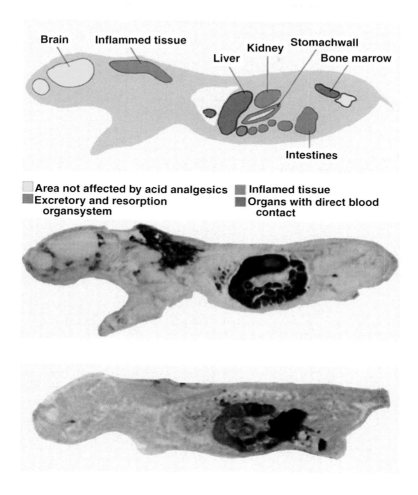

Fig. 3. Distribution of the nonsteroidal anti-inflammatory drugs (NSAIDs), phenylbutazone (acid) and phenazone (nonacid), as a consequence of their physicochemical properties. Radioautographs of rats treated with ^{3}H-labeled phenylbutazone and phenazone (from Graf, P., Glatt, M. and Brune, K. (1975) *Experientia* **31**, 951–954). Young rats (30 g body weight) were given 100 μCi (10 mg/kg) ^{14}C-labeled phenylbutazone or phenazone by stomach tube. At the same time inflammation was elicited by the injection of 0.05 mL of a 2% (w/v) suspension of carrageenan into the left hind-paw or 0.2 mL suspension plus 0.2 mL air into the subcutaneous tissue of the neck. Five hours later the animals were exsanguinated, deep frozen, and cut into thin (100 μm) slices which were mounted on X-ray film. After eight days of exposure, the resulting pictures were examined. The phenylbutazone treated animal (a) shows high activity in the inflamed tissue of the neck, the stomach wall, the liver, kidneys and blood, whereas the phenazone treatment (b) does not display high activity in the inflamed tissue or any compartment aside from the bladder and the large bowel (excreted metabolites). It is obvious that phenazone easily enters the CNS.

Table 3
Indications for Antipyretic Analgesics

Acidic antipyretic analgesics (antiinflammatory antipyretic analgesics, NSAIDs)[a]

Acute and chronic pain, produced by inflammation of different etiology:	High dose	Middle dose	Low dose
Arthritis: chronic polyarthritis (rheumatoid arthritis ankylosing spondilytis (Morbus Bechterew) acute gout attack)	diclofenac, indomethacin ibuprofen piroxicam (phenylbutazone)[b]	diclofenac, indomethacin ibuprofen piroxicam (phenylbutazone)[b]	no
Cancer Pain (e.g. bone metastatis)	indomethacin[c], diclofenac[c], ibuprofen[c], piroxicam[c],	indomethacin[c], diclofenac[c], ibuprofen[c], proxicam[c]	acetylsalicylic acid[d]
Active arthrosis (acute pain-inflammatory episodes)	no	diclofenac, indomethacin ibuprofen piroxicam	ibuprofen, ketoprofen
Myofascial pain syndromes (antipyretic analgesic are often prescribed but of limited value)	no	diclofenac ibuprofen piroxicam	ibuprofen, ketoprofen
Posttraumatic pain, swelling	no	indomethacin, diclofenac ibuprofen	acetylsalicylic acid ibuprofen[c]
Postoperative pain, swelling	no	indomethacin, diclofenac ibuprofen	ibuprofen

Nonacidic antipyretic analgesics

Acute pain and fever	Pyrazolinones (High Dose)	Pyrazolinones (Low dose)	Anilines (High dose is toxic)
Spastic pain (colics)	yes	yes	no
Conditions associated with high fever	yes	yes	no
Cancer pain	yes	yes	yes
Headache, migraine	no	yes	yes[f]
General disturbances associated with viral infections	no	yes[e]	yes

[a]Dosage range of NSAIDs and example of monosubstances (but note dosage prescribed for each agent).
[b]Indicated only in gout attacks.
[c]Compare the sequence staged scheme of WHO for cancer pain.
[d]Blood coagulation and renal function must be normal.
[e]If other analgesics and antipyretics are contraindicated, e.g., gastroduodenal ulcer, blood coagulation disturbances, asthma.
[f]In particular patients.

tions. A further consideration is that the marketed anti-inflammatory acids in particular, have very variable potency and pharmacokinetic properties. Both paramaters are summarized in Tables 1 and 2. Although there is no clear correlation between the plasma half-life of elimination and the duration of action of these drugs for chronic and intense inflammatory pain, drugs with a sufficiently high potency and slow rate of elimination such as the oxicams may be used with advantage (Table 1). Naturally, the higher risk of damage to the gastrointestinal tract and the kidneys must be taken into account. For acute pain that occurs regularly, e.g., at noon, in osteoarthrosis anti-inflammatory acids that are safe have a rapid onset of absorption but are also eliminated rapidly, such as ibuprofen or diclofenac in the form of solutions or effervescent tablets or in the form of a (soluble) salt, should be administered.

Basically, all antipyretic analgesics may be administered in postoperative, posttraumatic, rheumatic, and spastic pain. In life-threatening, painful conditions accompanied by anxiety, e.g., myocardial infarction, severe trauma, difficult surgery, and terminal cancer pain, where a euphoric, asedative, and detaching effect is required, opiates and opioids should be used. The selective use of analgesics can be especially helpful in cancer pain. If a tumor develops and produces painful bone metastases for example, then the best results are obtained with highly potent, long half-life, anti-inflammatory acids. If the patient realizes that his disease is not curable and becomes depressed, then suppplementary opiates must be introduced (or used exclusively). In this respect, the staged sequence scheme of the World Health Organization (WHO) complies with a logical, pharmacological-based approach to therapy. If the principles of this scheme are familiar to the therapist he will also select anti-inflammatory acids as required in the final phases of cancer, e.g., if inflammatory pain from bone metastases is present. Also, for early symptoms of pain, particularly if accompanied by anxiety, short-term opiate therapy may be chosen.

It has also to be pointed out that operative stress increases the vulnerability of the gastrointestinal tract mucosa, and that reduced renal function may lead to a greater risk of renal injury. Therefore, anti-inflammatory analgesic acids, which, all carry a certain risk of gastrointestinal tract, and renal toxiticity *(13)* should be administered as post or perioperative therapy only after minor surgery, in young patients, and if normal renal function in the postoperative period is guaranteed. It should also be mentioned that some anti-inflammatory acids reduce platelet aggregation for days (e.g., aspirin). The commonly used anti-inflammatory analgesic, ketorolac, at a dose of 30 mg im, also inhibits the aggregation of blood platelets for almost 48 hours *(14)*. However, metamizole, even in very large intravenous doses of 2.5 g, has a clearly shorter effect on blood coagulation *(14)*. Finally, azapropazone, another injectable acidic anti-inflammatory drug has a limited and rapidly reversible effect. Opioids and opiates show no effect on these organ systems. Certainly through inhibition of intestinal motility, nausea, vomiting, and inhibition of respiration, they may pose risks for the postoperative period. Some surgery-related pain conditions are not amenable to treatment with antipyretic or opioid analgesics.

REFERENCES

1. Schaible, H. -G. and Grubb, B. D. (1993) Afferent and spinal mechanisms of joint pain. *Pain* **55**, 5–54.
2. Brune, K. (1994) Spinal cord effects of antipyreti analgesics. *Drugs* **47**, 21–27.
3. Vane, J. (1994) Towards a better aspirin. *Nature* **367**, 215–216.
4. Jurna, I. and Yaksh, T. L. (1993) *Central mechanisms for Analgesia by Acetylsalicylic Acid and (Functionally) Related Compounds*. Gustav Fischer Verlag, New York.
5. Meller, S. T. and Gebhart, G. F. (1993) Nitric oxide (NO) and nociceptive processing in the spinal cord. *Pain* **52**, 127–136.
6. Neugebauer, V., Schaible, H. -G., He, X., Lücke, T., Gründling, P. and Schmidt, R. F. (1994) Electrophysiological evidence for a spinal antinociceptive action of dipyrone. *Agents Actions* **41**, 62–70.

7. Beiche, F., Scheuerer, St., Brune, K., Geisslinger, G. and Goppelt-Struebe, M. (1996) Up-regulation of cyclooxygenase-2 mRNA in the rat spinal cord following peripheral inflammation. *FEBS Lett.* **390**, 165–169.

8. Forster, C., Magerl, W., Beck, W., Geisslinger, G., Gall, T., Brune, K. and Handwerker, H. O. (1992) Differential effects of dipyrone, ibuprofen and paracetamol on experimentally induced pain in man. *Agents Actions* **35**, 112–121.

9. Lim, R. K. S. (1970) Pain. *Annu. Rev. Physiol.* **32**, 269–288.

10. Vane, J. (1971) Inhibition of prostaglandin synthesis as a mechanism of action for aspirin-like drugs. *Nature New Biol.* **231**, 232–237.

11. Brune, K., Rainsford, K. D., Wagner, K. and Peskar, B. A. (1981) Inhibition by anti-inflammatory drugs of prostaglandin production in cultured macrophages–Factors influencing the apparent drug effects. *Arch. Pharmacol.* **315**, 269–276.

12. Scheuren, N., Neupert, W., Ionac, M., Neuhuber, W., Brune, K. and Geisslinger, G. (1997) Peripheral noxious stimulation releases spinal PGE$_2$ during the first phase in the formalin assay of the rat. *Life Sci.* **60**, 295–300.

13. Henry, D., Lim, L., Rodriguez, L., Gutthann, S., Carson, J., Griffin, M., Savage, R., Logan, R., Moride, Y., Hawkey, Ch. and Hill, S. (1996) Variability in risk of gastrointestinal complications with individual non-steroidal anti-inflammatory drugs: results of a collaborative meta-analysis. *Br. Med. J.* **312**, 1563–1566.

14. Geissinger, G., Peskar, B. A., Pallapies, D., Sittl, R., Levy, M. and Brune, K. (1996) The effects on platelet aggregation and prostanoid biosynthesis of two parenteral analgesics: ketorolac tromethamine and dipyrone. *Thromb. Haemostasis* **76**, 592–597.

41 Dimethylheptyl-THC-11-oic Acid

A Nonpsychoactive Antiinflammatory Agent
with a Cannabinoid Template Structure

Robert B. Zurier, Ronald G. Rossetti, Joan H. Lane, John M. Goldberg, Sheila A. Hunter, and Sumner H. Burstein

Abstract

THC-11-oic acid, a non-psychoactive derivative of Δ^9-THC, inhibits cyclooxygenase and platelet-activating factors, which are the mechanisms of prostaglandin inhibition by the nonsteroid antiinflammatory drugs (NSAID's). A dimethylheptyl THC (DMH-11 Q synthetic derivative was effective in treating animal models of acute and chronic inflammatory pain. The dru administered per os was effective in doses of 0.1–0.2 mg/kg to suppress acute inflammgation induced by interleukin- 1β and tumor necrosis factor, in the subcutaneous air pouch model and reduce the chronic inflammatory response of adjuvant induced arthritis.

1. INTRODUCTION

1.1. Objective

To assess the anti-inflammatory activity of dimethylheptyl-THC-11-oic acid (DMH-11C), a nonpsychoactive synthetic derivative of tetrahydrocannabinol.

1.2. Methods

Acute inflammation was induced by injection of interleukin-1β and tumor necrosis factor α into subcutaneous air pouches formed on the backs of mice. Inflammation was quantified six hours later by pouch fluid leukocyte counts. Adjuvant-induced polyarthritis in rats was used as a model of chronic inflammation and joint tissue injury. Animals were either untreated, treated with safflower oil, or treated with DMH-11C in safflower oil. Arthritis was assessed by clinical observation and by histomorphologic evaluation of tibiotarsal joints.

From: *Marihuana and Medicine*
Edited by: G. G. Nahas et al.   © Humana Press Inc., Totowa, NJ

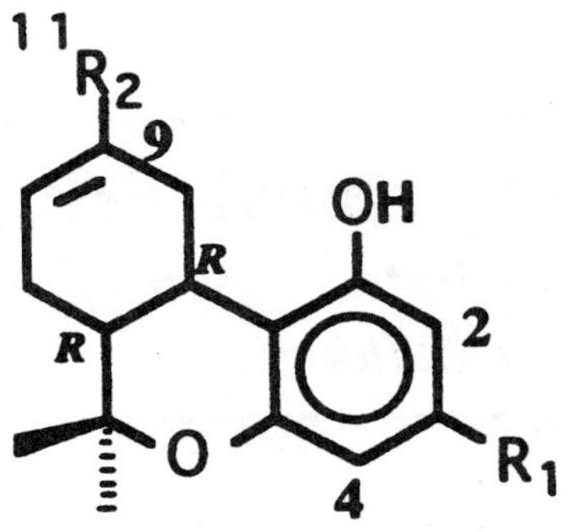

	R₁	R₂
THC	n-pentyl	methyl
THC-11 OIC ACID	n-pentyl	COOH
DMH-11 C	1',1'-dimethylheptyl	COOH

Fig. 1. Structures of the cannabinoids discussed in this report. R designates the absolute sterochemistry of the chiral centers in this series. THC = A'-tetrahydrocannabinol. THC-11-oic acid-A8_tetrahydrocannabinol-11-oic acid. DMH-11C = 1',I' dimethylihepty1Y-tetrahydrocannabinol-11-oic acid.

1.3 Results

Oral administration of DMH-11C reduced the accumulation of pouch fluid leukocytes and significantly reduced the severity of adjuvant-induced polyarthritis. Histopathologic studies of tibiotarsal joints showed that DMH-11C treatment attenuated pannus formation and joint tissue injury.

1.4. Conclusion

DMH-11C suppresses acute inflammation in the subcutaneous air pouch in mice and chronic joint inflammation characteristic of adjuvant disease in rats. These results demonstrate the potential use of this nonpsychoactive cannabinoid as an anti-inflammatory agent.

The *Cannabis* plant has been a source of medicinal preparations since the earliest written records on pharmacobotany. The Chinese emperor Shen-ming (c. 2000 BC), in a work called Pen-ts'ao Ching, noted many of the effects of *Cannabis* on the human body *(1)*. Among other properties, it was claimed that *Cannabis* "undoes rheumatism," suggesting possible anti-inflammatory effects. Throughout human history, cannabinoids have had a place in treating a variety of ailments. A major obstacle to broad acceptance of the drug has been its potent psychoactive effects. This problem has been studied in recent years in attempts to discover synthetic analogs that would retain their medicinal properties without the psychotropic effects. Despite preparation of hundreds of analogs, this goal has not been achieved.

A class of cannabinoids, the carboxy tetrahydrocannabinols, first described in 1972 *(2)*, shows potential as therapeutic agents that are free of cannabimimetic central nervous system activity. These substances, which are metabolites of tetrahydrocannabinol (THC), the psychoactive principle of *Cannabis*, do not produce behavioral changes in humans at doses several times greater than THC doses given to the same volunteers (3). The parent compound in this series, THC-11-oic acid (Fig. 1), is effective in animal models of inflammation and pain at oral doses of 20–40 mg/kg (4,5). THC-11-oic acid also blocks the actions of platelet-activating factor in mice (6), and suppresses both the cyclooxygenase and lipoxygenase activities of cells in tissue culture (6,7). However, a molecule more potent than THC-11-oic acid is needed for clinical use. It has been known for some time that certain modification of the pentyl side chain of THC increases its potency (8). Therefore, a derivative of THC-11-oic acid with a dimethylheptyl side chain was prepared and tested for analgesic and anti-inflammatory activity in several animal models (9). This analog, DMH-11C (Fig. 1), is more than two orders of magnitude more potent than the template molecule, THC-11-oic acid, in the rodent paw edema and hot plate assays.

We studied the effects of DMH-11C in two experimental models of inflammation: acute inflammation induced by interleukin-1β (IL-1β) and tumor necrosis factor α (TNFα) in the subcutaneous air pouch in the mouse, and chronic joint inflammation characteristic of adjuvant disease in the rat. The polypeptide mediators of inflammation IL-1β and TNF α are thought to be important in the initiation and propagation of joint tissue injury in patients with rheumatoid arthritis (10). Adjuvant disease in the rat includes a severe and persistent polyarthritis that appears 10–14 days after a single intradermal injection of Freund's complete adjuvant, and is widely accepted as a useful animal model of chronic inflammation (11). The results of these two sets of experiments indicate that DMH-11C has an anti-inflammatory effect in models of acute and chronic inflammation, and lend support to the view that this agent shows potential for development as an anti-inflammatory agent in humans.

2. MATERIALS AND METHODS

2.1. Reagents

DMH-11C was obtained from Organix (Woburn, MA). Its purity was monitored by comparison, on high-pressure liquid chromatography, with material previously synthesized (9). Indomethacin and A23187 were purchased from Sigma (St. Louis, MO). Recombinant human IL-1β (rHuIL-1β) was obtained from Boehringer Mannheim (Indianapolis, IN), and rHuTNFα was obtained from GIBCO BRL (Gaithersburg, MD). Purified cyclooxygenase 1 (COX-1) and COX-2 were obtained from Cayman Chemical (Ann Arbor, MI).

2.2. Induction of Acute Inflammation

Pouches were established on the backs of female Swiss (CD-1) mice by subcutaneous injection of 5 mL of air on three consecutive days. After six days, animals were treated with 0.1 or 0.2 mg/kg DMH-11C once daily for four days. Inflammation was induced on day 4 of treatment by injection, into the pouch cavity, of 10 ng rHuIL-1β plus 0.25 ng rHuTNFα in 3 cc of 1% carboxymethylcellulose (12). Inflammation was quantified six hours later by determination of pouch exudate leukocyte counts.

2.3. Induction of Chronic Inflammation

Chronic polyarthritis was induced in male Lewis rats (initial weight 125 g) by intradermal injection of Freund's complete adjuvant (2 mg Mycobacterium butyricum in 0.1 mL mineral oil). Arthritis in all four paws was assessed visually as described by Glenn and Gray (13). Each paw was scored clinically for degree of inflammation using a 0–4 scale (0 = normal; 1 = redness; 2 = redness, pain, slight swelling; 3 = redness, severe pain, severe swelling; 4 = ankylosis). Therefore, the maximum joint score was 16. Paws were evaluated by an examiner who had no knowledge of the treatment groups into which rats had been placed. Weight change was also recorded over the course of the experiment.

Animals were either untreated, treated with safflower oil, or treated with 0.1 mg/kg DMH-11C in a volume of 90–120 μL (adjusted for animal weight) each Monday, Wednesday, and Friday, beginning on day 3 after adjuvant injection. Compounds were administered with a 5-cm gavage needle. Animals were anesthetized on day 35 with sodium pentobarbital (50 mg/kg) and were killed by CO_2 asphyxiation. Hind limbs were then removed for histomorphologic examination.

2.4. Histologic Evaluation

Hind limbs of animals were fixed in 10% buffered formalin, then decalcified in 10% formic acid. Several sections of each tibiotarsal joint were stained with hematoxylin and eosin. Individual sections were studied without knowledge of the treatment groups into which animals had been placed.

2.5. Cells

BALB/c 3T3 cells were provided by the University of Massachusetts Medical Center cell-culture facility, and were grown in Dulbecco's modified Eagle's medium containing 10% calf serum. The cells were plated in 24-well culture dishes and grown to about 80–90% confluence. Serum-stimulated cells were obtained by changing to medium containing 20% calf serum four hours before exposure of cells to drugs. The cells were washed twice with serum-free medium immediately before each experiment; serum-free medium was also used for treatments with drugs.

2.6. Cyclooxygenase Measurements

The 3T3 cell culture medium concentrations of prostaglandin E (PGE) were measured by radioinummoassay as described previously (5,7). The antiserum used does not distinguish between PGE_1 and PGE_2; however, it shows little affinity for the other common eicosanoids. The experiments with purified COX-1 and COX-2 were performed at 37°C in 1 mL of 0.1 M Tris HCI buffer (pH 8.0) containing 1 unit of enzyme and 2 mM phenol. The reaction was initiated by the addition of ^{3}H-arachidonic acid (18,000 disintegrations per minute) and allowed to proceed with agitation for 10 minutes. After acidification to pH 3.0, the mixtures were extracted with ethyl acetate and the products determined by silica gel thin-layer radiochromatography using chloroform:methanol: acetic acid (90:6:6) as the eluent. The relevant zones were quantified by removal of the silica gel, followed by liquid scintillation chromatography.

2.7. Statistical Analysis

Data are expressed as the mean ± SD or mean ± SEM. Student's t-test was used for comparison of paired sets of data. P values less than 0.05 were considered significant.

3. RESULTS

3.1. Acute Inflammation

DMH-11C suppressed air pouch leukocyte counts in two separate experiments (Fig. 2). Cell counts in the pouch fluid were reduced by a mean of 42.3% in mice treated for four days with DMH-11C at 0.1 mg/kg/day, and by 65.5% in mice treated for four days with DMH-11C at 0.2 mg/kg/day. More than 90% of the cells were polymorphonuclear leukocytes.

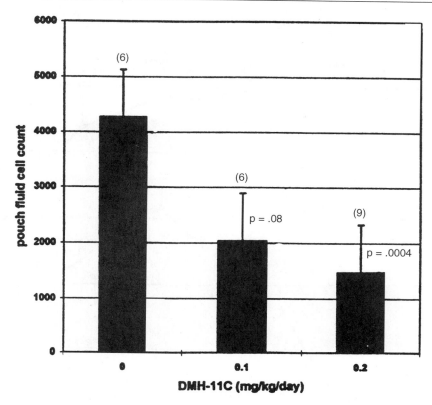

Fig. 2. Effect of dimethylheptyl-THC-11-oic acid (DMH-11C) treatment on inflammation in the mouse subcutaneous air pouch. Inflammation, induced by recombinant human interleukin-1 β plus recombinant human tumor necrosis factor α, was assessed by accumulation of leukocytes in the pouch. Values are the mean and SEM from two separate experiments; values in parentheses represent the number of animals. P values are versus control mice. The mean ± SEM baseline cell count in pouches injected with saline was 475 ± 122 ($n = 6$).

3.2. Chronic Inflammation

3.2.1. CLINICAL OBSERVATIONS

Severe polyarthritis developed in all untreated rats and in all rats treated with safflower oil. Since there was no difference in their joint scores, the data from these groups are combined and presented as control in Fig. 3. Most rats treated by gavage with 0.1 mg/kg DMH-11C three times weekly exhibited mild disease and remained active. Although they did not gain weight at the same rate as normal rats, they did not exhibit the weight loss seen between days 13 and 23 in the control rats with untreated arthritis (Fig. 4). Another measure of the anti-inflammatory effect of DMH-11C is illustrated by determination of the number of severely inflamed hind limb paws. On day 23 (the peak of disease activity), 17 of 18 hind paws in the control group had a clinical score of 4; 16 of 18 (88.9%) were still scored 4 on day 35. In contrast, 9 of 18 hind paws in the DMH-11C-treated group were scored 4 on day 23, but only 4 of 18 (22.2%) retained a clinical score of 4 on day 35.

3.2.2. HISTOPATHOLOGIC FINDINGS

Tibiotarsal joints from control rats on day 35 after adjuvant injection exhibited moderate-to-severe changes characteristic of subacute-to-chronic adjuvant-induced arthritis (14). These

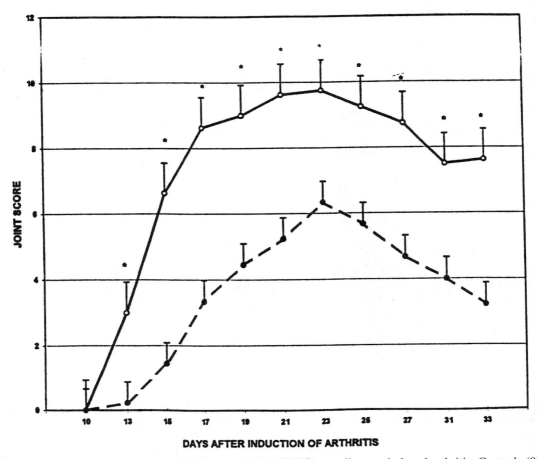

Fig. 3. Effect of dimethylheptyl-THC-11-oic acid (DMH-11C) on adj uvant-induced arthritis. Controls (0) included 5 rats treated with safflower oil and 4 untreated rats. Treated rats ($n \sim = 9$) (0) were given 0.1 mg/kg DMH-11C by gavage three times weekly, beginning on day 3 after adjuvant injection. Values are the mean and SEM joint score (*see* Subheading 2.)* $p < 0.001$ versus DMH-11C-treated animals.

included synovial hyperplasia with microvillus formation, mononuclear cell infiltration, par-mus formation, erosion of cartilage, erosion and remodeling of bone, and alteration of joint architecture. In contrast, only mild synovitis was seen in joints from rats treated with DMH-11C; however, the subsynovial adipose tissue was replaced by fibrous connective tissue. Ankylosis persisted on day 35 in four joints from DMH-11C-treated animals. In all four joints, only mild-to-moderate inflammatory changes were observed histomorphologically (Fig. 6), despite clinical scores of 4 and clinical documentation of ankylosis (no joint motion).

3.2.3. INHIBITION OF EICOSANOID SYNTHESIS

The expression of COX-2 in 3T3 cells in tissue culture can be stimulated by increasing the serum concentration from 10 to 20% (*15*). Under these conditions, a 65% increase in PGE production in 3T3 cells was completely prevented by exposure of cells to 2 μ*M* dexametha-sone (data not shown), an agent known to prevent the induction of COX-2 (*16*). In this model, DMH-11C at a concentration range of 1–10 μ*M* appeared to completely suppress

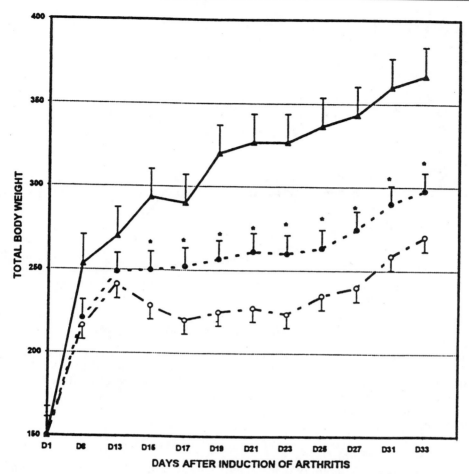

Fig. 4. Effect of dimethylheptyl-THC-11-oic acid (DMH-IIC) on the weight of rats with adjuvant-induced arthritis. ▲ normal rats ($n = 3$); O = control arthritic rats ($n = 9$); ● = DMH-II C-treated rats ($n = 9$). Values are the mean and SEM weight $p < 0.05$ versus other two groups.

COX-2 activity (Fig. 5). The residual activity, presumably due to COX-1, was abolished by treatment with indomethacin, a potent inhibitor of both COX-1 and COX-2 activities (17).

DMH-11C was also tested against a purified preparation of COX-2 obtained from sheep placental tissue, using a radiolabeled precursor assay to measure PGE production. The data in Fig. 6A show that DMH-11C suppressed COX-2 activity at the same 1–10 μM concentration range as was seen in the experiments with intact cells. As expected, the amounts of unreacted arachidonic acid precursor increased over the same concentration range (Fig. 6B). In contrast to its effect on COX-2, DMH-11C at concentrations of 0.25–25 μM caused no significant change in activity with a purified sample of COX-1 prepared from ram seminal vesicle (Fig. 6A).

4. DISCUSSION

Results of these studies indicate that DMH-11C, a synthetic nonpsychoactive derivative of THC, suppresses acute inflammation induced by IL-1β and TNFα in the subcutaneous air

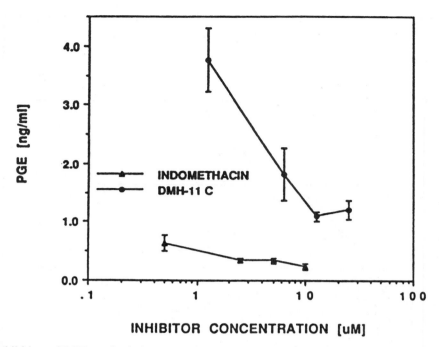

Fig. 5. Inhibition of PGE synthesis in serumstimulated 3T3 cells. Cells were grown as described in Subheading 2. Following two washes with fresh medium, the inhibitors dimethylheptyl-THC-II-oic acid (DMH-IIQ or indomethacin were added. After 15 minutes, the cells were challenged for 30 minutes with 3 p*M* calcium ionophore A23187. The media were then collected, centrifuged to remove particles, and analyzed for PGE by radioimmunoassay. Values are the mean ± SD of triplicate samples (vehicle control value 15.01–1.45 ng/ml).

pouch model, and reduces the more delayed and chronic inflammatory response in adjuvant-induced arthritis. The air pouch model is characterized by neutrophil infiltration, whereas tissue proliferation and degradation are the hallmarks of chronic inflammation. The subcutaneous air pouch simulates a synovial cavity by providing a blind connective tissue cavity without a mesothelial basement membrane; the pouch lining has the two cell types (fibroblasts and macrophage-like cells) common to synovia *(18)*. Comparison between the air pouch and the synovial space is limited, of course, but the pouch does provide a unique and convenient way to induce and monitor an inflammatory response. The response to IL-1β and TNFα is typical of an acute inflammatory reaction, with polymorphonuclear leukocyte infiltration of the pouch wall and cavity increasing in a dose-dependent manner *(19)*. The polyarthritis of adjuvant disease in the rat has been used extensively for evaluating anti-inflammatory and immunosuppressive drugs *(11)*.

The mechanisms by which DMH-11C exerts its anti-inflammatory effects are not clear, but several possibilities may be considered. Suppression of leukocyte adhesion by THC-11-oic acid *(20)* suggests that DMH-11C may reduce accumulation of neutrophils in the air pouch by interfering with adhesion of these cells to endothelial cells. Because DMH-11C is lipophilic and can accumulate in fat stores, we elected to use a three-times-per-week treatment regimen in the rats with chronic arthritis. The pattern of protection in the adjuvant-induced arthritis model (Figs. 3–6) suggests that DMH-11C may influence the activities of mediators of inflammation and of bone and cartilage destruction. Thus, although joint scores are not reduced completely by DMH-11C and weight gain is less than normal, the inflamma-

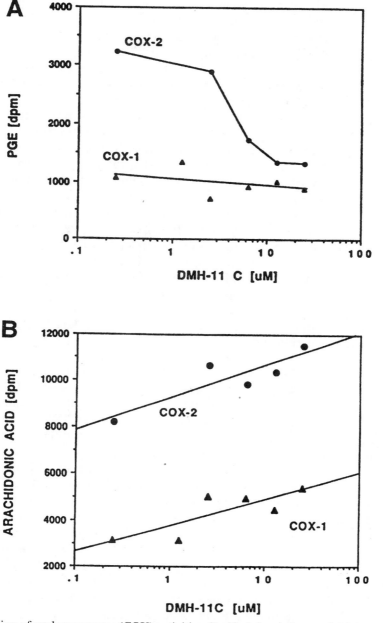

Fig. 6. Inhibition of cyclooxygenase (COX) activities. Purified sheep placental COX-2 and purified ram-seminal vesicle COX-1 were each incubated with dimethylheptyl-THC-11-oic acid (DMH-11C) as described in subheading 2, followed by the addition of ^{3}H-arachidonic acid to initiate synthesis of eicosanoids. After 10 minutes, the mixtures were acidified, extracted, and analyzed by thin-layer chromatography. Values are the mean of duplicate determinations. (**A**) Radioactivity in the PGE zone. (**B**) Remaining unreacted arachidonic acid.

tory response observed clinically in these animals resolves far more rapidly than in control rats. In addition, pannus formation and damage to cartilage and bone were diminished in intensity and extent in rats treated with DMH-11C. Histopathologic analysis showed replacement of the usual subsynovial adipose tissue with dense fibroconnective tissue. We suggest that this represents the residual of previous inflammation. It will be necessary to examine the histomorphology of joints at several defined intervals to determine critical stages in the course of disease which may be influenced by DMH-11C treatment.

In the control group, 17 of 18 hind paws were assigned a clinical score of 4 at the peak of the inflammatory response (day 23), and 16 of the joints (88.9%) remained immovable (ankylosed) on day 35. In contrast, in the DMH-11C-treated group, although 9 of 18 hind paws were given a clinical score of 4 on day 23, only 4 of those (22.2%) still had a score of 4 on day 35. Thus, the control group was 28 times (cross product ratio) more likely than the DMH-11C-treated group to maintain scores of 4 in the hind paws on day 35. Histomorphologic evaluation of the hind paws indicated that inflammation and pannus were attenuated in rats treated with DMH-11C even though the joints from those 4 paws remained clinically ankylosed. Therefore, we presume that, in contrast to the bony ankylosis seen in joints from rats in the control group, this ankylosis represents contracture as a residual of the intense periarticular swelling and inflammation in addition to synovial inflammation.

Ankylosis reflects an irreversible alteration in function subsequent to injury, disuse, tissue repair, or resolution of inflammation. The erosion of tendon, cartilage, and bone that accompanies inflammatory arthritis is mediated largely by collagenase and stromelysin, enzymes that are produced by synovial cells (21). Both enzymes belong to the gene family of metalloproteinases. Dexamethasone, which suppresses adjuvant-induced arthritis at doses similar to the dosage of DMH-11C used in this study (22), reduces gene expression of collagenase (23) and stromelysin (24). It will be important to determine whether DMH-11C has direct effects on metalloproteinase production and activity.

COX-1 is a constitutive enzyme thought to be responsible for production of eicosanoids that help maintain normal renal function, gastric mucosal integrity, and hemostasis (17). COX-2 is activated during inflammatory reactions such as those induced by IL-10 and TNFα (25), and is therefore thought to be responsible for production of eicosanoids that act as mediators of inflammation. The most compelling evidence that COX-2 is involved in the inflammatory response is the fact that its expression is inhibited by glucocorticoids (16). In contrast, glucocorticoids exert little influence on COX-1 expression.

Our data (Figs. 5 and 6) suggest that the anti-inflammatory action of DMH-11C may be caused in part by suppression of eicosanoid synthesis in inflamed tissue. In particular, DMH-11C appears to be a more effective inhibitor of COX-2 than of COX-1, both in intact cells and in preparations of pure enzymes. These findings are consistent with the observation that DMH-11C does not prevent arachidonic acid-induced aggregation of human platelets (Burstein, S and Friderichs, E, unpublished data). Human platelets appear to contain only COX-1 activity (26). THC-11-oic acid, the template molecule for DMH-11C, also did not inhibit platelet aggregation (Meyers, A. personal communication), suggesting that COX-2 selectivity may be a characteristic of cannabinoid acids in general. In support of this is the observation that THC-11-oic acid does not produce gastric lesions in an acute ulcerogenicity test in rats (27). Finally, DMH-11C suppresses leukotriene B$_4$ synthesis (median EC$_{50}$ dose 1.2 μM) in rat macrophages stimulated with calcium ionophore (Morgan D.W. personal communication), raising the possibility that DMH-11C may be a dual inhibitor of eicosanoid production. Of course, results of experiments performed in vitro allow only speculation about events in vivo. More definitive statements about the mechanisms of action of DMH-11C must await in vivo studies in humans.

The experimental evidence presented here suggests that DMH-11C holds promise as a safe therapeutic agent for inflammatory arthritis. Additional investigation is warranted to better define the molecular mechanisms whereby DMH-11C exerts its suppressive effects on inflammation and joint tissue injury, and to further characterize its antiinflammatory actions.

ACKNOWLEDGMENTS

The technical assistance of Tracy Wheeler is gratefully acknowledged, as is the secretarial support of Debra Roy.

Reprinted with permission from: Arthritis & Rheumatism, Vol. 41, No. 1, January 1998, pp. 163–170.

REFERENCES

1. Hui-Lin, L. (1975) The origin and use of cannabis in Eastern Asia. In: *Cannabis and Culture* (Rubin, V., ed.) The Hague, Mouton, pp. 51–62.
2. Burstein, S., Rosenfeld, J. and Wittstruck, T. (1972) Isolation and characterization of two major urinary metabolites of delta-1-tetrahydrocannabinol. *Science* **176**, 422–424.
3. Perez-Reyes, M. (1985) Pharmacodynamics of certain drugs of abuse. In: *Pharmacokinetics and Pharmaco-dynamics of Psychoactive Drugs.* (Barnett, G. and Chiang, N. C., eds). Foster City (CA): Biomedical Publishers, Foster City, CA, pp. 287–310.
4. Burstein, S. H., Hull, K., Hunter S. A. and Latham, V. (1988) Cannabinoids and pain responses: a possible role for prostaglandins. *FASEB J* **2**, 3022–3026.
5. Doyle, S. A., Burstein, S. H., Dewey, W. L. and Welch, S. P. (1990) Further studies on the antinociceptive effects of delta-6-THC-7-oic acid. *Agents Actions* **31**, 157–162.
6. Burstein, S. H., Audette, C. A., Doyle, S. A., Hull, K., Hunter S. A. and Latham V. (1989) Antagonism to the actions of PAF by a non psychoactive cannabinoid. *J. Pharmacol. Exp. Ther.* **251**, 531–535.
7. Burstein, S. H., Hunter, S. A., Latham, V. and Renzulli L. (1986) Prostaglandins and cannabis. XVI. Antagonism of delta-1-THC action by its metabolites. *Biochem. Pharmacol.* **35**, 2553–2558.
8. Loev, B, Bender, P. E., Dowalo, F., Macko, E. and Fowler, P. J. (1973) Cannabinoids: structure-activity studies related to 1,2-dimethylheptyl derivatives. *J. Med. Chem.* **16**, 1200–1206.
9. Burstein, S. H., Audette, C. A., Breuer, A, Devane, W. A., Colodner, S. and Doyle, S. A.. (1992) Synthetic non-psychotropic cannabinoids with potent antiinflammatory, analgesic and leukocyte antiadhesion activities. *J. Med. Chem.* **35**, 3135–3141.
10. Arend, W. P. and Dayer, J-M. (1995) Inhibition of the production and effects of interleukin-1 and tumor necrosis factor a in rheumatoid arthritis. *Arthritis Rheum* **38**, 151–160.
11. Taurog, J. D., Argentieri, D. C. and Reynolds, R. A. (1988) Adjuvant arthritis. *Methods Enzymol.* **162**, 339–355.
12. Rossetti, R. G., Seiler, C. M., Brathwaite, K. and Zurier, R. B. (1995) Effect of misoprosotol on acute and chronic inflammation. *Am. J. Ther.* **2**, 600–606.
13. Glenn, E. and Gray, J. (1964) Adjuvant induced polyarthritis in rats: biologic and histologic background. *Am. J. Vet. Res.* **26**, 1180–1194.
14. Pearson, C. M. and Wood, F. D. (1963) Studies of arthritis and other lesions induced in rats by the injection of mycobacterial adjuvant. VII. Pathologic details of the arthritis and spondylitis. *Am. J. Pathol.* **42**, 73–95.
15. Kujubu, D. A., Fletcher, S., Varnum, B. C., Lim, R. W. and Herschman, H. R. (1981) TIS10, a phorbol ester tumor promoter-inducible mRNA from Swiss 3T3 cells encodes a novel prostaglandin synthetase/cyclooxygenase homologue. *J. Biol. Chem.* **266**, 12,866–12,872.
16. Kujubu, D. A. and Herschman, H. R. (1992) Dexamethasone inhibits mitogen induction of the TIS10 prostaglandin synthase/cyclooxygenase gene. *J. Biol. Chem.* **267**, 7991–7994.
17. Griswold, D. E. and Adams, J. L. (1996) Constitutive cyclooxygenase (COX-1) and inducible cyclooxygenase (COX-2): rationale for selective inhibition and progress to date. *Med. Res. Rev.* **16**, 181–186.
18. Edwards, J. C., Sedgwick, A. D. and Willoughby, D. A. (1981) The formation of a structure with the features of synovial lining by subcutaneous injections of air: an in vivo tissue culture system. *J. Pathol.* **134**, 147–156.
19. Esser, R. E., Eyerman, M. C., Port, C. D. and Anderson, W. (1989) Proinflammatory effects of interleukin-1 in the rat air pouch. *Int. J. Tissue. React.* **XI**, 291–300.
20. Audette, C. A. and Burstein, S. (1990) Inhibition of leukocyte adhesion by the in vivo and in vitro administration of cannabinoids. *Life Sci.* **47**, 753–759.
21. Brinckerhoff, C. E. (1991) Joint destruction in arthritis: metalloproteinases in the spotlight. *Arthritis Rheum.* **34**, 1073–1075.
22. Pelegri, C., Franch, A., Castellote, C. and Castell, M. (1995) Immunohistochemical changes in synovial tissue during the course of adjuvant arthritis. *J. Rheumatol.* **22**, 124–132.

23. Clark, K. S. D., Kobayashi, D. K. and Welgus, H. G. (1987) Regulation of the expression of tissue inhibitor of metalloproteinases and collagenase by retinoids and glucocorticoids in human fibroblasts. *J. Clin. Invest.* **80**, 1280–1288.

24. Frisch, S. M. and Ruley, H. E. (1987) Transcription from the stromelysin promoter is induced by interleukin-1 and repressed by dexamethasone. *J. Biol. Chem.* **262**, 16,300–16,304.

25. Arias-Negrete, S, Keller K. and Chandee K. (1995) Proinflammatory cytokines regulate cyclooxygenase-2 mRNA expression in human macrophages. *Biochem. Biophys. Res. Commun.* **208**, 582–589.

26. DeWitt, D. L. (1991) Prostaglandin endoperoxide synthase: regulation of enzyme expression. *Biochim. Biophys. Acta* **1083**, 121–134.

27. Burstein, S. H. (1989) delta-1-THC-7-oic acid and analgesic and anti-inflammatory agents. US Patent 4,847,290. July 1989.

42

Analgesic Properties of THC and Its Synthetic Derivatives

Aron H. Lichtman and Billy R. Martin

Abstract

Cannabis has been used for thousands of years for the treatment of pain resulting from a wide range of disorders. Although clinical evaluations of *Cannabis* and its psychoactive constituent THC have not led to a general consensus regarding their analgesic effectiveness, THC and other synthetic cannabinoid analogs elicit antinociception in a variety of pain tests in laboratory animals. These antinociceptive effects are mediated through cannabinoid receptors in the central nervous system which, in turn, modulate the perception of painful stimuli. The endogenous ligand, arachinodyl-ethanolamine (anandamide), is also an effective antinociceptive agent in experimental models. The extent to which the endogenous cannabinoid system is involved in the modulation of pain is currently unknown. Coadministration of opioids and THC by the intrathecal route produces an additive antalgic effect. Recent work indicates that coadministration of opioids and cannabinoids produces at least an additive effect. The possibility exists that the analgesic effects can be optimized and untoward effects be minimized if agents from these two classes of drugs were coadministered for the treatment of painful conditions.

1. INTRODUCTION

Cannabis has been touted as a treatment for many maladies including pain for several centuries. A British army physician serving in India noted its analgesic properties and is credited with introducing *Cannabis* into Western medicine *(76)*. Subsequently, *Cannabis* was used for the treatment of psychiatric illnesses, insomnia, and appetite enhancement with no apparent addiction occurring. In addition, it had been used for treating opium addiction, chronic alcoholism, delirium tremens, and a large variety of painful disorders. *Cannabis* extracts were listed in the United States Pharmacopoeia in the late 1890s as treatments for neuralgia, gout, rheumatism, tetanus, hydrophobia, epidemic cholera, convulsions, chorea, hysteria, mental depression, delirium tremens, insanity, and uterine hemorrhage. It was removed from the

From: *Marihuana and Medicine*
Edited by: G. G. Nahas et al.   © Humana Press Inc., Totowa, NJ

United States Pharmacopoeia in 1942. Medical marihuana was again advocated in the United States after the widespread recreational use of *Cannabis* in the 1960s.

Several reasons may be suggested for the use of THC and of its synthetic analogs for the management of pain. First, THC may be capable of controlling pain that is refractory to other analgesics. Second, Δ^9-THC and synthetic cannabinoid derivatives may control pain by a mechanism distinct from that of opioids or nonsteroidal anti-inflammatory drugs (NSAID), thereby providing a new class of analgesics. The recent discovery of an endogenous cannabinoid system has provided further impetus for investigating the role of Δ^9-THC in pain modulation.

The development of a safe analgesic with limited abuse potential will be of great therapeutic value. In comparison to other areas of the brain, the brainstem medullary centers are practically devoid of cannabinoid receptors (36). Consequently, Δ^9-THC does not produce respiratory depression and there are no deaths directly attributable to use of *Cannabis* in humans. The high prevalence of marihuana use in the United States indicates that this drug is a positive reinforcer, however; in our opinion the preclinical data investigating the abuse liability of cannabinoids has been mixed. The self-administration paradigm in animals has been a valuable tool in predicting the abuse liabilities of drugs. In the case of THC, experimental self-administration of THC by animals has not been clearly observed. THC is an ineffective reinforcer in rhesus monkeys (35). Martellotta et al. observed self-administration of the synthetic cannabinoid agonist WIN 55,212–2 in drug-naive mice and reported that this effect was blocked by SR 141716A, though Δ^9-THC was not tested. Similar to attempts employing fixed ratio schedules, this study also failed to establish self-administration in laboratory animals. However, Fratta et al. observed strong self-administration of the synthetic cannabinoid agonist WIN 55,212–2 in drug-naive mice and reported that this effect was blocked by 141716 A. The apparent inability to establish THC as a reinforcer in the self-administration paradigm suggests either a limitation of this model to predict the abuse liability of drugs in humans or that THC has less of an abuse liability than opiates or major psychostimulants which is a general clinical observation.

Nonetheless, THC appears to act upon brain regions associated with reinforcement. Relatively high concentrations of cannabinoid receptors have been found in the nucleus accumbens, a brain area strongly implicated in drug-associated reinforcement (36). Moreover, THC appears to produce effects upon the mesotelencephalic dopamine reward pathway similar to other rewarding drugs (28). Δ^9-THC was found to reduce the amount of electric current required for self-stimulation in the medial forebrain bundle (29). In addition, systemic administration of Δ^9-THC was found to increase dopamine (DA) efflux in the nucleus accumbens, and this effect was blocked by naloxone (9). These effects are similar to those of other drugs that are reported to have rewarding effects in humans. THC also elicits various aversive effects and acts as an unconditioned stimulus in the taste-aversion paradigm (80) and an anxiogenic agent in the elevated plus maze (78). It may be hypothesized that these apparent adverse properties as well as feedback control on CRF, may mask the rewarding properties of cannabinoids and account for their failure to serve as positive reinforcers in the self-administration paradigm (11).

2. CANNABINOID-INDUCED ANTINOCICEPTION

To understand the mechanism by which psychoactive cannabinoids produce analgesia, it is important to understand pain, or nociception. The perception of a noxious stimulus is a complex sensory phenomenon that is dependent upon extrinsic factors including the type and intensity of the stimulus as well as intrinsic factor including which pain pathways are activated. Melzack and his colleagues have classified the concept of nociception into acute and chronic categories (70). Acute nociception has been further subdivided into phasic and tonic components (17). Phasic nociception can be elicited by a sharp, sudden, transient noxious stimulus and lasts as long as the noxious stimulus stimulates the nociceptors. The stimulus generally elicits withdrawal responses that are often reflexive and involves sensory or discriminatory processes. A tonic noxious stimulus involves affective, motivational processes and typically elicits an integrated response. Tonic nociception is often caused by tissue damage, is described as dull, throbbing, and aching, and has a more gradual onset than phasic nociception. Chronic pain, on the other hand, may occur long after healing has occurred and is associated with hypersensitivity to nonnoxious stimuli, a sensory abnormality termed allodynia. Several nociceptive tests that assess phasic nociception in laboratory animals include the tail-flick, paw-pressure, hot-plate, and tooth-pulp tests. Several tests that are used to elicit tonic nociception in laboratory animals include caustic agents such as *p*-phenylquinone (PPQ) or acetic acid that produce stretching when injected into the intraperitoneal cavity or carrageenan or formalin injected subcutaneously into a paw, the result of which is recuperative behavior directed at the inflicted paw. Several procedures for investigating chronic pain in laboratory animals include inducing an arthritic reaction using Freund's adjuvant or by ligation of the sciatic nerve or other nerves. THC has been used mostly in mice and rats, and was found to produce antinociception in some tests of pain to be described below. In mice, Waser oberved that Δ^9-THC had an analgesic effect in the writhing test, however, analgesic activity was not observed in the hot-plate test and there was large variability in doses of Δ^9-THC required by different authors to elicit an analgesic response (Table 1) (100a).

2.1. Antinociceptive Effects of Cannabinoids in Humans

During the past 25 years several investigators have studied *Cannabis* for the management of pain in humans. In a collection of self-reports *Cannabis* was described as an effective treatment for headache, migraine, menstrual cramps, and postsurgical pain (74). Two case studies were described in which smoking *Cannabis* relieved symptoms of low back pain and associated muscle spasms (81). Additionally, Grinspoon and Bakalar (33) reported anecdotal accounts of numerous individuals who claimed that smoking *Cannabis* alleviated chronic pain of mild to severe intensity.

Other studies that examined the use of smoked *Cannabis* for the management of pain in clinical controlled conditions have not corroborated anecdotal self-reports. An actual increase in pain sensitivity in subjects who smoked *Cannabis* containing 14 mg of Δ^9-THC was reported by Hill et al. (38,39). In a second report, Clark et al. (11) examined the effects of a thermal stimulus in subjects who smoked an average of 8.9–13.7 *Cannabis* cigarettes per day for four weeks, following which *Cannabis* decreased the threshold of pain perception. The authors of this study pointed out that changes in reported pain intensity following *Cannabis* exposure could be influenced by such factors as anxiety, mood, personality, and other subjective effects, and in order to account for all of these variables they used the sensory-decision theory to analyze the analgesic effects of Δ^9-THC. Noyes and Baram (74) concluded that *Cannabis* was at best a mild clinical analgesic whose effects were highly subject to both suggestion and expectation.

Some investigators have suggested that the analgesic properties could best be established by using the psychoactive constituents in *Cannabis* rather than THC itself. There are discrepancies among the conclusions of several controlled studies using Δ^9-THC to block pain. One study (Noyes et al., ref. 75) reported that orally administered Δ^9-THC (20 mg) and codeine (120 mg) had comparable efficacy in producing analgesia in cancer patients. But THC produced adverse effects including dizziness (97%), blurred vision (64%), and impaired think-

Table 1
Antinociceptive Activity of THC in Laboratory Animals

Test	Species	Route	Potency
Tail-flick	mice	i.p.	One-half as potent as morphine (7), very weak activity (34)
	rats	i.p.	Dose of 3 mg/kg produced analgesia (6), 10 mg/kg effective (72)
	mice	s.c.	ED_{50} = 197 (8), 55 (69), and 45 mg/kg (59)
	mice	i.v.	ED_{50} = 1.0 (59)
Hot plate	mice	i.p.	One-half as potent as morphine (7), ED_{50} = 39 mg/kg (34) and 50 mg/kg (23), 100% effect at 20 mg/kg (95)
	mice	p.o.	ED_{50} = 5.0 mg/kg (10), equipotent to morphine (96)
	mice	s.c.	ED_{50} = 9.6 (105), 178 (69), and 99 mg/kg (59)
Stretching	mice	i.p.	One-half as potent as morphine (7), partial agonist, high doses (23)
	mice	p.o.	Equipotent to morphine (96)
	mice	s.c.	ED_{50} = 5.1 (59) and 5.9 mg/kg (69)
	mice	i.v.	ED_{50} = 0.2 mg/kg (59)
Formalin	rat	p.o.	5 and 10 mg/kg effective analgesia (71)
paw pressure (Freund's adjuvant)	rat	i.p.	5 mg/kg produced antinociception in arthritic and nonarthritic rats (91)
Randall-Selitto Paw pressure	mice	p.o.	Equipotent to morphine (96)
Flinch jump	rat	s.c.	ED_{50} = 83 mg/kg (69)
Electroshock	rats	i.p.	Nondose-related effects in the range of 60–150 mg/kg (79)
Electrically stimulated sciatic nerve	rabbits	Not provided	One-half as potent as morphine (7)
Tooth pulp	dog	i.v.	400% effect with 1 mg/kg (47)
Skin-twitch reflex	dog	i.v.	Depressed the reflex (31)
Electro-acupuncture	rabbits	i.v.	Enhanced electroacupuncture (89)

ing (53%). In another experiment (73), elevation in mood and appetite stimulation were also reported, whereas 10 mg THC was better tolerated but not as effective as 60 or 120 mg codeine. However, Regelson and colleagues reported that Δ^9-THC neither alleviated pain in cancer patients nor decreased their need for pain medication (86). In an acute pain model (cold pressor test), Karniol et al. (46), found Δ^9-THC to be ineffective. Similarly, intravenous injection of high doses of Δ^9-THC in patients undergoing dental surgery failed to alter pain-detection thresholds (83), whereas low doses of drug produced increases in pain perception in some patients and some pain relief in others; marked tachycardia and anxiety were also reported.

There has also been a steady effort to develop synthetic cannabinoid derivatives that might be useful as analgesics. For example, Nabitan (a nitrogen analog of THC, benzopyranoperidine) failed to produce pain relief in cancer patients and there was some evidence for increased pain sensitivity (44). Conversely, others (97) reported that Nabitan elicited analgesia comparable to that of codeine in cancer patients. Levonantradol, another cannabinoid derivative, elicited some benefit for postoperative surgical pain but only at doses that produced significant behavioral disturbances (43).

2.2. Effects of Cannabinoids in Laboratory Animal Nociceptive Tests

The antinociceptive effects of Δ^9-THC as well as other cannabinoids have been investigated in rodent, canine, and primate species in a range of antinociceptive tests. As can be seen in Table 1, Δ^9-THC has been found to be effective in producing antinociception in phasic (e.g., tail-flick and hot-plate), tonic (e.g., stretching), and chronic (e.g., Freund's adjuvant and sciatic ligation) nociceptive tests. The antinociceptive potency of cannabinoids depends on several factors including the preparation of the drug, assay conditions, and, most notably, the route of administration (34). As can be seen in Table 1, administration route plays a critical role in determining the antinociceptive effects of THC. Specifically, THC exhibits a high degree of potency and efficacy, similar to that of morphine, when given via the intravenous route. In an early study, intravenous injection of hashish distillate was found to be equipotent to morphine (16). In contrast, the antinociceptive potency is considerably decreased when THC is administered via either subcutaneous or intraperitoneal routes. In fact, under certain circumstances intraperitonealy administered THC appears to act as a partial agonist. A physiochemical characteristic of the cannabinoids that also accounts for its high degree of variability is its highly lipophilic nature that precludes the use of aqueous vehicles for its administration. The use of a vehicle consisting of emulphor:ethanol:saline for preparation of injectable forms of cannabinoids (77) has provided a highly effective solvent system. This vehicle combined with intravenous administration, has demonstrated that Δ^9-THC produces potent analgesia reproducibly in several nociceptive assays (59).

The nociceptive test employed also plays a critical role in characterizing cannabinoid-induced antinociception. The fact that cannabinoids also elicit catalepsy and decrease spontaneous activity (56), raises the concern that increased tail-flick latencies arise indirectly from cannabinoid-induced motor impairment. However, the tail-flick test is a nociceptive assay that is highly resistant to impaired motor function. In particular, the antinociceptive and motor disruptive effects of cannabinoids can be pharmacologically dissociated. Intrathecal administration of the α_2-noradrenergic antagonist yohimbine (52), as well as the kappa-opioid antagonist nor-binaltorphimine (nor-BNI) (94) blocks cannabinoid-induced antinociception as assessed by the tail-flick test, without reducing cannabinoid-induced motor impairment. Conversely, intrastriatal administration of cannabinoids produced catalepsy (32), but failed to elevate tail-flick latencies (50). On the other hand, the apparent antinociceptive effects in other laboratory animal models of pain that require integrated responses, such as the hot plate or stretching tests, may be confounded by cannabinoid-induced motor impairment. Consequently, it is important to assess for motor impairment when these tests are employed.

Antinociceptive effects of synthetic cannabinoids in chronic nociceptive models have also been investigated. One recent report investigated the effects of WIN 55,212–2 on hyperalgesic responses following a chronic constriction injury of the sciatic nerve (37). They found that WIN 55,212–2 blocked the hyperalgesic responses to a thermal stimulus on the ipsilateral paw of the nerve ligation. The effect was dose-related and the inactive enantiomer was without effect. WIN 55,212–2 also alleviated the hyperalgesic responses in the afflicted paw to other stimuli including cold and a pin prick. In the case of a pin prick, however, WIN 55,212–2 also produced antinociception on the paw contralateral to the nerve ligation suggesting less specificity for a mechanical stimulus than for a thermal stimulus. Nonetheless, both antinociceptive responses were blocked by the cannabinoid antagonist SR 141716A.

Importantly, a moderate dose of WIN 55,212–2 (2.14 mg/kg) blocked thermal and mechanical hyperalgesia as well as mechanical allodynia with no side effects *(37)*. Another study employed an arthritic pain model using Freund's adjuvant *(91)*. A single dose of Δ^9-THC produced antinociception to a mechanical stimulus in both arthritic and nonarthritic rats. These two studies taken together may suggest that cannabinoids are more selective in alleviating hyperalgesia to a thermal stimulus than to a mechanical stimulus. The issue of whether this alleviation of hyperalgesia is modality specific can be better addressed by examining the entire dose-response relationship of the cannabinoid agonist.

One of the most notable features of the experimental studies summarized in Table 1 is that analgesic effects of Δ^9-THC are accompanied by prominent behavioral effects that would be intolerable if they were to occur in patients. The many behavioral effects produced by cannabinoids in a wide range of laboratory animals have been documented thoroughly *(22,84)*. Our laboratory has shown that at antinociceptive doses, Δ^9-THC also produces other behavioral effects that include sedation, hypothermia, and catalepsy in mice *(60)*. These observations are consistent with the clinical findings with Δ^9-THC and underscore the need to develop cannabinoid analgesics that lack undesired pharmacological effects. In addition, there are always concerns regarding the mechanism of action of an agent with multiple pharmacological effects. It is reasonable to ask whether the antinociceptive properties of Δ^9-THC are caused by a specific action in the central nervous system or a result of a general disruption of neuronal integration brought about by sedation. It is therefore crucial to understand the mechanism by which Δ^9-THC produces its analgesic effects.

3. THE CANNABINOID SYSTEM

3.1. Receptor Mechanism of Action

The hypothesis that the antinociceptive effects (as well as many other behavioral effects) of THC are mediated through a receptor mechanism of action is firmly supported. Early structure-activity relationship studies in which subtle changes in cannabinoid structure were found to greatly affect pharmacological potency provided initial line of experimental evidence indicating the existence of a functional cannabinoid receptor mechanism of action *(84)*. Moreover, the demonstration of enantioselectivity with highly pure enantiomers such as 11-OH-Δ^8-THC-dimethylheptyl, a highly potent crystalline THC analog *(57)* is consistent with a receptor mechanism of action.

Many structure-activity relationship studies have been established for the cannabinoids, in part because of the search for novel analgesics. Although it was initially assumed that an intact B ring (Fig. 1) was essential for pharmacological activity *(84)*, the synthesis of 9-*nor*-9β-hydroxyhexahydrocannabinol *(69)* that lacked the B ring entirely and had a dimethylheptyl side chain rather than the traditional pentyl group at the C3 position proved to have a pharmacological profile similar to that of Δ^9-THC. This synthetic approach led to the synthesis of CP 55,940 (Fig. 1) which was approximately 4 to 25 times more potent than Δ^9-THC depending upon the pharmacological measure *(14)*. Of importance, its (+)-enantiomer, CP 56,667, was inactive. Other analogs developed in this series *(45,68)* not only helped redefine many of the structural determinants of cannabinoid action but also resulted in extremely potent agonists, some of which were as much as 700 times more potent than Δ^9-THC *(56)*. Other potent analogs included 11-OH- Δ^8-THC-dimethylheptyl (DMH), 11-OH- Δ^9-THC-DMH *(61)*, and the hexahydro analog of the 11-OH-THC-DMH *(19)*.

Despite the apparent large structural differences between Δ^9-THC and CP 55,940, molecular modeling studies revealed striking similarities *(41)*. The structural diversity of the cannabinoids increased with the development of the aminoalkylindoles. The prototypical

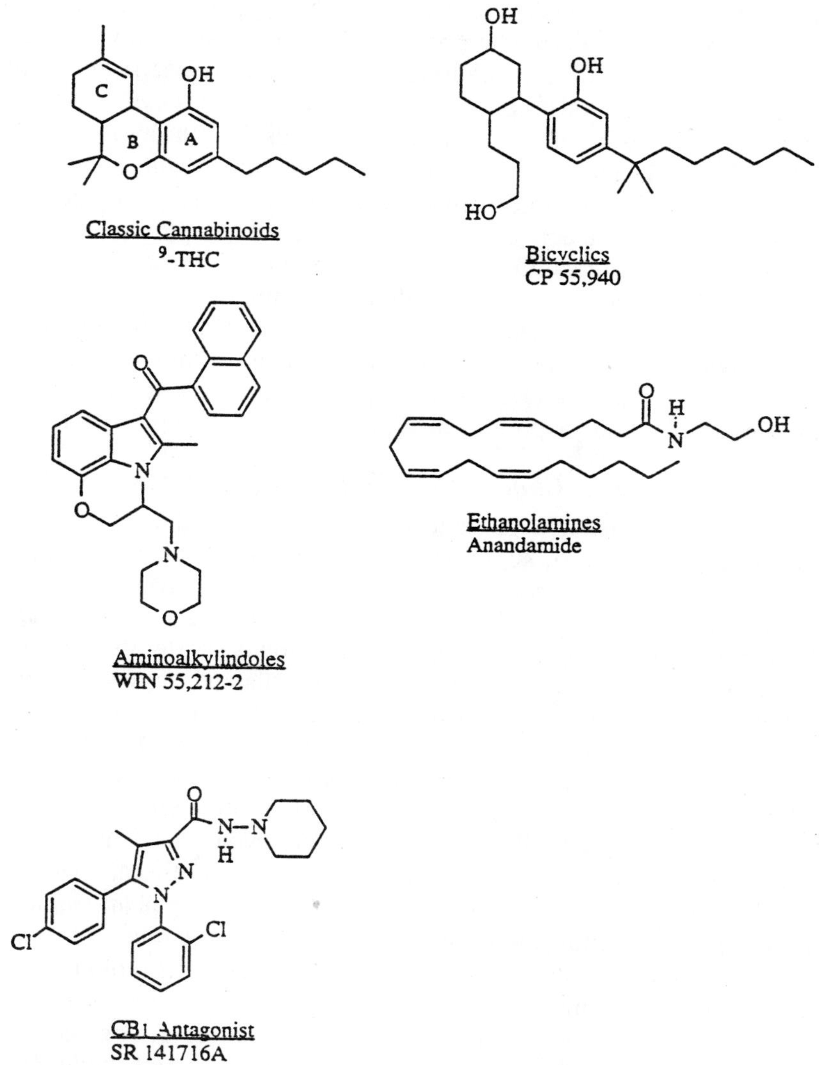

Fig. 1. Structures of selected compounds from different classes of cannabinoids including an endogenous ligand and an antagonist.

compound of this class WIN 55,212–2 (Fig. 1), which possesses a structure distinct from that of the traditional cannabinoids *(100)*. The pharmacological properties of the aminoalkylindoles share a common pharmacological profile with Δ^9-THC with the (+)-isomer exhibiting similar potencies as those of Δ^9-THC in producing hypoactivity, antinociception, hypothermia, and ring-immobility in mice *(13)*. Of importance, the (–)-isomer was inactive up to the highest dose tested. The observation that many compounds in the aminoalkylindole series produce potent antinociception has inspired a great deal of other structure-activity studies *(5,13,15,25,42,48)*.

Although structure-activity relationships provided compelling evidence that cannabinoid-induced antinociception was mediated via a receptor mechanism, the discovery of cannabinoid receptors offered definitive support. Howlett's group *(20)* was the first to characterize a brain receptor, now termed CB_1, using radiolabeled CP 55,940 and the subsequent cloning of this receptor *(66)* firmly established it existence. The discovery of cannabinoid receptors in brain and the relatively high correlation between antinociceptive activity and binding affinity of cannabinoids *(15,99)* as well as inhibition of adenylyl cyclase *(41)* provided compelling support for a receptor mechanism of action. Our laboratory has evaluated a large number of analogs in each of the different classes of cannabinoids for affinity to the CB_1 receptor and for antinociception in the tail-flick procedure following intravenous administration.

A major discovery to assess mechanism of action was the development of SR 141716A *(88)*, an antagonist that is selective for CB_1 cannabinoid receptors (Fig. 1). This antagonist has been demonstrated to block the antinociceptive effects of the prototypical cannabinoids Δ^9-THC, WIN 55,212–2, and CP 55,940 without affecting morphine-induced antinociception *(12,54,88)*. Consistent with these findings was that pretreatment with an antisense oligodeoxynucleotide to the brain cannabinoid receptor inhibited cannabinoid-induced antinociception *(24)*. Taken together these observations provide conclusive evidence that cannabinoid-induced antinociception is mediated via a CB_1 receptor mediation of action.

3.2. Endogenous Cannabinoid System

In addition to the existence of cannabinoid receptors, the discovery of endogenous cannabinoid ligands *(21,67,90)* suggests the existence of a functional cannabinoid system with physiological roles in the central and peripheral nervous systems. Exogenous administration of anandamide (Fig. 1) has been reported to produce antinociception in mice *(27,92)* and rats *(98)*. However, anandamide's duration of action is shorter than that of other cannabinoids *(92,98)* as a result of its rapid degradation in cells and tissues *(18)* and in whole animals *(104)*. Anandamide does not appear to be the only active endogenous cannabinoid as two other endogenous arachidonylethanolamides have been found to produce mild increases in hot-plate latencies in mice *(3)*. The antinociceptive effects of anandamide appear to be mediated by a different mechanism from the antinociceptive effects of other cannabinoids. Anandamide's antinociceptive effects endure *(27,92)* even after it is no longer detected in brain *(104)*. Although anandamide was effective via the intrathecal route of administration *(92)*, it failed to elicit antinociception or any other observable pharmacological effects following intracerebroventricular administration *(50)*. This apparent lack of effect following i.c.v. intracerebroventicular administration may be because of its rapid kinetics or inability to diffuse into the brain sites of action from the ventricles. Unlike a variety of other cannabinoids that are blocked by the kappa antagonist *nor*-binaltorphimine (*nor*-BNI) and several modulators of cAMP and potassium channels when given intrathecally, *(85,94,101)*, anandamide-induced antinociception was unaffected by these agents *(92,102)*. Most perplexing is that the cannabinoid antagonist, SR 141716A, failed to block the antinociceptive effects of anandamide in the tail-flick test in mice *(1)* and the paw-withdrawal test in rats *(91)*. The lack of antagonism by SR 141716A as well as by other modulators that block Δ^9-THC-induced antinociception and the lack of correspondence between anandamide's antinociceptive actions and brain levels suggest the possibility that anandamide-induced antinociception actions may be mediated by itself or metabolites at a non-CB_1 site. Despite the differences between anandamide and other cannabinoids, other evidence is consistent with a receptor mechanism of action. Specifically, anandamide binds to the cannabinoid receptor *(2)* and anandamide-induced antinociception exhibits cross-tolerance to the antinociceptive effects of Δ^9-THC *(26,102)*.

The fact that administered Δ^9-THC produces antinociception has been well documented; however, whether a putative anandamide system functions to modulate nociception remains to be determined. The observations that THC inhibits nociception *(50,64)* when injected into brain areas that are both known to modulate pain *(4)* and contain THC receptors *(36)* suggest that an anandamide system may function to modulate responsivity to pain. The cannabinoid receptor antagonist SR 141716A has been used to test the hypothesis that anandamides are tonically active to modulate nociception. The observations that low doses of intrathecally administered SR 141716A in mice elicited significantly decreased latencies in the hot-plate test *(87)* supports the hypothesis that anandamides may tonically modulate nociception. It should be noted though, that markedly low doses of SR 141716A were employed (ED_{50} = 0.0012 fmol) which would not be expected to antagonize the antinociceptive effects of exogeneously administered Δ^9-THC, and hyperalgesia was not observed at higher doses of intrathecal SR 141716A. In addition, hyperalgesia lasted less than 20 minute even though the antagonistic effects of SR 141716A are of a much longer duration *(88)*. Alternatively, the finding that SR 141716A decreased GTPγS binding when cannabinoid-receptor agonists stimulate the binding suggests that SR 141716A may be an inverse agonist *(49)*. Nonetheless, the observation that intrathecal administration of an antisense oligonucleotide complementary to the CB_1-receptor mRNA, which resulted in 60% decrease in binding sites, also elicited hyperalgesia in the hot-plate test is consistent with the notion that SR 141716A acts as CB_1-receptor antagonist. This hyperalgesic effect seems to involve the release of glutamate since competitive and noncompetitive NMDA antagonists blocked SR 141716A-induced hyperalgesia. Future studies will assess the dose dependancy of the hyperalgesic effects of SR 141716A, rule out nonspecific motor hyperexcitability, and determine whether the effects are modality specific. Moreover, electrophysiological studies can be used to determine whether SR 141716A elicits an increase in noxious stimulus-evoked activity in nociceptive neurons.

3.3. Cannabinoids Inhibit Electrophysiological Responses to Noxious Stimuli

Noxious stimuli are known to activate wide dynamic range (WDR) neurons in the dorsal horn of the spinal cord that transmit information regarding the intensity and location of noxious stimuli to rostral brain centers for nociceptive processing, predominantly through the spinothalamic tract *(82)*. Several recent electrophysiological studies have shown that THC blocks noxious stimulus-evoked activity in the central nervous system. WIN 55,212–2 administered intravenously selectively suppressed firing of the WDR neurons to a noxious pressure stimulus, but not stimulus-evoked activity of nonnociceptive neurons in the spinal cord *(40)*. The finding that the inactive stereoisomer, WIN 55,212–3, failed to suppress noxious-evoked firing of the WDR neurons is consistent with a receptor-mediated mechanism of action. WIN 55,212–2 also inhibited noxious stimulus-evoked activity of neurons in the ventrolateral posterior nucleus of the thalamus *(62)*, a major relay of the nociceptive pathway in the CNS *(82)*. Although these results demonstrated that THC suppresses the ascending nociceptive pathway, they did not address the site of THC action in the CNS. WIN 55,212–2 may have acted directly on the WDR neurons, on other spinal or supraspinal neurons that in turn inhibited the WDR neurons, or at a combination of these sites.

3.4. CNS Sites of Action

The simplicity of the tail-flick response, its resistance to impairment of motor function, in addition to the detailed understanding of the physiology of this test have made it very useful as a model of pain and analgesic action. In the tail-flick test, as well as other nociceptive tests, drugs produce antinociception either via direct spinal mechanisms *(108)*, at brain sites that activate descending monoaminergic analgesic pathways *(106)*, or through combined spinal and supraspinal mechanisms. Several studies have demonstrated that cannabinoids inhibit the tail-flick response through both spinal and supraspinal components of action. Surgical transection of the spinal cord has been used to delineate between spinal and supraspinal effects of analgesics since this response is a spinally mediated reflex that is modulated by supraspinal input. Consequently, an attenuation in the antinociceptive effects of a drug can implicate brain sites, whereas the occurrence of any antinociceptive effect in the spinally transected animals can be attributed to direct spinal action. Intravenous administration of either Δ^9-THC or CP 55,940 to spinally transected rats was found to reduce, but not eliminate, antinociception (53). On the other hand, spinal transection failed to attenuate the antinociceptive effects of intravenously administered Δ^9-THC in mice (93). These results suggest that there is a relevant supraspinal component to the Δ^9-THC antinociceptive effects of systemically administered THC in rats, but not necessarily mice.

Intrathecal administration of the cannabinoid analog levonantradol (107), CP 55,940 (53) to the lower lumbar level produced antinociception in rats. Similarly, intrathecally administered THC reliably produced antinociception in mice (55). Although the drugs were administered at the level of the spinal cord, intrathecally administered drugs can diffuse rostrally and thereby interact at the level of the brain. Moreover, given the failure of spinal transection to attenuate the antinociceptive effects of intravenously administered Δ^9-THC in mice (93), it was necessary to determine whether the cannabinoids remained at the spinal level or diffused to the brain. Biodisposition studies using [^{3}H]-CP 55,940 administered intrathecally to mice and rats revealed that the majority of drug remained at the site of injection, and only trace amounts of drug were detected in the brain (53,93). As the tail-flick response is mediated at the lumbar/sacral level of the spinal cord, drugs acting spinally would be expected to produce a greater effect when infused at the lumbar rather than the thoracic level. Consistent with a spinal component of action, CP 55,940 given into the lower lumbar area, but not the upper thoracic region (and therefore closer to the brain) produced antinociception (53).

Despite the fact that intrathecally administered cannabinoids produce antinociception at the spinal level, brain sites also contribute to this effect following systemic administration of cannabinoids in rats (53). Direct evidence implicating a supraspinal site of action were the observations that intracerebroventricular administration of WIN 55,212–2, CP 55,940, and Δ^9-THC produced antinociception (50,63). Assessment of the biodistribution of [^{3}H]-WIN 55,212–2 indicated that the majority of drug detected remained in the brain during the time of maximal effects with no detectable drug found in the spinal cord (63).

Direct administration of cannabinoids into brain sites containing cannabinoid receptors, and implicated in antinociception, has revealed interesting findings. The periaqueductal gray (PAG), a brain area that has been implicated in antinociception (4), and which has a much higher density of cannabinoid receptors than other brainstem structures (36), is a likely candidate to be involved in cannabinoid-induced antinociception. Intracerebral injections of WIN 55,212–2 into the dorsolateral PAG or dorsal raphe nucleus, but not the ventral PAG, medial septal area, lateral habenula, arcuate nucleus, or perihypothalamic area, produced a moderate antinociceptive effect (64). Conversely, CP 55,940 administered into the posterior ventrolateral area, in the region of the dorsal raphe produced antinociception and profound catalepsy (50). This effect exhibited regional specificity as drug administration into either the dorsolateral or anterior ventrolateral PAG sites or outside of the PAG borders failed to produce antinociception. Microinjection of CP 55,940 into other brain areas that contain a high concentration of cannabinoid receptors (36), but not generally associated with nociceptive processing, including the dorsal hippocampus and caudate putamen failed to produce antinociception (50,51). On the other hand, administration of WIN 55,212–2 and HU 210, but the inactive WIN 55,212–3, elicited antinociception when administered into the rostral ventromedial medulla, another brain region associated with antinociception (65). In addition, SR 141716A greatly attenuated the antinociceptive effects of HU 210. Although these findings suggest that direct administration of cannabinoids into the PAG or the rostral ventromedial medulla can elicit antinociceptive effects, they do not address the issue of whether these brain areas play necessary roles in the expression of cannabinoid-induced antinociception following its systemic administration. Similarly, these results do not rule out the involvement of other brain sites in the antinociceptive effects of systemically administered cannabinoids as in the case of morphine (109).

3.5. Interactions Between Cannabinoids and Opioids

Similarities between the opioids and THC include their antinociceptive properties. There is evidence that the combination of opioids and cannabinoids may be more effective in blocking pain than either agent alone. It has been shown that the antinociceptive effect of Δ^9-THC and morphine are additive following intravenous administration of both drugs, implying distinct mechanisms of action (30). Intrathecal administration of several cannabinoids leads to synergism with intrathecal and intracerebroventricular administered morphine in the production of antinociception in mice (103). Although pretreatment with morphine enhanced the effects of Δ^9-THC, pretreatment of the mice with naloxone (subcotaneously or intrathecally) failed to block the antinociceptive effects of the cannabinoids indicating that the cannabinoid-induced antinociception does not occur via interactions with the μ opioid receptor. Pretreatment of mice with Δ^9-THC significantly enhanced the potency of intrathecally administered morphine. Parallel shifts in morphine dose-response curves were produced not only with Δ^9-THC, but also with 11-OH-Δ^9-THC, Δ^8-THC and levonantradol, but not by CP-55,940. Thus, the antinociceptive effects of intrathecally administered morphine are enhanced by the pretreatment with some, but not all, cannabinoids active at the CB_1 receptor (103). At the present, there are no published reports that have examined the interaction between opioids and THC in managing pain and only one study has assessed the side effects of THC in the presence of an opioid. In this study (45a), all subjects were given a single dose of oxymorphone (11 mg/70 kg, intrathecally) followed by cumulative doses of THC (27–134 µg/kg. intravenously). Although significant increases in respiratory depression, heart rate, and cardiac index were reported following this drug combination, no firm conclusions can be made from this study because of the lack of controls for oxymorphone. Clearly, more work is needed to investigate possible interactions between THC and opioids for alleviating pain as well as characterizing potential side effects.

4. CONCLUSIONS

In conclusion, considerable controversy remains regarding the analgesic effectiveness of smoked *Cannabis* and oral THC in humans. It would appear that the etiology of pain is a determining factor in their effectiveness. Clearly, additional controlled studies are necessary before any conclusions can be made. On the other hand, there is compelling evidence that THC and its synthetic derivatives are effective in a wide range of antinociceptive tests in laboratory animals. In addition, there is overwhelming evidence that the antinociceptive effects of exogenously administered cannabinoids are mediated through cannabinoid receptors located in the CNS areas associated with the perception of pain. Despite the equivocal results obtained with clinical THC studies, there is a great potential to develop this novel class of analgesics for the clinical treatment of pain. One possible approach that has the potential to augment antinociception and decrease side effects is the coadministration of cannabinoids and opioids. Although there does appear to be an endogenous cannabinoid system, it remains to be established whether endogenous cannabinoids modulate pain, and if so, whether this system is tonically active or activated by conditions such as stress or chronic pain. The ongoing development of novel cannabinoids and other agents designed to manipulate the endogenous cannabinoid system will undoubtedly address these questions.

ACKNOWLEDGEMENTS

Portions of this work were supported by grants DA-03672, DA-05274, and DA-08387 from the National Institute on Drug Abuse.

REFERENCES

1. Adams, I. B., Compton, D. R. and Martin, B. R. (1998) Assessment of anandamide interaction with the cannabinoid brain receptor: SR 141716A antagonism studies in mice and autoradiographic analysis of receptor binding in rat brain. *J. Pharmacol. Exp. Ther.* **284**, 1209–1217.
2. Adams, I. B., Ryan, W., Singer, M., Thomas, B. F., Compton, D. R., Razdan, R. K. and Martin, B. R. (1995) Evaluation of cannabinoid receptor binding and in vivo activities for anandamide analogs. *J. Pharmacol. Exp. Ther.* **273**, 1172–1181.
3. Barg, J., Fride, E., Hanus, L., Levy, R., Matus-Leibovitch, N., Heldman, E., Bayewitch, M., Mechoulam, R. and Vogel, Z. (1995) Cannabimimetic behavioral effects and adenylate cyclase inhibition by two new endogenous anandamides. *Eur. J. Pharmacol.* **287**, 145–152.
4. Basbaum, A. I. and Fields, H. L. (1984) Endogenous pain control systems: brainstem spinal pathways and endorphin circuitry. *Annu. Rev. Neurosci.* **7**, 309–338.
5. Bell, M. R., D'Ambra, T. E., Kumar, V., Eissenstat, M. A., Herrmann, J. L., Wetzel, J. R., Rosi, D., Philion, R. E., Daum, S. J., Hlasta, D. J., Kullnig, R. K., Ackerman, J. H., Haubrich, D. R., Luttinger, D. A., Baizman, E. R., Miller, M. S. and Ward, S. J. (1991) Antinociceptive (aminoalkyl)indoles. *J. Med. Chem.* **34**, 1099–1110.
6. Bensemana, D. and Gascon, A. L. (1978) Relationship between analgesia and turnover of brain biogenic amines. *Can. J. Physiol. Pharmacol.* **56**, 721–730.
7. Bicher, H. J. and Mechoulam, R. (1968) Pharmacological effects of two active constituents of marijuana. *Arch. Int. Pharmacodyn.* **172**, 24–31.
8. Bloom, A. S. and Dewey, W. L. (1978) A comparison of some pharmacological actions of morphine and Δ^9-tetrahydrocannabinol in the mouse. *Psychopharmacology* **57**, 243–248.
9. Chen, J., Paredes, W., Li, J., Smith, D., Lowinson, J. and Gardner, E. (1990) Δ^9-Tetrahydrocannabinol produces naloxone-blockable enhancement of presynaptic basal dopamine efflux in nucleus accumbens of conscious, freely-moving rats as measured by intracerebral microdialysis. *Psychopharmacology* **102**, 156–162.
10. Chesher, G. B., Dahl, C. J., Everingham, M., Jackson, D. M., Merchant-Williams, H. and Starmer, G. A. (1973) The effect of cannabinoids on intestinal motility and their antinociceptive effect in mice. *Br. J. Pharmacol.* **49**, 588–594.
11. Clark, W. C., Janal, M. N., Zeidenberg, P. and Nahas, G. G. (1981) Effects of moderate and high doses of marihuana on thermal pain: a sensory decision theory analysis. *J. Clin. Pharmacol.* **21**, 299S–310S.
12. Compton, D., Aceto, M., Lowe, J. and Martin, B. (1996) In vivo characterization of a specific cannabinoid receptor antagonist (SR141716A): inhibition of Δ^9-tetrahdrocannabinol-induced responses and apparent agonist activity. *J. Pharmacol. Exp. Ther.* **277**, 586–594.
13. Compton, D. R., Gold, L. H., Ward, S. J., Balster, R. L. and Martin, B. R. (1992) Aminoalkylindole analogs: cannabimimetic activity of a class of compounds structurally distinct from Δ^9-tetrahydrocannabinol. *J. Pharmacol. Exp. Ther.* **263**, 1118–1126.
14. Compton, D. R., Johnson, M. R., Melvin, L. S. and Martin, B. R. (1992) Pharmacological profile of a series of bicyclic cannabinoid analogs: classification as cannabimimetic agents. *J. Pharmacol. Exp. Ther.* **260**, 201–209.
15. Compton, D. R., Rice, K. C., De Costa, B. R., Razdan, R. K., Melvin, L. S., Johnson, M. R. and Martin, B. R. (1993) Cannabinoid structure-activity relationships: correlation of receptor binding and in vivo activities. *J. Pharmacol. Exp. Ther.* **265**, 218–226.
16. Davies, R. L., Raventos, C. and Walpole, D. (1946) A method for the evaluation of analgesic activity using rats. *Br. J. Pharmacol.* **1**, 113–264.
17. Dennis, S. G. and Melzack, R. (1979) Comparison between phasic and tonic pain in animals. In: *Advances in Pain Research and Therapy* (Bonica, J. J., ed.) Raven, New York, p. 747–760.
18. Deutsch, D. G. and Chin, S. A. (1993) Enzymatic synthesis and degradation of anandamide, a cannabinoid receptor agonist. *Biochem. Pharmacol.* **46**, 791–796.

19. Devane, W. A., Breuer, A., Sheskin, T., Järbe, T. U. C., Eisen, M. S. and Mechoulam, R. (1992) A novel probe for the cannabinoid receptor. *J. Med. Chem.* **35**, 2065–2069.
20. Devane, W. A., Dysarz, F. A., Johnson, M. R., Melvin, L. S. and Howlett, A. C. (1988) Determination and characterization of a cannabinoid receptor in rat brain. *Mol. Pharmacol.* **34**, 605–613.
21. Devane, W. A., Hanus, L., Breuer, A., Pertwee, R. G., Stevenson, L. A., Griffin, G., Gibson, D., Mandelbaum, A., Etinger, A. and Mechoulam, R. (1992) Isolation and structure of a brain constituent that binds to the cannabinoid receptor. *Science* **258**, 1946–1949.
22. Dewey, W. L. (1986) Cannabinoid pharmacology. *Pharmacol. Rev.* **38**, 151–178.
23. Dewey, W. L., Harris, L. S. and Kennedy, J. S. (1972) Some pharmacological and toxicological effects of 1-trans- 8 and 1-trans- 9 -tetrahydrocannabinol in laboratory rodents. *Arch. Int. Pharmacodyn. Ther.* **196**, 133–145.
24. Edsall, S. A., Knapp, R. J., Vanderah, T. W., Roeske, W. R., Consroe, P. and Yamamura, H. I. (1996) Antisense oligodeoxynucleotide treatment to the brain connabinoid receptor inhibits antinociception. *NeuroReport* **7**, 593–596.
25. Eissenstat, M. A., Bell, M. R., D'Ambra, T. E., Alexander, E. J., Daum, S., Ackerman, J., Gruett, M., Kumar, V., Estep, K. G., Olefirowicz, E. M., Wetzel, J., Alexander, M. D., Weaver, J., Haycock, D., Luttinger, D., Casiano, F., Chippari, S., Kuster, J., Stevenson, J. and Ward, S. J. (1995) Aminoalkylindoles: structure-activity relationships of novel cannabinoid mimetics. *J. Med. Chem.* **38**, 3094–3105.
26. Fride, E. (1995) Anandamides: tolerance and cross-tolerance to Δ^9-tetrahydrocannabinol. *Brain Res.* **697**, 83–90.
27. Fride, E. and Mechoulam, R. (1993) Pharmacological activity of the cannabinoid receptor agonist, anandamide, a brain constituent. *Eur. J. Pharmacol.* **231**, 313–314.
28. Gardner, E. L. and Lowinson J. H. (1991) Marijuana's interaction with brain reward systems–update 1991. *Pharmacol. Biochem. Behav.* **40**, 571–580.
29. Gardner, E. L., Paredes, W., Smith, D., Donner, A., Milling, C., Cohen, A. and Morrison, D. (1988) Facilitation of brain stimulation reward by Δ^9-tetrahydrocannabinol. *Psychopharmacology* **96**, 142–144.
30. Gennings, C., Carter, W. H. and Martin, B. R. (1994) Response-surface analysis of morphine sulfate and 9-tetrahydrocannabinol interaction in mice. In: *Case Studies in Biom.* (Lange, N. ed.) Wiley, New York pp. 429–451.
31. Gilbert, P. E. (1981) A comparison of THC, nantradol, nabilone, and morphine in the chronic spinal dog. *J. Clin. Pharmacol.* **21**, 311S–319S.
32. Gough, A. L. and Olley, J. E. (1978) Catalepsy induced by intrastriatal injections of Δ^9-THC and 11-OH-Δ^9-THC in the rat. *Neuropharmacology* **17**, 137–144.
33. Grinspoon, L. and Bakalar, J. B. (1993) *Marihuana: The Forbidden Medicine* Yale University Press, New Haven, CT, p. 184.
34. Harris, L. S. (1971) General and behavioral pharmacology. *Pharmacol. Rev.* **23**, 285–294.
35. Harris, R. T., Waters, W. and McLendon, D. (1974) Evaluation of reinforcing capability of Δ^9-tetrahydrocannabinol in rhesus monkeys. *Psychopharmacologia* **37**, 23–29.
36. Herkenham, M., Lynn, A. B., Johnson, M. R., Melvin, L. S., de Costa, B. R. and Rice, K. C. (1991) Characterization and localization of cannabinoid receptors in rat brain: a quantitative in vitro autoradiographic study. *J. Neurosci.* **11**, 563–583.
37. Herzberg, U., Eliav, E., Bennett, G. J. and Kopin, I. J. (1997) The analgesic effects of *R* (+) WIN 55,212–2 mesylate, a high affinity cannabinoid agonist, in a rat model of neuropathic pain. *Neuro. Lett.* **221**, 157–160.
38. Hill, S. Y., Goodwin, D. W., Schwin, R. and Powell, B. (1974) Marijuana: CNS depressant or excitant? *Am. J. Psychiat.* **131**, 313–315.
39. Hill, S. Y., Schwin, R., Gooodwin, D. W. and Powell, B. J. (1974) Marihuana and pain. *J. Pharmacol. Exp. Ther.* **188**, 415–418.
40. Hohmann, A., Martin, W. J., Tsou, K. and Walker, J. M. (1995) Inhibition of noxious stimulus-evoked activity of spinal cord dorsal horn neurons by the cannabinoid win 55,212–2. *Life Sci.* **56**, 2111–2118.
41. Howlett, A. C., Johnson, M. R., Melvin, L. S. and Milne, G. M. (1988) Nonclassical cannabinoid analgetics inhibit adenylate cyclase: development of a cannabinoid receptor model. *Mol. Pharmacol.* **33**, 297–302.
42. Huffman, J. W., Dai, D., Martin, B. R. and Compton, D. R. (1994) Design, synthesis and pharmacology of cannabimimetic indoles. *Bioorg. Med. Chem. Lett.* **4**, 563–566.
43. Jain, A. K., Ryan, J. E., McMahan, F. G. and Smith, G. (1981) Evaluation of intra-muscular levonantradol in acute post-operative pain. *J. Clin. Pharmacol.* **21**, 3205–3265.
44. Jochimsen, P. R., Lawton, R. L., VerSteeg, K. and J. Noyes, R. (1978) Effect of benzopyranoperidine, a Δ^9-THC congener, on pain. *Clin. Pharmacol. Ther.* **24**, 223–227.

45. Johnson, M. R. and Melvin, L. S. (1986) The discovery of nonclassical cannabinoid analgetics. In: *Cannabinoids as Therapeutic Agents* (Mechoulam, R., ed.) CRC Press, Boca Raton, FL, pp. 121–144.

45a. Johnstone, R. E., Lief, P. L., Kulp, R. A. and Smith, T. C. (1975) Combination of Δ^9-tetrahydrocannabinol with oxymorphone or pentobarbital: effects on ventilatory control and cardiovascular dynamics. *Anesthesiology*, **42**, 674–684.

46. Karniol, I. G., Shirakawa, I., Takahashi, R. N., Knobel, E. and Musty, R. E. (1975) Effects of Δ^9-tetrahydrocannabinol and cannabinol in man. *Pharmacology* **13**, 502–512.

47. Kaymakcalan, S., Türker, R. and Türker, M. N. (1974) Analgesic effect of Δ^9-tetrahydrocannabinol in the dog. *Psychopharmacology* **35**, 123–128.

48. Lainton, J. A. H., Huffman, J. W., Martin, B. R. and Compton, D. R. (1995) 1-Alkyl-3-(1-naphthoyl)pyrroles: a new cannabinoid class. *Tetrahedron Lett.* **36**, 1401–1404.

49. Landsman, R. S., Burkey, T. H., Consroe, P., Roeske, W. R. and Yamamura, H. I. (1997) SR141716A is an inverse agonist at the human cannabinoid CB_1 receptor. *Eur. J. Pharmacol.* **331**, R1–R2.

50. Lichtman, A. H., Cook, S. A. and Martin, B. R. (1996) Investigation of brain sites mediating cannabinoid-induced antinociception in rats: evidence supporting periaqueductal gray involvement. *J. Pharmacol. Exp. Ther.* **276**, 585–593.

51. Lichtman, A. H., Dimen, K. R. and Martin, B. R. (1995) Systemic or intrahippocampal cannabinoid administration impairs spatial memory in rats. *Psychopharmacology* **119**, 282–290.

52. Lichtman, A. H. and Martin, B. R. (1991) Cannabinoid induced antinociception is mediated by a spinal α_2 noradrenergic mechanism. *Brain Res.* **559**, 309–314.

53. Lichtman, A. H. and Martin, B. R. (1991) Spinal and supraspinal mechanisms of cannabinoid-induced antinociception. *J. Pharmacol. Exp. Ther.* **258**, 517–523.

54. Lichtman, A. H. and Martin, B. R. (1997) The selective cannabinoid antagonist, SR 141716A, blocks cannabinoid-induced antinociception in rats. *Pharmacol. Biochem. Behav.* **57**, 7–12.

55. Lichtman, A. H., Smith, P. B. and Martin, B. R. (1992) The antinociceptive effects of intrathecally administered cannabinoids are influenced by lipophilicity. *Pain* **51**, 19–26.

56. Little, P. J., Compton, D. R., Johnson, M. R., Melvin, L. S. and Martin, B. R. (1988) Pharmacology and stereoselectivity of structurally novel cannabinoids in mice. *J. Pharmacol. Exp. Ther.* **247**, 1046–1051.

57. Little, P. J., Compton, D. R., Mechoulam, R. and Martin, B. R. (1989) Stereochemical effects of 11-OH-dimethylheptyl-Δ^8-tetrahydrocannabinol. *Pharmacol. Biochem. Behav.* **32**, 661–666.

58. Mansbach, R. S., Nicholson, K. L., Martin, B. R. and Balster, R. L. (1994) Failure of 9-tetrahydrocannabinol and CP 55,940 to maintain intravenous self-administration under a fixed-interval schedule in rhesus monkeys. *Behav. Pharmacol.* **5**, 219–225.

59. Martin, B. R. (1985) Characterization of the antinociceptive activity of intravenously administered Δ^9-tetrahydrocannabinol in mice, in: *Marihuana '84, Proceedings of the Oxford Symposium on Cannabis*, (Harvey, D. J., ed.) IRL Press, Oxford, UK, pp. 685–692.

60. Martin, B. R., Compton, D. R., Little, P. J., Martin, T. J. and Beardsley, P. M. (1987) Pharmacological evaluation of agonistic and antagonistic activity of cannabinoids. In: *Structure-Activity Relationships of Cannabinoids*, vol. NIDA Res. Monogr. Series #79, (Rapaka, R. S. and Makriyannis, A.) U. S. Govt. Printing Office, Washington, DC, pp. 108–122.

61. Martin, B. R., Compton, D. R., Thomas, B. F., Prescott, W. R., Little, P. J., Razdan, R. K., Johnson, M. R., Melvin, L. S., Mechoulam, R. and Ward S. J. (1991) Behavioral, biochemical, and molecular modeling evaluations of cannabinoid analogs. *Pharmacol. Biochem. Behav.* **40**, 471–478.

62. Martin, W. J., Hohmann, A. G. and Walker, J. M. (1996) Suppression of noxious stimulus-evoked activity in the ventral posterolateral nucleus of the thalamus by a cannabinoid agonist: correlation between electrophysiological and antinociceptive effects. *J. Neurosci.* **16**, 6601–6611.

63. Martin, W. J., Lai, N. K., Patrick, S. L., Tsou, K. and Walker, J. M. (1993) Antinociceptive actions of cannabinoids following intraventricular administration in rats. *Brain Res.* **629**, 300–304.

64. Martin, W. J., Patrick, S. L., Coffin, P. O., Tsou, K. and Walker, J. M. (1995) An examination of the central sites of action of cannabinoid-induced antinociception in the rat. *Life Sci.* **56**, 2103–2109.

65. Martin, W. J., Tsou, K. and Walker, J. M. (1998) Cannabinoid receptor-mediated inhibition of the rat tail-flick reflex after microinjection into the rostral ventromedial medulla. *Neurosci. Lett.* **33**, 242–36.

66. Matsuda, L. A., Lolait, S. J., Brownstein, M. J., Young, A. C. and Bonner, T. I. (1990) Structure of a cannabinoid receptor and functional expression of the cloned cDNA. *Nature* **346**, 561–564.

67. Mechoulam, R., Ben-Shabat, S., Hanus, L., Ligumsky, M., Kaminski, N., Schatz, A., Gopher, A., Almog, S., Martin, B., Compton, D., Pertwee, R., Griffin, G., Bayewitch, M., Barg J. and Vogel, Z. (1995) Identification of an endogenous 2-monoglyceride, present in canine gut, that binds to cannabinoid receptors. *Biochem. Pharmacol.* **50**, 83–90.

68. Melvin, L., Milne, G., Johnson, M., Subramaniam, B., Wilken, G. and Howlett, A. (1993) Structure-activity relationships for cannabinoid receptor-binding and analgesic activity: studies of bicyclic cannabinoid analogs. *Mol. Pharmacol.* **44**, 1008–1015.

69. Melvin, L. S., Johnson, M. R., Harbert, C. A., Milne, G. M. and Weissman, A. (1984) A cannabinoid derived prototypical analgesic. *J. Med. Chem.* **27**, 67–71.

70. Melzack, R. (1986) Neurophysiological foundations of pain, In: *The Psychology of Pain*, (Sternbach, K. A., ed.) Raven, New York, pp. 1–24.

71. Moss, D. E. and Johnson R. L. (1980) Tonic asnalgesic effects of Δ^9-Tetrahydrocannabinol as measured with the formailin test. *Eur. J. Pharmacol.* **61**, 313–315.

72. Novelli, G. P., Peduto, V. A., Bertol, E., Mari, F. and Pieraccioli E. (1983) Analgesic interaction between nitrous oxide and Δ^9-tetrahydrocannabinol in the rat. *Br. J. Anaesth.* **55**, 997–1000.

73. Noyes, J. R., Brunk, S. F., Avery, D. H. and Canter A. (1975) The analgesic properties of Δ^9-tetrahydrocannabinol and codeine. *Clin. Pharmacol. Ther.* **18**, 84–89.

74. Noyes, R. and Baram D. A. (1974) Cannabis analgesia. *Comp. Psych.* **15**, 531–535.

75. Noyes, R., Jr., Brunk, S. F., Baram, D. A. and Canter A. (1975) Analgesic effect of Δ^9-tetrahydrocannabinol. *J. Clin. Pharmacol.* **15**, 139–143.

76. O'Shaughnessy, W. B. (1842) On the preparation of Indian hemp and gunjah. *Trans. Med. Phys. Soc. Bombay* **8**, 421–461.

77. Olsen, J. L., Makhani, M., Davis, K. H. and Wall, M. E. (1973) Preparation of Δ^9-tetrahydrocannabinol for intravenous injection. *J. Pharm. Pharmacol.* **25**, 344.

78. Onaivi, E. S., Green, M. R. and Martin, B. R. (1990) Pharmacological characterization of cannabinoids in the elevated plus maze. *J. Pharmacol. Exp. Ther.* **253**, 1002–1009.

79. Parker, J. M. and Dubas, J. M. (1973) Automatic determination of the pain threshold to electroshock and the effects of Δ^9-THC. *Int. J. Clin. Pharmacol. Ther. Toxicol.* **7**, 75–81.

80. Parker, L. and Gillies, T. (1995) THC-induced place and taste aversions in Lewis and Sprague-Dawley rats. *Behav. Neurosci.* **109**, 71–78.

81. Petro, P. J. (1980) Marijuana as a therapeutic agent for muscle spasm or rigidity. *Psychosomatics* **21**, 81–85.

82. Price, D. D. and Dubner, R. (1977) Neurons that subserve the sensory-discriminative aspects of pain. *Pain* **4**, 307–338.

83. Raft, D., Gregg, J., Ghia, J. and Harris, L. (1977) Effects of intravenous tetrahydrocannabinol on experimental and surgical pain. Psychological correlates of the analgesic response. *Clin. Pharmacol. Ther.* **21**, 26–33.

84. Razdan, R. K. (1986) Structure-activity relationship in cannabinoids. *Pharmacol. Rev.* **38**, 75–149.

85. Reche, I., Fuentes, J. A. and Ruiz-Gayo, M. (1996) A role for central cannabinoid and opioid systems in peripheral 9-tetrahydrocannabinol-induced analgesia in mice. *Eur. J. Pharmacol.* **301**, 75–81.

86. Regelson, W., Butler, J. R., Schulz, J., Kirk, T., Peek, L., Green, M. L. and Zalis, M. O. (1976) Δ^9-Tetrahydrocannabinol as an effective antidepressant and appetite-stimulating agent in advanced cancer patients. In: *The Pharmacology of Marihuana* (Braude, M. C. and Sazara, S., eds.) Raven, New York, pp. 763–776.

87. Richardson, J. D., Aanonsen, L. and Hargreaves, K. M. (1997) SR 141716A, a cannabinoid receptor antagonist, produces hyperalgesia in untreated mice. *Eur. J. Pharmacol.* **319**, R3–R4.

88. Rinaldi-Carmona, M., Barth, F., Héaulme, M., Shire, D., Calandra, B., Congy, C., Martinez, S., Maruani, J., Néliat, G., Caput, D., Ferrara, P., Soubrié, P., Brelière, J. C. and Le Fur, G. (1994) SR141716A, a potent and selective antagonist of the brain cannabinoid receptor. *FEBS Lett* **350**, 240–244.

89. Shaofen, X., Xiaoding, C., Wanying, M., Zhenbang, X. and Yinying, P. (1989) Effect of combination of drugs with acupuncture on analgesic efficacy. *Acupuncture Electro-therapeutics Res. Int. J.* **14**, 103–113.

90. Shohami, E., Weidenfeld, J., Ovadia, H., Vogel, Z., Hanus, L., Fride, E., Breuer, A., Ben-Shabat, S., Sheskin, T. and Mechoulam R. (1996) Endogenous and synthetic cannabinoids recent advances. *CNS Drug Rev.* **2**, 429–451.

91. Smith, F. L., Fujimori, K., Lowe, J. and Welch, S. P. (1998) Characterization of Δ^9-tetrahydrocannabinol and anandamide antinociception in non-arthritic and arthritic rats. *Pharmacol. Biochem. Behav.* **60**, 1–9.

92. Smith, P. B., Compton, D. R., Welch, S. P., Razdan, R. K., Mechoulam, R. and Martin, B. R. (1994) The pharmacological activity of anandamide, a putative endogenous cannabinoid, in mice. *J. Pharmacol. Exp. Ther.* **270**, 219–227.

93. Smith, P. B. and Martin, B. R. (1992) Spinal mechanisms of Δ^9-tetrahydrocannabinol-induced analgesia. *Brain Res.* **578**, 8–12.

94. Smith, P. B., Welch, S. P. and Martin, B. R. (1993) *nor*-Binaltorphimine specifically inhibits Δ^9-tetrahydrocannabinol-induced antinociception in mice without altering other pharmacological effects. *J. Pharmacol. Exp. Ther.* **268**, 1381–1387.

95. Sofia, R. D. and Barry, H. III (1983) The effects of SKF 525-A on the analgesic and barbiturate-potentiating activity of Δ^9-tetrahydrocannabinol in mice and rats. *Pharmacology* **27**, 223–236.

96. Sofia, R. D., Vassar, H. B. and Knobloch, L. C. (1975) Comparative analgesic activity of various naturally occurring cannabinoids in mice and rats. *Psychopharmacology* **40**, 285–295.

97. Staquet, M., Gantt, C. and Machin B. (1978) Effect of a nitrogen analog of tetrahydrocannabinol on cancer pain. *Clin. Pharmacol. Ther.* **23**, 397–401.

98. Stein, E. A., Fuller, S. A., Edgemond, W. S. and Campbell W. B. (1996) Physiological and behavioural effects of the endogenous cannabinoid, arachidonylethanolamide (anandamide), in the rat. *Br. J. Pharmacol.* **119**, 107–114.

99. Thomas, B. F., Compton, D. R. and Martin B. R. (1990) Characterization of the lipophilicity of natural and synthetic analogs of Δ^9-tetrahydrocannabinol and its relationship to pharmacological potency. *J. Pharmacol. Exp. Ther.* **255**, 624–635.

100. Ward, S. J., Baizman, E., Bell, M., Childers, S., D'Ambra, T., Eissenstat, M., Estep, K., Haycock, D., Howlett, A., Luttinger, D. and Miller, M. (1991) Aminoalkylindoles (AAIs): a new route to the cannabinoid receptor? In: *Problems of Drug Dependence 1990: Proceedings of the 52nd Annual Scientific Meeting* vol. NIDA Res. Monogr. Series #105, (Harris, L. S., ed.) U. S. Gov. Printing Office, Washington, DC, pp. 425–426.

101. Welch, S. P. (1993) Blockade of cannabinoid-induced antinociception by *nor*-binaltorphimine, but not N,N-diallyl-tyrosine-aib-phenylalanine-leucine, ICI 174,864 or naloxone in mice. *J. Pharmacol. Exp. Ther.* **256**, 633–640.

102. Welch, S. P., Dunlow, L. D., Patrick, G. S. and Razdan, R. K. (1995) Characterization of anandamide- and fluoroanandamide-induced antinocicepton and cross-tolerance to Δ^9-THC following intrathecal administration to mice: blockade of Δ^9-THC-induced antinociception. *J. Pharmacol. Exp. Ther.* **273**, 1235–1244.

103. Welch, S. P. and Stevens, D. L. (1992) Antinociceptive activity of intrathecally administered cannabinoids alone, and in combination with morphine, in mice. *J. Pharmacol. Exp. Ther.* **262**, 10–18.

104. Willoughby, K. A., Moore, S. F. Martin, B. R. and Ellis, E. F. (1997) The biodisposition and metabolism of anandamide in mice. *J. Pharmacol. Exp. Ther.* **282**, 243–247.

105. Wilson, R. S. and May E. L. (1975) Analgesic properties of the tetrahydrocannabinols, their metabolites, and analogs. *J. Med. Chem.* **18**, 700–703.

106. Yaksh, T. L. (1979) Direct evidence that spinal serotonin and noradrenaline terminals mediate the spinal antinociceptive effects of morphine in periaqueductal gray. *Brain Res.* **160**, 180–185.

107. Yaksh, T. L. (1981) The antinociceptive effects of intrathecally-administered levonantradol and desacetyllevonantradol in the rat. *J. Clin. Pharmacol.* **21**, 3345–3405.

108. Yaksh, T. L. and Rudy, T. A. (1977) Studies on the direct spinal action of narcotics in the production of analgesia in the rat. *J. Pharmacol. Exp. Ther.* **202**, 411–428.

109. Yaksh, T. L., Yeung, J. C. and Rudy, T. A. (1976) Systematic examination in the rat of brain sites sensitive to the direct application of morphine: observation of differential effects within the periqueductal gray. *Brain Res.* **114**, 83–103.

43

Barbiturate Potentiating, Temperature Reducing, Analgesic, and Behavioral Effects of Some Synthetic Tetrahydrocannabinol Derivatives in Comparison with Δ^9-Tetrahydrocannabinol

Peter G. Waser and Anne Martin

Abstract

Four synthetic THC derivatives (Δ^9, 11-8-hydroxy-THC (A), Δ^{7-8}-9-hydroxy-THC (B), $\Delta^{8,9}$-3 (1′ dimethyl-3′ aza-4′keto)-THC (C), and $\Delta^{8,9}$-1′dimethyl-THC (D) were investigated for their pharmacological activity with reference to barbiturate potentiation, temperature reduction, and analgesic properties and were compared with Δ^9-THC.

All four substances were qualitatively more or less similar to Δ^9-THC. However, there were obvious quantitative differences. Substance D, a dimethylated compound on alpha-C of the side chain, displayed on action that was at least 10 times greater than that of Δ^9-THC in all experiments. The other substances, in comparison with Δ^9-THC, proved to be either less, or at most, equally effective. Whether, in fact, Δ^9-THC and the four derivates do have analgesic action is questionable from the results of the tests carried out. Δ^9-tetrahydrocannabinol (1 mg/kg) had no effect on avoidance learning of rats in a symmetrical Y maze, whereas 3 and to a lesser extent 9 mg/kg produced more rapid acquisition, with a significantly better performance compared with controls. Avoidance learning under Δ^9-THC was shown to be state dependent; also, behavioral tolerance to this drug developed rapidly. The synthetic THC derivatives B, C, and D had similar effects on behavior, showed similar development of tolerance, and made the rats cross-tolerant to Δ^9-THC. Compound D was again the most active.

From: *Marihuana and Medicine*
Edited by: G. G. Nahas et al.   © Humana Press Inc., Totowa, NJ

1. INTRODUCTION

Δ^9-tetrahydrocannabinol (THC), the natural main active substance of hashish and marihuana, is commonly known to potentiate barbiturate action *(1–3)* and reduce body temperature *(12,13)*. Information about the possible analgesic properties of Δ^9-THC is, on the other hand, not consistent *(4–6)*.

In this chapter the pharmacological activity and behavioral effect, especially on learning, of four synthetic THC derivatives are investigated and compared with the effect of Δ^9-THC. The substances–denoted A, B, C, and D in the text–were two hydroxy compounds (A and B) and two derivates of Δ^8-THC, modified in the side chain (C, D) (Fig. 1). These compounds were synthesized and given to us by T. Petrzilka, Department of Organic Chemistry, Federal Institute of Technology (ETH), Zürich. The synthesis of the hydroxy derivatives was an obvious step because it is thought that the first metabolite of Δ^9-THC, 11-hydroxy-THC, is more effective than Δ^9-THC, and is in fact an active form of Δ^9-THC *(7)*. For the compounds D and C, there was the interesting possibility of strengthening the analgesic components by the introduction of one quaternary C atom neighboring the phenol ring.

Although substance D is known to induce changes in the electroencephalogram *(8)*, there is no information available at all for the substances A, B, and C.

2. METHODS

2.1. Animals

The experiments were carried out with mice of the C3H/He/Gif COB strain from the Animal Breeding Institute at the Veterinary Medicine Faculty, University of Zürich. Male animals were used for all experiments except for the hot-plate test.

2.2. Solutions

The substances A, B, C, and D, as well as Δ^9-THC, which served as the reference substance, were suspended in a 2% Tween-20, 98% saline solution. The substance being tested was combined shortly before the experiment with a corresponding amount of Tween-20 and was then made up to the required volume with saline solution.

The amount injected was 0.1 mL per 10 g mouse.

2.3. Determination of the Barbiturate Potentiating Effect

Ten mice were given the substance to be tested intraperitoneally, and one hour later were injected i.p. with 40 mg/kg pentobarbital. After losing consciousness, the animals were placed on their backs, and the time taken for spontaneous awakening was measured. The experiment was conducted at a room temperature of 22 to 23°C with each animal kept alone in a small cage. The percentage increase in the length of sleeping time was calculated in comparison with the length of sleep of the control animals ($n = 30$), which were injected only with the solvent and 1 hour later with 40 mg/kg pentobarbital (control = 100%). The dosages were for Δ^9-THC, 5, 10, 25, and 50 mg/kg; for the substances A, B, and C, 25 and 50 mg/kg; and for substance D; 0.5, 1, 2.5, and 5 mg/kg.

2.4. Determination of the Hypothermic Effect

The rectal body temperature of the mice was measured before i.p. injection of the substance ($n = 10$) or solvent ($n = 60$). The first temperature reading was taken 30 minutes, and the second 1 hour, after injection. Four or five further readings were taken at hourly intervals. The dosages were for Δ^9-THC, 25, 50, and 100 mg/kg and for substance D, 2.5, 5, and 10

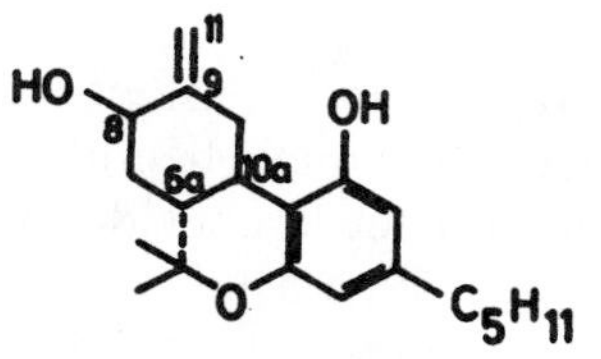

compound A

(-)-$\Delta^{9,11}$-6a,10a- trans-8-hydroxy-
tetrahydrocannabinol

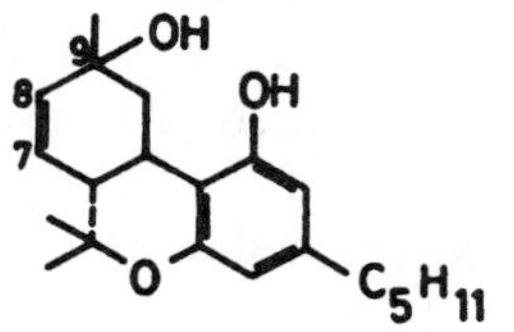

compound B

(-)-$\Delta^{7,8}$-6a,10a- trans-9-hydroxy-
tetrahydrocannabinol

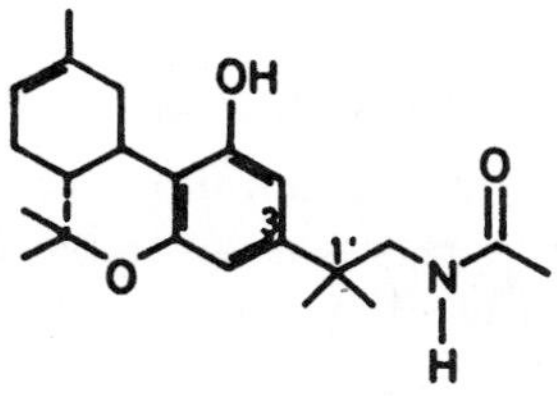

compound C

(-)-$\Delta^{8,9}$-6a,10a- trans,3 (1'- dimethyl-
3'aza-4'keto)-
tetrahydrocannabinol

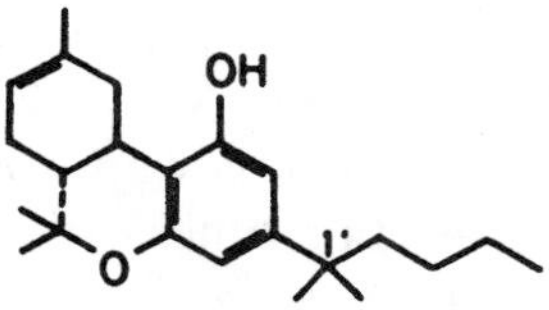

compound D

(-)$\Delta^{8,9}$-6a,10a- trans-(1'-dimethyl)-
tetrahydrocannabinol

Fig. 1. Structural formulas of A9-THC and derivatives A, B, C, and D. (Courtesy of T. Petrzilka).

mg/kg. The measurements, which were carried out at a room temperature of 22 to 23°C, were taken with a thermoelement inserted 2.5 cm into the rectum.

2.5. Determination of the Analgesic Effect

2.5.1. WRITHING TEST

For this experiment (14) 10 mice were injected intraperitoneally with the substance to be tested and 10 mice with the solvent. One hour later, 0.25 mL of an 0.7% acetic acid solution was administered intraperitoneally. During the 15 minutes following the acetic acid injection, the number of cramps caused by the acetic acid in the animals was counted. The percentage reduction of the cramps, as compared with the number in the control group, was taken as an estimation of the analgesic effectiveness of the substances. The dosages were for morphine-HCl, 2.5, 5, and 10 mg/kg; for Δ^9-THC, 2.5, 3.5, 5, and 10 mg/kg; for substances A, B, and C, 10, 20, and 40 mg/kg; and for substance D, 0.5, 0.75, 1, 5, and 10 mg/kg.

2.5.2. HOT-PLATE TEST

In this test *(15)* mice were placed on a plate that was kept at a constant temperature of 64°C. In response to the painful stimulation of their feet, the animals begin to jump after a certain length of time. The increase in the time taken to react is considered a measurement of the analgesic effectiveness of the substance. Ten female mice were first tested twice with an interval of 30 minutes between the tests. The mean reaction time of the two measurements served as the base value (0 value). Then the substance to be tested or the solution (control) were injected (10 mice per experimental and 37 mice in control group, all female). The next measurements on the hot plate were taken after 30, 60, 90, 120, and 180 minutes. The mean reaction times were compared with the 0 value of the group, and the increase or decrease in latencies was calculated as percentage values. The experiment with Δ^9-THC was replicated with 10 male mice in each experimental and 8 in the control group. The dosages were for morphine-HCl, 5, 10, and 20 mg/kg; for Δ^9-THC, 10 and 20 mg/kg; for substances A, B, and C, 20 mg/kg; and for substance D, 1, 2, and 5 mg/kg.

2.6. Conditioning Experiments with Rats

The influence of Δ^9-THC and derivatives A, B, C, and D, administered intraperitoneally one hour before session, on learning and behavior of rats was investigated using a condition avoidance response test (CAR) over a 25- to 35-week period that included two experimental sessions per week. Four groups of 9–10 10 rats of the CFN-COBS strain were trained in a symmetrical Y maze for the acquisition of the CAR *(9)*. The rats learned, upon onset of a light and tone (conditioned stimuli), to go to the lit compartment of the Y maze, and thereby to avoid the unconditioned electric shock stimulus delivered through the grid floors in the two incorrect compartments. The number of trials per session was increased from 15 in the first to 30 in the fourth and later sessions. The percentage of correct responses per session provided the avoidance rate. Once the rats were conditioned, effects of the compound on the CAR response and average reaction time (time from onset of the conditioned stimulus to obtainment of the correct response) were determined.

3. RESULTS

3.1. Barbiturate Potentiating Effect

Δ^9-THC and the substances A, B, C, and D lengthened the duration of barbiturate-induced sleep of the mice, depending on the dosage. Substance D proved to be the most effective, and produced in doses of 0.5–5 mg/kg the same increase in the duration of sleep as 5–50 mg/kg of Δ^9-THC. In contrast, Δ^9-THC, in doses of 25–50 mg/kg, was two to four times more active than compounds A, B, and C (*see* Table 1).

3.2. Lowering of Rectal Body Temperature

All of the substances investigated (Δ^9-THC and the compounds A, B, C, and D) produced a lowering of the rectal temperature (Fig. 2 A–C), which was dependent on the dose. The maximal reduction in temperature was reached after 30 minutes to one hour for substances Δ^9-THC, A, B, and C, but only after about four hours with substance D. In doses of 50–100 mg/kg, Δ^9-THC and substances A and B produced a reduction in temperature of 5–7°C; substance C was slightly less effective (3–5°C reduction). Substance D proved to be extremely powerful: 2.5, 5, and 10 mg/kg (i.e., one-tenth of the THC dose) produced maximum temperature reductions of 5, 7, and 9°C, respectively.

Table 1
Duration of Pentobarbital Sleep in the Mouse pretreated with Δ^9-THC and Compounds A, B, C, and D.

Substance[a]	Dosage mg/kg	Duration of sleep min ± SD	Percent increase in duration of sleep compared with control
Control	–	49.4 ± 9.3	–
Δ^9-THC	5	73.1 ± 22.1	48
	10	80.4 ± 17.5	63
	25	113.9 ± 22.9	130
	50	127.8 ± 33.5	158
A	25	69.0 ± 15.7	40
	50	84.5 ± 16.1	71
B	25	64.2 ± 23.0	30
	50	89.2 ± 20.8	81
C	25	66.5 ± 23.0	35
	50	84.9 ± 20.0	72
D	0.5	65.7 ± 13.6	33
	1.0	82.1 ± 15.5	66
	2.5	106.0 ± 18.0	115
	5.0	130.7 ± 39.1	165

Control group $n = 30$, experimental groups $n = 10$.
[a] The substance to be tested was injected i.p. and one hour later 40 mg/kg pentobarbital was also injected i.p.

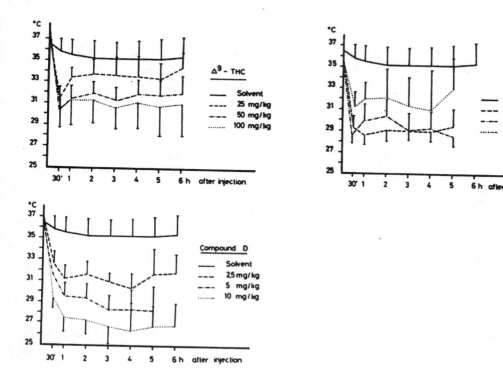

Fig. 2. (A–C) Lowering of rectal body temperature of mice after i.p. administration. Ambient temperature, 22°C to 23°C; control animals, $n = 60$; experimental groups for each dose, $n = 10$).

Table 2
Analgesic Activity of Δ^9-THC and Compounds A, B, C, and D
in Comparison with Morphine-HCI in the Writhing Test

Compound	Dosage mg/kg	Number of cramps in 15 minutes of each 10 animals	Percent analgetic activity with reference to control
Control (Tween-20/phys. NaCl)	0.1 mL/kg	112	0
Morphine-HCI	2.5	81	28
	5.0	40	64
	10.0	16	86
Δ^9-THC	2.5	123	0
	3.5	83	26
	5.0	23	80
	10.0	0	100
A	10.0	101	10
	20.0	46	59
	40.0	44	61
B	10.0	88	22
	20.0	42	63
	40.0	12	89
C	10.0	84	25
	20.0	93	17
	40.0	40	65
D	0.5	70	42
	0.75	37	69
	1.0	0	100
	5.0	0	100
	10.0	0	100

3.3. Analgesic Activity

The two test procedures gave strikingly different results. In the acetic acid test (Table 2) Δ^9-THC in doses of 2.5–10 mg/kg produced an effect similar to that of morphine; 10 mg/kg of Δ^9-THC supressed writhing caused by the acetic acid by 100%. The activity was somewhat less with substances A, B, and C; for a dosage of 40 mg/kg it was similar to that of 5–10 mg/kg of morphine and Δ^9-THC, respectively. The effects of substance D were 10 times greater than those of both morphine and Δ^9-THC; 1 mg/kg of D immediately suppressed all cramps. In contrast to the acetic acid test, the hot-plate experiment gave no indications of analgesic properties of Δ^9-THC and the THC derivatives (Table 3). Whereas 10–20 mg/kg of morphine produced a considerable lenghening of the reaction time (1150–1550%, respectively, 30 minutes after injection), the measurements for 10 and 20 mg/kg of Δ^9-THC and 1 and 2 mg/kg of substance D remained close to those of the control animals; they even showed a tendency to shorten the reaction time. For both substances there was considerable reaction of the animals to the heat stimulus, which was so great with a dosage of 5 mg/kg of D that further measurements were not possible. In addition pronounced catalepsy occurred, especially with substance D, which impeded the animals' move ment and made jumping impossible. Substances A, B, and C caused a slight but not significant (t-test) lengthening in the reaction time. The increase in sensitivity to stimulation and the catalepsy were less pro-

Table 3

Analgesic Activity of Δ^9-THC and Compounds A, B, C, and D in Comparison with Morphine-HCI in the Hot-Plate Test

Average reaction time in seconds ±SD and percent increase in reaction time compared with 0 value

Compound mg/kg		0 value (before injection) 100%	Time in minutes after injection				
			30	60	90	120	180
Control solution		3.0 ± 2.6	4.0 ± 3.5 33%	5.1 ± 5.1 70%	6.4 ± 5.2 113%	8.3 ± 5.9 176%	10.9 ± 11.3 263%
Morphine-HCI	5	4.4 ± 4.2	13.5 ± 12.1 207%	16.5 ± 12.4 275%	15.3 ± 19.8 248%	16.7 ± 16.7 280%	18.9 ± 20.3 330%
	10	2.3 ± 2.4	28.4 ± 27.6 1150%	23.2 ± 24.0 910%	22.6 ± 22.0 890%	13.0 ± 10.5 465%	7.8 ± 7.6 239%
	20	3.1 ± 2.6	51.2 ± 18.0 1550%	35.3 ± 27.3 1,040%	44.8 ± 24.7 1,350%	23.7 ± 21.1 662%	9.4 ± 12.9 203%
Δ^9-THC	10	5.5 ± 6.7	4.5 ± 4.7 −18%	3.0 ± 3.7 −46%	3.0 ± 3.7 −46%	3.1 ± 2.6 −49%	6.2 ± 5.2 −13%
	20	2.5 ± 2.1	4.9 ± 3.8 96%	4.7 ± 2.5 88%	2.8 ± 2.2 11%	3.3 ± 2.7 33%	4.3 ± 2.7 72%
A	20	4.7 ± 5.6	8.9 ± 11.4 83%	8.6 ± 11.1 82%	10.4 ± 14.3 117%	8.7 ± 8.2 83%	14.5 ± 14.4 205%
B	20	3.0 ± 3.1	8.3 ± 5.9 200%	9.1 ± 10.2 219%	7.1 ± 5.7 154%	8.5 ± 9.4 207%	12.2 ± 9.5 341%
C	20	3.5 ± 3.5	7.0 ± 9.6 100%	5.7 ± 7.6 63%	7.1 ± 6.5 103%	12.3 ± 13.3 250%	8.1 ± 5.2 132%
D	1	5.8 ± 6.9	8.3 ± 9.0 43%	12.8 ± 11.6 121%	9.3 ± 7.9 60%	10.2 ± 9.8 76%	11.1 ± 9.0 91%
	2	2.6 ± 2.9	6.7 ± 10.3 116%	3.0 ± 2.7 15%	5.0 ± 3.6 93%	3.7 ± 2.2 42%	5.3 ± 5.6 104%

Controls $n = 37$, experimental groups $n = 10$.

nounced with these substances. In order to see whether the sex of the animals had any influence on the results, an additional experiment with 10 and 20 mg/kg of Δ^9-THC and a control experiment were carried out, using male animals. There were no differences in the results between male and female animals.

3.4. General Behavioral Effects of Substances A, B, C, and D on Mice

The changes in the behavior of the animals brought about by the four derivatives were, apart from quantitative differences, basically the same as those seen with Δ^9-THC. The two-phase THC effect, stimulation and sedation, was similar. Usually, a period of stimulation occurred shortly after the injection and was followed by a period of sedation that lasted from four to six hours and was accompanied by ataxia. This last stage was disturbed, as with Δ^9-THC, by external stimuli such as noises or touching. As far as the changes in behavior are concerned, 5–20 mg/kg of Δ^9-THC had an effect comparable with that of substances A, B, and C in doses of 20–50 mg/kg. Substance D produced the same or even more pronounced reactions with doses that were 10 times lower than those of Δ^9-THC. Most remarkable was the strong cataleptic effect, which with doses of merely 5 mg/kg, prevented measurements on the hot plate; with doses over 2.5 mg/kg the animals moved in a peculiar crawling manner. At the same time an increased sensitivity to stimuli and a state of excitation, which lasted from three to four hours, were observed in the animals.

3.5. Influence of Δ^9-THC and Compounds A, B, C, and D on the Behavior and Learning of Rats

3.5.1. EFFECT ON ACQUISITION OF AN AVOIDANCE RESPONSE

The acquisition of an active avoidance response in a Y maze was not influenced by 1 mg/kg Δ^9-THC, but was facilitated with doses of 3 and 9 mg/kg (Fig. 3). The variance analysis for the period from experimental days 1–20 showed for the 3-mg/kg THC group a significantly better performance ($p < 0.0001$) than that of the control group. The avoidance rate of the 9-mg/kg group fluctuated considerably and their performance was significantly better ($p < 0.01$) only from days 5–20 of trials. Both groups eventually attained an avoidance rate of over 80%. The withdrawal of Δ^9-THC on the 26th day of the experiment produced in all groups a remarkable drop in the avoidance rate, which was most pronounced in the 9-mg/kg group (Fig. 3). Already in the next session, without THC, the rate increased again, and was recovered by Δ^9-THC application on the 28th day.

The rats in the 1-mg/kg group were excited and made frequent errors in finding the right compartment. The animals of the 3-mg/kg group were sedated and sleeping at the beginning of the experiments, but afterward became alert, and efficiently learned the flight and avoidance reactions. Irritability was strongest in the animals of the 9-mg/kg group. These animals occasionally fought and exhibited a high sensitivity to electric shock. After one hour they became heavily sedated and ataxic. In all groups, the gross behavioral effects of THC gradually became attenuated with repeated injections, and after 20 injections the animals appeared to be tolerant to THC.

3.5.2. EFFECT ON AVOIDANCE RESPONSE OF CONDITIONED RATS

If Δ^9-THC was replaced by compound D (0.1, 0.3, 0.9 mg/kg) in trained rats the avoidance rate was not changed, except when the experiment was run 1.5 hours after the injection instead of one hour (Fig. 4, day 6) as in the 9-mg/kg group. Withdrawal (days 9 and 11) of compound D resulted in a dose-dependent decrement in the avoidance behavior, which readily improved again on the 10th day upon reinjection for all groups. In the following days

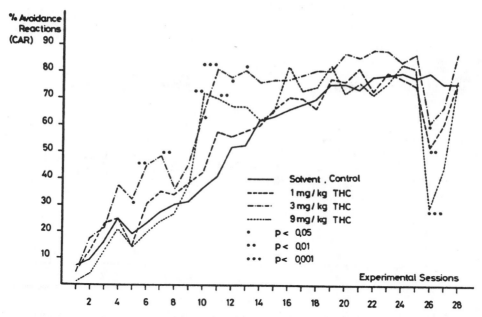

Fig. 3. Conditioning of rats. Acquisition of conditioned avoidance reaction (CAR ordinate) during consecutive training sessions (abscissa). The i.p. injection was given one hour before sessions, omitted before sessions 26 and 27.

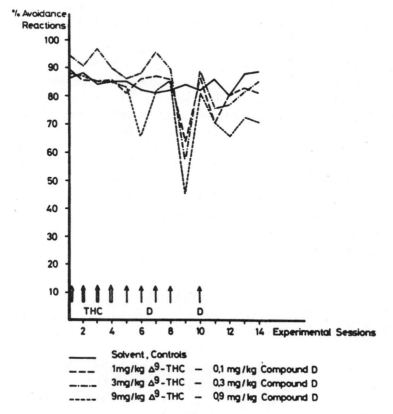

Fig. 4. Cross-tolerance in conditioned avoidance response between A9-THC and compound D. Control group, $n = 9$; experimental groups, $n = 10$.

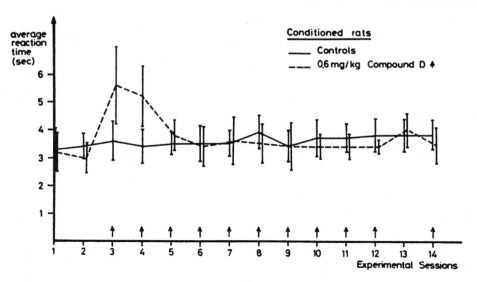

Fig. 5. Average reaction time (seconds) influenced by compound D. Signs of tolerance and withdrawal reaction after application during 10 days. Control group, $n = 9$; compound D, 0.6 mg/kg, $n = 9$.

(11–14) again only the solvent without compound D was given. All groups, and especially the 9-mg/kg group, showed disturbed avoidance behavior, which then slowly approached the control value. The similarity of this effect to THC tolerance and withdrawal indicates cross-tolerance between compound D and Δ^9-THC.

3.5.3. Effect on Average Reaction Time of Conditioned Rats

The reaction time of conditioned rats was significantly increased by 0.6 mg/kg of compound D given intraperitoneally on the first two days of administration ($p < 0.01$) because of sedation and catatonia, but not afterward when the animals became tolerant and less sedated (Fig. 5). Withdrawal on 13 day produced only a small increase in reaction time. Compounds B and C at 10-to 30-mg/kg doses had similar influences on the behavior of conditioned rats. The reaction time was prolonged by one to two second after the first injection, and then returned to normal, within five to seven injections, probably because of tolerance. Cross tolerance with Δ^9-THC (5–10 mg/kg) was demonstrated for both compounds.

The general behavior of the rats treated with compounds A, B, C, and D was biphasic (exciting-sedating), as with Δ^9-THC. The action of 5–20 mg/kg Δ^9-THC was comparable with 20–50 mg/kg A, B, and C. However, D was 20 times stronger, and with doses of 2.5–5 mg/kg produced catalepsia and increased sensitivity for three to four hours.

4. DISCUSSION

Δ^9-THC acted in our investigations exactly according to the information in the literature. The derivatives A, B, C, and D displayed basically the same action profile as Δ^9-THC. No qualitative differences could be established, but there were quantitative ones. The dimethylation in the side chain of the Δ^8-THC molecule (substance D) produced an increase in activity that was approximately 10 times greater than that of Δ^9-THC. It may be assumed that the methylation in the alpha position of the side chain has a protective effect against possible oxidative metabolism in this position. Some other mono- and dimethyl derivatives of Δ^9-THC (1′-methyl-THC, 1′, 2′-dimethyl-5-ethyl THC) and Δ^8-THC (1′-methyl-THC and 1′, 2′-

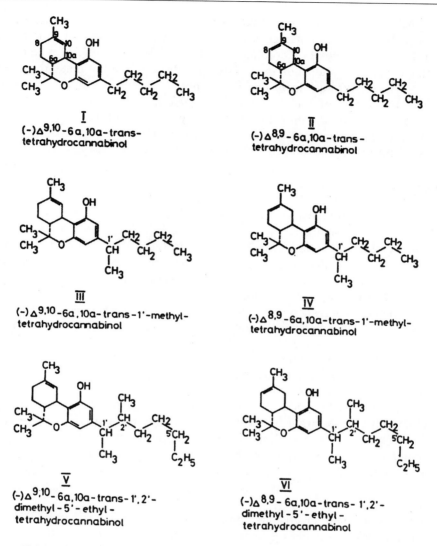

Fig. 6. Structural formulas of some side-chain methylated compounds of Δk and Δ⁹-THC.

dimethyl-5′-ethyl-THC), carrying one or two vicinal methyl groups in the side chain (Fig. 6), produced, after intraperitoneal injection of 120 mg/kg, excitation followed by sedation or hypnosis, and sometimes catatonia for 6–24 hours. They were generally more active than the natural tetrahydrocannabinols, but some produced at first convulsions, followed by strong sedation (Waser and Baumann, unpublished).

On the other hand the introduction of a polar group such as an acetamido group in the dimethylated side chain (compound C in Fig. 1) results in a substantial reduction of activity. This may be explained by the increase in solubility and the resulting accelerated elimination. The hydroxylation in positions 8 and 9 of the ring system (substances A and B) diminishes activity.

As far as the analgesic effectiveness of Δ⁹-THC and the four THC derivates is concerned, one must question whether it is, in fact, true analgesia. The evidence found in the literature on the analgesic action of THC is not consistent. Using the relatively nonspecific hot-plate test with rats, Buxbaum (5) obtained a result comparable with that of morphine; in mice, however, THC was less active. According to Bicher and Mechoulam (4), who obtained good results with the acetic acid test and inconsistent results with the hot plate, the mechanism of action of Δ^9-THC is different from that of morphine. They were able to demonstrate that under direct stimulation of the formatio reticularis the threshold value for the arousal response is, in contrast to morphine, lowered by Δ^9-THC; the fall in blood pressure caused by pain (stimulation of the sciatic nerve) is not affected by THC.

Henriksson and Järbe (10) refer to the considerable sensitivity of Δ^9-THC-treated animals to touch. According to Harris (6), the analgesic properties of Δ^9-THC depend largely on the method of investigation and the species of animals used. The action profile differs from that of other analgetics.

In our experiments with the acetic acid test, Δ^9-THC had an action that was nearly as great as that of morphine; substance D was approximately 10 times more active, whereas derivatives A, B, and C were much less effective. In contrast, the experiments carried out with the hot plate produced results that were not comparable with morphine. In the cases of Δ^9-THC and substance D an even greater shortening of the reaction time was seen, due, obviously, to the pronounced sensitivity to stimulation and the high excitability of the animals (4). It is questionable whether analgesic properties can be recognized on the basis of the writhing test alone. Chernov, Wilson, Fowler, and Plummer (11) point out that even nonanalgesic substances, such as physostigmine and pilocarpine, can produce positive results in this test. With Δ^9-THC it is possible that sedation, ataxia, or catalepsy counteracted the cramps produced by the acetic acid, and thereby stimulated analgesia.

The conditioned avoidance learning of rats was improved by 3–9 mg/kg Δ^9-THC, whereas 20 and 100 pg/kg LSD slowed the rate of acquisition of an active avoidance response (9). Both effects might be the result of increased sensitivity to stimulation, with THC combined with sedation leading to better discrimination of stimuli. After LSD there is predominantly excitation and an inability to distinguish between different stimuli. Δ^9-THC produces state-dependent learning, and tolerance to the drug develops rapidly. With LSD the final rate of avoidance was higher (> 90%) and state dependent, but no tolerance was observed.

Compounds B, C, and D changed behavior in the same way as Δ^9-THC, i.e., they increased the reaction times and made animals rapidly tolerant. Cross-tolerance is based on the similar chemical structure of all compounds, of which only D is much stronger and probably more slowly eliminated. Fine differences in the behavior of animals were not seen and will be studied in man.

5. POSTSCRIPT

Since the initial animals studies were reported, I have been able to conduct various other experiments with compound D, using myself as the subject. This I have done on several occasions and at varying dose levels. The oral doses were 0.15, 0.5, 1.5, and 2.0 mg compound D on sugar, ingested with water. Signs of psychotropic action were first noticed one to two hours after ingesting 1.0 mg. Stronger effects were noted after 2.0 mg. The symptoms consisted of sedation combined with a feeling of warmth, dizziness, general gaiety, confusion, hyperacusis (near auditory hallucinations) (no visual hallucinations), a strong feeling of hunger, and contractions of the stomach and the esophagus. After two hours, I was very tired. Later on I had a long sleep with no recall of dreams, and a hangover the next day.

Now that we know the limiting dose for psychotropic action, we plan to investigate the compound carefully and study its behavioral effects in man.

ACKNOWLEDGMENTS

We gratefully acknowledge the financial assistance of the Swiss National Research Foundation (Grant No. 3.692.71) and the technical help and advice of J. Huston, Isabelle Baumann, E. Pichler, H. Körber, and E. Kreis. Our special thanks belong to T. Petrzilka for his gift of the THC derivatives mentioned in the text.

Reprinted with permission from The Pharmacology of Marihuana, (M. C. Braude and S. Szara, eds.) Raven Press, New York, 1976, pp. 313–327.

REFERENCES

1. Bose, B. C., Saiti, A. Q. and Bhagwat, A. W. (1963) Effects of cannabis indica on hexobarbital sleeping time and tissue respiration of the rat brain. *Arch. Int. Pharmacodyn. Ther.* **141**, 520–524.
2. Garriott, J. C., King, L. J., Forney, R. B. and Hughes, F. W. (1967) Effects of some tetrahydrocannabinols on hexobarbital sleeping time and amphetamine induced hyperactivity in mice. *Life Sci.* **6**, 2119–2128.
3. Kubena, R. K. and Barry, H. III (1970) Interactions of Δ^9-tetrahydrocannabinol with barbiturates and methamphetarnine. *J Pharmacol. Exp. Ther.* **173**, 94–100.
4. Bicher, H. L. and Mechoulam, R. (1968) Pharmacological effects of two active constituents of marihuana. *Arch. Int. Pharmacodyn. Ther.* **172**, 24–31.
5. Buxbaum, D. M. (1972) Analgesic activity of Δ^9-tetrahydrocannabinol in the rat and mouse. *Psychopharmacologia* **25**, 275–280.
6. Harris, L. S. (1971) General and behavioral pharmacology. *Pharmacol. Rev.* **23**, 285–295.
7. Christensen, H. D., Freudenthal, R. J., Gidley, J. T., Rosenfeld, R., Boegli, G., Testine, L., Brine, D. R., Pitt, C. G. and Wall, M. E. (1971) Activity of Δ^8- and Δ^9-tetrahydrocannabinol and related compounds in the mouse. *Science* **172**, 165–167.
8. Lipparim, F., Scotti de Carolis and Longo, V. G. (1969) A neuropharmacological investigation of some transtetrahydrocannabinol derivatives. *Physiol. Behav.* **4**, 527–532.
9. Waser, P. G., Martin, A. and Heer-Carcano, L. (1977) The effect of Δ^9-tetrahydrocannabinol and LSD on the acquisition of an active avoidance response in the rat. *Psychopharmacologia*.
10. Henriksson, B. G. and Jarbe, T. (1971) Cannabis-induced vocalisation in the rat. *J. Pharm. Pharmacol.* **23**, 457–458.
11. Chernov, H. J., Wilson, D. E., Fowler, F. and Plummer, A. J. (1967) Non-specifity of the mouse writhing test. *Arch. Int. Pharmacodyn. Ther.* **167**, 171–178.
12. Holtzman, D., Lovell, R. A., Jaffe, J. H. and Freedman, D. X. (1969) 1-Δ^9-tetrahydrocannabinol: neurochemical and behavioral effects in the mouse. *Science* **163**, 1464–1467.
13. Haavik, C. O. and Hardman, H. (1973) Evaluation of the hypothermic action of tetrahydrocannabinols in mice and squirrel monkeys. *J. Pharmacol. Exp. Ther.* **187**, 568–574.
14. Koster, R., Anderson, M. and de Beer, E. J. (1959) Acetic acid for analgesic screening. *Fed. Proc.* **18**, 412.
15. Woolfe, G. and McDonald, A. D. (1944) The evaluation of the analgesic action of pethidin hydrochloride (Demerol). *J. Pharmacol. Exp. Ther.* **80**, 300–307.

44

Hyperalgesia and Response Bias Following Chronic Marihuana Smoking

W. Crawford Clark

Abstract

Fourteen habitual marihuana users were kept under surveillance in a research ward for three months. During the first and third month, the subjects were drug-free; during the second month, they smoked marihuana cigarettes containing 20 mg of THC. The subjects rated 180 thermal stimuli of nine different intensities between 30°C and 50°C. The data were analyzed according to sensory decision theory (SDT). This psychophysical model yields two measures of perceptual performance: *discriminability,* the subject's ability to discriminate among stimuli of different intensities, and hence, an index of neurosensory function, and the *response criterion,* which reflects attitudinal and emotional factors influencing report bias. The results for the lower-dose group, particularly at the noxious stimulus intensities, demonstrated the following. During weeks 3 and 4 of smoking (12.5 cigarettes a day), and for up to four weeks postsmoking, the subjects increased their ability to discriminate among the stimulus intensities, higher P(A), and lowered their pain report criterion, B, more pain reports. The conjoint changes in P(A) and B indicate that smoking had increased neurosensory activity mediating pain. That is, marihuana possesses hyperalgesic activity. The results for the higher-dose group (18.5 cigarettes a day) showed a slight decrease in P(A) during weeks 3 and 4 of smoking, but because it was unaccompanied by a change in criterion B, it may be concluded that heavy smoking, which induced dysphoria and tolerance, had no effect on the amount of pain experienced. In both groups changes in criterion, B, occurred without a parallel change in discriminability P(A). The lower-dose group reported more pain, lower B, during the weeks 1 and 2 of smoking; and the higher-dose group reported less pain, higher B, during the three to four weeks after smoking stopped. Since discriminability, P(A), was not altered on these occasions, changes in the criterion, B, represent response bias changes based on expectation.

From: *Marihuana and Medicine*
Edited by: G. G. Nahas et al.   © Humana Press Inc., Totowa, NJ

1. INTRODUCTION

1.1. Substantive Research Findings

The purpose of this paper is to review and reinterpret previously reported studies by Clark et al. (1,2) on the putative analgesic effect of marihuana smoking in the light of recent advances concerning its mode of action in the CNS. The folklore surrounding the use of various preparations of *Cannabis sativa* such as marihuana and hashish suggests that cannabinoids possess analgesic properties. However, the evaluation of possible analgesic properties of psychoactive substances such as marihuana that possess marked mood-altering characteristics presents a particularly difficult problem, since, as Clark et al. (3) have demonstrated by cluster analysis, pain is a complex mixture of sensations and emotions. Accordingly, as Dray et al. (4) emphasize, a change in pain report, and hence pain threshold, could be caused not only by altered sensory sensitivity but by changes in mood and expectation. Changes in pain report do not necessarily reflect a change in pain sensation. This is particularly true for clinical pain in which a patient's report of less pain following the administration of a psychoactive drug (or a placebo for that matter), may be merely the result of expectation, euphoria, reduced anxiety, or decreased nausea rather than a specific analgesic effect. The problem of response bias, which is inherent in the almost universally used method of limits, may be resolved by resorting to the sensory decision theory (SDT) model used in the study discussed here.

Recent animal studies (*see* refs. 5–7), demonstrate that cannabinoids act on receptors in the CNS, including regions that mediate pain (e.g., substantia gelatinosa) and memory (e.g., hippocampus). There are at least two types of receptors, CB_1 and CB_2, which are distributed in different regions of the CNS. Some CB_1 receptors are located on presynaptic nerve terminals where they can lead to suppression of the release of neurotransmitters and there are endogenous receptor agonists and antagonists. In spite of these advances in animal research and the finding by Jain et al. (8) that a cannabinoid-related substance, levonantrol, has an analgesic effect in humans, the possible role of marihuana as an analgesic in humans remains controversial.

Clinical trials that claim that marihuana produces analgesia are seriously flawed. According to Hollister (9) and others there is no question that cannabinoids reduce nausea and vomiting caused by chemotherapy for cancer. But analgesia is another matter. Noyes et al. (10) and Chang et al. (11) found that cancer patients undergoing chemotherapy and given THC reported less pain than those given a placebo. However, the patients' ratings on the pain (10) or comfort (11) scale presented to them (unfortunately they were not given a nausea scale) could readily have been influenced by a general feeling of well-being following the reduction in nausea and vomiting. It cannot be concluded from these studies that a specific analgesic effect had been produced. Nor can one rule out a placebo effect, the patients' expectation that the treatment would help. Given the psychotropic effect of marihuana, they could easily have peeked through the "double blind." Studies that do not involve the treatment of nausea have failed to find an analgesic effect. Gregg et al. (12) found no evidence of an analgesic effect on painful stimuli (injections, bone and tooth sectioning) associated with oral surgery; indeed, retrospectively, some of the THC patients reported greater awareness of surgical pain on THC trials than on placebo or diazepam trials.

Because of the problems associated with the measurement of clinical pain, human experimental, or "laboratory," pain models are helpful in understanding pain mechanisms. Although laboratory pain cannot duplicate the emotions experienced in the clinical setting, it has the following advantages: (i) reproducible activation of nociceptive afferents in specific sensory modalities; (ii) the intensity and duration of the noxious stimuli are known exactly;

(iii) greater homogeneity in the subject population permits a smaller sample size and lower costs; (iv) laboratory pain studies form a critical link between concepts derived from animal experiments and (v) clinical pain in humans; and laboratory pain has been successfully used to test in an objective manner the analgesic efficacy of drugs used in the management of pain.

A number of investigators have studied the effect of marihuana on the verbal response to calibrated noxious stimulation in human volunteers. However, they have yielded conflicting results. A double-blind study by Milstein et al. *(13)* showed a significant increase in the ability to tolerate pain among those who had smoked marihuana. On the other hand, Harris et al. *(14)* were not able to confirm the analgesic effect of THC. Gregg et al. *(12)* found no evidence that THC influenced the pain-tolerance threshold to noxious periosteal pressure and electrocutaneous stimulation. However, the lower-intensity pain sensitivity thresholds were slightly raised. In sharp contrast to those who reported either analgesia or no effect, Hill et al. *(15)* found that a dose of 12 mg of THC made the subjects more sensitive to painful electrical stimulation, that is, it actually decreased the pain threshold. This result is consistent with reports of heightened sensitivity or 'perceptual sharpening' described by Tart *(16)* in the auditory, taste, and olfactory modalities, and with the visual flicker fusion threshold described by Schwin et al. *(17)*. In this regard, Hill et al. *(14)* insightfully noted that the decrease in threshold they obtained may have been caused not by drug-induced physiologic changes but by the subject's expectation that pain sensitivity would be enhanced by marihuana.

1.2. Psychophysical Measurement: Method of Limits

The major reason for the confusion in the literature is the psychophysical procedure used: the ascending method of limits, or serial exploration. In this method the subject responds to a series of calibrated stimuli that steadily increase in intensity. As portrayed in Table 1, the observer on the left has a high threshold; faint pain is reported to a thermal stimulus of 48°C. This high threshold is generally interpreted as demonstrating sensory insensitivity to noxious stimulation (possibly he/she is suffering diabetic neuropathy, or has received an analgesic). In contrast, the observer on the right has a low threshold of 40°C and is considered very sensitive to pain (possibly he/she is suffering causalgia). However, the commonly held view that the threshold is a pure sensory measure is mistaken; it is equally possible that both observers are experiencing the same amount of pain, but that the subject on the left is simply more stoic, whereas the subject on the right is more squeamish.

Table 1
Pain Detection Thresholds by the Ascending Method of Limits or Serial Exploration

Stimulus	Response	
Temperature °C	High Threshold (48°C) (Stoic? Neuropathy?)	Low Threshold (40°C) (Squeamish? Causalgia?)
50	Pain ***	Withdraw
46	Very hot	Severe pain
42	Hot	Faint pain ***
38	Very warm	Very hot
34	Warm	Very warm
30	Nothing	Warm

*** Represents the interpolated method of limits threshold.

The problem with the method of limits is that it is impossible to distinguish between a neurosensory difference and an attitudinal, or response bias difference. Clark *(18)*, Clark and Goodman *(19)*, and Clark and Bennett, Clark *(20)* have demonstrated that pain thresholds may be: increased by a placebo described as an analgesic, either increased or decreased by changing the subjects' expectation, and, may vary with ethnocultural differences in stoicism. In brief, the method of limits fails to distinguish between pain sensation and pain report. The magnitude of these threshold changes can be as great or greater than that obtained with morphine. In addition to unmeasured response bias, the method of limits suffers another defect. Since the stimuli are presented in a regular ascending series, two errors unrelated to sensory function may occur. These are the error of anticipation: the subject, knowing that intensity is increasing, reports a stimulus as more intense even though it feels the same, and the error of habituation: if in doubt, the subject repeats the previous response. The habituation and anticipation problems may be avoided by using the method of constant stimuli in which the various stimulus intensities are presented in a random order. Here the threshold is the intensity at which 50% of the reports are "pain." However, the problem of response bias contamination of this threshold remains the same as with the method of limits. It may be necessary for the clinician to use the method of serial exploration at the bedside, but it is inexcusible to use it as a research instrument.

1.3. Psychophysical Measurement: Sensory Decision Theory

The confusion of sensory sensitivity and response bias inherent in the traditional psychophysical procedures has been solved by the SDT model. As described by Swets *(21)*, this model, as well as the Medical Decision Making model that applies decision theory to clinical judgments, is based on SDT. Clark *(22,23)* has reviewed its applications to problems in pain measurement. The intent of the model is to isolate the effect of the observer's idiosyncratic placement of the decision criterion (the intensity that the subject decides to call painful) so that a pure measure of discrimination is obtained.

SDT partitions the traditional threshold into two independent indices of observer performance. The sensory measure, d', P(A) or P_r (the indices are similar, but are based on slightly different assumptions), employs error rate to estimate the subject's ability to discriminate between stimuli of two different intensities. It reflects neurosensory function. For example, Gybels et al. *(24)* demonstrated a close relation between discriminability, P(A), based on the subject's rating of sensations to noxious thermal stimuli, and the concurrent spike discharge rate of C-fibers in the subject's superficial radial nerve. Yang et al. *(25)* and Clark and Yang *(26)* have demonstrated that morphine and partial carbocaine nerve block decreases P(A), presumably because the amount of sensory information reaching higher centers is attenuated. Clark *(22)* has reviewed a number of studies demonstrating that the discrimination index is not influenced by nonsensory variables (e.g., expectation, placebos, anxiety). The other SDT parameter, the report criterion, Lx, B, or B_r, quantifies the subject's criterion for reporting pain, that is, his tendency to report or to deny the presence of pain. A series of studies by Clark and associates *(22)* have shown that the pain report criterion can be altered by a placebo, instructions, age, ethnicity, and so on, without influencing the discriminability index.

A brief introduction to SDT follows. More details may be found in Green and Swets *(27)* and McNicol *(28)*. The stimulus-response matrix of sensory decision theory appears in Fig.1. In the binary decision case, stimuli of two intensities are presented randomly, and the subject responds "high" or "low," or "painful" or "not painful." Dozens of stimuli are randomly presented and judged. The report of high or pain to the higher-intensity stimulus yields the hit rate; a report of pain or high to the lower-intensity stimulus yields the false alarm or false affirmative rate.

RESPONSES

		"Pain"	"No Pain"
S T I	48°C	HITS .90	Misses .10
M U		(P_r=.5)	
L I	46°C	FALSE ALARMS .40	Correct Rejection .60
		(B_r= -.65)	

Fig. 1. Simple sensory decision theory measures of discriminability, P_r, and criterion B_r. Discriminability: Hit rate *minus* false affirmative rate measures the subject's ability to distinguish between higher and lower stimulus intensities, P_r =0.5. Criterion: The average of hit rate *plus* false affirmative rate measures the subject's response bias, B_r= -0.65. A low or liberal criterion (hence the minus sign) reflects a relatively large proportion of pain reports, whereas a high value identifies a stoic. In the present study the raw data were analyzed by McNicol's procedure to yield P(A) and B, analogous to P_r and B_r.

The readily understood SDT model devised by Snodgrass and Corwin *(29)* serves as a means of exposition here, since the basic concepts underlying the discriminability and criterion parameters, respectively, for the Gaussian (d′, L_x), the nonparametric (P(A),B) and the Snodgrass (P_r,B_r) models are similar. As shown in Fig. 1, the discriminability parameter, P_r = 0.5, is the hit rate minus the false alarm rate; it measures the ability of the subject to distinguish between two stimulus intensities. Good discrimination is defined by a combination of high hit rates and low false alarm rates, that is, a low error rate. Conversely, poor discriminability is defined by low hit rates and high false alarm rates. Obviously, when the difference between hits and false alarms equals zero, the observer is performing at chance level and P_r = 0. The other index of perceptual performance is the criterion, B_r = −0.65; it is the average of the hit and false Affirmative rates and measures the response bias of the subject, the tendency to favor one response category over the other. (The addition of the minus sign keeps values of B_r in conformity with L_x and B.) A low or liberal criterion reflects a large proportion of pain reports to both stimulus intensities, whereas a high value identifies a stoic who seldom reports pain. It is clear that values of P_r and B_r can vary independently of each other.

The advantages of the SDT approach are illustrated by four possible patterns of perceptual performance shown in Fig. 2. According to traditional psychophysics, subject-1 (S-1) with a pain response or hit rate of 0.90 to the 48°C stimulus appears to be much more sensitive (lower threshold) to noxious stimulation than S-2 with a hit rate of only 0.60. However, SDT analysis takes into account the false alarm rates, 0.40 and 0.10 for S-1 and S-2, respectively, and determines that P_r = 0.5 for both subjects. Thus, according to SDT, S-1 and S-2 are equal in their ability to discriminate between the 48°C and the 46°C stimuli. This suggests that equal amounts of neurosensory information are reaching higher decision-making centers. It also is obvious that S-3 and S-4, with their lower hit and higher false affirmative rates, are poorer discriminators than S-1 and S-2; in both instances their P_r = 0.1. Again, note that according to the traditional threshold measure, S-2 with fewer pain reports (hits = 0.60)

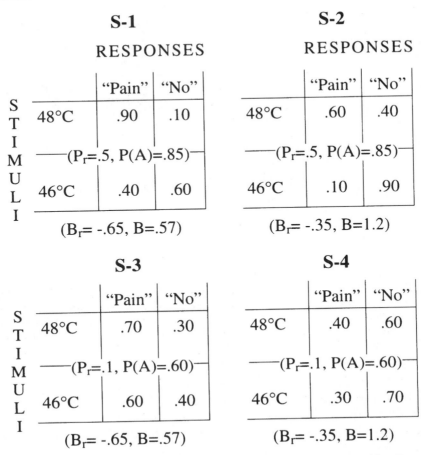

Fig. 2. Responses of four subjects with different discriminability, P_r, and report bias, B_r, to two intensities of thermal stimulation. The equivalent values of discriminability, P(A), and criterion, B, for McNicol's nonparametric SDT model also appear.

would be considered less sensitive to noxious stimulation than S-3 (hits = 0.70); however, SDT draws the opposite conclusion: S-3 is a far poorer discriminator than S-4.

The measure of response bias, the report criterion, is the other SDT index of perceptual performance. S-1 and S-3 with a large number of pain reports to both the low and high intensity stimuli exhibit a low pain-report criterion; for both subjects the criterion is $B_r = -.65$. In contrast, S-2 and S-4 with few pain reports manifest a high or stoical criterion, $B_r = -0.35$. The discrepancy between the SDT and the threshold analyses of the data is because the traditional procedures do not, and indeed cannot, take into account the influence of response bias on the threshold.

2. PROCEDURES

The present study will use McNicol's model to compute the discrimination and criterion measures P(A) and B in place of P_r and B_r, because the procedure is well-established in pain research, and is superior when treating rating scale data. (The rating-scale, which appears in Table 2, is similar to the example in Fig. 1 because the scale may be dichotomized serially between each response category.)

Table 2
Subject's Response Category Scale and Criterion, B

14	13	12	11	10	9	8	7	6	5	4	3	2	1
Nothing	Maybe something	Faint warmth	Warm	Hot	Very hot	Very faint pain	Faint pain	Pain	Very painful	**Withdrawal times(s)**			
										2.8	2.5	2.3	<2.0

The numbers associated with the response categories represent values of B. They and the mean withdrawal times less than 3.0 seconds do not appear on the scale given to the subject.
B represents the median category on the scale, half of the responses are above and half below. A high value of B indicates few reports of pain; a low value indicates many pain reports and withdrawals.

The purpose of the present study is to improve on earlier marihuana studies of laboratory pain in four ways: by examining the effect of chronic rather than single doses; by comparing higher and lower levels of consumption; by providing cigarettes assayed for cannabinoid content; and, most important, by using the SDT model instead of the method of limits to measure separately the effect of marihuana on pain sensation and pain report. According to SDT, if marihuana is an analgesic, it should decrease discriminability, P(A), and raise the pain report criterion, B. On the other hand, if marihuana enhances pain perception, it should increase P(A) and lower B. Furthermore, if there is a change in expectation without a change in neurosensory activity, then B would be raised or lowered without a change in P(A).

Detailed description of the results for both the sensory and memory studies and details of procedures, including recruitment, rules for exclusion, and so on, appear elsewhere (1,2). In the present report, the effects of high and low levels of consumption are examined, and the posttest data are treated in greater detail.

Fourteen males, 18–30 years old, who were regular users of marihuana but not other drugs, were admitted to the Drug Abuse Research Ward of the New York State Psychiatric Institute. The subjects were under 24-hour surveillance, were paid for participating in the study, and signed an informed consent form. The study was in three parts: a three- to four-week presmoking period, a four-week smoking period, and a four-week postsmoking period. Subjects smoked marihuana cigarettes prepared by the National Institutes of Drug Abuse, standardized to contain 2% Δ^9-tetrahydrocannabinol (20 mg per cigarette). At the end of the study the subjects were divided into higher- and lower-consumption groups. The average number of cigarettes smoked daily during each period appears in Table 3.

The subjects were administered the thermal pain test approximately every one to two weeks for a period of approximately three months. A modified Hardy-Wolff dolorimeter was used to present 120 thermal stimuli on each occasion. The stimuli were presented randomly with respect to intensity and focused in turn (to allow cooling) on 12 spots of India ink on the volar surface of each forearm. The calibrated stimulus intensities were: 108, 225, 270, 315, 360, and 405 mcal/sec/cm^2. These values approximated temperatures of: 30, 32, 35, 37, 39, 41, 43, 45, 48, and 50°C. The subjects responded from the category scale shown in Table 2.

3. RESULTS

Values of P(A) and B were computed for each subject for each of the nine pairs of stimulus intensities from 30–32°C to 48–50° C. Analyses of variance (ANOVA) were performed separately at each intensity pair for P(A) and B, and have been reported in detail elsewhere (1,2). The results, summarized over intensity, for discriminability, P(A), and criterion, B, including its related verbal response category, are presented in Table 3. For thermal discrim-

Table 3
Discriminability, P(A), and Criterion, B, Averaged Over Pairs of Thermal Stimuli
from 30–32°C to 48–50°C

		Smoking			
				Post 1	Post 2
		Weeks	Weeks	Weeks	Weeks
Session	Pre	1 and 2	3 and 4	5 and 6	7 and 8
Lower-dose group					
Cigarettes[a]	0	5.5	12.5	0	0
P(A)	0.69	0.70	0.72[c]	0.73[c]	0.73[c]
Criterion, B	9.5	8.6[c]	8.7[c]	8.3[c]	8.4[c]
Median Category[b]	H/VH	VH/VFP	VH/VFP	VFP	VFP
Higher-dose group					
Cigarettes[a]	0	8.5	18.5	0	0
P(A)	0.71	0.69	0.68[c]	0.69	0.70
Criterion, B	8.7	8.6	8.5	9.4	9.7[c]
Median category	VH/VFP	VH/VFP	VH/VFP	H/VH	H

V, very; H, hot; FP, faint pain.
[a]Mean number of cigarettes smoked daily.
[b]The median response category is determined from values of B, *see* Table 2.
[c]$p < .05$, difference from presmoking period.

inability, there was a significant session-by-group interaction, $F = 2.98$, $df = 4.48$, $p < 0.03$. According to the *posthoc* Tukey Honestly Significant Differences test (HSD), $q(5) = 4.04$, $df = 48$, $p \leq 0.05$, for a critical difference ≥ 0.03. Overall intensities discriminability for the more moderate consumers increased over the presmoking period during Weeks 3 and 4 and remained higher during the two postsmoking sessions. On the other hand, discriminability for the high-consumption smokers showed little change throughout except for a slight decrease in P(A) during weeks 3 and 4. The session-by-stimulus intensity interaction, $F = 1.84$, $df = 32,384$, $p < 0.004$, demonstrated that P(A) at the three noxious intensity stimulus pairs from 41–43°C to 48–50°C increased during weeks 3 and 4 of smoking and during postsmoking weeks 5 and 6 and 7 and 8, whereas discriminability for the innocuous intensity pairs from 39–41°C to 30–32°C to showed little change.

ANOVA for the report criterion, B, revealed a significant triple interaction for session-by-group-by-intensity, $F = 3.49$, $df = 32,384$, $p < 0.001$. According to the HSD test, $q(5) = 3.86$, $df = 32,384$, $p < 0.05$, for a critical difference of ≥ 1.2. This interaction was caused by differences between the moderate and heavy smokers in criterion values at different stimulus intensities over the various sessions.

4. DISCUSSION

The lower-consumption group, particularly at the noxious intensities above 41°C, demonstrated the most striking finding (Table 3). Compared to the presmoking period, both the increase in discriminability, P(A), and the decrease in B (more pain reports and withdrawals) during weeks 3 and 4 and the two postsmoking periods demonstrated that marihuana smoking had increased the sensitivity to noxious stimulation. According to the criterion, during the presmoking period fewer than half of the reports were in the painful region, whereas in the latter sessions over half of the reports ranged from very painful to severe pain and withdrawal. The parallel increase in discriminability, P(A), which indicates that more sensory information reached higher centers, also confirms that more pain was experienced.

There was absolutely no indication of an analgesic effect in the lower-dose group. These results confirm those of Hill et al. (15). It might be argued that the effects of mild analgesics cannot be demonstrated by cutaneous thermal stimulation. However, the finding of a significant hyperalgesic effect means that the measurement technique used can detect changes in sensory sensitivity and that the failure to find a decrement in discriminability, P(A), demonstrates that no analgesia resulted from marihuana smoking in the lower-dose group.

The high-dose group during weeks 1 and 2 showed a slight decrement in P(A); however, since it was unaccompanied by an increment in the pain report criterion (fewer pain reports) the decrease in P(A) probably does not reflect an analgesic effect. The heavy dose may have had a different pharmacological effect, since tolerance and marked dysphoria occurred in this group. Or the high dose may have clouded the subjects' consciousness and, hence, their ability to discriminate. In this regard, they performed somewhat more poorly on the memory and attention tests that were given as part of this study (2); this might have interfered with their sensory decision-making.

The concomitant changes found in P(A) and B may be interpreted in the light of earlier SDT studies (25,26). The administration of an analgesic and a partial local-nerve block were found to decrease P(A), led to poorer discrimination, and to raise the pain report criterion, B, with fewer pain reports. Conversely, a substance that increases discriminability and decreases the criterion must be enhancing the pain. Thus, it may be concluded from application of the SDT model that the lower-dose marihuana smokers experienced a hyperalgesic effect. In view of the well-established lipophilic quality of THC, it is not surprising that the effect on P(A) and B persisted for at least three to four weeks after cessation of smoking.

On two occasions the criterion changed without a change in P(A). The lower-dose group lowered their criterion during weeks 1 and 2, but P(A) was not altered. The lack of change in P(A) indicates that the amount of pain experienced was unchanged, whereas the lower criterion suggests that the subjects' expectation that marihuana would sharpen the pain experience, caused them to report more pain (lower criterion). The high-dose group set its presmoking criterion between very hot and very faint pain, and unlike the low-dose group, did not vary it until the Post 2 period when they raised their criterion and stoically described the stimuli as merely hot, but not painful.

Changes in the SDT criterion measure in the absence of a change in P(A) reflect only psychological or attitudinal changes; Clark and Goodman (19) demonstrated that the subject's expectation that more pain would be felt resulted in a lowered pain-report criterion, and that the expectation that less pain would be felt raised the criterion. In the present study, the lower-dose group lowered its report criterion during weeks 1 and 2, without a change in P(A); this suggests that the subjects expected that marihuana smoking would increase pain, the well-known marihuana "perceptual sharpening" effect. This finding of a lower report criterion is in agreement with the lower thresholds reported following an acute dose of THC by Hill et al. (15) and Schwin et al (17). The relationship between threshold and criterion has been demonstrated by Yang et al (25) and Clark and Goodman (19) who found that high and low method of limits thresholds are correlated, respectively, with high and low criteria measures of SDT. Our participants provided anecdotal evidence for the "sharpening" interpretation. In accordance with their beliefs, they avoided marihuana while suffering a headache or toothache because they felt that it increased the pain. Nor, in our study, did they smoke before being venipunctured for blood samples, a procedure they found very painful.

The high-dose group showed no criterion effect until the period when the raised criterion indicated a more stoic attitude. The failure to find a lower criterion in the heavy smokers may have been caused by the marked tolerance to marihuana that developed in the heavy smokers. Unlike the more moderate smokers, during the latter part of the study they were no longer getting a "high." They became angry and aggressive and vigorously complained that the investigators were providing them with placebo cigarettes; for this group nothing was enhanced, not even pain.

The effect of marihuana smoking on the clinical pain threshold is in opposite direction to sharpening, patients report less pain. However, patients suffering clinical pain are particularly ready to believe that any new treatment should be helpful and ameliorate pain. Expectation can of course cause the pain-report criterion to move in either direction (19). Clark (18) demonstrated that a placebo described as a potent analgesic raised the pain-report criterion without changing P(A). If interpreted according to the method of limits, this decrease in pain report would falsely suggest an analgesic effect. Thus, the reputed analgesic effect of marihuana in patients receiving treatment for cancer pain reported by Noyes et al. (10) probably caused by such a placebo effect. Much of the confusion in the literature is undoubtedly caused by the beliefs held by the subject. Habitual smokers expect sharpening, and report more pain, whereas naive subjects, who probably have read about marihuana's supposed analgesic properties, will report less pain.

P(A) and B are mediated by different neural systems. The decision criterion, B, is a cognitive variable mediated by neocortical and limbic system activity; for example, Tanda et al. (30) have shown that THC influences mesolimbic dopamine transmission through a opioid receptor mechanism located in the ventral mesencephalic tegmentum. In contrast, thermal discriminability, P(A), the neurosensory component, is mediated via spinothalamic tracts and the sensory cortex. Pharmacologic effects, including tolerance, could occur at different doses in these various compartments and affect P(A) and B either congruently (the low-dose group) or independently (the high-dose group). Obviously, a unitary neural mechanism cannot explain the dose differences found. The presence of such complex mechanisms may account for much of the confusion in the clinical literature, as well as for the discrepancy between our data and animal studies.

At first glance, there appears to be a wide discrepancy between animal studies that demonstrate that cannabinoids inhibit activity in neural systems known to mediate pain and the results of the studies on humans described here. However, there are a number of factors that may account for this. Neural and receptor subsystems (typically spinal) are studied, not the total organism; pure compounds are used, not marihuana "joints" that may contain up to 300 compounds; dose levels given to animals are often higher, and are difficult to compare across species; motor responses usually are studied, not verbal report; additional neuronal pathways and receptor subtypes mediating and inhibiting pain especially in the brain remain to be discovered. Note the recent finding of a nonopioid analgesic, based on a compound from the skin of a frog, which acts through a receptor for the neurotransmitter acetylcholine (31).

5. CONCLUSIONS

The studies presented here should make obvious the superiority of the SDT model over traditional threshold procedures. SDT quantifies two parameters of perceptual behavior, discriminability and response bias, which are inextricably mixed in the threshold measure. The threshold is not a pure sensory measure, but can be greatly influenced by shifts in the observer's attitude or responses bias set. If thresholds are wanted they can easily be computed from data collected by the SDT procedure (22). It is clear that further marihuana studies of the effect of calibrated noxious stimulation on humans should be pursued. Stimulus modalities other than heat, such as focal pressure, focal cold, tourniquet, and cold pressor (ice-water) pain should be studied, and detailed dose–response studies undertaken. The effect of marihuana on persistent clinical pain should be studied using pain questionnaires such as the Multidimensional Affect and Pain Survey (MAPS) that assess simultaneously the sensory and emotional components of pain *(3)*.

ACKNOWLEDGMENTS

This study was supported in part by grants from NIH GMNS (26461) and NIDA (5R010A00894). The author wishes to thank M. Janal, R. R. Goetz, R. H. McCarthy, B. Bemporad, and S. Bennett Clark for their assistance with data collection, analysis, and manuscript preparation.

REFERENCES

1. Clark, W. C., Goetz, R. R., McCarthy, R. H., Bemporad, B., and Zeidenberg, P.(1979) Effects of marihuana on pain and verbal memory: a sensory decision theory analysis. In: *Marihuana: Biological Effects* (Nahas, G. G. and Paton, W. D. M., eds.) Pergamaon, Oxford, UK, pp. 665–680.
2. Clark, W. C., Janal, M. N., Zeidenberg, P., and Nahas, G.G.(1981) Effects of moderate and high doses of marihuana on thermal pain: a sensory decision theory analysis. *J. Clin. Pharmacol.* **21**,299S–310S.
3. Clark, W. C., Janal, M. N., and Carroll, J. D.(1995) Hierarchical clustering of 270 pain/emotion descriptors: toward a revision of the McGill Pain Questionnaire. In: *Pain and the Brain* (Bromm, B. and Desmedt, J., eds.), Raven, New York, pp. 310–330.
4. Dray, A., Urban, L., and Dickenson, A.(1994) Pharmacology of chronic pain. *Trends Pharmacol. Sci.* **15**,2–10.
5. Pertwee, R. G.(1977) Pharmacology of cannabinoid CB_1 and CB_2 receptors. *Pharmacol. Ther.* **74**,129–180.
6. Durnett-Richardson, J., Aanonsen, L., and Hargreaves, K. M.(1997) Hypoactivity of the spinal cannabinoid system results in NMDA-dependent hyperalgesia. *J. Neurosci.* **18**,451–457.
7. Martin, W. J., Hohmann, A. G., and Walker, J. M.(1996) Suppression of noxious stimulus-evoked activity in the ventral posterolateral nucleus of the thalamus by a cannabinoid agonist: correlation between electrophysiological and antinociceptive effects. *J. Neurosci.* **16**,6601–6611.
8. Jain, A. K., Ryan, J. R., McMahon, G., and Smith, G.(1981) Evaluation of intramuscular levanantradol and placebo in acute postoperative pain. *J. Clin. Pharmacol.* **21**,320S–326S.
9. Hollister, L. E.(1986) Health aspects of cannabis. *Pharmacol. Rev.* **38**,1–20.
10. Noyes, R., Brunk, S. F., Baram, D. A., and Canter, A. (1975) Analgesic effect of delta-9-tetrahydrocannabinol. *Clin. Pharmacol.* **15**,134–143.
11. Chang, A. E., Shiling, D., Stillman, R. C., Goldberg, N. H., Seipp, C. A., Barofsky, I., Simon, R. M., and Rosenberg, S. A. (1979) Delta-9-tetrahydrocannabinol as an antiemetic in cancer patients receiving high-dose methotrexate. *Ann. Int. Med.* **91**,819–824.
12. Gregg, J. M., Small, E. W., Moore, R., and Raft, D. (1976) Emotional response to intravenous delta-9-tetrahydrocannabinol during oral surgery. *J. Oral Surg.* **34**,301–313.
13. Milstein, S. L., MacCannell, K., Karr, G., and Clark, S.(1975) marihuana produced changes in pain tolerance: experienced and nonexperienced subjects. *Int. Pharmacopsychiatry (Basel)* **10**,177–182.
14. Harris, L. S. (1976) Analgesic and antitumor potential of the cannabinoids. In: *The Therapeutic Potential of marihuana* (Cohen, S. and Stillman, R. C., eds.), Plenum, New York, pp. 299–312.
15. Hill, S. Y., Schwin, R., Goodwin, D. W., and Powell, B. J.(1974) marihuana and pain. *J. Pharmacol. Exp. Therap.* **188**,415–418.
16. Tart, C. T. (1970) marihuana intoxication common experiences. *Nature* **226**,701–704.
17. Schwin, R., Hill, S. Y., Goodwin, D. W., and Powell, B. J.(1974) marihuana and critical flicker fusion. *J. Nervous Mental Behav.* **138**,142–144.
18. Clark, W. C. (1969) Sensory decision theory analysis of the placebo effect on the criterion for pain and thermal sensitivity (d'). *J. Abnorm. Psychol.* **74**,363–371.
19. Clark, W. C. and Goodman, J. S. (1974) The effect of suggestion on d' and C for pain detection and pain tolerance. *J. Abnorm. Psychol.* **83**,364–372.
20. Clark, W. C and Bennett Clark, S. (1980) Pain responses in Nepalese porters. *Science* **209**,410–412.
21. Swets, J. A (1998) *Signal Detection Theory and ROC Analysis in Psychology and Diagnostics.* Erlbaum, Mahwah, NJ.

22. Clark, W. C. (1994) The *Psyche* in the psychophysics of pain: an introduction to sensory decision theory. In: *Touch, Temperature and Pain in Health and Disease: Mechanisms and Assessment, Progess in Pain Research and Management,* vol 3 (Boivie, J., Hansson, P. and Lindblom, U., eds), International Association for the Study of Pain Press, Seattle, WA, pp. 41–62.
23. Clark, W. C. (1998) Somatosensory and pain measurement by signal detection theory, in *Encyclopedia of Neuroscience* 2nd ed. (Adelman, G. and Smith, B., eds.), Elsevier, Amsterdam, CD-ROM and in press.
24. Gybels, J., Handwerker, H. O., and Van Hees, J. (1979) A comparison between the discharges of human nociceptive nerve fibres and the subject's ratings of his sensations. *J. Physiol.* **292,**193–206.
25. Yang, J. C, Clark, W. C, Ngai, S. H, Berkowitz, B. A, and Spector, S. (1979) Analgesic action and pharmacokinetics of morphine and diazepam in man: an evaluation by sensory decision theory. *Anesthesiology* **61,**495–502.
26. Clark, W. C. and Yang, J. C. (1974) Acupunctural analgesia? Evaluation by signal detection theory. *Science* **184,**1096–1098.
27. Green, D. M. and Swets, J. A. (1966) *Signal Detection Theory and Psychophysics* Wiley, New York.
28. McNicol, D. A. (1972) *A Primer of Signal Detection Theory* Allen & Unwin, London.
29. Snodgrass, J. G. and Corwin, J. (1988) Pragmatics of measuring recognition memory. *J. Exp. Psychol.* **117,**34–50.
30. Tanda, G., Pontieri, F., and Di Chiara, G. (1997) Cannabinoid and heroin activation of mesolimbic dopamine transmission by a common u_1 opioid receptor mechanism. *Science* **276,**2048–2054.
31. Bannon, A. W., Decker, M. W., Holladay, P., Curzon, D., Donnelly-Roberts, D., Puttfarcken, P. S., Bitner, R. S., Diaz, A., Dickenson, A. H., Porsolt, R. D., Williams, M., and Arneric, S. P. (1998) Broad-spectrum, nonopiod analgesic activity by selective modulation of neuronal nicotinic acetylcholine receptors. *Science* **279,**77–80.

45 Levonantradol

B. Kenneth Koe

Abstract

The analgesic activity of Δ^9-THC was enhanced considerably by removing unsaturation at C9 and replacing 9-methyl with 9β-hydroxy to obtain HHC. This finding prompted an extensive discovery program from 1975 to 1980 to synthesize novel and potent nonopiate analgesic agents. One such compound, levonantradol, entered clinical trials and showed analgesic effects in postoperative pain and antiemetic effects in cancer patients on chemotherapy. The synthetic program also afforded the bicyclic compounds, (-)-CP-55,940 and (-)-CP-55,244, that both have nontraditional cannabinoid structures yet exert potent analgesic activity. These bicyclics played important roles in the advances achieved in cannabinoid pharmacology, such as characterization of the brain cannabinoid receptor (CB_1) and the cloning of rat and human CB_1 receptors.

A new monograph on *Therapeutic Uses of Cannabis* (British Medical Association [1997] Harwood, Amsterdam, The Netherlands) offers the following suggestion in the last chapter on summary and recommendations:

"Pharmaceutical companies should undertake basic laboratory investigations and develop novel cannabinoid analogues which may lead to new clinical uses."

This report is a brief account of the cannabinoid research project at Pfizer Central Research from 1975 to 1980, which led to levonantradol. This project was a continuation of a research effort to discover nonopiate analgesic agents. The stage was set for a cannabinoid project by availability of chemists from a prostaglandin project (Ross Johnson, Larry Melvin), return of George Milne (chemist turned pharmacologist, and now President of Pfizer Central Research) from a sabbatical in analgesia pharmacology with William Dewey at the Medical College of Virginia, and the National Institutes of Health (NIH) disclosure of a new Δ^9-THC derivative, 9-nor-9β-hydroxyhexahydrocannabinol (HHC), with the analgesic potency of morphine *(1)*.

The development of structure-activity relationships and progress of this discovery project rested entirely on synthesizing pure compounds and testing them in vivo in well-known whole-animal assays for antinociception (Table 1). Contrast this "old-fashioned" pharmacological approach with much of current discovery research in the pharmaceutical industry. In

From: *Marihuana and Medicine*
Edited by: G. G. Nahas et al.   © Humana Press Inc., Totowa, NJ

Table 1
Methods for Studying Analgesia

Pain of Chemical Origin
   induction of abdominal stretching (writhing) in mouse by intraperitoneal injection of
   p-phenyl benzoquinone *(PBQ test)*

Pain of Thermal Origin
   on mouse paw *(hot plate test)*
   on mouse tail *(tail flick test)*

Pain of Electrical Origin
   stimulation of rat paws by variable electrical charges *(flinch–jump test)*

Pain of Mechanical Origin
   constant pressure applied to base of tail of young rat *(rat tail pinch test)*

many programs today a strong emphasis is placed on screening vast numbers of chemicals or mixtures of substances derived from high-speed synthesis, combinatorial chemistry, or natural product extracts in high throughput assays using cloned receptors, cloned transporters, and other gene products expressed in various isolated cell systems.

Compound HHC, in which the C9 double bond of Δ^9-THC was removed and 9β-hydroxy replaced 9-methyl, was the starting point for synthesizing new analgesic cannabinoids (Fig. 1A). The Lilly Laboratories independently synthesized canbisol, a HHC with dimethyl-heptyl, an alkyl side chain well-known to increase potency, in place of pentyl. We chose to replace the pentyl with a 5-phenyl-2-pentoxy group and made CP-42,096. Both canbisol and CP-42,096 showed better analgesic potency than HHC (Table 2). It is interesting to note that Lilly Laboratories opted to develop nabilone (9-oxo in place of 9β-hydroxy in canbisol). In analgesic tests nabilone was less potent than canbisol but equivalent to HHC (Table 2).

Next, Pfizer researchers replaced the pyran oxygen with nitrogen, deleted a methyl group, and obtained nantradol. The phenolic OH in nantradol is also acetylated to improve stability, but this ester is readily hydrolyzed in vivo to desacetylnantradol. Nantradol showed broad analgesic efficacy in mice and rats *(2)*. Peak activity was reached in 1 hour with a duration of action of 3–6 hours. Nantradol did not bind to the opiate receptor, and its analgesic activity was not reversed by naloxone. Although nantradol was 10 times as active as Δ^9-THC in a rat drug discrimination paradigm *(3)*, the analgesic potency of nantradol was 100–200 times that of Δ^9-THC in the rat tail-pinch assay *(2)*. As a result, it was concluded that analgesic efficacy could be achieved without encountering the subjective effects of Δ^9-THC. Nantradol was advanced into clinical trials in 1977.

Nantradol itself is made up of four stereoisomers that form two racemic pairs of enantiomers, A and B (Fig. 2). A was more active than B *(2,3)*. Separation of A into the constituent enantiomers gave levonantradol and dextronantradol. Analgesic activity resided in levonantradol, whereas considerably less activity was observed for dextronantradol (Table 2). In 1979 levonantradol replaced nantradol in the clinical trials. The derivative, *N*-methyllevonantradol, was more potent in analgesic tests (Table 2) and showed a longer duration of action with possibly better toleration in animals. The chemical modifications involved in enhancing analgesic potency by about 1000-fold in going from Δ^9-THC to HHC to *N*-methyllevonantradol is summarized in Table 3A.

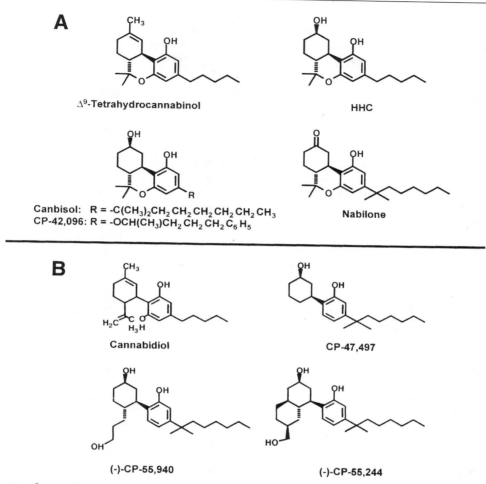

Fig. 1. (A) Δ^9-Tetrahydrocannabinol and synthetic tricyclic cannabimimetics. **(B)** Cannabidiol and synthetic bicyclic cannabimimetics.

The bicyclic compound cannabidiol is devoid of cannabimimetic properties (Fig. 1B). In the course of introducing ring alterations to the HHC molecule, the 3-(2-hydroxyphenyl) cyclohexanol, CP-47,497, was found to have the analgesic potency of morphine. An extensive study of structure-activity relationships in the bicyclic series led to (-)-CP-55,940 and (-)-CP-55,244, compounds showing potent activity in analgesic tests (Table 2). These bicyclics demonstrated that elimination of the pyran ring from Δ^9-THC yielded not only no loss but a gain in cannabinoid agonist potency. As with dextronantradol (+)-CP-55,940 and (+)-CP-55,244 were much less active than the respective levorotatory enantiomer. The approximately 1000-fold increase in analgesic potency achieved in going from Δ^9-THC to (-)-CP-55,244 and the chemical changes involved are summarized in Table 3B.

(-)-CP-55,940 and (-)-CP-55,244 had the potential of replacing levonantradol in the clinical program because of their marked analgesic activity. The potency differences between levo and dextro bicyclic enantiomers are also evident in vitro (Table 4). The (-) and (+) enantiomers of CP-55,940 and CP-55,244 and the radioligand [^{3}H]-(-)-CP-55,940 came to play significant roles in the advances made in cannabinoid pharmacology by helping to establish

Table 2
Analgesic Activity in Mice

Compound	MPE$_{50}$ Time min	Tail flick mg/kg sc	Time min	PBQ mg/kg sc
Δ9-THC	30	55	20	9.1
			60	5.9
			60	5.4
Cannabidiol		not tested	60	>56
HHC	30	2.5	20	0.63
	60	9.1		
Canbisol	30	0.46	20	0.06
Nabilone	30	3.8	20	0.48
			60	0.20
CP-42,096	30	0.32	20	0.07
			60	0.07
Nantradol	60	0.7	20	0.4
Levonantradol	30	0.11	20	0.08
	60	0.21	60	0.10
	120	0.20		
Dextronantradol	60	> 56	60	6.5
N-Methyllevonantradol	60	0.033	60	0.012
CP-47,497	30	5.6	60	1.0
	60	4.4		
	60	6.8		
(-)-CP-55,940	60	0.32	60	0.059
	120	0.50	60	0.07
	120	0.42		
(+)-CP-55,940		not tested	60	14.6
(-)-CP-55,244	60	0.070	60	0.007
	60	0.060	60	0.016
	120	0.053		
	120	0.026		
(+)-CP-55,244		not tested	60	>100
Morphine	30	2.9	20	0.91
	60	5.7	30	1.8
			60	0.9

MPE$_{50}$ is best estimate of the dose at which 50% of the maximum possible effect is observed.
95% Confidence limits are omitted for clarity; cf. Koe, B.K. et al. (1985) *Eur. J. Pharmacol.* **109**, 201–212.

For potencies in other antinociceptive tests, cf. ref. 2; also Johnson, M.R. et al. (1981) *J. Clin. Pharmacol.* **21**, 271s–282s; Howlett, A.C. et al. (1988) *Mol. Pharmacol.* **33**, 297–302; Melvin, L.S. et al. (1993) *Mol. Pharmacol.* **44**, 1008–1015; Melvin, L.S. et al. (1995) *Drug Design Disc.* **13**, 155–166.

the existence and localization of a brain cannabinoid receptor and in the cloning of the rat and human CB$_1$ receptors (4).

In clinical trials, levonantradol (dose range: 0.5–4 mg/intramuscular dose; 0.5–2 mg/oral dose) showed analgesic efficacy in postoperative pain and antiemetic and antinausea effects in cancer patients receiving chemotherapy (Table 5; summary in ref. 2). Side effects included somnolence, dysphoria, dizziness, thought disturbance, hypotension, pain at injection site,

Diastereoisomer A

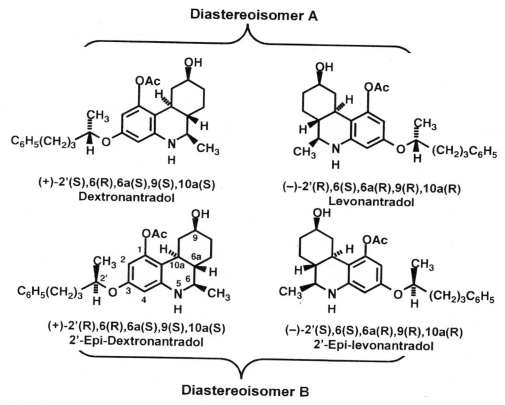

(+)-2'(S),6(R),6a(S),9(S),10a(S)
Dextronantradol

(−)-2'(R),6(S),6a(R),9(R),10a(R)
Levonantradol

(+)-2'(R),6(R),6a(S),9(S),10a(S)
2'-Epi-Dextronantradol

(−)-2'(S),6(S),6a(R),9(R),10a(R)
2'-Epi-levonantradol

Diastereoisomer B

Fig. 2. The four stereoisomers comprising nantradol.

dry mouth, and urinary retention. The dose-limiting side-effects contributed to the decision to discontinue the project. (-)-CP-55,940 and *N*-methyllevonantradol had been recommended as back-up clinical candidates. Preclinical and clinical studies on levonantradol to date were presented at a 1980 symposium, and the proceedings were published in 1981 (Table 6).

Since the levonantradol project more than 20 years ago, remarkable advances have occurred in cannabinoid research, not the least of which are the discoveries of entirely unrelated chemical structures with affinity for the cannabinoid receptor, such as agonist WIN 55,212-2, putative endogenous ligand arachidonylethanolamide (anandamide), and antagonist SR 141716A *(4)*. These new discoveries along with the cloning of the cannabinoid receptors promise momentum in the understanding of the workings of the cannabinoid system in brain. Will this new knowledge also spawn new therapeutic agents? Enthusiasm about such prospects is tempered by the fact that the varied behavioral and pharmacological effects of cannabinoid agonists are strongly correlated with their affinity for the CB_1 receptor, including the subjective effects in rats and human *(5)*. Thus, their potency in rat drug discrimination (Δ^9-THC) and human behavior (psychoactivity) also correlate with affinity for the CB_1 receptor *(5)*, indicating that the discriminative cue is mediated by the latter *(6)*. In view of the clinical experience with levonantradol, these correlations would hinder commercial interest in new drug development. Cannabinoid-derived structures (HU-210, levonantradol, (-)-CP-55,940) and anandamide on the one hand, and WIN 55,212-2 (and related naphthoylaminoalkylindoles, naphthoylalkylindoles) on the other, are postulated to have different "docking" sites in the transmembrane helices of the CB_1 receptor *(7,8)*, which might translate to differential agonist

Table 3
Structural Modifications that Increase Analgesic Activity

		Increase in potency	
(A) *Structure evolution*	*New change*	*Tail flick*	*PBQ*
Δ^9-THC→HHC[a]	9β-OH	~10-fold	~10-fold
HHC[a]→canbisol/CP-42,096	Side-chain	~10-fold	~10-fold
Canbisol/CP-42,096→levonantradol	NH for pyran O, demethyl, 1-acetoxy	~2-fold	None
Levonantradol→*N* methyllevonantradol	*N*-methyl	~10-fold	~10-fold

[a]HHC equivalent to morphine in analgesic potency.

		Increase in potency	
(B) *Structure evolution*	*New change*	*Tail flick*	*PBQ*
Δ^9-THC→CP-47,497[a]	"9"β-OH, side-chain, absence of pyran ring	~10-fold	~5–10-fold
CP-47,497→(-)-CP-55,940[b]	Hydroxypropyl	~10-fold	~20-fold
(-)CP-55,940→(-)-CP-55,244[c]	Hydroxypropyl part of rigid ring	~10-fold	~10-fold

[a]CP-47,497 equivalent to HHC/morphine in analgesic potency.
[b](-)-CP-55,940 equivalent to levonantradol in analgesic potency.
[c](-)-CP-55,244 equivalent to *N*-methyllevonantradol in analgesic potency.

Table 4
Enantiomeric Selectivity In Vitro

Enantiomer	CB_1 binding, K_i nM[a]	Adenylate cyclase, K_i nM[b]
Levonantradol	c	100
Dextronantradol	c	> 5000
Desacetyllevonantradol	0.621	7
Desacetyldextronantradol	> 1000	c
(-)-CP-55,940	0.137	25
(+)-CP-55,940	12	>5000
(-)-CP-55,244	0.11	5
(+)-CP-55,244	> 1000	>10000

[a][^{3}H]-(-)-CP-55,940, Melvin, L. S. et al. (1995) *Drug Design Disc.* **13**, 155–166.
[b]Howlett, A. C. et al. (1988) *Mol. Pharmacol.* **33**, 297–302.
[c]Not tested.

actions via different receptor conformational changes. However, WIN 55,212-2 and metabolically stable (R)-methanandamide and 2-methylarachidonyl-2'-fluoroethylamide, with dissimilar docking sites, all substitute (cue) for Δ^9-THC *(9–11)*. Even the putative anandamide transport inhibitor, AM404 [*N*-(4-hydroxylphenyl)anandamide *(12)*], by extension could evoke the subjective effects of CB_1 agonists. New therapeutics based on Δ^9-THC's multiple

Table 5
Levonantradol Studies in Human Subjects

Study	Reference
Postoperative pain	Jain, A.K. et al. (1981) *J. Clin. Pharmacol.* **21,** 320s–326s.
Emesis	Citron, M.L. et al. (1983) *Proc. Am. Assoc. Cancer Res.* **24,** 165.
Emesis	Citron, M.L. et al. (1985) *Cancer Treat. Rep.* **69,** 109–112.
Emesis	Cronin, C.M. et al. (1981) *J. Clin. Pharmacol.* **21,** 43s–50s.
Emesis	Diaso, R.B. et al. (1981) *J. Clin. Pharmacol.* **21,** 81s–85s.
Emesis	Earhart, R.H. et al. (1983) *Proc. Am. Assoc. Cancer Res.* **24,** 163.
Emesis	Gerhartz et al. (1983) *Klin. Wochenschr.* **61,** 719–721.
Emesis	Heim, M.E. et al. (1981) *J. Clin. Pharmacol.* **21,** 86s–89s.
Emesis	Heim, M.E. et al. (1982) *Onkologie* **5,** 94–96.
Emesis	Heim, M.E. et al. (1984) *Cancer Chemother. Pharmacol.* **13,** 123–125.
Emesis	Higi, M. et al. (1982) *Dtsche. Med. Wochenschr.* **107,** 1232–1234.
Emesis	Hutcheon, A.W. et al. (1983) *Eur J. Cancer Clin. Oncol.* **19,** 1087–1090.
Emesis	Joss, R.A. (1982) et al. *Cancer Chemother. Pharmacol.* **9,** 61–64.
Emesis	Kenny, J.B. et al. (1982) *Clin. Oncol.* **8,** 335–339.
Emesis	Lazlo, J. et al. (1981) *J. Clin. Pharmacol.* **21,** 51s–56s.
Emesis	Lucraft, H.H. et al. (1982) *Clin. Radiol.* **33,** 621–622.
Emesis	Sheidler, V.R. et al. (1984) *J. Clin. Pharmacol.* **24,** 155–159
Emesis	Stambaugh, J.E. et al. (1984) *J. Clin. Pharmacol.* **24,** 480–485.
Emesis	Stuart-Harris, R.C. et al. (1983) *Clin. Oncol.* **9,** 143–146.
Emesis	Tyson, L.B. et al. (1985) *Am. J. Clin. Oncol.* **8,** 528–532.
Emesis	Welsh, J. et al. (1983) *Cancer Chemother. Pharmacol.* **11,** 66–67.

Table 6
Pfizer Cannabinoid Project

1975	Discovery project was initiated (chemical synthesis and testing for analgesic activity).
1977	Nantradol was advanced to clinical trials for postoperative pain and emesis
1979	Levonantradol replaced nantradol in clinical trials.
1980	(-)-CP-55,940 was recommended for clinical evaluation.
1980	*N*-Methyllevonantradol was recommended for clinical evaluation.
1981	Publication in the *Journal of Clinical Pharmacology,* vol. 21, of the proceedings of Symposium on "Therapeutic Progress in Cannabinoid Research," held at University of Connecticut at Avery Point, October 20–21, 1980.

effects may have to wait until exploration of the cannabinoid-receptor system unravels the pathways that lead to selectivity of action. The antagonist SR 141716A also exhibits inverse agonist activity *(4)* and may elicit actions opposite to those of CB_1 agonists, e.g., SR 141716A can effect memory improvement in rodents *(13)* but anxiety in rats *(14)* and hyperalgesia in mice *(15)*.

REFERENCES

1. Wilson, R. S., May, E. L., Martin, B. R., and Dewey, W. K. (1976) 9-Nor-9β-hydroxyhexahydrocannabinols. Synthesis, some behavioral and analgesic properties, and comparison with tetrahydrocannabinols. *J. Med. Chem.* **19,** 1165–1167.

2. Johnson, M.R. and Melvin, L.S (1986) The discovery of nonclassical cannabinoid analgetics, In: *Cannabinoids as Therapeutic Agents* (Mechoulam, R., ed.), CRC Press, Boca Raton, FL, pp. 121–145.

3. Browne, R.G. and Weissman, A. (1981) Discriminative stimulus properties of Δ^9-tetrahydrocannabinol: mechanistic studies. *J. Clin. Pharmacol.* **21**, 227s–234s.

4. Pertwee, R.G. (1997) Pharmacology of cannabinoid CB_1 and CB_2 receptors. *Pharmacol. Ther.* **74**, 129–180.

5. Compton, D.R., Rice, K.C., De Costa, B.R., Razdan, R.K., Melvin, L.S., Johnson, M.R., and Martin, B.R. (1993) Cannabinoid structure-activity relationships: correlation of receptor binding and in vivo activities. *J. Pharmacol. Exp. Ther.* **265**, 218–226.

6. Perio, A., Rinaldi-Carmona, M., Maruani, J., Barth, F., Le Fur, G. and Soubrie, P. (1996) Central mediation of the cannabinoid cue—activity of a selective CB1 antagonist, SR 141716A. *Behav. Pharmacol.* **7**, 65–71.

7. Huffman J. W. and Lainton, J. (1996) Recent developments in the medicinal chemistry of cannabinoids. *Curr. Med. Chem.* **3**, 101–116.

8. Song, Z. H. and Bonner, T. I. (1996) A lysine residue of the cannabinoid receptor is critical for receptor recognition by several agonists but not WIN55212-2. *Mol. Pharmacol.* **49**, 891–896.

9. Compton, D. R., Gold, L. H., Ward, S. J., Balster, R. L., and Martin, B. R. (1992) Aminoalkylindole analogs: cannabimimetic activity of a class of compounds structurally distinct from Δ^9-tetrahydrocannabinol. *J. Pharmacol. Exp. Ther.* **263**, 1118–1126.

10. Burkey, R. T. and Nation, J. R. (1997) (R)-methanandamide, but not anandamide, substitutes for delta 9-THC in a drug discrimination procedure. *Exp. Clin. Psychopharmacol.* **5**, 195–202.

11. Wiley, J. L., Golden, K. M., Ryan, W. J., Balster, R. L., Razdan, R. K., and Martin, B. R. (1997) Evaluation of cannabimimetic discriminative stimulus effects of anandamide and methylated fluoroanandamide in rhesus monkeys. *Pharmacol. Biochem. Behav.* **58**, 1139–1143.

12. Beltrano, M., Stella, N., Calignano, A., Lin, S. Y., Makriyannis, A., and Piomelli, D. (1997) Functional role of high-affinity anandamide transport, as revealed by selective inhibition. *Science* **277**, 1094–1097.

13. Terranova, J.-P., Storme, J.-J., Lafon, N., Perio, A., Rinaldi-Carmona, M., Le Fur, G., and Soubrie, P. (1996) Improvement of memory in rodents by the selective CB_1 cannabinoid receptor antagonist, SR 141716. *Psychopharmacology* 126, 165–172.

14. Navarro, M., Hernandez, E., Munoz, R. M., del Arco, I., Villanua, M. A., Carrer, M. R. and Rodriguez de Fonseca, F. (1997) Acute administration of the CB1 cannabinoid receptor antagonist SR 141716A induces anxiety-like responses in the rat. *Neuroreport* **8**, 491–496.

15. Richardson, J. D., Aanonsen, L., and Hargreaves, K. M. (1997) SR 141716A, a cannabinoid receptor antagonist, produces hyperalgesia in untreated mice. *Eur. J. Pharmacol.* **319**, R3–4.

46 Nabilone

A Synthetic Cannabinoid of Medicinal Utility

Louis Lemberger

Abstract

Nabilone is a synthetic cannabinoid. It was discovered and developed at the Lilly Research Laboratories as the first modern day cannabinoid to achieve the distinction of obtaining regulatory approval for use in the treatment of patients. Earlier work with Δ^9-THC revealed that it was ITS metabolite, 11-hydroxy-Δ^9-THC which accounted for the psychoactive properties. Further studies with this compound and with DMHP led to the synthesis and discovery of nabilone. Nabilone has undergone extensive clinical pharmacologic testing and its physiologic and drug abuse potential were studied. It was found to be an effective agent in the treatment of nausea and vomiting secondary to cancer therapy. In well-controlled studies it was superior to placebo and prochlorperazine. It appeared to be especially effective in children, a group that experiences lesser side effects. Nabilone has also been studied in early phase II trials as an agent for lowering intraocular pressure, as an antianxiety agent, and as a drug for producing bronchodilation. These other indications were not vigorously pursued because nabilone either had undesired side effects in these populations, or it was not better than current standard therapy. Nabilone was marketed in the United States, Canada, the United Kingdom, and several other countries under the trade name Cesamet.

1. INTRODUCTION

It has been stated that *Cannabis sativa* has been used medicinally since as early as 3000 BC, when Emperor Chen Nung mentioned its use in a medical formulary. In the early 1900s through 1927, *Cannabis* was widely used therapeutically for a variety of ailments and diseases. It was marketed alone and in combination with a number of other medicinal agents. With the passage of the Marihuana Tax Act in 1937, it became illegal to prescribe any preparations containing this plant.

The search for synthetic cannabinoids, to be utilized for medicinal purposes, dates back to the early 1940s, when Todd *(1)* and Adams *(2)* studied a series of cannabinoid derivatives. Since that time, several major pharmaceutical companies have undertaken research programs

From: *Marihuana and Medicine*
Edited by: G. G. Nahas et al.   © Humana Press Inc., Totowa, NJ

to attempt to develop agents based upon this unique chemical structure, i.e., a centrally active compound that is devoid of a nitrogen substituent. The firms involved in this endeavor included Hoffmann LaRoche; Smith, Kline and French; Abbott; Pfizer; and Eli Lilly.

I first became interested in the pharmacological activity of *Cannabis* while a researcher at the National Institutes of Health (NIH) in Bethesda, Maryland. It was here that Drs. Axelrod, Kopin, and I studied the physiologic disposition of radiolabeled Δ^9-tetrahydrocannabinol (Δ^9-THC), the psychoactive constituent of marihuana *(3)*, in humans. We administered C-14-Δ^9-THC and demonstrated that the drug had a long half-life in humans and was metabolized by the liver microsomal enzymes to a hydroxylated compound that we identified as 11-hydroxy-Δ^9-THC *(4)*. Further studies in our laboratory suggested that this metabolic product might be responsible for the psychoactive effects *(5)*.

In 1971, I moved to Indianapolis and joined the research group at the Lilly Laboratory for Clinical Research of Eli Lilly and Co. and became a faculty member at the Indiana University School of Medicine. Here I continued to investigate the activity of cannabinoids, and my colleagues and I administered 11-hydroxy-Δ^9-THC to humans and reported on its almost instantaneous onset of action after intravenous administration *(6)*. We then conducted a double blind placebo controlled experiment comparing C-14-Δ^9-THC, tritiated 11-hydroxy-Δ^9-THC, and placebo in a crossover design to a series of healthy volunteers who had a history of mild to moderate cannabis usage. We demonstrated that the psychotomimetic effects of Δ^9-THC were related to its conversion to 11-hydroxy-Δ^9-THC, which was in fact the active constituent. These findings were further supported by the demonstration that the physiologic disposition of delta-9-THC after its administration to humans was almost identical to that seen after the administration of 11-hydroxy-Δ^9-THC *(7)*.

Upon my arrival at Eli Lilly I was pleased to learn that the company had also been engaged in a synthetic cannabinoid research program under the direction of Robert Archer. Archer and his colleagues in the chemical group were actively synthesizing compounds, and they were collaborating with Paul Stark, a pharmacologist, who was testing these compounds in a variety of animal models. With my expertise as a clinical pharmacologist also interested in this research, we soon developed a close friendship and collaboration and a desire to find a useful medicinal agent from the chemical group known as cannabinoids.

To further study the pharmacology and mechanism of action of the cannabinoids as they relate to their physiologic disposition, I convinced Archer to synthesize radiolabeled

Δ-6a,10a-dimethylheptyl benzopyran (DMHP), a cannabinoid analog (DMHP has a double bond in the 6a,10a position and a dimethyl heptyl side chain) that had been studied extensively as a psychotomimetic at the Edgewood Arsenal in Maryland. We administered this drug to humans and studied its pharmacologic activity as well as its physiologic disposition *(8)*.

Based upon our studies with DMHP and our earlier studies with 11-hydroxy-Δ^9-THC, Archer, Stark, and I felt that an ideal candidate cannabinoid drug might contain an oxygen substituent at the top of the A ring analogous to 11-hydroxy-Δ^9-THC and a side chain similar to that present in the DMHP molecule. After synthesizing and testing a large number of compounds with these characteristics, we selected a compound whose laboratory name was compound 109514, and whose generic name was nabilone. Nabilone chemically consists of the basic cannabinoid nucleus with a ketone function in the A ring and a dimethyl heptyl side chain. However, in contrast to DMHP, the 2 methyl groups are attached to the same carbon. We elected to proceed through the preclinical toxicology with this compound with the hopes that it would pass this safety assessment and we would thus feel comfortable administering it to humans.

The initial 90-day toxicologic studies in both rats and dogs was without significance, and thus initial clinical pharmacologic studies were conducted in normal volunteers. The early phase I studies consisted of several protocols. The first introduction of nabilone (9) to humans was in a single-dose, -dose ranging study in which doses ranging from 0.1. to 5 mg were administered. This was followed by a multiple dose study with either 1 mg. or 2mg. being administered twice daily for seven days. As a result of this study it was concluded that that tolerance developed to the cardiovascular effects (i.e., postural hypotension) of nabilone. Thus a protocol was designed to specifically address the issue of tolerance development. It clearly indicated that tolerance developed to the effect of nabilone on postural hypotension and also to the psychologic high (i.e., euphoria) produced by nabilone.

After completion of the phase I studies we embarked upon a variety of early phase II efficacy studies (both open labeled and controled) in a number of therapeutic areas. This was based upon a number of original articles and reviews that espoused the alleged therapeutic effects attributed to marihuana (10). These included studies assessing marihuana or Δ^9-THC as an antiemetic secondary to cancer chemotherapy in cancer patients receiving emetogenic oncolytic drugs (11); as an anxiolytic in patients suffering from anxiety (12); for the pulmonary effects of nabilone as a bronchodilator in normal subjects and in asthmatic patients (13); as an agent for lowering intraoccular pressure in patients with glaucoma (14).

2. ANTIEMETIC STUDIES

Nabilone was first studied as a potential antiemetic because this area was felt to be the simplest, quickest and most fruitful based on the studies with marihuana and Δ^9-THC. Open-labeled studies were initially conducted by Larry Einhorn at Indiana University and by Herman and Jones at the University of Arizona. These early studies at both sites revealed that, indeed, nabilone was a safe and effective drug. They expanded these studies and published them as a lead article in the *New England Journal of Medicine (15)*. The results indicated that nabilone was superior to placebo and prochlorperazine (Compazine) as an antinauseant and antiemetic. The side effect profile for nabilone was more pronounced, yet it was acceptable considering the therapeutic benefits. Similar results were reported by Steele et al. (16) and Levitt (17). Since these initial studies, and after nabilone was marketed, numerous studies conducted in adult cancer patients have confirmed the drug's efficacy and substantiated its side effect profile. Pomeroy (18) stated that nabilone was superior to domperidone in the control of cytotoxin induced emesis, whereas Crawford and Buckman (19) reported that oral nabilone was equieffective as intravenous metoclopramide as an antiemetic. Niiranen and Mattson (20) studied nabilone alone, and in combination with dexamethasone. The combination was found to be more effective and the side effects were also reduced when the drugs were given together. Studies conducted with nabilone in children found it to be superior to prochlorperazine (21) and when administered at lower doses, nabilone exhibited the same efficacy and there were minimal side effects. Dalzell et al. (22) found nabilone superior to domperidone in children, although it exhibited a higher degree of side effects. However, they were acceptable to most patients.

Other antiemetic studies showed nabilone to be effective in patients undergoing abdominal hysterectomy who had nausea and vomiting after anesthesia (23) and in patients receiving radiation therapy (24). While these antiemetic studies were being conducted, a variety of other clinical studies were being conducted as well.

3. ANXIOLYTIC STUDIES

Several investigators studied nabilone as an antianxiety agent. Hollister and colleauges (25) demonstrated that diazepam was more effective than nabilone in reducing anxiety in normal volunteers subjected to an experimental model of anxiety, whereas Glass et al. (26) found a single oral doses (1–2 mg) of nabilone administered to anxious volunteers had no significant antianxiety effect, although a small percentage seemed to improve. In contrast, Fabre and McLendon *(27)* who studied the effect of nabilone in anxious outpatients reported a dramatic improvement compared to placebo.

4. BRONCHODILATOR EFFECTS

Tashkin and colleagues *(28)* studied the effect of nabilone and terbutaline in healthy and asthmatic subjects. They found terbutaline to have superior bronchdilatory effects, and at times found nabilone to precipitate bronchospasm in asthmatic subjects.

5. EFFECT ON INTROCCULAR PRESSURE

Since marihuana and Δ^9-THC are known to reduce intraocular pressure in animals, normal volunteers, and patients with glaucoma, it was of interest to determine what effect nabilone might exhibit on intraocular pressure. Newell et al. at the University of Chicago *(29)* reported that the oral administration of nabilone to patients with open-angle glaucoma, (0.5–2 mg), resulted in an average 28% reduction in introccular pressure in these patients. However, in this elderly population the side effects of nabilone were perceived as dysphoric and negatively affected the patients' desire to receive additional courses of drug treatment.

6. CONCLUSIONS

Following the conclusion of the phase II studies, it was determined that the area of greatest potential for the development of nabilone as a marketable drug was as an antiemetic secondary to cancer chemotherapy. Phase III clinical trials were conducted comparing nabilone to either placebo therapy or Compazine, the currently available standard treatment for emesis at that time. The intention of these studies was to obtain sufficient clinical data to support the submission of the nabilone data to the United States Food and Drug Administration (FDA), The Committee on Safety and Medicines in the United Kingdom, and the Canadian regulatory authority, as well as other regulatory bodies worldwide.

Nabilone was approved by the FDA in the United States, but unfortunately, the Drug Enforcement Agency (DEA) insisted on scheduling it as a class II narcotic, a label that was totally unjustified based on the scientific data generated with nabilone. They completely ignored the scientific data *(30,31)* regarding the abuse potential of nabilone which clearly indicated that it had only a small and limited abuse liability. This served as a deterrent, and thus the drug never became a viable product in the United States because of its perception of being unable to generate significant sales because it was a controlled drug. As a result, when the FDA asked that the pharmaceutical formulation be subjected to additional bioavailability tests, the company elected not to pursue these studies and allowed the NDA to become inactive. This essentially determined the fate of nabilone and resulted in its removal from the marketplace and its demise in the United States.

The Committee on Safety and Medicines in the United Kingdom took a totally different approach to nabilone. They approved nabilone for use as an antiemetic without any restrictions. After considering the scientific data, they decided to wait and see if any serious drug abuse, addiction, or diversion occurred then decided if it would be controlled as a narcotic. As a result of this more realistic approach, nabilone has been in continual usage as an antiemetic for over two decades in the United Kingdom without any special controls, and to date no drug abuse problems have arisen.

In conclusion, the journey that started as a study to investigate the pharmacologic actions and mechanism of action of marihuana and Δ^9-THC concluded in the development of a useful drug for the symptomatic treatment of nausea and vomiting in cancer patients taking chemotherapeutic drugs. In some instances these antiemetic drugs are life saving, since without them certain patients refuse to continue their life-sustaining albeit toxic chemotherapy.

REFERENCES

1. Todd, A. R.(1942) The chemistry of hashish. *Soc.J.Roy.Coll. Sci.* **12,** 37.
2. Adams,R. (1941) Marihuana, Harvey Lectures **37,** 168.
3. Mechoulam, R. and Ganoi, Y. (1967) The absolute configuration of delta-1-tetrahydrocannabinol, the major active constiuent of hashish. *Tetrahedron Lett.* **12,** 1109.
4. Lemberger, l., Silberstein,S., Axelrod, J., and Kopin. I.J. (1970) Marihuana: Studies on the disposition and metabolism of Δ^9-tetrahydrocannabinol in man. *Science* **170,** 1320
5. Lemberger, L., Weiss, J. L., Watanabe, A. M. et al. (1972) Delta-9-tetrahydrocannabinol: temporal correlation of the psychological effects and blood levels after various routes of administration. *N.Engl.J.Med.* **286,** 685.
6. Lemberger, L., Crabtree, R. E., and Rowe, H. M. (1972) 11-hydroxy-delta-9-tetrahydrocannabinol: Pharmacology, disposition and metabolism of a major metabolite of marihuana in man. *Science* **177,** 62.
7. Lemberger, L.,Martz.R, Rodda, B. et al. (1973) Comparative pharmacology of delta-9-tetrahydrocannabinol and its metabolit, 11-hydroxy-delta-9-tetrahydrocannabinol. *J. Clin. Invest.* **52,** 2411.
8. Lemberger, L., McMahon, R., Archer, R., et al. (1974) Pharmacologic effects and physiologic disposition of delta-6a,10a-dimethyl heptyl tetrahydrocannabinol (DMHP) in man. *Clin. Pharmacol. Therap.* **25,**380.
9. Lemberger, L. and Rowe, H. M. (1975) Clinical pharmacology of nabilone, a cannabinol derivative. *Clin. Pharmacol. Therap.* **18,** 720.
10. Lemberger, L.(1980) Potential therapeutic usefulness of marihuana.*Ann. Rev. Pharmacol. Toxicol.* **20,** 151.
11. Sallan, S. E., Zinberg, N. E. and Frei, E. (1975) Antiemetic effect of delta-9-tetrahydrocannabinol in patients receiving cancer chemotherapy. *N. Engl.J.Med.* **293,** 796.
12. Hollister, L. E.(1971) Hunger and appetite after single doses of marihuana, ethanol and dextroamphetamine. *Clin. Pharmacol. Therap.* **12,**44.
13. Tashkin, D. P., Shapiro, B. J.and Frank, I. M.(1973) Acute pulmonary physiologic effects of smoked marihuana and oral delta-9-tetrahydrocannabinolin healthy young men. *N. Engl. J. Med.* **289,** 336.
14. Hepler, R. S., Frank, I. M. (1971) Marihuana smoking and intraocular pressure. *JAMA* **217,** 1392.
15. Herman, T. S. Einhorn, L. H., Jones, S.E. et al. (1979) Superiority of nabilone over prochlorperazine as an antiemetic in patients receiving cancer chemotherapy. *N.Engl. J. Med.* **300,** 1295.
16. Steele, N., Gralla, R. J., and Braun, D. W. (1980) *Cancer Treat. Rep.* **64,** 1054.
17. Levitt, M. (1982) Nabilone v.s. placebo in the treatment of chemotherapy-induced nausea and vomiting in cancer patients. *Cancer Treat. Rev.* **9(suppl)**
18. Pomery, M., Fennelly, J. J. and Towers, M.(1986) Nabilone versus domperidone in the treatment of cytotoxic induced emesis. *Cancer Chemothert. Pharmacol.* **17,** 625.
19. Crawford, S. M. and Buckman, R. (1986) Nabilon and metoclopramide in the treatment of nausea and vomiting due to cisplatinum: a double blind study. *Med. Oncol. Tumor pharacotherapy.***3,** 242.
20. Niiranen, A. and Mattson, K. (1985) A cross-over comparison of nabilone and perchloro perazine for emesis induced by cancer chemotherapy. *Am. J. Clin. Oncol.* **8,** 336.
21. Chan, H. S., Correia, J. A. and McLeod, S. M. (1987) Nabilone versus prochlorperazine for control of cancer chemotherapy-induced emesis in children:a double blind crossover trial. *Pediatrics* **79,** 946.
22. Dalzell, A. M., Bartlett, H. and Lilleyman, J.S. (1986) Nabilone: an alternative antiemetic for cancer chemotherapy. *Arch. Dis. Child.* **61,** 50.
23. Lewis, I. H., Campbell, D. N. and Barrowcliffe, N. (1994) Effect of nabilone on nausea and vomiting after total abdominal hysterectomy. *Br. J. Anaesth.* **73,** 24.
24. Preistman, S. G., Preistman, T. J. and Canney, J.(1987) A double blind randomized cross-over comparison of nabilone and metoclopramide in the control of radiation-induced nausea. *Clin. Radiol.* **38,** 543.
25. Nakano, S., Gillespie, H. K. and Hollister, L. (1978) A model for evaluation of antianxiety drugs with the use of experimentally induced stress: comparison of nabilone and diazepam. *Clin. Pharmacol. Therap.* **23,** 54.
26. Glass, R. M., Uhlenhuth, E. H., and Hartel, F. W. (1980) A single dose study of nabilone, a synthetic cannabinoid. *Psychpharmacology* **71,** 13.
27. Fabre, L. F. and McLendon, D.(1981) The efficacy and safety of nabilone (a synthetic cannabinoid) in the treatment of anxiety. *J. Clin. Pharmacol.* **21,** 8.
28. Gong, H. jr., Tashkin, D. P., and Calvarese, B.(1983) Comparison of bronchial effects of nabilone and terbutaline in healthy and asthmatic subjects. *J. Clin. Pharmacol.* **23,** 12.

29. Newell, F. W., Stark, P. and Jay, W. M. (1979) Nabilone: a pressure-reducing synthetic benzopyran in open-angle glaucoma. *Ophthalmology* **86,** 156.

30. Lemberger, L., Rubin, A., Wolen, R. et al. (1982) Pharmacokinetics, metabolism and drug-abuse potential of nabilone. *Cancer Treat. Rev.* **9: (supp B)** 17–23.

31. Mendelson, J. H. and Melo, N. K.(1984) Reinforcing properties of oral delta-9-tetrahydrocannabinol, smoked marihuana, and nabilone: influence of previous marihuana use. *Psychopharmacology* **83,** 36.

47

Clinical Experience of the Synthetic Cannabinoid Nabilone for Chronic Pain

William Notcutt, Mario Price, Patrick Blossfeldt, and Glen Chapman

Abstract

Sixty patients were treated with nabilone while in the pain relief service of James Paget Hospital. Eighteen have obtained useful benefit, and 15 have been equivocal or have experienced significant side-effects. Twenty-seven have obtained no benefit. A 30% success rate would be considered poor by many standards. However, these patients suffered from the worst pain problems of our service and do not respond to placebos.

1. INTRODUCTION

Chronic pain is widespread and its treatment can be one of the most challenging areas of modern medical practice. Patients may have a complex of biological, psychological, and social problems. Their pain is commonly longstanding, and has often been poorly diagnosed and managed. They have usually been to a large number of doctors, had a large number of tests, and have often lost faith with modern medicine.

Whereas there have been many advances in pain management there have be no radically new drugs in this field for more than a decade. Most advances have come in novel delivery modes or systems (e.g. patient controlled analgesia, transdermal fentanyl, etc.).

Clinicians specializing in the management of chronic pain have become skilled in the use of a variety of drugs, many of which are not traditionally considered to be analgesics, such as antidepressants.

2. THE USE OF NABILONE AT JAMES PAGET HOSPITAL

The Pain Relief Service at the James Paget Hospital, Great Yarmouth, United Kingdom, has a small staff of two consultant anesthetists, three nurses, and one psychologist (part-time). It functions in a multidisciplinary mode by working closely with other services (e.g., orthopedics, physical therapy) and supports all pain relief activity within the hospital and out

From: *Marihuana and Medicine*
Edited by: G. G. Nahas et al.   © Humana Press Inc., Totowa, NJ

into the community. The usual problems of high referral rate, rapid turnover, and limited resources are a normal part of everyday practice.

Faced with patients who were untreatable by conventional therapy, one of the authors (W. N.) started using synthetic cannabinoid, nabilone, in a selected group of patients. This as a result of anecdotal reports that *Cannabis* can relieve the pain of multiple sclerosis (MS) and other painful problems such as chronic osteoarthritis. Nabilone was the only prescribable cannabinoid in the United King until 1997. It is only licenced for use for antiemesis in chemotherapy.

All patients who have been considered for treatment with nabilone have received extensive pain management in the past. This has been found to be either inadequate, unsuccessful, or in some cases unavailable. The patients were at "the end of the line," and there were no other options. As experience has grown, we have started to consider the possibility of nabilone at an earlier stage.

Patients with a history of drug abuse or significant recreational use of *Cannabis* have not been treated with nabilone, although we have discovered a number of patients attending our clinics who self medicate with *Cannabis* for their pain. Advising on its use can be part of the pharmacological management of pain nowadays. In large cities this is becoming a normal and regular part of practice. The real drug abusers (heroin, etc.) remain almost impossible to treat for chronic pain.

3. PRESCRIBING NABILONE

We have evolved a method of using nabilone. Initially we prescribe it at night-time so that any drowsiness merely enhances sleep. Most of the patients were suffering from significant sleep disturbance from their pain. The dose required seems to be variable. Sometimes we found that the 1 mg capsule was too much. We therefore would reduce the dose to 0.25 mg for some patients. As the patient's confidence in the drug was achieved, we would introduce it during the daytime as necessary. The highest dose that we have reached is 3 mg/day.

All patients who have perceived some benefit from nabilone have been subjected to a "start–stop–start" regime to establish whether the benefits are real. This would be the normal clinical practice when introducing any other drug to a patient for the management of chronic pain. No placebos were used. No formal trial has yet been undertaken.

Sixty patients have been studied. The age range of most patients lies between 30 and 50 years. More females than males were treated, reflecting the sex difference in a group of patients with multiple sclerosis. The patients have been divided into six groups for presentation. There is overlap between the groups, but from a clinical perspective it is easier to view them in this way.

3.1. Multiple Sclerosis

About 50% of patients with MS present with a variety of pain problems caused by the widespread and variable damage that they suffer in the central nervous system. Although pain management can be relatively easy in the early stages, it can become progressively harder and a few patients become unresponsive to conventional analgesic practice. When combined with other physical disabilities, life can become miserable for this group of patients.

Sixteen patients with advanced MS have been treated with nabilone after the failure of conventional analgesic practice. Six patients have received benefit and three have continued to use nabilone for up to three years. Two have a cluster of pains including neurogenic and retro-orbital pain and problems with muscle spasm. The third experienced mainly searing leg pains. Two of the three have deteriorated significantly from their MS. And one of these has recently discontinued nabilone, finding that she no longer needed it. The benefits for these patients have been analgesia, muscle relaxation, and sleep improvement.

Three patients gained benefit but discontinued nabilone. Two found that *Cannabis* provided better symptom relief both in quality of analgesia and dose control. A third obtained excellent pain control but developed a supraventricular tachycardia (she had experienced this spontaneously in the past). The final 10 patients with a variety of pain problems from MS obtained no useful benefit and some developed the usual side effects of dysphoria and drowsiness.

From the experience of this group of patients, we realized that further studies will require a much greater analysis of the different types of pain to establish what benefits there are.

3.1.1. Aetiology of Pain in MS

1. Central neuropathic caused by damage to pain pathways.
2. Somatic muscle spasm caused by damage to pathways controlling muscle tone.
3. Visceral muscle spasm (e.g., bladder, see above).
4. Mechanical (mainly spinal) caused by loss of muscle function, strength and coordination.
5. Other.
6. Unrelated to MS.

All of these symptoms may be aggravated by a multitude of psychosocial factors including depression, loss of mobility, increased dependence, terminal illness and so on. Therefore, a much more detailed analysis of the pain problems will be essential for future studies of cannabinoids in multiple sclerosis.

3.2. Central Neurogenic Pain

Some are of the most impressive records of the effects of cannabinoids on pain seem to be in the area of central neurogenic pain. Such patients have usually experienced substantial damage to the central nervous system and their pain is commonly very difficult to control.

A 62 year-old woman with de-afferentation pain secondary to a radiofrequency denervation for uncontrolled pain on the right side of her face. This was classical anesthesia dolorosa. She had had a range of assessments including neurological and psychiatric. She had a range of treatments including conventional antidepressant and anticonvulsant therapy. The trial of nabilone achieved good control of the pain and she was able to reduce her use of antidepressants. After nine months of nabilone she was able to discontinue with no return of her pain. Unfortunately she was found at the same time to have a carcinoma of the kidney with significant destruction of the body of L1 by a metastasis. The malignancy was considered to be entirely coincidental. She underwent nephrectomy and radiotherapy (*see* Subheading 4.2).

A variety of other central neurogenic problems have been less successful. A tetraplegic patient obtaining pain control for his legs found nabilone of no use even though *Cannabis* was highly effective. This was probably dosage related. An amputee following a brachial plexus avulsion has obtained temporary benefit, losing all his phantom pain yet continuing to work as a computer engineer. A third patient with a complex regional pain syndrome involving his chest and arm obtained significant relief and was prepared to accept some dysphoria as a trade off. Five other patients have not obtained significant help (cervical myelopathy, central cord injury, and thalamic pain).

3.3. Peripheral Neuropathic Pain

Pain from peripheral neuropathies can be very difficult to treat successfully. They are usually poorly responsive to opioid analgesics and only some patients respond to anticonvulsants and tricyclic antidepressants.

Two patients with diabetic neuropathy and two with surgical nerve damage have been helped, although one found the side effects of nabilone intolerable. A variety of other neuropathies have been tackled in four patients without success (sensorimotor neuropathy, postherpetic neuralgia, postchemotherapy neuropathy, and complex regional pain syndrome of arm).

3.4. Malignancy

The pain of malignancy has become a comparatively easy problem to treat nowadays. The few patients now seen by the pain management service are those with the most complex problems. A 45-year-old male with an advanced bronchial carcinoma that had formed a tracheo-esophageal fistula was experiencing severe upper anterior chest pain, partially relieved by morphine and other standard adjuvant therapy. Nausea and vomiting was also a major problem. He had had extensive surgery and was unwilling to go through any more invasive treatment. As a previous occasional user of *Cannabis* he agreed to try nabilone. He obtained significant improvement in his symptoms, allowing him to cope better with his pain and circumstances. This enabled him to be managed at home for the last few weeks of life.

A 63-year-old woman who had previously used nabilone for anesthesia dolorosa (*see* Subheading 3.2) had developed a renal carcinoma with spinal secondaries. Surgery and radiotherapy had left her with the pain of a partially collapsed L1 vertebra. This pain was only partially controlled with morphine. She requested a further trial of nabilone. One milligram at night has acted as an adjuvant to her analgesics and she maintains a good level of activity some two years after her original diagnosis. From an experience of five patients it is difficult to draw conclusions. However, we have little doubt that cannabinoids may be an adjuvant to the well-established range of analgesics and other drugs that are used to control the pain of malignancy. They may avoid the need for expensive implanted analgesic systems for some patients.

3.5. Spinal Problems

Spinal pain is the commonest problem presenting to all standard pain management services. Out of this group the patients diagnosed as "failed back" (in whom surgery has not led to cure) are the most daunting. They may have a combination of nociceptive and neuropathic pain complicated by major psychosocial disturbances.

Of 15 patients treated, 10 probably obtained benefit with five continuing to use nabilone for up to 2.5 years. Overall this group had the highest incidence of previous *Cannabis* use and all preferred this to nabilone. However, it must be pointed out that these patients had turned to *Cannabis* for assistance but were not previous extensive recreational users.

A wide range of benefits (*see* Subheading 5) has been seen but no specific tendencies could be identified, reflecting the heterogeneity of the group. Improvement in sleep and ability to cope has been more dominant than real analgesia.

3.6. "Heartsink Patients"

Every pain management service has it share of "Heartsink" patients, whose pain and psychosocial circumstances are so bizarre, distorted, and dysfunctional that conventional therapy is wholly ineffective. Such patients can become substantial consumers of clinical time and there is a great temptation to offer them any new therapy that comes along in a desperate attempt to "do something."

Eight such patients have been treated with nabilone. Although three perceived some short-term improvement, there was no continuing therapy in any patient beyond an initial short trial. The temptation to use cannabinoids in this group should be resisted at this stage of knowledge.

4. SUMMARY OF THE RESULTS OF PATIENTS TREATED WITH NABILONE

Sixty patients were treated with nabilone in the Pain Relief Service of James Paget Hospital. Eighteen have obtained useful benefit, and 15 have been equivocal or have experienced significant side effects. Twenty-seven have obtained no benefit. A 30% success rate would be considered poor by many standards. However, these patients suffered from the worst pain problems of our service and do not respond to placebos.

5. SUMMARY OF THE BENEFITS OF NABILONE

This group of patients has been very heterogenous and it is difficult to draw many conclusions. Certain benefits of nabilone were seen and most patients experienced more than one:

1. Relief of pain.
2. Distancing of the patient from his pain, "compressing" the pain.
3. Improvement in sleep.
4. Relief of muscle spasm.
5. Relief of bladder spasms.
6. Relief of constipation.
7. Relaxation and relief of anxiety.
8. Relief of misery, life more tolerable, relief of depression.
9. Mild euphoria

This list of benefits defines the main symptoms that need to be studied in the next generation of clinical trials of cannabinoids for chronic pain.

All patients who have tried smoked cannabis as well as nabilone have found the former to be better. The quality of pain control and the ability to titrate the amount of drug have been the key issues.

6. SUMMARY OF THE ADVERSE EFFECTS OF NABILONE

A large proportion of the patients we have treated have experienced side effects. Drowsiness and dysphoria have been the commonest and are the reason why many have discontinued the drug in spite of obtaining a benefit. The intrinsic properties of nabilone, the difficulty of controlling the bioavailability, and the inability to titrate the drug against fluctuations of pain through the day are all possible reasons for this. However, to set this within the context of chronic pain, these symptoms and problems are part of the normal spectrum of adverse effects that a physician will see from the analgesics, anticonvulsants, antidepressants, and other drugs used for pain management.

Dependency is a major concern. However, we have only seen it occur in one patient. He gets mild withdrawal symptoms on discontinuation of nabilone. These are far less in intensity than is seen with therapeutically used opiates and are also much less of a problem than those seen from benzodiazepine use. The only cardiovascular problem has been the precipitation of a supraventricular tachycardia in a patient susceptible to this condition.

7. FUTURE STUDIES

Patients with chronic pain are a heterogeneous group. Therefore the classical double-blind, placebo-controlled studies are going to prove very difficult. Other techniques such as open crossover studies using each patient as his or her own control ($n = 1$) will probably be the next step forward. Studies of other drugs in chronic pain such as amitriptylline may be appropriate models to follow. The success of future trials will depend heavily not only on a satisfactory range of cannabinoids and cannabinoid mixtures (i.e., plant extracts) but also on a range of delivery modes and systems (e.g., oral slow acting, inhaled rapid acting, suppository, parenteral, and soon). However, clinical studies on the analgesic properties of smoked *Cannabis* are unnecessary, scientifically almost impossible to conduct, and medically unacceptable.

8. CONCLUSION

This experience with nabilone adds to a large body of anecdotal information on the use of cannabinoids for the management of pain. Although it produces no absolute proof, our evidence indicates that cannabinoids may well have a place in pain management and thus provides some sign posts for the way ahead. Further clinical trials are essential to establish the place of this potentially very valuable group of drugs. The medical use of cannabinoids is a medical issue and should remain entirely with clinicians and scientists who can best determine the true therapeutic place of these agents.

48 Cannabinoids in the Treatment of Pain
An Overview

Michel Dubois, Gabriel Nahas,
and Kenneth Sutin

The mechanisms of the analgesic properties of marihuana and cannabinoids anecdotally reported until this day have never been clearly defined in pharmacology or in clinical medicine. The purpose of the session devoted to "Cannabinoids and the treatment of pain" was to discuss the clinical reports of marihuana use as an analgesic in the light of the pharmacological and molecular mode of action of this drug on pain mechanisms.

SUMMARY OF PAPERS

The papers presented described the effects of THC and of its psychoactive derivatives, parenterally administered on the expression of pain clinically reported or experimentally induced. The two major pathways that modulate pain perception, the endorphin receptors and prostaglandin biosynthesis, were first described.

Terenius summarized the mechanisms of action of centrally acting "analgesics" mediated by opioid receptors. He described the role of different neuronal systems of the dorsal horn of the spinal cord and of the brain, primarily the opioid receptor and their modulation by $\alpha 2$ adrenergic agents and NMDA. Interactions of THC with the endorphin system of the brain and spinal cord were suggested, though the reported antinociceptive effects of the drug are not blocked by naltrexone. The overall fundamental role of the opioid system in the control of acute pain was emphasized.

Brune reported his studies on the mechanisms of action of NSAID's, which inhibit biosynthesis of prostaglandins by cyclooxygenase inhibition. This inhibitory effect of cyclooxygenase on prostaglandins occurs in peripheral tissues as a result of inflammation or trauma, but also in the dorsal root of the spinal cord. NSAIDs have therefore besides their peripheral antinociceptive properties a central nervous analgesic effect *(1)*.

From: *Marihuana and Medicine*
Edited by: G. G. Nahas et al.   © Humana Press Inc., Totowa, NJ

Martin reviewed the experimental studies performed on rodents exposed to acute pain (tail flick or hot plate test) or inflammatory pain (acetic acid administration). He reported significant antinociceptive effects of THC in both models of pain. The most effective mode of administration of THC was intravenously or intrathecally. His studies indicated that the AEA-G protein receptor which is the target of THC mediates the antinociceptive effect of the drug since AEA synthetic agonists have a similar antinociceptive effect and AEA synthetic antagonists suppress it.

The review of Dray (2) on chronic pain summarizes the manifold changes occurring in this unfortunate condition, including neurochemical cellular alterations and morphological rearrangement in the nervous system. The management of these alterations remains problematic and difficult, requiring special care. A range of medications targeted to specific molecular sites of the central and autonomic nervous system are tailored to individual patients.

Koe reviewed the experimental studies and clinical trials up to phase II of Levonantradol, a synthetic cannabinoid developed by Pfizer in the 1970s. The drug proved to have effective antinociceptive properties similar to that of morphine, but its psychoactive side effects prevented its clinical acceptance and its development was discontinued. A similar decision was taken in the United States for Nabilone, a drug developed by Lilly under the direction of L. Lemberger. Nabilone was mostly used as an antiemetic.

However, Nabilone is still available for medical prescription in the United Kingdom. Notcutt reported clinical studies using Nabilone capsules (0.5 –1 mg) for the management of chronic pain. Administration of the drug resulted in a 30% positive outcome for the management of chronic refractory pain in various conditions such as multiple sclerosis, central neurogenic pain and malignancy. Large clinical controlled trials of Nabilone and THC for the management of chronic pain are now being considered.

The only controlled clinical trial of marihuana smoking to assess its antalgic property was reported by Clark. Clark updated his previous observations on 16 heavy marihuana smokers studied under controlled conditions over a 2-yr period in a hospital environment. He used the sensory decision methodology that allows one to distinguish between discriminability and response criteria in reference to thermal pain. The statistical analysis of his studies concluded that smoked marihuana lowers the pain threshold by an increase in sensory perception. This controlled study was never duplicated but clinical observations have reported limited analgesia associated with side effects and less effectiveness than morphine (3).

DISCUSSION

It would appear that cannabinoids exert their antalgic properties by interacting with the two major biochemical pathways that control pain: the endorphin pathway (targeted by the opiates) for acute pain (4) and the prostaglandin pathway (targeted by the NSAID's) for inflammatory pain (1). Effects of THC on acute pain have been attributed to a G protein coupled mechanism, and the effects of THC on inflammatory pain on a bilipid layer membrane mediated effect.

Cannabinoids and the Opiate Pathway: A Receptor Mediated Effect?

Effects of THC and other psychoactive natural or synthetic cannabinoids in relieving pain have been documented in rodents by Martin, especially when he used the i.v. and intrathecal route of administration (5). However, Waser and Martin (6), using the hot plate test on mice, reported that THC has no antalgic effect when compared to similar doses of morphine. In man, the use of THC for the control of acute pain has given equivocal results (3). THC is not as effective as codeineand presents unwanted side effects *(7)*. The combination of opiates (dihydromorphine) andTHC when used clinically as preanesthetic medication significantly increases the undesirable side effects of both medications in a dose-related fashion (8), and this combination should not be prescribed.

The reported analgesic effects of cannabinoids in acute pain would be mediated like its psychoactive effects by the AEA–G-protein-coupled receptor of THC. The main suggested effector mechanism of this AEA–G-protein-coupled receptor is decreased cyclic AMP. This mechanism has not been directly related to a decrease in pain perception. The mechanism of action of the AEA–G-protein-coupled receptor mediated effect on acute pain remains to be clarified, but it does not seem to be dominant, since THC has a limited clinical antalgic effect on acute pain.

Should the analgesic effect of THC be mediated by the AEA–G-protein-coupled receptor, it would not be possible to dissociate analgesia from psychoactivity, which is the stated goal of the search for medications based on THC and its psychoactive derivatives *(9)*.

Conversely, THC and cannabinoids exert a significant effect on inflammatory pain, which is mediated by cyclooxygenase inhibition of prostaglandins.

Cannabinoids in Inflammatory Pain

THC releases prostaglandins *(10)* and its 11 THC oic acid derivative inhibits cyclooxygenase and prostaglandin biosynthesis *(11)*. Therefore, cannabinoids exert a dual promoting and inhibiting effect on prostaglandin biosynthesis. THC 11 oic acid and its synthetic derivatives are effective in relieving inflammatory pain in rodents, which confirms an observation made by Waser and Martin *(6)* who reported that THC in doses of 3.5–10 mg i.p. was as effective as morphine in the writing test (acetic acid injection).

A clinical comparison of nonpsychoactive cannabinoids (11-THCoic acid derivatives) with NSAID's in the treatment of inflammatory pain remains to be performed.

Cannabinoids: "Partial" Analgesics

For acute pain (surgical pain) THC and psychoactive cannabinoids exert a limited analgesic effect, inseparable from their euphoriant effect. Nonpsychoactive cannabinoids lack analgesic effect.

In inflammatory pain, primarily synthetic nonpsychoactive cannabinoids, which release prostaglandin and inhibit cyclooxygenase, exert antalgic properties which must still be clinically assessed.

By comparison, the opiates and NSAID's are targeted specifically to the major mechanisms that mediate pain (endorphin system in acute pain, and cyclooxygenase inhibition in inflammatory pain) and produce dose-related effects. The combination of both opiates and NSAID's increases their antalgic properties. In addition, infiltration of tissue with local anesthetics offers another therapeutic intervention to relieve acute pain by a direct action on pain fibers. THC does not have local anesthetic effects.

Cannabinoids might be considered "partial" analgesics for inflammatory pain. The AEA–G-protein receptor, dubbed the "cannabinoid receptor," has not proven to be the site of an independent new pathway for the control of pain, comparable to the endorphins or cyclooxygenase.

THC and Smoked Marihuana

Anecdotal accounts report patient claims that smoked marihuana is more effective in relieving their symptoms than THC (marinol) administered by mouth. The rapid euphoriant

RECEPTOR AND NON-RECEPTOR MEDIATED ANTALGIC EFFECTS OF THC

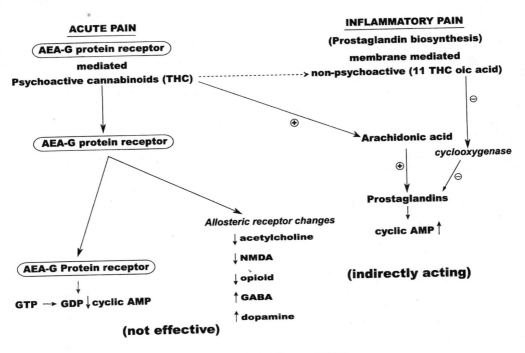

Fig. 1. Receptor- and nonreceptor-mediated antalgic effects of THC.

property of marihuana smoke could act as a reinforcer, which may be compared to the psychopharmacological effect of alcohol or benzodiazepines. This euphoriant property of marihuana smoke would be an asset if it were not associated with an inherent toxicity to the lung (12). Marihuana smoke in addition to its toxic components (aldehydes, phenols, carcinogens, and carbon monoxide) also contains, besides THC, sixty cannabinoids in varying concentration according to the origin of the cannabis plant (13). Psychoactive cannabinoids like CBN or CBD, which are present in significant concentration in marihuana smoke, have properties that are antagonistic to THC (14). Presently there are no standardized marihuana cigarettes containing uniform THC and cannabinoid concentrations. These will vary from one batch to another (15).

It is not possible to compare the effects of marihuana smoke, a composite mixture of cannabinoids, with the effects of ingested pure THC for methodological limitations (16).

Smoking marihuana is neither a practical nor a harmless mode of drug delivery, especially in the hospital where smoking is prohibited and an open flame unsafe. Marihuana has adverse interactions with other approved therapeutic drugs. It has multiple pharmacological effects and causes adverse psychoactive effects at doses required to achieve a therapeutic endpoint. It is contraindicated in older patients and patients with cardiac disease or pulmonary insufficiency. As discussed in this monograph (17), the deregulation of membrane signaling mechanisms by THC and marihuana accounts for its partial and discordant therapeutic effects (Fig. 1).

Physicians have a variety of safe, highly selective short or long acting (slow release) analgesic drugs which effectively produce analgesia, sedation, sleep, or anxiolysis.

REFERENCES

1. Brune, K. (1998) Antipyretic analgesic drugs, in *Marihuana and Medicine* (Nahas, G., et al., ed.), Humana Press, Totowa, New Jersey.
2. Dray, A. (1998) Pharmacology of chronic pain, in *Marihuana and Medicine* (Nahas, G., et al., ed.), Humana Press, Totowa, New Jersey.
3. Sutin, K., Nahas, G. (1998) Interactions of marihuana (THC) and other drugs with special reference to anesthesia, in *Marihuana and Medicine* (Nahas, G., et al., ed.), Human Press, Totowa, New Jersey.
4. Terenius, L. (1998) Central mechanisms of pain and analgesia, in *Marihuana and Medicine* (Nanas, G. ed.), Humana Press, Totowa, New Jersey.
5. Martin, B., Lichtman, A. (1998) Analgesic properties of "cannabinoids" and anandamides, in *Marihuana and Medicine* (Nahas, G., et al., ed.), Humana Press, Totowa, New Jersey.
6. Waser, P., Martin, A. (1998) Analgesic and behavioral effects of delta-9-THC and some of its synthetic derivatives, in *Marihuana and Medicine* (Nahas, G., et al., ed.), Humana Press, New Jersey.
7. Noyes, R., Jr., Brunk, S.F.nol , Avery, D.A.H., Canter, A.C. (1975) The analgesic properties of delta-9-tetrahydrocannabiand codeine. *Clin Pharmacol Ther.* **18,** 84–89.
8. Johnstone, R.E., Lief, P.L., Kulp, R.A., Smith, T.C. (1975) Combination of delta–9 tetrahydrocannabinol with oxymorphone or pentobarbital: Effects on ventilatory control and cardiovascular dynamics. *Anesthesiology.* **42,** 674–684.
9. Mechoulam, R., Devane, W., Glaser, R. (1998) Cannabinoid geometry and biological activity, in Marihuana and Medicine (Nahas, G., et al., ed.), Humana Press, Totowa, New Jersey.
10. Burstein, S., Hunter, S., Sedor, C., Shulman, S. (1982) Prostaglandins and cannabis IX. Stimulation of PGE-2 synthesis in human lung fibroblasts by delta- 1 -THC. *Biochem Phannacol.* **31,** 2361–2365.
11. Zurier, R.B., Rossetti, R.G., Lane, J.H., Goldberg, J.M., Hunter, S.A., Burstein, S.H.(1998) Dimethylheptyl-THC-11 oic acid: a nonpsychoactive anti inflammatory agent with a cannabinoid template structure, in *Marihuana and Medicine* (Nahas, G., et al., ed.), Humana Press, New Jersey.
12. Tashkin, D. (1998) Marihuana and the lung, in *Marihuana and Medicine* (Nahas, G., et al., ed.), Humana Press, Totowa, New Jersey.
13. Turner, C. (1998) About science and politics, in *Marihuana and Medicine* (Nahas, G., et al., ed.), Humana Press, Totowa, New Jersey.
14. Trouve, R., Nahas, G. (1998) Marihuana and the cardiovascular system, in *Marihuana and Medicine* (Nahas, G., et al., ed.), Humana Press, Totowa, New Jersey.
15. Thomas, B., Parker, V., Caddell, L., Jones, L., Sabharwal, S., McDaniel, A., Keimowitz, A., S, Scheffler, N., Hart, E., Mitchell, J., Davis, K. (1998) Composition and stability of a standard marihuana cigarette, in *Marihuana and Medicine* (Nahas, G.,et al., ed.). Humana Press, Totowa, New Jersey.
16. Frick H., Pace N., Sutin, K., Rosenthal M., Manger W., Hyman, G., and Nahas, G. (1998) Marihuana for Medicine in perspective, in Marihuana and Medicine (Nahas, G., et al ed), Humana Press, Totowa, New Jersey
17. Nahas, G., Harvey D., Sutin K., and Agurell S. Receptor and non-receptor membrane mediated effects of THC and cannabinoids, in Marihuana and Medicine (Nahas, G. et al Ed.) p. 781, Humana Press, Totowa, New Jersey

VI Marihuana and Glaucoma

49

Marihuana and Intraocular Pressure
Possible Mechanisms of Action

Keith Green

Abstract

An objective scientifically based overview is presented of clinical and basic data on intraocular pressure (IOP) and other ocular effects of marihuana or cannabinoids. All data indicate that marihuana or cannabinoid inhalation, and oral cannabinoids, reduce IOP in 60 to 65% of normal or glaucoma volunteers. Animal studies reveal that the IOP reduction occurs via a primary effect on ocular fluid outflow pathways. The rapid rate of change of IOP would indicate a pathway for fluid exit of other than conventional outflow. Recent data indicate that the IOP reduction may not be mediated by cannabinoid receptors. Pursuit of individual cannabinoids or related agents with IOP-reducing capacity coupled with low euphoria induction as topical or oral agents for glaucoma treatment should be undertaken. Smoking of marihuana *per se* as a treatment modality for glaucoma appears to present unfavorable conditions for the medical therapy of this disease.

1. GENERAL MEDICAL EFFECTS

Several marihuana health hazards have been identified *(1–3)*. Some responses cannot be exclusively ascribed to marihuana because of the intermittent patterns of human marihuana intake; the use of marihuana in younger age groups who are usually in better health than an elderly population; the absence of defined, controlled marihuana intake; and the difficulty in separating marihuana effects from those associated with the parallel use of alcohol, tobacco, and other drugs.

Acute marihuana effects have been documented as increased pulse rate, orthostatic hypotension, euphoria, conjunctival hyperemia, and reduction in intraocular pressure (IOP) *(4–8)*. Long-term clinical effects in humans are mainly related to respiratory, hormonal, and reproductive toxicity *(9–13)*. Marihuana smoking leads to emphysema-like changes as a result of cannabinoids or the release of tars, carcinogens, and other volatiles as found with tobacco smoke *(12)*. Of concern are the marihuana-induced cognitive effects that assume greater significance with chronic repetitive exposure especially in the age group in which glaucoma occurs *(14,15)*.

From: *Marihuana and Medicine*
Edited by: G. G. Nahas et al.   © Humana Press Inc., Totowa, NJ

Each of these factors must be considered when their potential use on a chronic basis is examined as a treatment modality. This is especially true for glaucoma where continued use would be necessary to control this 24-hour-a-day disease with between 2200 and 3600 marihuana cigarettes per year.

The ubiquitous effects of the cannabinoids, and marihuana, on many biological systems have been attributed to one of several modes of action. These include direct effects on intracellular biochemical processes, perturbations of cell membranes, or interaction with one of the two cannabinoid receptors. CB_1 is located in the CNS, whereas CB_2 receptors occur in systemic immune system tissues (16,17). Through the use of cannabinoid agonists such as WIN 5512-2, and methanandamide and others such as HU211, the identification of cannabinoid receptors, and their role in reflecting the biological activity of the cannabinoids, a better overview of the effects of these compounds has occurred (18–20).

2. OCULAR EFFECTS

In humans, smoking marihuana, inhalation of cigarette smoke containing Δ^9-tetrahydrocannabinol (Δ^9-THC), intravenous cannabinoids, or oral intake of Δ^9-THC or marihuana leads to conjunctival hyperemia and decreased lacrimation (21–36). Ocular side effects include diplopia, impairment of accommodation, photophobia, nystagmus, and blepharospasm. It is difficult to identify a priori a common pharmacological mechanism to account for all of these changes. While only little is known, the ocular effects of chronic marihuana inhalation appear to be the same as those for acute administration (26,30). Different pupillary effects have been reported that appear to depend to some degree upon the circumstances of marihuana intake (37,38).

Different cannabinoids reduce IOP in about 60 to 65% of humans when given intravenously (25). Marihuana and Δ^9-THC (whether inhaled or taken orally) also decrease IOP in 60–65% of nonglaucomatous volunteers (21–24,27,32,33,35) and in the same percentage of volunteer glaucoma patients (27,28,31,33,35,36). Orthostatic hypotension and decreased lacrimation occur quickly after smoking 2% Δ^9-THC cigarettes, as has been noted with a synthetic THC homolog (34).

Individual responses vary widely in nonglaucoma volunteers and patients after marihuana smoking. Nevertheless, an apparent dose-response relationship occurred between cannabinoids, or marihuana smoking, and IOP when groups were evaluated. It is of interest to note that increased dose leads to a greater maximal IOP fall but no prologation of logevity of the response. The major difficulty with smoking marihuana was an inability to separate IOP fall from euphoria. The IOP fell by about 25%, with a range from –45 to +5% after smoking 2% marihuana through a water-cooled pipe (21). A further study revealed a 50% decrease in tear flow (27). The IOP fall duration was about 3–4 hours, by which time IOP approached the presmoking level (21–24,26–28,31–36).

Further studies in primary open-angle glaucoma (POAG) patients also revealed a fall in IOP in 60–65% of the population after either smoking marihuana or ingestion of Δ^9-THC (27,28,31,34,36). Seven of 11 patients in one study showed a fall in IOP of about 30% after smoking 2% marihuana cigarettes (28). This was confirmed later with either smoking or oral Δ^9-THC (33).

In a meta-analysis of published data, about 300 volunteers (nonglaucomatous subjects or POAG patients) were examined for acute ocular effects of marihuana smoking or cannabinoid use (topical, oral, or intravenous). Since the largest group consisted of about 40 persons, a broad spectrum of situations existed under which marihuana or one of its constituents reduced IOP.

The IOP fall is of therapeutic interest because of the relationship between IOP and glaucomatous eye damage. Glaucoma often consists of an increased IOP, decreased visual field (with irreversible defects), and a change in the color and appearance of the optic disc. Because IOP offers a quantitative measurement, it is frequently used as a marker of the efficacy of glaucoma drug effects. This may or may not be appropriate, depending upon the simultaneous determination of visual fields and photographic documentation of the optic disc.

3. ANIMAL STUDIES

Following the initial report of an IOP fall in man after smoking marihuana (21), a series of animal studies was undertaken. Intravenous Δ^9-THC reduced rabbit IOP (39) at dose levels akin to those in human plasma after smoking a marihuana cigarette. Others reported a 30% fall in rabbit IOP after 100 to 200 µg Δ^9-THC per kilogram body weight (40), with a time-course of a maximal fall at 1 hour and return to baseline by 3 hours.

Elsohly and coworkers (41,42) reported that intravenous Δ^8-THC, Δ^9-THC, cannabinol, and nabilone reduced rabbit IOP and reduced monkey IOP after oral administration. These results supported others reported after either intravenous or topical cannabinoids in rabbits (43,44). Structure-activity relationships have been explored (41–44). Rabbits exposed to marihuana smoke showed an IOP fall of 30 to 40% with the maximum at 1–2 hours (27). Topical solutions of 1 and 2% Δ^9-THC in sesame oil reduced rabbit IOP (27,44) as did suspensions of Δ^9-THC in carboxymethylcellulose (45). Mechoulam and coworkers (46) found that Δ^8-THC and cannabinoid acetate reduced IOP in a rabbit glaucoma model.

The IOP effects of various cannabinoids have been examined when administered as a topical drop (44–54). There is a strong influence of the adrenergic nervous system in the modulation of cannabinoid effects in the rabbit (49,55), although this is absent in the cat (56). Both rabbit and cat results indicate that the cannabinoid effect on IOP is realized through an effect primarily on the outflow pathways for aqueous humor from the eye (39,47,57–59). There is a small, but distinguishable, effect on inflow of fluid into the eye (39). Inflow and outflow balance regulates IOP; hence changes in the rate of fluid entry or egress alter IOP.

The rate of aqueous humor flow (µL/min) through the anterior chamber of the eye can be described as:

$$\text{Aqueous humor flow rate} = (\text{IOP} - \text{Pev}) \, C$$

where IOP is intraocular pressure, Pev is episcleral venous pressure (the drainage site for aqueous humor into the circulation; the pressure in these veins is normally 7 mmHg), thus (IOP - Pev) is the pressure head for fluid outflow from the eye (in mmHg); C = outflow facility (µL fluid/mmHg/min), or 1/resistance to outflow.

Normally the equation is approximately:

$$2.5 \, \mu L/min = 10 \, mmHg \times 0.25 \, \mu L/mmHg/min$$

Thus, if IOP decreases and aqueous flow is constant, then outflow facility must increase to maintain balance at steady state. Aqueous humor flow rate is readily measured noninvasively using fluorophotometry thereby providing a means of determining the cause of an alteration in IOP.

A regulatory aspect of Δ^9-THC effects on IOP involving the central nervous system has been examined through the infusion of cannabinoids into conscious rabbit cerebral ventricles (60,61). No effects occurred after intraventricular injection of up to 1 mg Δ^9-THC, suggesting that the ocular hypotensive effect does not lie in the central nervous system.

4. PHARMACOLOGY

The speed of onset of the IOP effect and the underlying change in fluid egress from the eye strongly imply that the marijuana/cannabinoid effects are not modulated via conventional outflow pathways, namely, the trabecular meshwork. It is known that effects in this fluid pathway are controlled to a large extent by the composition of the glycosaminoglycan matrix of the trabecular meshwork. Agents that influence this pathway, e.g., steroids, usually reveal effects only after continued use over a several week duration (62–65). Another pathway for fluid exit from the eye is the uveoscleral (66,67), or uveovortex (68,69) route, where fluid passes rearwards through the root of the iris to the suprachoroidal space and hence exits the eye via transscleral or vortex vein routes. Recent studies have identified several pharmacological agents that reduce IOP through effects on the latter pathway (70–75).

Several years ago we identified that intravenous ^{9}-THC suppressed the substantial ocular IOP and other responses to 2% arachidonic acid, but not prostaglandin E_2 (PGE_2), indicating that THC antagonized the in vivo production of prostaglandin from arachidonic acid (76). The quantities of arachidonic acid (2%) and PGE_2 (10 μg) used were high. More recent information has been obtained to show that very low quantities of prostaglandin analogs (0.001–0.005%; 0.5–2.5 μg) significantly reduce IOP in test animals as well as normal and glaucomatous human populations (77–83). THC and other cannabinoids are known to stimulate arachidonic acid biosynthesis that results, in different species and in different tissues, in a cascade of prostaglandins and related compounds (84–88). It is possible, therefore, that the effects of marijuana/cannabinoids on IOP are the result of enhancement of the arachidonic acid metabolic cascade that further leads to effects revealed on the unconventional outflow pathways. The latter is known to respond rapidly to pharmacological stimuli and perhaps offers an explanation for the IOP effects. Such a hypothesis would be easily tested by determining IOP responses to cannabinoids in the presence or absence of known inhibitors (e.g., indomethacin and other NSAIDs) of the arachidonic acid cascade.

5. TOPICAL CANNABINOIDS IN HUMANS

Topical Δ^9-THC was examined in rabbits, dogs, and primates both for pharmacological activity (27,43–54) as well as toxicology (89) prior to being tested in humans (90–93). The lipophilic cannabinoids represent a challenge in terms of local drug delivery to the eye. The best vehicle identified in the early 1980s (50) (light mineral oil) has been superseded in the late 1990s by technological advancements that allow solubilization of lipid-soluble compounds with chemicals that are themselves water-soluble (e.g., cyclodextrins). Other approaches have used a prodrug approach with water-soluble esters of a maleate salt of a Δ^9-THC-related compound (54). The development of nonpsychoactive drugs also has resulted in separation of IOP reduction from euphoric effects in experimental animal tests (94,95). In humans, Δ^9-THC drops using mineral oil vehicle were ineffective in reducing IOP in either single or multiple drop studies because of the induction of ocular irritation (92,93).

6. ADDITIONAL DRUGS

The development of compounds such as HU211 that show a complete absence of euphoric effects, whereas retaining IOP-reducing activity (94) is a major advance. HU211 also reduces IOP through an effect on outflow of fluid from the eye (96). This compound also shows a lack of binding to the CB_1 receptor (95). Increasing knowledge concerning cannabinoid receptor behavior and their relationship to pharmacological events will allow exploration of different structural analogs. Such studies may identify compounds and ligands that reduce IOP when given topically to rabbit or monkey eyes and thus might be efficacious as potential glaucoma medications *(48,97–105)*. Topical administration has the clinical advantage of allowing the use of a low drug mass per delivery volume. Oral administration of cannabinoid-related compounds that lack psychoactive effects, but will reduce IOP could be a significant addition to the ophthalmic armamentarium against glaucoma.

Because cannabinoids and related substances are readily characterized chemically, they represent an area in which a focus should be made in the future. Compounds could be identified which have no, or minimal, euphoric effects. Use of these chemicals would provide drugs that reduce IOP by specific interactions with receptors or other membrane components. Furthermore, the cannabinoid-related compounds could be additive to other currently available glaucoma medications that act on aqueous humor inflow or conventional outflow pathways.

7. CONCLUSION

The reasons for the selection of cannabinoids versus marihuana are compelling for glaucoma studies. Such a maneuver would allow a focus on individual chemicals rather than on a nonstandardized plant material *(106)*. The latter has no possibility, because of the inherent variability and the plant versatility, of reaching the standards required by the FDA, or equivalent agencies in other countries or alliances, in terms of chemical identity, purity, or characterization. Furthermore, use of modalilties other than smoking reduce the exposure of a cannabinoid user to undersirable side effects including smoke as well as other drugs within its plant material.

8. ACKNOWLEDGMENTS

Supported in part by an unrestricted departmental award from Research to Prevent Blindness, New York, NY. The author is a Senior Scientific Investigator Awardee from Research to Prevent Blindness. I thank Brenda Sheppard for her valuable secretarial assistance.

REFERENCES

1. Hollister, L. E. (1986) Health aspects of cannabis. *Pharmacol. Rev.* **38**, 1–20.
2. Nahas, G. G., ed. (1984) Marihuana in Science and Medicine, Raven, New York.
3. Agurell, S., Dewey, W. L., and Willette, R. E., eds. (1984) *The Cannabinoids: Chemical, Pharmacologic and Therapeutic Aspects,* Academic, New York.
4. Hollister, L. E. (1971) Actions of various marihuana derivatives in man. *Pharmacol. Rev.* **23**, 349–357.
5. Dewey, W. L. (1986) Cannabinoid pharmacology. *Pharmacol. Rev.* **38**,151–178.
6. Klonoff, H. (1983) Acute psychological effects of marihuana in man, including acute cognitive, psychomotor, and perceptual effects in driving, In: *Adverse Health and Behavioral Consequences of Cannabis Use* (Fehr, K.O. and Kalant, H., eds.), Addictive Research Foundation, Toronto, pp. 433–474.
7. Perez-Reyes, M., Lipton, M. A., Timmons, M. C., Wall, M. E., Brine, D. R., and Davis, K. H. (1973) Pharmacology of orally administered Δ^9-tetrahydrocannabinol. *Clin. Pharmacol. Therap.* **14**, 48–55.
8. Green, K. (1979) The ocular effects of cannabinoids, In: *Current Topics in Eye Research, Vol. I* (Zadunaisky, J.A. and Davson, H., eds.) Academic, New York, pp. 175–215.
9. Munson, A. E. and Fehr, K. O. (1983) Immunological effects of cannabis, In: *Adverse Health and Behavioral Consequences of Cannabis Use* (Fehr, K. O. and Kalant, H., eds.), Addictive Research Foundation, Toronto, pp. 257–353.
10. Bloch, E. (1983) Effects of marihuana and cannabinoids on reproduction, endocrine function, development, and chromosomes, In: *Adverse Health and Behavioral Consequences of Cannabis Use* (Fehr, K. O. and Kalant, H., eds.), Addictive Research Foundation, Toronto, pp. 355–432.
11. Rosenkrantz, H. (1983) Cannabis, marihuana, and cannabinoid toxicological manifestations in man and animals, In: *Adverse Health and Behavioral Consequences of Cannabis Use* (Fehr, K. O. and Kalant, H., eds.) Addictive Research Foundation, Toronto, pp. 91–175.

12. Tashkin, D. P., Shapiro, B. J., Ramanna, L., Taplin, G. V., Lee, Y. E., and Harper, C. E. (1976) Chronic effects of heavy marihuana smoking on pulmonary function in healthy young males, In: *The Pharmacology of Marihuana* (Braude, M. C. and Szara, S., eds.), Raven, New York, pp. 291–295.

13. Dornbush, R. L. and Kokkevi, A. (1976) The acute effects of various cannabis substances on cognitive, perceptual, and motor performance in very long-term hashish users, In: *The Pharmacology of Marihuana* (Braude, M. C. and Szara, S., eds.), Raven, New York, pp. 421–427.

14. Fletcher, J. M., Page, J. B., Francis, D. J., Copeland, K., Naus, M. J., Davis, C. M., Morris, R., Krauskopf, d., and Satz, P. (1996) Cognitive correlates of long-term cannabis use in Costa Rican men. *Arch. Gen. Psych.* **53**,1051–1057.

15. Solowij, N., Michie, P. T., and Fox, A. M. (1995) Differential impairments of selective attention due to frequency and duration of cannabis use. *Biol. Psych.* **37**, 731–739.

16. Howlett, A. C. (1995) Pharmacology of cannabinoid receptors. *Ann. Rev. Pharmacol. Toxicol.* **35**, 607–634.

17. Lynn, A. B. and Herkenham, M. (1994) Localization of cannabinoid receptors and nonsaturable high-density cannabinoid binding sites in peripheral tissues of the rat: implications for receptor-mediated immune modulation by cannabinoids. *J. Pharmacol. Exp. Therap.* **268**, 1612–1623.

18. Mechoulam, R., Feigenbaum, J. J., Lander, N., Segal, M., Jarbe, T. U., Hiltunen, A. J., and Consroe, P. (1988) Enantiomeric cannabinoids: Stereospecificity of psychotropic activity. *Experientia* **44**,762–764.

19. Howlett, A. C., Champion, T. M., Wilken, G. H., and Mechoulam, R. (1990) Stereochemical effects of 11-OH- Δ^8-tetrahydrocannabinol-dimethylheptyl to inhibit adenylate cyclase and bind to the cannabinoid receptor. *Neuropharmacology* **29**, 161–165.

20. Fride, E. and Mechoulam, R. (1993) Pharmacological activity of the cannabinoid receptor agonist, anandamide, a brain constituent. *Eur. J. Pharmacol.* **231**, 313–314.

21. Hepler, R. S. and Frank, I. M. (1971) Marihuana smoking and intraocular pressure. *JAMA* **217**, 1392.

22. Purnell, W. D. and Gregg, J. M. (1973) Δ9-tetrahydrocannabinol, euphoria and intraocular pressure in man. *Ann. Ophthalmol.* **7**, 921–923.

23. Flom, M. C., Adams, A. J., and Jones, R. T. (1975) Marihuana smoking and reduced pressure in human eyes. Drug action or epiphenomenon. *Invest. Ophthalmol.* **14**, 52–55.

24. Cooler, P. and Gregg, J. M. (1976) The effect of delta-9-tetrahydrocannabinol on intraocular pressure in humans, In: *The Therapeutic Potential of Marihuana* (Cohen, S. and Stillman, R.C., eds.), Plenum, New York, pp. 77–87.

25. Perez-Reyes, M., Wagner, D., Wall, M. E., and Davis, K. H. (1976) Intravenous administration of cannabinoids on intraocular pressure, In: *The Pharmacology of Marihuana* (Braude, M.C. and Szara, S., eds.), Raven, New York, pp. 829–832.

26. Jones, R. T. and Benowitz, N. (1976) The 30-day trip: Clinical studies of cannabis tolerance and dependence, In: *The Pharmacology of Marihuana* (Braude, M. C. and Szara, S., eds.), Raven, New York, pp. 627–642.

27. Hepler, R. S., Frank, I. M., and Petrus, R. (1976) Ocular effects of marihuana smoking, In: *The Pharmacology of Marihuana* (Braude, M. C. and Szara, S., eds.), Raven, New York, pp. 815–824.

28. Hepler, R. S. and Petrus, R. (1976) Experiences with administration of marihuana to glaucoma patients, In: *The Therapeutic Potential of Marihuana* (Cohen, S. and Stillman, R. C., eds.), Plenum, New York, pp. 63–75.

29. Green, K. and Bowman, K. A. (1976) Effect of marihuana derivatives on intraocular pressure, In: *The Pharmacology of Marihuana* (Braude, M. C. and Szara, S., eds.), Raven, New York, pp. 803–813.

30. Dawson, W. W., Jiminez-Antillon, C. F., Perez, J. M., and Zeskind, J. A. (1977) Marihuana and vision after ten years' use in Costa Rica. *Invest. Ophthalmol.* **16**, 689–699.

31. Crawford, W. J. and Merritt, J. C. (1979) Effects of tetrahydrocannabinol on arterial and intraocular hypertension. *Int. J. Clin. Pharmacol. Biopharm.* **17**, 191–196.

32. Merritt, J. C., Crawford, W. J., Alexander, P. C., Anduze, A. L., and Gelbart, S. S. (1980) Effect of marihuana on intraocular and blood pressure in glaucoma. *Ophthalmology* **87**, 222–228.

33. Merritt, J. C., McKinnon, S. M., Armstrong, J. R., Hatem, G., and Reid, L. A. (1980) Oral Δ^9-tetrahydrocannabinol in heterogeneous glaucomas. *Ann. Ophthalmol.* **12**, 947–950.

34. Tiedeman, J. S. Shields, M. B., Weber, P. A., Crow, J. W., Cocchetto, D. M., Marris, W. A., and Howes, J. F. (1981) Effect of synthetic cannabinoids on elevated intraocular pressure. *Ophthalmology* **88**, 270–277.

35. Merritt, J. C., Cook, C. E., and Davis, K. H. (1982) Orthostatic hypotension after Δ9-tetrahydrocannabinol marihuana inhalation. *Ophthalmic Res.* **14**, 124–128.

36. Green, K. (1984) Marihuana effects on intraocular pressure, In: *Glaucoma: Applied Pharmacology in Medical Treatment* (Drance, S. M. and Neufeld, A. H., eds.), Grune & Stratton, Orlando, FL, pp. 507–526.

37. Hepler, R. S., Frank, I. M., and Ungerleider, J. T. (1972) Pupillary constriction after marihuana smoking. *Am. J. Ophthalmol.* **74**, 1185–1190.

38. Brown, B., Adams, A. J., Halgerstrom-Portnoy, G., Jones, R. T., and Flom, M. C. (1977) Pupil size after use of marihuana and alcohol. *Am. J. Ophthalmol.* **83**, 350–354.

39. Green, K. and Pederson, J. E. (1973) Effect of Δ^1-tetrahydrocannabinol on aqueous dynamics and ciliary body permeability in the rabbit. *Exp. Eye Res.* **15**, 499–507.

40. Cool, S. J., Kaye, S., and Cullen, A. P. (1974) Topical and intravenous dosage of Δ^9-THC: Effects on blood pressure and intraocular pressure. *Invest. Ophthalmol.* **13 (suppl.),** 22.

41. El-Sohly, M. A., Harland, E. C., Benigni, D. A., and Waller, C. W. (1984) Cannabinoids in glaucoma II, The effect of different cannabinoids on intraocular pressure of the rabbit. *Curr. Eye Res.* **3,** 841–850.

42. Waller, C. W., Benigni, D. A., Harland, E. C., Bedford, J. A., Murphy, J. C., and El-Sohly, M. A. (1984) Cannabinoids in glaucoma III: The effects of different cannabinoids on intraocular pressure in the monkey, In: *The Cannabinoids: Chemical, Pharmacologic and Therapeutic Aspects* (Agurell, S., Dewey, W. L., and Willette, R. E., eds.), Academic, New York, pp. 871–880.

43. Green, K., Symonds, C. M., Oliver, N. W., and Elijah, R. D. (1982/83) Intraocular pressure following systemic administration of cannabinoids. *Curr. Eye Res.* **2,** 247–253.

44. Green, K., Wynn, H., and Bowman, K. (1978) A comparison of topical cannabinoids on intraocular pressure. *Exp. Eye Res.* **27,** 239–246.

45. Dren, A. T. (1976) Preclinical neuropharmacology of three nitrogen-containing heterocyclic benzopyrans derived from the cannabinoid nucleus, In: *The Therapeutic Potential of Marihuana* (Cohen, S. and Stillman, R. C., eds.), Plenum, New York, pp.439–455.

46. Mechoulam, R., Lander, N., Dikstein, S., Carlini, E., and Blumenthal, M. (1976) On the therapeutic possibilities of some cannabinoids, In: *The Therapeutic Potential of Marihuana* (Cohen, S. and Stillman, R. C., eds.) Plenum, New York, pp. 35–45.

47. Green, K., Kim, K., and Bowman, K. (1976) Ocular effects of Δ9-tetrahydrocannabinol, In: *The Therapeutic Potential of Marihuana* (Cohen, S. and Stillman, R. C., eds.) Plenum, New York, pp. 49–62.

48. Green, K. and Kim, K. (1977) Acute dose response of intraocular pressure to topical and oral cannabinoids. *Proc. Soc. Exp. Biol. Med.* **154,** 228–231.

49. Green, K., Bigger, J. F., Kim, K., and Bowman, K. (1977) Cannabinoid action on the eye as mediated through the central nervous system and local activity. *Exp. Eye Res.* **24,** 189–196.

50. Green, K., Bigger, J. F., Kim, K., and Bowman, K. (1977) Cannabinoid penetration and chronic effects in the eye. *Exp. Eye Res.* **24,** 197–205.

51. Merritt, J. C., Peiffer, R. L., McKinnon, S. M., Stapleton, S. S., Goodwin, T., and Risco, J. M. (1981) Topical Δ^9-tetrahydrocannabinol on intraocular pressure in dogs. *Glaucoma* **3,** 13–16.

52. Merritt, J. C., Whitaker, R., Page, C. J., Peace, J. J., Grimson, R. C., Olsen, J. L., Peiffer, R. L., and Davanzo, R. (1982) Topical Δ^8-tetrahydrocannabinol as a potential glaucoma agent. *Glaucoma* **4:**253–255.

53. Howes, J. F. (1984) Antiglaucoma effects of topically and orally administered cannabinoids, In: *The Cannabinoids: Chemical, Pharmacologic and Therapeutic Aspects* (Agurell, S., Dewey, W. L., and Willette, R. E., eds.), Academic, New York, pp. 881–890.

54. Mechoulam, R., Lander, H., Srebnik, M., Zamir, I., Brever, A., Shalita, B., Dikstein, S., Carlini, E. A., Leice, J. R., Edeny, H., and Porath, G. (1984) Recent advances in the use of cannabinoids as therapeutic agents, In: *The Cannabinoids: Chemical, Pharmacologic and Therapeutic Aspects* (Agurell, S., Dewey, W. L., and Willette, R. E., eds.), Academic, New York, pp. 777–793.

55. Green, K. and Kim, K. (1976) Mediation of ocular tetrahydrocannabinol effects by adrenergic nervous system. *Exp. Eye Res.* **23,** 443–448.

56. Colasanti, B. K. and Powell, S. R. (1985) Effect of Δ^9-tetrahydrocannabinol on intraocular pressure after removal of autonomic input. *J. Ocular Pharmacol.* **1,** 47–57.

57. Green, K., Wynn, H., and Padgett, D. (1978) Effect of Δ^9-tetrahydrocannabinol on ocular blood flow and aqueous humor formation. *Exp. Eye Res.* **26,** 65–69.

58. Colasanti, B. K. and Powell, S. R. (1985) Factors involved in the intraocular pressure lowering effect of Δ^9-tetrahydrocannabinol (Δ^9-THC) in the cat. *Invest. Ophthalmol. Vis. Sci.* **26(suppl.),** 232.

59. Colasanti, B. K. and Gong, H. (1987) Cannabinoid effects on aqueous humor dynamics in the cat. *Invest. Ophthalmol. Vis. Sci.* **28(suppl.),** 12.

60. Liu, J. H. K. and Dacus, A. C. (1987) Central nervous system and peripheral mechanism in ocular hypotensive effect of cannabinoids. *Arch. Ophthalmol.* **105,** 245–248.

61. Liu, J. H. K. and Neufeld, A. H. (1985) Study of central regulation of intraocular pressure using ventriculocisternal perfusion. *Invest. Ophthalmol. Vis. Sci.* **26,** 136–143.

62. Becker, B. (1965) Intraocular pressure response to topical corticosteroids. *Invest. Ophthalmol.* **4,** 198–205.

63. Armaly, M.F. (1965) Statistical attributes of the steroid hypertensive response in the clinically normal eye. I. The demonstration of three levels of response. *Invest. Ophthalmol.* **4,** 187–197.

64. Green, K., Phillips, C.I., Gore, S.M., Elijah, R.D., Bowman, K.A., and Cullen, P. (1985) Ocular fluid dynamics response to topical RU486, a steroid blocker. *Curr. Eye Res.* **4,** 605–612.

65. Green, K., Phillips, C.I., Cheeks, L., and Slagle, T. (1988) Aqueous humor flow rate and intraocular pressure during and after pregnancy. *Ophthalmic Res.* **20,** 353–357.

66. Nilsson, S.F. (1997) The uveoscleral outflow routes. *Eye* **11,** 149–154.

67. Bill, A. (1989) Uveoscleral drainage of aqueous humor: Physiology and pharmacology. *Prog. Clin. Biol. Res.* **312,** 417–427.

68. Sherman, S.H., Green, K., and Laties, A.M. (1978) The fate of anterior chamber fluorescein in the monkey eye. 1. The anterior chamber outflow pathways. *Exp. Eye Res.* **27,** 159–173.

69. Green, K., Sherman, S.H., Laties, A.M., Pederson, J.E., Gaasterland, D.E., and MacLellan, H. (1979) The fate of anterior chamber tracers in the living monkey eye with evidence for uveo–vortex flow, In: The Intraocular Fluids (Cant, J.S., ed.) Headley Brothers, Oxford, pp. 731–739

70. Kanno, M., Araie, M., Tomita, K., and Sawanbori, K. (1998) Effects of topical nipradilol, a beta-blocking agent with alpha-blocking and nitroglycerin–like activities, on aqueous humor dynamics and fundus circulation. *Invest. Ophthalmol. Vis. Sci.* **39,** 736–743.

71. Wang, R.F., Lee, P.Y., Mittag, T.W., Podos, S.M., and Serle, J.B. (1997) Effect of 5-methyluropidil, an alpha 1 α-adrenergic antagonist and 5-hydroxytryptamine 1α-agonist, on aqueous humor dynamics in monkeys and rabbits. *Curr. Eye Res.* **16,** 769–775.

72. Stern, F.A. and Bito, L.Z. (1982) Comparison of the hypotensive and other ocular effects of prostaglandin E_2 and $F_2\alpha$ on cat and rhesus monkey eyes. *Invest. Ophthalmol. Vis. Sci.* **22,** 588–598.

73. Toris, C.B., Gleason, M.L., Camras, C.B., and Yablonski, M.E. (1995) Effects of brimonidine on aqueous humor dynamics in human eyes. *Arch. Ophthalmol.* **113,** 1514–1517.

74. Serle, J.B., Stein, A.J., Podos, S.M., and Severin, C.H. (1984) Corynanthine and aqueous humor dynamics in rabbits and monkeys. *Arch. Ophthalmol.* **102,** 1385–1388.

75. Wang, R.F., Lee, P.Y., Taniguchi, T., Becker, B., Podos, S.M., Serle, J.B., and Mittag, T.W. (1993) Effect of oxymetazoline on aqueous humor dynamics and ocular blood flow in monkeys and rabbits. *Arch. Ophthalmol.* **111,** 535–538.

76. Green, K. and Podos, S.M. (1974) Antagonism of arachidonic acid–induced effects by Δ1-tetrahydrocannabinol. *Invest. Ophthalmol.* **13,** 422–429.

77. rawford, K. and Kaufman, P.L. (1987) Pilocarpine antagonizes prostaglandin F_2 alpha-induced ocular hypotension in monkeys. Evidence for enhancement of uveoscleral outflow by prostaglandin F_2 alpha. *Arch. Ophthalmol.* **105,** 1112–1116.

78. Nilsson, S.F., Samuelsson, M., Bill, A., and Stjernschantz, J. (1989) Increased uveoscleral outflow as a possible mechanism of ocular hypotension caused by prostaglandin F_2 alpha-1-isopropylester in the cynomolgus monkey. *Exp. Eye Res.* **48,** 707–716.

79. Gabelt, B.T. and Kaufman, P.L. (1989) Prostaglandin F2 alpha increases uveoscleral outflow in the cynomologus monkey. *Exp. Eye Res.* **49,** 389–402.

80. Poyer, J.F., Gabelt, B., and Kaufman, P.L. (1992) The effect of topical PGF_2 alpha on uveoscleral outflow and outflow facility in the rabbit eye. *Exp. Eye Res.* **54,** 277–283.

81. Fristrom, B. and Nilsson, J.F. (1997) A double masked comparison of the intraocular pressure reducing effect of latanaprost 0.005% and 0.001% administered once daily in open angle glaucoma and ocular hypertension. *Br. J. Ophthalmol.* **81,** 867–870.

82. Watson, P.G. (1998) Latanaprost. Two years experience of its use in the United Kingdom. Latanoprost Study Group. *Ophthalmology* **105,** 82–87.

83. Resul, B., Stjernschantz, J., Selen, G., and Bito, L. (1997) Structure-activity relationships and receptor profiles of some ocular hypotensive prostanoids. *Surv. Ophthalmol.* **41(suppl 2),** S47–S52.

84. Bhattacharya, S.K. (1986) delta-9-tetrahydrocannabinol (THC) increases brain prostaglandins in the rat. *Psychopharmacology* **90,** 499–502.

85. Burstein, S., Hunter, S.A., and Ozman, K. (1983) Prostaglandins and cannabis. XII. The effect of cannabinoid structure on the synthesis of prostaglandins by human lung fibroblasts. *Mol. Pharmacol.* **23,** 121–126.

86. Reichman, M., Nen, W., and Hokin, L.E. (1987) Effects of delta-9-tetrahydrocannabinol on prostaglandin formation in brain. *Mol. Pharmacol.* **32,** 686–690.

87. Hunter, S.A. and Burstein, S.H. (1997) Receptor mediation in cannabinoid stimulated arachidonic acid mobilization and anandamide synthesis. *Life Sci.* **60,** 1563–1573.

88. Burstein, S., Hunter, S.A., Latham, V., Mechoulam, R., Melchior, D.L., Renzulli, L., and Tefft, R.E., Jr. (1986) Prostaglandin and cannabis. XV. Comparison of enantiomeric cannabinoids in stimulating prostaglandin synthesis in fibroblasts. *Life Sci.* **39,** 1813–1823.

89. Green, K., Sobel, R. E., Fineberg, E., Wynn, H. R., and Bowman, K. A. (1981) Subchronic ocular and systemic toxicity of topically applied Δ9-tetrahydrocannabinol. *Ann. Ophthalmol.* **13,** 1219–1222.

90. Merritt, J. C., Olsen, J. L., Armstrong, J. R., and McKinnon, S. M. (1981) Topical Δ^9-tetrahydrocannabinol in hypertensive glaucoma. *J. Pharm. Pharmacol.* **33,** 40–41.

91. Merritt, J. C., Perry, D. D., Russell, D. N., and Jones, B. F. (1981) Topical Δ^9-tetrahydrocannabinol and aqueous dynamics in glaucoma. *J. Clin. Pharmacol.* **21,** 467S–471S.
92. Green, K. and Roth, M. (1982) Ocular effects of topical administration of Δ^9-tetrahydrocannabinol in man. *Arch. Ophthalmol.* **100,** 265–267.
93. Jay, W. M. and Green, K. (1983) Multiple-drop study of topically applied 1% Δ^9-tetrahydrocannabinol in human eyes. *Arch. Ophthalmol.* **101,** 591–593.
94. Beilin, M., Aviv, H., Friedman, D., Vered, M., Belkin, M., Neumann, R., Amselem, S., Schwarz, J., and Bar-Zlan, A. (1993) HU211, a novel synthetic, non-psychotropic cannabinoid with ocular hypotensive activity. *Invest. Ophthalmol. Vis. Sci.* **34(suppl),** 1113.
95. Little, P. J., Compton, D. R., Mechoulam, R., and Martin, B. R. (1989) Stereochemical effects of 11-OH-Δ8-THC-dimethylheptyl in mice and dogs. *Pharmacol. Biochem. Behav.* **32,** 661–666.
96. Beilin, M., Neumann, R., Belkin, M., Green, K., and Bar-Ilan, A (1998) Pharmacology of the intraocular pressure (IOP) lowering effect of systemic HU-211, a non-psychotropic cannabinoid. *J. Ocular Pharmacol. Therap.* Submitted for publication.
97. Newell, F. W., Stark, P., Jay, W. M., and Schanzlin, D. J. (1979) Nabilone: A pressure reducing synthetic benzopyran in open angle glaucoma. *Ophthalmology* **86,** 156–160.
98. Mechoulam, R., Lander, N., Varkony, T. H., Kimmel, I., Recker, O., Ben-Zvi, Z., Edery, H., and Parath, G. (1980) Stereochemical requirements for cannabinoid activity. *J. Med. Chem..* **23:** 1068–1072.
99. Lemberger, L. (1980) Potential therapeutic usefulness of marihuana. *Ann. Rev. Pharmacol. Toxicol.* **20,** 151–172.
100. Weber, P. A. and Howes, J. F. (1981) Lowering of intraocular pressure in normotensive human volunteers by naboctate. *Invest. Ophthalmol. Vis. Sci.* **20(suppl),** 196.
101. Razdan, R. K. (1986) Structure-activity relationships in cannabinoids. *Pharmacol. Rev.* **38,** 75–149.
102. Sugrue, M. F., Funk, H. A., Leonard, Y., O'Neill-Davis, L., and Labelle, M. (1996) The ocular hypotensive effects of synthetic cannabinoids. *Invest. Ophthalmol. Vis. Sci.* **37(suppl),** 831.
103. Pate, D. W., Jarvinen, K., Urtti, A., Harho, P., and Jarvinen, T. (1995) Arachidonylethanolamide decreases intraocular pressure in normotensive rabbits. *Curr. Eye Res.* **14,** 791–797.
104. D. W. Pate, Jarvinen, K. Urtti, A., Jarho, P., Fich, M., Mahareran, V., and Jarvinen, T. (1996) Effects of topical anandamides on intraocular pressure in normotensive rabbits. *Life Sci.* **58:**1849–1860.
105. Hodges, L. C., Reggio, P. H., and Green, K. (1997) Evidence against cannabinoid receptor involvement in intraocular pressure effects of cannabinoids in rabbits. *Ophthalmic Res.* **29,** 1–5.
106. Green, K. (1998) Marihuana smoking vs. cannabinoids for glaucoma therapy. *Arch. Ophthalmal.* submitted.

50

Marihuana and the Treatment of Glaucoma

Max Forbes

Abstract

Glaucoma is a group of diseases in which elevated intraocular pressure (IOP) in conjunction with unknown aberrant neural factors causes a specific type of progressive optic-nerve degeneration and loss of vision. To date, reduction of IOP, whether by means of medications, or laser or invasive surgery, constitutes the only principle of treatment of proven efficacy. Marihuana inhalation or Δ^9-THC administered intravenously, or orally, reduces IOP in glaucoma. This effect is of short duration and undetermined mechanism. It has not yet been elicited by topical administration. Neither marihuana nor any cannabinoids thus far tested could meet the standards of approval by the United States Food and Drug Administration (FDA) for treatment of glaucoma. Further investigation of the mechanism of action of marihuana in glaucoma should be pursued. Meanwhile, a trial on oral dronabinol (Δ^9-THC), which is available as a Shedule II narcotic agent under the Controlled Substances Act, might be considered for patients with glaucoma in whom all approved methods of treatment, including surgery, have failed to stop progressive visual deterioration.

1. INTRODUCTION

Marihuana is currently being used by some individuals as a treatment for their glaucoma. However, the evidence available at this time is insufficient to determine whether or not a legitimate FDA-approved pharmaceutical agent for such treatment can be derived from marihuana. To date, all methods of treating glaucoma involve reduction of IOP, an effect that can be produced by smoking marihuana (1–3). Since glaucoma is a chronic condition that requires long-term around-the-clock pressure control in predominantly elderly and middle-aged patients, it is quite obvious that marihuana smoking cannot help to accomplish that goal without unacceptable side effects (4). Efforts have therefore been made to develop an acceptable pharmaceutical product from Δ^9-THC and other cannabinoids in marihuana that mediate

From: *Marihuana and Medicine*
Edited by: G. G. Nahas et al.   © Humana Press Inc., Totowa, NJ

591

the IOP-lowering effect *(5–8)*. The current standard for success is a topical agent that reduces IOP by at least 25–30% for 12 hours or longer (once or twice per day instillation) with minimal, if any, adverse local or systemic side effects. Nothing related to marihuana has yet been found to approach that standard, but the effort should continue because there is considerable room for improvement in the management of glaucoma.

2. THE GLAUCOMA PROBLEM

For many years glaucoma was regarded as a group of ocular diseases in which increased IOP caused typical patterns of optic-nerve degeneration and associated visual-field impairment. It was classified into four major categories: primary open-angle glaucoma, (POAG), primary angle-closure glaucoma, primary congenital glaucoma, and the secondary glaucomas in accordance with the various mechanisms of obstruction of aqueous humor outflow that cause increased IOP. Although that general classification is still operative, our understanding of POAG, the predominant form of glaucoma which accounts for at least 80% of cases in the United States, has been revised. Clinical and epidemiological investigations have demonstrated conclusively that optic-nerve damage in POAG can develop and progress at statistically normal IOP levels *(9–12)*. Damage is therefore a consequence of interaction of the IOP with optic-nerve structure and hemodynamics, though at sufficiently high levels pressure alone would suffice.

For pharmacological considerations, it is appropriate to take POAG as the prototype for glaucoma because of its numerical preponderance and because it is the testing ground for development of new medications. POAG is defined as a chronic bilateral optic-nerve degeneration in which the obstruction to aqueous humor outflow is not clinically discernible (open angle of the anterior chamber) and elevated IOP is the major risk factor rather than the cause. Reduction of IOP, whether elevated or not, is still the fundamental goal of treatment. Concerted efforts are underway to find neuroprotective agents, but none are yet available.

POAG is a public health problem of considerable magnitude. It is estimated that two million Americans have POAG, 80,000 are legally blind, and 5–10 million are at risk because of increased IOP *(13)*. Treatment consists of varying combinations of medications, laser applications to the trabecular meshwork, and surgical procedures deployed in accordance with severity of the disease. None of these methods permanently eliminates the submicroscopic trabecular obstruction. Six classes of topical medications are used, three adrenergic agents and a carbonic anhydrase inhibitor that decrease aqueous humor formation, a cholinergic agent that improves outflow through the obstructed trabecular meshwork, and a recently introduced prostaglandin analog that enhances outflow through the secondary uveoscleral pathway.

Difficulties with compliance, cost, local and systemic side effects, and limited efficacy constitute significant impediments to medical management of POAG. Laser therapy is essentially an adjunct to medical therapy of temporary benefit. Filtration surgery, which creates a bypass to the intrinsic drainage system, is not uniformly successful and may result in serious complications. In view of these considerations there is ample reason to seek new treatment modalities.

3. MARIHUANA AND CANNABINOIDS

Interest in marihuana began in 1971 when Hepler and Frank reported that smoking of a product containing 0.9% Δ^9-THC reduced IOP by 31% in 9 of 11 normal volunteers *(1)*. That effect was confirmed by subsequent reports involving patients with glaucoma as well as additional volunteers *(2,3,6)*. It was also shown that the marihuana effect on IOP could be duplicated by oral or intravenous administration of Δ^9-THC *(2,6,7)*. However, topical instillation of Δ^9-THC, although effective in animals *(14,15)*, failed to reduce IOP in human eyes *(16)*. That failure seemed to be caused by inadequate corneal penetration of the highly lipid soluble cannabinoid molecule, and it remained unclear whether the effect on IOP was caused by local or systemic action of Δ^9-THC. Since Δ^9-THC and other cannabinoids increase arachidonic acid biosynthesis leading to a cascade of prostaglandins, it is possible that their effect on IOP might be prostaglandin-mediated via enhanced uveoscleral outflow.

Derivatives of Δ^9-THC and other cannabinoids have also been tested, some of which succeeded in lowering IOP by the oral route. Nabilone, a synthetic cannabinoid developed by Eli Lilly Company reduced IOP in glaucoma by 27.9%, but psychotropic effects and orthostatic hypotension occured in some individuals. Clinical trials of nabilone in glaucoma were discontinued when neurotoxicity was noted in dogs after two months of exposure *(17,18)*. A single oral dose of BW146Y, a derivative of Δ^1-THC, reduced IOP by 25–40% at peak action when given in adequate dosage to patients with elevated IOP, but this agent also caused psychotropic effects and orthostatic hypotension in some of them. One patient experienced a syncopal episode. In this study there was no correlation between lowering of blood pressure and reduction of IOP *(19)*.

Of special interest is a small group of patients with glaucoma, each of whom obtained an individual compassionate Investigational New Drug (IND) waver from the FDA for medical treatment with marihuana. These patients have received their marihuana cigarettes from the National Institute on Drug Abuse free of charge. Although the program was terminated in 1992, there are still eight remaining participants who continue to be supplied with marihuana. The ophthalmologist of one of these patients, Dr. Paul Palmberg, has provided significant clinical data regarding her response to cannabinoids (personal communication). She has been in the program since 1988. Her baseline untreated IOP is 50mm Hg. It is reduced to 30 mmHg by instillation of timolol 0.5% after which smoking a 3% Δ^9-THC marihuana cigarette produces still further pressure reduction to a normal level of 15mm Hg within 30 minutes, but lasting only two hours. This patient smokes 10 marihuana cigarettes daily with no superficially evident side effects. The IOP-lowering effect of marihuana has not diminished over a period of several years, and it is additive to dorzolamide as well as timolol. Oral ingestion of Δ^9-THC produces essentially the same result as marihuana inhalation.

Canisol, a topical derivative of marihuana, was developed on the island of Jamaica by Manley West of the University of the West Indies in collaboration with Albert Lockhart of Dallas, Texas. According to West (personal communication) it is a water-soluble extract of marihuana that contains no cannabinoids, but nevertheless decreases aqueous humor formation by 55% within 15 minutes for a duration of three to four hours by the action of an α-adrenergic agonist. Canisol has been approved for treatment of glaucoma by the Ministry of Health of Jamaica. It is available there by prescription and an attempt is being made to obtain similar approval in some European countries. This information concerning canisol appears to be contradictory to all of the studies which have attributed the IOP-lowering action of marihuana to cannabinoids, especially Δ^9-THC. Perhaps this discrepancy can be resolved by independent clinical studies and publication of peer-reviewed data.

4. CONCLUSION

Inhalation of marihuana and oral administration of certain cannabinoids can produce a significant reduction of IOP in glaucoma. To date the mechanism and site of action are still unknown. Neither marihuana cigarettes nor any of the oral cannabinoids thus far tested could qualify for FDA approval in glaucoma because of the short duration of action and frequency of unacceptable systemic side effects, On the other hand one would like to have the opportunity to try this type of treatment in special desperate situations, namely the subgroup of patients with glaucoma, perhaps 2–3%, who are threatened with blindness because of failure to respond to conventional therapeutic methods, including surgery.

Widespread utilization of the marihuana effect in glaucoma would require development of a topical derivative that can penetrate the cornea in adequate concentration to exert its influence within the eye. It has been suggested that a submicron emulsion might facilitate such penetration *(20)*. But local activity would probably require a peripheral cannabinoid receptor *(21)* to mediate the desired effect on IOP and no such receptor has yet been found in ocular tissue. Beyond these considerations are potential problems in connection with duration and side effects. Nevertheless research in this area should continue because of persistent difficulties in treating glaucoma.

It should be evident that success in this endeavor, although beneficial, will not produce a cure for glaucoma. That type of breakthrough is more likely to follow discovery of the cause of dysfunction on a molecular level.

REFERENCES

1. Hepler, R. S. and Frank, I. R. (1971) Marihuana smoking and intraocular pressure. *J. Amer. Med. Assn.* **272**, 1392.
2. Hepler, R. S. and Petrus, R. J. (1976) Experiences with administration of marihuana to glaucoma patients. In: *The Therapeutic Potential of Marihuana* (Cohen, S. and Stillman, R. C., eds.) Plenum Press, New York, pp. 6–75.
3. Merritt, J. C., Crawford, W. J., Alexander, P. C., Anduze, A. L., and Gelbart, S. S. (1980) Effect of marihuana on intraocular and blood pressure in glaucoma. *Ophthalmology* **87**, 222–228.
4. Goldberg, I., Kass, M. A., and Becker, B. (1979) Marihuana as a treatment for glaucoma. *Sight Sav. Rev.* **48**, 147–155.
5. Green, K. (1979) The ocular effects of cannabinoids. In: *Current Topics in Eye Research,* vol.I (Zadunaisky, J. A. and Davson, H., eds.) Academic Press, New York, pp.175-215.
6. Cooler, P. and Gregg, J. M. (1976) The effect of delta-9-tetrahydrocannabinol on intraocular pressure in humans. In: *The Therapeutic Potential of Marihuana* (Cohen, S. and Stillman, R. C., eds.) Plenum Press, New York, pp. 77-87.
7. Perez-Reyes, M., Wagner, D., Wall, M. E., and Davis, K. H. (1976) Intravenous administration of cannabinoids and intraocular pressure. In: *The Pharmacology of Marihuana* (Braude, M. C. and Szara, S., eds.) Raven, New York, pp. 82
8. Adler, M. W. and Geller, E. B. (1986) Ocular effects of cannabinoids, In: *Cannabinoids as Therapeutic Agents* (Mechoulam, R., ed.) CRC Press, Boca Raton, FL, pp. 51–70.
9. Sommer, A. (1989) Intraocular pressure and glaucoma (editorial). *Am. J. Ophthalmol.* **107**, 186–188.
10. Sommer, A., Tielsch, J. M., Katz, J., Quigley, H. A., Gottsch, J. D., Javitt, J. and Singh, K. (1991) Relationship between intraocular pressure and primary open-angle glaucoma among white and black Americans: the Baltimore Eye Survey. *Arch. Ophthalmol.* **109**, 1090–1095.
11. Sommer, A. (1996) Doyne Lecture Glaucoma: facts and fancies. *Eye.* **10**, 295–304.
12. Dielemans, I., Vingerling, J. R., Wolfs, R. C. W., Hofman, A., Grobbee, D. E. and deJong, P. T. V. M. (1994) The prevalence of primary open-angle glaucoma in a population-based study in the Netherlands. The Rotterdam Study. *Ophthalmology* **101**, 1851–1855.
13. Quality of Care Committee, Glaucoma Panel. (1992) Primary Open-Angle Glaucoma. Preferred Practice Pattern. American Academy of Ophthalmology, San Francisco, p.4.
14. Green, K. and Kim, K. (1977) Acute dose response of intraocular pressure to topical and oral cannabinoids. *Proc. Soc. Exp. Biol. Med.* **154**, 228–231.
15. Green, K., Bigger, J. F., Kim, K., and Bowman, K. (1977) Cannabinoid penetration and chronic effects in the eye. *Exp. Eye Res.* **24**, 197–205.
16. Jay, W. M. and Green, K. (1983) Multiple-drop study of topically applied 1% Δ9-tetrahydrocannabinol in human eyes. *Arch. Ophthalmol.* **101**, 591–593.
17. Newell, F. W., Stark, P., Jay, W. M. and Schanzlin, D. J. (1979) Nabilone: a pressure-reducing synthetic benzopyran in open-angle glaucoma. *Ophthalmology* **86**, 156–160.

18. Newell, F. W., Jay, W. M. and Sternberg, P. (1979) Use of cannabinoid derivatives in glaucoma. *Trans. Ophthalmol. Soc. U. K.* **99,** 269–271.

19. Tiedeman, J. S., Shields, M. B., Weber, P. A., Crow, J. W., Cocchetto, B. S., Harris, M. A. and Howes, J. F. (1981) Effect of synthetic cannabinoids on elevated intraocular pressure. *Ophthalmology* **86,** 270–277.

20. Muchtar, S., Almog, S., Torracca, M. T., Saettone, M. F., and Benita, S. (1992) A submicron emulsion as ocular vehicle for delta-8-tetrahydrocannabinol: effect on intraocular pressure in rabbits. *Ophthalmic Res.* **24,** 142–149.

21. Munro, S., Thomas, K. L. and Abu-Shaar, M. (1993) Molecular characterization of a peripheral receptor for cannabinoids. *Nature.* **365,** 61–65.

VII Marihuana, Cannabinoids, and the Nervous System

51

Cannabinoids and the Control of Chemotherapy-Induced Nausea and Vomiting

Richard J. Gralla

Abstract

The major progress in controlling chemotherapy-induced emesis benefits thousands of patients each day. Antiemetic efficacy is found with agents of many different classes, including phenothiazines, butyrophenones, cannabinoids, corticosteroids, substituted benzamides, and serotonin receptor antagonists. To date, the most effective antiemetic regimens are combinations of serotonin-receptor antagonists with corticosteroids.

Most antiemetic studies with cannabinoids have methodological difficulties and can be difficult to interpret. If one concentrates on the better-conducted trials, however, it is clear that cannabinoids possess antiemetic properties in patients receiving cancer chemotherapy. The degree of antiemetic activity demonstrated by cannabinoids is not as high as that seen with several other classes of agents. The side effects associated with cannabinoid use are tolerable, but greater that those seen with other classes of agents.

Studies have not demonstrated an advantage of one tested cannabinoid over another. Results of trials with synthetic cannabinoids, such as levonantradol or nabilone, do not indicate a superior therapeutic index over naturally occurring cannabinoids. Only limited data from well-designed trials can be found comparing inhalant marihuana with other cannabinoids. From that which exists, there is no clear advantage for either inhalant marihuana or for oral THC. Additionally, there is no demonstration that the inhalant agent results in an improved pharmacokinetic profile, an advantage in self titration, or in a different pattern of side effects.

Further studies with cannabinoids, using accepted methodology, could more accurately outline their activity. Decisions should be made whether or not the current moderate degree of efficacy and moderate amount of associated side effects with all tested cannabinoid antiemetics warrant such trials in the context of substantially more active agents that have more favorable toxicity profiles.

From: *Marihuana and Medicine*
Edited by: G. G. Nahas et al.   © Humana Press Inc., Totowa, NJ

Table
Drugs With Antiemetic Activity

Class of agent	Example	Other uses
Phenothiazines[a]	Prochlorperazine	Major tranquilizer
Butyrophenones	Haloperidol	Major tranquilizer
CCannabinoids[a]	Dronabinol	Antidiarrheal[b]
Corticosteroids[a]	Dexamethasone	Anti-inflammatory
Substituted benzamides[a]	Metoclopramide	Prokinetic agent
Serotonin-receptor antagonists[a]	Ondansetron	Antiemetic with general anesthesia
Neutrokinin-1-receptor antagonists	Investigational agents	

[a] Demonstrated to be a more effective antiemetic than placebo in randomized trials
[b] Use of *Cannabis sativa* in the 19th century

1. INTRODUCTION AND BACKGROUND

The development of effective strategies to control the emesis induced by many chemotherapeutic agents is a major goal in the supportive care of patients with cancer. Chemotherapy use has become more frequent as trial results indicate benefit in an increasing number of settings, both curative and palliative.

Studies have investigated the emphasis that patients place on the problems of nausea and vomiting. Such surveys reported 15 years ago and more recently indicate the continuing prominence of patient concerns. Of over 70 potential concerns, patients rated nausea and vomiting at the top of the list in the 1983 study *(1)*. Recently, a similar report noted marked progress in that vomiting was no longer among the five highest patient concerns; however, nausea still rated directly after hair loss at the top of the list *(2)*. This study could be criticized for less than optimal use of antiemetics and for surveying a group that is atypically predisposed to experience emesis. In spite of these problems, it underscores the continuing need for improving the control of emesis.

Progress in controlling emesis has been striking, but the need for further improvement is clear. As an example, when cisplatin was first introduced in the 1970s, more than 99% of patients experienced acute vomiting, with 10 as the median number of emetic episodes *(3)*. Currently, large, multicenter, randomized trials report complete control with cisplatin in the 60%–80% range, with the mean number of episodes as less than one *(4)*. Cisplatin is an important guide to efficacy. To date, when antiemetics are effective with cisplatin, they are at least as effective with other chemotherapy agents. The public is largely unaware of this progress.

New classes of agents with antiemetic properties have emerged over the last 10 years, as outlined in Table 1. Additionally, the activities of older agents have been more accurately defined. Many classes of available agents possess antiemetic activity with chemotherapy, and include serotonin-type 3 receptor antagonists, substituted benzamides, corticosteroids, butyrophenones, and phenothiazines (Table 1). Among the agents with efficacy in the prevention of emesis in patients receiving cancer chemotherapy, are the cannabinoids.

Several cannabinoids have been tested as antiemetics. These include semisynthetic agents (nabilone, levonantradol), the constituent of marihuana, Δ^9-tetrahydrocannabinol (THC), and inhalant marihuana *(5–14)*. Public awareness of the use of cannabinoids for chemotherapy-induced emesis is higher than that seen for other agents. This is likely because of repeated media coverage of this use of cannabinoids, as opposed to the sparse publicity for the improved control of emesis with chemotherapy as a problem for many people.

2. NEUROPHARMACOLOGY AND THE CONTROL OF EMESIS

The mechanism by which chemotherapy induces emesis is still not completely understood, although the studies of Borison *(15)* and of others *(16)*, as has recently been reviewed *(17,18)*, have been revealing. Questions that remain include: Is it the chemotherapy drug itself, a metabolite, or a neurotransmitter that stimulates a receptor and causes emesis? Why is there a delay from the administration of chemotherapy to the onset of emesis, which is not present with such chemicals as apomorphine? and Why do different chemotherapy agents that have similar intracellular effects have such varying potentials for inducing emesis?

Studies support the hypothesis that chemotherapy-induced emesis is caused by stimulation of neurotransmitter receptors in the central nervous system or in the gastrointestinal tract. Receptor areas have been identified that affect a proposed vomiting center in the lateral reticular formation of the medulla, which then coordinates the act of vomiting. An important area is also located in the medulla is the chemoreceptor trigger zone (CTZ), in the area postrema *(15)*. This receptor region is sensitive to chemical stimuli from both the blood and the cerebrospinal fluid. Chemotherapeutic agents, their metabolites, or a neurotransmitter may stimulate receptors in the CTZ. Impulses generated in the CTZ and transmitted to the vomiting center may then lead to the initiation of emesis. Relevant neuroreceptors are also located in the gastrointestinal tract *(16)*. Vagal afferents from the gut to the vomiting center, may also play a role in chemotherapy-induced nausea and vomiting. Antiemetic agents that block neuroreceptors in the CTZ, the vomiting center, or in the gastrointestinal tract may be useful in preventing or controlling emesis.

Initially, antiemetic research focused on agents capable of blocking dopamine receptors in the medulla, because of the high concentration of these receptors and to the availability of candidate agents. The success of high doses of metoclopramide led to further analysis of the accepted neuropharmacology. Metoclopramide binds with great affinity to dopamine receptors; the superior efficacy seen with high doses would more likely be caused by involvement of receptors other than dopamine in that binding to these receptors should have been maximal at lower metoclopramide doses. Preclinical studies indicated that metoclopramide indeed blocked serotonin receptors (5-hydroxytryptamine receptors, type 3 or 5-HT$_3$) *(16)*. The efficacy of metoclopramide may be mediated via 5-HT$_3$ receptors, whereas its toxicity may be caused by its interaction with dopamine receptors. The serotonin-receptor antagonist antiemetics are highly selective for the 5-HT$_3$ receptors and are active without the toxicities seen with metoclopramide. The specific mechanism of cannabinoid antiemetic effects has not been carefully established.

3. METHODOLOGY: TESTING ANTIEMETIC EFFECTIVENESS

A critical step in improving the control of emesis was the establishment of proper methodology for measuring nausea and vomiting *(3,19)*. Whereas there are many factors of importance related to the control of emesis, it is paramount that the degree of emesis itself be accurately determined.

Older trials often used a variety of differing response criteria to evaluate efficacy of agents. These criteria included reduction of emesis from a prior chemotherapy experience, reduction of the number of vomiting episodes to half of that reported with prior chemotherapy, or simply reporting of improvement without any specific or objective parameters *(20)*. Whereas any of these may represent some degree of improvement, each is subject to error. First, there can be variation from one chemotherapy treatment to the next, without the use of antiemetics. Second, reduction to half the number of emetic episodes can leave control as highly unsatisfactory (as an example, the reduction of vomiting episodes from 35 to 17). Third, confounding factors, such as more attentive care, can improve a chemotherapy experience without reducing the degree of emesis.

Clearly, the most desired end point for an antiemetic is to control emesis completely. This has become the primary standard in testing new agents. Patients recall the number of emetic episodes accurately, even with antiemetics that are sedating or affect memory. Patients are exact in reporting whether or not emesis has occurred at all (21). This makes the endpoint of complete control more than just a desirable goal: It is also a highly reliable method of evaluation. In most studies, nausea occurs more often than vomiting (4,22,23), but the control of nausea as reported by patients correlates strongly with the control of vomiting (24). The degree of nausea is accurately measured through the use of established visual analog scales (3,21,24).

Several other factors contribute to making trials more accurate and reliable, especially in comparison studies. Controlling for factors such as the influence of prior chemotherapy and balancing predisposing factors (such as gender, age, and prior heavy alcohol usage) between study groups is vital for accuracy. The risk of emesis varies from highly unlikely for many chemotherapeutic agents, to certain for cisplatin. Ascertaining that the emetic stimulus (the chemotherapy) is the same for all patients in a comparison is necessary if the results are to be useful. Accepted randomization and blinding techniques are requirements in an objective evaluation of the control of vomiting and nausea.

The quality and usefulness of antiemetic studies depend on adherence to the considerations outlined above. Methodology problems are common in many of the cannabinoid clinical experiences. Such problems are particularly prominent in the state-run cannabinoid programs. It must be realized that these programs were established more for drug distribution than for formal study; little attention was applied to study methodology, and programs were rarely funded to cover the expenses occurred when carefully monitoring antiemetic trials. Although these problems exist, useful conclusions can be drawn from several trials.

4. CANNABINOIDS AND THE CONTROL OF EMESIS

4.1 Trials Comparing THC with Placebo and with Agents of Low Efficacy

Earlier formal trials tested the question of whether cannabinoids had antiemetic efficacy. The agent most frequently studied was THC. This cannabinoid was first made available for trials and then for individual patient use by the National Cancer Institute (see Table 2 for a summary of these trials).

When THC was tested against placebo, the majority of studies indicated superior results for THC. As seen in Table 2, the chemotherapy varied in most of the trials, and some of the studies included a small number of patients. In one study, THC was found to be superior in patients receiving chemotherapy with methotrexate, an agent of low potential to induce emesis (8). When the same investigators studied THC in a small number of patients receiving chemotherapy more likely to cause emesis (anthracyclines), the antiemetic effect was poor (9). In spite of the methodological limitations, a trend toward efficacy with THC emerges (7–10).

Other trials outlined in Table 2 compare the efficacy of THC with prochlorperazine (10–12). The prochlorperazine is typically administered orally in these studies. At the time of these studies, prochlorperazine was considered to be one of the more effective antiemetics. Although it was felt to be among the best available antiemetics, it was the lack of satisfactory efficacy of prochlorperazine that led to a search for better agents. Results from the trials comparing THC with prochlorperazine are mixed. In general, THC and the phenothiazine are

Table 2
Randomized Studies with Oral Delta-9-Tetrahydrocannabinol (THC)
vs Placebo or Oral Prochlorperazine

Author (Reference)	Patients	Chemotherapy	Results
Sallan 1975 (7)	20	Various	THC > placebo
Chang 1979 (8)	15	Methotrexate	THC > placebo
Chang 1981 (9)	8	Cyclophosphamide/ doxorubicin	THC = placebo
Frytak 1979 (10)	116	5-Fluorouracil/ methyl-CCNU	THC > placebo THC = prochlorperazine
Sallan 1980 (11)	84	Various	THC > prochlorperazine
Orr 1980 (12)	55	Various	THC > prochlorperazine

reported to have a similar degree of efficacy in these studies that often use various chemotherapeutic agents. These results further contribute to the interpretation that THC possesses antiemetic efficacy, but they also suggest that the degree of efficacy is not high.

4.2 The Comparison of THC with High-Dose Metoclopramide

In the early 1980s, it was found that very high doses of metoclopramide (2–3 mg/kg, intravenously) were more effective than the same agent given at low doses (10–20 mg, orally) (5,25,26). Studies conducted with patients receiving cisplatin revealed superiority with significant differences when high-dose metoclopramide was compared with placebo or with parenteral prochlorperazine (3,27). With these results, and with the developing picture of efficacy with THC, a comparison of high-dose metoclopramide with THC was planned (14).

Measures were taken in the THC versus metoclopramide trial to control for several variables. No patient had previously received chemotherapy, so that anticipatory emesis would not be a factor. All received the same dose of the same chemotherapy (cisplatin at 120 mg/m2), which invariably induces nausea and vomiting if an effective antiemetic is not given (3,14,26). The study was double-blinded and randomized. Patients were observed for the number of vomiting episodes and completed visual analog scales to assess nausea. Patients were given the doses of the antiemetics that had been most effective in prior trials (2 mg/kg of metoclopramide every 2 hours, and 10 mg/m2 of THC every 3 hours). The results demonstrated significant differences, favoring the group randomized to metoclopramide. Complete control of emesis was 47% for those receiving metoclopramide, as opposed to 13% for those assigned to THC (major control—2 or fewer episodes—was 73% with metoclopramide and 27% with THC, $p = 0.02$). The median number of emetic episodes was 2 and 8 ($p = 0.01$), respectively, as shown in Table 3 (14).

4.3 Inhalant Marihuana Studies: An Open Trial and a Trial in Comparison with THC

With THC studies showing that this agent is superior to placebo, at least equivalent to oral prochlorperazine, and inferior to high-dose metoclopramide, a reasonable question concerns the activity of inhaled marihuana. Among the efforts to study this cannabinoid treatment is an open single-arm study conducted in New York State (20). In this survey, patients receiving a variety of chemotherapeutic agents were asked to rate the effectiveness of marihuana compared with prior chemotherapy cycles. The results showed that 34% of patients indicated that

Table 3
Randomized Studies with Oral Delta-9-Tetrahydocannabinol (THC)
vs Inhalant Marihuana or Intravenous High-Dose Metoclopromide

Author (Ref.)	Patients	Chemotherapy	Results
Levitt 1984 *(13)*	20	Cisplatin (60%)[a]	Complete control of vomiting (all patients): 25%
Study Design: Double-blinded, randomized, crossover		Cyclophosphamide (75%)[a]	Complete control of nausea (all patients): 15%
		Doxorubicin (85%)[a]	
Oral THC Capsules + placebo cigarette vs Inhalant marihuana + oral placebo			Patient preference: None expressed: 45% THC capsules: 35% Inhalant marihuana: 20%
Gralla 1984 *(14)*	30	Cisplatin (100%)[a]	Major control of vomiting (0–2 emetic episodes):
Study Design: Double-blinded, randomized			THC capsules: 27% *p*=0.02 Metoclopramide: 73%
Oral THC Capsules + placebo IV infusion vs IV metoclo-pramide + oral placebo			Median number of voiting episodes: THC capsules: 8 *p*=0.01 Metoclopramide: 2

[a] Percent of patients receiving the indicated chemotherapy.

the marihuana had been "highly effective." The authors concluded that marihuana had antiemetic efficacy, but its relative value was difficult to determine in that no control group was used and the patient population was varied *(20)*.

A Canadian group conducted a double-blinded study comparing inhalant marihuana with oral THC *(13)*. To achieve blinding, all 20 patients received either placebo capsules or a placebo cigarette, with the appropriate cannabinoid. Patients were assigned to each treatment arm by random assignment, and then were crossed over to the opposite treatment arm on the next cycle of chemotherapy in this double-blinded study. End points include: patient preference between the two types of cannabinoids, with each patient having received one cycle of each cannabinoid; complete control of emesis; and a pharmacokinetic evaluation of blood levels of cannabinoid metabolites to see if differences were found between the two dosing forms. All patients received anthracyclines or cyclophosphamide (agents with a moderate likelihood of inducing emesis), and 60% received the highly emetogenic agent cisplatin, in addition.

The Canadian THC versus marihuana study is outlined in Table 3. The results indicated a similar degree of antiemetic control, with 25% of patients having complete control, overall. The double-blinded study revealed a slight preference for the THC over the marihuana (35 vs 20%), but a larger number of patients expressed no preference for either agent (45%). Pharmacokinetic determinations did not show higher levels of either THC or the 11-nor-9-COOH-THC metabolite in the treatment cycle in which patients received the inhalant marihuana *(13)*.

Table 4
Commonly Reported Side Effects with Cannabinoids in Antiemetic Trials[a]

Toxicity[b]	THC	Navilone	Levonantradol	Marihuana
Dizziness	80%	36%	60%	39%
Dry mouth	80%	25%	63%	77%
Hypotension	53%	17%	40%	
Sedation (Moderate):	13%	47%	91%	
Confusion				13%
Anxiety				11%
Euphoria/dysphoria	20%	21%	30%	

[a] See refs.: 5–14.

[b] Not all toxicity parameters measured in each study; different criteria used to assess or grade criteria in various trials.

4.4 Trials Using Semisynthetic Cannabinoids: Nabilone and Levonantradol

Neither nabilone nor levonantradol is commercially available in the United States at this time (nabilone was withdrawn from the market several years ago). Both agents were tested in a variety of settings, with results apparently similar to THC. Although efficacy was observed in several trials (5,6), there never emerged either an efficacy or side effect advantage for these agents. As with the THC and marihuana trials, efficacy was apparent, but the degree of efficacy generally was not seen as being particularly greater than that seen with available agents that were not felt to be satisfactory in moderately to highly emetogenic settings.

A review of the trials of the semisynthetic agents is helpful in confirming the image of cannabinoids in possessing a degree of antiemetic efficacy. There does not appear to be interest in future investigations with these agents.

4.5 Side Effects of Cannabinoids in Antiemetic Trials

Antiemetics are supportive-care agents in cancer chemotherapy. The most desirable supportive-care drugs are free of side effects. This ideal may not be achieved with most supportive-care agents, but those with few side effects that will not further complicate chemotherapy administration are important factors in selecting among available choices.

The cannabinoid trials in the setting of cancer chemotherapy are helpful in outlining the toxicity profile of these agents. Table 4 lists the more frequent side effects documented in several trials. Disagreement exists as to whether psychoactive effects correlate with antiemetic activity. In the prospective double-blinded trial evaluating THC and metoclopramide, complete antiemetic control occurred independent of mood alteration, euphoria or dysphoria(14), whereas patients with these effects (20%) may have had poor control of emesis. Other investigators believe that such effects are more often found with improved antiemetic control (11). Both dysphoria and euphoria have been reported with cannabinoids in the emetic setting (5–14). Most investigators believe that dysphoric effects are more common among patients who have not had prior experience with cannabinoids.

Table 4 outlines several autonomic effects observed in patients receiving THC or marihuana with cancer chemotherapy. The effects are not unexpected with the cannabinoids. Perhaps the most troubling side effects are orthostatic hypotension and dizziness. In that agents such as cisplatin are renally cleared, lower blood pressure could lead to decreased renal blood flow and a potential for additional toxicity. This is particularly a consideration for patients receiving chemotherapy on an outpatient basis in that they will have to be ambulatory. Side effects such as dry mouth and sedation, although not desirable, are generally not a major concern to most patients.

An important and unexpected problem was encountered in the New York State open trial with marihuana. Nearly one-quarter of the patients were unable to tolerate the administration method of the inhalant marihuana *(20)*. It has been suggested that this is largely a function of inexperience with inhaled marihuana among many adults. Whatever the cause, this is an important consideration in that no other antiemetic has a feasibility problem associated with its administration.

4.6 Blinding of Antiemetic Trials

An important consideration in randomized comparison studies in which both objective and subjective factors are measured, is the concept that neither the patients nor the investigators are aware of which agent was given. In many antiemetic studies, such as those comparing different serotonin-receptor antagonists, blinding is not difficult to maintain. These latter agents are not psychoactive, and it is not unexpected that blinding is achieved. In contrast, maintaining a double-blind with cannabinoids may be more difficult.

In the study discussed above in which high-dose metoclopramide and THC are compared *(14)*, both patients and the treating staff were blinded. When asked, the majority of the patients were unsure which agent they had been given, even though a high dose of THC (10 mg/m$_2$ per dose, for five doses) was administered. This may be because of the inexperience of most of the patients with prior usage of cannabinoids in this largely older age group, which is typical of the majority of patients with cancer. A marked difference in efficacy occurred in this trial, favoring the metoclopramide. The treating nurses, familiar with the efficacy of metoclopramide, based their guesses as to which agent the patients received on antiemetic activity rather than on psychoactive effects, and were quite accurate in their identifications.

The Canadian trial comparing oral THC with inhalant marihuana in a crossover design, in which all patients also received a placebo of the alternate delivery form, is interesting concerning the question of blinding *(13)*. In that both forms of cannabinoid administration produce similar psychoactive side effects, could patients tell the difference between the two? Did the placebo cigarette maintain the blind, especially in the setting of receiving oral THC? Is blinding different among age groups or by prior cannabinoid experience? It appears that these questions were not part of the trial. Additionally, it is not clear that the placebo adequacy of the cigarettes has been tested.

5. THE CURRENT STATUS OF THE CONTROL OF EMESIS

5.1 Control Rates with Cancer Chemotherapy

The complete control of emesis is regularly achieved in the majority of patients receiving cancer chemotherapy likely to induce emesis. Many useful antiemetics are in frequent clinical use, have few side effects when given on a short-term basis, and are convenient in a variety of clinical settings.

The most effective of the commonly used antiemetics are the serotonin-receptor antagonists and the corticosteroids. Large clinical studies have documented the efficacy of these drugs as single agents and in combination *(4,22,23,28,29)*. As outlined in Table 5, these trials show that complete control of acute cisplatin-induced emesis is achieved in about 70–80% of patients when the combination of dexamethasone and a serotonin antagonist is used. Control as high as 90% is achieved in patients receiving these combinations with chemotherapy of moderate risk, as opposed to only 70% when single antiemetic agents are given *(28)*.

Table 5
Complete Control Rates of Acute Chemotherapy-Induced Emesis
with the Most Effective Antiemetic Regimens[a]

Antiemetic Regimen	Emetric Risk	Complete Control of Emesis
Serotonin-receptor antagonist plus a corticosteroid	Severe or high	70–80%
	Moderate	80–90%
High-dose metoclopramide plus a corticosteroid	Severe or high	60–75%
	Moderate	70–80%

[a] See refs. 3,4,21–,23,28–32, and 36.

Older trials comparing high-dose metoclopramide with serotonin-receptor antagonists showed somewhat better efficacy for the latter agents, with fewer side effects (29). As outlined above, high-dose metoclopramide was more effective with fewer side effects than THC (14). To date, trials with cannabinoids have not indicated the degree of control that is easily achieved and frequently reported with serotonin-receptor antagonist regimens.

5.2 Route of Administration and Convenience

Trials have indicated that the more effective antiemetics are not schedule dependent. Single-dose regimens, given prior to chemotherapy, are as active as multiple-dose regimens, and allow these agents to be given in a convenient fashion (22,23,30,31).

Do antiemetics need to be given intravenously? Several recent large random-assignment double-blinded studies addressed this issue. The results have consistently shown that similar results are achieved with single-dose oral serotonin-receptor antagonist regimens (with or without corticosteroids) when compared with intravenous treatment, in patients receiving cisplatin or chemotherapy of moderate emetic risk (22,23). These trials illustrate how easily effective antiemetics can be administered. These findings also suggest the potential of cost savings.

5.3 Costs and Controlling Emesis

The cost of effective antiemetic regimens can vary markedly depending on the agent, the dose, the schedule, and the route of administration. With the demonstration that single-agent regimens are as useful as multiple doses, and that oral regimens are equal to intravenous, less costly treatment is available in many settings.

Oral regimens are less costly because of lower pharmacy and administration costs, as well as lower acquisition costs in many countries. Regimens costing (to the pharmacy) as low as 0–35 have been shown to be effective (32). These costs reflect the treatment of acute emesis and delayed emesis, with the use of generic agents where available. Using equally effective, low side-effect, convenient regimens that save costs are important if the most active regimens are to be made available to all patients receiving cancer chemotherapy likely to induce emesis.

5.4 Improving Emetic Control and New Directions

Whereas better antiemetic control could be achieved by staff education and universal usage of the best established regimens, a fundamental change requires discovery of agents that work by a unique mechanism of action.

Among the proposed new agent pathways, agents that involve the neurokinin receptors (NK-1 antagonists) appear to be the most promising. There are three well-described neurokinin receptors; the type 1 receptor, or NK-1 receptor, is stimulated by substance P *(33)*. In animal models, agents that block the NK-1 receptor prevent cisplatin-induced emesis. Additionally, these agents prevent emesis by a variety of known emetogenic chemicals, giving the NK-1-receptor antagonists the broadest range of activity of all antiemetics, in preclinical studies.

Clinical trials with NK-1-receptor antagonists are now being conducted. To date, these are phase II or small phase III comparison studies. Preliminary results have indicated that these agents are safe to administer orally, and that they appear to have useful activity in both acute and delayed chemotherapy-induced emesis *(33–35)*. Confirmatory trials are needed, as are studies to see if these agents are superior to currently available agents, and to find if they add to the efficacy of the best combination regimens.

6. CONCLUSIONS

The major progress in controlling chemotherapy-induced emesis benefits thousands of patients each day. Well-designed and conducted studies have documented this progress. As examples, patients receiving the most difficult to control emetic agents, now have a 70–80% likelihood of being free of acute emesis *(4)*. This is in contrast to the nearly 100% risk of vomiting in the 1970s *(3,27)*. Additionally, patients given agents such as cyclophosphamide with anthracyclines (commonly used in breast cancer and in lymphoma) may have as high as a 90% chance of not vomiting with the best available antiemetic regimens *(28)*.

It is interesting that this degree of progress is largely unknown by the general public, indicating that common sources of information have not accurately informed our society. The control of emesis is an important factor for patients and families involved in cancer care. In contrast, antiemetics are not a major issue in health care and public awareness of recent advances is low. Nonetheless, it is also likely that most citizens are not well-informed about major cancer-related progress, including the high cure rates regularly obtained in childhood leukemia, testicular cancer, or Hodgkin's disease. The outcome of an incompletely or inaccurately informed public is illustrated in attempts to approve new drugs through popular referenda rather than through scientific drug evaluation.

Most antiemetic studies with cannabinoids have methodological difficulties and can be difficult to interpret. If one concentrates on the better-conducted trials, however, it is clear that cannabinoids possess antiemetic properties in patients receiving cancer chemotherapy. It must be noted that some degree of antiemetic efficacy is found with agents of many different classes. This activity includes phenothiazines, butyrophenones, corticosteroids, substituted benzamides, serotonin-receptor antagonists, and other classes, as well.

The degree of antiemetic activity demonstrated by cannabinoids to date is not as high as that seen with several other classes of agents (especially with substituted benzamides, corticosteroids, and serotonin-receptor antagonists). The side effects associated with cannabinoid use are tolerable, but greater than those seen with these other classes of agents. Even mild or moderate side effects are important in that antiemetics are supportive-care agents given to reduce toxicities, not to result in more problems in a population of patients who already deal with difficulties related to many organ systems.

Studies have not demonstrated an advantage of one tested cannabinoid over another. Results of trials with synthetic cannabinoids, such as levonantradol or nabilone, do not indicate a superior therapeutic index over naturally occurring cannabinoids. Only limited data from well-designed trials can be found comparing inhalant marihuana with other cannabinoids. From that which exists, there is no clear advantage for either inhalant marihuana or for oral THC. Additionally, there is no demonstration that the inhalant agent results in an improved pharmacokinetic profile, an advantage in self titration, or in a different pattern of side effects.

The theoretical potential exists that oral THC added to more effective regimens could enhance activity, in that the mechanism of cannabinoid action appears to be different than that of the serotonin-receptor antagonists and corticosteroids. Such combinations should aim to be as convenient as possible, yet have few added side effects.

Further studies with cannabinoids, using accepted methodology, could more accurately outline their activity. Decisions should be made whether or not the current moderate degree of efficacy and moderate amount of associated side effects with all tested cannabinoid antiemetics warrant such trials in the context of substantially more active agents that have more favorable toxicity profiles.

REFERENCES

1. Coates, A., Abraham, S., Laye, S. B., et al. (1983) On the receiving end-patient perception of the side-effects of cancer chemotherapy. *Eur. J. Cancer Clin. Oncol.* **19,**203–208.
2. Griffin, A. M., Butow, P. N., Coates, A. S., et al. (1996) On the receiving end V: patient perceptions of the side effects of cancer chemotherapy in 1993.*Ann. Oncol.* **7,**189–195.
3. Gralla, R. J., Itri, L. M., Pisko, S. E., et al. (1981) Antiemetic efficacy of high dose metoclopramide: randomized trials with placebo and prochlorperazine in patients with chemotherapy-induced nausea vomiting. *N. Engl. J. Med.* **305,**905–909.
4. Roila, F., Tonato, M., Cognetti, F., et al. (1991) Prevention of cisplatin-induced emesis: a double-blind multicenter randomized crossover study comparing ondansetron and ondansetron plus dexamethasone. *J. Clin. Oncol.* **9,** 674–678.
5. Steele, N., Gralla. J., and Braun, D. W., Jr.(1980) Double-blind comparison of the antiemetic effects of nabilone and prochlorperazine on chemotherapy-induced emesis. *Cancer Treat. Rep.* **64,**219–224.
6. Tyson, L. B., Gralla, R. J., Clark, R. A., et al. (1985) Phase I trial of levonantradol in chemotherapy-induced emesis. *Am. J. Clin. Oncol.* **8,**528–532.
7. Sallan, S. E., Zinberg, N. E., and Frei, E. (1975) Antiemetic effect of delta-9-tetrahydrocannabinol in patients receiving cancer chemotherapy. *N. Engl. J. Med.* **293,**795-797, 1975.
8. Chang, A. E., Shiling, D. J., Stillman, R. C., et al. (1979) Delta-9-tetrahydrocannabinol as an antiemetic in patients receiving high-dose methotrexate: a prospective, randomized evaluation. *Ann. Intern. Med.* **91,**819–824.
9. Chang, E. A., Shiling, D. J., Stillman, R. C., et al. (1981) A prospective evaluation of delta-9-tetrahydrocannabinol as an antiemetic in patients receiving adriamycin and cytoxan chemotherapy. *Cancer* **47,**1746–1751.
10. Frytak, S., Moertel, C. G., O'Fallon, J., et al. (1979) Delta-9-tetrahydrocannabinol as an antiemetic in patients treated with cancer chemotherapy: a double comparison with prochlorperazine and a placebo. *Ann. Intern. Med.* **91,**825–830.
11. Sallan, S. E., Cronin, C. M., Zelen, M., et al. (1980) Antiemetics in patients receiving chemotherapy for cancer: a randomized comparison of delta-9-tetrahydrocannabinol and prochlorperazine. *N. Engl. J. Med.* **302,**135–138.
12. Orr, L. E., McKerman, J. F., and Bloone, B. (1980) Antiemetic effect of tetrahydrocannabinol. *Arch. Intern. Med.* **140,**1431–1433.
13. Levitt, M., Faiman, C., Hawks, R., et al: (1984) Randomized double blind comparison of delta-9-tetrahydrocannabinol (THC) and marihuana as chemotherapy antiemetics. *Proc. Am. Soc. Clin. Oncol.* 3,91.
14. Gralla, R. J., Tyson, L. B., Borden, L. B., et al. Antiemetic therapy: a review of recent studies and a report of a random assignment trial comparing metoclopramide with delta-9-tetrahydrocannabinol. Cancer Treat Rep 68:163-172, 1984.
15. Borison, H. L., Mc Carthy, L. E. (1983) Neuropharmacology of chemotherapy induced emesis. *Drugs* **25,**8–17.
16. Fozard, J. R. (1984) Neuronal 5-HT receptors in the periphery. *Neuropharmacology* **23,**1473–1486.
17. Andrews P. L. R., and Davis CJ. The physiology of emesis induced by anti-cancer therapy. IN: *Serotonin and the Scientific Basis of Anti-Emetic Therapy. (Reynolds, D. J. M., Andrews, P. L. R., and Davis, C. J., eds.) Oxford Clinical Communications, Oxford, UK, 1995, pp. 25–49.*

18. Davis C.J. Emesis research: a concise history of the critical concepts and experiments. In: Serotonin and the Scientific Basis of Anti-Emetic Therapy. (Reynolds D. J. M., Andrews, P. L. R., Davis, C. J., eds.) Oxford Clinical Communications, Oxford, UK, 1995, pp.9–24.

19. Gralla, R. J., Clark, R. A., Kris, M. G., and Tyson, L. B.: (1991) Methodology in anti-emetic trials. *Eur. J. Cancer* **27,** S5–8.

20. Vinciguerra, V., Moore, T., and Brennan, E. (1988) Inhalation marihuana as an antiemetic for cancer chemotherapy. *NY State J. Med.* **10,525–527.**

21. Kris, M. G., Gralla, R. J., Clark, R. A., et al. (1987) Antiemetic control and prevention of side effects of anti-cancer therapy with lorazepam or diphenhydramine when used in combination with metoclopramide plus dexamethasone: a double-blind randomized trial. *Cancer* **60**2816–2822.

22. Perez, E. A., Chawla, S. P., Kaywin, P. K., et al. (1997) Efficacy and safety of oral granisetron versus IV ondansetron in prevention of moderately emetogenic chemotherapy-induced nausea and vomiting. *Proc. Am. Soc. Clin. Oncol.* **16** 43.

23. Gralla, R. J., Navari, R. M., Hesketh, P. J., et al. (1998) Single-dose oral granisetron has equivalent antiemetic efficacy to intravenous ondansetron for highly emetogenic cisplatin-based chemotherapy. *J. Clin. Oncol.* **16 1–7.**

24. Clark, R. A., Tyson, L. B., and Frisone, M. (1985) A correlation of objective and subjective parameters in assessing antiemetic regimens. *Proc. Tenth Ann. Cong. Oncol. Nurs. Soc.* **2,**96.

25. Gralla, R. J., Braun, T. J., Squillante, A., et al. Metoclopramide: initial clinical studies of high dosage regimens in cisplatin-induced emesis. In: Poster D, ed. The treatment of nausea vomiting induced by cancer chemotherapy. New York, N.Y.: Masson Publishing; 167-176, 1981.

26. Gralla, R. J. (1983) Metoclopramide. A review of antiemetic trials. *Drugs* **25:**163–73.

27. Homesley, H. D., Gainey, J. M., Jobson, V. N., et al. (1982) Double-blind placebo-controlled study of metoclopramide in cisplatin-induced emesis.*N. Engl. J. Med.* **307**250–251.

28. The Italian Group for Antiemetic Trials (1995) Dexamethasone, granisetron, or both for the prevention of nausea and vomiting during chemotherapy for cancer. *N. Engl. J. Med.* **332**–337.

29. DeMulder, P. H. M., Seynaeve, C., Vermorker, J. B., et al. (1990) Ondansetron compared with high-dose metoclopramide in prophylaxis of acute and delayed cisplatin-induced nausea and vomiting. A multicenter, randomized, double-blind, crossover study. *Ann. Inter. Med.* **113,**834–840.

30. Beck, T. M., Hesketh, P. J., Madajewicz, S., et al. (1992) Stratified, randomized, double-blind comparison on intravenous dose regimens in the prevention of cisplatin-induced nausea and vomiting. *J. Clin. Oncol.* **10(12),**1969–75.

31. Kris, M. G., Gralla, R. J., Tyson, L. B., et al. (1985) Improved control of cisplatin-induced emesis with high-dose metoclopramide and with combinations of metoclopramide, dexamethasone and diphenhydramine: results of consecutive trials in 255 patients. *Cancer* **55,**527–534.

32. Gralla, R. J., Rittenberg, C. N., Lettow, L. A., et al. (1995) A unique all-oral, single-dose, combination antiemetic regimen with high efficacy and marked cost saving potential. *Proc. Am. Soc. Clin. Oncol.* **14,**526.

33. Kris, M. G., Radford, J. E., Pizzo, B. A., et al. (1997) Use of an NK-1 receptor antagonist to prevent delayed emesis following cisplatin. *J. Natl. Cancer Inst.* **89,** 817–818.

34. Hesketh, P. A., Gralla, R. J., Webb, R. T., et al. (1998) Randomized Phase II Study of the Neurokinin-1 Antagonist CJ-11,974 for the Control of Cisplatin-Induced Emesis. *Proc. Am. Soc. Clin. Oncol.* **17**

35. Navari, R. M., Gralla, R. J., Hesketh, P., Kris, M. G., et al. (1998) MK-869, A selective neurokinin-1 antagonist, reduces cisplatin-induced acute and delayed emesis. *Proc. Am. Soc. Clin. Oncol.* **17**

36. Tyson, L. B., Clark, R. A., and Gralla, R. J. (1982) High-dose metoclopramide: control of dacarbazine-induced emesis in a preliminary trial. *Cancer Treat. Rep.* **66,**2108.

52

Clinical and Experimental Reports of Marihuana and Cannabinoids in Spastic Disorders

Paul Consroe

Abstract

Recently, the subject of medical marihuana has received an extraordinary amount of attention. This issue has been discussed and scrutinized in the lay media and at several medical and scientific venues in the United States and United Kingdom. Many of the purported uses of marihuana or cannabinoids are for neurological symptoms associated with spastic disorders such as multiple sclerosis and spinal cord injury. The present report provides a review the clinical literature on this topic. In the basic research of cannabinoids, there have been many important discoveries that are relevant to therapeutic concerns. The present report also selectively examines these findings for clues as to the possible therapeutic mechanisms of action of marihuana and cannabinoids. It appears that marihuana and Δ^9-THC likely provide symptomatic improvement of spasticity, pain, ataxia, and tremor, and additional clinical studies are warranted. The spasmolytic and analgesic effects of Δ^9-THC and other brain cannabinoid (CB_1) receptor agonists may involve gamma-aminobutyric acid (GABA), glutamate, N-methyl-D-aspartate (NMDA), and noradrenergic mechanisms at spinal and supraspinal sites. More basic research is needed to discover the functional roles of cannabinoid receptors and their endogenous ligands as major keys for possible therapeutic applications.

1. INTRODUCTION

In 1996, the USA states of Arizona and California "legalized" marihuana for medical use. For many reasons, including that marihuana is still illegal in Federal law, these voter-initiated bills resulted in unprecedented legal, political, and scientific repercussions. As one result, several notable scientific meetings were held in 1997 to examine the issue of medical marihuana. The meetings (and the Internet addresses for further information) were: the United States National Institutes of Health (NIH) Workshop on the Medical Utility of Marihuana (http://www.nih.gov/news /medmarijuana/ MedicalMarijuana.htm); the United States National

From: *Marihuana and Medicine*
Edited by: G. G. Nahas et al.   © Humana Press Inc., Totowa, NJ

Academy of Sciences Institute of Medicine Assessment of the Science Base of the Medical Use of Marihuana (http:// www2.nas.edu/medical-mj); and, the International Cannabinoid Research Society Symposium on Medical Marihuana (http://129.49.19.42/ICRS/Abs97.html). There was also a meeting on the Therapeutic Applications of Cannabinoids sponsored jointly by the Royal Pharmaceutical Society of Great Britain and the Multiple Sclerosis Society of Great Britain and Northern Ireland (see *The Pharmaceutical Journal*, 1997, vol. 259, pp. 104–105). One outcome was the establishment of a cannabinoid group that will facilitate clinical trials with marihuana and cannabinoids in the United Kingdom.

Marihuana continues to be used illegally for self medication of several conditions, although the extent of this use is unknown. Dronabinol (Δ^9-THC; Marinol; available in the United States, Canada, Europe, and Australia) and nabilone (Cesamet; discontinued in the United States in 1989, but available in Canada, Europe, and Australia) are oral prescription drugs for treatment of nausea and vomiting associated with cancer, and loss of appetite and weight associated with AIDS. These drugs have been used occasionally in clinical trials as treatments for some other disorders. In the preclinical area, discoveries of brain cannabinoid receptors and their endogenous ligands and other cannabinoid mechanisms have fueled speculation that cannabinoids could be developed as novel therapeutic drugs. The present report will review the clinical and experimental reports of marihuana and cannabinoids as potential treatments for neurological disorders with spasticity.

2. CANNABINOID RECEPTORS, LIGANDS, AND DRUGS

The identity and location of the mutually exclusive brain (CB_1) and peripheral (CB_2) cannabinoid receptor are now well-established *(1)*. The CB_1 receptor is found in greatest abundance in the substantia nigra pars reticulata (SNr), globus pallidus, cerebellum, and hippocampus. However, CB_1 receptors are distributed throughout the brain and spinal cord, in a heterogenous fashion *(2)*. Similarly, the endogenous CB_1-receptor ligands (eicosanoids known as endocannabinoids), notably anandamide and 2-arachidonoylglycerol, are well confirmed *(3,4)*. In humans, anandamide has been found (from highest to lowest concentration) in hippocampus, parahippocampal cortex, thalamus, striatum (caudate nucleus and putamen), and cerebellum. A mechanistic classification of cannabinoids has been made difficult by the more recent findings of novel effects of several standard cannabinoids. One general finding is that full agonists can act as partial agonists, and (neutral) antagonists can act as inverse agonists depending on the cell, tissue, or pharmacological system under study *(5)*. In these regards, nabilone, CP 55,940, HU-210, WIN 55,212-2, and 2-arachidonylglycerol frequently are considered to be full CB_1 receptor agonists, whereas Δ^9-THC and anandamide are usually considered to be partial agonists. Partial agonists are also partial antagonists and as such, they can inhibit the responses produced by full agonists. Furthermore, the competitive CB_1 receptor blockers, SR141716A and 6-iodopravadoline (AM630), are also inverse agonists at the CB_1 receptor. This means that when given alone, they can produce effects opposite to those of cannabinoid agonists and marihuana. Another intriguing finding *(6)* is that cannabinoid efficacies in brain (CP 55,940 > HU-210 > anandamide > Δ^9-THC) are quite different than their potencies (HU-210 >> CP 55,940 = Δ^9-THC >> anandamide). Lastly, there are cannabinoids, such as cannabidiol (CBD) and HU-211 (the + isomer of HU-210), which have therapeutic-related effects but they do not act upon cannabinoid receptors *(1)*.

3. SPASTICITY AND SPASTIC DISORDERS

Spasticity is a specific type of muscle hypertonia that develops after supraspinal or spinal lesions in descending corticospinal (pyramidal) or other motor pathways *(7,8)*. In the spinal

Table 1
Clinical Effects of Marihuana and Cannabinoids in Multiple Sclerosis and Spinal Cord Injury

Disorder	Drug	Study design or report type	Major effect	Ref.
MS and SCI	Marihuana smoking	Anecdotal (many patients)	↓ Spasticity, tremor, pain	10–14
MS and SCI	Marihuana smoking	Three anonymous surveys (10 SCI patients; 43 SCI patients; 112 MS patients)	↓ Spasticity, tremor, pain	15–17
MS	Marihuana smoking	Open label (1 patient)	↓ Spasticity, tremor, ataxia	18
MS	Marihuana smoking	Double blind, placebo control (10 patients)	↓ Balance in marihauna group	19
MS	Δ^9-THC orally	Three studies: double blind, placebo control (9 patients); single blind, placebo control (8 patients); double blind, placebo control, crossover (13 patients)	↓ Spasticity in Δ^9-THC group; ↓ tremor (2 of 8 Δ^9-THC patients); ↓ only subjective spasticity in Δ^9-THC group	20–22
SCI	Δ^9-THC orally	Two studies: double blind, placebo control crossover (5 patients); double blind, placebo control (1 patient)	↓ Spasticity (2 of 5 Δ^9-THC patients); ↓ spasticity and pain	23–24
MS	Nabilone orally	Double blind, placebo control crossover (1 patient)	↓ Spasticity	25
MS and SCI	Δ^9-THC orally or rectally	Open label (1 MS patient; 1 SCI patient)	↓ Spasticity and rigidity	26

Abbreviations: MS, multiple sclerosis; SCI, spinal cord injury; Δ^9-THC, Δ^9-tetrahydrocannabinol.

cord, there is increased activity of alpha motoneurons and excitatory interneurons, and decreased activity of inhibitory interneurons (9). This results in facilitation of excitatory glutamate neurons, and inhibition of inhibitory GABA neurons (8,9). A separate ceruleus-spinal projection also modulates the activity of spinal motor neurons via a noradrenergic mechanism (8). Spasticity, along with flexor and extensor spasms, clonus, cerebellar limb and gait ataxia and intention tremor, and acute, chronic, and paroxysmal pains are often features of multiple sclerosis (MS) and/or spinal cord disease or injury (7). Baclofen, a $GABA_B$-receptor agonist, and tizanidine, an alpha$_2$ receptor agonist, are commonly used spasmolytic drugs. There are no good treatments for ataxia, intention tremor and chronic pain (7). Antiepileptic drugs especially carbamazepine, baclofen, or surgery are the most common treatments of the paroxysmal pains such as trigeminal neuralgia (7).

4. MARIHUANA AND CANNABINOIDS IN SPASTIC DISORDERS

Table 1 presents an brief synopsis of the clinical reports on the effects of marihuana and cannabinoids in patients with MS or spinal cord disease or injury (10–26). Reviews and critiques of the clinical literature on this topic have been published (13,14,27). The bulk of the marihuana reports are anecdotal, and all of the clinical trials have few subjects and other defects. Whereas none of these reports singly would be considered conclusive, the totality of the reports suggest that marihuana, Δ^9-THC, and nabilone likely have beneficial symptomatic activity in conditions with spasticity. Few reports cite any side effects. One study (19) reported that smoked marihuana adversely affected balance in 10 MS patients when assessed by sophisticated electronic equipment and videotaping, but not when assessed by the standard neurological exam. This is not surprising, since sensitive equipment rather than routine clinical exams are often required to detect neurological deficits in normal subjects given marihuana or THC (13). A few of the studies (22,23,26) reported that Δ^9-THC produced adverse effects. This is not unexpected since these effects (dizziness, mental clouding, dry mouth, weakness) are typical subjective side effects of the drug. Anecdotal reports (e.g., 11,12,17) indicate that when subjects have had experience with both drugs, smoked marihuana usually is preferred over oral Δ^9-THC.

Symptomatic improvement of spasticity, intention tremor, ataxia, trigeminal neuralgia, and chronic pain would be uniquely important attributes of marihuana and cannabinoids. A controlled comparative study of marihuana, oral Δ^9-THC, and (smoked and oral) placebos given for at least 6 months in a sufficient number of patients with spasticity, tremor, ataxia and pain would do much to promote closure of the contentious debate about efficacy and safety of these drugs.

5. PRECLINICAL EFFECTS OF CANNABINOIDS

Over 30 years ago it was demonstrated that a Δ^9-THC analog, and Δ^9-THC and cannabis extract, could depress the polysynaptic linguomandibular reflex in the cat (28) and dog (29), respectively. This effect is mediated at some supraspinal level and is consistent with spasmolytic activity (28). However in the spinal cord, Δ^9-THC was found to increase excitatory postsynaptic potentials (EPSP) and decrease inhibitory postsynaptic potentials (IPSP) at cat spinal motor neurons (30). These effects might tend to oppose spasmolytic activity. Interestingly, CBD was found to decrease EPSP and increase IPSP at cat spinal motoneurons (31).

More recently, other findings have emerged that indicate that CB_1 receptor agonists can have a major influence on the activity of the SNr. Specifically, WIN 55,212-2 (32,33) and CP 55,940 (33) increased the firing rate of neurons in the SNr, and WIN 55,212-2 (32) antagonized the inhibition of firing in the SNr by electrical stimulation of the striatum. Furthermore, WIN 55,212-2 blocked the increase in the firing rate of SNr neurons induced by chemical stimulation of the subthalamic nucleus (34). The SNr is a major output nuclei of the basal ganglia (8), and is the site of the greatest abundance of CB_1 receptors in the brain (2). In genetically spastic rats, the SNr was identified as a major supraspinal site of action for the muscle-relaxing effects of baclofen and tizanidine (35). This appears to be a promising lead for future study with CB_1-receptor agonists.

There are many data that indicate that CB_1-receptor agonists enhance GABA function in the brain (36,37). Moreover, there is evidence that the behavioral motor inhibition produced by Δ^9-THC or anandamide may be mediated through $GABA_B$-receptor activation (38). It is generally accepted that CB_1-receptor agonists can reduce transmitter release, via decreasing calcium-channel conductance, and decrease action potential generation, via increasing potassium-channel conductance (1). Also, CB_1-receptor agonists have been found to inhibit presynaptic glutamic acid release in rat hippocampal cultures (39). If these cannabinoid effects act in tandem, and act in the appropriate sites in brain and cord, then they would be analogous to the purported spasmolytic mechanism of action of baclofen (9). That is, activation of postsynaptic $GABA_B$ receptors by baclofen results in increased potassium conductance, neuronal hyperpolarization, and subsequent presynaptic inhibition. Activation of presynaptic $GABA_B$

receptors by baclofen decrease calcium-channel conductance which in turn inhibits the release of glutamic acid.

The effects of CB_1-receptor agonists also may resemble those of tizanidine. One study has reported that an alpha$_2$ noradrenergic antagonist (yohimbine) given intrathecally at lumbar spinal level blocked the antinociceptive response (mouse tail flick) of Δ^9-THC given intravenously (40). The authors concluded that cannabinoids activate descending noradrenergic neurons, resulting in antinociception via the stimulation of alpha$_2$ adrenergic receptors. Tizanidine stimulates alpha$_2$ adrenergic receptors, resulting in both a direct impairment of glutamate release from spinal interneurons, and a concomitant inhibition of the excitatory ceruleus-spinal pathway (9,41). The connection between the spasmolytic and analgesic activities is that tizanidine also has antinociceptive activity, and this effect like its spasmolytic activity is caused by an alpha$_2$ adrenergic receptor mediated inhibition of spinal interneuronal activity (41).

As an important extension of the analgesic and glutamate effects discussed above, recent evidence has been presented in mice indicating that there is a tonic modulation of nociceptive thresholds by spinal cannabinoid systems (42). Further, these spinal cannabinoid systems made hypoactive by injections of antisense to the CB_1 receptor mRNA or by SR 141716A resulted in an NMDA-dependent hyperalgesia (42). Presumably this hyperalgesia was caused by release of glutamate which subsequently activated the NMDA receptor (42). Hyperalgesia and allodynia (pain elicited by normally nonpainful stimuli) are characteristic features of the chronic and paroxysmal pains of MS and also of the chronic neuropathic pains of other conditions (7). In one rat model of neuropathic pain (chronic sciatic nerve constriction injury), hyperalgesia and allodynia were greatly reduced by WIN 55,212-2 (43). These effects appear to be mediated by CB_1 receptors since the inactive enantiomer of WIN 55,212-2 was inactive in this model (43). Curiously, in the only other reported model of neuropathic pain, HU-211 was shown to significantly reduce a rat behavior of self-mutilation following neuronal denervation (44). HU-211, which does not act on CB_1 or CB_2 receptors (1), presumably produced this effect by a stereospecific, noncompetitive blockade of the NMDA receptor (45).

The two other major features of MS that are potential targets for therapy by cannabinoids are intention tremor and ataxia. Yet, a major puzzle is that marihuana and Δ^9-THC appear to ameliorate these signs of MS, and yet they appear to cause these signs in laboratory animals and humans (13). Whereas the clinical descriptions of cerebellar ataxia and intention tremor caused by MS (7) and the ataxia and tremor caused by marihuana or Δ^9-THC (13) appear to differ significantly, there still are no animal or human data to resolve directly this important paradox. Lastly, Δ^9-THC (or Δ^8-THC) was found to reduce histological and clinical features of experimental autoimmune encephalomyelitis (EAE) and experimental autoimmune neuritis (EAN) in experimental animals (46–48). EAE is the commonly used animal model for MS, whereas EAN is a commonly used animal model for Guillain-Barre Syndrome (47). Both of these disorders have in common a possible immunological etiology, and a focal demyelinating pathology (7). Current drug treatments to reduce acute exacerbations or to prevent worsening of these diseases consist of various immunosuppressant therapies (7). Δ^9-THC has immunosuppressant effects, presumably by acting on primarily CB_2 receptors located in the immune system (1). These findings suggest that cannabinoid-receptor agonists might affect the underlying disease process of MS.

ACKNOWLEDGMENT

This work was supported by a grant from the Arizona Disease Research Control Commission.

REFERENCES

1. Pertwee, R. G. (1997) Pharmacology of cannabinoid CB1 and CB2 receptors. *Pharmac. Ther.* **74,** 129–180.
2. Glass, M., Dragunow, M., and Faull, R. L. M. (1997) Cannabinoid receptors in the human brain: a detailed anatomical and quantitative autoradiographic study in the fetal, neonatal and adult human brain. *Neuroscience* **77,** 299–318.
3. Di Marzo, V. and De Petrocellis, L. (1997) The endogenous cannabinoid signaling system: chemistry, biochemistry and physiology. *Internet J. Sci. Biol. Chem.* **http://www.netsci-journal.com/97v1/97007/index.htm.**
4. Stella, N., Schweitzer, P., and Piomelli, D. (1997) A second endogenous cannabinoid that modulates long-term potentiation. *Nature* **388,** 773–778.
5. Consroe, P. (1998) Brain cannabinoid systems as targets for the therapy of neurological disorders, *Neurobiology of Disease,* vol. 5, No 6, to be published.
6. Burkey, T. H., Quock, R. M., Consroe, P., Ehlert, F. J., Hosohata, Y., Roeske, W. R., and Yamamura, H. I. (1997) Relative efficacies of cannabinoid receptor agonists in the mouse brain. *Eur. J. Pharmacol.* **336,** 295–298.
7. Adams, R. D., Victor, M., and Ropper, A. H., eds. (1997) *Principles of Neurology*, 6th ed. McGraw-Hill, New York, NY.
8. Gilman, S. and Newman, S. W., eds. (1996) *Manter and Gatz's Essentials of Clinical Neuroanatomy and Neurophysiology*, 9th ed. F.A. Davis, Philadelphia, PA.
9. Noth, J. (1991) Trends in the pathophysiology and pharmacotherapy of spasticity. *J. Neurol.* **238,** 131–139.
10. Petro, D. J. (1980) Marihuana as a therapeutic agent for muscle spasm or spasticity. *Psychosomatics* **21,** 81–85.
11. Randall, R. C., ed. (1991) *Muscle Spasm, Pain & Marihuana Therapy*. Galen Press, Washington, DC.
12. Grinspoon, L. and Bakalar, J. B., eds. (1993) *Marihuana the Forbidden Medicine*. Yale University Press, New Haven, CT.
13. Consroe, P. and Snider, S.R. (1986) Therapeutic potential of cannabinoids in neurological disorders, In: *Cannabinoids as Therapeutic Agents* (Mechoulam, R., ed.), CRC Press, Boca Raton, FL, pp. 21–49.
14. Consroe, P. and Sandyk, R. (1992) Potential role of cannabinoids for therapy of neurological disorders, in *Marihuana/Cannabinoids: Neurobiology and Neurophysiology* (Bartke, A. and Murphy, L., eds.), CRC Press, Boca Raton, FL, pp. 459–524.
15. Dunn, M. and Davis, R. (1974) The perceived effects of marihuana on spinal cord injured males. *Paraplegia* **12,** 175.
16. Malec, J., Harvey, R. F., and Cayner, J. J. (1982) Cannabis effect on spasticity in spinal cord injury. *Arch. Phys. Med. Rehab.* **63,** 116–118.
17. Consroe, P., Musty, R., Rein, J., Tillery, W., and Pertwee, R. (1997) The perceived effects of smoked cannabis on patients with multiple sclerosis. *Eur. Neurol.* **38,** 44–48.
18. Meinck, H. M., Schonle, P. W. A., and Conrad, B. (1989) Effect of cannabinoids on spasticity and ataxia in multiple sclerosis. *J. Neurol.* **236,** 120–122.
19. Greenberg, H. S., Werness, SAS, Pugh, J. E., Andrus, R. O., Anderson, D. J., and Domino, E. F. (1994) Short-term effects of smoking marihuana on balance in patients with multiple sclerosis and normal volunteers. *Clin. Pharmacol. Ther.* **55,** 324–328.
20. Petro, D. J. and Ellenberger, C. (1981) Treatment of human spasticity with Δ^9-tetrahydrocannabinol. *J. Clin. Pharmacol.* **21 (suppl),** 413s–416s.
21. Clifford, D.B. (1983) Tetrahydrocannabinol for tremor in multiple sclerosis. *Ann. Neurol.* **13,** 669–671.
22. Ungerleider, J. T., Andrysiak, T., Fairbanks, L., Ellison, G. W., and Myers, L. W. (1987) Delta-9-THC in the treatment of spasticity associated with multiple sclerosis. *Advan. Alcohol Substance Abuse* **7,** 39–50.
23. Hanigan, W. C., Destree, R., and Truong, X.T. (1986) The effect of Δ^9-THC on human spasticity. *Clin. Pharmacol. Ther.* **39,** 198.
24. Maurer, M., Henn, V., Dittrich, A., and Hofmann, A. (1990) Delta-9-tetrahydrocannabinol shows antispastic and analgesic effects in a single case double-blind trial. *Eur. Arch. Psychiat. Clin. Neurosci.* **240,** 1–4.
25. Martyn, C. N., Illis, L. S., and Thom, J. (1995) Nabilone in the treatment of multiple sclerosis. *Lancet* **345,** 579.
26. Brenneisen, R., Egli, A., Elsohly M. A., Henn, V., and Spiess, Y. (1996) The effect of orally and rectally administered delta-9-tetrahydrocannabinol on spasticity: a pilot study with 2 patients. *Int. J. Clin. Pharmacol. Ther.* **34,** 446–452.
27. Pertwee, R. G. (1997) Cannabis and cannabinoids: pharmacology and rationale for clinical use. *Pharmaceut. Sci.* **3,** 539–545.
28. Boyd, E. S. and Meritt, D. A. (1965) Effects of a tetrahydrocannabinol derivative on some motor systems in the cat. *Arch. Int. Pharmacodyn.* **153,** 1–12.

29. Sampaio, C. A., Lapa, A. J., and Valle, J. R. (1967) Influence of cannabis, tetrahydrocannabinol and pyrahexyl on the linguomandibular reflex of the dog. *J. Pharm. Pharmacol.* **19,** 552–554.

30. Turkanis, S. A. and Karler, R. (1983) Effects of delta-9-tetrahydrocannabinol on cat spinal motoneurons. *Brain Res.* **288,** 283–287.

31. Turkanis, S. A. and Karler, R. (1986) Cannabidiol-caused depression of spinal motoneuron responses in cats. *Pharmacol. Biochem. Behav.* **25,** 89–94.

32. Miller, A. S. and Walker, J. M. (1995) Effects of a cannabinoid on spontaneous and evoked neuronal activity in the substantia nigra pars reticulata. *Eur. J. Pharmacol.* **279,** 179–185.

33. Tersigni, T. J. and Rosenberg, H. C. (1996) Local pressure application of cannabinoid agonists increases spontaneous activity of rat substantia nigra pars reticulata neurons without affecting response to iontophoretically-applied GABA. *Brain Res.* **733,** 184–192.

34. Sanudo-Pena, M. C. and Walker, J. M. (1997) Role of the subthalamic nucleus in cannabinoid actions in the substantia nigra of the rat. *J. Neurophysiol.* **77,** 1635–1638.

35. Turski, L., Klockgether, T., Schwarz, M., Turski, W. A., and Sontag, K. H. (1990) Substantia nigra: a site of action of muscle relaxant drugs. *Ann. Neurol.* **28,** 341–348.

36. Pertwee, R. G. (1987) The central neuropharmacology of psychotropic cannabinoids. *Pharmac. Ther.* **36,** 189–261.

37. Maneuf, Y. P., Crossman, A. R., and Brotchie, J. M. (1996) Modulation of GABAergic transmission in globus pallidus by the synthetic cannabinoid WIN 55,212-2. *Synapse* **22,** 382–385.

38. Romero, J., Garcia-Palomero, E., Fernandez-Ruiz, J. J., and Ramos, J. A. (1996) Involvement of GABA$_B$ receptors in the motor inhibition produced by agonists of brain cannabinoid receptors. *Behav. Pharmacol.* **7,** 299–302.

39. Shen, M., Piser, T. M., Seybold, V. S., and Thayer, S. A. (1996) Cannabinoid receptor agonists inhibit glutamatergic synaptic transmission in rat hippocampal cultures. *J. Neurosci.* **16,** 4322–4334.

40. Lichtman, A. H. and Martin, B. R. (1991) Cannabinoid-induced antinociception is mediated by a spinal alpha-2-noradrenergic mechanism. *Brain Res.* **559,** 309–314.

41. Coward, D. M. (1994) Tizanidine: neuropharmacology and mechanism of action. *Neurology* **44 (suppl. 9),** S6–S11.

42. Richardson, J. D., Aanonsen L., and Hargreaves, K. M. (1998) Hypoactivity of the spinal cannabinoid system results in NMDA-dependent hyperalgesia. *J. Neurosci.* **18,** 451–457.

43. Herzberg, U., Eliav, E., Bennett, G. J., and Kopin, I. J. (1997) The analgesic effects of R(+)-WIN 55,212-2 mesylate, a high affinity cannabinoid agonist, in a rat model of neuropathic pain. *Neurosci. Lett.* **221,** 157–160.

44. Zeltser, R., Seltzer, Z., Eisen, A., Feigenbaum, J. J., and Mechoulam, R. (1991) Suppression of neuropathic pain behavior in rats by a non-psychotropic synthetic cannabinoid with NMDA receptor-blocking properties. *Pain* **47,** 95–103.

45. Nadler, V., Mechoulam, R., and Sokolovsky, M. (1993) Blockade of 45Ca^{2+} influx through N-methyl-D-aspartate receptor ion channel by the non-psychoactive cannabinoid HU-211. *Brain Res.* **622,** 79–85.

46. Lyman, W. D., Sonett, J. R., Brosnan, C. F., Elkin, R., and Bornstein, M.B. (1989) Δ^9-Tetrahydrocannabinol: a novel treatment of experimental autoimmune encephalomyelitis. *J. Neuroimmunol.* **23,** 73–81.

47. Lyman, W. D. (1991) Drugs of abuse and experimental autoimmune diseases, In: *Drugs of Abuse, Immunity and Immunodeficiency* (Friedman, H., Specter, S., and Klein, T.W., eds.), Plenum, New York, pp. 81–92.

48. Wirguin, I., Mechoulam, R., Breuer, A., Schezen, E., Weidenfeld, J., and Brenner, T. (1994) Suppression of experimental autoimmune encephalomyelitis by cannabinoids. *Immunopharmacology* **28,** 209–214.

53

Marihuana: Effects on Neuronal Excitability and Seizure Threshold

Elisabeth Gordon and Orrin Devinsky

Abstract

In the late 19th century, British neurologists found that cannabis had a limited role in epilepsy therapy. Cannabinoid receptors are found in the brainstem, limbic and neocortical areas that modulate seizure activity. The recent studies of the effects of THC, CBD, and related cannabinoids in animal models of epilepsy reveal that (1) the effects vary significantly in different models, in different species, and for the different derivatives; (2) the mechanisms by which the cannabinoids exert their anti- or proconvulsant effects is not well-defined; and (3) the effects of acute administration (e.g., increasing seizure threshold) may be followed, in certain models, by a rebound effect (e.g., decreasing seizure threshold).

No well-controlled studies have evaluated cannabinoids in the treatment of epilepsy patients. However, clinical anecdotes and single case reports suggest that marijuana may reduce seizure frequency or, conversely may provoke seizure activity in select cases, while in most instances it has no significant effect on seizure activity. Several clinical studies have examined the efficacy of CBD on seizure frequency. These studies found either some reduction in seizure frequency or no statistically significant reduction compared to placebo. The few epidemiological studies that have been conducted suggest that marijuana use may protect against seizures induced by illicit drugs such as heroin and cocaine. The limited evidence therefore suggest that marijuana and the cannabinoids may have antiepileptic effects in man, but these effects may be specific to partial or tonic-clonic seizures.

1. INTRODUCTION

The use of *Cannabis* for the treatment of neurological problems, including epilepsy and motor disorders, probably predates Western records. The *Herbal*, the equivalent of the United States pharmacopoeia, written in approximately 450 BC, documents ancient medicinal uses of *Cannabis sativa (1)*. Drs. Russell Reynolds *(2)* and William Gowers *(3)*, two of the most

From: *Marihuana and Medicine*
Edited by: G. G. Nahas et al.   © Humana Press Inc., Totowa, NJ

prominent late 19th century British neurologists, both reported on the role of *Cannabis* in epilepsy therapy, in their separate monographs on epilepsy.

> *Indian hemp I have administered in many cases, and with the effect of delaying the paroxysms and mitigating their severity in some individuals. Thus in one case an habitual series of 17 severe attacks was reduced to three of slight severity; in other cases intervals have been prolonged; whereas in a still larger number I have obtained no beneficial result. The dose given has varied form one-third of a grain to one grain of the alcoholic extract, prepared by Squire, three to four times daily. In several cases of convulsions, from either eccentric irritation, such as gonorrhea, etc., or cerebral congestion, I have seen not only marked improvement, but permanent relief.[2]*
>
> *Cannabis indica, which was first recommended in epilepsy by Dr. Reynolds, is sometimes, though not very frequently, useful. It is of small value as an adjunct to the bromide, but is sometimes of considerable service given separately. It may be noted that the action of Indian hemp presents many points of resemblance to that of belladonna; it is capable of causing also delirium and sleep, first depression and then acceleration of the heart, and also dilates the pupil. The cerebral excitement is relatively more marked, and the effect on the heart and pupil much less than in the case of belladonna.*
>
> *In the following case its effect was far more decided than that of bromide:*
>
> *John K., age 40, came under treatment in 1868, having suffered from fits for 25 years. They occurred during both sleeping and waking, at intervals of a fortnight. There was a brief warning, vertigo, then loss of consciousness, and tonic and clonic spasm followed by some automatism; — [then he] acts strangely and cannot dress himself. The attacks ceased for a time on bromide, but recurred when he discontinued attendance. He came again in October 1870; scruple doses of bromide of potassium three times a day had now no effect, and the fits, at the end of four months' treatment, were as frequent as ever. Ext. Cannabis indicae gr. 1/6, three times a day, was then ordered; the fits ceased at once, 'a wonderful change,' the patient declared. He had no fit for six months, and then, having discontinued attendance, the fits recurred, but were at once arrested by the same dose of Indian hemp. He continued free from fits for some months, until, during my absence, bromide was substituted for the Indian hemp; the fits immediately recurred, and he left off treatment. He returned to the hospital in six months' time, and on Indian hemp passed two months without an attack. In the third month another fit recurred, and the patient again ceased to attend, and did not return.*

Despite the clinical observation that cannabis could help control seizures in selected patients, and the passing notice given to *Cannabis* in some early texts on epilepsy and neurology (4), its use for epilepsy received little attention and *Cannabis* was not mentioned in early North American texts on epilepsy (5,6) or neurology (7). The introduction of phenobarbital in 1912 and phenytoin in 1937 for epilepsy, together with the 1937 Federal Marihuana Tax Act, effectively shut the door for further interest or exploration into the therapeutic potential of marihuana in epilepsy. The more recent medical literature has focused on Δ^9-tetrahydrocannabinol (THC), and other cannabinoids in animal models of epilepsy, as well as anecdotal reports in which marihuana could prevent or induce seizures.

2. MECHANISM OF ACTION OF CANNABINOIDS: RELEVANCE TO EPILEPSY AND TO MOVEMENT DISORDERS

Cannabinoid (CB_1) receptors are found in greatest density in subcortical regions such as the substantia nigra pars reticulata, corpus striatum, cerebellum, hippocampus (CA1 and CA3 regions, and dentate gyrus) and neocortex.

2.1. Substantia Nigra Pars Reticulata

Cannabinoid receptors are most densely concentrated in the nondopaminergic cells of the substantia nigra pars reticulata. This structure is one of the relay output stations of the basal ganglia; it transforms and carries the neuronal activity towards implementation of spinal motor activity *(8)*. The substantia nigra pars reticulata is a site of anticonvulsant activity of the GABA-mimetic drugs in genetic, electroshock, and chemoshock animal models of epilepsy *(9)*. Thus, this structure may modulate epileptogenic activity. Activation of GABA receptors and the subsequent activation of the GABA-ergic nigrocollicular pathways inhibit the spread of both generalized tonic-clonic and absence seizures *(9,10)*. These mechanisms may contribute to the anticonvulsant activity of cannabinoids in animal models, which appear to inhibit seizure spread in the CNS.

2.2. Corpus Striatum

The corpus striatum (i.e., the globus pallidus, putamen, and caudate nucleus) have a high density of cannabinoid receptors. The internal operation of the corpus striatum is an interplay of four neurotransmitters: dopamine (DA), L-glutamate, GABA, and acetylcholine (ACh). The major output of the striatum is to the motor cortex. Dopamine and ACh have opposing effects. Low levels of GABA potentiate the effect of DA, whereas high levels have an anti-DA effect. Also, L-glutamate from the cerebellum exerts phasic control over nigrostriatal dopamine neurotransmission and modulates ACh and GABA activities *(11)*, as well as producing excitotoxicity and neuronal degeneration. Cortical projections more directly control the activity of the lower motor neurons via descending pyramidal and extrapyramidal pathways. However, the corpus striatum modulates motor cortex and subcortical areas that influence motor activity. The striatum is integral for the normal physiology of movement.

2.3. Cerebellum

Although the density of cannabinoid receptors is lower in the cerebellum than in the pars reticulata or striatum, they are relatively abundant within the cerebellum *(12)*. The cerebellum modulates motor function, with various neurological disorders resulting from abnormalities involving the functional and anatomic connections between the cerebellum, substantia nigra striatum, ventral midbrain regions, and limbic system *(13,14)*. Inputs from the cerebral cortex, hypothalamus, and locus ceruleus to the cerebellum regulate the process of motor activity. Further, the cerebellum has efferent connections to the reticular, vestibular, and red nuclei, and the motor cortex *(8)*. Norepinephrine, serotonin, GABA, and L-glutamate are key neurotransmitters regulating cerebellar functions. The cerebellum phasically modulates nigrostriatal DA transmission through L-glutamate/NMDA-receptor activity.

There are functional implications for the cerebellum in epilepsy. Chronic cerebellar stimulation in humans has been used to treat epilepsy *(15)* with therapeutic effects possibly mediated by release of striatal dopamine *(16)*. However, the effectiveness of cerebellar stimulation for any disorder remains controversial.

2.4. Hippocampus and Neocortex

In addition to helping to account for the effects of cannabinoids on memory and cognition *(12)*, the presence of the cannabinoid receptors in the hippocampus and neocortex suggest a potential effect of cannabinoids on seizure activity *(17)* and can also explain their effects on memory and cognition *(12)*. Further, the question of a possible functional connection between the mechanisms of action of the cannabinoid and the NMDA receptors is raised since the two receptors are colocalized in many of the same brain areas.

Enhancing NMDA-receptor-mediated excitatory actions produces epileptiform activity in experimental models, and, conversely, decreasing excitatory synaptic efficacy (e.g., blocking NMDA receptors) produces antiepileptic effects in most animal models and human patients. It has also been shown that antagonists of NMDA receptors effectively suppress seizures in hippocampal slices *(18,19)* and in in vitro hippocampal preparations, NMDA antagonists prevented the development of electrographic seizures that followed repeated electrical stimulation of the CA3 regions *(20)*. Thus, hyperfunction of NMDA receptors or of the receptor agonist (L-glutamate) are likely involved in the pathophysiology of epilepsy. Therefore, cannabinoids may have important potential antiepileptic effects since, not only are the cannabinoid and NMDA receptors colocalized, but also in preparations of rat cortical membranes, the (+) enantiomer of HU-210 was found to be a functional antagonist of the NMDA receptor *(21)*.

2.5. Thalamocortical Activity

Electrophysiological studies reveal that cannabinoids influence thalamocortical projections, which could alter the seizure threshold or cause sensory illusions induced by cannabinoids *(22)*. A dose-dependent effect of cannabinoids on CNS excitability occurs, with low doses producing activation and higher doses reducing electrical activity. These dose-dependent electrophysiological changes may underlie the biphasic effects of cannabinoids, including effects on the seizure threshold *(23)*.

2.6. Catecholaminergic Effects

THC and other cannabinoids influence activity levels of major catecholaminergic transmitters such as dopamine and norepinephrine, possibly by exerting a presynaptically mediated anticholinergic effect in the cerebral cortex, hippocampus, and striatum *(22,24)*. These transmitters can modulate seizure and motor activity. In preparations of rat cortical membranes, the (+) enantiomer of HU-210 is a functional antagonist of the NMDA receptor *(21)*. This may have therapeutic implications since stimulation of NMDA receptors can lower the seizure threshold *(11)*. NMDA receptors tonically excite and exert phasic control over dopaminergic transmission in the nigrostriatum, probably by an action within the cerebellum *(13)*.

3. CANNABINOIDS STUDIED FOR POTENTIAL ANTISEIZURE EFFECTS

Approximately 60 cannabinoids and 260 noncannabinoid constituents of marijuana have been identified *(25)*. In addition, many hundreds of natural and synthetic analogs have been synthesized *(26)*. Unfortunately, most pharmacological research on cannabinoids has focused on relatively few constituents. This is especially true for the possible antiseizure effects of cannabinoids, with most of this research studying the effects of (−)Δ^9-tetrahydrocannabinol, commonly referred to as Δ^9-THC (THC), the main psychoactive constituent of marihuana, and with cannabidiol (CBD) another naturally occurring but nonpsychoactive, constituent. Also, limited investigations explored the antiepileptic effects of several derivatives of CBD, Δ^8-THC, and (−)-HU-210, a crystalline THC of absolute stereochemical purity *(27–29)*.

4. ANIMAL STUDIES OF THE EFFECTS OF CANNABINOIDS ON EPILEPSY

Δ^9-Tetrahydrocannabinol (THC), cannabidiol (CBD), and related derivatives were studied in several animal models to assess their effect on seizure threshold and kindling *(28–43)*. These studies reveal that: effects vary significantly in different models, in different species, and for different derivatives; the mechanisms by which THC, CBD, and related compounds exert their anticonvulsant or proconvulsant properties are not clearly defined; and the effects of acute administration (e.g., increasing seizure threshold) may be followed in certain models by a rebound effect (e.g., decreasing seizure threshold).

The pharmacological effects of THC are stereospecific; only the (–) enantiomer has an effect on seizure threshold (31). However, the actual effects of THC on seizure threshold vary widely, with various studies providing directly conflicting evidence. (29,33) THC has both proconvulsant and anticonvulsant effects, depending on dose, seizure model, and factors of seizure initiation versus seizure spread. (32).

An anticonvulsant effect from THC is observed in cases with rapidly evoked tonic discharges, utilizing posttetanic potential for recruitment. In animal models of epilepsy, THC is effective against some forms of both complex partial seizures and generalized maximal seizures. However, in animal models of genetic epilepsy, simple partial, complex partial, and absence seizures, THC has excitatory or proconvulsant effects. Several studies indicate that the convulsant effect of THC results from hypersynchronous neuronal discharges (34). Thus, with slowly propagating seizure discharges, a convulsant effect of THC may result from drug-induced hypersynchrony (34).

Since THC has sedating and anticonvulsant effects in several animal models, THC-mediated GABA-agonist activity has been postulated but has not been supported by animal studies (35), although further study is warranted. Synthetic cannabinoids can functionally block NMDA receptors (21) suggesting that an effect on these receptors may contribute to anticonvulsant effects of THC.

The anticonvulsant properties of THC were compared with phenytoin (PHT), phenobarbital (PB), and chlordiazepoxide (CDP) using several seizure models in mice (i.e., maximal electroshock [MES], pentylenetetrazol [PTZ], strychnine, and nicotine) (38). In the MES test, THC was the least potent and PHT the most potent blocker of hind-limb tonic extensor convulsions, whereas THC was the most potent and PHT the least potent in increasing the latency to this response and in preventing mortality. Seizures and mortality induced by PTZ or by strychnine were enhanced by THC and PHT but were blocked by PB and CDP. None of the four agents prevented nicotine-induced seizures. Only PHT failed to increase latency; THC and DPH were less potent than PB and CDP in preventing mortality. THC most closely resembled DPH in tests with chemical convulsant agents.

In the kindling model of epilepsy in mice, THC enhanced kindling to electroconvulsive therapy (ECT), PTZ, and picrotoxin. This enhancement of kindling persisted after the cannabinoid was withdrawn. With ECT and PTZ, but not picrotoxin, a single exposure to THC facilitated subsequent kindling. With electrical kindling, the cannabinoid decreased the convulsion threshold. Because the threshold was not lowered to all kindling stimuli, however, other mechanisms are probably involved. Even a single dose of THC can cause long-lasting elevations of CNS excitability (33).

The antiepileptic and prophylactic effects of THC and Δ^8-THC were examined in rats that developed generalized seizures in the kindling model using intermittent electrical stimulation of the amygdala. In direct contrast to the studies cited above, both isomers of THC can acutely suppress kindled seizures, but consistent antiepileptic effects were obtained only with high, toxic dosages. Tolerance to the antiepileptic effects of THC developed rapidly when the drugs were given repeatedly, and repeated administration of high doses of Δ^9-THC may induce acute physical dependence. Tolerance to THC effects may reflect biochemical and cellular, rather than pharmacological changes. Receptor downregulation caused by chronic agonist treatment underlie tolerance (29). Administration of the isomers of THC during seizure development suppressed kindling, suggesting a prophylactic effect. The rate of rekindling after drug withdrawal was not significantly different from that of control rats. Thus a true prophylactic effect was not obtained (39).

An autosomal recessive condition in New Zealand White rabbits results in convulsions following intravenous injections of THC and other psychoactive cannabinoids of marijuana (36,37). Ontologically, postnatal days of nonsusceptibility were (15–23), partial susceptibility (24–38), and complete susceptibility (39–548) were found.

The complex effects of THC on seizure threshold remain to be more fully defined in terms of specific epilepsy model, species, doserelated effects, acute versus withdrawal effects, and tolerance. CBD and its derivative analogs, including both the (+) and (–) enantiomers, have anticonvulsant properties without stimulatory or convulsant properties. The parent molecules, not their metabolites, appear to alter seizure threshold. In animal models of epilepsy, cannabinoids are effective in (1) blocking or reducing the spread of generalized seizures induced by maximal electroshock or GABA-inhibiting drugs; (2) blocking simple partial seizures produced by the topical application of convulsant metals on the cortex (e.g., cobalt-induced simple partial seizures); and (3) increasing the seizure threshold for electrical kindling of limbic structures (44). CBD and the derivative analogs are not effective against animal models of generalized absence epilepsy (44). Further, these compounds increase the potency of antiepileptic drugs in animal models of partial and generalized motor seizures, yet inhibit the action of antiepileptic drugs in animal models of generalized absence seizures (30).

A pharmacological comparison between cannabidiol (CBD) and four CBD derivatives (II–V), was carried out in mice by Carlini and colleagues (28). CBD, CBD-II, CBD-III, and CBD-IV were active in protecting mice against electroconvulsive shock at doses of 100–200 mg/kg, although at the larger-dose CBD and compound II were the most effective.

More research is needed to define the potential role of CBD as an antiepileptic drug or as an adjunctive therapy to increase the potency of other antiepileptic drugs.

4.1. Rebound Hyperexcitability to Cannabinoids

Several animal studies document a rebound effect to both THC and to CBD. In mice, a single exposure to THC resulted in a rebound hyperexcitability in the CNS manifested by increased susceptibility to electrically induced convulsions. The magnitude of the hyperexcitability was dose-related. The time-course of the effect was maximal at 24 hours after administration of the drug, with a duration lasting up to 196 hours. The time course of the rebound hyperexcitability to THC was compared to that for PB, which peaked at 48 hours after administration of the drug and returned to the control value by 96 hours. Tolerance developed rapidly to the motor-toxic effect of THC, but after 23 days of daily treatment there was no tolerance to the rebound hyperexcitability. The functional significance of the hyperexcitable state was assessed in two tests: electrical kindling to minimal convulsions was enhanced, even when the kindling procedure was initiated 120 hours after exposure to the drug; and the anticonvulsant activity of PHT was blocked when mice were treated with the anticonvulsant 96 hours after a single exposure to THC. The results suggest that the rebound response from a single exposure to THC represents a functionally significant prolonged increase in CNS excitability (40).

The effects of CBD on electrically evoked kindled seizures were studied in conscious, unrestrained rats with chronically implanted cortical and limbic electrodes, and the results were compared with those of THC, PHT, and ethosuximide (ESM). All drugs were anticonvulsant, but there were marked differences in their effects on afterdischarge (AD) threshold, duration, and amplitude. CBD, like PHT and Δ^9-THC, elevated the AD threshold; in contrast, ESM decreased the threshold but suppressed AD spread. CBD, however, also resembles ESM since both drugs decrease AD duration and amplitude. Electrophysiologically, the antiseizure effects of CBD resemble a combination of those of PHT and ESM. These effects may account for the observation that CBD was the most efficacious drug tested against limbic ADs and convulsions. Compared with Δ^9-THC, CBD is a more attractive anticonvulsant without potential motor toxicity. CBD also lacks the CNS excitatory effects produced by Δ^9-THC, PHT, and ESM. These characteristics, combined with its apparently unique set of electrophysiological properties, support the suggestion that CBD has therapeutic potential as an antiepileptic (42).

The anticonvulsant activity of CBD and the central excitation of THC were investigated electrophysiologically with conscious, unrestrained cobalt-induced epileptic rats. The conventional antiepileptics, trimethadione (TMO), ESM and PHT, were included as reference drugs. Spontaneously firing, epileptic potentials from a primary focus on the parietal cortex were directly measured and convulsions were monitored visually. ESM and TMO decreased the frequency of focal potentials, but PHT and CBD exerted no such effect. Although CBD did not suppress the focal abnormality, it abolished jaw and limb clonus and had no excitatory effects. In contrast, THC markedly increased the frequency of focal potentials, evoked generalized bursts of polyspikes, and produced convulsions. 11-OH-Δ^9-THC, the major metabolite of THC, only produced bursts of polyspikes. Thus, in this model of focal epilepsy, CBD blocked the motor manifestations of convulsions and THC had proconvulsant effects, although the mechanisms remains uncertain (43).

The effects of subacute treatment with CBD, THC, PHT, and PB on anticonvulsant activity and on withdrawal excitability in mice were compared in three electrically induced seizure-threshold tests. In the MES test, subacute treatment did not alter the anticonvulsant activity of CBD, PHT, or PB, but tolerance developed to THC. In the 60-Hz electroshock-threshold test, THC and CBD activity did not change, but tolerance developed to PB, and there was an increase in sensitivity to PHT. In the 6-Hz electroshock-threshold test, there was an increase in sensitivity to both THC and CBD, tolerance to PB, and the PHT activity was unchanged. Although tolerance developed in some of the seizure-threshold tests to THC and PB, tolerance to CBD and PHT did not develop in any of the tests. In the case of tolerance to the effects of THC, biochemical, or cellular changes seem to be responsible, not pharmacological changes. Hyperexcitability followed withdrawal from only THC (6 and 60-Hz electroshock-threshold tests) and PB (maximal electroshock-threshold and 60-Hz electroshock-threshold tests). The THC withdrawal hyperexcitability suggests that marihuana use could provoke withdrawal seizures in susceptible patients (41).

Comparative studies of the anticonvulsant properties of the cannabinoids and prototype antiepileptic drugs in numerous animal seizure models suggest the following: (1) as an anticonvulsant, CBD, in contrast to THC, is relatively selective for CNS depressant and excitatory properties; (2) the potency of CBD, unlike PHT and PB, varies greatly between species; (3) the large potency difference between the cannabinoids and the AEDs in the mouse may reflect dispositional differences, because brain concentrations of all the drugs are similar; (4) tolerance to the anticonvulsant properties of cannabidiol is not a prominent feature since in three seizure models, tolerance developed in one, but reverse tolerance developed in the other two; (5) and the results of a study of the electrophysiologic mechanisms of action indicate that cannabidiol produces some unique effects and that its spectrum of antiepileptic activity may be different from that of the prototype drugs. The anticonvulsant nature of CBD suggests that it has a therapeutic potential in at least three of the four major types of epilepsy: tonic-clonic, focal motor, and complex partial seizures (41).

5. CLINICAL STUDIES OF CANNABINOIDS AND EPILEPSY

Few clinical studies have investigated the effects of THC and other cannabinoids on epilepsy in humans. No large double-blind or controlled studies have evaluated marihuana,

THC, CBD, or other cannabinoids in the treatment of epilepsy patients. Clinical anecdotes and single case reports suggest that marihuana may reduce seizure frequency or, conversely, may provoke seizure activity in select cases, whereas in most instances it has no significant effect on seizure activity.

Our personal experience and interviews with more than 300 patients with active epilepsy who have used marihuana intermittently or regularly is that the majority have failed to identify a relationship between marihuana use and seizure frequency or severity. Three of our patients reported that regular marihuana use decreased or controlled seizures. None of our patients reported that marihuana use or withdrawal led to increased seizure activity. However, these patients were not asked to chart marihuana use and seizure activity, and the interviews represented retrospective recollections in a population with frequent short-term memory impairments. Several colleagues have informally reported to us that patients with primary generalized epilepsy, particularly juvenile myoclonic epilepsy, have had seizures associated with marihuana use. Many of these patients may have also consumed alcohol and been subjected to sleep deprivation near the time of marihuana consumption, complicating interpretation of this anecdotal data. The greatest experience to date probably remains that of Reynolds and Gowers (see Subheading 1.)

Keeler and Reifler *(45)* described a young man who had been seizure free for six months. After smoking marihuana seven times within three weeks, he had three generalized seizures. However, none of these recurrent seizures occurred during or immediately after consumption *(45)*. Another case report indicated that marihuana use was necessary for seizure control *(46)*. Also, Ellison and colleagues *(47)* reported on an adult male in whom regular use of marihuana seemed to suppress complex partial seizures, which repeatedly recurred when he stopped using marihuana. This patient had a history of alcoholism and bipolar affective disorder, and was on psychotropic medications (lithium, trifluoperazine, benztropine, disulfiram, lorazepam, or clonepam, and/or carbamazapine). The difficulty with individual case reports is highlighted by a patient in whom marihuana use was implicated as the cause of new-onset seizures, but an infectious etiology was subsequently documented *(48)*.

Although no studies explored the antiepileptic efficacy of THC in humans, several examined the effects of CBD on seizure frequency. These studies found either some reduction of seizure frequency *(49–51)*. or no statistically significant reduction compared to placebo *(51,52)*.

A double-blind study examined CBD in addition to standard antiepileptic drugs in nine patients with refractory partial epilepsy and secondarily generalized seizures with temporal foci. Among the four patients who received CBD, two showed clinical improvement (i.e., no convulsions) over the three months on the drug, one showed partial improvement, and one had no improvement. There was no change in seizure frequency in any of the five patients on placebo *(49)*. In 1980, a study of 16 patients with poorly controlled complex partial or secondarily generalized seizures tested the efficacy of orally administered CBD over 4.5 months in a double-blind, placebo-controlled, randomized, add-on trial. CBD initially increased epileptiform activity on the EEG, but not the clinical symptoms of seizure activity. However, after 4.5 months, seven of the eight patients on CBD were seizure-free with no EEG evidence of epileptiform activity, compared to only one of the eight controls. The results suggested that CBD at 200–300 mg/day was an effective adjunctive therapy for epilepsy *(50)*. In both of these studies CBD may have potentiated the effects of other antiepileptic drugs or acted itself as an effective antiepileptic drug.

Two other studies found no statistically significant difference between epilepsy patients on CBD and those on placebo. The first study examined the effects of oral CBD at doses of 200–300 mg/day, over four weeks, in 12 patients as adjunctive therapy *(52)*. The second study was longer, administering CBD as adjunctive therapy (one or more standard antiepileptic drugs at baseline) to 10 medically refractory patients with generalized tonic-clonic, simple-partial motor, or complex-partial seizures over two years. After a three-month baseline and six months of single-blind placebo, patients entered a six-month double-blinded treatment period with placebo or 300 mg/day CBD, followed by another three-month baseline period. In those patients taking CBD, a consistent blood level of 20–30 ng/mL was maintained. There were no significant differences between CBD and placebo-treatment groups for seizure pattern, frequency, or character, neuropsychological test results, or hematological studies (51). The same group conducted an open trial of CBD, at doses of 900–1200 mg/day for 10 months, in a patient with refractory epilepsy. This patient had a significant decrease in seizure frequency. Blood levels of CBD in this patient were higher than those in the double-blind, placebo-controlled study, averaging approximately 150 ng/mL. The authors suggested that CBD at larger doses might have an anticonvulsant effect and CBD deserves further investigation despite the results of the larger study (51).

To summarize, the limited evidence suggests that marihuana and its active cannabinoid metabolites may have antiepileptic activity in humans, but these effects may be specific to partial or tonic-clonic seizures. CBD may not possess clinical antiepileptic activity, at least at doses of 200–300 mg/day. However, further study of its pharmacological effects at higher doses is warranted.

Epidemiololgic studies suggest that marihuana may protect against seizures induced by illicit drugs such as heroin or cocaine. Heroin, marihuana, and cocaine use was studied before the onset of a first seizure in 308 patients with seizures and 294 controls at Harlem Hospital Center, New York City, between 1981 and 1984. Heroin use, both past and present, was a risk factor for all first seizures (adjusted odds ratio 2.8), with the greatest risk for heroin use within 24 hours of hospitalization. Marihuana use appeared to be a protective factor against first seizures in men. For men with unprovoked seizures, the adjusted odds ratio was 0.42 (95% CI 0.22–0.82) for marihuana use at any time and 0.36 (95% CI 0.18–0.74) for marihuana use within 90 days of hospitalization. For men with provoked seizures, respective adjusted odds ratios were 1.03 (95% CI 0.36–2.89) and 0.18 (95% CI 0.04–0.84). Cocaine use, although common among study subjects, was not a significant risk factor either for all first seizures or for subgroups of seizures, regardless of the time of last use (53). In another study of 49 patients with presumed drug-induced seizures, none had seizures following use of only marihuana (54). Five of the 49 patients had recently used marihuana, but all of these subjects had also used concomitant drugs such as heroin or cocaine.

Few studies have explored the mechanisms of action of marihuana in humans. Knowledge of the effects of marihuana on neurotransmitter systems are predominantly based on animal studies that have been previously cited. One study showed that marihuana decreases alpha amplitude and frequency (55). Additional research on the mechanisms of action of cannabinoids in humans is needed.

REFERENCES

1. Grinspoon, L. (1971) *Marijuana Reconsidered.* Harvard University Press, Canbridge, MA, p. 1.
2. Reynolds, J. R. (1861) *Epilepsy: Its Symptoms, Treatment, and Relation to Other Chronic Convulsive Diseases.* Churchill, London, UK p. 321.
3. Gowers, W. R. (1881) *Epilepsy and Other Chronic Convulsive Disorders.* Churchill, London, pp. 223–224.
4. Binswanger, O. Epilepsie. A. Holder: Wien, 1913, p. 418.
5. Escheverria, M. G. (1870) On Epilepsy: Anatomo-Pathological and Clinical Notes. New York
6. Spratling, W. P. (1904) *Epilepsy and Its Treatment* W. B. Saunders, New York.
7. White, W. A. andc Jelliffe, S. E. (1913) *The Modern Treatment of Nervous and Mental Diseases* Lea & Febiger, Philadelphia.

8. Gillman, S. and Newman, S. W. (1989) *Manter and Gatz's Essentials off Clinical Neuroanatomy and Neurophysiology*, 7th ed., F. A. Davis, Philadelphia.

9. Iadarola, M. J., and Gale, K. (1982) Substantia nigra: site of anticonvulsant ctivity mediated by gamma-aminobutyric acid. *Science* **218**, 1237.

10. Depaulis, A., Vergnes, M., Lui, Z., Kempf, E., and Marescaux, C. (1990) Involvement of the nigral output pathways in the inhibitory control of the substantia nigra over generalized non-convulsive seizures in the rat. *Neuroscience*, **39**, 339.

11. Olney, J. W. (1989) Excititory amino acids and neuropsychiatric disorders. *Biol. Phsychiatry.* **26**, 505.

12. Herkenman, M., Lynn, A. B., Little, M. D., Johnson, M. R., Melvin, L. S., de Costa B. R., and Roce, K. C. (1990) Cannabinoid receptor localization in the brain. *Proc. Natl. Acad. Sci. USA* **87**, 1932.

13. Rao, T. S., Cler, J. A., Mick, S. J., Emmett, M. R., Farah, J. M., Contreras PC, Iyengar, S., and Wood, P. L. (1991) Neurochemical interactions of competitive *N*-methyl-*D*-aspartate antagonists with dopaminergic neurotransmission and the cerebellar cyclic GMP system: functional evidence for a phasic glutamatergic control of the nigrostriatal dopaminergic pathway. *J. Neurochem.* **56**, 907.

14. Snider, R. S., Maiti, A, and Snider, S. R. (1976) Cerebellar pathways to ventral midbrain and nigra. *Exp. Neurol.* **53**, 714.

15. Cooper, I. S., Amin, I., and Riklin, M. (1976) Chronic cerebellar stimulation in epilepsy. *Arch. Neurol.* **33**, 559.

16. Tabbador, K., Wolfson, L. I., and Sharples, N. S. (1978) Ventricular fluid homovanillic acid concentrations in patients with movement disorders. *Neurology* **28**, 1249.

17. Deadwyler, S. A., Heyser, C. J., Michaelis, R. C., and Hampson, R. E. (1990) The effects of delta 9-THCon mechanisms of learning and memory. *NIDA Res. Monogr.* **97**, 79–93.

18. Dingeldine, R., McBain, C. J., and McNamara, J. O. (1990) Excitatory amino acid receptors in epilepsy. *TIPS*, **11**, 334–338.

19. Herron, C. E., Williamson, R., and Collingridge, G. L. (1985) A selective N-methyl-D-aspartate antagonist depresses epileptiform activity in rat hippocampal slices. *Neurosci. Lett.* **61**, 255–260.

20. Stacheff, S. F., Anderson W. W., Clark S., and Wilson W. A. (1989) NMDA antagonists differentiate epileptogenisis from seizure expression in an *in vitro* model. *Science* **245**, 648–651.

21. Feigenbaum, J. J., Bergmann, F., and Richmond, S. A. (1989) Nonpsychotropic cannabinoid acts as a functional N-methyl-D-aspartate receptor blocker. *Proc. Natl. Acad. Sci. USA* **86**, 9584–9587.

22. Pertwee, R. G. (1988) The central neuropharmacology of psychotropic cannabinoids. *Pharmacol. Ther.* **36**, 189.

23. Feldman, R. G. and Pippenger, C. E. (1976) The relation of anticonvulsant drugs to complete seizure control. *Journal of Clinical Pharmacology* **16 (1)**, 51–59.

24. Miller and Branccouier

25. Turner, C. E., ElSohly, M. A., and Boeren, E. G. (1980) Constituents of cannabis sativa L. XVII. A review of the natural constituents. *J. Nat. Products.* **43**, 169.

26. Razdan, R. (1986) Structure-activity relationships in cannabinoids. *Pharmacol. Rev.* **38**, 75.

27. Mechoulam, R., Lander, N., Srebnik, M., Breuer, A., Segal, M., Feigenbaum J. J., Jarbe, TUC, and Consroe, P. (1987) Stereochemical requirements for cannabimimetic activity. In: *Structure-Activity Relationships of Cannabinoids* (Rapaka RS, and Makriyannis A, eds.) NIDA Research Monograph 79, National Institute on Drug Abuse, Rockville, MD, 108.

28. Carlini, E. A., Mechoulam, R., and Lander, N. (1975) Anticonvulsant activity of four oxygenated cannabidiol derivatives. *Res. Commun. Chem. Pathol. Pharmacol.* **12**, 1–15.

29. Abood, M. E. and Martin, B. R. (1996) Molecular neurobiology of the cannabinoid receptor. *Int. Revi. Neurobiol.* **39**, 197–221.

30. Consroe, P. F., and Sandyk, R. (1992) Potential role of cannabinoids for therapy of neurological disorders In: *Marijuanal Cannabinoids: Neurobiology and Neurophysiology.* (Murphy L and Bartke A., ed.) CRC Press, Ann Arbor, MI, pp. x to x.

31. Consroe, P. F., and Mechoulam, R. (1987) Anticonvulsant and neurotoxic effects of tetrahydrocannabinol stereoisomers. In: *Structure Activity Relationships of the Cannabinoids* (Rapaka R. S., Makriyanis A, eds) NIDA Research Monograph 79, National Institute on Drug Abuse, Rockville MD, p. 59.

32. Consroe, P. and Snider, S. R. (1986) Therapeutic potential of cannabinoids in neurological disorders. In: *Cannabinoids as Therapeutic Agents*, (Mechoulam R, ed.) CRC press, Boca Raton, FL, p. 21.

33. Karler, R., Calder, L. D., Sangdee, P, and Turkanis, S. A. (1984) Interaction between delta-9-tetrahydrocannabinol and kindling by electrical and chemical stimuli in mice. *Neuropharmacology* **23**, 1315–1320.

34. Feeney, D. M. (1978) Marihuana and epilepsy: paradoxical anticonvulsant and convulsant effects. *Adv. Biosci.* **22–23**, 643–657.

35. Pertwee, R. G., Browne, S. E., Ross, T. M., and Stretton, C. D. (1991) An investigation of the involvement of GABA in certain pharmacological effects of delta9-tetrahydrocannabinol. *Pharmacol. Biochem. Behav.* **40**, 581–585.

36. Fish, B. S., consroe, P., and Fox, R. R. (1981) Inheritance of delta 9-tetrahydrocannabinol seizure susceptibility in rabbits. *J. Hered.* **72**, 215–216.
37. Fish, B. S., Consroe, P., and Fox, R. R. (1983) Convulsant-anticonvulsant properties of delta-9-tetrahydrocannabinol in rabbits. *Behaviour Genetics* **13(2)**, 205–211.
38. Sofia, R. D., Solomon, T. A., and Barry, H 3rd. (1976) Anticonvulsant activity of delta-9-tetrahydrocannabinol compared with three other drugs. *Eur. J. Pharmacol.* **35**, 7–16.
39. Corcoran, M. E., McCaughran, J. A., Jr, and Wada, J. A. (1978) Antiepileptic and prophylactic effects of tetrahydrocannabinols in amygdaloid kindled rats. *Epilepsia* **19**, 47–55.
40. Karler, R., Calder, L. D., and Turkanis, S. A. (1986) Prolonged CNS hyperexcitability in mice after a single exposure to delta-9-tetrahydrocannabinol. *Neuropharmacology* **25**, 441–446.
41. Karler, R. and Turkanis, S. A. (1981) The cannabinoids as potential antiepileptics. *J. Clin. Pharmacol.* **21 (8–9 Suppl)**, 437S–448S.
42. Turkanis, S. A., Smiley, K. A., Borys, H. K., Olsen, D. M., and Karler, R. (1979) An electrophysiological analysis of the anticonvulsant action of cannabidiol on limbic seizures in conscious rats. *Epilepsia* **20**, 351–363.
43. Chiu, P., Olsen, D. M., Borys, H. K., Karler, R., and Turkanis, S. A. (1979) The influence of cannabidiol and delta 9-tetrahydrocannabinol on cobalt epilepsy in rats. *Epilepsia* **20**, 365–375.
44. Consroe, P., Benedito, M. A. C., Leite, J. R., Carlini, E. A., and Mechoulam R. (1982) Effect of cannabidiol on behavioural seizures caused by convulsant drugs or current in mice. *Eur. J. Pharmacol.*, 83: 293.
45. Keeler, M. H. and Reifler, C. B. (1967) Grand mal convulsions subsequent to marijuana use. *Diseases of the Nervous System.* **28**, 474–475.
46. Consroe, P. F., Wood, G. C., and Buchsbaum, H. (1975) Anticonvulsant nature of marihuana smoking. *JAMA* **234**, 306–307.
47. Ellison, J. M., Gelwan, E., and Ogletree, J. (1990) Complex partial seizure symptoms affected by marijuana abuse. *Clin. Psychiatry* **51**, 439–440.
48. Cohen M. R. (1997) Stymied by seizures. When the clues point to the wrong path. *Postgrad. Med.* **101**, 289–292.
49. Mechoulam, R., and Carlini, E. A. (1978) Towards drugs derived from cannabis. [Review] [48 refs] *Naturwissenschaften*, **65(4)**, 174–179.
50. Cunha, J. M., Carlini, E. A., Pereira, A. E., Ramos, O. L., Pimental, C., Gagliardi, R., Sanvito, W. L., Lander, N., and Mechoulam, R. (1980) Chronic administration of cannabidiol to healthy volunteers and epileptic patients. *Pharmacology* **21**, 175.
51. Trembly, B. and Sherman, M. (1990) Double-blind clinical study of cannabidiol as a secondary anticonvulsant, paper presented at Marijuana '90 Int. Conf. on Cannabis and Cannabinoids, Kolympari (Crete), July 8–11.
52. Ames, F. R. (1986) Anticonvulsant effect of cannabidiol. *S. Afr. Med. J.* **69**, 14.
53. Ng, S. K., Brust, J. C., Hauser, W. A., and Susser, M. (1990) Illicit drug use and the risk of new-onset seizures. *Am. J. Epidemiol.* **132**, 47–57.
54. Alldredge, B. K., Lowenstein, D. H., and Simon, R. P. (1989) Seizures associated with recreational drug abuse. *Neurology* **39**, 1037–1039.
55. Hughes, J. R. (1996) A review of the usefulness of the standard EEG in psychiatry. *Clin. Electroencephalogr.* **27**, 35–39.

54 Marihuana Use in Multiple Sclerosis

Gordon S. Francis

Abstract

Marihuana has received considerable attention as a potential therapy for symptoms of spasticity, ataxia, tremor, pain, and bladder dysfunction in patients with multiple sclerosis. However controlled clinical studies are either lacking, inconclusive, or not supportive of benefit. Ataxia and tremor appear to worsen with marihuana. Bladder dysfunction results are too limited to draw conclusions. Spasticity is probably not favorably affected, but may warrant further investigation with objective, standardized assessment techniques in a rigorous, double-blind, placebo-controlled fashion.

1. INTRODUCTION

Multiple sclerosis is a chronic neurologic disease that is classified as a demyelinating disorder of the central nervous system (1). The disease typically has an age of onset between 20 and 40 and is characterized, at least initially, by relapses and remissions. A relapse is defined as the new onset of neurologic symptoms that generally proceeds over several days to a few weeks with subsequent resolution of symptoms with total or partial recovery. The vast majority of patients start with relapsing-remitting disease but eventually a very high proportion of these patients develop the more steady and insidious progressive form of illness. Disability accumulates gradually over the years at a variable rate. Some patients become massively disabled in a short time, whereas others can live their entire lives with only minimal or no disability.

The etiology of multiple sclerosis (MS) remains unknown, although data implicates a role for genetic factors, environmental influences, and the immune system. Cases of familial MS, a higher rate of MS in family members of affected cases (2), a high rate of concordance in monozygotic twins (3), and certain racial predilections all argue for the role of genetics in susceptibility to MS. The genetic influence however is probably polygenic and represents only a susceptibility to develop MS (4), because even in identical twins the concordance rate is only 30%. Other factors must also be important.

Evidence for environmental factors includes data from migration studies indicating a change in prevalence with a change in geographic location (5). In addition, the worldwide distribution of so-called MS epidemics (6), suggests an environmental effect exists. As stated

From: *Marihuana and Medicine*
Edited by: G. G. Nahas et al.   © Humana Press Inc., Totowa, NJ

above, the fact that 70% of identical twins are discordant also suggests that some external factor must be at work.

What is accepted is the fact that the immune system is very important in disease causation (7–9). Presumably based on a genetic predisposition and some external triggering event, the immune system is primed to direct an immune attack against the central nervous system (CNS) myelin. It is felt that this priming occurs in the systemic circulation and that activated cells migrate across the blood–brain barrier to enter the CNS. Once within the CNS, such activated T cells initiate an immune-mediated inflammatory process when faced with similar epitopes that can result in demyelination and even axonal damage producing the neurologic symptoms in MS patients (8).

Clinically the manifestations of MS are highly variable but typically can involve visual loss, double vision, ataxia and incoordination, motor weakness, sensory loss, sphincter dysfunction, and cognitive impairment. Any portion of the CNS myelin may be affected, resulting in widespread and varied neurologic symptoms. The peripheral nervous system myelin is unaffected.

Therapy in multiple sclerosis can be divided into two categories; therapy for disease activity and symptomatic therapy for MS-related problems. For disease-modifying therapy, the typical treatment for acute relapses is corticosteroid therapy (10–12), which may reduce relapse duration, but does not affect eventual outcome. There is however new attention being directed towards acute-relapse therapy in the form of antiadhesion molecules to try to prevent the migration of activated lymphocytes into the nervous system and thus reduce the severity and duration of attack-related symptoms.

Two types of drugs have now been approved as therapy for multiple sclerosis; the β interferons and glatiramer acetate. Both types of compounds have been shown to reduce the attack frequency in multiple sclerosis (13–16), with some impact on the progression of disability. These agents currently are approved only for relapsing-remitting patients but recent unpublished results also suggest benefit for the progressive form of MS.

Symptomatic therapy refers to treatment of residual symptoms that result from MS-related injury. Such persistent symptoms include fatigue, spasticity, urinary urgency and frequency, tremor, ataxia, paroxysmal symptoms, and pain. Fatigue occasionally responds to amantadine (17) or pemoline (18), whereas spasticity is treated with a variety of drugs, including baclofen, benzodiazepines, tizanidine, botulinum toxin, and dantrolene (19–23). Urinary sphincter urgency and frequency is treated with oxybutynin, whereas failure to empty can be treated with cholinergic agents or intermittent catheterization (24). Pain syndromes respond best to medication such as carbamazepine, phenytoin, baclofen, or amitriptyline (25). Ataxia and tremor have proven exceedingly resistant to any form of therapy in MS patients.

2. POTENTIAL USES OF MARIHUANA IN MS

Quite frequently MS patients themselves are the source of potential new therapies for their disease. This is not surprising given the relative lack of therapeutic agents for MS patients and the chronicity and disabling nature of the disease. This prompts a large number of anecdotal therapies to be explored and publications exist on literally hundreds of such therapies (26). Marihuana might best be considered in the anecdotal category of therapy for MS. Symptoms that have been suggested as potentially amenable to marihuana therapy include spasticity, ataxia, tremor, and urinary dysfunction.

3. MARIHUANA AS THERAPY OF SPASTICITY IN MS

Spasticity is defined as a velocity-dependent increase in tone produced by lesions at a number of sites (20). The final common pathway appears to be enhancement of the alpha and/or gamma motor tone at the segmental level, resulting in increased resistance to passive stretch of muscle and tendon (27). Lesions at a variety of sites including the spinal cord, brain stem, subcortical structures, and cortex can all result in spasticity. Agents commonly used, such as baclofen and benzodiazepines, appear to have an action at the spinal-cord (20) level, whereas dantrolene acts directly on muscle (20). Agents such as clonidine and tizanidine function as alpha$_2$ noradrenergic agonists with inhibitory influences on spinal motor neurons and on descending facilitating coerulospinal pathways (21). Most of the antispasticity products are less effective on spasticity caused by cerebral lesions than spinal causes. The site of action of antispasticity products in the cord appears to be at the presynaptic level to enhance inhibition of the spinal-cord motor neuron. The supposed site of action of marihuana in spasticity is unclear but it is interesting to note that the cannabinoid receptors are quite sparse within the spinal cord and thus if THC is effective in spasticity it is presumably at a suprasegmental level much higher than the site of action of the most effective currently available antispasticity agents.

One of the first indications of potential benefit for marihuana derives from writings by Reynolds in the 19th century (28) in which he reports on extensive use of *Cannabis indica* administered as an alcohol extract tincture. He describes it as effective for the spasms of spinal sclerosis as well as for a syndrome that sounds consistent with trigeminal neuralgia. The report is clearly anecdotal but was quite positive in its recommendations for this product in general. Contrasted with this enthusiasm is the position of the Multiple Sclerosis Society in their publication on Therapeutic Claims in Multiple Sclerosis (26). Their assessment is that there is no generally accepted scientific basis for use of this therapy.

Data in support of the efficacy of marihuana or derivatives for spasticity are relatively limited. An early report by Petro and Ellenberger (29) used either 5 or 10 mg oral THC in nine marihuana-naïve MS patients and assessed a change in a composite motor/spasticity score after administration of placebo or THC. Although treatment assignment was blinded, the same examiner did all assessments and the general exam as well as collecting information on side effects. Benefit was reported for THC (as mean change by group) and was statistically significant. Individual data is not presented. Meinck and colleagues (30) reported in 1989 the results of single-dose, unblinded observations on one patient who had previously reported benefit with marihuana. According to the investigators, multiple signs and symptoms were improved in the patient within a short time of ingestion of THC and furthermore, the effect was prolonged with some of the symptoms being alleviated for two or three days. A somewhat larger study by Ungerleider et al. (31) examined neurologic symptoms of weakness, spasticity, coordination, gait impairment, and reflexes as well as asking patients for self-assessments of spasticity and side effects while using THC. Doses ranged from 2.5 to 15 mg and 13 patients were enrolled in the study by random assignment with drug administered in a double-blind fashion using a crossover study design. The physician ratings of all of the outcome measures were unchanged with either placebo or THC although the patients self-report was that spasticity was significantly improved with THC. The authors state that the patient assessment was probably more reliable since it was based on the total functioning over 24 hours versus the one-time postdosing assessment by the neurologist. Additionally they felt that the neurologic assessment by the clinicians was somewhat less sensitive than the patient's own perceptions. Even accepting the possible benefit as experienced subjectively by patients, the authors found that 7.5 mg was a minimal effective dose of THC and yet at this dose, unpleasant side effects were fairly prominent and patients declined to stay on the THC as a form of therapy subsequent to the study.

Benefit was also reported in a patient with a non–MS-related spinal cord origin spasticity (32). This individual patient had been disabled by a spinal cord tumor. The authors found that

5 mg of THC was the best dose in an open dose-finding phase and then proceeded to study the effects of THC versus codeine versus placebo in random, blinded, assignment multiple times over 5 months. Outcome was self-reporting on a visual-analog scale by the patient. No objective assessments were performed. The authors report that there was subjective improvement of spasticity, pain, bladder function, sleep, concentration, and mood when using THC.

A well-designed, double-blind, randomized, placebo-controlled study was conducted on 10 MS patients and 10 normal controls (*33*). These patients were given a single marihuana cigarette or placebo (an alcohol extracted marihuana cigarette) and were tested after a 10-minute smoking session. The patients were tested on 3 separate days, 2 with drug and 1 with placebo, and on each day patients underwent 20 different trials on a balance platform with either eyes open or eyes closed. The main outcome was to assess whether balance was affected (*see* Subheading 4). With respect to spasticity, however, patients underwent a pre- and postdosing assessment. According to the evaluators, there was no change in the objective assessment of spasticity after therapy.

In another single case report of a patient with MS, investigators provided the patient with nabilone 1 mg daily or placebo for a week at a time with random allocation of treatment for four different time periods (*34*). The assignment of treatment was double-blind, but the assessments were self-report by the patient on symptoms of nocturia and muscle spasms. The patient reported a reduction in nocturia and muscle spasm coincident with mood elevation that correlated with drug ingestion (as opposed to placebo). The issue of potential unblinding based on the nabilone side effects is relevant as the patient improvement coincided with mood elevation and the outcome was patient self report.

Finally Consroe et al. reported in 1997 the results of a questionnaire survey of 255 patients known to have used marihuana for treatment of MS symptoms (*35*). Response rate was only 57% and the total number of usable questionnaires was only 112 of the 255 sent out. The patient distribution was skewed towards higher levels of disability which is fairly typical of the patients who use marihuana for symptom management. Over 70% of the respondees indicated that symptoms of spasticity, pain, tremor, and emotional dysfunction were improved with marihuana therapy. A striking finding was the extent of marihuana use by these patients with the average duration of use being 6 years and the average frequency of marihuana ingestion being 2.7 times per day and 5.6 days per week.

The data indicating a benefit on spasticity of marihuana or its derivatives is quite limited. A biological mechanism of action is lacking given the paucity of receptors in the spinal cord, which is the site at which most drugs are effective if they do in fact reduce spasticity. From the studies reporting the use of THC in MS patients with spasticity, the better-designed studies failed to demonstrate objective improvement. However, the number of patients is small and the assessment of spasticity tended to be subjective. One could consider readdressing the issue of benefit in spasticity by using some of the newer techniques available for spasticity assessments that can objectively measure response or lack thereof (*36*). This must however be balanced by the fact that a number of agents are currently available that are quite effective for spasticity with fewer side effects than effective doses of THC.

4. MARIHUANA AS THERAPY FOR ATAXIA
AND TREMOR IN MS

Tremor and ataxia in multiple sclerosis patients can be caused by to lesions at various sites including the afferent spinocerebellar pathways from the spinal cord, the brain stem-cerebellar connections, cerebellar hemisphere, cerebellar nuclei, or the efferent pathways from the cerebellum. Lesions typically result in a large amplitude tremor with titubation and truncal ataxia. Several therapies effective in other forms of tremors have been found to be ineffective in multiple sclerosis including benzodiazepines, propanolol, and other β-blockers, primidone, INH, and ondansetron (37–40). This lack of specific therapy often prompts the anecdotal use of other therapies.

The only two studies that report sufficient details on the benefit of cerebellar dysfunction in MS are the studies by Ungerleider (31) and Greenberg (33). The study by Ungerleider found no objective change in gait dysfunction, coordination, or ataxia in patients treated with THC. The study by Greenberg using a stability platform paradigm examined the ability of patients to correct for randomly administered shifts in posture before and after dosing. The investigators found that MS patients did worse than normal controls both before and after therapy but more significantly, the deterioration was greater in MS patients following inhalation of marihuana than the deterioration seen in normal controls. Furthermore, only the MS patients demonstrated an increased delay in the onset of corrective response in the eyes-closed position which was not noticed in the normal controls following inhalation of marihuana. This study indicates that marihuana did not help the incoordination and, in fact, worsened the dysfunction in MS patients. No objective changes in the standard neurologic examinations were noted apart from these test-related findings. There is a single report on tremor specifically related to MS using THC therapy by Clifford involving 8 patients (41). Half of these patients had been previous users of THC and all patients were quite severely disabled. Patients were given single-blinded THC versus placebo with a THC dose of 5–15 mg given orally. Five of the eight patients reported some mild subjective improvement, whereas only two of the eight had any objective improvements. The authors comment that because of significant toxicity, the use of such a product may be limited.

The data reported would indicate that there is little if any support for use of THC for cerebellar ataxia and that in fact the drug may worsen ataxia. There is some very mild evidence that it may improve tremor, but only in a small proportion of patients and at what is probably unacceptable toxicity. Other evidence of support for tremor comes only from anecdotal uncontrolled observations.

This clinical data correlates with what is found in animal models. The cerebellum appears to have a high density of cannabinoid receptors, but when THC or similar products are administered to animals, they develop a cerebellar ataxic syndrome (42,43). Thus, the animal data and the best clinical studies suggest that the cerebellum is adversely effected by THC therapy.

5. MISCELLANEOUS SYMPTOMS TREATED WITH MARIHUANA

Various other symptoms have been reported as improved by marihuana but only in anecdotal fashion. These include pain syndromes, mood and behavioral changes, and sphincter dysfunction. There is insufficient information on which to base the use of THC as therapy for any of these symptoms apart from the pain syndromes. Pain syndromes have been studied in diseases other than MS and appear to be somewhat benefited by THC, although the benefit on pain versus the benefit derived by mood alteration or elevation is difficult to distinguish. In fact, it would appear that the psychotropic manifestations of THC are virtually inseparable from the analgesic properties (44). This will again limit the usefulness of THC as does the availability of other effective agents for use in pain syndromes such as amitriptyline, carbamazepine, phenytoin, and neurontin.

6. CONCLUSION

As with many other areas of clinical efficacy of THC in medicine, the controlled, rigorously obtained data is limited. The controlled data that is available generally indicates a lack of benefit or possibly even a deleterious effect. The area that has been studied the most is spasticity, but here the benefit has not been clearly demonstrated. Spasticity assessment has improved recently and might be amenable to further investigation should nontoxic congeners of THC become available for testing.

REFERENCES

1. Francis, G. S., Duquette, P., and Antel, J. P. (1995) Inflammatory demyelinating diseases of the CNS, In: *Neurology in Clinical Practice*, 2nd ed. (Bradley W. G, Daroff, R. B., Fenichel, G. M., Marsden, C. D., eds), Butterworth, Newton, MA, pp. 1307–1343.
2. Ebers, G. C., Sadovnick, A. D., Risch, N. J., and Canadian Collaborative Study Group. (1995) A genetic basis for familial aggregation in multiple sclerosis. *Nature* **377**, 150.
3. Ebers, G. C., Bulman, D. E., and Sadovnick, A. D. (1986) A population-based study of multiple sclerosis in twins. *N. Engl. J. Med.* **315**, 1638–1642.
4. Ebers, G. C. and Sadovnick A. D. (1994) The role of genetic factors in multiple sclerosis susceptibility. *J. Neuroimmunol.* **54**, 1–17.
5. Sadovnick, A. D. and Ebers G. C. (1993) Epidemiology in multiple sclerosis: a critical overview. *Can. J. Neurol. Sci.* **20**, 17–29.
6. Kurtzke, J. F. and Hyllested, K. (1986) Multiple sclerosis in the Faroe Islands. II. clinical update, transmission and the nature of MS. *Neurology* **36**, 307–328.
7. Hafler, D. A. and Weiner, H. L. (1995) Immunologic mechanisms and therapy in multiple sclerosis. *Immunological Rev.* **144**, 75–107.
8. Hohlfeld, R. (1997) Biotechnological agents for the immunotherapy of multiple sclerosis: principles, problems and perspectives. *Brain* **120**, 865–916.
9. Steinman, L. (1996) Multiple sclerosis: a coordinated immunological attack against myelin in the central nervous system. *Cell* **85**, 299–302.
10. Goodin, D. S. (1991) The use of immunosuppressive agents in the treatment of multiple sclerosis: a critical review. *Neurology* **41**, 980–985.
11. Menken, M. (1989) Consensus and controversy in neurologic practice: the case of steroid treatment in multiple sclerosis. *Arch. Neurol.* **46**, 322.
12. Oliveri, R. L., Valentino, P., Russo, C., Sibilia, G., Aguglia, U., Bono, F., Fera, F., Gambardella, A., Zappia, M., Pardatscher, K., and Quattrone, A. (1998) Randomized trial comparing two different high doses of methylprednisolone in multiple sclerosis. *Neurology*, **50**, 1833–1836.
13. IFNB Multiple Sclerosis Study Group. (1993) Interferon beta-1b is effective in relapsing-remitting multiple sclerosis. I. Clinical results of a multicenter, double-blind, placebo-controlled trial. *Neurology* **43**, 655–661.
14. IFNB Multiple Sclerosis Study Group, University of British Columbia MS/MRI Analysis Group. (1995) Interferon beta-1b in the treatment of multiple sclerosis: final outcome of the randomized controlled trial. *Neurology* **45**, 1277–1285.
15. Jacobs, L. D., Cookfair, D. L., Rudick, R. A., and Herndon, R. M. (1996) Intramuscular interferon Beta-1a for disease progression in relapsing multiple sclerosis. *Ann. Neurol.* **39**, 285–294.
16. Johnson, K. P., Brooks, B. R., Cohen, J. A., Ford, C. C., Goldstein, J., Lisak, R. P., Myers, L. W., Panitch, H. S., Rose, J. W., Schiffer, R. B., Vollmer, T., Weiner, L. P., Wolinsky, J. S., and Copolymer1 Multiple Sclerosis Study Group (1995) Copolymer 1 reduces relapse rate and improves disability in relapsing-remitting multiple sclerosis: results of a phase III multicenter, double-blind, placebo-controlled trial. *Neurology* **45**, 1268–1276.
17. Krupp, L. B., Coyle, P. K., Doscher, C., Miller, A., Cross, A. H., Jandorf, L., Halper, J., Johnson, B., Morgante, L., and Grimson, R. (1995) Fatigue therapy in multiple sclerosis: results of a double-blind, randomized, parallel trial of amantadine, pemoline and placebo. *Neurology* **45**, 1956–1961.
18. Weinshenker, B. G., Penman, M., Bass, B., Ebers, G. C., and Rice, G. P. A. (1992) A double-blind, randomized, crossover trial of pemoline in fatigue associated with multiple sclerosis. *Neurology* **42**, 1468–1471.
19. Nance, P. W., Sheremata, W., Lynch, S., Vollmer, T., Hudson, S., Francis G. S., O'Connor, P., Cohen J., Shapiro, R. T., Whitham, R., and Wolinsky, J. (1997) Relationship of the antispasticity effect of tizanidine to plasma concentration in patients with multiple sclerosis. *Arch. Neurol.* **54**, 731–736.
20. Young, R. R. (1994) Spasticity: a review. *Neurology* **44(suppl 9)**, S12–S20.
21. Coward, D. M. (1994) Tizanidine: neuropharmacology and mechanism of action. *Neurology* **44(suppl. 9)**, S6–S11.
22. Snow, B. J., Tsui, J. K. C., Bhatt, M. H., Varelas, M., Hashimoto, S. A., and Calne, D. B. (1990) Treatment of spasticity with botulinum toxin: A double-blind study. *Ann. Neurol.* **28** 512–515.

23. Coffey, R. J., Cahill, D., Steers, W., Park, T. S., Ordia, J., Meythaler, J., Herman, R., Shetter, A. G., Levy R., and Gill, B. (1993) Intrathecal baclofen for intractable spasticity of spinal origin: results of a long-term multicenter study. *J. Neurosurg.* **78**, 226–232.

24. Fowler, C. J. (1998) Bladder dysfunction in multiple sclerosis: causes and treatment. *Int. MSJ.* **1**, 99–107.

25. Moulin, D. E., Foley, K. M., and Ebers, G. C. (1988) Pain syndromes in multiple sclerosis. *Neurology* **38**, 1830–1834.

26. Sibley, W. A. (1996) Symptomatic treatments affecting spasticity, In: *Anonymous Therapeutic Claims in Multiple Sclerosis*, 4th ed. (Sibley, W. A., ed.) USA: Demos Vermande, New York, pp. 124.

27. Brown, P. (1994) Pathophysiology of spasticity. *J. Neurol Neurosurg. Psychiat.* **57**, 773–777.

28. Reynolds, J. R. (1890) Therapeutical uses and toxic effects of cannabis indica. *Lancet* **1**, 637–638.

29. Petro, D. J. and Ellenberger, C. (1981) Treatment of human spasticity with delta-9-tetrahydrocannabinol. *J. Clin. Pharmacol.* **21**, 413S–416S.

30. Meinck, H. M., Schonle, P. W., Conrad, B. (1989) Effect of cannabinoids on spasticity and ataxia in multiple sclerosis. *J. Neurol.* **236**, 120–122.

31. Ungerleider, J. T., Andrysiak, T., Fairbanks, L., Ellison, G. W., and Myers, L. W. (1987) Delta-9-THC in the treatment of spasticity associated with multiple sclerosis. *Ad. Alcohol Substance Abuse* **7**, 39–50.

32. Maurer, M., Henn, V., Dittrich, A., and Hofmann, A. (1990) Delta-9-tetrahydrocannabinol shows antispastic and analgesic effects in a single case double-blind trial. *Eur. Arch. Psychiatr. Neur. Sci.* **240**, 1–4.

33. Greenberg, H. S., Werness, A. S., Pugh, J. E., Andrus, R. O. Anderson, D. J., and Domino, E. F. (1994) Short-term effects of smoking marihuana on balance in patients with multiple sclerosis and normal volunteers. *Clin. Pharmacol. Ther.* **55**, 324–328.

34. Martyn, C. N., Illis, L. S., and Thorn, J. (1995) Nabilone in the treatment of multiple sclerosis. *Lancet* **315**, 579.

35. Consroe, P., Musty, R., Rein, J., Tillery, W., and Pertwee, R. (1997) The perceived effects of smoked cannabis on patients with multiple sclerosis. *Eur. Neurol.* **38**, 44–48.

36. Nance, P. W., Bugaresti, J., Shellenberger, K., Sheremata, W., Martinez-Arizala, A., and North American Tizandine Study Group. (1994) Efficacy and safety of tizanidine in the treatment of spasticity in patients with spinal cord injury. *Neurology* **44(suppl 9)** S44–S52.

37. Sabra, A. F., Hallett, M., Sudarsky, L., and Mullally, W. (1982) Treatment of action tremor in multiple sclerosis with isoniazid. *Neurology* **32**, 912–913.

38. Rice, G. P. A. and Ebers, G. C. (1995) Ondansetron for intractable vertigo complicating acute brainstem disorders. *Lancet* **345**, 1182–1183.

39. Duquette, P., Pleines, J., and du Souich, P. (1985) Isoniazid for tremor in multiple sclerosis: a controlled trial. *Neurology* **35**, 1772–1775.

40. Hallet, M., Lindsay, J. W., Adelstein, B. D., and Riley, P. O. (1985) Controlled trial of isoniazid therapy for severe postural cerebellar tremor in multiple sclerosis. *Neurology* **35**, 1374–1377.

41. Clifford, D. B. (1983) Tetrahydrocannabinol for tremor in multiple sclerosis. *Ann. Neurol.* **13**, 669–671.

42. Fernandez-Guardiola, A., Salgado, A., Contreras, C. M., Gonzalez-Estrada, T., Solis, H., Calvo, J. M., and Ayala, F. (1976) Multiunit activity and polygraphic recordings of the pharmacological effects of delta-9-tetrahydrocannabinol, In: *The Pharmacology of Marihuana* (Braude, M. C. and Szara, S., eds.) Raven, New York, pp. 335–43. Vol. 1.

43. Segal, M. (1978) The effect of SP-111, a water-soluble THC derivative, on neuronal activity in the rat brain. *Brain Res.* **139**, 263–.

44. Consroe, P., Snider, S. R. (1986) Therapeutic potential of cannabinoids in neurological disorders. In: *Cannabinoids as Therapeutic Agents* (Mechoulam, R., ed.), CRC, Boca Raton, FL, pp. 21–49.

55

Recreational and Medical Uses of Marihuana in Latin America

F. Raúl Jerí

Abstract

Cannabis was introduced to Latin America by the black slaves brought by the Spanish and Portuguese conquistadores. During four centuries its use was limited to particular areas and populations of Mexico, the Carribean, and Brazil. In the 1960s, an extensive epidemic of marihuana use spread from the United States to all Central and South American countries.

Although the harmful effects of excessive cannabis use has been known for over 2000 years, its psychotic disorders were only recently fully and scientifically documented. Medical uses of marihuana have not been very popular in Latin America in the past. Recently, small groups have demanded liberalization and legalization of the drug for recreational use, but not for therapeutic purposes.

1. INTRODUCTION

By the end of the 15th century, the Portuguese and Spanish conquistadors introduced cannabis to the New World through the slave trade. The portuguese had imported slaves from Africa to Europe since the year 1444. They established factories (trading ports) for that purpose on the coast of Guinea. Black slaves were imported in ever-increasing numbers into southern Portugal and neighboring Spanish regions, thus Seville became an important slave market.

During the "discovery" of America, Spaniards and Portuguese incorporated black slave labor. This occurred in large part because of the considerable mortality among the Arawack and other Caribbean Indians due to disease, overwork, and slaughter by the Europeans.

An early advocate for the American Indians, Bartolomé de las Casas (1517) sought permission from the Emperor Charles I for slaves to be brought from Africa to spare the Indians. The Africans would replace the Indians as the New World slaves. Consequently, Africans were introduced in great numbers to the Caribbean islands and later to South America. Similar events occurred in Brazil after the coast of that country fell under Portuguese domination.

From: *Marihuana and Medicine*
Edited by: G. G. Nahas et al.   © Humana Press Inc., Totowa, NJ

West African slaves brought *Cannabis* to those lands, and soon the practice of hemp smoking was incorporated into the rituals of some indigenous groups accustomed to smoking tobacco. Since then marihuana, named maconha by the natives, has been cultivated and used in recreational and religious activities by the Brazilian coastal inhabitants.

Jamaica, during Spanish and British domination, received many waves of "ebony pieces," and they also grew *Cannabis* in a soil well-suited for its cultivation. In 1840, indentured laborers from India were brought to the island. They introduced the practice of smoking "ganga," the Indian word for a marihuana preparation. In Mexico, *Cannabis* was grown immediately after the first foray of Hernan Cortez; Pedro Caudrado, one of the conquistadores, probably introduced the plant. It seems that the natives, already knowledgable about peyote, ololiuqui, and psilocbe, soon discovered the mind-altering properties of the transplanted herb. By 1550, an ordinance had been passed prohibiting the cultivation of *Cannabis*. This ordinance was not obeyed to the fullest extent *(1)*. During the ensuing four centuries, hemp smoking occurred commonly within very particular sectors of the general population of Mexico, Brazil, and the Caribbean. This began to change during the 19th century because of intellectual, economic, and social forces exerted from abroad. After Jacques Joseph Moreau popularized hashish eating in Paris during the 19th century, a Peruvian physician enthusiastically wrote that "medicine has today the glory to convert a pleasure instrument into a lever for health," and he recommended *Cannabis* for neuralgia, chorea, and cholera *(2)*. By the end of the 19th century the *Cannabis* plant was smoked extensively in Jamaica and Costa Rica by imported "coolies" working in the plantations and the railroads *(3)*. Marihuana was introduced to Colombia through the Atlantic ports in the 1920s, especially through Barranquilla. It was the marginalized classes, living and working around the docks, who began consuming *Cannabis*, usually by smoking it. The habit became so troublesome that laws prohibiting cultivation and use of cannbis *(4)* were passed in 1939 and 1946.

In Mexico, smoking marihuana was common during the 19th century. Pancho Villa, the famous revolutionary, forced his men to smoke *Cannabis* before combat so that they might go into battle without fearing death. However, at other times *Cannabis* was rigorously forbidden *(5)*. As is well-known, cannabis was introduced to the United States during the 1920s through the East Coast (from Jamaica), and the West Coast (from Mexico) *(6)*.

2. THE EPIDEMIC

During the first half of the 20th century, apart from marginalized groups, the larger Latin American populations did not consume marihuana. The intellectual and "Bohemian" figures such as the poet Porfirio Barba Jacob (1883–1942) were notable exceptions. Jacob, a heavy user of marihuana, possessed a complex personality and exhibited hypersexual, homosexual, hypomanic, and hyperkinetic tendencies. It was presumed that he used the drug as auto medication for his excessive activity *(7)*.

In Brazil, marihuana smoking, which was mainly restricted to the Northeast, suddenly increased enormously. Becoming prevalent in jails, bars, dancing halls, schools, and favelas, *Cannabis* abuse became a national scourge *(8)*.

The greatest increase of marihuana abuse occured during the 1960s, largely, due to the influence of the United States drug subculture. In recent years, research into marihuana use in Latin America has yielded interesting observations. For instance, in Argentina, marihuana emergencies had become common in general hospitals *(9)*. and *Cannabis* use sometimes precipitated asthma caused by *Aspergillus fumigatus* commonly found in marihuana cigarettes *(10)*.

In Bolivia, smoking coca paste is replacing marihuana smoking, but *Cannabis* is still used freely by a considerable number of the inhabitants in the country's three major cities *(11)*. In Brazil, it is said that prisoners with "abnormal personalities" abuse hashish very frequently, though researchers believe that familial, social, and economical factors were also considered important factors shaping patterns of cannabis abuse *(12)*. Marihuana abuse continues among many university students *(13)*. Smoking *Cannabis in* Colombia has been frequently associated with the ingestion of coca paste (bazuco), and the diverse symptoms of that dual chronic intoxication, described by us 20 years ago *(14)*, have since been confirmed in Caldas *(15)* and Medellin *(16)*. Yet, according to most surveys, marihuana abusers still outnumber coca paste smokers *(17)*.

Since 1968, Chile has also reported a massive increase in the consumption of hemp *(18,19)*. Notably, the frequent use of psychoactive drugs became slightly higher among affluent adolescents *(20)*. One investigator has claimed a significant increase in the number of adolescents who abused *Cannabis (2)*. In high schools, 38–60% of students of varying ages (and differing social strata) smoke marihuana *(22)*. Research done in three major cities of Ecuador revealed that of all the patients seen at special units for drug dependence, 49.3% were marihuana abusers *(23)*. Mexico has a chronic problem with production and abuse of *Cannabis* and opium. According to studies done in homes *(24)*. in schools, and in city sectors, marihuana is always the major drug of abuse *(25)*.

During the 1970s, marihuana was the main drug consumed in Lima, but in the decade that followed, investigators documented a rapid shift towards smoking coca paste among drug abusers. Significantly, two-thirds of these addicts first abused marihuana before trying the more potent, or "harder," drugs. Often drug abusers began ingesting drugs in a variety of combinations, since coca paste abusers, for example, experienced different physiological and psychological effects when they combined cocaine with tobacco or with cannabis *(28)*. When epidemiological investigations were done in cities of Peru, the evidence indicated that *Cannabis* continued to be the primary drug of substance abusers *(29)*, although coca paste became the drug of choice in later years. Likewise in the same period in Colombia, marihuana *(31)* increasingly gave way to coca paste (bazuco) as the drug of choice *(32)*. Elsewhere, *Cannabis* was the drug most seized by customs officers in Venezuela *(33)*. In other studies concentrating on a breakdown of drug preferences among specific age groups, researchers found that inhalants, such as glue, were popular among preadolescent drug abusers; adolescents preferred marihuana, cocaine, and bazuco *(34)*. Again, the "introductory" drug was marihuana *(35)*.

The use of cannabis has become widespread and endemic in Jamaica, especially in the lowest socioeconomic strata *(36)*. Interestingly, in the Bahamas, those deemed to be "delinquents" consumed marihuana seven times more than high school students of presumably good standing *(37)*.

In conclusion, it can be said that during the 1970s, marihuana consumption was extensive in Guatemala, Belize, Jamaica, Venezuela, Chile, Paraguay, Argentina, Brazil, and Mexico. Since 1974, coca paste smoking began to increase in Peru, Bolivia, and Colombia, gradually surpassing the use of marihuana in later years *(38)*. There appear to be contradictions existing in the literature considering the causes of *Cannabis* abuse. Some studies seem to suggest that the existing socioeconomic structures help predispose certain classes of people, usually the marginalized, to the abuse of *Cannabis* and other drugs, as seems to be the case in Venezuela and the Bahamas. Yet, that *Cannabis* abuse became so prevalent among university students and others who belong, ostensibly, to the better-placed strata of Latin American societies, indicates that structuralized inequities probably do not in themselves determine the causes and contours of illicit drug use throughout Latin America.

3. INTOXICATION

The harmful effects of excessive *Cannabis* use have been known for at least 2000 years *(39)*. In South America the toxicity of *Cannabis* has been related to dose,resin content, and various states of the substance's preservation and modes of preparation. Also, interplaying factors governing an individual's physical and psychological characteristics may predispose him or her to abnormal reactions, psychoses, and addiction when using the drug. Some users have developed schizophrenic disorders after abusing hemp *(8)*. In Bahia, abuse of hashish, which had often begun in a user's late childhood, was practiced mainly by people with one or more personality disorders, perhaps strongly conditioned by environmental factors. The addict's reactions seem to have been affected by the qualities of the ingested plant itself, as well as the method of smoking, not to mention the addict's own physical and mental condition at the time of his or her ingestion of the drug *(12)*.

In Peru, children and adolescents had been referred to psychiatric units for behavior disturbances, compulsive drug use, acute psychotic intoxications, anxiety attacks, and suicide attempts. All used marihuana by itself, or marihuana combined with LSD, or even with alcohol. The group as a whole suffered various behavioral disorders, and what was diagnosed as paranoid schizophrenia or paranoid psychoses *(26)*. Some years later, research on another group of drug abusers, in a military setting, showed that most were males (86%), young (79.7%) were 15–20 years, and most came from "stable" homes (94.9%). The great majority used marihuana (86%), alone or combined with other drugs *(27)*. Of 158 coca paste abusing patients, 75.3% began using drugs by experimenting with cannabis *(14)*. The literature reveals a number of striking parallels between North America and Latin America *vis-à-vis* marihuana abuse.

In New York, psychological disorders were also documented in children and adolescents soon after they used *Cannabis*. These disorders also included psychotic reactions *(40)*. In light of these observations, authorities proposed a new pharmacological classification of toxic drugs, based on a quantitative scale, since the evidence strongly suggested that marihuana could produce neurological, psychological, and somatic signs *(41)*. The mental state of psychotic men with high urinary cannabinoid levels indicated significantly more hypomania and agitation, and significant less affective flattening, incoherence of speech, and hysteria than did those diagnosed as classic schizophrenics *(42)*.

After one week, the group that had used *Cannabis* (presumably) before the onset of their symptoms, having abstained from use during hospitalization, showed marked improvement, particularly in the psychotic syndromes. Investigators came to the conclusion that a high intake of cannabis may be related to a rapidly resolving psychosis, manifesting marked hypomanic features, though often appearing as a schizophrenia-like illness *(42)*.

Research suggests that impairment of short-term memory and lingering deficit in psychomotor performance, are two of the acute *Cannabis* intoxication components that may have long-term consequences for users, because the first affects learning and the latter interferes a users ability to act and react as external stimuli will demand. For instance, a marihuana user will impair his or her ability to safely handle transport vehicles, industrial machinery, or precision instruments. The most frequently observed complication includes a short-term acute psychological disturbance with symptoms of panic, paranoid apprehension, and personality disorganization. The psychiatric consequences of chronic use have included residual cognitive deficit, lethargic symptoms, and *Cannabis* psychosis *(43)*.

Returning the focus to Latin America, one study has indicated that among 16,000 Ecuadorian out patients, marihuana abuse was second only to coca paste (bazuco), and it was believed responsible for 15.3% of cases of psychoses induced by drugs, as opposed to 4.2%

of alcohol-induced psychoses *(31)*. According to other researchers, it is the continuous ingestion of substantial amounts of *Cannabis* that increases the emergence of pathological changes caused by the accumulation of Δ⁹-tetrahydrocannabinol (THC) in the body. Tolerance and physical dependence, as well as the aforementioned effects of *Cannabis* abuse have all been observed. Extensive and chronic use of marihuana in the Caribbean, for example, is associated with undefined dysfunction and mental disorder in its users *(36)*.

Experienced marihuana smokers who participated in experimental sessions in which they smoked only one or two cigarettes containing 2.57% THC, at different times, showed slightly impaired performance in a circular lights task in all subjects. Performance was also impaired (decreased accuracy and increased response time) on serial addition, substraction, and digital recall tasks. These results forcefully suggest that *Cannabis* adversely affects complex human performance up to 24 hours after its ingestion by smoking *(44)*.

Elsewhere, researchers found that in group of 100 young Venezuelan addicts (less then 26 years old), all started drug use with marihuana before age 16; interestingly, from a sociological perspective, most of the addicts had little education. They were "unstable" at work, and though they had extensive experience operating various types of motor vehicles, these same individuals evinced difficulties maintaining control while driving *(35)*. These patients with psychotic symptoms, and *Cannabis*-positive urine analysis, were mostly single, poorly educated, and had histories of psychotic episodes. They were more often male, Afro-Caribbean, with histories of criminal convictions, and compulsory hospital admissions. The most common initial diagnosis was schizophrenia. A short-lived psychotic episode followed by a clearing consciousness was observed after *Cannabis* intoxication, but chronic *Cannabis* use that induced psychosis was not found in this group of 61 subjects *(45)*.

In yet another study, acute marihuana administration (2 mg THC intravenous) produced in 11 of 19 subjects a pleasant experience; 4 reported minimal effects, but 3 became extremely anxious and paranoid. There was consistent increase in cerebellar metabolism, which correlated with the plasma concentration of THC. Marihuana abusers showed less of a cerebellar response upon THC administration, but they also demonstrated increased metabolic activity in the prefrontal cortex after ingesting the THC. In this way, the study suggests that chronic marihuana affects brain functions. It is well known that the cerebellum is related to motor coordination, perception, and learning *(46)*.

The results of a number of studies on *Cannabis* abuse abroad compare favorably with those done in Latin America. In Morocco, 104 male patients admitted to a psychiatric ward were found to have smoked cannabis before their hospitalization. Of those, 44 suffered from a progressive and structured psychopathology, from schizophrenic-like symptoms to paranoid psychosis, lasting 14 days to 7 months. Sixty patients evinced acute undifferentiated psychiatric symptoms, mostly "acute toxic psychosis," which lasted less than two weeks *(47)*. In Northern Europe, more than 50,000 Swedish conscripts were followed up in the national register for psychiatric care. The relative risk of developing schizophrenia was six times greater among high consumers of *Cannabis* (more than 50 occasions) compared to nonusers. According to the author of this study, the evidence suggests a causal relationship between *Cannabis* abuse and schizophrenia. In other words, *Cannabis* may trigger schizophrenia in certain individuals *(48)*. In Amsterdam, schizophrenic patients who abused marihuana were compared with schizophrenic patients who did not use it. Results showed significantly more and earlier psychotic relapses in the *Cannabis*-abusing group. The researchers concluded that *Cannabis* abuse, and particularly heavy abuse, might be a stress that elicits relapses in patients with schizophrenia and related disorders *(49)*.

Next to tobacco and alcohol, *Cannabis* and cocaine are often the substances readily abused by schizophrenic individuals. The prevalence of marihuana abuse is probably caused by a number of environmental conditions impacting upon the innate physiological traits that are specific to its users. If researchers have not reached a clear consensus on why schizophrenic individuals abuse *Cannabis*, and other drugs, they are far more certain about how marihuana and cocaine actually act upon their users. Cocaine and *Cannabis* stimulate the dopaminergic activity of the brain, whereas *Cannabis* also decreases central acetylcholine turnover. These latter drugs increase the frequency and intensity of the psychophysiological symptoms. Therefore, the psychiatric patient with a history of *Cannabis* abuse often requires more therapeutic interventions, responds less well to antipsychotics, but becomes less lethargic and anhedonic, increasing his or her motivation to abuse drugs *(50)*.

4. THE MEDICINE

The oldest known therapeutic description of the plant was recorded in China, ca. 2000 B.C.. He prescribed cannabis for beri-beri, constipation, "female weakness," gout, malaria, and absent mindedness. In Egypt 2000 B.C., *Cannabis* was used for "eye problems," perhaps glaucoma. In India, prior to the 10th century B.C., *Cannabis* was used as an anesthetic and antiphlegmatic. The religious use of *Cannabis* in India is thought to have preceded its medical use; *Cannabis* users believed that the drug freed the mind from worldy distractions so that one could concentrate his or her thoughts on the Supreme Being *(51)*. The hemp plant was mentioned in the *Athavaveda* as a protector. It was thought that the plant could protect all animals and properties. Indra gave the *Cannabis* deity 1000 eyes and conferred upon it the property of driving away all diseases and killing all monsters. *Cannabis* users praised marihuana as the best of medicines, often wearing a segment of the plant as a precious talisman. Its effects on humans were described as excitant, warming. It was also astringent. *Cannabis* was said to destroy phlegm, expel flatulence, induce costivness, sharpen the memory, and stimulate the appetites. However, warnings about its damaging effects after prolonged use were recorded.

In the fifth chapter of Menu, a prohibition appears that suggests sociological implications: Brahmins are prohibited from using *Cannabis*. According to colonial British physicians in later centuries, *Cannabis* remained one of the curses of India: "if its use is persisted in, it leads to indigestion, wasting of the body, cough, melancholy, impotence, and dropsy. After a time the user becomes an outcast from society, and his career terminates in crime, insanity, and idiocy"*(39)*. Nevertheless, it remained one of the important drugs in the *Indian Materia Medica* from the XVIII century until 1945. *Cannabis* was widely used in the rural areas for asthma and bronchitis *(51)*. For millennia in India, *Cannabis* has been cited as a medicine for almost any ailment: to ameliorate catarrh, to relieve hemorrhoids, gonorrhea, asthma, "stitches on the side," and diarrhea. It was cited as aphrodisiac, and in Persia, a remedy for strangulated hernia.

During the Europe's age of empire, French and British doctors used hemp to treat tetanus, hydrophobia, neuralgia, neuritis, migraine, locomotor ataxia, gout, and epilepsy "due to organic nerve centre lesions." However in tonic spasms, such as torticollis, "writers-cramp," chorea, genuine epilepsy, paralysis agitans, trismus, tetanus, and the spastic movements caused by spinal lesions, *Cannabis* proved absolutely useless *(39)*. As already mentioned, in Peru, *Cannabis* was for a time recommended as a remedy for neuralgia, chorea, and cholera *(2)*. As most of these medical applications were proved false under scientific scrutiny, *Cannabis sativa* gradually disappeared from the text books of materia medica, pharmacology, and therapeutics *(5)*.

Be this as it may, throughout the world individuals continue to use marihuana as an "alternative" medication for anxiety, depression, schizophrenia, and personality disorder, as well as for problems in marriage, family, work, and the stress of life in prison. In many forums and television talk shows throughout Latin America, young people and addicts demand the legalization of marihuana for recreational use. Yet, in contrast to the United States and Europe, few in Latin America advocate dispensing *Cannabis* as a treatment for glaucoma, nausea caused by cancer chemotherapy, wasting as a result the acquired immunodeficiency disease (AIDS), or muscle spasms.

REFERENCES

1. Ardila, F. Aspectos médicolegales y médicosociales de la marihuana. Tesis de Doctorado, Madrid, 1965.
2. Corpancho, M. N. (1856) Fantasía Poética producida por hashish. *Gacet. Med. Lima* **1**, 2–4.
3. Stewart, W. Keith and Costa Rica, Univ. New Mexico Press, Albuquerque, 1964.
4. Reales, E. Marihuana, en Memorias del Primer Seminario de Actualización en Prevención de Drogadicción. Vol. 4, *Drogas de Abuso.* pp. 41–47, CEDA (Colombia), 1989.
5. Zapata, V. Farmacología y sus aplicaciones en Terapéutica, 2da. Edición, pp 102–105, Talleres S. Valverde, Lima, 1960.
6. Nahas, GG. (1992) *Keep off the Grass*, Pergamon Press, Eriksson, VT.
7. Roselli, H. (1986) Barba-Jacob y la historia de la marihuana. *Acta Psiquiat Psicol. Am. Lat.* **32**, 259–270.
8. Pacheco, E., Silva, A. C. (1959) Intoxicación crónica en América Latina. *Rev. Psiquiat. Peruan.* **2**, 159–181.
9. Miguez, H. A. and Grinson, R. W. (1989) Consultas por abuso de substancias psicoactivas en Hospitales de Buenos Aires. *Bol. Of. Sanit Panamer.* **107**, 296–306.
10. Portes, R. Marihuana y Asma. (1990) *Arch. Argent. Alergia Inmunol. Clin.* **21**, 136–139.
11. De la Quintana, M. Situación nacional de la fármacodependencia en Bolivia y los problemas derivados de la misma. Grupo Consult. En Farmacodepend; Convenio H. Unanue, pp. 1–38, Quito, 1986.
12. Pires de Veiga, E. and Rabin do Pinho, A. (1962) Contribucao ao estado do maconhismo na Bahia. *Neurologia* **25**, 38–68.
13. Magalhaes, M. P., Silva, R. Oliviera, R. (1989) Padroes de frequencia do uso de maconha por estudantes universitarios. *Revista ABP-APAL* **11**, 35–40.
14. Jerí, F. R., Sánchez, C. C., Del Pozo, T. and Fernández, M. (1978) El sindrome de la pasta de coca. Observaciones en un group de 158 pacientes del área de Lima. *Rev. Sanid. Minist. Int.* **39**, 1–18.
15. Verhelst, R., Amesquita, M. E., Giraldo, L. (1983) Observaciones y medidas preventivas sobre los síntomas producidos por fumar pasta de coca. *Med. Caldas* **5**, 251–260.
16. Velásquez, E., Torres, Y., Sánchez, M. M., et al. (1985) Estudio epidemiológico de uso de drogas en la población general de Medellín. *Rev. Colomb. Psiquiat.* **14**, 116–153.
17. Torres, Y. and Murelle, L. (1989) Consumo de substancias que producen dependencia en Colombia. *Bol. Ofic. Sanit. Panamer.* **107**, 485–494.
18. Richard, P. El consumo de marihuana. Un problema social en Chile. Inst. Social, Univ. Católica, Chile, Santiago, 1971.
19. Florenzano, R., Madrid, V., Martini, A. M. (1981) Prevalencia y características del consumo de algunas sustancias químicas en estudiantes de enseñanza media en Santiago. *Rev. Med. Chile* **109**, 1051–1059.
20. Maddaleno, M., Florenzano, R., Alvo, D. (1987) Estructura de movilidad de adolescentes consultantes en el sector Oriente de Santiago. *Rev. Chilen. Pediat.* **58**, 164–168.
21. Murillo, G. A. (1988) Consideraciones antropológicas acerca del uso de drogas en el adolescente chileno. *Rev. Psiquiat. Hosp. Horwitz* **5**, 13–17.
22. Florenzano, R. (1989) Alcoholismo y abuso de otras drogas. Programa de prevención en Santiago. *Biol. Ofic. Sanit. Panamer.* **107**, 577–589.
23. Samaniego, N. Desarrollo de los Programas de atención de f#aarmacodependientes en el Ecuador. *Grupo Consult. Farmacodepend. Conv. H. Unanue*, Quito, 1986; pp. 1–16.
24. Medina, M. E., Tapia, C. R., Rascon, M. L., et al. (1989) Situación epidemiológica del abuso de drogas en México. *Bol. Of. Sanit. Panamer.* **107**, 475–484.
25. Ortiz, A. (1989) Desarrollo del sistema de registro de información sobre drogas en México. *Bol. Ofic. Sanit. Panamer.* **107**, 523–530.
26. Jerí, F. R., Carbajal, C. and Sánchez, C. C. (1971) Uso de drogas por adolescentes y escolares. *Rev. Neuropsiquiat.* **34**, 243–273.
27. Jerí, F. R., Sánchez, C. C., and Del Pozo, C. C., (1976) Consumo de drogas peligrosas por miembros y familiares de la Fuerza Armada y de la Fuerza Policial Peruana. *Rev. Sanid. Minist. Int.* **37**, 104–112.
28. Del Pozo, C. C., (1987) Pasta de coca. Efectos de la mezcla de pasta de coca con tabaco y de pasta de coca con marihuana. *Rev. Sanid. Fuerz. Polic.* **48**, 138–141.

29. Jutkowitz, J. M., Arellano, R., Castro, R., et al. Uso y abuso de drogas en el Perú. *Tall. Graf.* Tarea, Lima, 1987.
30. Ferrando, D. Uso de drogas en las ciudades del Perú. *Encuesta en hogares*, Cedro, Lima, 1990.
31. Olivares, A. Informe de Colombia, Consejo Consult. *Farmacodepend. Conv. H. Unanue*, Quito, 1986, pp. 1–6.
32. 1997 Centro de Estudios de la Fundación Santa Fé de Bogotá: II Estudio de consumo de substancias psicoactivas en Colombia. *Coloquio* **5**, 31–47.
33. Roge, R. A. (1986) Informe de la República de Venezuela. *Reun Grupo Consult. Farmacodep. Conv. Unanue*, Quito, 1986, pp. 1–23.
34. Kramer, S. II National Survey on Drug Abuse among high school students in Venezuela. *Epidem. Trends Drug Abuse.* pp II (68–74), June 1990, NIDA, Rockville.
35. Hueso, H., Lara, E. and Cuervo, F. (1991) Estudio exploratorio de 100 pacientes fármacodependientes. *Arch. Venez. Psiquiat. Neurol.* **37**, 15–20
36. Wray, S. R. and Murthy, N. V. A. (1989) Review of the effects of cannabis on mental and physiological functions. *West Ind. Med. J.* **36**, 195–268
37. Smart, R and Patterson, S. D. (1989) Comparación del abuso de alcohol, tabaco y drogas entre estudiantes y delincuentes en las Bahamas. *Bol. Ofic. Sanit. Panamer.* **107**, 514–522.
38. Florenzano. R. (1986) Uso de drogas en América Latina y en el Caribe. *Bolet. Vigilancia Epidemiol de Chile* **13**, 266–273.
39. Dymock, W., Warden, C. J. H. and Hooper, D. (1893) *Pharmagraphia Indica.* Vol III Kegan Ltd; London, 1893, pp. 318–337
40. Milman, D. Effect on children and adolescents of mind altering drugs with special reference to cannabis. In, Drug Abuse in the Modern World (ed. Nahas, G.), Pergamon Press, New York, 1981, pp 47–56
41. Nahas, G. G. (1981) Clasificaión farmacológica de las drogas toxicomanígenas. *Bol. Estuperfac.* **33** 1–20.
42. Rottamburg, D., Robins, AH., Ben-Arie, O., et al. (1982) Cannabis associated psychosis with hypomanic features. *Lancet* **2**, 1364–1366.
43. Negrete, J. C. Efectos del canabismo sobre la salud. (1983) *Acta Psiquiat. Psicol. Amer. Lat.* **29**,
44. Heishman, S. J., Huestis, M. A., Hennielfield, J. E., et al (1990). Acute and residual effects of marihuana. Profiles of plasma THC levels. Physiological, subjective and performance measures. *Pharmacol. Biochem. Behav.* **37**, 561–565
45. Mathers, D. C. and Ghodse, A. M. (1992) Cannabis and psychotic illness. *Br. J. Psychiat.* **161**, 648–653.
46. Volkow, N. D. and Fowler, J. S. (1993) Use of position tomography to study drugs of abuse. In: *Cannabis* (Nahas, GG and Latour, C, eds), CRS Press, Boca Raton, FL 1993, pp. 21–43.
47. Chkili, T. and Ktiouet, J. E. (1993) *Prospective study of 104 psychiatric cases associated with cannabis use in a Moroccan medical center. In:* Cannabis (Nahas, GG and Latour, C eds), CRC Press, Boca Raton, Fl, pp. 101–104.
48. Allebek, S. (1993) Schizophrenia and cannabis: cause-effect relationship? In: *Cannabis* (Nahas, GG and Latour, C, eds), CRS Press, Boca Raton, FL, pp. 113–117.
49. Linszen, D. H., Dingemans, P. H. and Lenior, M. E. (1994). Cannabis abuse and the cause of recent onset schizophrenic disorders. *Arch. Gen. Psychiat.* **51**, 273–279.
50. Negrete, J. (1994) Cannabinisme et cocainisme chez le schizophrene. Aspects cliniques et physiopathologiques, in III eme Colloque *Scientifique International sur les drogues illectes*, Mairie de Paris, pp. 91–98.
51. Pradhan, S. N. (1977) Marijuana, In: *Drug Abuse.* Mosby, St, Louis, Mo, pp. 148–149.

VIII MARIHUANA AND PSYCHIATRY

56

The Neuropsychiatric Syndrome of Δ^9-Tetrahydrocannabinol and *Cannabis* Intoxication in Naive Subjects

A Clinical and Polygraphic Study During Wakefulness and Sleep

C. A. Tassinari, G. Ambrosetto, M. R. Peraita-Adrado, and H. Gastaut

Abstract

Summing up our study in naive subjects, we can draw two main conclusions. First, heavy (0.7–1 mg/kg) single oral doses of Δ^9-THC in alcohol or in oily solution lead to effects similar to oral doses of hashish containing a similar amount of Δ^9-THC; in both cases a severe intoxication occurs with a typical psychic and neurological (abnormal movements and hyperflexial) syndrome. Second, Δ^9-THC intoxication is also responsible for significant changes in nocturnal sleep with disappearance of REM stages and a decrease of slow sleep.

When comparing the dramatic effects observed in our naive subjects and the effects observed with similar heavy doses of cannabis in chronic users one should admit that tolerance is likely to be the main factor responsible for such extreme differences.

1. INTRODUCTION

We began a series of studies on the effect of marihuana in humans in 1969. Our approach consisted of three stages.

At first, we studied the effect of usual doses taken by inhalation and corresponding to the effect of 2–10 mg of Δ^9-tetrahydrocannabinol (THC). The results of this study have been partially published *(1,2)*.

In a second series we undertook the study of the effect of higher doses of hashish or oily solution of Δ^9-THC given orally in doses corresponding to 10–40 mg of Δ^9-THC *(3,4)*.

From: *Marihuana and Medicine*
Edited by: G. G. Nahas et al.   © Humana Press Inc., Totowa, NJ

In this work, we report the findings of a third series of experiments focused on the effect of a heavy single dose of Δ^9-THC or hashish given to naive subjects. At the doses used, both the Δ^9-THC and the hashish were found responsible for an intoxication leading to a quite uniform and constant neuropsychiatric syndrome, which will be described from the neurological and neurophysiological point of view.

2. MATERIALS AND METHODS

2.1. Group A: Subjects and Doses

Seven young volunteers (21–25 years old) were given one single oral dose of Δ^9-THC, in alcoholic solution; the doses varied from 0.7 to 1 mg of Δ^9-THC/kg. The subjects were university students who had never before used *Cannabis* or other psychoactive drugs.

2.2. Group B: Subjects and Doses

Group B was composed of four young subjects (21–25 years old) of which two received 10 g of hashish given in cachets taken orally. The doses corresponded to 1 and 1.4 mg/kg.

Two other subjects received 0.7 and 0.9 mg/kg oral doses of Δ^9-THC in oily solutions.

The subjects, usually lying or sitting in bed, were under direct clinical control and observed on a closed-circuit TV system with tape recorder. The recording apparatus was in an adjacent room. The electroencephalogram (EEG) was taken by the conventional technique, the head electrodes being fixed by collodion, and placed according to a 10–20 system. The effects of intermittent light stimuli, acoustic stimuli, and hyperventilation were studied at various intervals before, during, and after Δ^9-THC intoxication.

Electromyograms (EMG) of different muscles were taken by surface electrodes. The horizontal oculogram, the electromyogram of the mylohyoid muscle, respiratory movements, and the electrocardiogram (EKG) were constantly monitored. A full neurological examination was carried out at different periods of the experiment (before, during, and after Δ^9-THC intoxication). The EMG of the right quadriceps was usually monitored in order to quantify the amplitude of the patellar reflexes, and arterial pressure was measured at various intervals.

The different parameters were recorded on a polygraph and on an FM 1300 Ampex tape recorder for subsequent analysis (average evoked potentials; quantification of the EEG and EMG responses).

2.3. Polygraphic Recordings

Polygraphic recordings of the subjects of group A started at 3:00 to 5:00 PM and the Δ^9-THC was given in the evening between 7:00 and 9:00 PM. The subjects subsequently lay or sat in bed, free to do what they liked (read, turn the light on or off, steep, listen to music, drink [water], etc.). The recording was continued until 7:00 AM of the following day. The subjects were under medical observation in the hospital or at home for the subsequent two days.

Recordings of the subjects of group B started at noon, and the hashish or Δ^9-THC in oily solution was given between 3:00 and 5:00 PM.

2.4. Sleep Recordings

The seven subjects of group A slept in the laboratory for a total of 26 nights. Ten nights served as a control before Δ^9-THC absorption (four subjects for one night, three subjects for two nights each; all subjects had previously slept in the laboratory in order to exclude the "first night effect;" three subjects received a placebo). The subjects slept in the laboratory for the seven nights of the same day during which they received the Δ^9-THC. Four subjects were recorded for the nine nights immediately after Δ^9-THC ingestion (three subjects slept two consecutive nights and one subject slept three consecutive nights). The three remaining subjects were not available for the night studies after Δ^9-THC ingestion because of their lack of cooperation.

3. RESULTS: THE NEUROPSYCHIATRIC SYNDROME

3.1. Group A

The seven naive subjects (group A) who received one single oral dose of 0.7–1 mg/kg of Δ^9-THC in an alcohol solution all presented a neuropsychiatric syndrome that included as constant symptoms severe psychic disturbances and a progressively increasing lowering of the level of vigilance leading to sleep. Frequent but not constant associated symptoms were the appearance of a neurological syndrome characterized by abnormal movements and increased deep tendon reflexes.

The symptoms appeared at a variable delay after Δ^9-THC ingestion but in a quite constant sequence, after the appearance first of tachycardia. The psychic disturbances appeared first, followed by the neurological symptoms with abnormal movements, and then by episodes of drowsiness leading to sleep.

3.1.1. PSYCHIC SYMPTOMS

In all cases these were the first clinical manifestations. In three cases there was a sudden modification of mood, with dysphoria and bursts of spontaneous laughter appearing after a delay of 30 to 45 minutes after Δ^9-THC ingestion; in two cases anxiety was the first clinical symptom, appearing 30 minutes and one hour after Δ^9-THC ingestion.

A full description of the psychic symptoms would be too lengthy to include here. We will stress only the following effects:

1. Psychic symptoms lasted from one to three hours and in our clinical setting, usually ended with sleep onset.
2. Onset of the dysphoric symptoms, and to some extent their intensity, seemed very much triggered by and related to the environment, the symptoms appearing or increasing with the presence of the examiner, during tests, and so on.
3. Dysphoria usually was the predominant symptom during the first hour. Anxiety subsequently became the most distressing one, requiring the continuous assistance by doctors and better still by reassuring friends.
4. Consciousness was never affected, even when anxiety, visual imagery, and paresthesias were at their height. No hallucinations were reported.
5. Anxiety and mood changes, often with rapid transition from laughter to crying, were extremely important and quite unpredictable. They usually prevented getting full cooperation from the subjects who, however, never become aggressive or violent, even when repeatedly requesting a stop to the experience.

Anxiety and panicky reactions were observed in all subjects but became the most striking features in two cases who both tried to escape from the laboratory. One subject described below succeeded.

A 22-year-old student had 0.9 mg/kg of Δ^9-THC at 8:00 PM; 45 minutes later he reported pleasant visual imageries (colored pictures in fast succession). He had slight temporal disorientation. Suddenly, at 9:30 PM. while performing on request a Valsalva maneuver, he tore off the electrodes from his scalp, got out of bed, and apparently calmly announced his *definite intention to stop the study. He approached the laboratory door and suddenly started to run out of the lab, vainly pursued throughout the garden (150 m), to reach the main street, where, naked, he kept running (100 m), shouting "help, I have been drugged" and trying to stop the oncoming cars. Then back in the lab, he could not lay in bed, was extremely agitated and anxious ("what has been done to me?" "will I recover"?). Heart rate was 162. This unpleasant situation lasted more than one hour and progressively the subject fell asleep.*

In the morning, he remembered correctly the events but did not recognize some people who had participated in his pursuit and capture. He could recall that when he tore off the electrodes he had most unpleasant imageries of "burned and hacked people" and himself was feeling "burning and electric discharges" all over.

In addition to mood changes and anxiety, the subjects reported various associations of pleasant (in two cases) or unpleasant (two cases) visual imageries, as well as paresthesias and burning sensations predominant over the extremities or around the point of attachment of the electrodes; three subjects had a sensation of cold and one subject of heat. Two subjects reported "having hands that were transparent" and "not feeling any more my eyes and tongue." Four cases reported "heart palpitation or irregularity in the heart rate," a feeling which was in two subjects a source of severe anxiety ("Is it [the heart] going to stop?").

Systematic testing of psychomotor performances could not be carried out because of the impossibility of obtaining reliable and continuous cooperation from the subjects during the height of the intoxication. Some tests (illustrated in Figs. 1A and b, and 2A, B, and C) showed a clear-cut deterioration of performance.

One subject, in the evening of the following day, experienced for approximately one hour an intense feeling of anxiety, and complained that the "effects were back again." There was slight tachycardia, no conjunctival hyperemia, and the neurological examination was normal. After adequate reassurance from the doctor, the subject progressively returned to normal; he refused, however, to sleep in the laboratory.

3.1.2 Neurological Symptomatology–Abnormal Movements and Hyperflexia

The abnormal movements appeared in four subjects after a delay of from 50 minutes to two hour (Figs. 3 and 6, below). The movements varied in different subjects and from moment to moment in the same subject.

Clinically, they consisted of shivering and tremor-like movements associated with variable hypertonia and myoclonias.

The electromyographic patterns of these abnormal movements could vary from time to time in the same subject and could not be corrected with any of the best known abnormal movement patterns observed, for example, in extrapyramidal disorders. They can, however, be described as consisting mainly of two types.

The first is irregular tonic activity with superimposed rhythmic bursts of synchronous potentials usually of 2 to 4 cps (but at times up to 6 cps), clinically corresponding to a resting irregular tremor. The bursts could involve both antagonist and agonist muscle effect or only one of these. The movements were more frequent on the upper extremities where they could be continuous for minutes.

The second is myoclonias, consisting of brief (100–200 msec) phasic potentials of various (100–200 pV but at times up to 700 pV) amplitude, at times synchronous over different muscles, at times and most often asynchronous and arhythmic. The myoclonias were responsible for clinical manifestations of various intensity, from subclinical twitches to evident jerks (Fig. 4).

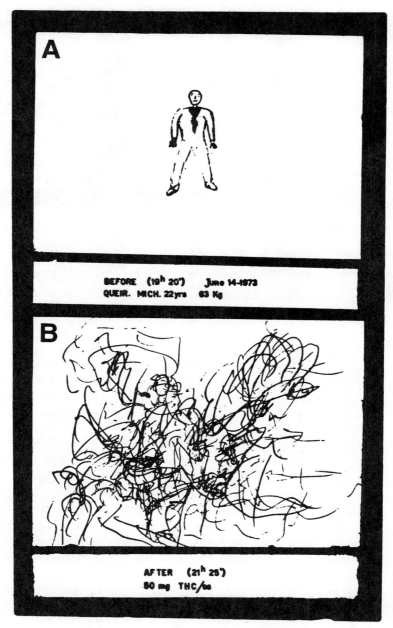

Fig. 1. Drawing of a man: before, during, and after Δ^9-THC intoxication.

The abnormal movements were most evident at rest, but could persist during voluntary movements of mild intensity. The duration of the abnormal movements varied from 45 minutes to two hours and decreased progressively in number and intensity with the gradual appearance of drowsiness; the abnormal movements disappeared during sleep.

Startle-like reactions, occurring apparently spontaneously, were observed during wakefulness in four subjects, during the periods when the abnormal were present. In four subjects unexpected visual and auditory stimuli were given in order to test the startle responses; these

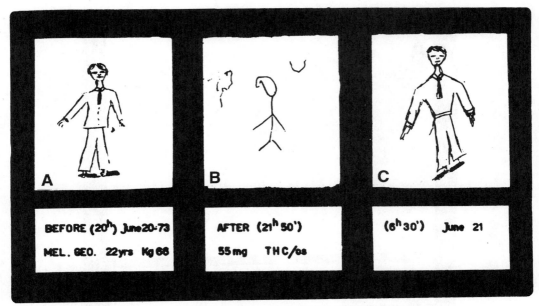

Fig. 2. Drawing of a man: before, during, and after Δ^9-THC intoxication.

were similar to those evoked before Δ^9-THC ingestion. Two cases, however, had repeated startle response on light, unexpected tactile contacts during the neurological examination.

Increased deep tendon reflexes under the influence of Δ^9-THC was a clear-cut finding in five out of seven subjects. Four of these five subjects were also those who had abnormal movements.

Increased tendon reflexes had a similar evolution as the abnormal movements and the hyperflexia, which varied widely from time to time in the same subjects, often in relation to variations in the vigilance leading to sleep (Fig. 3).

We did not observe any other neurological abnormalities during Δ^9-THC intoxication. Polysynaptic reflexes (abdominal, plantar) were unchanged as well as the blinking reflex by corneal stimulation. There was no nystagmus or ataxia (as we have reported previously, a subject could run, and quickly too, at the height of the drug effect). Strength was normal. Voluntary movements were also normal except in one case, where clear-cut tremors at rest persisted during voluntary movements.

Pupil size did not change significantly. Reaction to light was normal in all cases, except in one that showed intermittent hyppus (Fig. 3). Conjunctival hyperhernia was a constant finding.

Drowsiness and sleep were manifestations appearing in all subjects two to three hours after Δ^9-THC ingestion. If the subjects were not allowed to sleep and were kept aroused by testing, they became incoherent and finally went to sleep anyway.

The episodes of drowsiness, whether occurring in the afternoon or leading to nocturnal sleep onset, showed on the EEG the usual transitions in stages I and II of sleep as under normal conditions (see below).

3.1.3 POLYGRAPHIC DATA

On visual inspection, the EEGs during Δ^9-THC intoxication were quite similar to those before intoxication.

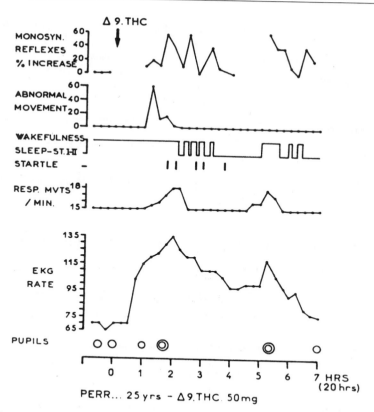

Fig. 3. Evolution of various physiological parameters after an oral dose of 0.7 mg/kg of Δ^9-THC in alcohol solution (group A). There is at first a progressive appearance of abnormal movements (arbitrary units), increased tendon reflex, and later episodes of drowsiness leading to stages I and II sleep. In this particular case, there was some increase in respiratory movements. Note the disappearance of abnormal movements with sleep onset and the variability of deep tendon reflexes in relation to changes from wakefulness to sleep. Startle indicates occurrence of apparently spontaneous startle responses. Pupil size, usually not modified, showed transient mydriasis and hyppus in this particular case.

Alpha activity was always present, four cases showing a slight amplitude increase and decrease in frequency of 1/2 cps. Reactivity of the alpha to eye opening was unchanged except in two cases, which showed a poor reactivity or a persistence of the alpha activity with the eyes opened. The subjects were at that time very drowsy.

Physiological posterior slow waves, lambda waves, and fast activity over the anterior head region, when present, did not show any significant change at any time after Δ^9-THC intoxication.

The responses to intermittent light stimulation and to hyperventilation were not modified by Δ^9-THC ingestion.

It should be noted that one of our normal subjects had in the control EEG diffuse, isolated, medium voltage slow waves with a sharp component that were either not modified or at time slightly more frequent after Δ^9-THC ingestion (Fig. 10 below).

Visual-evoked responses in three subjects showed an increased amplitude and slowing of the late after-discharge when the eyes were closed (two to four hours after Δ^9-THC).

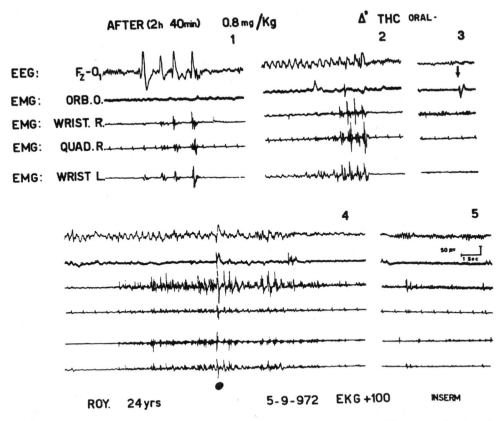

Fig. 4. Abnormal movements after Δ^9-THC (group A). 1 and 2: Repeated diffuse myoclonias of various intensity involving almost simultaneously the extensor of the right and left wrist and the right quadriceps. 3: An unexpected noise (arrow) evokes only physiological blinking recorded on the orbicularis oculi. 4: Prolonged bursts of myoclonias, asynchronous and arhythmic, over different muscles. The dot indicates a spontaneous startle-like reaction. 5: Note the normal posterior background activity on the EEG. In the other sequences from 1 to 4, different movement artifacts document the presence of head involuntary movements due to myoclonias of the neck muscles.

In four subjects the average of the visual-evoked responses and in all subjects the average of the somesthetic potential subsequent to median nerve electric stimulation could not be evaluated because of the lack of cooperation of the subjects under the influence of Δ^9-THC.

An increased EKG rate, as is well known, was the first (delay between 20 and 30 minutes) and constant modification signaling the onset of the drug effects. Maximal mean increase was observed between one and two hours. Maximal increase occurred in two subjects.(who were given 0.9 and 1 mg/kg of Δ^9-THC, respectively), who had severe panicky reactions (beats/minute increased from 72 to 90 in the control period up to a miximum of 156 and 168, respectively, during Δ^9-THC intoxication).

Respiratory movements did not change significantly in frequency except in one case, in which an increase was observed.

The electrodermogram, measured as the Tarchanoff effect, was not significantly modified after Δ^9-THC ingestion in the two cases in which quantification of the phenomena was possi-

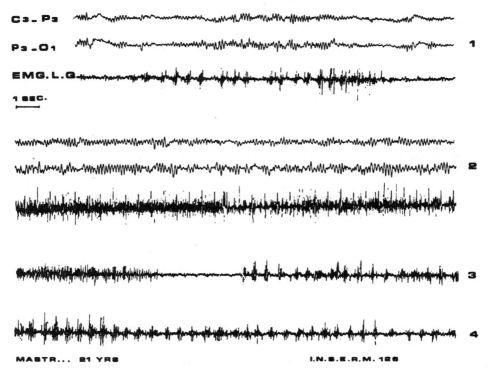

C3 - P3

P3 - O1   **1**

EMG. L.Q.

1 SEC.

2

3

4

MASTR... 21 YRS   **I.N.S.E.R.M. 126**

Fig. 5. Abnormal movements after hashish. Subject from group B, four hours after a 1.4 mg/kg oral dose of hashish. 1 and 2: EEG (C3-P3; P3-01) and electromyogram of the left quadriceps (L.Q.). Burst of grouped potential at 2–3 cps is a tremor-like phenomena, which became associated in two with irregular tonic activity. 3 and 4: EMG of the L.Q. showing prolonged tremor-like activity. Strips 2,3, and 4 are continuous. Note the normal EEG.

ble. Taansient orthostatic hypotension occurred in two subjects three and five hours after receiving Δ^9-THC, leading to transient loss of consciousness in one subject.

3.1.4. SLEEP AFTER Δ^9-THC INTOXICATION

The results of the sleep study are summariezed in the histograms (Fig.8) and in Fig. 9.

From these data, it can be concluded that a single oral dose of Δ^9-THC, given between 5:00 and 8:00 PM, is responsible for every significant modification of sleep organization and percntage of stages.

Two findings stand out as being the most significant: a complete or almost complete suppression of REM sleep and an increase of stage II sleep (from 59 to 83%), with a decrease of slow (stages III to IV) sleep.

3.2 Group B: Hashish and Δ^9-THC (in Oily Solution) Intoxication

Hashish in a single oral dose (10 mg) was given to two subjects, one naive and the other a marihuana smoker for two years (one or two joints every week). The corresponding doses of Δ^9-THC were 1 mg/kg for the naive subject and 1.4 mg/kg for the marihuana smoker.

After a delay of 60 to 80 minutes, there appeared in both cases a very pronounced dysphoric syndrome, severe anxiety, and abnormal movements. These were very important symptoms. The myoclonias and the tremor-like movements were at times subcontinuous (*see* Figs. 5 and 6). Both cases showed a clear-cut increase of deep tendon reflexes (Fig. 7).

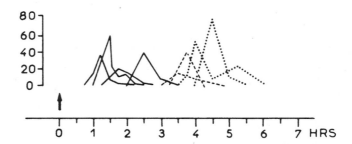

Fig. 6. Histogram showing the evolution and number (ordinate, arbitrary units) of abnormal movements after Δ^9-THC in (solid line) four subjects of group A compared with four subjects of group B receiving oral doses of hashish (dotted line) or Δ^9-THC in oily solution (broken line). Abnormal movements seem more frequent, are of higher intensity, and appear after a longer delay in group B as compared with group A.

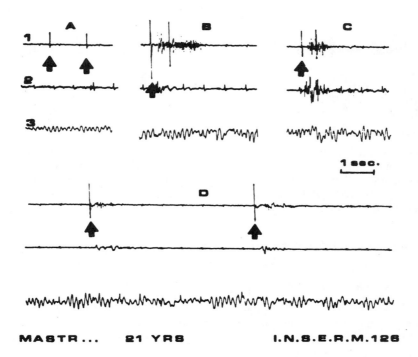

Fig. 7. Increased monosynaptic reflexes (patellar reflexes) shown on the EMG of the right (1) and left (2) quadriceps. Right patellar stimulation (arrow) evokes after Δ^9-THC ingestion higher responses (in B, C, and D) as compared with before (A). Note (B and C) that after the direct response there is a late startle-like response, diffuse and recorded here over both quadriceps. Note on the EEG (3) the persistence or even increase in amplitude of the alpha rhythm.

The subject who received hashish at the equivalent dose of 1.4 mg/kg of Δ^9-THC was unable to stand and had a drop of temperature of 1°C from the third to sixth hour after the oral doses; lipothymias occurred immediately upon standing.

This subject slept from 8:00 AM to noon of the following day. She had little food at noon and felt dizzy and depressed. Neurological examination was normal. The subject went to sleep again from 1:00 to 6:00 PM and on awakening, she was mildly depressed, felt dizzy, but

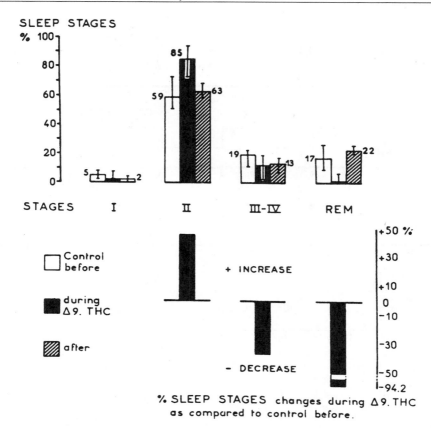

Fig. 8. Top: Percentage of mean night sleep stages (ordinate) and range of the variations in seven subjects of group A. White areas, mean of 10 nights in seven subjects before intoxication. Black areas, mean of seven nights in seven subjects during Δ^9-THC intoxication, Hatched areas, mean of nine nights in four subjects immediately after intoxication. Bottom: Mean percent changes of stage II, III to IV, and REM sleep observed during the night of intoxication compared with the night before.

was otherwise normal. She went to sleep again from 9:00 PM to 8:00 PM of the following day. After this experience and up to now (9 months later) she did not smoke again.

Δ^9-THC in oily solution was given orally to two naive subjects at doses of 0.7 and 0.9 mg/kg.

Neurological, EEG, and psychic phenomena were similar to those for the subjects of group A. Both subjects had abnormal movements consisting mainly of myoclonias and spontaneous startle-like responses (Fig. 6). A clear-cut increase of deep tendon reflexes was observed in one case.

Sleep EEGs were recorded during the whole night only in the subject who had hashish at the equivalent dose of 1.4 mg of Δ^9-THC. The subject slept only in stage II sleep and no REM or slow sleep stages were observed.

4. DISCUSSION

The findings presented in our study lend themselves to little, if any, comparison and discussion with the data available in the literature because of two essential points: first and most

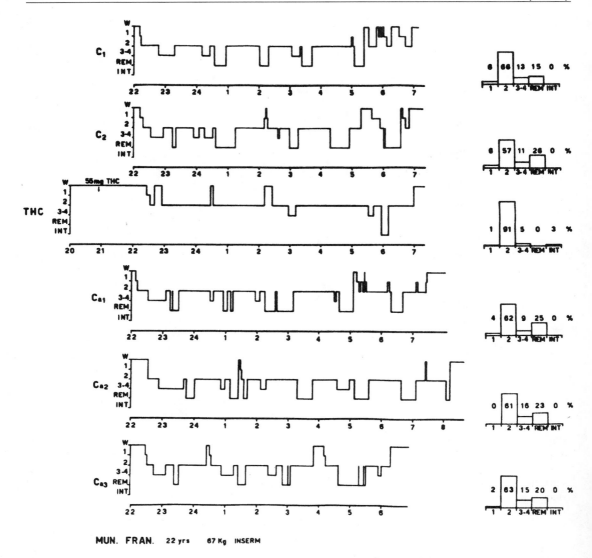

MUN. FRAN. 22 yrs   67 Kg INSERM

Fig. 9. Histograms of the night sleep before (C_1 and C_2), during Δ^9-THC intoxication, and of the three subsequent nights (C_{a1}, C_{a2}, C_{a3}). On the right column, the corresponding percentages of sleep stages. Intermediate (INT) refers to possible atypical REM periods. Note the typically prolonged stage II, the absence of REM, and decrease of slow (stage III to IV) sleep during the night of Δ^9-THC.

important, all but one of our subjects were naive subjects who never had *Cannabis* in any form before our experience; in addition, they never had experience with any other psychoactive drug (amphetamine, mescaline, and soon). For this reason, direct comparison between our results and those in the literature with nonnaive subjects would not be appropriate. The second point is the route of administration and the dose utilized. The heavy doses given resulted in such severe intoxication with clinical and neurological manifestations that our study could hardly be compared with others in the literature. There are, however, common clinical and polygraphic findings in our study and those already described in the literature. These include tachycardia and psychic symptoms, with a mixture of dysphoria associated with anxiety, and

AWAKE

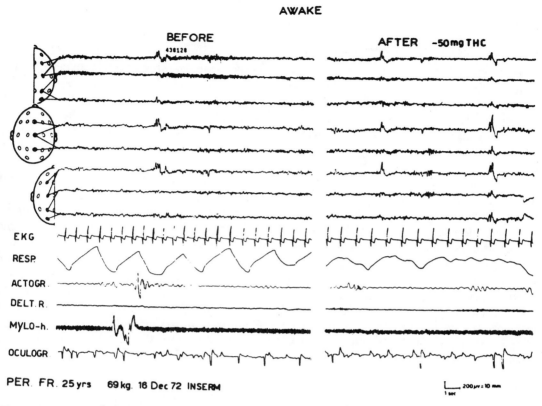

BEFORE

AFTER ~50mg THC

EKG

RESP.

ACTOGR.

DELT.R.

MYLO-h.

OCULOGR.

PER. FR. 25 yrs   69 kg. 16 Dec 72 INSERM

200 μV ≈ 10 mm
1 sec

Fig. 10. Effect of Δ^9-THC (0.8 mg/kg per os) on atypical isolated sharp waves observed in a 25-year-old normal subject. The diffuse sharp waves are predominant over the anterior head regions, and were not modified or slightly more numerous during Δ^9-THC intoxication (on the right).

finally the drowsiness leading to sleep. One should stress in our case the intensity of the psychic syndrome with the extreme anxiety and protracted and severe panicky reactions.

Psychomotor performance was clearly impaired, even if difficult to test because of the lack of subject cooperation. It should be noted that consciousness was always normal.

The subjects could analyze their feelings correctly and never reported hallucinations. Progressively, however, because of increased drowsiness and later quite incoherent sleepiness, contact with the subjects became more and more difficult.

Orthostatic hypotension, which could lead to loss of consciousness, occurred in two subjects who tried to stand up. This happened in the late stage of intoxication, when the subjects were drowsy or were awakened from sleep. It is likely that if the subjects had been systematically checked for orthostatic hypotension, this could have been a more common finding.

Overall, the subjects judged the experience as extremely unpleasant and none was willing to repeat it.

The EEGs, on visual inspection, even at the peak of drug effect, were always normal, namely, the alpha rhythm was well preserved or even increased in amount and amplitude. A slowing of 1/2 cps of the alpha frequency, as already reported by others, and the poor reactivity or even the persistence of the alpha activity with the eyes opened was observed in two subjects. This could be the result of either a specific effect of the drugs, or an unspecific effect caused by drowsiness, or both. In our study the latter factor seemed to us the most likely in explaining the lack of reactivity of alpha activity.

In conclusion, it seems clear, however, that *Cannabis*, at heavy doses, does not lead, in naive subjects, to an EEG "desynchronization" (i.e., decrease of the alpha reactivity and appearance of fast activity) as observed after effective doses of other psychoactive drugs such as mescaline or LSD *(5)*. As previously reported in naive subjects with smaller doses *(34)* visual evoked responses did not show significant changes during the intoxication in our present study. The only findings were an increase in amplitude and a slowing of the late (after 200 msec) after-discharge with the eyes closed, a predictable finding if, as we think, this component corresponds to alpha waves, which were increased on visual inspection of the EEG.

In nonnaive subjects, Rodin, Domino, and Porzak *(6)* did not find significant changes in the visual evoked responses, whereas Lewis, Dustman, Peter, Straight, and Beck *(7)* observed latency changes of the early visual-evoked components. In our study the early components were not adequately studied mainly because of the impossibility of obtaining the necessary cooperation and muscular relaxation of the subjects at the height of the intoxication.

The effects of hyperventilation and of intermittent light stimulation at various frequencies were not significantly modified by drug intoxication, at least as judged by visual inspection of the EEG. Paroxysmal generalized sharp waves, occurring spontaneously on the EEG in one normal subject, were not modified by Δ^9-THC; at times they were slightly more frequent, probably because of the drowsiness. They were similarly represented during nocturnal light sleep stages (stages I and II) in both control sleep and sleep after Δ^9-THC. Further studies are obviously needed in order to assess in man the effects, if any, of cannabis on paroxysmal discharges and epilepsy.

As seen from the EEG, drowsiness and the episodes of light sleep after Δ^9-THC were accompanied by the normal physiological patterns of light sleep. We would like to stress that the recurrent episodes of drowsiness, particularly those of brief duration (1 or 2 seconds), can be evaluate only by the EEG recordings, where they became evident well before they could be detected clinically. They appear as a transient decrease of alpha activity when the subjects keep their eyes closed, or as a brief burst of low voltage theta waves when the subjects have their eyes opened. These subclinical episodes of "microsleep," which become progressively more frequent (as observed in sleep-deprived subjects), should always and carefully be looked for on the EEG and taken into account when quantifying the EEG with computing techniques, when examining for visual evoked potentials, when testing psychomotor performances, and soon.

The abnormal movements observed in our study constitute a frequent (8 out of 11 subjects) finding. In our experience the threshold for the appearance of abnormal movements in naive subjects is approximately 0.7 mg/kg of Δ^9-THC. They were observed in subjects taking Δ^9-THC in alcohol (group A) or oily solution (group B) or taking hashish orally (group B of this study and in other studies, i.e. refs. *(3,4)*. Severe abnormal movements were also observed in our only marihuana smoker who had a single oral dose of hashish equivalent to 1.4 mg/kg of Δ^9-THC.

The abnormal movements constitute a mixture of various involuntary movements occurring at rest, which are subcontinuous or occur in isolated bursts, are clearly decreased by drowsiness, and disappear during sleep. Their topography is variable: they are diffuse and involve the neck and trunk muscles as well as the limbs; they rarely affect the face. When evident and intermittent in the upper extremities, they persist during voluntary movements. Schematically, we could distinguish from clinical and polygraphic recordings of the various muscles the following patterns.

4.1. Myoclonias

Following the classification of Gastaut *(8)*, myoclonias were found in the following forms. Partial, intermittent, asynchronous myoclonias of very brief duration (100 msec or less) occurred asymmetrically with or without displacement of the segments involved in the myoclonias. Therefore, when the myoclonias involved the wrist or the finger muscles, they were responsible for twitches with sudden finger or wrist movements. These myoclonias can be compared with those observed in various degenerative diseases in man, for example, in the progressive myoclonus epilepsy with Lafora bodies. At times, and this was the prominent feature in one subject, the myoclonus involved mainly the trunk, neck and shoulder muscles and particularly the pectoral and abdominal muscles, which were subcontinuously shaken, as in a belly dance.

Segmentary myoclonus was responsible for a sudden displacement of an extremity, most usually a leg or a limb. These segmentary myoclonias could at times be evoked by unexpected stimuli.

Massive myoclonus involved all the musculature, and was similar to that observed in a startle response or "jumping-like" reaction. As for the segmentary myoclonus, the massive myoclonus could be spontaneous or evoked by unexpected tactile stimuli, and also less frequently, by a sudden noise or by simply requesting something of the subject.

4.2. Tremors

Irregular tremors of 3–5 eps could be observed, with shifting frequencies of up to 6 to 8 cps. The tremor, appearing at rest, did not have the regularity, frequency, and the alternation over agonist and antagonist muscles as observed in the parkinsonian tremor. Its slow frequency remind us of the tremor observed in the red nucleus syndrome and in Wilson's disease. On the other hand, when the tremor was faster, at 6–8 cps, it could be similar to a shivering tremor, whose frequency in man varies from 7–13 cps. When well evident, the tremor could persist during a voluntary movement; it disappeared during sleep.

4.3. Hypertonia

Hypertonia of variable degree and intensity appeared in the EMG as subcontinuous. The tonic activity greatly fluctuated in intensity and topography and was often associated with the previously described tremor. No clinical or polygraphic evidence, however, was found of hypertonus of the pyramidal or extrapyramidal type.

We are unable to explain the mechanism responsible for these abnormal movements as well as why they have been, up to now, observed only by us (perhaps because the subjects were naive and doses were high).

4.4. Increased Tendon Reflexes

Hyperreflexia was the other neurological finding not previously described in the literature and appeared more or less concomitantly with the abnormal movements. As for the abnormal movements, the threshold for the appearance of hyperreflexia was around 40 mg of Δ^9-THC *(3,4)*, tendon reflexes could increase to such an extent as to give polycynetic responses. It should be noted that we did not find any other evidence of neurological abnormalities. In particular, polysynaptic reflexes were unchanged and there was no evidence of other "pyramidal" signs, or of cerebellar or vestibular clear disturbances. As for the abnormal movements, further studies are needed in man in order to assess the origin of the increased tendon reflexes after heavy doses of Δ^9-THC and hashish.

4.5. Sleep

As evidence from our nocturnal polygraphic recordings, it is unquestionable that in naive subjects heavy doses of Δ^9-THC or hashish suppress REM stage and decrease slow (stages III and IV) sleep.

Data in the literature concerning the effects of cannabis on sleep are somewhat contradictory. A decrease of slow sleep while REM sleep was unchanged was reported by Barrat, Breaver, and White *(9)* after the smoking of 0.2 mg/kg of THC before bedtime; Feinberg et al. *(10)* observed a large decrease of REM sleep in chronic use of large doses of cannabis.

Obviously, these variable results reflect differences of doses utilized, differences between subjects, the experimental setting of the study, etc.

On the nights immediately following Δ^9-THC intoxication, we observed a relatively small REM rebound; unfortunately, only three subjects were available for the night studies after the intoxication. One could, however, suggest that the rebound was small because of the persistence, one day later, of the effects of Δ^9-THC.

ACKNOWLEDGMENTS

This work was supported by Contract DGRST 1970–1973–70–7–2558 and Grant At 71–5–529–15 from INSERM.

The Pharmacology of Marihuana, edited by M. C. Braude and S. Szara. Raven Press, New York, 1976

REFERENCES

1. Tassinari, C. A., Charpy, J. P., Guey, N. and Saier, J. (1970) Marihuana: effetti psicofisiologici nell'uomo. In: Gli Stati di Conscienza, Bologna, Gaggi. pp. 97–109.
2. Charpy, J. P. and Guey, N. (1973) Approche expérimentale et clinique des effets du cannabis. *Cah. Psych.* **16**, 31–56.
3. Tassinari, C. A., Ambrosetto, G. and Gastaut, H. (1973) Effects of marihuana and Δ^9-THC at high doses in man. *Electroencephalogr. Clin. Neurophysiol.* **34**, 760.
4. Tassinari, C. A., Ambrosetto, G., Peraita-Adrados, M. R. and Gastaut, H. (1973) Neurophysiological effects of high doses of marihuana in man. *Electroencephalogr. Clin.* Neurophysiol. **35**, 404–405.
5. Gastaut, H., Ferrer, S. and Castelli, C. (1953) Action de la diéthylamide de l'acide D-lysergique (LSD 25) sur les fonctions psychiques et l'électroencé phalogramme. *Confin. Neurol.* **13**, 224–236.
6. Rodin, E. A., Domino, E. F. and Porzak, J. P. (1970) The marihuana-induced "social high": neurological and electroencephalographical concomitants. *JAMA* **213**, 1300–1302.
7. Lewis, E. G., Dustman, R. E., Peters, B. A., Straight, R. C. and Beek, E. C. (1973) The effects of varying doses of Δ^9-tetrahydrocannabinol on the human visual and somatosensory evoked response. *Electroencephalogr. Clin. Neurophysiol.* **35**, 347–354.
8. Gastaut, H. (1968) Séméiologie des myoclonies et nosologie analytique des syndromes myocloniques. *Rev. Neurol.* **119**, 1–30.
9. Barrat, E. S., Bayer, W. and White, R. (1974) The effects of marijuana on human sleep patterns. *Biol. Psychiat.* **8**, 47–54.
10. Feinberg et al. (1975) Effects of a chronic high dosage of delta-9-THC on sleep patterns in man. Quoted by "Marihuana and Health. IV report 1974." *Clin. Pharm. Ther.* **17**, 458–466

57 Cannabis and Psychiatric Syndrome

Peter Allebeck

Abstract

It has long been known that cannabis consumption may cause a number of psychopathological reactions. Mental effects of cannabis range from acute intoxication to long-standing psychiatric disorders. Research on the association between cannabis and psychiatric disorders is difficult, since there are a number of confounding factors and since many persons with psychiatric disorders use cannabis. Thus the causal pathways linking cannabis to psychiatric disorders are particularly difficult to elucidate. Although it is clear that cannabis may precipitate or aggravate psychotic reactions, it has been debated whether cannabis is an independent risk factor for schizophrenia. The paper summarizes the major psychiatric syndromes that may be associated with cannabis consumption and also Swedish studies that give support to the hypothesis that cannabis is a risk factor for schizophrenia.

1. INTRODUCTION

It happened during the Olympic games in Nagano, Japan, 1998, that a winner in the snowboard games lost his gold medal since a blood test revealed that he had used cannabis. The case was given widespread attention, and after serious deliberations, the authorities of the olympic games found that the regulation of doping agents was unclear with regard to cannabis. Thus, the gold medal was given back to the snowboard winner. The reactions of mass media was interesting; it was argued that cannabis could not be considered a doping agent since it did not increase the capacity of performing sports, it could only reduce it. Besides the fact that the same argument could be made with regard to opiates or many other substances on the doping list, the mental effects of cannabis are complex, and it is quite possible that for some sports and in some persons, cannabis might indeed have an effect that enhances the chances of winning a game. As one of the first observers of the mental effects of cannabis, the French doctor Joseph Moreau de Tours, pointed out in 1845, "There is no single manifestation of psychiatric disorder that is not to be found among those mental states that are caused by cannabis, from slight excitement to complete confusion, from the weakest impulse to the most irresistible drive, the wildest delirium, the most varied types of emotional disturbances."

From: *Marihuana and Medicine*
Edited by: G. G. Nahas et al.   © Humana Press Inc., Totowa, NJ

Table 1
ICD-10 Category F12: Mental and Behavioral Disorders Due to Use of Cannabinoids

F12.0	Acute intoxication
F12.1	Harmful use
F12.2	Dependency syndrome
F12.3	Withdrawal state
F12.4	Withdrawal state with delirium
F12.5	Psychotic disorder
F12.6	Amnesic syndrome
F12.7	Residual and late-onset psychotic disorder
F12.8	Other mental and behavioral disorder
F12.9	Unspecified mental and behavioral disorder

The case of the Nagano gold medal illustrates the controversy between the concept that cannabis is a harmless drug, perhaps even more harmless than alcohol or nicotine, and the concept that cannabis is a narcotic drug with strong mental and addictive effects. The controversy might have been easy to solve if the effects of cannabis were directly dose dependent, as are basically the effects of alcohol and nicotine, but this is not the case. Depending on genetic, psychological, and environmental factors, a given dose of cannabis can have a variety of effects in different persons as well as the same person on different occasions.

Another problem common in clinical settings is the distinction between mental effects caused by cannabis intoxication and symptoms of mental disorders in persons using cannabis. Anxiety reactions, psychotic reactions, and delirum are examples of possible components of cannabis intoxication that can also be part of a psychiatric syndrome. Furthermore since many psychiatric patients use cannabis, the role of cannabis in the psychiatric disorder is indeed difficult to sort out—the causal pathways can go in different directions and with different mechanisms.

The standard classification of psychopathological manifestation of cannabis abuse is given in the International Classification of Diseases (ICD-10). This classification has a common format for mental and behavioral disorders caused by substance abuse, and the text explicitly says that all subcategories in the table are applicable to all substances, and the code F12 refers to cannabis (Table 1).

Space does not permit an overview of all these disorders, and it can also be questioned whether this general format is well suited to describe psychiatric effects of cannabis abuse. Many of the effects in different categories are related, and some of them (e.g., intoxication) comprise a variety of different mental disorders. I will limit myself to discuss three of the main categores in the table: acute intoxication; psychotic disorder, and residual and late-onset psychotic disorder; and one unspecified disorder, amotivational syndrome.

2. ACUTE INTOXICATION

Anxiety reactions and panic attacks are the most common effects of cannabis intoxication. They may include restlessness, depersonalization, sense of loss of control, panic, and other related syndromes. These effects may cause anxiety by themselves, depending on the psychological and social background of the subject and the mental "set" during the time of use. Thomas (1) pointed out that there is a gray zone between desired effects of the drug and adverse, anxiety-provoking reactions, and that the user's experiences and expectations are strong determinants of the reactions provoked.

Table 2
Classification of Cannabis-related Psychotic Disorders According to Thornicroft (4)

Acute and subacute confusional states (293.0, 293.1)
Pathological drug intoxication (292.2)
Paranoid and/or hallucinatory states induced by drugs (292.1)
Clear affective or schizophrenic psychoses and their usual ICD code
Cannabis dependence, withdrawal, nondependent use (304.3, 292.0, 305.2)

Although alterations in thought processes are frequently reported by users, and vividly described in literature and arts since the middle of the 19th century, auditory and visual hallucinations are less often reported, but documented by several authors (2,3).

Flashbacks may occur days after the drug use has been discontinued. They are usually described as a re-experience of the sensations the subjects had during intoxication. but sometimes with strong adverse reaction. They may be difficult to distinguish from psychotic episodes, described below. They are thought to be caused by accumulation of THC in fat depots with slow release of psychoactive metabolites.

3. PSYCHOTIC DISORDER

The association between cannabis and psychosis has been the subject of much debate, as reviewed by, e.g., Thornicroft (4) and Thomas (1). The term "cannabis psychosis" has frequently been used in clinical settings and case reports, and Thornicroft convincingly pointed out that there is no support for a separate clinical diagnosis of "cannabis psychosis." He suggested the following classification of cannabis related psychotic disorders according to ICD-9 (Table 2).

The first category can also be termed acute organic reactions or "toxic psychoses." They may include disorientation, confusion, and auditory and visual hallucinations of different types and severity. Among the more severe types is the acute delirium, a confusional state with perceptual distortions, memory loss, and sometimes psychomotor agitation and violent behavior. It has been reported among soldiers with cannabis abuse during the Vietnam War, who were otherwise physically and mentally healthy. These confusional states are limited in time, they may last hours to days, but have a good outcome provided drug intake is discontinued.

Other psychotic states are more similar to schizophrenic or functional psychoses, comprising paranoid and/or hallucinatory states. They are distinguished from schizophrenia by their shorter duration and more benign course. Examples can be found in the case series described by Chopra and Smith (5) Thacore and Shukla (6) and Pålsson et al (7).

An important aspect of the association between cannabis and psychosis is the fact that many schizophrenics use cannabis, as part of their lifestyle or as a form of self-medication to relieve symptoms. The theory of self medication is however poorly supported by research. Negrete (8) found that the severity of psychotic symptoms in a group of 137 schizophrenics was positively associated with the extent and recency of cannabis use. Although the causal association is hard to establish, it is possible that cannabis might aggravate psychotic symptoms among schizophrenics. Treffert (9) described cases of schizophrenia in which marijuana use caused exacerbation and deterioration of the disease, and suggested that marijuana use is a clear hazard to schizophrenics.

Table 3
Types of Association Between Cannabis and Psychosis

1. Cannabis causes psychosis
2. Cannabis triggers latent psychosis
3. Cannabis causes relapse of previous psychosis
4. Psychotic disorder causes cannabis abuse
5. Spurious association—confounding
6. No association

4. RESIDUAL AND LATE ONSET PSYCHOTIC DISORDER

As Negrete *(10)* pointed out, "The true existence of severe mental illness caused by cannabis, and existing beyond a period of acute intoxication, remains one of the most controversial issues in the discussion of the psychiatric complications of this drug." One reason for the difficulty in assessing this association is that a number of different types of causal associatons may exist, and that there are important methodological problems in assessing the nature of an association found. Research in this area requires assessment of exposure to cannabis (dose and duration of use), correct assessment of the type of psychotic disorder, analysis of the cause-effect relation and control for potential confounding factors (Table 3).

We were able to address this issue in a followup of a 50,000 men who conscripted for military training in 1969–70. We had data on use of cannabis as well as other potential confounding factors. By followup in the national psychiatric register, we identified 246 cases of schizophrenia in this cohort during a 14 year period. Even after control for confounding factors we found a threefold increased risk for schizophrenia among conscripts who reported use of cannabis more than 50 times *(11)*.

There were methodological problems in the study, e.g., the validity of the diagnosis schizophrenia and the question of whether the subjects also had used other substances besides cannabis. We addressed these issues by a scrutiny of medical records among cases of schizophrenia with prior cannabis use and cases of schizophrenia without such history *(12)*. We found that cannabis was indeed the dominating drug used by conscripts who later became schizophrenic, that the DSM-III criteria for schizophrenia were fulfilled and that there was no evidence of psychiatric disorder prior to the onset of substance abuse.

5. OTHER MENTAL AND BEHAVIORAL DISORDERS

The so called "amotivational syndrome" is probably the most well-known chronic effect of cannabis use. It was described by the previously mentioned French authors of the 19th century, and information on this long term effect has been widely spread in the public information on cannabis. It is characterized by apathy, lethargy, and a lack of drive and ambition to carry out tasks. Although the phenomenon is indeed common among regular users of cannabis, its clinical background remains unclear. It could be a toxic effect causing psychological deficit, it could be physical fatigue because of the drug use, or it could be part of a lifestyle or even personality disturbance that had contributed to development of cannabis abuse. Although the concept has been questioned *(13)*, it does represent a clinical reality that is hard to ignore when summarizing the psychopathological effects of cannabis.

REFERENCES

1. Thomas, H. (1993) Psychiatric symptoms in cannabis users. *Br. J. Psychiatr.* **163,** 141–149.
2. Keeler, M., Ewing, J., and Rouse, B. (1971) Hallucinogenic effects of marijuana as currently used. *Am. J. Psychiatr.* **128,** 213–216.
3. Tart, C. (1970) Marijuana intoxication: common experiences. *Nature* **226,** 701–704.
4. Thornicroft, G. (1990) Cannabis and psychosis. Is there epidemiological evidence for an association? *Br. J. Psychiatr.* **157,** 25–33.
5. Chopra, G. and Smith, J. (1974) Psychotic reactions following cannabis use in East Indians. *Arch. Gen. Psychiatr.* **30,** 24–27.
6. Thacore, V. R., and Shukla, S. (1976) Cannabis psychosis and paranoid schizophrenia. *Arch. Gen. Psychiatr.* **33,** 383–386.
7. Pålsson, A., Thulin, S., and Tunving, K. (1982) Cannabis psychosis in South Sweden. *Acta Psychiatr. Scand.* **66,** 311–321.
8. Negrete, J., Knapp, W., Douglas, D., and Smith, W. (1986) Cannabis affects the severity of schizophrenic symptoms: results of a clinical survey. *Psycholog. Med.* **16,** 515–520.
9. Treffert, D. A. (1978) Marijuana use in schizophrenia: a clear hazard. *Am. J. Psychiatr.* **135,** 1213–1215.
10. Negrete, J. (1983) Psychiatric effects of cannabis use, in *Cannabis and health hazards* (Fehr, K. and Kalant. H.), Toronto: Addiction Research Foundation, pp. 577–616.
11. Andréasson, S., Allebeck, P., Engström, A., and Rydberg, U. (1987) Cannabis and schizophrenia: a longitudinal study of Swedish conscripts. *Lancet* **ii,** 1483–1485.
12. Andréasson, S., Allebeck, P., and Rydberg, U. (1989) Schizophrenia in users and non-users of cannabis: a longitudinal study of Swedish conscripts. *Acta Psychiatr. Scand.* **79,** 505–590.
13. Comitas, L. (1976) Cannabis and work in Jamaica: a refutation of the amotivational syndrome. *Ann. NY Acad. Sci.* **282,** 24–32.
14. Solowij, M., Michie, P. T., Fox, M. (1995) A differential impairment of selective attention due to frequency and duration of cannabis use. *Bio Psych.* **37,** 731–734.

58

Cannabis and Schizophrenia
An Overview of the Evidence to Date

Juan C. Negrete and Kathryn Gill

1. INTRODUCTION

The issue of *Cannabis* use and abuse on the part of persons with schizophrenia has attracted the attention of both epidemiologists and clinicians for some time. Their interest is motivated by the likely possibility of a significant interaction between a drug–which at sufficient doses can cause measurable psychodysleptic changes *(1)*–and a disease process with similar effects on psychic function. Some observations have been reported consistently by different authors in separate settings, and have thus become part of the current "factual knowledge" base in the field of clinical psychiatry. Others have been rather inconsistent and their interpretation remains unconvincing or frankly controversial. Of course, all the findings registered to date in the *Cannabis*/schizophrenia literature derive from the study of naturalistic conditions (i.e., the spontaneous use of the drug within the population in case) for ethical considerations preclude the experimental administration of this drug to individuals suffering from schizophrenia.

The present discussion will address the aspects that most often have been the subject of research until now: an excess prevalence of *Cannabis* use among schizophrenics; *Cannabis* use as a trigger of the clinical manifestation of schizophrenia; the effects of *Cannabis* on different symptoms of the illness; the impact of *Cannabis* use on the clinical course of schizophrenia, on therapeutic response, and on service utilization; and some hypotheses about the mechanisms of the *Cannabis*/schizophrenia interaction. Both, findings published in the scientific literature and the authors' own work on the subject will be referred to in support of the comments expressed here. The latter includes a prospective clinical outcome survey of schizophrenics attending a continuing care program ($n = 90$), 37.7% ($n = 34$) of whom reported a lifetime occurrence of regular *Cannabis* use (defined as no less than once a week for at least one year). This study is ongoing, but the data collected for the baseline assessment provides information relevant to the issues discussed here.

From: *Marihuana and Medicine*
Edited by: G. G. Nahas et al.   © Humana Press Inc., Totowa, NJ

Table 1
Reported Number of Days Using Other Substances in the Last Month

Cannabis Use	Alcohol	Tobacco
Yes ($n = 34$)	4.1 ± 5.9^a	24.8 ± 10.3^a
No ($n = 52$)	1.1 ± 2.5	13.6 ± 14.8

$^a p = 0.0001$

2. PREVALENCE ISSUES

The rates of *Cannabis* use among schizophrenics have been found to be higher than in the population at large. They have also been shown to be higher for schizophrenia than for other psychiatry diagnostic groups. Similar observations have been recorded repeatedly across different societies such as the United States *(2)*, Canada *(3)*, France *(4)*, Switzerland *(5)*, Germany *(6)*, Sweden *(7)* and Israel *(8)*. Both surveys of community samples and of patients attending psychiatric treatment facilities demonstrate an excess lifetime prevalence of cannabism in subjects who qualify for a diagnosis within the schizophrenia-spectrum disorders. The Epidemiological Catchment Area study *(9)*, for instance, has revealed that the probability of *Cannabis* abuse in persons with schizophrenia is five times the one shown by the population without such diagnosis; and also that the risk of occurrence among them is significantly higher than in persons who report a history of affective or anxiety disorders.

It becomes apparent then, that although there is an increased risk of *Cannabis* abuse associated with the presence of any psychiatric diagnosis at all, the odds ratio for schizophrenics is greater than for any such illness, with the exception of antisocial personality disorder *(9)*.

The schizophrenics' high affinity for *Cannabis*, however, cannot be said to be specific, because an excess prevalence of abuse is also observed with most of the intoxicating substances currently available, including alcohol, cocaine, and the opiates. In fact, if accessible, cocaine seems to attract this specific population more readily, for the probability of abuse is 13 times the one found in the population at large *(9)*. However, because of the smaller numbers involved, the overall rates for cocaine abuse are still much lower than for nicotine, *Cannabis*, or alcohol.

Cannabis is one of the three substances most frequently abused by schizophrenics, second only to nicotine and often ahead of alcohol *(10,11)*; but this drug is rarely consumed by itself; the most common pattern being one of multiple drug use, with the combination nicotine, alcohol and *Cannabis* reported by a significant number of subjects *(see* Table 1).

Another important finding is the large percentage of schizophrenics who did use *Cannabis* but no longer practice the habit when they reach their mid-30s. This, of course, is the pattern in the general population as well, but the rate of quitting among schizophrenics appears to be quicker *(12)*. Research shows that among individuals who will eventually receive the diagnosis of schizophrenia, the number who become involved in *Cannabis* smoking is larger than in the rest of the population *(13)*. This evidence suggests the existence of a premorbid vulnerability, or an increased need for the drug at the prodromal stages of the illness. Past 40 years of age, however, the percentage of schizophrenics who use the drug is no different than the one in the general population. A progressive decline in mental and social performance abilities could conceivably render these patients less capable of maintaining the habit in the later stages of the illness. There are other possible explanations that have not been satisfactorily explored as yet, for instance: Do schizophrenics quit smoking *Cannabis* more readily because of some specific aversive effects? *(14)*; do they do it because of the extinction of the drug's reinforcing effects in the more advanced phases of the psychotic disorder? These are but two examples of epidemiological research questions that could be better addressed through the study of prevalence of use in relation to age and stage of illness; an aspect that has not been studied sufficiently to date.

3. TRIGGER EFFECT

Andreasson et al. *(13)*, from data pertaining to a cohort of nearly 45,000 subjects, noted that a history of *Cannabis* use predicted the risk of hospital admissions for schizophrenia, and concluded that the effects of this drug in the brain should be seen as a "stressor," capable of precipitating the clinical occurrence of the illness. This is an assertion of considerable significance, which has been questioned by some *(15)*, and endorsed by others *(16,17)*. A major challenge to this interpretation is the fact that the incidence of schizophrenia has not increased over the last 30 years, the period in which the use of *Cannabis* has expanded considerably. For instance, in the United States, where the rates of cannabism in the population most at risk for schizophrenia (age group 15–45) have shown a considerable growth from the mid 1960s to 1979 *(18)*, and stayed consistently higher than in the first half of the century to the present, the point prevalence of schizophrenia, elicited through several successive surveys, has remained stable at approximately 10 per 1000 adults *(19)*. Not only has the widespread use of *Cannabis* in recent years not been accompanied by an increase in the number of people diagnosed with schizophrenia, but there are authors who suggest that this illness is even less prevalent now than it was in the past *(20)*.

That inconsistency notwithstanding, other research evidence would seem to support the "trigger effect" hypothesis. One such finding is the earlier age of onset for schizophrenia in persons with a history of *Cannabis* use *(21,22)*. With a few exceptions *(23,24)* this observation has been made time and again, including by the present authors, in the survey they are currently conducting: the schizophrenics who reported regular *Cannabis* use had their first psychiatric treatment an average of 4.7 years earlier than the nonusers (age 20.0 ± 7.5 vs 24.7 ± 8.4, $p = 0.007$); and they experienced their first admission to a psychiatric in-patient facility at a younger age (25.1 ± 7.5 vs 27.7 ± 8.1). These findings do suggest that *Cannabis* might contribute to advance the manifestation of the disorder in individuals who already have the conditions to develop it. Consistent with this interpretation is a study of family background, which elicited similar rates of psychosis among the relatives of schizophrenics who used *Cannabis* and those who did not *(25)*. The fact that the genetic diathesis profile does not seem to differ between those two groups of patients would suggest that rather than causing schizophrenia *de novo*, the abuse of *Cannabis* may simply precipitate the earlier clinical expression of an illness that most probably would have occurred anyway.

4. EFFECTS ON SYMPTOMS

Most clinicians today would assume that *Cannabis* use causes a worsening in the symptoms of schizophrenia. This is what has been learned from case reports and clinical studies in the last 30 years. The examples are multiple: Treffert *(26)*, for instance, published a detailed description of four cases under his care whose psychotic symptoms intensified every time they resumed the use of the drug. These were *bona fide* schizophrenics who had responded favorably to the neuroleptic therapy with which they were compliant. The clinical setbacks reported by this author involved symptoms which are designated presently as of the positive type (i.e. delusions, agitation, bizarre behavior, and hallucinations). Negrete et al. *(27)* surveyed the clinical condition of schizophrenics in treatment over a period of six months and also found that the current use of *Cannabis* was associated with increased hallucinatory and

Table 2
Correlation Coefficients in Schizophrenics Aged 35 Years or Younger ($n = 40$)

Scores	Days Using Cannabis Last Month	Years of Cannabis Use History
SCL-90 GSI	.38[a]	.44[a]
Psychoticism	.32[b]	.46[a]
Anxiety	.38[a]	.44[a]
Paranoid ideation	.27	.44[a]

[a] $p = 0.01$
[b] $p = 0.05$.

delusional activity. Another study (28) which was conducted in part to test the validity of those observations, did not elicit significant differences in average symptom scores when comparing groups of schizophrenics on the basis of Cannabis use. It did nonetheless demonstrate a significant positive correlation between quantity of current Cannabis use and the scores on positive symptom scales; a finding that is consistent with the previous reports. Similarly, a survey of psychotic patients hospitalized for treatment in England (29), established significant differences in the severity of some positive symptoms depending on the presence of cannabinoids in the urine screening performed at admission. These differences had dissipated at a follow-up rating completed while the patients were still in hospital, and the authors concluded that the initial higher severity in the cannabis-positive group was the result of the acute effects of the drug.

Self-reports of drug effects also confirm that Cannabis enhances the positive symptoms of schizophrenia; patients consistently state that the drug makes them feel less trustful, more suspicious, and delusional (30,31). In the authors' own survey, the scores obtained in the relevant subscales of the Symptom Check List (SCL-90)—which is a self-rated scale of current psychological distress—do correlate strongly with the number of days Cannabis was used in the last month and, interestingly, with the overall duration of Cannabis use history (see Table 2).

The negative symptoms, on the other hand, have not been found to be adversely affected by the use of Cannabis. On the contrary, most observations record a lesser severity of such symptoms in schizophrenics who smoke Cannabis: Dixon et al. conducted a self-report study (30) in which the subjects attributed to Cannabis beneficial effects on "depression" and "energy;" and a survey of expectations and motives for using drugs among schizophrenics (32) found that the ones who qualified for a clinical diagnosis of Cannabis use disorder (i.e., dependence/abuse), report using this drug for "social and sexual facilitation" and for "cognitive enhancement" in statistically significant numbers. Peralta and Cuesta (28), in their comparative, cross-sectional assessment with the Positive (SAPS) and Negative (SANS) symptom scales, found that Cannabis-abusing schizophrenics received lower scores in the latter, and concluded that the drug might in fact improve negative symptoms. The present authors are also finding a variance of the sort in their current study; schizophrenics with a history of regular Cannabis use do receive lower negative symptom scores at the Positive and Negative Symptoms Scale (PANSS) examination, but the intergroup difference is accounted for entirely by the subjects aged 35 years or less. In fact, older users and nonusers, in this sample of chronic cases attending a continuing care clinic, do not appear to differ in this clinical parameter (see Table 3).

Several interpretations could be given to the evidence that emerges from these data; one of them is that Cannabis use is more likely to be reported by subjects who are able to take the initiative required to procure and consume the drug (i.e. social contacts, securing of funds to pay for it). That is, precisely, those schizophrenics who are less handicapped by negative symptoms such as social withdrawal, lack of energy, anhedonia, or alogia. Cannabis use then

Table 3
PANSS Negative Symptoms Ratings[a]

Cannabis History	Total Sample[b]	Younger	Older
Yes	16.0 ± 6.2	15.1 ± 4.7	17.3 ± 8.0
	(n = 34)	(n = 21)	(n = 13)
No	18.4 ± 5.7	21.2 ± 6.1	16.7 ± 4.8
	(n = 52)	(n = 19)	(n = 33)

[a] group averages ± SD,
[b] $p = 0.03$.

could be expected to involve patients who are more "functional" and capable of engaging in it, and the findings mentioned above would result not from the drug's therapeutic effects on negative symptoms but from a selection factor. This interpretation is supported by the conclusions of several authors who have noted that substance-abusing schizophrenics in general could be said to exhibit higher levels of premorbid adjustment *(33,34)*, and to be less impaired socially and interpersonally than their nonuser counterparts *(35)*.

The age-effect portrayed in Table 3 suggests that if *Cannabis* has any impact on negative symptoms, this beneficial effect is noticeable mostly in the early phases of the illness. The drug, it would appear, loses its remedial properties as the abuse becomes more chronic, or when the schizophrenic disorder reaches a more advanced stage. Of course, the age differences observed may be totally unrelated to *Cannabis* use, reflecting rather a tendency for all schizophrenics to develop a similar degree of negative symptom deterioration in the more chronic phases; a sort of "ceiling" effect with everyone obtaining equally high scores. Chronicity-related changes in symptom scores have been reported in the schizophrenia literature *(36–38)*, but the present authors cannot ascertain that such is the case with this sample, for the PANSS scores given to these subjects do not seem to vary as a function of age or chronicity of illness (MANOVA results = NS).

Thus, the adverse effects of *Cannabis* on the positive symptoms of schizophrenia would appear to be fairly well established. Whether this is caused by an "additive" process whereby a toxic psychosis simply compounds the picture of the illness, as some authors suggest *(39–41)*, or to the drug's enhancement of the neurobiological mechanisms that produce those symptoms, is a question that awaits elucidation. The effects on negative symptoms are much less clear; *Cannabis* may indeed contribute to reduce their severity, but a possible selection bias in drug users still needs to be ruled out more conclusively.

5. EFFECTS ON THERAPEUTIC RESPONSE AND CLINICAL OUTCOME

The literature does contain convincing evidence that *Cannabis* use contributes to a poorer clinical outcome for schizophrenics in treatment. A major effect is the precipitation of earlier relapse in individuals who had shown a satisfactory recovery with active treatment. Linszen et al. *(42,43)*, in an elegant prospective outcome study, demonstrated that the use of *Cannabis* following discharge from an index admission was the single most important factor that predicted relapse during the first year. These authors were also interested in the role of "expressed emotion" as a risk factor–a higher level of emotional interaction in the patient's immediate environment contributes to decompensation–and were able to establish that, among subjects exposed to this particular stressor, it was the *Cannabis* users who presented the highest probabilities of relapsing.

Another 12 months follow-up study *(44)* elicited similar findings, *Cannabis* users were significantly overrepresented among the patients who relapsed during the observation period. In this case, however, the use of *Cannabis* was associated with another important risk factor: poor compliance with the prescribed pharmacotherapy.

This is another feature of the substance-abuse problem in schizophrenics; it is associated frequently with poor treatment compliance, not only in the case of *Cannabis*, but also alcohol and other drugs *(45)*. It is not justifiable, therefore, to draw conclusions about a specific *Cannabis* effect on medication-taking behavior or on exclusive drug interactions that would explain this attitude toward treatment. It is widely assumed that schizophrenics intensely dislike the CNS side effects of neuroleptic medications, and that they may turn to certain non-medical drug practices in an attempt to relieve such discomfort *(46,47)*. It may be, too, that the schizophrenics who engage in substance abuse are precisely the ones who tolerate side effects the least–particularly the anhedonia resulting from dopamine-receptor blockade–and would consequently be less compliant with treatment.

Nonetheless, the literature reports some intriguing findings with respect to the interaction between *Cannabis* and the antipsychotic drugs. Knudsen and Vilmar *(48)* concluded that the pharmacotherapy of schizophrenia is less successful in the presence of *Cannabis* use because the latter "antagonizes" its therapeutic effectiveness through an anticholinergic action in the hippocampus. Another, more recent study *(49)* reports that both tobacco and *Cannabis* smoking increase the clearance of chlorpromazine, whereas alcohol consumption does not. It is not clear however if this negative pharmacokinetic effect would not be observed also in the case of other drug-smoking practices (i.e. a nonspecific effect on drug metabolism of gas and particle components of smoke).

Finally, a study of risk factors for tardive dyskinesia (TD) *(50)*–a well-known complication of long-term neuroleptic treatment–concluded that *Cannabis* use was the strongest predictor of TD occurrence, through a multiple regression analysis in which it was compared hierarchically with other traditional predictors such as tobacco smoking, caffeine consumption, and neuroleptic dose. This finding is puzzling, and the authors offer no pharmacological interpretation; but it is tempting to suggest that *Cannabis* may exert similar effects on receptor hypersensitivity to the ones ascribed to nicotine *(46)*.

Given both its relapse-provoking effects and the possible interference with the effectiveness of antipsychotic pharmacotherapy, it is not surprising that *Cannabis* abuse has been found to be associated with an increased demand for health and social services. Schizophrenics who actively engage in it are significantly more likely to be seen at emergency rooms and tend to require more frequent interventions *(27,51)*. It must be said, however, that personality factors may also play a significant role in their service-utilization profile, and that this aspect has been brought to general attention only recently. There are authors who contend that the increased difficulties psychiatric services experience managing substance-abusing schizophrenics are due to character pathology as much as to the negative effects of drug use *(52,53)*. Personality disorders, of course, are quite prevalent in the drug-using population at large; these authors simply point out that schizophrenics are not exempt from such epidemiological selection profile.

6. MECHANISMS

The last ten years have witnessed an accelerated progress in the knowledge of *Cannabis* pharmacology. The identification of the first cannabinoid receptor subtype (CB_1) in 1988 opened the field for a very productive decade of neurobiological research *(54,55)*. Of the two protein receptor structures–seven-transmembrane spaning type–described so far *(56)*, only CB$_1$ appears to mediate the CNS action of *Cannabis*, for CB$_2$ is not found in the brain but in peripheral tissues such as spleen, lymph nodes, and testes. These are G-protein-coupled receptors that exert an inhibitory effect on adenylate cyclase and on Ca^{2+} channels. Endogenous ligands have been found (57,58); and a powerful synthetic antagonist has been developed (59), whose administration to laboratory animals chronically exposed to *Cannabis* precipitates a significant withdrawal state (60). It has been also suggested that the highly lipophilic cannabinoids may have effects that are not receptor mediated, and which result from their interaction with proteins and enzymes associated with biological membranes (61).

Receptor autoradiographic studies have revealed that CB$_1$ is located densely in the basal ganglia, the cerebellum, the olfactory bulb, and the hippocampus. Less dense concentrations are observed in the rest of the forebrain; and the receptor is practically non detectable in the brainstem and spinal cord, an evidence that may explain the relatively low lethality of *Cannabis*.

The localization of cannabinoid receptors in the hippocampus and forebrain is relevant to an explanation of the drug's effects on learning and memory (62); and their presence in the cerebellum does point to the reasons for the impairment in movement and coordination which is part and parcel of the *Cannabis* intoxication picture. Laboratory animals present rather specific responses to the administration of *Cannabis*. Rodents, for instance, display a tetrad of pharmacological effects (i.e., inhibition of activity, antinociception, hypothermia, and catalepsy) so consistent and predictable that its presence permits one to conclude that the agent employed possesses definitive cannabinoid properties (57).

Despite the tremendous progress in the science of *Cannabis*, the knowledge of the mechanisms that underlie its effects on higher psychic functions is still quite limited. This drug causes an altered state of consciousness with euphoria, disinhibition, purposeless laughter, loosening of associations, aimless reverie, and feelings of lassitude, as well as cognitive distortions such as impaired attention, memory, and time perception. Occasionally–i.e, when used in high doses or by vulnerable individuals–*Cannabis* may cause severe dysphoria or even psychotic symptoms: panic anxiety, paranoid apprehension, derealization, depersonalization, delusional perceptions, and hallucinations (1,63). The neurophysiology of the cannabinoid system is not known sufficiently yet to provide an explanation for those psychic changes. A critical question, of course, is whether the endogenous ligands act as neurotransmitters in their own right, or exert a modulating action on the other systems whose relation with psychic phenomena is better established (e.g., dopamine).

Although a full understanding of the neurobiological basis of schizophrenia is still very much in the future, much has been learned since the introduction of the first effective antipsychotics and the knowledge base is expanding at an accelerated pace (64). The earliest and still most common interpretation of the pathophysiology at play, is an abnormality or disregulation of dopaminergic function, with an excess activity being suggested as responsible for the emergence of positive symptoms (65). This hypothesis is largely supported by the pharmacological evidence that demonstrated that drugs that block dopamine transmission are effective in the treatment of the illness. It is further confirmed by the fact that dopamine-function enhancers, such as amphetamine and cocaine, are capable of causing paranoid thinking and hallucinations (66).

More recently, abnormalities in other neurotransmitter systems are thought to play a significant role as well: glutamate (67), serotonin (68), and opioid peptides (69). These hypotheses are also based on pharmacological evidence, for example, the psychotogenic properties of glutamate-receptor antagonist drugs such as PCP and ketamine; the hallucinogenic effects of LSD and other 5-HT$_2$ stimulants; the powerful antipsychotic properties of clozapine, a

proven 5-HT$_2$-receptor antagonist; and the improvement of negative symptoms of schizophrenia after the administration of opioid-receptor antagonists.

These findings suggest that if a derangement in neurotransmission is a significant factor in
the pathophysiology of schizophrenia, it is probably not limited to a single system but
involves rather a pathogenic interaction between several of them (64). One major result of
such complex dysfunction is believed to be an increased dopaminergic activity in the
mesolimbic area, leading to the emergence of productive psychotic symptoms. *Cannabis*, it
has been shown (70), excites dopamine neurons in areas relevant to such pathophysiology. It
is therefore permissible to suggest that such action of *Cannabis* might be a major reason for
the observed worsening of delusional and hallucinogenic activity in schizophrenics who use
it. The dopamine hyperactivity effect could be enhanced by the drug's interference with other
systems, such as the cholinergic and serotonergic ones (48,68) that are believed to exert a
regulatory effect on dopamine function.

Dopaminergic stimulation in the prefrontal cortex, if in fact *Cannabis* does cause it, could
in turn explain its beneficial effects on some negative symptoms. For a dopamine deficit in
that area is thought to be one of the main causes of such clinical phenomena.

The hypotheses that view schizophrenia as the result of neurodevelopmental or neu-
rostructural deficiencies (71), provide grounds for additional considerations about the possible mechanisms for a *Cannabis*-schizophrenia interaction. Katsulos et al. (72) draw attention
to the cerebellum as a possibly significant site, and argue that the role of this organ in higher
cognitive and affective functions remains under investigated. They note that the structural
and functional deficits in limbic/paralimbic regions–generally seen as the basis of the schizophrenic disorder–are associated with a failure of the integrative and associative functions;
which, these authors contend, is what leads to a distorted interpretation of external reality.
The cerebellum, of course, is also one of the main foci of cannabinoid activity in the brain.

Both schizophrenia and *Cannabis* appear to cause similar alterations in cognitive functions: Studies of event-related potentials in *Cannabis* users (62) and schizophrenics (71) have
put in evidence comparable defects in P300 responses evoked by auditory cues. These alterations reflect a diminished ability to recognize and process irrelevant stimuli in a speedy and
accurate fashion, and a recent study by Emrich et al. (73) has found that both neuroleptic-
naive schizophrenics and healthy volunteers under the influence of *Cannabis*, present the
same disturbance at a depth-perception test. The abnormality is quite peculiar in that the subjects tended to view concave objects as convex, a binocular depth inversion which represents
an illusion of visual perception. Whereas the specificity of this finding has not been demonstrated–there were no comparisons made with subjects exposed to other substances–this
study does show that *Cannabis* intoxication causes a schizophrenia-like perceptive disturbance. Once again, a greater understanding of the function of the cannabinoid system in the
brain is needed in order to ascertain the nature of the relation between the two conditions.

REFERENCES

1. Negrete, J. C. (1983) Psychiatric effects of cannabis use, in *Cannabis and Health Hazards* (O'Brien Fehr, K.
   and Kalant, H., eds.), Addiction Research Foundation, Toronto, Ontario, pp. 577–601.
2. Mueser, K. T., Yarnold, R. R., Levinson, D. F., Mueser, K. T., Yarnold, P. R., Levinson, D. F., Singh, H., Bel-
   lack, A. S., Kee, K., Morrison, R. L., and Yadalam, K. G. (1990) Prevalence of substance abuse in schizophrenia: demographic and clinical correlates. *Schizophr. Bull.* **16**, 31–42.
3. Bland, R. C., Newman, S. L. and Orn, H. (1987) Schizophrenia: lifetime co-morbidity in a community sample. *Acta Psychiatr. Scand.* **75**, 383–391.
4. Verdoux, H., Mury, M., Besancon, G., Verdoux, H., Mury, M., Besancon, G., and Bourgeois, M. (1996) Comparative study of substance dependence comorbidity in bipolar, schizophrenic and schizoaffective disorders.
   Encephale **22**, 95–101.

5. Modestin, J., Nussbaumer, C., Angst, K., Modestin, J. Nussbaumer, C., Angst, K., Scheidegger, P., and Hell, D. (1997) Use of potentially abusive psychotropic substances in psychiatric inpatients. *Eur. Arch. Psychiatry Clin. Neurosci.* **247(3)**, 146–153.

6. Hambrecht, M. and Häfner, H. (1996) Substance abuse and the onset of schizophrenia. *Biol. Psychiatry* **40:11**, 1155–1163.

7. Tunving, K. (1995) Psychiatric effects of cannabis use. *Acta Psychiatr. Scandi.* **72**, 133–136.

8. Silver, H. and Abboud, E. (1994) Drug abuse in schizophrenia: comparison of patients who began drug abuse before their first admission with those who began abusing drugs after their first admission. *Schizophr. Res.* **13(1)**, 57–63.

9. Regier, D. A., Farmer, M. E., Rae, D. S., Regier, D. A., Farmer, M. E., Rae, D. S., Locke, B. Z., Keith, S. J., Judd, L. L., and Goodwin, F. K. (1990) Comorbidity of mental disorders with alcohol and other drug abuse. Results from the Epidemiological Catchment Area (ECA) study. *JAMA* **264**, 2511–2520.

10. Schneier, F. R. and Siris, S. G. (1987) A review of substance use and abuse in schizophrenia: patterns of drug choice. *J. Nerv. Ment. Disord.* **175**, 641–652.

11. DeQuardo, J. R., Carpenter, C. F. and Tandon, R. (1994) Patterns of substance abuse in schizophrenia: nature and significance. *J. Psychiat. Res.* **28(3)**, 267–275.

12. Negrete, J. C. (1993) Effects of cannabis on schizophrenia, in *Cannabis: Physiopathology, Epidemiology, Detection* (Nahas, G. G. and Latour, C., eds.), CRC, Boca Raton, FL, pp. 105–112.

13. Andreasson, S., Allebeck, P., Engstrom, A., Andreasson, S., Allebeck, P., Engstrom, A., and Rydberg, U. (1987) Cannabis and schizophrenia: a longitudinal study of swedish conscripts. *Lancet* **2**, 1483–1486.

14. Negrete, J. C. and Kwan, M. W. (1975) Relative value of various etiological factors in shortlasting, adverse psychological reactions to cannabis smoking. *Int. Pharmacopsychiatry* **7**, 249–259.

15. Castle, D. J. and Ames, P. R. (1996) Cannabis and the brain. *Austr. and New Zealand J. of Psychiatry* **30**, 179–183.

16. Longhurst, J. G., Boutros, N. N. and Bowers, M. B. (1997) Cannabis-induced chronic psychosis–an under acknowledged disorder. *Austr. and New Zealand J. of Psychiatry* **31**, 305–306.

17. Negrete, J. C. (1989) Cannabis and schizophrenia. *Br. J. of Addict.* **84(4)**, 349–351.

18. Kandel, D. B. (1993) Social demography of drug use, in *Drug Policy, Illicit Drugs in a Free Society* (Bayer, R. and Oppenheimer, G. M., eds.), Cambridge University Press, Cambridge, UK, pp. 24–77.

19. Karno, M. and Norquist, G. S. (1989) Schizophrenia: epidemiology, in *Comprehensive Textbook of Psychiatry*, vol., 4th ed. (Kaplan, H. I. and Sadock, B. J. eds.), Williams & Wilkins, Baltimore, pp. 699–704.

20. Eaton, W. W. (1985) Epidemiology of schizophrenia. *Epidemiol. Rev.* **7**, 105–122.

21. Cleghorn, J. M., Kaplan, R. D. and Szechman, B. (1991) Substance abuse in schizophrenia: effect on symptoms but not on neurocognitive function. *J. Clin. Psychiatry* **52**, 26–30.

22. Smith, J. and Hucher, S. (1994) Schizophrenia and substance abuse. *Br. J. Psychiatry* **165**, 13–21.

23. Kovasznay, B., Bromet, E., Schwartz, J. E., Kovasznay, B., Bromet, E., Schwartz, J. E., Miller, A. D., and Fleisher, J. (1993) Substance use and onset of psychotic illness. *Hosp. Community Psychiatry* **44**, 567–571.

24. Cuffel, B. J., Helthoff, K. A. and Lawson, W. (1993) Correlates of patterns of substance abuse among patients with schizophrenia. *Hosp. Community Psychiatry* **44**, 247–251.

25. McGuire, P. K., Jones P., Harvey, I., McGuire, P. K., Jones, P., Harvey, I., Williams, M., McGuffin, P., and Murray, R. M. (1995) Morbid risk of schizophrenia for relatives of patients with cannabis-associated psychosis. *Schizophr. Res.* **15(3)**, 277–281.

26. Treffert, D. A. (1978) Marijuana use in schizophrenia: a clear hazard. *Am. J. Psychiatry* **135(10)**, 1213–1215.

27. Negrete, J. C., Knapp, W. P., Douglas, D. E. Negrete, J. C., Knapp, W. P., Douglas, D. E., and Smith, W. B. (1986) Cannabis affects the severity of schizophrenic symptoms: results of a clinical survey. *Psychological Med.* **16**, 515–521.

28. Peralta, V. and Cuesta, M. J. (1992) Influence of cannabis abuse on schizophrenic psychopathology. *Acta Psychiatr. Scand.* **85(2)**, 127–130.

29. Mathers, D. C. and Ghodse, A. H. (1992) Cannabis and psychotic illness. *Br. J. Psychiatry* **161**, 648–653.

30. Dixon, L., Haas, G., Weiden, P. J. Dixon, L., Haas, G., Weiden, P. J., Sweeney, J., and Frances, A. J. (1991) Drug abuse in schizophrenic patients: clinical correlates and reasons for use. *Amer. J. Psychiatry* **148**, 224–230.

31. Baigent, M., Holme, G. and Hafner, R. J. (1995) Self reports of the interaction between substance abuse and schizophrenia. *Austr. N. Z. J. Psychiatr.* **29**, 69–74.

32. Mueser, K. T., Hishith, P., Tracy, J. I., Mueser, K. T., Nishith, JIT., DeGirolamo, J., and Molinaro, M. (1995) Expectations and motives for substance use in schizophrenia. *Schizophr. Bull.* **21(3)**, 367–378.

33. Arndt, S., Tyrrell, G., Flaum, M., Arndt, S., Tyrrell, G., Flaum, M. and Andreasen, N. C. (1992) Comorbidity of substance abuse and schizophrenia: the role of pre-morbid adjustment. *Psychological Med.* **22**, 379–387.

34. Breakey, W. C., Goodell, H., Lorenz, P. C. Breakey, W. C., Goodell, H., Lorenz, P. C., and McHugh, P. R. (1974) Hallucinogenic drugs as precipitants of schizophrenia. *Psychological Med.* **4**, 255–261.

35. Dixon, L., Haas, G., Weiden, P. J. et al. (1990) Acute effects of drug use in schizophrenia patients: clinical observations and patient self-reports. *Schizophr. Bulletin* **16**, 69–79.

36. Sandyk, R. (1993) Positive symptoms and chronicity of illness in schizophrenia. *Int. J. Neurosci.* **70(1–2)**, 65–67.

37. Addington, J. and Addington, D. (1991) Positive and negative symptoms of schizophrenia. Their course and relationship over time. *Schizophr. Res.* **5(1)**, 51–59.

38. Rosenthal, R. N., Hellerstein D. J. and Miner, C. R. (1994) Positive and negative syndrome typology in schizophrenic patients with psychoactive substance use disorders. *Compr. Psychiatry* **35(2)**, 91–98.

39. Solomons, K., Neppe, V. M. and Kuyl, J. M. (1990) Toxic cannabis psychosis is a valid entity. *S. Afr. Med. J.* **78(8)**, 476–481.

40. Saxena, S. (1993) Cannabis-induced psychosis' may obscure paranoid schizophrenia. *Natl. Med. J. India* **6(2)**, 78–79.

41. Boutros, N. N. and Bowers, M. B. (1996) Chronic substance-induced psychotic disorders: state of the literature. *J. Neuropsychiatry* **8(3)**, 262–269.

42. Linzen, D. H. Kingemans, P. M. and Lenior, M. E. (1994) Cannabis abuse and the course of recent-onset schizophrenic disorders. *Arch. Gen. Psychiatry* **51**, 273–279.

43. Linzen, D. H., Dingemans, P. M., Nugter, M. A. Linzen, D. H., Dingemans, P. M., Nugter, M. A., Van der Does, A. J. W., Scholte, W. F., and Lenior, M. A. (1997) Patient attributes and expressed emotion as risk factors for psychotic relapse. *Schizophr. Bulletin* **23(1)**, 119–130.

44. Martinez-Arevalo, M. J., Calcedo-Ordonez, A. and Varo-Prieto, J. R. (1994) Cannabis consumption as a prognostic factor in schizophrenia. *Br J Psychiatr.* **164(5)**, 679–681.

45. Owen, R. R., Fischer, E. P., Booth, B. M. Owen, R. R., Fischer, E. P., Booth, B. M., and Cuffel, B. J. (1996) Medication noncompliance and substance abuse among patients with schizophrenia. *Psychiatr. Serv.* **47(8)**, 853–858.

46. Levin, M. R., Siris, S. G. and Mason, S. E. (1996) What is the clinical importance of cigarette smoking in schizophrenia? *Amer. J. on Addict.* **5**, 189–208.

47. Rosenthal, R. N. (1998) Is schizophrenia addiction prone? *Curr. Opinion in Psychiatry* **11**, 45–48.

48. Knudsen, P. and Vilmar, T. (1984) Cannabis and neuroleptic agents in schizophrenia. *Acta Psychiatr. Scand.* **69**, 162–174.

49. Chetty, M., Miller, R. and Moodley, S. V. Smoking and body weight influence the clearance of chlorpromazine. *Eur. J. Clin. Pharmacology* **46(6)**, 523–526.

50. Zaretsky, A., Rector, N. A., Seeman, M. V., Zaretsky, A., Rector, N. A., Seeman, M. V. and Fornazzari, X. (1993) Current cannabis use and tardive dyskinesia. *Schizophr. Res.* **11(1)**, 3–8.

51. Turner, W. M. and Tsuang, M. T. (1990) Impact of substance abuse on the course and outcome of schizophrenia. *Schizophr. Bull.* **16(1)**, 87–95.

52. Mueser, K. T., Drake, R. E., Ackerson, T. H., Mueser, K. T., Drake, R. E., Ackerson, T. H., Alterman, A. I., Miles, K. M., and Noordsy, D. L. (1997) Antisocial personality disorder, conduct disorder, and substance abuse in schizophrenia. *J. Abnorm. Psychol.* **106(3)**, 473–477.

53. Van Ammers, E. C., Sellman, J. D. and Mulder. R. T. (1997) Temperament and substance abuse in schizophrenia: is there a relationship? *J. Nerv. Ment. Dis.* **185(5)**, 283–288.

54. Musty, R. E., Reggio, P. and Consroe, P. (1995) A review of recent advances in cannabinoid research. *Life Sciences* **56**, 1933–1940.

55. Howlett, A.C. (1995) Pharmacology of cannabinoid receptors. *Annu. Rev. Pharmacol. Toxicol.* **35**, 607–634.

56. Abood, M. and Martin, B. R. (1996) Molecular Neurobiology of the cannabinoid receptor. *Int. Rev. of Neurobiol.* **39**, 197–221.

57. Mechoulam, R., Shabat, B. and Ilanus, S., Mechoulam, R., Shabat, B., Ilanus, S., Fride, E., Bayewitch, M., and Vogel, Z. (1996) Endogenous cannabinoid ligands, in *AIDS, Drugs of Abuse and the Neuroimmune Axis* (Friedman, H, ed.), Plenum Press, New York, pp. 95–101.

58. Stella, N., Schweitzer, P. and Piomelli, D. (1997) A second endogenous cannabinoid that modulates long-term potentiation. *Nature* **388**, 6644, 773–778.

59. Rinaldi-Carmona, Barth, M., Heaulme, F. Rinaldi-Carmona, M., Barth, F., Heaulme, M., Shire, D., Calandra, B., Congy, C., Martinez, S., Maruani, J., Neliat, G., Caput, D., Ferrar, P., Soubrie, P., Breliere, J. C., and Fur, G. L. (1994) SR 141716A, a potent and selective antagonist of the brain cannabinoid receptor. *FEBS Letters* **350**, 240–244.

60. Aceto, M. D., Scates, S. M. and Lowe, J. A., Aceto, M. D., Scates, S. M., Lowe, J. A., and Martin, B. R. (1995) Cannabinoid precipitated withdrawal by selective cannabinoid receptor antagonist, SR 141716A. *Eur. J. Pharmacol.* **282**, R1–R2.

61. Makriyannis, A. and Rapaka, R. S. (1990) The molecular basis of cannabinoid activity. *Life Sciences* **47**, 173–184.
62. Solowij, N. (1995) Do cognitive impairments recover following cessation of cannabis use? *Life Sciences* **56**, 2119–2126.
63. Edwards, G. (1983) Psychopathology of a drug experience. *Brit. J. Psychiatry* **143**, 509–512.
64. Weinberger, D. R. (1997) The biological basis of schizophrenia: new directions. *J. Clin. Psychiatr.* **58(suppl 10)**, 22–27.
65. Hietala, J. and Syvälahti, E. (1996) Dopamine in schizophrenia. *Ann. Med.* **28(6)**, 557–561.
66. Mirin, S. (1986) The relevance of laboratory studies in animals and humans to an understanding of the relationship between addictive disorders and psychopathology, in *Psychopathology and Addictive Disorders* (Meyer, R. E., ed.), Guildford Press, New York, pp. 199–237.
67. Gonzalez-Garcia, G. and Gonzalez Torres, M. A. (1997) The glutamatergic hypothesis of schizophrenia: an update. *Psiquis* **18**, 440–448.
68. Abi-Dargham, A., Laruelle, M., Aghajanian, G. K., Abi-Dargham, A., Laruelle, M., Aghajanian, G. K., Charney, D., and Krystal, J. (1997) The role of serotonin in the pathophysiology and treatment of schizophrenia. *J. Neuropsychiatr. Clin. Neurosci.* **9**, 1–17.
69. Welch, E. B. and Thompson, D. F. (1994) Opiate antagonists for the treatment of schizophrenia. *J. Clin. Pharm. Ther.* **19**, 279–283.
70. French, E. D., Dillon K. and Wu, X. (1997) Cannabinoids excite dopamine neurons in the ventral tegmentum and substantia nigra. *Neuroreport* **8(3)**, 649–652.
71. Javitt, D. C. (1997) Psychophysiology of schizophrenia. *Curr. Opinion in Psychiatry* **10**, 11–15.
72. Katsulos, C. D., Hyde, T. M. and Herman, M. M. (1997) Neuropathology of the cerebellum in schizophrenia-an update: 1996 and future directions. *Biol. Psychiatry* **42**, 213–224.
73. Emrich, H. M., Leweke, F. M., and Schneider, U. (1997) Toward a cannabinoid hypothesis of schizophrenia: cognitive impairments due to dysregulation of the endogenous cannabinoid system. *Pharmacol. Biochem. Behav.* **56(4)**, 803–807.

59

Detection of Cannabis in Victims of Violent Death in Stockholm (1987–1994)

Jovan Rajs and Anna Fugelstad

Abstract

During the eight-year period of 1987–1994, *Cannabis* was detected in 58 medicolegal postmortem investigations in Stockholm. In 17 cases, *Cannabis* was the only drug detected; in 41 instances it was combined with alcohol, heroin, or amphetamine. 54 of 58 deaths (93%) were violent. The percentage of suicides and homicides (i.e., intentional deaths) was highest among persons in whom only cannabis was detected (76.4%). By comparison, there were 22% suicides, 2% homicides, and 23% accidental death in all forensic autopsies in Sweden (47%). In *Cannabis*-related car accidents, reckless driving of cars at high speed and collision with other vehicles was the main cause of accidents. Violence directed toward other persons was not premeditated, and was carried out with intent to kill with whatever weapon was found, as a single stab or shot. Suicides related to *Cannabis* use were more violent and impulsive than suicides associated with other illicit drug use.

1. INTRODUCTION

There have been anecdotal reports about potential links between the use of marihuana and aggression. Both retrospective and experimental studies in human beings have failed to yield evidence that marihuana use leads to increased aggression. Most of these studies suggest quite the contrary effect. Marihuana appears to have a sedative effect, and it may reduce somewhat the intensity of angry feelings and the probability of interpersonal aggressive behavior (1–6). However, marihuana use has been associated with delinquent behavior such as drug trafficking and stealing. Furthermore, as Abel (7) stated, "while *Cannabis* does not precipitate violence, there are certain individuals, and certain situations of set and setting in which marihuana use may result in violence." Mendelson et al. (8) reached a similar conclusion.

From: *Marihuana and Medicine*
Edited by: G. G. Nahas et al.   © Humana Press Inc., Totowa, NJ

Medicolegal death investigations have always been an important source of knowledge of the factors that contribute to violence, in turn leading to injuries and death of the involved persons. Information about the circumstances of death and about alcohol and drugs in connection with violent acts can often be obtained from medicolegal files. We have reported previously data from our department concerning the association between *Cannabis* use and violent death *(9)*. This review reports additional cases of violent death observed in subjects in whom *Cannabis* was detected on autopsy.

2. Patients and Methods

The study was based on medicolegal death investigations made at the Government Institute for Forensic Medicine in Stockholm, Sweden during an eight-year period (1987–1994). In accordance with Swedish regulations, a medicolegal investigation must be made on deceased persons who have died as a result of obvious or suspected violence. This includes poisoning, alcohol and/or substance abuse, sudden deaths without previously known fatal disease, or unclear and suspicious circumstances. These regulations were changed in the middle of the study period, July 1, 1991; resulting in a marked reduction of autopsies of unclear but probably natural deaths occurring in elderly persons.

During these eight years, a total of 20,661 medicolegal autopsies were made in Stockholm on persons of all ages. Information about deceased persons was obtained from police reports and was supplemented with information from medical journals, family members, friends, and social workers whenever possible.

Toxicological analyses were made with the purpose of disclosing the presence of alcohol and medicinal and illicit drugs; as suggested by autopsy findings, past history, police records, or circumstances at death. Toxicological analyses were also carried out whenever information concerning the circumstances of death was insufficient, e.g., cases of violent death or inconclusive postmortem findings, or when information about irregular behavior or symptoms was available. Chemical analyses were made at the National Laboratory of Forensic Chemistry in Linköping in accordance with the methods described previously *(9)*.

Determination of tetrahydrocannabinol (THC) in blood and other cannabinoids in urine was introduced as a routine laboratory method at the end of the 1980s. Out of the total of 20,661 autopsies, toxicological analyses with regard to alcohol, medicinal, and illicit drugs were made in 17,438 (84.4%) instances. The analyses regarding illicit drugs mostly concerned opiates (found in 440 cases, i.e. 2.13%) and central stimulants (found in 214 cases, i.e. 1.03%), but in a total of 1897 cases (9.1%) analyses for the detection of THC and/or other cannabinoids were made. Among these 186 positive results were obtained (0.9% of the total number of autopsies and 9.8% of the directed analyses).

Results obtained were classified in four groups. Group I comprised deaths in which THC or other cannabinoids were found ($n = 17$). Deaths of subjects who did not use drugs but who were killed by *Cannabis* users or died in accidents caused by *Cannabis* users were not included in this study. Group II comprised deaths in which THC and alcohol or heroin and amphetamine were detected ($n = 41$). Group III comprised deaths in which heroin was detected ($n = 94$). Group IV comprised deaths in which amphetamine was detected ($n = 32$). The number of deaths with findings of cocaine was too small to categorize (Table 1).

The autopsies were made by several forensic pathologists, and there were no strict rules for indications for toxicological examinations. Consequently, in some instances, the pathologist was satisfied with information about *Cannabis* use and had not requested toxicological confirmation. Such cases were not included in this study. For the same reason, the manner of death, i.e. whether it was of accidental, homicidal, suicidal, or undetermined origin, was reascertained by the authors in all drug-related deaths according to the criteria described previously *(10,11)*.

Table 1
**Findings of *Cannabis* and Other Illicit Drugs in Medicolegally Autopsided Violent
and Natural Deaths in Stockholm 1987–1994.**

Drugs	Suicides n (%)	Homicides n (%)	Accidents n (%)	Natural n (%)	Unknown or undetermined n (%)
Cannabis, no alcohol n = 17	9 (52.9)	4 (23.5)	2 (11.8)	2 (11.0)	0
Cannabis and alcohol n = 41	13 (31.7)	4 (9.8)	22 (53.7)	2 (4.9)	0
Cannabis and heroin n = 94	5 (5.3)	0	86 (91.4)[a]	0	3 (3.2)
Cannabis and amphetamine n = 32	3 (9.4)	7 (21.9)	20 (62.5)	1 (3.1)	1 (3.1)

[a]79 (84.0%) sudden deaths upon heroin administration.

3. RESULTS

During the eight-year period of 1987–1994, *Cannabis* was found in postmortem samples of 58 cases; in 17 of these, without alcohol; in 41 instances combined with alcohol and/or medicinal drugs. There were 55 males and 3 females, 20–43 years of age (mean age 29.6 years).

As shown in Table 1, 54 of 58 *Cannabis*-related deaths (93%) were violent. The percentage of suicides and homicides (i.e., intentional deaths) was highest among those persons in whom *Cannabis*, but no alcohol, was found at autopsy (76.4%). The percentage of suicidal deaths was lower when, besides *Cannabis*, amphetamine or heroin metabolites could also be detected (9.4% and 5.3%, respectively).

In all forensic autopsies in Sweden there were 22% suicides, 2% homicides, 23% accidents, 4% with undetermined cause of death, 45% natural deaths, and 3% with unknown cause of death.

In addition to the quantitative differences described, there were qualitative ones. These differences were also seen when behavioral patterns and types of injuries of accidental and homicidal deaths related to the use of *Cannabis* were evaluated and compared to those related to other drugs of abuse.

3.1. Accidental Death

Fifteen of 24 *Cannabis* users who died in accidents were killed in car accidents, eight as drivers of motor vehicles, and five as passengers (with *Cannabis*-influenced drivers). In one of the automobile accidents, high speed (exceeding the speed limit threefold through central Stockholm) preceded collision with another car; in an other case, the *Cannabis*-influenced driver passed another car, at twice the speed limit, and just continued to drive on the left side of the road until he collided with a car coming from the opposite direction. In other cases, the drivers were not able to keep their cars on the road in a minor curve; and in yet another, the car was simply driven into a ditch.

The nine other accidents comprised four cases of drowning, four cases of intoxication, and one boat accident. In eight of the nine cases, the victims had ingested considerable amounts of alcohol, which probably contributed to the fatal outcome.

3.2. Homicides

Eight out of 58 *Cannabis* users were murdered, seven males and one female, ranging in age from 22 to 37 years (mean age 26.6 years). A knife was the dominating murder weapon, used in six instances, whereas a firearm was used in two.

Two *Cannabis* users were murdered by their fiancé, who were *Cannabis* users as well. The settings were similar: Emotional relationships existed between the future victim and the perpetrator, and a sudden stabbing to death resulted from a short quarrel over trivial matters. In one of these cases, the murderer was shocked and regretful; in the other, the murderer was confused and disoriented upon arrival of the police. Three of the five remaining victims of solved homicides were also killed by *Cannabis* users. One or two stabs or shots ended the life of a close friend in four out of eight homicides; in the remaining cases, the killing continued in "overkill" inflicting numerous additional severe injuries.

3.3. Suicides

There were 22 suicides among the 58 deaths. Suicides were more common among those who have died with only THC in their bodies than among those where other illicit drugs also were found (cf. Table 1). Both THC and alcohol were found in 13 suicidal deaths, and in 9 cases only THC. Twenty one of the deceased were males and only one was female.

Still more notable than the variation in suicidal rate is the great qualitative difference between the groups in the type of suicide and the methods used when committing the suicide.

We have divided the suicide methods into three groups according to the degree of violence in the used methods:

1. Nonviolent suicides: Intoxication by pharmaceutical or illicit drugs or by alcohol.
2. Low violence suicides: Drowning, hanging, gassing, and so on.
3. Violent suicides involving physical trauma: Shooting, stabbing with a sharp instrument, jumping from high places or in front of a train.

The suicide methods in the 22 *Cannabis*-related cases were compared with those suicides involving amphetamine and heroin but not *Cannabis,* 33 and 51 cases, respectively, that were found at autopsy during the same period.

Suicidal techniques of persons presenting *Cannabis*, amphetamine, or heroin in their body fluids are presented in Fig. 1.

The violent suicides dominated among deaths in which *Cannabis* but no other illicit drug was found in the blood. Such suicides were not as common in the other groups, especially not among heroin-related deaths.

In three cases, the suicides occurred among persons who had been treated for a toxic *Cannabis*-related psychosis shortly before death. In all these cases, hospital records of the respective treatment period were available. All three persons had fallen sick in connection with a period of intensive *Cannabis* smoking, all suffering from very dramatic symptoms, in one case leading to compulsory treatment. All of them recovered very rapidly and could be discharged from the hospital and committed suicide by jumping from high places. The suicides occurred very soon after the discharge, in connection with relapse into *Cannabis* smoking. THC (but no alcohol) was present in the blood of all three persons. One of these persons had been treated for a *Cannabis*-related psychosis on several occasions over nine years. He

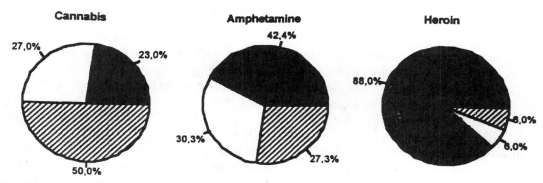

Fig. 1. Modes of execution among suicide victims in whom the presence of cannabis, amphetamine or heroin was detected. (1) Suicides involving intoxication by pharmaceuticals, illicit drugs, or alcohol: ■; (2) suicides involving drowning, hanging, or gassing: □; (3) suicides involving shooting, stabbing, plunging to one's death or mjumping in front of a train: ▨.

recovered very rapidly when admitted to the hospital, but always relapsed into drug abuse after discharge, necessitating a new admittance. In spite of intensive treatment efforts, it was not possible to contain his misuse; finally he committed suicide by jumping from a high cliff while on a temporary leave from the hospital.

Four persons committed suicide by jumping from high places. None of them had been treated for a *Cannabis*-related psychosis or any other psychiatric disease. The suicides seemed to be unplanned and impulsive. In all three cases, the *Cannabis* user behaved in a very aggressive way toward relatives or other close persons who were present but unable to prevent the suicides.

In four cases, male subjects committed suicide by hanging and gassing themselves immediately after their wives or girlfriends had left them. The suicides occurred as an immediate reply to the separation, without any intervening period of depression. In another case, a man reacted very violently to a doctor who told him to go back to work after a leave of absence although he did not feel well.

There were two cases of murder/suicides among *Cannabis*-related deaths. Murder/suicides are very uncommon in Sweden (only a few cases each year).

In the remaining nine cases, there was no sufficient anamnestic information. The majority of these cases did not seem to be violent or impulsive; the persons were rather depressed or tired of life. In one case there was a farewell note. It is uncertain if the use of *Cannabis* was related to these suicides.

3.4. THC concentration in the blood

The number of *Cannabis*-related deaths in this series was still too low to supply an adequate basis for statistical analyses, especially when subdivisions were made relating to causes and manners of deaths, or activities at the time of death. Median THC concentration among the eight car drivers was 11 ng/g blood (range 1–40); in six cases alcohol was also involved. THC concentrations were low (< 3 ng/g blood) among natural deaths caused by various intercurrent diseases, like complications of chronic alcoholism and arteriosclerotic heart disease or perforated gastric ulcer conditions which could not be related to *Cannabis* use.

4. DISCUSSION

The methods for detection and quantitative analysis of *Cannabis* and other metabolites in the body, though improved, are still complicated and expensive, and a screening for *Cannabis* has still not been included in all forensic examinations.

The autopsy frequency of drug addicts in Stockholm is rather high. A recent study *(10)* of hospitalized drug addicts in Stockholm reported that 80% of the deceased addicts were examined in the department of forensic medicine. *Cannabis*-related violent deaths in Stockholm could be reported on as a significant sample.

It was found that 93% of the deaths of subjects in whom *Cannabis* was detected were violent. This compares with 51% of all forensically examined deaths in Sweden which were of a violent nature. The incidence of *Cannabis*-related violent death was also related to the concurrent presence of amphetamine or heroin in the victims. Amphetamine seems to have had an "additive" effect, whereas heroin a "subduing" effect. When alcohol was a cofactor with *Cannabis*, the violent deaths appeared to occur according to an accidental, unintentional mode (53.7 vs 11.8% when *Cannabis* alone was detected in the victim).

Our case records also indicate qualitative differences in patterns of violent behavior and types of injuries related to *Cannabis* detection in victims. Typical of *Cannabis*-related car accidents is the reckless driving of cars at high speed, and head-on collisions with other vehicles.

Notable is the occurrence of impulsive intentional "*Cannabis*-related" violent deaths. When violence was directed toward other persons, the killing seems to have been committed without premeditation, carried out with any available weapon as a single stab or a shot (sometimes also as overkill). *Cannabis*-related deaths seem different from deaths related to alcohol, amphetamine, cocaine, heroin, and anabolic androgenic steroids *(12–14)*.

Cannabis-related suicides appeared to be more violent and impulsive than suicides related to other illicit drugs. We have attempted to describe the circumstances under which the suicides were made and the degree of violence that was used. There were three main groups of suicides:

1. Suicides committed with violent methods by patients previously treated for *Cannabis*-related psychotic episodes and who had relapsed into *Cannabis* abuse.
2. Impulsive and violent suicides by patients who had shown violent behavior against close friends or relatives immediately before their suicide.
3. Impulsive suicides by persons who were slighted or insulted such as males who had been rejected by wives or girlfriends.

Several studies have reported that patients who have presented *Cannabis*-related psychosis often recover quite rapidly after a period of *Cannabis*-free hospitalization. Their psychiatric illness does recur when they resume their smoking of cannabis *(15–17)*. One of the victims in the present study had been treated at several occasions during a nine-year period but could not refrain from relapsing into *Cannabis*-smoking. It is well known that the risk of suicide is very high in psychotic patients.

REFERENCES

1. Hemphill, R. E. and Fisher, W. (1980) Drugs, alcohol and violence in 604 male offenders referred to inpatient psychiatric assessment. *S. Afr. Med. J.* **57**, 243–247.
2. McGuire, J. S. and Megaree, E. I. (1974) Personality correlates of marihuana use among youthful offenders. *J. Consult. Clin. Psychol.* **42**, 124–133.
3. Salzman, C., Van Der Kolk, B. A. and Shader, R. I. (1976) Marihuana and hostility in a small-group setting. *Am. J. Psychiatry* **133**, 1029–1033.
4. Taylor, S. P., Vardaris, R. M., Rawtich, A. B., et al. (1976) The effects of alcohol and Δ^9-THC on human physical aggression. *Aggressive Behav.* **2**, 153–161.

5. Tinklenberg, J. R. (1974) Marihuana and human aggression, In *Marihuana: Effects on Human Behavior* (Miller, L. L., ed.) Academic, New York, pp. 339–357.

6. Tinklenberg, J. R., Roth, W. T., Kopell, B. S. and Murphy, P. (1976) Cannabis and alcohol effects on assaultiveness in adolescent delinquents. *Ann. NY Acad. Sci.* **282**, 85–94.

7. Abel, E. L. (1977) The relationship between cannabis and violence: a review. *Psychol. Bull.* **84**, 193–211.

8. Mendelson, J. H., Rossi, A. M. and Meyer, R. E., eds. (1974) *The Use of Marihuana: A Psychological and Physiological Enquiry*, Plenum, New York.

9. Rajs, J., Fugelstad, A. and Jonsson, J. (1993) Cannabis-associated deaths in medicolegal postmortem studies. Preliminary report. Cannabis, physiopathology, epidemiology, detection. From the Proceedings of the Second International Symposium organized by the National Academy of Medicine, April 8–9, 1992. (Nahas, G. G. and Latour, C., eds.) CRC Press, Boca Raton, FL, pp. 123–133.

10. Fugelstad, A., Annell, A., Rajs, J. and Ågren, G. (1997) Mortality and causes and manner of death among drug addicts in Stockholm during the period 1981–1992. *Acta Psychiatr. Scand.* **96**, 169–175.

11. Adamsson Wahren, C., Allebeck, P. and Rajs, J. (1997) Unnatural causes of death among drug addicts in Stockholm: an analysis of health care and autopsy records. *Subst. Use Misuse* **32**, 2163–2183.

12. Marzuk, P. M., Tardiff, K. et al. (1995) Fatal injuries after cocaine use as a leading cause of death among young adults in New York City. *N. Engl. J. Med.* **332**, 1753–1757.

13. Spunt, B., Goldstein, P., Brownstein, H. and Fendrich, M. (1994) The role of marihuana in homicide. *Int. J. Addict.* **29**, 195–213.

14. Thiblin, I., Kristiansson, M. and Rajs, J. (1997) Anabolic androgenic steroids and behavioural patterns among violent offenders. A medicolegal and psyhiatric study. *J. Forensic Psychiatry* **8**, 299–310.

15. Ramström, J., ed. (1997) Skador av hasch och marihuana. *SoS-Rapport* **16**.

16. Rottanburg, D., Robins, A. H., Ben-Arie, O., Teggin, A. and Elk, R. (1982) Cannabis-associated psychosis with hypomanic features *Lancet* **2**, 1364–1366.

17. Rolfe, M., Tang, C. M., Sabally, S., Todd, J. E., Sam, E. B. and Hatib N'Jie, A. B. (1993) Psychosis and cannabis abuse in the Gambia. A case-control study. *Br. J. Psychiatry* **163**, 798–801.

IX MARIHUANA AND AIDS MANAGEMENT

60

Pathogenesis of Malnutrition in HIV Infection

Donald P. Kotler

1. INTRODUCTION

Malnutrition is common in HIV infection and plays an independent and significant role in its morbidity and mortality. Malnutrition was one of the earliest complications of AIDS to be reported and has been one of the most common AIDS-defining diagnoses. There have been major advances in the understanding of the role of malnutrition in HIV infection, including several studies that have documented the ability to improve nutritional status. The potential for providing clinical benefit to patients using nutritional therapies justifies their development and application.

The aim of this presentation is discuss the pathogenesis of nutritional alterations in HIV-infected individuals. The body composition changes associated with HIV infection will be described. The specific pathogenic mechanisms will be presented through the demonstration of clinical-pathologic correlations of specific disease complications. The heterogeneity of potential mechanisms underlying wasting will be emphasized. The interrelationships among the various pathogenic mechanisms and weight loss will be discussed. Recent trends in nutritional status of HIV infection will be discussed, including the syndrome of truncal obesity. The potential role of cannabinoids in the treatment of malnutrition in HIV infection will be reviewed.

2. EFFECT OF HIV INFECTION AND AIDS ON BODY COMPOSITION

The earliest reported nutritional studies were performed in hospitalized AIDS patients between 1981 and 1983 *(1)*. Significant weight loss to an average of 80% of ideal was a universal finding as was evidence of visceral and somatic protein depletion. Several other studies also documented significant weight loss in AIDS patients.

Sophisticated measurements of body composition using high-precision techniques were initiated in 1984. A cross-sectional study in hospitalized, clinically ill AIDS patients with active disease complications demonstrated significant weight loss to 82% of ideal body weight plus a disproportionate loss of body cell mass, to <70% of control *(2)*. The magnitude of body

From: *Marihuana and Medicine*
Edited by: G. G. Nahas et al.   © Humana Press Inc., Totowa, NJ

cell mass depletion was notable, since body fat content was not severely depressed, at least in men. These studies also documented altered distribution of body waters. Total body water and intracellular water volumes were decreased, consistent with the loss of lean mass, which is composed of about 70% water. However, extracellular water volume often was normal or even increased, and the ratio of extracellular-to-intracellular water was often markedly elevated, similar to previous observations in kwashiorkor or severely stressed states.

Further studies demonstrated that the loss of total body potassium was accompanied by depletion of total body nitrogen, a quantitative indicator of protein depletion (3). Skeletal-muscle-modeling studies using CT scans were performed (4) and the results showed that more than one-half of the weight difference between HIV-infected and control men could be ascribed to differences in skeletal muscle mass.

These cross-sectional studies framed the issue of malnutrition in HIV infection for over a decade. However, many of these studies were performed prior to the advent of effective anti-retroviral agents. As such, they represent the natural history of untreated HIV infection and AIDS. More recent studies have shown lesser depletion of body-cell mass, an undoubted consequence of improvements in the medical management of HIV-infected individuals (5). However, the results of these studies likely reflect the situation in much of the world, especially in developing countries, which have not been able to take advantage of treatment developments.

Body composition analyses also were applied to the question of differing pathogenic mechanisms (see below). Starvation and cachexia represent the two major classes of malnutrition. Either may exist in HIV-related wasting syndrome, and they may coexist. Starvation is defined as deprivation of food, either voluntary or involuntary, that leads to weight loss. Nutrient malabsorption, which may occur in HIV-infected individuals, can be viewed as a form of starvation. Metabolic adaptations limit the loss of lean mass during uncomplicated starvation. In contrast, cachexia is characterized by a disproportionate loss of lean body mass that results from specific alterations in intermediary metabolism. These metabolic alterations are an integral part of the body's defense as they provide energy and substrate needed to fuel the body's response to illness or injury. The key distinguishing factor between starvation and cachexia is that the effects of starvation can be reversed by providing food, while the nutritional alterations associated with cachexia are resistant to the effects of feeding.

The relative effects of malabsorption and systemic infection upon body composition were analyzed. The relative depletion of total body potassium and total body nitrogen were compared in patients (3). Both subgroups were significantly depleted of potassium and nitrogen. However, the patients with malabsorption had markedly greater relative losses of potassium than of nitrogen, reflecting the excess losses of electrolytes as a consequence of intestinal dysfunction. Studies also examined the effect of pathogenic mechanism upon hydration status (3a). Wasting was associated with a decrease in intracellular water volume as shown previously. The patients with malabsorption had greater depletion of total body water, compared to HIV-positive subjects without malabsorption and to controls. The hydration coefficient (TBW/FFM), which varies over a very narrow range in a variety of mammals, was calculated. The results showed that subjects with systemic infections were overhydrated, as shown previously. In contrast, patients with malabsorption had significant decreases in TBW/FFM, indicating chronic dehydration.

Other studies have extended these cross-sectional observations. Body composition studies, using bioimpedance analysis, showed that the depletion of body-cell mass preceded the progression to AIDS, implying that malnutrition may be a consequence of the underlying viral infection and inflammatory response, rather than accompany the complications of AIDS (6). In contrast, clinical stability may be associated with nutritional stability (7). Weight loss often is episodic and related to an acute event, often a specific disease complication (8).

Emerging data suggests that sex, race, environment, and comorbid diseases also affect body composition. Malnutrition in children is manifested as growth failure, that is a decrease in the rate of increase in linear height.

3. PAHOGENIC MECHANISMS UNDERLYING WASTING

Many studies have shown that the development of malnutrition in HIV infection is multifactorial. Pathogenic mechanisms vary as a function of disease stage as well as specific disease complications. The pathogenesis of malnutrition in such patients is related to specific pathologic processes that affect either nutrient intake, nutrient absorption, or intermediary metabolism.

There are many causes of decreased food intake, including oropharyngeal and esophageal pathology; psychosocial and economic factors; fatigue; focal or diffuse neurological diseases; and anorexia caused by medications, malabsorption, or systemic infection. Food avoidance also may be due to fear of fecal incontinence. Active systemic infections are associated with profound anorexia that is believed to be mediated by proinflammatory cytokines and acts at central and peripheral levels (9). Intestinal dysfunction with malabsorption also may be associated with decreased food intake (10).

Intestinal dysfunction with nutrient malabsorption is a common and important cause of wasting, especially in late-stage patients. Intestinal injury and malabsorption are related more to specific disease complications that to the underlying HIV infection or immune deficiency per se (11). Chronic infection with an enteric pathogen can be detected in a majority of such patients (12). Malabsorption may occur as a result of several types of intestinal injury causing malabsorption by distinct pathogenic mechanisms. The most common cause of malabsorption is due to decreased intestinal epithelial surface area as a result of primary enterocyte infections by the protozoa, *Cryptosporidia, Isospora,* and *Microsporidia.*

Exudative enteropathy is another type of malabsorption found in AIDS patients, and is most often caused by *Mycobacterium avium* (MAC). Intestinal damage is the result of infiltration of macrophages containing mycobacterial organisms into the intestinal lamina propria, and intestinal lymphatics, with resulting lymphatic blockade (13). Malabsorption, particularly of fats, is the result of this process. In addition, enteric protein losses, especially from chylomicrons, may be increased. A third type of malabsorption is the result of ileal dysfunction, which has been associated with a chronic bacterial enteropathy caused by adherence of pathogenic strains of *E. coli (14)* as well as by protozoa.

Several studies have documented metabolic abnormalities in HIV-infected individuals. Most studies have found resting energy expenditure to be elevated (15,16). Protein turnover may be increased in clinically ill patients (17) but normal in clinically stable subjects (18). Other metabolic alterations include hypertriglyceridemia and decreased serum cholesterol concentrations (19). Elevations in serum cortisol concentration with loss diurnal rhythm have been reported (20). Serum testosterone and dihydroepiandosterone (DHEA) concentrations are low in many HIV-infected patients, a prevalence that increases with disease progression (21). Deficiencies in endogenous anabolic factors may promote protein depletion.

4. RELATIVE ROLES OF ALTERED FOOD INTAKE AND ENERGY EXPENDITURE IN PROMOTING WASTING

As noted above, mechanisms underlying wasting are different in people who are starving or who have cachectic diseases. The situation is complicated, since decreased food intake may accompany other diseases. Systemic infections also may lead to alterations in gastrointestinal physiology, with an adverse impact upon absorption. Furthermore, the body undergoes adaptive responses in response to malnutrition, which may moderate the observed changes. However, regardless of the underlying mechanism, weight loss ultimately is a consequence of negative caloric balance. For macronutrient status to be stable, total energy intake and total energy expenditure (TEE) must be equal (accounting for the efficiency of nutrient absorption). TEE is the sum of resting energy expenditure (REE), also known as basal metabolic rate, voluntary energy expenditure, and energy expended in digestion.

Grunfeld and his colleagues compared the effects of caloric intake and REE upon short-term weight change (one month) in HIV-infected subjects at various disease stages and in controls (22). The study groups included HIV-positive non-AIDS, asymptomatic AIDS, and AIDS plus a secondary infection. The AIDS patients with secondary infections lost weight, whereas the other groups had stable weights. Food intake was decreased in the AIDS patients with infections and normal in the other groups. In contrast, REE was equally elevated in asymptomatic AIDS patients and in AIDS patients with infections. Short-term weight change was significantly correlated with food intake and not with REE.

The results of this important study were confirmed by Macallan and his colleagues (22a). In this longitudinal study, weight-stable patients had adequate energy intake, whereas weight-losing patients had decreased intake. The investigators extended these observations by making measurements of total energy expenditure. They reasoned that calorie balance is directly related to TEE and not to REE, and made measurements of both REE and TEE, the latter by the double-labeled water technique. They found an increase in REE in HIV-infected subjects whether or not they were losing weight. However, TEE was reduced in patients undergoing weight loss, whereas TEE was normal in patients who had either stable weight or weight gain. Thus, weight loss was caused by decreased food intake and not to excess energy expenditure. In addition, since REE was elevated or normal in weight-losing subjects, the reduction in TEE could be attributed primarily to a reduction of voluntary energy expenditure. Fatigue and lethargy are physical correlates of decreased voluntary energy expenditure in HIV infection. Weight loss occured because the decrease in food intake exceeded the decrease in energy expenditure. A major promoting factor was the lack of a fall in REE during weight loss, a characteristic of uncomplicated starvation (23).

5. TRUNCAL OBESITY IN PATIENTS TREATED WITH COMBINATION ANTIRETROVIRAL THERAPIES

Advances in the antiviral treatment of HIV infection coupled with developments in the prophylaxis and therapy of opportunistic infections have changed the outlook for long-term health of HIV-infected individuals. Death rates have halved and the incidence rates of serious complications, including malnutrition have fallen markedly. Yet, nutritional status does not return to normal in many people. Weight gain is variable, and an uncertain percentage of people notice a striking increase in waist size. A variety of metabolic alterations also are being reported, with uncertain relationship to the weight gain. It is widely believed to be a side effect of protease inhibitor therapy. Its significance and consequences are unknown.

The first patients were recognized about 18 months ago because of a sudden increase in waist size (truncal obesity), or because of the development of a fatty mass (Buffalo hump) at the back of the neck. These developments occured several months after starting combination therapy. A report from the FDA noted reports of diabetes mellitus in patients receiving protease inhibitors soon followed. Other patients were found to have hypertriglyceridemia, though this abnormality was first reported more than 8 years ago to be associated with HIV infection, in the presence or absence of disease complications. Patients with hypertriglyceridemia prior to starting therapy appear to have an exacerbation of the abnormality while on therapy, rather than returning to normal. In other patients, serum cholesterol concentrations rise, though rarely to dangerously high levels. Some patients developed hypertension. Low serum testosterone concentrations developed or preexisting hypogonadism persisted.

The body composition changes in the syndrome are more related to the regional distribution of fat than to the absolute amounts of fat and lean tissue. The most visible alteration is an increase in waist size. Other visible changes include thinning of the skin on the arms and legs, and increased wrinkling of the face, especially in the nasolabial folds. As noted above, a Buffalo hump (dorsocervial fat pad) or enlarged supraclavicular fat pads may be noted. Females also are affected by the syndrome, and the most notable changes in addition to increased waist size are narrowing of the hips and breast enlargement. An Australian group documented increased truncal fat in a majority (64%) of a group of subjects receiving protease inhibitors, using the technique of dual X ray absorptiometry. In contrast, a cross-sectional studies from New York found a prevalence of truncal obesity of only 2–5%, though no sophisticated measurements were made. A group from the NIH evaluated patients with truncal obesity using a CT scanning technique and found that fat accumulation occured in the intraperitoneal (visceral) compartment, rather than in the subcutaneous compartment. Associations among increased visceral fat, hypertriglyceridemia, and hypercholesterolemia were found in this study. We also have found increased visceral fat, plus pelvic and perinephric fat using a whole-body MRI technique.

Whereas patients superficially resemble those with Cushing's disease, serum cortisol concentration typically is normal, though 24-hour urinary free cortisol may be moderately elevated (unpublished data). Dexamethasone suppression tests have ruled out Cushing's disease in all cases reported. Several studies have documented insulin resistance in patients receiving protease inhibitor therapy, despite good virologic and immunologic effects. In contrast, the incidence of clinical diabetes mellitus is low.

The cause for these changes is unknown. There are two main possibilities. The changes represent a side effect of protease inhibitor therapy. The changes could be unmasked by some effect of protease inhibitors, such as abolishing viral replication.

The Australian study referred to above included studies to identify a possible molecular mechanism for the changes noted. An amino acid sequence in the catalytic site of HIV protease was found to have a significant homology with a low-density-lipoprotein receptor-like protein. This finding suggests a direct effect of the agent upon fat metabolism. The major weakness in the hypothesis that the changes represent a toxic, metabolic effect of protease inhibitors is that some patients with the syndrome are not taking protease inhibitors. Investigators from San Francisco reported that the development of a Buffalo hump was not limited to patients receiving protease inhibitor therapy. We also have observed several patients with the syndrome who were not taking protease inhibitors. Their plasma viral burdens were low. We also have been evaluating the ability of anthropometric measurements to detect the alterations in fat distribution, since data are available on large number of HIV-positive and control subjects studied since 1984. There is preliminary evidence of altered fat distribution was a common phenomenon in HIV-infected subjects studied in the past, prior to the availability of protease inhibitors. However, a few patients were seen in the past who were identical to those being seen currently. At the time, they were one group of "long-term survivors." It is possible that both mechanisms are operative.

A similar syndrome of truncal obesity and metabolic abnormalities has been described in HIV-negative subjects, and is termed Syndrome X. Clinical descriptions of the syndrome sound strangely like those with the HIV-associated syndrome, including the body composition changes in both men and women, glucose intolerance, hyperlipidemia, and hypertension, but also mild elevations in cortisol secretion, and subnormal serum testosterone concentration.

One prominent hypothesis states that the abnormality represents a hypersensitivity of the hypophyseal-pituitary-adrenal axis leading to excess cortisol secretion and insulin resistance. A common thread in the two conditions appears to be the presence of a chronic stress response. The similarities in the findings in HIV-infected individuals are those with Syndrome X is worrisome, since that syndrome is associated with accelerated cardiovascular disease.

6. POTENTIAL ROLE OF CANNABINOIDS IN THE TREATMENT OF HIV-ASSOCIATED MALNUTRITION

Given the current state of knowledge about malnutrition in HIV infection, it is unlikely that cannabinoids would be a primary therapy for this condition. Specifically, the purported mechanism of action, increasing food intake, likely would be ineffective in promoting an increase in body-cell mass or skeletal muscle mass, given the published studies of other strategies designed to increase caloric intake. However, the therapy could find use as adjunctive therapy, i.e., as part of a combination of therapies. For example, appetite stimulation might be of assistance in patients with diminished appetite who are undergoing exercise therapy or anabolic agent therapy.

There is little published information about the potential effectiveness of cannabinoids, which is limited to a synthetic THC (dronabinol). Short-term (6 weeks) and long term (1 year) therapy with dronabinol was associated with an increase in appetite, as determined by a visual analog scale, but not with weight gain (24,25). A randomized, open label study comparing dronabinol and megestrol acetate, alone or in combination, upon body weight (26). Dronabinol was not associated with weight gain, whereas high-dose megesterol acetate promoted weight gain. No studies have formally evaluated any other cannabinoid preparation.

Evaluation of the effect of THC or other cannabinoids upon nutritional status in HIV-infected people will have to be done starting with phase *I* studies, evaluating safety, efficacy, and dose-responsiveness for each specific preparation. Given the potential for cannabinoids to alter people's perceptions, objective as opposed to subjective endpoints will be needed.

CONCLUSION

Knowledge of the pathogenic mechanisms has grown steadily over the past five years. Understanding of the complex changes that occur are important in designing effective nutritional therapies. The knowledge gained from studies in HIV infection also might be extrapolated to other states of malnutrition with similar pathogenic mechanisms.

REFERENCES

1. Kotler, D. P., Gaetz, H. P., Klein, E. B., Lange, M., and Holt, P. R. (1984) Enteropathy associated with the acquired immunodeficiency syndrome. *Ann. Intern. Med.* **101,** 421–428.
2. Kotler, D. P., Wang, J., and Pierson, R. N. (1985) Studies of body composition in patients with the acquired immunodeficiency syndrome. *Am. J. Clin. Nutr.* **42,** 1255–1265.
3. Kotler, D. P., Tierney, A. R., Dilmanian, F. A., Kamen, Y., Wang, J., Pierson, R.N. Jr, and Weber, D. (1991) Correlation between total body potassium and total body nitrogen in patients with acquired imunodeficiency syndrome. *Clin. Res.* **39,** 649A.
3a. Babameto, G., Kotler, D. P., Burastero, S., Wang, J., and Pierson, R. N. (1994) Alterations in hydration in HIV-infected individuals. *Clin. Res.* **42,** 279A.
4. Wang, Z. M., Visser, M., Ma, R., Baumgartner, R. N., Kotler, D. P., Gallagher, D., and Heymsfield, S. B. (1996) Skeletal muscle mass: Validation of neutron activation and dual energy X-ray absorptiometry methods by computerized tomography. *J. Appl. Physiol.* **80,** 824–831.
5. Mulligan, K., Tai, V. W., and Schambelan, M. (1997) Cross-sectional and longitudinal evaluation of body composition in men with HIV infection. *J. Acquir. Immunodefic. Syndr.* **15,** 43–48.

6. Ott, M., Lambke, B., Fischer, H., Jagre, R., Polat, H., Geier, H., Rech, M., Staszeswki, S., Helm, E. B., and Caspary, W.F. (1993) Early changes of body composition in human immunodeficiency virus-infected patients: tetrapolar body impedance analysis indicates significant malnutrition. *Am. J. Clin. Nutr.* **57**, 15–19.

7. Kotler, D. P., Tierney, A. R., Brenner, S. K., Couture, S., Wang, J., and Pierson, R. N. Jr. (1990) Preservation of short-term energy balance in clinically stable patients with AIDS. *Am. J. Clin. Nutr.* **57**, 7–13.

8. Macallan, D. C., Noble, C., Baldwin, C., Foskett, M., McManus, T., and Griffin, G. E. (1993) Prospective analysis of patterns of weight change in stage IV human immunodeficiency virus infection. *Am. J. Clin. Nutr.* **58**, 417–424.

9. Moldawer, L. L., Anderson, C., Gelin, J., and Lundholm, K. G. (1988) Regulation of food intake and hepatic protein synthesis by recombinant-derived cytokines. *Am. J. Physiol.* **254**, G450–456.

10. Sclafani, A., Koopmans, H. S., Vasselli, J., and Reichman, M. (1978) Effects of intestinal bypass surgery on appetite, food intake, and body weight in obese and lean rats. *Am. J. Physiol.* **234**, E389–398.

11. Kotler, D. P., Reka, S., Chow, K., and Orenstein, J. M. (1993) Effects of enteric parasitoses and HIV infection upon small intestinal structure and function in patients with AIDS. *J. Clin. Gastro.* **16**, 10–15.

12. Kotler, D. P. and Orenstein, J. M. (1994) Prevalence of intestinal microsporidiosis in HIV-infected individuals referred for gastroenterological evaluation. *Am. J. Gastroenterol.* **89**, 1998–2002.

13. Roth R. I., Owen, R. L., Keren, D. F., and Volberding, P. A. (1985) Intestinal infection with *Mycobacterium avium* in acquired immunodeficiency syndrome (AIDS): histological and clinical comparison with Whipple's disease. *Dig. Dis. Sci.* **30**, 497–500.

14. Kotler, D. P., Giang, T. T., Thiim, M., Nataro, J. P., Sordillo, E. M., and Orenstein, J. M. (1995) Chronic bacterial enteropathy in patients with AIDS. *J. Infect. Dis.* **171**, 552–558.

15. Hommes, M. J. T., Romijn, J. A., Godfried, M. H., Eeftinck Schattenkerk, J. K. M., Buurman, W. A., Endert, E., and Sauerwein, H. P. (1990) Increased resting energy expenditure in human immunodeficiency virus-infected men. *Metabolism* **39**, 1186–1190.

16. Melchior, J-C., Salmon, D., Rigaud, D., Leport, C., Bouvet, E., Detruchis, P., Vilde, J-L., Vachon, F., Coulaud, J-P., and Apfelbaum, M. (1991) Resting energy expenditure is increased in stable, malnourished HIV-infected patients. *Am. J. Clin. Nutr.* **53**, 437–441.16.

17. Macallan, D. C., McNurlan, M. A., Milne, E., Calder, A. G., Garlick, P. J., and Griffin, G. E. (1995) Whole body protein turnover from leucine kinetics and the resopnse to nutrition in human immunodeficiency virus infection. *Am. J. Clin. Nutr.* **61**, 818–826.

18. Salbe, A. D., Kotler, D. P., Soave, R., Matthews, D. E., Wang, J., Ma, R. M., Pierson, R. N., and Campbell, R. G. (1995) Protein turnover and resting metabolic rate (RMR) are normal in asymptomatic, HIV-infected men. *Clin. Res.* **43**, 370A.

19. Grunfeld, C., Kotler, D. P., Hamadeh, R., Tierney, A., Wang, J., Pierson, R. N. Hypertriglyceridemia in the acquired immunodeficiency dyndrome. *Am. J. Med.* **86**, 27–31.

20. Villette, J. M., Bourin, P., Doinel, C., Mansour, I., Feit, J., Boudou, P., Dreux, C., Roue, R., Debord, M., and Levi, F. (1990) Circadian variations in plasma levels of hypophyseal, adrenocortical and testicular hormone in men infected with human immunodeficiency virus. *J. Clin. Endocrinol. Metab.* **70**, 572–577.

21. Coodley, G. O., Loveless, M. O., Nelson, H. D., and Coodley, M. K. (1994) Endocrine function in the HIV wasting syndrome. *J. Acq. Immunodefic. Syndr.* **7**, 46–51.

22. Grunfeld, C., Pang, M., Shimizu, L., Shigenaga, J. K., Jensen, P., and Feingold, K. R. (1992) Resting energy expenditure, caloric intake, and short-term weight change in human immunodeficiency virus infection and AIDS. *Am. J. Clin. Nutr.* **55**, 455–460.

22a. Macallan, D. C., Noble, C., Baldwin, C., Jebb, S. A., Prentice, A. M., Coward, W. A., Sawyer, M. B., McManus, T. J., and Griffin, G. E. (1995) Energy expenditure and wasting in human immunodeficiency virus infection. *N. Engl. J. Med.* **333**, 83–88.

23. Heshka, S., Yang, M. U., Wang, J., Burt, P., and Pi-Sunyer, F. X. (1990) Weight loss and change in resting metabolic rate. *Am. J. Clin. Nutr.* **52**, 981–986.

24. Beal J. G., Olson, R., Laubenstein, L., et al. (1995) Dronabinol as treatment for anorexia associated with weight loss in patients with AIDS. *J. Pain Symptom Manag.* **10**, 89–97.

25. Beal JG, Olson R, Lefkowitz L, et al. (1997) Long term efficacy and safety of dronabinol for acquired immunodeficiency syndrome-associated anorexia. *J. Pain Symptom Manag.* **14**, 7–14.

26. Timpone, J. G., Wright, D. J., Li, N., Egorin, M. J., Enama, M. E., Mayers, J., and Galetto, G. (1997) The safety and pharmacokinetics of single-agent and combination therapy with megestrol acetate and dronabinol for the treatment of HIV wasting. *AIDS Res. Hum. Retroviruses.* **13**, 305–315.

61

The Safety and Pharmacokinetics of Single-Agent and Combination Therapy with Megestrol Acetate and Dronabinol for the Treatment of HIV Wasting Syndrome

Joseph G. Timpone, David J. Wright, Ning Li, Merrill J. Egorin, Mary E. Enama, Jacqueline Mayers, Giorgio Galetto, and the DATRI 004 Study Group *

Abstract

This randomized, open-labeled, multicenter study was designed to assess safety and pharmacokinetics of dronabinol (Marinol) tablets and megestrol acetate (Megace) micronized tablets, alone and in combination, for treatment of HIV wasting syndrome. Weight and quality-of-life data were also collected. Fifty-two patients (mean CD4+ count, 59 cells/mL) were randomized to one of four treatment arms: dronabinol 2.5 mg twice/day (D); megestrol acetate 750

* DATRI 004 Study Group includes the following:
Suzanne Gagnon, M.D., Jeri Vargo, R.N., University of Kansas School of Medicine, Wichita, Kansas.
Keith Chirgwin, M.D., Adrien Marcel, M.D., State University of New York Health Science Center, Brooklyn, New York.
David Cohn, M.D., Beverly Hopkins, R.N., Denver Public Health Administration and Disease Control, Denver, Colorado.
Michael Dudley, Pharm.D., Sandra Geletko, Pharm.D., University of Rhode Island College of Pharmacy, Providence, Rhode Island.
Harold Standiford, M.D., Karen Cervino, R.N., University of Maryland School of Medicine, Baltimore, Maryland.
David M. Mushatt, M.D., M.P.H., Debra Greenspan, R.N., Tulane University School of Medicine, New Orleans, Louisiana.
William Powderly, M.D., Mark Meyers, R.N., Washington University School of Medicine, St. Louis, Missouri.
James H. Sampson, M.D., Gregory McMillan, P.A., The Research and Education Group, Portland, Oregon.
Richard Novak, M.D., Luiz Moreira, M.D., University of Illinois-Chicago, Illinois.

From: *Marihuana and Medicine*
Edited by: G. G. Nahas et al.   © Humana Press Inc., Totowa, NJ

mg/day (M750); megestrol acetate 750 mg/day+dronabinol 2.5 mg twice/day (M750+D); or megestrol acetate 250 mg/day+dronabinol 2.5 mg twice/day (M250+D). After therapy initiation, 47 patients returned for at least one visit, and 39 completed the planned 12 weeks of study visits. Occurrence of adverse events, drug discontinuation, new AIDS-defining conditions, or $CD4^+$ T-lymphocyte changes were not statistically significant different among arms. Serious adverse events related to dronabinol included CNS events (e.g., confusion, anxiety, emotional lability, euphoria, hallucinations) and those related to megestrol acetate included dyspnea, liver enzyme changes, and hyperglycemia. The mean weight change ± SE over 12 weeks was as follows: D, −2.0 ± 1.3 kg; M750, + 6.5 ± 1.1 kg; M750 + D, +6.0 ± 1.0 kg; and M250+D, −0.3 ± 1.0 kg (difference among treatment arms, p = 0.0001). Pharmacokinetic parameters measured after two weeks of therapy for M750 were C_{max} = 985 ng/mL and AUC = 22,487 ng × h/mL, and for dronabinol and its active metabolite (HO-THC), respectively, were C_{max} = 2.01; 4.61 ng/mL and AUC = 5.3; 23.7 ng × h/mL. For megestrol acetate, but not dronabinol, there was a positive correlation at week 2 between both C_{max} and AUC with each of the following: weight change, breakfast visual analog scale for hunger (VASH) score, and dinner VASH score.

1. INTRODUCTION

The course of the acquired immunodeficiency syndrome (AIDS) is complicated, in approximately 18% of cases, by HIV wasting syndrome (1). The presence of anorexia, profound involuntary weight loss, unexplained fever, diarrhea, weakness, and multiple nutrient deficiencies is of particular concern in that they may exacerbate the primary illness, decrease survival, and decrease the quality of life (2). Analysis of weight loss as a function of time before death suggests that, in the presence of HIV wasting syndrome, body weight at death extrapolates to about 66% of ideal body weight (3). The pathophysiologic mechanism for this syndrome is not known although a number of putative mechanisms have been described (4). In the presence of AIDS, the relationship between caloric intake and energy expenditure is disturbed (5,6), and it has been observed that in HIV wasting there may be loss of body cell mass with little loss of fat (3). Among the pharmacologic remedies in use by patients with AIDS to offset weight loss and improve caloric intake are megestrol acetate and dronabinol.

Megestrol acetate is a synthetic progestational drug, first approved for use as a palliative treatment for advanced carcinoma of the breast or endometrium. The weight gain observed in cancer clinical trials of megestrol acetate (7–9) stimulated interest in this agent as a treatment for HIV-associated cachexia. Its use for this indication has been reviewed by Von Roenn (10) and two large placebo-controlled studies of megestrol acetate in the treatment of HIV wasting syndrome (11,12) have shown that, compared to placebo, there was a statistically significant weight gain in those receiving 400 mg/day (11) or 800 mg/day (11,12). In 1993, megestrol acetate oral suspension was approved by the Food and Drug Administration (FDA) for the treatment of anorexia, cachexia, or an unexplained significant weight loss in patients with a diagnosis of AIDS.

Δ^9-Tetrahydrocannabinol (THC; dronabinol), a component of marijuana, was first developed for treatment of nausea and vomiting associated with cancer chemotherapy and it is administered over a dose range of 2.5 to 20 mg/day in divided doses *(13)*. Studies in patients with cancer-related cachexia provided the basis for the dronabinol doses selected for studies in AIDS patients *(13,14)* and small studies of dronabinol in patients with HIV infection suggested a trend toward weight stabilization and enhanced appetite and mood *(15,16)*. A larger placebo-controlled trial in patients with AIDS indicated the dronabinol group had significantly greater improvement in appetite and nausea than the placebo group and showed a trend toward weight stabilization *(17)*. In 1992, dronabinol received FDA approval for treatment of anorexia associated with weight loss in patients with AIDS.

In this era of prophylaxis for multiple opportunistic pathogens, it is expected that the incidence of HIV wasting syndrome will increase. Therefore, it is imperative to explore additional pharmacologic approaches to the treatment of this complication. Megestrol acetate increases fat synthesis and appears to act on the central nervous system (CNS) as an appetite stimulant (reviewed in ref. *4*). Dronabinol acts on the CNS as an appetite stimulant and antiemetic (reviewed in ref. *4*). The two drugs have different mechanisms of action and the most frequent side effects of each are nonoverlapping. We undertook a clinical trial of these two drugs, alone and in combination, in persons with HIV wasting syndrome. The objectives of this study were to obtain data on the safety of administering megestrol acetate and dronabinol as single agents or in combination to patients with HIV wasting syndrome; to obtain preliminary data on the efficacy of single-agent and combination therapy with megestrol acetate and dronabinol with regard to weight gain, appetite increase, and quality of life in this patient population; and to obtain steady-state pharmacokinetics data when megestrol acetate and dronabinol are administered as single agents and in combination.

2. MATERIALS AND METHODS

2.1. Study Design

This multicenter, open-label, randomized study was designed to assess the safety and pharmacokinetics of megestrol acetate (Megace; Bristol-Myers Squibb, Princeton, NJ) and dronabinol (Δ^9-tetrahydrocannabinol, Marinol; Unimed,/Roxane Laboratories, Columbus, OH) when given alone and in combination to patients with HIV wasting syndrome. Megestrol acetate was provided in the form of 250-mg micronized tablets and dronabinol was provided as 2.5-mg tablets. At the time the study was developed, these drugs were not yet approved by the FDA for HIV-associated cachexia and anorexia, and the megestrol acetate 250-mg micronized tablets were not commercially available. The study was therefore conducted under an Investigational New Drug application (IND) filed with the FDA, Division of Pilot Drugs.

The major criteria for patient eligibility was a clinical diagnosis of HIV wasting syndrome with anorexia and no severe diarrhea. The weight criterion for patient eligibility was either at least 10% weight loss, as compared to a prior documented weight, or a body mass index (BMI) that was low with respect to an age-based suggested range. If the BMI criterion was used, patients had to be 20.5 kg/m^2 for age 18–34 years or 22.5 for age 35 years. The suggested BMI ranges are 19–24, 20–25, 21–26, and 22–27 kg/m^2 for age categories 18–24, 25–34, 35–44, and 45–54 years, respectively *(18)*. Other inclusion criteria were as follows: HIV infection, 18 years of age or older, a diagnosis of HIV wasting syndrome with anorexia but no severe diarrhea, Karnofsky performance status 60%, life expectancy greater than four months, adequate organ function as measured by specified laboratory parameters, able to tolerate oral intake, and stable dose of any concomitant medications (four weeks for antiretroviral therapy or one week for all other medications). Exclusion criteria were as follows: hospitalization in the prior two weeks, major opportunistic infections in the prior two months, dronabinol or megestrol acetate therapy in the prior two months, marijuana use in the prior one month, anabolic steroid use in the prior three months, pregnancy, active neoplasms (except cutaneous Kaposi's sarcoma or localized skin carcinoma), history of allergy to either study drug, history of psychiatric disorders (except depression), history of thromboembolic events, current drug or alcohol abuse, cardiac arrhythmias, congestive heart failure, diabetes, clinical ascites, uncontrolled hypertension, or requirement for anticonvulsants.

Patients were sequentially enrolled, and the study was performed in an outpatient setting. All subjects signed an informed consent prior to study entry. After enrollment, patients were randomly assigned to one of four open-label treatment arms for 12 weeks of therapy. The study plan called for following patients for 12 weeks, even if study therapy was modified or discontinued. The four treatment arms were as follows:

Arm 1: dronabinol, 2.5 mg twice per day (D).

Arm 2: megestrol acetate, 750 mg once per day (M750).

Arm 3: megestrol acetate, 750 mg once per day and dronabinol, 2.5 mg twice per day (M750+D).

Arm 4: megestrol acetate, 250 mg once per day and dronabinol, 2.5 mg twice per day (M250+D).

In accordance with treatment assignment, patients were instructed to take dronabinol one hour before lunch and one hour before supper; and to take megestrol acetate one hour before lunch. Arm 4 was included to elucidate whether any benefit that might be observed with combination therapy could also be achieved with a lower dose of megestrol acetate. M250 alone was considered a subtherapeutic dose for appetite stimulation and was not included as an arm because the protocol was intended to provide all patients with a therapeutic regimen based on best available knowledge of the drugs at that time.

2.2. Clinical and Laboratory Evaluations

Baseline evaluations included a complete medical history and physical examination (including height, weight, and vital signs), Karnofsky performance status, complete blood count (CBC) with differential and platelets, $CD4^+$ T-lymphocyte count, chemistry panel, visual analog scale for hunger (VASH) three times per day before meals, visual analog scale for mood (VASM) at noon, visual analog scale for nausea (VASN) at noon, and functional assessment for HIV (FAHI) questionnaire. The visual analog scales were completed at home on two weekdays and one weekend day and the FAHI was completed in clinic. Patients were clinically evaluated and weighed every two weeks.

Sites were instructed to record all adverse events regardless of relationship to study therapy. Each adverse event was assigned a severity grade (NIAID Table for Grading Severity of Adult Adverse Experiences) and a COSTART term (*Coding Symbols for Thesaurus of Adverse Reaction Terms*, Food and Drug Administration, 3rd Ed., 1989). Deaths, grade 4 adverse events, and lower-grade adverse events with possible, probable, or definite relation to study drugs were promptly assessed through the IND adverse events reporting system. CBC, $CD4^+$ T-lymphocyte count, and chemistry profile were performed every four weeks. Quality-of-life assessment was accomplished by the following: Karnofsky evaluation every two weeks; completion of VASH, VASM, and VASN three days/week throughout the study; and completion of the FAHI questionnaire every four weeks. After two weeks of therapy, patients who had not missed the last dose prior to the session and had not missed more than one dose of study medication in the five previous days were eligible for a pharmacokinetic evaluation. The assigned study drug(s) were administered in clinic, followed by lunch one hour later. Plasma samples were collected before study drug administration, and 0.5, 1,2,3,4,6,8,12, and 24 hours after administration. Patients taking dronabinol received only one dose on the day of the pharmacokinetic sample collection. For megestrol acetate, blood was collected in tubes with heparin anticoagulant. Plasma was promptly separated by centrifugation and frozen in cryovials. For dronabinol and its active metabolite, blood was collected in tubes with EDTA anticoagulant. Plasma was promptly separated by centrifugation and frozen in silylated glass tubes.

2.3. Determination of Plasma Drug Concentration

Δ^9-tetrahydrocannabinol, its active metabolite, 11-hydroxy-Δ^9-tetrahydrocannabinol, and megestrol acetate were measured simultaneously in human plasma. The procedure included solid-phase extraction and trimethylsilylation of all three compounds, and analysis by capillary gas chromatography combined with positive-ion chemical ionization and selective-reaction monitoring of daughter ions formed by collision-induced dissociation of the protonated molecules of each of the analytes. Deuterated analogs of each compound were added to plasma as internal standards (19). The analyses were performed by Northwest Toxicology, (Salt Lake City, UT) on a Finnigan MAT TSQ 700 tandem mass spectrometer coupled to a Varian model 3400 gas chromatography fitted with a 5% phenylmethylsilicone fused silica capillary column (12.5 × 0.20 mm ???i.d. with a 0.33-mm film thickness).

The measured concentrations were determined by dividing the peak area of the production for each analyte by the peak area of the corresponding internal standard production, and comparing the ratio to a calibration curve generated by fortifying drug-free plasma with known concentrations of each analyte.

The measured concentrations were linear from 0.1 to 20 ng/mL for THC and HO-THC, and from 2.0 to 200 ng/mL for megestrol acetate. Plasma samples that gave quantitative values above the limit of linearity were diluted with drug-free plasma and reanalyzed. The within-run and between-run precision determined at low, medium, and high concentrations gave coefficients of variation of less than 10% for all three analytes.

2.4. Pharmacokinetics Modeling

Pharmacokinetic models were fit to the data of individual patients using an ADAPT II software package (20,21). For each patient receiving megestrol acetate, both one- and two-compartment models were fit to the pharmacokinetic data. Modeling employed least-squares estimation, weighted with linear inverse variance of the output error. Model discrimination was based on Akaike's information criteria (22). For each patient receiving dronabinol, a drug-metabolite model was necessary because the metabolite is active and both drug and metabolite were measured. Modeling of the THC and HO-THC data employed the maximum likelihood estimation method. Individual patients with data that were substantially incomplete or that were not collected with reasonable adherence to protocol were not included in the analysis. On the basis of the individual model used, the pharmacokinetic parameters calculated were the area under the concentration × time curve (AUC), maximum plasma concentration (C_{max}), plasma half-life ($t_{1/2}$), and time to maximum plasma concentration (T_{max}).

2.5. Statistical Methods

Binary outcomes were compared using the Chi-square test of association. The Poisson test for rates was used for counts per unit of time (e.g., number of adverse events per week). Non-parametric tests, such as the Kruskal-Willis test and Spearman rank correlation, were used for continuous or categorical variables, as appropriate.

Laboratory values, weight, and quality of life measures were obtained at multiple times over the study treatment period. A logarithmic transformation was made for most of these variables to provide either variance stabilization or approximate normality. Repeated measures data analyses were used to compare the four treatment arms over time (23). The treatment effect compares the averages of the four arms over all time points, and the time effect tests if the measurement changes over the course of the protocol. The time by treatment interaction then tests the differences among the four treatment-response profiles. All statistical analyses were performed with the use of the SAS system (24).

The FAHI questionnaire is composed of subscale and perception scores in six categories (physical well-being, social/family well-being, relationship with doctor, emotional well-being, fulfillment/contentment, and additional concerns). Scores were calculated according to the method of Cella et al. (25) and evaluated for treatment arm and time effects as noted above.

Given that many significance tests were performed among sets of variables possibly related to toxicity and efficacy, some were likely to achieve nominal levels of statistical significance because of chance alone. Critical values for statistical tests were not adjusted using multiple comparison techniques, because had they been used, the chance of recognizing some clinically important associations would have been reduced. Rather, results of significance tests were considered simply as indicators for covariates that would be candidates for confirmation in studies with larger sample sizes (26).

2.6. Participating Sites

This study was conducted by the Division of AIDS Treatment Research Initiative (DATRI), National Institute of Allergy and Infectious Diseases (NIAID), National Institutes of Health (NIH), Bethesda, Maryland at the nine clinical sites noted in the DATRI 004 Study Group list. The study was approved by the institutional review board (IRB) of each site and was conducted in accordance with the human experimentation guidelines of the U.S. Department of Health and Human Services.

3. RESULTS

3.1. Accrual and Baseline Characteristics

A total of 52 patients, from nine clinical sites, were enrolled in the study and randomized to one of four treatment arms. Owing to a pharmacy dispensing error, one patient who was randomized to M750 was incorrectly issued M250+D for the entire duration of study participation. This patient's results are analyzed as treated. Fifty patients completed the baseline evaluations; the two noncompletions of baseline were because of failure to appear for scheduled appointments by one patient and prohibition against use of dronabinol by a drug-abuse rehabilitation program for another patient.

The characteristics for the 50 patients who completed the baseline evaluations are shown in Table 1. The patient population was composed predominantly of white men, whose self-reported risk factor for HIV infection was homosexuality. The mean $CD4^+$ T-lymphocyte count ($\pm$ SD) for patients entering this study was 59 ± 95 cells/mL. There were no statistically significant differences among arms for any of the measured baseline characteristics. As the study allowed different options for establishing weight eligibility, it is important to note that 26 patients had documented 10% weight loss and 24 had low BMI with respect to the normal suggested range. At baseline 17 of the 26 patients were enrolled using the weight loss criterion and 1 of the 24 patients enrolled using the low BMI criterion were within the age-based suggested ranges for BMI. Forty-three of the 50 patients were receiving a stable dose

Table 1
Baseline Characteristics of Study Participants[a]

Characteristic	D (n = 12)	M750 (n = 12)	M759 + D (n = 13)	M250 + D (n = 13)	Overall (n = 50)
Gender					
Percent male	83	83	92	92	88
Percent female	17	17	8	8	12
Age (years)	39 (7)	46 (7)	38 (8)	40 (9)	40 (8)
Race					
Percent white	58	58	92	46	64
Percent black	34	42	8	39	30
Percent other	8	0	0	15	6
Weight (kg)	61.2 (9.0)	60.7 (10.7)	63.3 (12.8)	63.2 (11)	62.2 (10.7)
Body mass index, BMI (kg/m^2)	20.5 (2.7)	19.1 (2.1)	20.3 (2.9)	20.2 (2.9)	20.0 (2.7)
Weight criteria used[b]					
Percentage of patients ≥10% weight loss	42	33	62	69	52
Percentage of patients low BMI	58	67	38	31	48
Karnofsky					
Percentage of patients ≥90	50	33	39	46	42
Percentage of patients ≤80	50	68	62	54	58
CD4 (cells/μl)	56 (74)	123 (154)	21 (20)	40 (49)	59 (95)
Hemoglobin (g/dl)	11.5 (1.4)	11.4 (1.7)	11.0 (1.9)	11.0 (2.5)	11.2 (1.9)
Albumin (g/dl)	3.8 (0.5)	3.8 (0.8)	3.9 (0.4)	3.9 (0.4)	3.9 (0.6)
AST (SGOT) (IU/liter)	47 (26)	61 (28)	42 (16)	46 (35)	49 (27)
ALT (SGPT) (IU/liter)	42 (34)	47 (30)	37 (15)	31 (23)	39 (26)
Cholesterol (mg/dl)	145 (46)	143 (32)	155 (46)	153 (46)	149 (42)
Antiretroviral use					
Percent yes	83	83	85	92	86
Percent no	17	17	15	8	14

[a]Results given a percentage or mean (standard deviation).
[b]Weight eligibility was either documented ≥ 10% weight loss or low BMI (defined as ≤20.5 for age 18–34 years: ≤22.5 for aged ≥35 years). All patients had anorexia and a clinical diagnosis of HIV wasting.

of antiretroviral therapy at study entry. This included zidovudine (n = 24), didanosine (n = 12), zalcitabine (n = 6), and stavudine (n = 1). There was no difference across arms with respect to concomitant antiretroviral use.

3.2. Study Therapy Modifications and Discontinuations

Two patients who completed baseline evaluations did not initiate study therapy owing to development of a contraindicating condition by one patient and refusal to accept arm assignment by another. Of the 48 patients who started assigned therapy, 47 patients completed one or more study visits after baseline. Thirty-nine patients completed study visits through week 12. Among the 39 patients who completed the week 12 visit, 28 patients were receiving the assigned doses of study medications, six were receiving a modified dose of study medications, and five had discontinued therapy. Nine patients discontinued study visits prior to week 12. Reasons for study therapy modifications and discontinuations are shown by treatment arm and study completion status in Table 2.

3.3. Patient Safety and Adverse Events

There were no statistically significant differences among arms in the occurrence of adverse events when analyzed by body system, COSTART term, or total number of events of

Table 2
Study Therapy Modifications and Discontinuations by Treatment Arm

| | Reported reason (number of patients) | | | |
Modification/ discontinuation	D (n = 11)	M750 (n = 11)	M750 + D (n = 13)	M250 + D (n = 13)
Study therapy modified; completed study visits through week 12	Confusion[a]/ emotion lability (1)		Anxiety/depression[a] (1) Confusion[a] (1)	Euphoria[a] (1) Anxiety[b] (1) Not specified[b] (1)
Discontinued therapy; completed study visits through week 12		Dyspnea (1)	Cryptosporidiosis[b] (1)	Seizure (1) Dyspnea (1) Tuberculosis[b] (1)
Discontinued therapy; did not complete study visits through week 12	Lymphoma (1) Hallucinations (1) Tuberculosis[b] (1) Somnolence[b] (1) Not specified[b] (1)	Lymphoma (1)	Unable to locate (1) Candida esophagitis[b] (1)	Unable to locate (1)

[a]These grade 3 reported terms are counted under the coded term "mental status change" in Table 3.
[b]In these cases, continuation of assigned therapy was permitted on the basis of type or low-grade severity of event, but the patient requested that therapy by modified or discontinued.

Table 3
Number of Patients with Grade 3 or 4 Adverse Events by Treatment Arm

Event	D (n = 11)	M750 (n = 10)[a]	M750 + D (n = 13)	M250 + D (n = 13)
Asthenia	2	1	5	7
Nausea	0	1	0	1
Vomiting	0	0	0	1
Diarrhea	0	0	1	1
Dyspnea	0	0	1	1
Headache	1	1	0	2
Myasthenia	1	0	1	5
Psychosis	0	1	0	0
Mental status change	1	1	2	1
Hallucinations	1	0	0	0
Seizures	0	0	0	1
All neurological events	2	2	3	3
Deep vein thrombosis	0	0	0	1
Hyperglycemia	0	1	0	0
Leukopenia	2	1	3	2
Anemia	1	1	3	2
AST (SGOT) increase	0	1	1	1
ALT (SGPT) increase	0	0	1	1
Overall (all body systems combined)	7	8	11	11

[a]TEleven patients started therapy on M750, but only 10 returned for 1 or more study visits.

severity grade 3 or higher; however, the study was not adequately powered to detect small differences in the rate of adverse events. Overall, 37 of the 47 (79%) patients who returned after baseline experienced one or more adverse events of grade 3 or 4 severity (*see* Table 3). All of the patients experienced one or more adverse events of grade 1 severity (data not shown). Table 3 shows, by treatment arm, the total number of patients with grade 3 or 4 adverse events, for categories that were frequently reported or sometimes assessed as related to one of the study drugs.

Signs and symptoms of particular concern were analyzed for event rate (severity grade 3) by taking into account the number of weeks each patient was observed. A Poisson test showed no statistically significant difference in the event rate among treatment arms for nausea, vomiting, diarrhea, headache, total neurological events, and total adverse events.

Central nervous system adverse events are known to be associated with dronabinol *(17)*. In this study, 10 patients experienced neurological events of severity grade 3 or 4 (Table 3). Of these, seven were CNS events that required immediate assessment through the IND adverse events reporting system. These events (treatment arm) were reported as follows: confusion and emotional lability (D), hallucinations and somnolence (D), psychosis (M750), anxiety and depression (M750+D), confusion in a patient who also had amblyopia (M750+D), euphoria (M250+D), and seizure (M250+D). The psychosis was noted at the week 12 study visit and assessed as unrelated to megestrol acetate. The seizure was assessed as unrelated to both drugs because the patient was diagnosed with cryptococcal meningitis. The other five CNS events (all grade 3) were assessed as probably related to dronabinol. In response to these events, one patient discontinued all study therapy, whereas four patients had resolution of symptoms following study therapy modification, and completed the study on the modified dose (*see* Table 2).

Hypertension, dyspnea, deep vein thrombosis (DVT), and edema are potential adverse events related to megestrol acetate. A repeated-measures analysis for mean arterial pressure showed no statistical difference among treatment arms over the course of the study. Two episodes of dyspnea (M750, grade 2; M250+D, grade 3) were reported as possibly related to megestrol acetate. In both cases all study therapy was discontinued (*see* Table 2). The only DVT (M250+D) was considered a complication of hospitalization for cryptococcal meningitis. There was one report of edema (M750+D, grade 1).

There were no statistically significant differences among treatment arms over the study period for any laboratory parameter (repeated-measures analysis applied to hemoglobin, white-blood-cell count, absolute neutrophil count, platelet count, glucose, bilirubin, AST, ALT, albumin, total protein, cholesterol, triglycerides, amylase, blood urea nitrogen, and creatinine). Three patients developed liver function changes that met criteria requiring assessment through the IND adverse events reporting system. One patient (M750) developed grade 3 AST elevation and grade 2 ALT elevation at week 8, which resolved when megestrol acetate was discontinued but recurred by week 12 after rechallenge. This was assessed as probably related to megestrol acetate. One patient (M750+D) developed grade 3 AST and ALT elevations at week 12, which was assessed as possibly related to both study drugs. One patient (M250+D) developed grade 3 elevations of alkaline phosphatase and g-glutamyl transpeptidase, which were assessed as unlikely to be related to study drugs owing to study drug noncompliance and potentially hepatotoxic concomitant medications. One other laboratory change assessed as probably related to megestrol acetate (M750) was grade 3 hyperglycemia.

A repeated-measures analysis was applied to the CD4$^+$ T-lymphocyte counts. There were large variations in CD4$^+$ T-lymphocyte counts throughout the study, but there were no statistically significant changes from baseline overall or differences among treatment arms over the 12 weeks of study. On the basis of the repeated-measures analysis, the mean ($\pm$ SD) CD4$^+$ T-lymphocyte count was 57 $\pm$ 108 cells/mL at week 12.

3.4. AIDS-Defining Conditions and Patient Deaths

An analysis of AIDS-defining conditions was performed using the Poisson test. There were no statistically significant differences in the event rate among the four treatment arms. Twenty-two new AIDS-defining events in 19 patients were diagnosed between the start of therapy through week 12. These included *Candida* esophagitis ($n = 5$), disseminated *Mycobacterium avium* complex ($n = 4$), bacterial pneumonia ($n = 4$), *Mycobacterium tuber-*

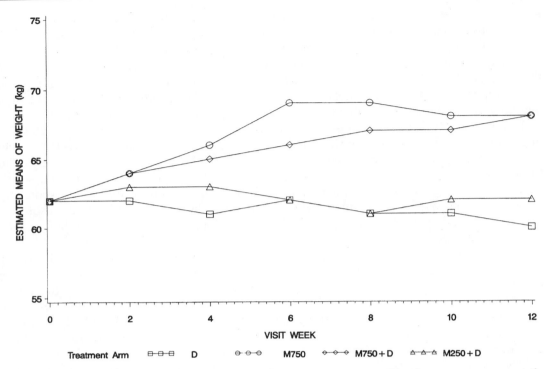

Fig. 1. Estimated mean weight by study visit week and treatment arm: The four curves represent the repeated measures estimates of weight by visit week based on all available weight data ($n = 47$). The four treatment arms are as follows: D, dronabinol 2.5 mg BID ($n = 11$); M750, megestrol acetate 750 mg QD ($n = 10$); M750+ D, megestrol acetate 750 mg QD and dronabinol 2.5 mg BID ($n = 13$); M250+13, megestrol acetate 250 mg QD and dronabinol 2.5 mg BID ($n = 13$).

culosis ($n = 2$), systemic cytomegalovirus ($n = 2$), and one case each of herpes bronchitis, cryptosporidiosis, cryptococcal meningitis, toxoplasmosis of the CNS, and lymphoma. In addition, two patients were diagnosed with an AIDS-associated malignancy after enrollment, but before initiation of study therapy. These were one patient each with Kaposi's sarcoma and lymphoma. This latter case of lymphoma was in a patient (randomized to M750) who died from a fulminant course without completing any study visits after baseline. Another death occurred within the 30 days after last study therapy. This was a patient who completed week 12 on the M750+D arm, was hospitalized with a diagnosis of adult respiratory distress syndrome about one week later, and died of respiratory failure two weeks after completion of study participation. Both deaths were assessed as unrelated to study therapy.

3.5. Weight Change

Weight was measured at every clinic visit following standard clinical practice. Figure 1 shows the repeated measures analysis of weight, which takes into account all weight measurement on all 47 patients who had at least one weight measurement after starting study therapy. There are statistically significant differences in average weight change among the four treatment arms ($p = 0.0001$). Patients receiving M750 or M750+D, on average, gained weight, and patients receiving D or M250 + D, on average, did not gain weight. The mean weight change ± standard error by treatment arm was as follows: D = –2.0 ± 1.3 kg; M750 =

+6.5 ± 1.1 kg; M750+D = +6.0 ± 1.0 kg; and M250+D = –0.3 ± 1.0 kg. The increase in weight on the M750 and M750+D arms was most rapid in the first six weeks and slowed or remained stable for the remainder of the trial. Because normal patient weight varies by height, a repeated measures analysis of body mass index (BMI) was also performed. For the M750 and M750+D treatment arms the mean increase in BMI was 2 kg/m^2 from the baseline mean BMI of 20 kg/m^2. Finally, if viewed as a percentage weight gain, there was an average 11% weight gain for patients receiving M750 or M750+D.

3.6. Quality-of-Life Measures

A repeated-measures analysis was applied to the Karnofsky performance status score, FAHI questionnaire data, and visual analog data. Karnofsky performance status scores indicated no statistically significant change from baseline or difference among arms (data not shown). Repeated-measures analysis for each FAHI subscale and perception score did not demonstrate a statistically significant difference among the four treatment arms for any subscale or perception score over the course of the study. Since no differences among arms were demonstrated, the four treatment arms are assumed to have the same response profile. The study population (all arms combined) did show some statistically significant changes from baseline for two of the perception scores, but not for any of the subscale scores. For this study population, the perception score means (on a scale of 0 to 10) showed improvement at week 4 for the categories social/family (baseline = 6.8, week 4 = 7.8; p = 0.005), and additional concerns affecting quality of life (baseline = 7.0, week 4 = 8.0; p = 0.003). These values showed no statistically significant change from the week 4 values for the remainder of the study period.

Visual analog scales for mood and nausea showed no statistically significant difference among arms or change over time for the study population. The visual analog scale for hunger was analyzed as the cumulative weekly score for each meal, in which the possible weekly score ranged from 0 (extremely hungry) to 330 (not hungry at all). There was no statistically significant difference among treatment arms; however, for the study population, after one week of therapy, the VASH showed an improvement in the weekly sum score for breakfast from 170 to 133 (p = 0.0002), for lunch from 193 to 112 (p = 0.0001), and for dinner from 192 to 114 (p = 0.0001). These values showed no statistically significant change after week 1.

3.7. Pharmacokinetics

On the three megestrol acetate-containing arms, 34 of the 37 patients who initiated therapy participated in pharmacokinetic sessions. For 30 patients, a one-compartment model, with first-order absorption and excretion, was most appropriate. For the other four patients (M750+D = 3 and M250+D = 1), a two-compartment model with first-order absorption provided a better fit. The data for five patients (M750 = 2 and M250+D = 3) were excluded from the analysis because of inadequate adherence to protocol. Table 4 shows the pharmacokinetic parameters for the 29 evaluable patients by treatment arm. The $t_{1/2}$ value for megestrol acetate could not be determined accurately, as the sampling period of 24 hours is shorter than the $t_{1/2}$ of about 30 hours, reported by others (27,28). Shown for comparison are data from another study in which nine male, cachectic patients with AIDS were evaluable for steady-state pharmacokinetic parameters after receiving megestrol acetate oral suspension 800 mg/day for 21 days (27).

When M750 and M750+D data are compared, there are no statistically significant differences for any of the pharmacokinetic parameters (data not shown), suggesting that concomitant dronabinol therapy does not alter the metabolism or exposure to megestrol acetate. Comparison of the AUC and C_{max} values associated with M250+D to that associated with

Table 4
Pharmacokinetics Parameters for Megestrol Acetate Micronized Table
with Comparison to Oral Suspension

Patient group	C_{max} (ng/ml)	T_{max} (hr)	$T_{1/2}$ (hr)	AUC (ng × hr/ml)
Megestrol acetate micronized tablet				
M750 ($n = 8$)	985.0 (± 538.5)	3.1 (± 1.7)		22,487 (± 17,207)
M750 + D ($n = 12$)	1457.5 (± 1796.8)	5.1 (± 3.2)		24,067 (± 19,199)
M250 + D ($n = 9$)	393.3 (± 365.5)	4.8 (± 2.4)		8200 (± 5344.2)
Megestrol acetate oral suspension, 800 mg/day ($n = 9$)[a]	828 (± 513)	3.6 (± 2.5)	30 (± 9.9)	11,250 (± 7305)

[a]See Graham et al.[27]

Table 5
Pharmacokinetic Parameters (Median and Range) for Dronabinol
and Its Primary Active Metabolite

	C_{max} (ng/ml)	T_{max} (hr)	$T_{1/2}\beta$ (hr)	AUC (ng × hr/ml)
Dronabinol (THC)[a]	2.01 (0.58–12.48)	2.07 (0.66–8.26)	1.45 (0.60–42.1)	5.3 (2.7–35.4)
Metabolite (HO-THC)[a]	4.61 (0.52–37.5)	2.07 (0.49–8.00)	2.11 (0.16–7.9)	23.7 (3.8–63.5)

[a]Data from 20 patients (D = 4, M750 + D = 9, M250 + D = 7).

M750 or M750+D indicates a dose proportionally for megestrol acetate over the dose-range tested.

On the three dronabinol-containing arms, 31 (D = 8, M750+D = 12, and M250+D = 11) of the 37 patients who initiated therapy participated in pharmacokinetic sessions. Prior to the pharmacokinetic session, patients on all three arms received dronabinol, 2.5 mg twice per day. On the day of the pharmacokinetic session, only a single dose was given for the 24-hour period. Three patients (one from each arm) had incomplete datasets. Eight patients (D = 3, M750+D = 2, and M250+13 = 3) had inadequate adherence to protocol. The data from these 11 patients were excluded from the analysis. A three-compartment model with first-order absorption was applied. The median pharmacokinetic data for THC and its active metabolite, HO-THC, from the remaining 20 patients (D = 4, N1750+D, and M250+D = 7) are shown in Table 5. There were no statistically significant differences among the three arms when comparison of the pharmacokinetic parameters was conducted using a Kruskal-Wallis test.

3.8. Pharmacodynamics

Correlation analyses (Spearman correlation method) were performed for megestrol acetate, THC, and HO-THC pharmacokinetic parameters with weight gain and VASH scores. There was no correlation between baseline weight and any pharmacokinetic parameter. There was a positive correlation between megestrol acetate AUC and C_{max} with both absolute weight gain (AUC, $p = 0.03$; C_{max} $p = 0.008$) and percentage change in weight (AUC, $p = 0.02$; C_{max} $p = 0.006$) at week 2. This result implies that megestrol acetate exposure is an important factor in weight gain. Similarly, there was a positive correlation between megestrol acetate AUC and C_{max} with both VASH score for breakfast (AUC, $p = 0.04$; C_{max} $p = 0.004$) and VASH score for dinner (AUC, $p = 0.02$; C_{max}, $p = 0.03$). That is, there is a statistically significant correlation between megestrol acetate exposure and improved appetite at breakfast and dinner.

4. DISCUSSION

HIV wasting syndrome continues to be an important complication in persons with AIDS. In this study, we investigated two agents, megestrol acetate and dronabinol, in an effort to obtain safety data, pharmacokinetic parameters, and preliminary efficacy data with regard to weight gain and quality of life. This study of single-agent and combination therapy includes consideration of pharmacokinetics and pharmacodynamics. Both megestrol acetate and dronabinol are now FDA approved for the patient population studied; however, the 250-mg micronized tablets of megestrol acetate are not commercially available at this time.

This open-label, randomized study enrolled participants with mean CD4+ T-lymphocyte counts of 59 cells/mL, consistent with the advanced disease state that is characteristic of patients with HIV wasting syndrome. The baseline characteristics of the population enrolled are representative of the AIDS population in general. Because the study was primarily designed to evaluate pharmacokinetics and safety, the efficacy results discussed are limited by several factors. These include relatively small sample size, weight eligibility criteria adapted (*see* Subheading 2. and Table 1) to allow enrollment of patients clinically considered to have HIV-associated wasting, but who lacked the documented prestudy weight measures necessary to calculate percent weight loss, and weight data collection by standard clinical practice rather than with rigorous controls (e.g., monitoring of scale calibration, controlling weight measurement with regard to time of day, time from last meal time, and amount of clothing worn).

There were no statistically significant differences across the four treatment arms with regard to study medication discontinuation; however, only 28 (58.3%) of 48 patients who initiated study medications were receiving the full dose at the end of 12 weeks. There were no statistically significant differences across the four treatment groups with respect to frequency of adverse events. Overall, 37 (79%) of the 47 patients with safety data experienced at least one adverse event of severity grade 3 or higher. These events were not necessarily related to study medication. The overall high rate of adverse events reflects the underlying advanced state of HIV infection in the study population. Although our study was not adequately powered to detect small differences across the four treatment groups, there does not appear to be any increased or additive toxicity when megestrol acetate and dronabinol are given in combination.

Among the 37 patients receiving dronabinol alone or in a combination, 5 patients (14%) experienced grade 3 CNS events (confusion, anxiety, emotional lability, euphoria, hallucinations) that were assessed as related to dronabinol. In a trial for AIDS-related anorexia and weight loss, Beal et al. *(17)* reported treatment-related nervous system events in 35% of patients treated with dronabinol, 2.5 mg twice per day, compared to 9% of patients receiving placebo ($p < 0.001$). The nervous system events were categorized as moderate or severe in 24% of the patients receiving dronabinol and 6% of those receiving placebo.

With regard to known side effects of megestrol acetate, there was no evidence of a hypertensive effect or significant edema, and the single episode of DVT was not attributed to megestrol acetate. Two patients discontinued therapy because of dyspnea attributed to megestrol acetate. Von Roenn and colleagues *(11)* noted one case of DVT, an increase or new onset of edema in the 400-mg dose arm, and a 12% incidence of impotence in the 800-mg dose arm. Impotence was not reported in our study; however, this information was not specifically requested in the case report forms. Two patients did develop AST/ALT abnormalities that were judged to be possibly or probably related to megestrol acetate. Larger, randomized, placebo-controlled trials of megestrol acetate have not reported an increased incidence of hepatic toxicity. *(11,12)*.

Nineteen (40%) of 47 patients with safety data developed one or more new AIDS-defining conditions after initiation of study therapy. This high incidence is again consistent with the advanced disease state of the study participants. It has been suggested that HIV wasting syndrome is associated with profound immunologic deterioration and might independently contribute to disease progression *(4)*.

The efficacy results of this study are limited by the factors discussed above, but are consistent with previously published placebo-controlled efficacy trials of each agent. In our study, statistically significant weight gain occurred only in the two treatment arms that included high-dose megestrol acetate (750 mg/day micronized tablets). In previous studies of megestrol acetate, which enrolled patients with at least 10% weight loss, a 400-mg/day *(11)* or 800-mg/day *(11,12)* oral suspension was associated with statistically significant weight gain compared to low-dose megestrol acetate *(11)* or placebo *(11,12)*. A placebo-controlled study of dronabinol, which enrolled patients with AIDS-related anorexia and 2.3 kg weight loss at baseline, suggested a trend toward weight stabilization with dronabinol compared to placebo, but did not demonstrate a statistically significant weight gain *(17)*. In our study, there does not appear to be any additive weight gain effect when dronabinol was given in combination with megestrol acetate or any weight gain effect of dronabinol when given alone. Our data indicate that megestrol acetate at 750 mg/day is associated with an average 11% weight increase over the 12-week study period, and that weight gain should be evident by approximately six weeks after initiation of therapy. We do not have data on body composition and therefore cannot comment on whether the weight gain was associated with increased lean body mass.

With regard to the quality-of-life data, there was no statistically significant difference among the four treatment arms. By one week after initiating therapy, there was a statistically significant improvement overall as compared to baseline for the visual analog scale for hunger. This is consistent with the previously cited studies of dronabinol and megestrol acetate monotherapy *(11,12,17)*.

A complete discussion of the pharmacokinetics modeling for megestrol acetate and dronabinol is beyond the scope of this article; however, a few comments are warranted. The pharmacokinetics data for megestrol acetate were applied to a standard model without difficulty. The dronabinol pharmacokinetics analysis proved to be more complicated. No previous study was identified in the literature in which data for both THC and its active metabolite HO-THC have been simultaneously incorporated into a metabolite model. Different compartmental models were applied to the dronabinol data, and it was found that a three-compartment model with first-order absorption fit most of the data well.

The values for the pharmacokinetic parameters C_{max}, T_{max}, and AUC reported for the micronized tablets of megestrol acetate, in a dose of 750 mg/day, are compatible with parameters previously reported for this formulation *(28)* and show them to provide comparable, and possibly improved, drug exposure when compared with the 800-mg/day oral suspension (*see* Table 4). The pharmacokinetics parameters obtained for THC are similar to those reported in the literature *(29)*. For example, the median β-phase half-life reported for THC ranges from 0.95 to 2.37 hours and our data indicate 1.45 hours. Because samples were collected at steady state for only 24 hours after a dose, the model is limited to alpha and β phases. No drug–drug interactions were obvious when megestrol acetate and dronabinol were administered concomitantly, although the power to detect interactions in this study is low.

The pharmacodynamic data indicate that there is a positive correlation between drug exposure to megestrol acetate and weight gain, as well as improvement in hunger score as measured by the VASH. Previously, weight gain and improvement in well-being were noted to be dose dependent by Von Roenn et al. *(11)* and a relationship between megestrol acetate exposure (i.e., percentage of 24-hour period in which megestrol acetate concentration exceeded 300 ng/ml) and increase in body weight was noted by Graham et al *(27)*. Our data are consistent with these studies and provide further evidence of the pharmacologic basis for response to megestrol acetate. A lack of response to megestrol acetate may be related to problems with drug absorption or rapid clearance. This study, however, does not define an optimal dose, C_{max} or AUC that would result in weight gain. In this study, no pharmacodynamic relationship was noted for dronabinol at a dosage of 5 mg/day. Furthermore, there was no evidence of an enhanced effect on weight gain or the quality-of-life measurements when dronabinol was given in combination with megestrol acetate. This statement is limited by the fact that our study only tested a 5-mg/day dose of dronabinol. Higher doses of dronabinol are unlikely to be well tolerated in this patient population, however, because of the neurological side effects, that were observed in this study and are reported in the literature *(13,17)*.

Weight loss associated with HIV infection continues to be a perplexing problem for both clinicians and patients. Taking into consideration the results of the placebo-controlled trials of monotherapy with the two study agents *(11,12,17)*, our data do not support the need for a large trial of combination megestrol acetate and dronabinol therapy. The use of these drugs as monotherapies serves a palliative role. Both of these agents are appetite stimulants, but in this and cited studies *(11,12)* only high-dose megestrol acetate was associated with statistically significant weight gain. It may be more appropriate to combine one of these agents with an anabolic agent, such as human growth hormone, or a cytokine inhibitor *(4)*. It is hoped that a better understanding of the pathophysiology of HIV wasting syndrome will result in non-toxic, cost-effective pharmacologic approaches to this condition.

ACKNOWLEDGMENTS

This study was supported by NIAID, NIH contract N01–A115123. Bristol-Myers Squibb Company provided the megestrol acetate and Unimed,/Roxane Laboratories provided the dronabinol for this trial. We gratefully acknowledge the study volunteers, the site support staff, and the reviews of the manuscript by Steven Schnittman (Division of AIDS, NIAID, NIH) and Jonas Ellenberg (Westat). Northwest Toxicology performed the chemical analysis of plasma concentrations of megestrol acetate, THC, and HO-THC. Ogden Bioservices (Rockville, MD) managed the DATRI specimen and investigational drug repository.

Reprinted from: AIDS Research and Human Retroviruses, 13(4):305–315, 1997. Mary Ann Liebert, Inc.

REFERENCES

1. Nahlen, B. L., Chu, S. Y., Nwanyanwu, O. C., Berkelman, R. L., Martinez, S. A. and Rullen, J. V.: (1993) HIV wasting syndrome in the United States. *AIDS* **7**, 183–188.
2. Chlebowski, R. T. (1985) Significance of altered nutritional status in acquired immunodeficiency syndrome (AIDS). *Nutr. Cancer* **7**, 85–91.
3. Kotler, D. P., Tierney, A. R., Wang, J. and Pierson, R. N., Jr (1989) Magnitude of body cell-mass depletion and the timing of death from wasting in AIDS. *Am. J. Clin. Nutr.* **50**, 444–447.
4. Weinroth, S. E., Parenti, D. M. and Simon, G. L. (1995) Wasting syndrome in AIDS: pathophysiologic mechanisms and therapeutic approaches *Infect Agents Dis.* **4**, 76–94.

5. Grunfeld, C. and Feingold, K. R. (1992) Metabolic disturbances and wasting in the acquired immunodeficiency syndrome. *N. Engl. J. Med.* **327(5)**, 329–337.

6. Macallan, D. C., Noble, C., Baldwin, C., Jebb, S. A., Prentice, A. M., Coward, A., Sawyer, M. S., McManus, T. J. and Griffen, G. E. (1995) Energy expenditure and wasting in human immunodeficiency virus infection. *N. Engl. J. Med.* **333(2)**, 83–88.

7. Ansfield, F. J., Kailas, G. J. and Singson, J. P. (1982) Clinical results with megestrol acetate in patients with advanced carcinoma of the breast. *Surg. Gynecol. Obstet.* **155**, 888–890.

8. Alexieva-Figusch, J., van Gilse, H. A., Hop, W. C. J., Phoa, C. H., Blonkvon der Wijst, J. and Treurniet, R. E. (1980) Progestin therapy in advanced breast cancer: megestrol acetate-an evaluation of 160 treated cases. *Cancer* **46**, 2369–2372.

9. Tchekmedyian, N. S., Tait, N., Moody, M. and Aisner, J. (1987) High dose megestrol acetate: possible treatment for cachexia. *JAMA* **257(9)**, 1195–1198.

10. Von Roenn, J. H. (1993) Pharmacologic interventions for HIV-related anorexia and cachexia. *Oncology* **7(11 Suppl.)**, 95–99.

11. Von Roenn, J. H., Armstrong, D., Kotler, D. P., Cohn, D. L., Klimas, N. G., Tchekmedyian, N. S., Cone, L., Brennan, P. J. and Weitzmann, S. A. (1994) Megestrol acetate in patients with AIDS-related cachexia. *Ann. Intem. Med.* **121(6)**, 393–399.

12. Oster, M. H., Enders, S. R., Samuels, S. J., Cone, L. A., Hooten, T. M., Browder, 21 H. P. and Flynn N. M. (1994) Megestrol acetate in patients with AIDS and cachexia. *Ann. Intern. Med.* **121(6)**, 400–408.

13. Plasse, T. F., Gorter, R. W., Krasnow, S. H., Lane, M., Shepard, K. V. and 22. Wadleigh, R. G. (1991) Recent clinical experience with dronabinol. *Pharmacol. Biochem. Behav.* **40**, 695–700.

14. Regelson, W., Butler, J. R., Schulz, J., Kirk, T., Peek, L., Green, M. L. and Zalis, M. O. (1976) Tetrahydrocannabinol as an effective antidepressant and appetite-stimulating agent in advanced cancer patients in: *The Pharmacology of Marihuana: A Monograph of the National Institute on Drug Abuse* (Braude, M. C. and Szara, S., eds.). Raven, New York, pp. 763–776.

15. Struwe, M., Kaempfer, S. H., Geiger, C. J., Pavia, A. T., Plasse, T. F., Shepard, K. V., Ries K. and Evans T. G. (1993) Effect of dronabinol on nutritional status in HIV infection. *Ann. Pharmacother.* **27**, 827–831.

16. Gorter, R., Seefried, M. and Volberding, P. (1992) Dronabinol effects on weight in patients with HIV infection. *AIDS* **6**, 127.

17. Beal, J. E., Olson, R., Laubenstein, L., Morales, J. P., Bellman, P., Yangco, B., Lefkowitz, L., Plasse, T. F. and Shepard, K. V. (1975) Dronabinol as a treatment for anorexia associated with weight loss in patients with AIDS. *J. Pain Symptom Manage* **10(2)**, 89–97.

18. Bray, G. (1987) Overweight is risking fate–definition, classification, prevalence and risks. *Ann. NY. Acad. Sci.* **499**, 14–28; and the resulting chart "Suggested Weights for Adults" in the National Institutes of Health, Nutrition Department, Standards of Care-May 1991.

19. Nelson, C. C., Fraser, M. D., Wilfahrt, J. K. and Foltz, R. L. (1993) Gas chromatography/tandem mass spectrometry measurement of Δ^9-tetrahydrocannabinol, naltrexone, and their active metabolites in plasma. *Therapeutic Drug Monogr.* **15(6)**, 557–562.

20. D'Argenio, D. Z. and Schurmitsky, A. (1979) A program package for simulation and parameter estimation in pharmacokinetic systems. *Comput. Prog. Biochern* **9**, 115–134.

21. D'Argenio, D. Z. and Schumitsky, A. (1990) *ADAPT II User's Guide*. Biomedical Simulations Resource, University of Southern California, Los Angeles, Cal.

22. Akaike, H. (1974) A new look at the statistical model identification. *IEEE Trans. Automatic Control* **19**, 716–723.

23. Crowder, M. J. and Hand, D. J. (1990) *Analysis of Repeated Measures*. Chapman & Hall, London, UK.

24. SAS Institute. (1990) *SAS/STAT User's Guide*, version 6. SAS Institute, Inc., Cary, NC.

25. Cella, D. F., Tulsky, D. S., Gray, G., Sarafian, B., Linn, E., Bonomi, A., et al. (1993) The functional assessment of cancer therapy scale: development and validation of the general measure. *J. Clin. Oncol.* **11**, 570–579.

26. Mantel, N. and Haenszel, W. (1959) Statistical aspects of the analysis of data from retrospective studies of disease. *J. Natl. Cancer. Inst.* **22**, 719–749.

27. Graham, K. K., Mikolick, D. J., Fisher, A. E., Posner, M. R. and Dudley, M. N. (1994) Pharmacologic evaluation of megestrol acetate oral suspension in cachectic AIDS patients. *J. AIDS* **7**, 580–586.

28. Gaver, R. C., Pittman, K. A., Reilly, C. M., Goodson, P. J., Breault, G. O. and Fenzl, E. (1986) Evaluation of two new megestrol acetate tablet formulations in humans. *Biopharm. Drug Dispos.* **7**, 35–46.

29. Ohlsson, A., Lindgren, J-E., Wahlen, A., Agurell, S., Hollister, L. E. and Gillespie, H. K. (1980) Plasma delta-9-tetrahydrocannabinol concentrations and clinical effects after oral and intravenous administration and smoking. *Clin. Pharmacol. Ther.* **28(3)**, 409–415.

62

Marihuana for AIDS Wasting

A Critique of the Data

William M. Bennett and Sandra S. Bennett

1. INTRODUCTION

Cachexia, weight loss, and muscular wasting are characteristics of advanced infection with the human immunodeficiency virus (HIV). Death usually occurs when 20% of total body weight is lost. Usually, when an individual develops this syndrome, commonly known as AIDS wasting, it is a poor prognostic sign for survival. The impact of modern treatments for AIDS infections with antiretroviral drugs and protease inhibitors has had a positive impact to increase long-term survival with the disease. AIDS wasting is now becoming much less common. The pathogenesis of AIDS wasting involves poor appetite, inefficient use of caloric intake because of intercurrent diseases, medication-induced gastrointestinal problems (nausea, vomiting, and diarrhea), and the effect of HIV infection itself on muscle and tissue breakdown *(1,2)*.

The association of increased appetite with smoking of *Cannabis sativa* has led to the anecdotal use of smoked crude marihuana in an attempt to prevent or treat AIDS wasting. This would only be justified if the therapeutic intervention was actually shown to be effective. Obviously, the adverse effects of smoking either *Cannabis sativa* or tobacco, particularly in an already immunosuppressed host, raise serious safety questions. Much of the literature in this area is anecdotal and therefore, subject to the bias of placebo effects and self reporting *(3)*. As an example a study reported in 1970 showed that 91% of moderate-to-heavy marihuana users reported eating each time they smoked the drug. Eighty-five percent thought that their intake of food increased to greater quantities when under the influence of the drug than when they did not smoke, with two-thirds of the patients indicating that they would eat even though they were no longer hungry. Others have reported that smoked marihuana inhibits the sensation of satiety *(3)*. Some controlled studies indicate an appetite-stimulating property of marihuana in healthy subjects and in patients with cancer *(4,5)*, although other studies could not confirm this *(6)*. Thus, the application of smoked crude marihuana as a treatment of AIDS wasting would need to be proven by a controlled study since the disadvantages of such therapy in terms of increased risk of pulmonary infection, interaction with other drugs, and other side effects are obvious.

From: *Marihuana and Medicine*
Edited by: G. G. Nahas et al.   © Humana Press Inc., Totowa, NJ

Because there are no scientifically acceptable data regarding smoked marihuana, this book reviews the evidence that bears on this issue from studies using oral Δ^9-tetrahydrocannabinol (dronabinol), which is approved by the Food and Drug Administration (FDA) for AIDS wasting.

The difficulty of studying the appetite-stimulating and cachexia-sparing use of smoked marihuana is admittedly daunting. Appetite increases may be dependent on the user's familiarity with marihuana smoking and the accompanying social aspects often facilitated by its use in groups. These social conditions may not be available for the majority of those patients who try smoking marihuana for AIDS wasting. It has been shown that individuals who respond with increased food intake after marihuana were those who socialized with other marihuana smokers as opposed to those who smoke the drug by themselves (7,8). In addition, marihuana appears to be less effective as an appetite stimulant in older patients or those who are not familiar with marihuana smoking prior to its use as "therapy" (9). Dronabinol, on the other hand, is variably absorbed from the gastrointestinal (GI) tract and its effect on appetite stimulation is also variable, possibly related to complex drug pharmacokinetics (10,11). Patients using Δ^9-THC have reported a very high prevalence of side effects, including sedation, dry mouth, delusions, and inability to carry out the daily functions of life. The optimum dose regimen for appetite stimulation has not been evaluated, and this is important since low doses stimulate intake, whereas higher doses actually inhibit intake (11). Most studies have shown that the stimulation of appetite is dependent on obtaining a subjective feeling of intoxication, although some studies have shown that lower doses of 2.5 mg of tetrahydrocannabinol twice a day may produce benefits even when subjective sensations are minimal. Smoked marihuana leads to higher plasma THC levels with more subjects reporting subjective "high" effects and more reliably increasing appetite compared to oral administration (11). This has not been studied or confirmed in patients with HIV infections or AIDS. Rectal administration in the form of a suppository has been proposed by Mattes et al., and this route is promising for clinical use (3). In the studies of Mattes et al., oral administration of 10–15 mg of Δ^9-THC versus placebo in relatively healthy adult light marihuana users showed increased caloric intake (3). Following chronic dosing by rectal suppository, but not by the oral capsules, there was actual weight gain relative to controls. There was no evidence of impairment of satiety by any route of Δ^9-THC administration and there was no correlation between food intake and age, reported psychological high, or plasma pharmacokinetics (3).

2. STUDIES ON Δ^9-THC IN PATIENTS WITH AIDS WASTING

As mentioned above, much of the information about the utility of marihuana in AIDS wasting is based on anecdotes and the characteristics noted above of the associaton of smoked marihuana with increased food intake. There are some data using the approved drug dronabinol, a pharmacologic oral preparation of Δ^9-THC, which is formulated in 2.5-mg capsules. Gorter et al. showed an increased weight gain in AIDS patients using dronabinol in a short-term study, although there were no control groups in the study and most of the patients had previously been habitual marihuana smokers (12).

Beal et al. carried out a randomized double-blind placebo-controlled appetite stimulation study in 18 centers throughout the United States to evaluate the effect of dronabinol on appetite and weight (13). One hundred thirty-nine patients were enrolled. These patients had to have lost five pounds from their normal body weight and needed to have one AIDS-defining event prior to enrollment in the study. They also had to be able to feed themselves and to consume a normal diet. Retroviral medicines were allowed if the patient had tolerated the medication for at least four weeks prior to the study and the dose was stable at least two weeks prior to the start of the study. Patients who had smoked marihuana within 30 days were not eligible for the study and the participants all agreed not to use marihuana throughout the course of the trial. Of the 139 patients who met enrollment criteria, 72 patients were randomized to receive an oral dose of dronabinol of 2.5 mg orally, administered one hour before lunch and one hour before supper. Sixty-seven patients received a matching placebo. The duration of the study was six weeks. There were no differences in baseline characteristics between patients treated with dronabinol versus placebo. The outcome measurement was a visual analog scale for appetite, as well as a similar scale for nausea and mood. These tests were done at baseline and three times a week after that. A zero score represented no appetite, no nausea, and poor mood, and a 100 score represented the maximum beneficial response. Weight was measured at baseline and twice weekly thereafter. To be included in the results, the patients had to be observed at least four weeks and to have taken 75% of the planned medication regimen and to be free of protocol violations (mainly smoking marihuana). Of 139 patients entered, 63 percent were evaluable. Of these, there was an equal percentage in the dronabinol and placebo groups. The most common reason for being unevaluable was the presence of cannabinoids in the urine of placebo patients. Of 10 such patients, nine reported a worsening of appetite during the course of the study despite the presumed use of marihuana as indicated by the urine specimens. Of the evaluable patients, 38% noted an increase in appetite versus 8% of the placebo group, and this difference reached statistical significance by two weeks (13). Mood is measured by the visual analog scale was improved at all timepoints in the dronabinol group versus no change or worse in the placebo group (14). Although this did not reach statistical significance, there was a tendency in that direction. Nausea, which was generally mild at baseline, was improved in dronabinol-treated patients by 22% compared to 4% in the placebo group. After the blinded trial, there was an open-label follow-up study for patients who had completed six weeks of treatment with dronabinol or placebo. The previous placebo patients were eligible to enter the follow-up study as were patients who had discontinued the double-blind trial prematurely. Ninety-four patients were enrolled and received an oral dose of dronabinol 2.5 mg twice daily or once daily in the evening. Dosage could be titrated up as needed for efficacy, or down for side effects, but not greater than a maximum of 20 mg. Therapy was continued for up to one year unless side effects not improve by dosage reduction occurred. The visual analog scale for hunger was used as an outcome measure. Of the 94 patients enrolled, 46 had received dronabinol previously and 48 had received placebo. They were predominantly male (93% and Caucasian 84%) . Their mean age was 37 years and their mean weight loss at the start of the open study was 9.2 kg. Of the 93 patients evaluable for efficacy, 24% completed the full 12-month course of treatment and 76% were terminated early. The primary reason for early termination was intercurrent illness and drug toxicity. The data suggested that the increase in appetite experienced after dronabinol treatment in the 24% was sustained for the 12-month duration of the studies and patients did not develop tolerance to the appetite-stimulation effect, although only 22 patients actually completed one year of therapy. Twenty-five percent of all the patients who completed this study achieved a weight gain of 5 pounds or more (14). Adverse effects, as expected, were related to the central nervous system. Anxiety, confusion, dizziness, euphoria, somnolence, or thinking abnormalities occurred in 35 of the 93 patients, or 38% of those enrolled in the study. In half of these patients, this led to withdrawal or early discontinuation of the study. There was no evidence of drug interactions between dronabinol and other medications used to treat HIV infection.

The safety and pharmacokinetics of dronabinol with or without megestrol acetate was examined by Timpone and associates (15). This was an open-randomized, open-label, multicenter study designed to assess the safety and pharmacokinetics of dronabinol and megestrol alone and in combination for HIV wasting syndrome. Fifty-two patients were entered into one of four treatment arms. Their mean CD4 count was 59 cells per microliter prior to study. The four treatment arms were dronabinol 2.5 mg twice a day, megestrol acetate 750 mg per day, megestrol acetate 750 per day plus dronabinol 2.5 mg twice a day, or megestrol acetate 250 mg per day plus dronabinol 2.5 mg twice a day. After the initiation of therapy, 47 of the 52 patients returned for at least one visit, and 39 patients completed the planned 12-week study visits. The occurrence of adverse effects, although different between groups, were not statistically different in total number among the variety of treatment arms. Drug discontinuation, new AIDS-defining conditions or significant changes in CD4 T-lymphocyte count were not different. Dronabinol-induced side effects included confusion, anxiety, emotional lability, euphoria, and hallucinations, and those thought to be caused by megestrol included shortness of breath, liver enzyme changes, and high blood sugar. The results showed that the mean weight change over 12 weeks was negative 2 kg with dronabinol alone, increased by 6.5 kg with megestrol, and megestrol 750 mg dose plus dronabinol, and approximately stable in patients taking dronabinol plus megestrol. These differences between treatment arms were highly statistically significant. For megestrol, but not dronabinol, there was a positive correlation between the area under the drug concentration curve, weight change, and the visual analog scale for hunger. Based on these data, it appears that megestrol is more effective for treatment of AIDS wasting in terms of hunger and weight gain than is dronabinol. However, the metabolic effects of megestrol are troubling for long-term use, since hyperglycemia, increases in body fat, and other metabolic changes may be adverse for patients staying on this type of drug on a chronic basis, particularly in the current era, in which effective AIDS treatments allow long-term survival. Thus, cardiovascular disease, as in the rest of American society, will become an important factor in risk of death.

3. CONCLUSION

Whereas anecdotal information and case reports suggest that smoked crude marihuana is beneficial for treatment of AIDS patients with profound wasting syndromes, there are no data that support this use. The studies with oral dronabinol, which are the only controlled studies in this area *(13—15)*, are disappointing. The hazards of smoking marihuana on the immune system, the risk of opportunistic infections, and the risk of neoplasia at the current time outweigh any benefits alleged by anecdotal data to date.

REFERENCES

1. Kotler, D. P., Tierney, A. R., Wang J., and Pierson, R. N., Jr. (1989) Magnitude of body cell-mass depletion and the timing of death from wasting in AIDS. *Am. J. Clin. Nutr.* **50,**444–447.
2. Macallan, D. C., Noble, C., Baldwin, C., Jebb, S. A., Prentice, A. M., Coward, A., Sawyer, M. S., McManus, T. J., and Griffen, G. E. Energy expenditure and wasting in human immunodeficiency virus infection. *New Engl. J. Med.* **333(2),** 83–88.
3. Mattes, R. D., Engelman, K., Shaw, L. M., and Elsohly, M. A. (1994) Cannabinoids and appetite stimulation. *Pharmacology Biochem. Behavior* **49,** 187–195.
4. Regelson, W., Butler, J. R., Schulz, J., Kirk, T., Peek, L., Green M. L., and Zalis, M. O. (1976) Δ⁹-Tetrahydrocannabinol as an effective antidepressant and appetite-stimulating agent in advanced cancer patients. In: *The Pharmacology of Marijuana* (Braude, M. C., and Szara, S., eds.) Raven Press, New York, 763–776.
5. Sallan, S. E., Cronin, C., Zelen, M., and Zinberg, N. E. (1980) Antiemetics in patients receiving chemotherapy for cancer: a randomized comparison of delta-9-tetrahydrocannabinol and prochlorperazine. *N. Engl. J. Med.* **30,**135–138.
6. Chang, A. E., Shiling, D. J., Stillman, R. C., Goldberg, N. H., Seipp, C. A., Barofsky, I., Simon, R. M., and Rosenberg, S. A. (1979) Δ⁹-tetrahydrocannabinol as an antiemetic in cancer patients receiving high-dose methotrexate: a prospective, randomized evaluation. *Ann. Int. Med.* **91,**819–824.

7. Haines, L., and Green, W. (1970) Marijuana use patterns. *Br. J. Addict.* **65,** 347–362.
8. Kelly, T. H., Foltin, R. W., Emurian, C. S., and Fischman, M. W. (1990) Multidimensional behavioral effects of marijuana. *Prog. Neuropsychopharmacol. Biol. Psychiatry* **14,** 885–902.
9. Foltin, R. W., Fischman, M. W., and Byrne, M. R. (1988) Effects of smoked marijuana on food intake and body weight of humans living in a residential laboratory. *Appetite* **11,**1–14.
10. Plasse, T. F., Gorter, R. W., Krasnow, S. H., Lane, M., Shepard, K. V., and Wadleigh, R. G. (1991) Recent clinical experience with dronabinol. *Pharmacol. Biochem. Behav.* **40,** 695–700.
11. Agurell, S., Halldin, M., Lindgren, J. E., Ohlsson, A., Widman, M., Gillespie, H., and Hollister, L. (1986) Pharmacokinetics and metabolism of Δ1-tetrahydrocannabinol and other cannabinoids with emphasis on man. *Pharmacol. Rev.* **38,** 21–43.
12. Gorter, R., Seefried, M., and Volberding, P. (1992) Dronabinol effects on weight in patients with HIV infection. *AIDS* **6,** 127.
13. Beal, J. E., Olson, R., Laubenstein, L., Morales, J. P., Bellman, P., Yangco, B., Lefkowitz, L., Plasse, T. F., and Shepard, K. V. (1995) Dronabinol as a treatment for anorexia associated with weight loss in patients with AIDS. *J. Pain Symptom Manage* **10(2),** 89–97.
14. Beal, J. E., Olson, R., Lefkowitz, L., Laubenstein, L., Bellman, P., Yangco, B., Morales, J. O., Murphy, R., Powderly, W., Plasse, T. F., Mosdell, K. W., and Shepard, K. V. (1997) Long-term efficacy and safety of dronabinol for acquired immunodeficiency syndrome-associated anorexia. *J. Pain Symptom Manage.* **14(1),** 7–14.
15. Timpone, J. G., Wright, D. J., Li N., Egorin, M. J., Enama, M. E., Mayers, J., Galetto, G., and the DATRI 004 Study Group. (1997) The safety and pharmacokinetics of single-agent and combination therapy with megestrol acetate and dronabinol for the treatment of HIV wasting syndrome. *AIDS Research and Human Retroviruses* **13,**305–315.

X   MARIHUANA AND MEDICINE, PUBLIC HEALTH, AND PUBLIC POLICY

63 *Cannabis* and Alcohol
The Green and the Red

Franz Rosenthal

The historian conversing with scientists is at a disadvantage. His presumed facts and the conclusions based upon them cannot be either proved or disproved by constantly renewable experiments. They depend upon fossilized sources that are often limited, more often than not the result of fallible observations and hazardous transmission. And then, they are subjected to the vagaries of the combinatory powers of the human mind, which are even more fallible. On the other hand, historians can give free play to their creative imagination because of the limitations inherent in the character of their information. This makes possible an arrangement of the available data in such a way as to allow for the emergence of a clear and instructive picture of the historical impact on human society of the subject under study.

In the past, the means of written communication were much more expensive and difficult to access than they are today. Scholars and writers had to be vastly more selective with respect to what they chose to write down. The ordinary human experiences of daily life were often taken for granted and little commented upon. This was true of many matters that appear to us to be fundamental for an understanding of society. One such example is the use of drugs for sensory stimulation. At certain periods in history–and our own is one of them–such use causes noticeable and unusual societal problems.

Such a period occurred in the Muslim world in the late twelfth or early thirteenth century when the use of hashish became a social problem in the far-flung regions dominated by Islam. It has remained one ever since. From Central Asia, the use of hashish worked its way rapidly and relentlessly westward until it reached Muslim Spain. "The herb," "the green one," "the morsel of thought" could not be stopped. Its many other nicknames were used as terms of endearment and also of mystification, but with increasing frequency it came to be called "the evil herb" or "Satan's own food." For the benefit of latter-day scholars, the calamity became so marked that the literature of the time could no longer overlook the existence of hashish.

With respect to its effect upon society, the use of hashish should be considered under three aspects, each very different in nature and significance: first, its use for purely medical applications; second, its sporadic and haphazard consumption for nonmedical purposes; and third, its spread from casual use by individuals to wide-spread consistent use by society at large.

From: *Marihuana and Medicine*
Edited by: G. G. Nahas et al.   © Humana Press Inc., Totowa, NJ

The knowledge of a possible medicinal use for *Cannabis* passed from classical antiquity to the physicians and pharmacologists of Muslim civilization. Although the historic references are few, a small number of allegedly beneficial applications are mentioned. Problems of language and terminology, however, constantly interfere with our understanding; less so, perhaps, in the strictly medical and pharmaceutical literature than in general reports on hashish. Sometimes drugs other than *Cannabis*, or in addition to it, may have been involved in a so-called medicinal use. In some instances, there is no way of knowing what the confection referred to as "hashish" really was; in others there is no doubt. Furthermore, there is no clear indication from medieval times that *Cannabis* was ever smoked. Apparently the smoking of it began about the same time that tobacco cigarettes were introduced from the New World. Before that, hashish was eaten as a confection, usually made up of a variety of ingredients.

No matter how much or how little the literature has to say about *Cannabis*, it was always present in the Muslim pharmacopoeia, just as it had been known and used by Galen and Dioscurides long before the appearance of Islam.

The use of hemp leaves was recommended in a large number of ailments: to stimulate the appetite, to dissolve flatulence, as a diuretic, to clean up dandruff, to clear the brain, for soothing pain of the ears. It was also "good for digestion," and one report claims its usefulness in epilepsy.

That hashish was also used as a stimulant–or, to translate the Arabic term literally, as an "intoxicant"–by some individuals in the Muslim world between the seventh and twelfth centuries remains a conjecture. There is no information in the historical sources. In Islamic society, it was of no concern to public authorities what an individual did in the privacy of his or her home, especially if, as in the case of hashish, no explicit statement against its use existed in the authoritative religious texts. As long as individual action did not come to public attention and cause a public nuisance, it was likely to be disregarded.

There are many who feel today that what an individual does in private is indeed no matter of public concern. But when sufficiently large numbers of individuals all do the same thing, it will inevitably provoke public scrutiny and, if necessary, some kind of public action.

In the case of hashish use in Muslim society, from the twelvth century on it became obvious that it was a problem for society and that action was called for. But what kind of action, and how to justify it in a society held together by one thing only–the religious law of Islam? The prophet Muhammad and the early Muslims could not be credited with an express statement declaring hashish unlawful. Because hashish use had not been a problem in the early years of Islam, there had been no reason to take note of it. In contrast, the consumption of alcohol was a different matter. Well known for its effects, it was forbidden in Muslim law on the basis of the Holy Qur'ân. Thus, legal scholars used as their principal argument for control of hashish the assumed similarity of its effects with those of wine and other alcoholic beverages. Unfortunately, just as it is true today, the factual situation was ambiguous, and the necessary legal reasoning was therefore compromised. Already the jurists had to contend with problems concerning the prohibition of wine, and any comparison of hashish with alcohol was troublesome because their effects were not identical.

Not only did the jurists compare hashish with wine, but also poets who used the terms the "green one" and the "red one." Even though wine was forbidden and illegal, it was enjoyed by many, in particular by the upper classes who could afford it. Since poetry about wine was extremely popular, with the advent of hashish, its rich repertory of poetic images and rhetorical figures could be transferred easily. In Islam, every educated individual (and many of those with little formal education) was a poet, so verses on hashish provided new sensations for the jaded tastes of the connoisseurs.

Another literary convention of the writers from Near Eastern times as well as classical antiquity was the highly esteemed form of the playful exposition of the merits or faults of two comparable objects. For example, different kinds of animals, flowers, human occupations, and cities were often compared. In Muslim civilization this form of poetry reached new pinnacles of artistry. Quite naturally, as soon as the hashish habit had insinuated itself into wider social groups, writers of the day applied the literary form to an alleged rivalry between hashish and wine.

Such was the case with a poet who lived in Syria from 1222 to 1258, and who exercised his considerable wit and poetic skill by composing a long rhymed debate between imaginary prohashish and prowine parties. Characteristically, he does not reveal his own preference nor does he make any moral judgements about either hashish or wine. Whether poets approved or disapproved of the moral practices they used for themes in their poetry remains a mystery. Personal experience or opinion counted for little, linguistic and literary virtuosity was their goal. And yet, this medieval Syrian poet presents in his poem the main arguments that have been repeated over and over again in popular discussions for and against the use of hashish.

First, the word is given to the pro-hashish party:

1. *Greetings, my friend! Don't listen to the critics*
   And don't condemn without a legal basis!
2. *You wish to know about wine and the green stuff.*
   Thus listen to the words of a true expert!
3. *Hashish has qualities that wine cannot boast of.*
   Can wine be drunk in mosque and Sufi Convent?
4. *You can obtain the green stuff without haggling.*
   You do not need much gold and silver for it.
5. *No! Unlike wine, it is a gift. It's gratis,*
   Yes truly indispensable though cheap it may be.
6. *It grows in meadows green like heavenly gardens,*
   Whereas their wine is like a Hellish firebrand.
7. *Their wine makes you forget all meanings. Our herb*
   Recalls the mysteries of godly beauty.
8. *The secret of hashish lifts up the spirit*
   In an ascent of disembodied thinking.
9. *It is the spirit pure. Free are its confines*
   From worries. Only the elect may taste it.
10. *No feet have trampled on it, nor has black pitch*
    Been used for sealing casks and made them dirty.
11. *The body is not tired eliminating*
    And vomiting like an inflated wine-skin.
12. *No one will think of you as void of reason,*
    Nor call you a corrupter of religion.
13. *Tucked in a handkerchief it can be carried.*
    No cup is needed if you wish to use it.
14. *Hashish involves no sin. You are not punished.*
    There's no disgrace, no quarrelsome companions.
15. *In times both good and bad you can enjoy it.*
    It is no hindrance to nights of devotions.
16. *There is no danger of raids by policemen.*
    The government will not unjustly fine you.

17. *You find yourself clean, virtuous, and witty,*
    Bright, too, and free from all annoying dullness.
18. *You find you have no enemies to hate you.*
    You always have a lot of friends around you.
19. *The beloved, tasting it, will sneak away from*
    Invidious chaperones and come unbidden.
20. *Another thing: it's good for your digestion.*
    But all its many virtues cannot be mentioned.
21. *They're all there when my company at eating*
    Hashish is a gazelle like a willow slender!
22. *She treats me to a pretty poem, singing,*
    Her voice putting to shame the cooing pigeon.
23. *She flirts with me demurely with her big eyes,*
    And when she smiles shows rows of brilliant white teeth.
24. *When critics talk about hashish, don't listen!*
    Their aim is to deter you. Don't obey them!

Then it is the turn of the champions of wine:

25. *Now, dear companion whom I love so dearly,*
    Accept right guidance to preserve your pleasure!
26. *Would you by eating grass that is not juicy*
    Want to be like a dumb beast without reason?
27. *Please disregard the views of bestial people!*
    Just pass around the starry, shining jewel!
28. *'Tis wine I mean. A traveler lost is guided*
    At night back to the right path by its brilliance.
29. *Their herb brings shame upon a decent person*
    So that he slinks about just like a killer.
30. *It reproduces on his cheeks a green sheen.*
    His face seems darkish, like pale dust its color.
31. *When his friend thinks of him at night, he shudders.*
    It is like morning turning into dark night.
32. *Our wine brings honor to the lowly person*
    And dignity so that none is his master.
33. *When wine appears, it banishes all worry.*
    The drinker's thirsty heart is fully sated.
34. *When wine appears, the drinker's secret gets out*
    And gladdens him, his rosy cheek wine-colored.
35. *Unlike hashish, its qualities are useful.*
    Speak out! Count and describe wine's many meanings!
36. *That other substance is harmful to mankind.*
    Thus tell us all about the evil in it!
37. *No caliph surely ever tasted hashish,*
    Nor did a king in full command and power.
38. *No poet ever seriously praised it*
    In words as artful as the singer's, Ma'bad.
39. *No strings were ever plucked in praise of hashish.*
    The roseate drink alone can make this happen.
40. *Whatever else but wine can tinge the hands that*
    Holding a cup of wine reflect its color?

41. Drunk the beloved turns and bends down, swaying
    Gracefully like the bent branch of a willow,
42. Giving you wine like wine in her saliva,
    The white teeth in her mouth agleam and brilliant.
43. She hesitates no more to join her lover.
    Then she forgets all on the day that follows.
44. Who would refrain from something of this nature?
    I was not well advised to give up drinking.
45. But for those meddlers I would ne'er be sober,
    Nor would I listen to the critics' comments.
46. Drink wine! Don't listen to censorious people,
    Though wine may be outlawed in our religion!

Note that the poet was writing at a time when the hashish wave was still in its early stages and probably had not yet engulfed urban life. Perhaps this is why he can afford to give the impression of a certain objectivity. Nonetheless, his arguments are very familiar. He begins triumphantly with a fanfare: Hashish has not been proved illegal. He continues with the trump card of addicts: It is used by the representatives of true religious fervor–the mystics. It is even eaten in mosques. It involves no sin, no legal danger, no penalties. It is easily carried and consumed. Above all, it is cheap, much cheaper than wine, and everyone can afford it. But the poet describes only briefly the physical and mental deterioration caused by hashish, because the wine lovers are only too glad to make their most important point, namely, that in contrast to wine, hashish means low social status and reduces its users to the dregs of society and culture. But the hashish addicts think of themselves as an elite group. They claim beautiful experiences in the realm of pure spirit, experiences that set them apart from the rest of the common herd of the uninitiated. They are alone and withdrawn, but they have many friends. They believe that the drug makes them peaceful, and they feel that by using it, they become especially lovable individuals.

The poet permits each side to claim that its favorite intoxicant is a powerful aid to seduction. His poem, like so many others, was meant to appeal to erotic fancy. In fact, hashish use was often declared detrimental to sexual activity, but it was also described, in the same way as in the above poem, as a means to obtain sexual satisfaction from a lover unaware of being under the influence of the drug and whose inhibitions were weakened by its use.

Poets in later times continued to compose short "jeux d'ésprit" exalting the alleged virtues of hashish. Whether or not they were serious is difficult to determine. Quite often, it seems, they reflected the positive attitude toward the drug that was characteristic of certain members of the upper class intellectuals. For them, hashish is a thing of true beauty; it gives them irrepressible joy and repose and provides them with relief from worries and anxiety. It reveals to them secrets and opens to them new meanings. It increases their understanding and enlarges their imaginative perceptions. An affinity of the hashish eater to music was occasionally reported. No truly violent actions directed against other persons under the influence of hashish are mentioned in these stories; but the prohashish faction never comes to grips with the points raised by the attackers.

These scholars compiled a long list of the mental and physical ill effects caused by the drug: reddening of the eye, dryness of mouth, excessive sleeping, and heaviness in the head when the drug takes possession of the brain, as well as numbness of the extremities. Prolonged use dries up the semen (already noted by Galen) and cuts off the desire for sexual intercourse, cuts short the reproductive capacity, brings forth hidden disease, harms the intestine, makes the limb inactive, causes a shortage of breath, diminishes vision in the eye and increases pensiveness in the imagination after initially causing joy; hashish produces narcosis, laziness, stupor, weakening of sense perception, foul breath, and ruination of color and complexion.

Hashish is mind changing and personality changing, causing "insanity in the habitual user," "changes the mind making it absent from reality."

Habituation to hashish is also stated. "Among the greatest physical harm caused by it is the fact that habitual users of it are hardly ever able to repent of it because of the effect it has upon their temper" says al-Zakarshi, and al-Badri concurs: "The user cannot separate from it and leave it alone."

Hashish is stated consistently by its adversaries to be something that saps the user's energy and ability and willingness to work. Implicitly this was considered its greatest danger to the social fabric.

Finally, a holyman, Sheikh al-Hariri described what may be the lingering effect of chronic hashish usage. He claimed that abstinence for a long period was necessary to overcome the long-term action of the drug in the organism. "One has to give it up for 40 days, until the body is free from it, and 40 more days until he is rested from it after becoming free." The jurists also used on occasion the persuasive form of rhyme to speak about hashish. Their attitude was extremely negative, as one from their ranks put it:

All the destructive effects of wine
Are found in hashish many times over.

They tried to fight hashish or assumed the official posture against the drug, but they were waging an uphill struggle. Even though they were successful in arguing for the illegality of hashish, they proved decidedly unsuccessful in devising effective means for curtailing its use. On the contrary, it appears that eventually they became resigned to letting matters take their course.

The similarity of views and arguments, then and now, is the most striking feature of the medieval debate. The dilemma still exists between the rights of individuals (which in our view, if not the Muslim, may extend to self-debasement and self-destruction) and the needs of society. It is no closer to being solved. The same romantic claims to beauty and spiritual release and other benefits derived from hashish use, and on the other hand, the same strong statements about its generally harmful effects are heard today. The most appropriate course for society to take is still mired in the same kind of helplessness and confusion. Many things have changed, of course, yet the only really new element to appear in the picture is the scientific ability modern society now possesses to understand and measure objectively the properties and effects of the drug. This is a very recent development. Until a decade ago, it was not possible to discover any satisfactory scientific literature on *Cannabis*.

Perhaps the current efforts of scientists can be translated soon into beneficial social action. Even though the historian, familiar with the character of man and society through the ages, is not inclined to believe in the coming of the millennium in our own day, still that unscientific component of man's mind called "hope" constantly raises its small voice to say: "Maybe it will."

64

The Distribution of Consumption of Alcohol and Marihuana

Gabriel Nahas, Renaud Trouvé, and Colette Latour

Abstract

Ledermann reported in 1956 that the distribution of consumption of alcohol in different populations could be related as a first approximation to a normal logarithmic mode. In the present study, the distribution of alcohol consumption (in decaliters per week) in a group of 180 oil rig workers was computed using probability logarithmic scales. A cumulative distribution of rates was established by calculating the proportion in the population that used alcohol in increasing amounts. The weekly consumption of alcohol in this population (1983) follow a log normal distribution similar to that reported by Ledermann on a group of 93 consumers (the slope of the two curves are –0.75 and –0.73 respectively). The same method was used to analyze the cumulative frequency of marihuana use among American high school seniors during the period 1975–1981. When plotted on probability logarithmic scale, the fit of a straight line is excellent for frequency of marihuana use among those who had ever used marihuana The percentage of daily marihuana smokers represent 12–17% of the population of consumers. Other studies of lifetime prevalence of *Cannabis* use in French or Canadian adolescents also display a log normal distribution. The weekly consumption of *Cannabis* among the male population over age 15 in three Jamaican villages follow a log normal distribution with 64% of the sample of 418 smokers consuming 4–10 g a day of the drug. A survey of coca leaf chewing among Peruvian miners reports that over 90% of them chew the leaf and 80% are daily chewers consuming 40–60 g of leaves (400–600 mg cocaine base). These data suggest the consumption of psychoactive euphoriant drugs more potent than alcohol (*Cannabis*, cocaine) may be associated with a significantly higher rate of intake (daily intoxicating dose) when they are socially acceptable and freely available.

From: *Marihuana and Medicine*
Edited by: G. G. Nahas et al.   © Humana Press Inc., Totowa, NJ

1. INTRODUCTION

A knowledge of the actual rates of consumption of dependence-producing drugs in a population is most useful in order to predict the medical or social risk associated with their use. Such information is fragmentary, except for alcohol.

The French mathematician Sully Ledermann was the first epidemiologist to study the frequency distribution of individual consumption of alcohol in France *(1)*. His fundamental observation was that diverse frequencies did not occur randomly, but that their distribution could be related as a first approximation to the statistical law known as the normal logarithmic law: The distribution curve is sharply skewed–the average consumption does not divide the population into two equal groups, one consuming less than the average, the other more; in France, the distribution of consumption is roughly two-thirds below and one-third above.

Ledermann also noted in studying different groups of consumers, that if the average consumption is 10 L per year, the proportion of daily consumers of 200 mL or more ("excessive consumers") will be 1.5% of the population of users. If average consumption is 30 L of pure alcohol per year the percentage of "excessive consumers" will be 7%. Within the range of average consumption considered, the proportion of excessive consumers "alcoholics," tends to increase geometrically rather than arithmetically. Ledermann concluded that there was covariance between average "reasonable" consumption and heavy "unreasonable" consumption, associated with pathology. Therefore, average and heavy consumption are not independent from each other, and an increase or a decrease in average consumption should be associated with parallel changes in heavy consumption. Roughly, the percentage of heavy drinkers in a population of alcohol consumers remains constant and is related to the total number of consumers.

Since Ledermann's pioneering work, additional data on the distribution of alcohol consumption were analyzed for a number of populations in North America and Europe *(2,3)*. These distributions are for the most part reasonably approximated by a log normal curve. In all cases, they exhibit a single mode and are markedly skewed to the right, with the top 10% of drinkers consuming 40–50% of the total consumption. Other authors *(4,5)* expressed their conclusions in terms of tendencies rather than precise mathematical relationships, but still concluded that a substantial increase in mean consumption of alcohol is likely to be accompanied by an increased prevalence of heavy users. All of the conclusions strongly suggest "that a close link exists between the mean consumer's drinking level and the consumption level of the consumer at the 90 through 95th percentile of the distribute" *(6)*.

Other studies extended the Ledermann analysis to the consumption of dependence-producing drugs, such as marihuana, among Canadian and British university students *(7,8)*, and in a randomly selected sample of subjects from Kansas *(9)*. In these later studies, based on questionnaires instead of amount of drug used, prevalence or frequency of intake within a year was computed. The authors reported that the frequency of drug intake "could be plotted on a normal logarithmic curve."

In the present study we have analyzed the distribution of alcohol consumption in a sample of alcohol consumers recently reported *(10)* and compared it to the distribution computed earlier by Ledermann in 1956. We have also used the same method to analyze the frequency of use of marihuana reported by Jonhston *(11)* among American high school students and in other populations of consumers *(12,13)*.

2. METHODS

We have used the method suggested by Paton *(14)* and plotted the data on logarithmic-probability scales. accumulative distribution of rates was established by calculating the proportion in a population that used alcohol or marihuana in increasing amounts or frequency within a certain time frame. These proportions of the population were then plotted against the rates of use. A probability scale (probit) was used on the ordinate for the cumulated percentage of the different groups of consumers and a logarithmic scale was used on the abcissa for the quantities consumed at a given rate or higher.

If a straight line runs across the plotted points, the distribution is log normal. The intercept of the curve with a perpendicular passing through the point corresponding to 50% of the population will give the median, and the slope of the curve gives the standard deviation. We have selected decaliters of pure alcohol consumed per week as the units for alcohol consumption. For marihuana we have used the frequency of consumption, per week, month, or year, or the life-time prevalence.

3. RESULTS

The weekly consumption of alcohol in a group of 180 oil rig workers in the North Sea (10) (out of a total sample of 213) follows a log normal distribution. This distribution is very similar to that reported by Ledermann in 1956 in a group of 93 consumers. In this case, the consumption of alcohol originally reported in liters per year was converted to decaliters per week. The slopes of these two curves are –0.75 and –0.73 respectively.

The cumulative frequency of marihuana use among American high school seniors during the period 1975–1981 was computed from the data reported by Jonhston et al. When plotted on probability logarithmic scale, the fit of a straight line to the data is excellent for frequency of marihuana consumption among those who had ever used marihuana. The percentage of daily users of marihuana represents 12–17% of the population of consumers.

Life-time prevalence of hashish use among 109 French adolescents 14–18 years old reported by Kandel (12) and yearly prevalence among 3723 Canadian students studied by Smart (13) also display a log normal distribution. In these two studies the highest frequency of use was reported in 20% of the consumers. Finally, monthly consumption of marihuana was reported by Gallegos (15) in a group of 82 urban youth from Lima (average age 20); 3 in this group the frequency of daily use is 29%.

4. DISCUSSION

The two samples of consumers of alcohol analyzed in this study were reported by different authors in different populations, Scotland and France, and at 27-year intervals. The fitted straight lines, based on a coarse grouping of weekly alcohol consumption in the two groups have similar slopes and ran very close to each other. In both cases, consumption of 7 decaliters of pure alcohol or more a week (a consumption that has been associated with alcohol intoxication) is observed among 7–8% of the consumers. This percentage of "heavy" users of alcohol is comparable to that observed in the United States.

Another survey (16) concludes: "Out of 394 American physicians who took the self-administered alcoholism screening test, 12% were abstinent. Among the 350 who consumed alcohol, 8.6% were classified as 'possible alcoholics' ... This proportion was similar to that prevailing in a non-physician general medical patient population."

The relative constancy of the percentage of heavy consumers of alcohol in different populations might indicate that proneness to alcohol abuse is present in certain individuals. However, the unimodal distribution of consumption does not permit one to define statistically two populations of "moderate" and heavy drinkers. If there were two distinct groups, a discontinuity in the distribution would appear. The log normal analysis does not eliminate the proneness to alcohol use, it suggests that such a feature is not limited to a sharply defined group but randomly distributed to the whole population. Such an interpretation would account for the fact that an increase in average consumption of alcohol is accompanied by an increase in heavy use. Ledermann (1) did suggest that the log normal distribution of alcohol consumption did result from a snowball, recruiting effect that was a function of two factors, one biologically related to the action of the drug on the individual and the other environmentally related to the sociocultural milieu. The log normal distribution of alcohol consumption would be another example of a nature-nurture interaction.

One would therefore expect that a similar log normal distribution might be observed with other dependence-producing drugs as was suggested by Paton (14). Consumption of these drugs is related to sociocultural factors, and also have a reinforcing effect on brain and behavior.

The frequency of marihuana use in the populations studied also follows a log normal distribution with a rather high incidence of daily or frequent intoxication among high school seniors and adolescents (12–29%), depending on its availability and social acceptance. The present data does not permit one to relate frequency of consumption to amount consumed, and to perform a quantitative analysis of the distribution of consumption of marihuana similar to that of alcohol. However, frequency of consumption of marihuana is related to a similar frequency of the psychoactive, intoxicating effect after each exposure to the drug. There is also some data concerning the amounts of Cannabis consumed in parts of Jamaica where the drug is freely available and has wide social acceptability. The weekly consumption of "ganja" (Cannabis) among the male population over the age of 15 in three Jamaican villages (17) indicates that 64% of the sample of 418 smokers of ganja were heavy daily users. They consumed four or more "spliffs" a day which equals 4 to 10 g of Cannabis (ganja) equivalent to 60–120 mg Δ^9-tetrahydrocannabinol (THC).

On the basis of the data presently available, it would appear that easy access and social acceptance of marihuana as prevailing in Jamaican rural villages are associated with a high proportion of heavy use (over 50% in the population of consumers). This proportion is significantly greater than that observed among consumers of alcohol. THC, the psychoactive substance in marihuana, has been reported to induce pleasant euphoric experiences (18), and to interact with limbic structures (19) associated with pleasure reward (20). Such reinforcing psychopharmacological properties might account for its heavy use in a climate of social acceptability.

The consumption of other dependence-producing drugs has not been systematically reported in a fashion that could be analyzed according to the log normal distribution. However, many clinical observations indicate that the proportion of heavy users of opium and cocaine is very high among the consumers of these drugs. And a survey of coca leaf chewing among miners and farm in Peru (21) reports that 96 and 92% of them chewed the coca leaf and 88 and 82% were daily chewers ("acullicadores"), consuming 40–60 g of coca leaves (corresponding to 400–600 mg of cocaine base). Blood levels exceeding 500 ng/mL of cocaine have been measured on these subjects, concentrations that produce psychoactive effects. This data would indicate that the more potent dependence-producing psychoactive drugs are associated with a higher frequency of consumption. Such tentative conclusions should be confirmed by systematic epidemiologic studies of the distribution of consumption of dependence-producing drugs in different populations. Selected well-studied, relatively small samples of a few hundred subjects reporting consumption over a period of one month in different populations should yield meaningful information.

These studies will provide a clearer definition of the magnitude of vulnerable groups: those with a consumption greater than some limit. The log normal distribution of consumption gives a concise description of an entire distribution because it may be defined by only two parameters, the mean and standard deviation. Given the value of those parameters, one may compare the results of different studies. Furthermore, the general effects of intervention methods may be quantitatively expressed. The log normal distribution also defines more clearly the choices confronting those who wish to control the use of dependence-producing drugs and limit their spread: namely, either to steepen the slope of the k-line by reducing consumption at high rates, or to reduce the overall rate of use at all levels. So far the latter solution, though fraught with controversy, has been the only one that has been proven to be effective.

ACKNOWLEDGMENT

The authors acknowledge with thanks the valuable assistance of Joseph Fleiss, Professor of Biostatistics, at the College of Physicians and Surgeons of Columbia University.

REFERENCES

1. Ledermann, S., Alcool, alcoolisme et alcoolisation. Presses Universitaires de France, vol. 1 and 2, 1956 and 1964.
2. De Lint, J. E. and Schmidt, W. (1970) Estimating the prevalence of alcoholism from consumption and mortality data. *Quart. J. Stud. Alc.*, **31**, 957–964.
3. Bruun, K., Griffith, E., Lumio, M., Makela, K., Pan, L., Popham, R. E., Room, R., Schmidt, W., Skog, O. J., Sulkinen, P. and Osterberg, E. (1975) *Alcohol Control Policies in Public Health Perspective* Rutgers University Center of Alcohol Studies, New Brunswick, NJ.
4. Skog, O. G. (1983) The collectivity of drinking cultures: a c-theory of the distribution of alcohol consumption. National Institute for Alcohol Research, Oslo, Norway.
5. Popham, I. L. E. and Schmidt, W. (1979) Words and deeds: the validity of self-report data on alcohol consumption. *J. Stud. Alc.* **42**, 355–358. (In the same volume: comments by J. de Lint, Merton M. Hyman, H. A. Mulford, J. L. Fitzgerald and Henri Weschler.)
6. Moore, M. H. and Gerstein D. R. eds. (1981) *Alcohol and Public Policy: Beyond the Shadow of Prohibition.* National Academy Press, Washington, DC, p. 67.
7. Smart, R. G. and Whitehead, P. C. (1973) The prevention of drug abuse by lowering per capita consumption: distribution of drug use in samples of Canadian adults and British university students. *Bull. Narc.* **XXV**, 4955.
8. Smart, R. G. (1978) The distribution of illicit drug use correlations between extent of use, heavy use and problems. *Bull. Narc.* **XXX**, 34–41.
9. McDermott, D. and Scheurich, I. (1977) The logarithmic normal distribution in relation to the epidemiology of drug abuse. *Bull. Narc.* **XXIX**, 13–19.
10. Aiken, G. J. M. and Lance, C. (1983) Alcohol consumption by offshore oil-rig workers. U.S.N. *Sci. News* **37**, 195–196.
11. Johnston, L. D., Bachman, J. G. and Malley, P. M. (1982) Drugs and the nation's high school students. *N.I.D.A.* Rockville, MD.
12. Kandel, D., Adler, I. and Sudit, M. (1981) The epidemiology of adolescent drug use in France and Israel. *Am. J. Public Health* **71**, 256–265.
13. Smart, R. G., Goodstadt, M. S. and Sheppard, M. A. (1981) Preliminary report of alcohol and other drug use among Ontario students in 1981. Alcoholism and Drug Addiction Research Foundation, Toronto.
14. Paton, W. D. M. (1975) The uses and implications of the log-normal distribution of drug use. In *Cannabis and Man: Psychological and Clinical Aspects and Patterns of Use.* (Connell and Dorn, eds.) Churchill Livingstone.
15. Gallegos, M. F. (1982) The problem of drugs in Peru. Historical and Epidemiological Consultations Symposium on Alcoholism and Drug Dependence, Sao Paolo, Peru.
16. Niven, R. G., Hurt, R. D., Morse, R. M. and Swenson, W. M. (1984) Alcoholism in physicians. *Mayo Clin. Proc.* **59**, 12–16.
17. Dreher, M. (1982) *Working Men and Ganja*, I.S.H.I., Philadelphia, PA, p. 34.
18. Moreau, L. (1844) *Hashish and Mental Illness* translated (1973) Raven, New York, p. 27.

19. Olds, J. (1977) *Drives and Reinforcements* Raven, New York.
20. Heath, R. G. (1972) Marihuana: effects on deep and surface electroencephalograms of man. *Arch. Gen. Psychiat.* **26**, 577–584.
21. Carter, W. E., Parkerson, P. and Mamani, M. (1980) Traditional and changing patterns of coca use in Bolivia. In *Cocaine, Proceedings of the Intra-American Seminar on Coca and Cocaine*, (Jeri, F. R., ed.) Lima, Peru, pp. 159–164.

65

Drug Abuse and the Law

Prosecution or Persecution?

James A. Moss

I have always admired the unflagging confidence doctors seem to have in their professional opinions. My admiration probably dates back to the time I first heard the story about a sickly, young boy who was taken by his mother to be examined by their family physician. Although the doctor concluded that the child was suffering from pneumonia, the mother was not so sure. She told the doctor about cases she had heard of where people were treated for pneumonia, but died of typhoid fever. The physician became irate. "Madam," he said, "when I treat a patient for pneumonia, he dies of pneumonia."

The more deeply involved I become in the field of drug abuse, however, the more apparent it becomes that many important medical questions about the physiological and psychological effects of psychotropic drugs have not been answered with the same firm conviction displayed by the doctor in my story. For example, public opinion is genuinely divided on the question of whether marihuana is a harmless alternative to alcohol, or instead poses a serious health hazard. This division exists in part because your profession has not yet spoken in one authoritative voice about the effects of marihuana *(1)*. The same may be said of the public's conception about many of the other stimulants, depressants, narcotics, and hallucinogens that are currently regulated by federal criminal statutes.

I make this observation not for the purpose of criticizing the medical profession. Notable efforts are being made by the profession to resolve unanswered questions and to separate fact from fiction in the area of drug use and drug abuse. Symposiums, such as this one, are a testament to those efforts. But because many questions about drugs remain unanswered (at least in the public's mind) a vigorous debate has persisted on the very question which I have been asked to address this afternoon: Is there any justification for curtailing an individual's use of mind-altering drugs? Put another way, does the community as a whole have the right to prevent its members from using such drugs if they freely choose to do so? Or is the individual's right to choose his own destiny paramount?

From: *Marihuana and Medicine*
Edited by: G. G. Nahas et al.   © Humana Press Inc., Totowa, NJ

When I was first asked to discuss this topic with you, it occurred to me that it might be a waste of our time to explore the philosophical basis for controlling drug use. The legislatures in every state of the union have exercised the power to control drug use and the courts have upheld that power–whether the exercise of that power is philosophically justified or not. Why then should we occupy ourselves discussing the philosophy of such regulation?

After some reflection, I have come to welcome the opportunity to philosophize about the drug laws. For I believe that the present scheme for the regulation of psychotropic drugs (at least in the federal practice with which I am familiar) is a thoughtful, pragmatic approach to this country's drug problem. The philosophy underlying this approach strikes a reasonable balance between the views of libertarians who would safeguard individual freedom of choice at all cost, and those who recognize in society a right to control individual action for the good of the community.

Almost 60 years ago, the Supreme Court of the United States recognized the power of Congress and of the states to regulate the use of dangerous drugs. Justice Day wrote for a unanimous court:

> *"There can be no question of the authority of the State in the exercise of its police power to regulate the administration, sale, prescription and use of dangerous and habit-forming drugs ... The right to exercise this power is so manifest in the interest of the public health and welfare, that it is necessary to enter upon a discussion of it beyond saying that it is too firmly established to be successfully called in question."* Whipple v. Martinson, 256 U.S. 41, 45 (1921) (2).

The concept of the "police power" has been distilled into a very simple, almost-trite formula: the right to swing your arm ends at the point where someone else's nose begins. No one member of society may inflict harm upon another; none may breach the peace, or cause the breakdown of the orderly interaction among people that the community requires for its collective survival. In the context of our discussion here, no one may inflict upon others the debilatation that results from drug dependency; nor may anyone cause society as a whole to suffer the disabilities that result from widespread drug addiction.

The "police power" has also been exercised to mean that society may prevent individuals from inflicting harm even upon themselves, if in so doing they cause harm to the structure of society. That is to say, a person's right to swing his arm may end at the point where *his own* nose begins. This is what the Supreme Court tells us when it recognizes that legislatures may prescribe not only the distribution of dangerous drugs to others, but they may make it a crime for an individual to use those drugs himself. And all of this in the name of the public good.

The stauncher libertarians may rail at this suggestion, choosing instead to adhere to the notion that individuals ought to be free "to choose their own road to hell if that is where they want to go" *(3)*. However, my view and, more importantly, the prevailing view in my profession is that society must retain the right to restrict individual freedom, at least where the widespread exercise of that freedom threatens to disrupt the public health. Nowhere is this clearer than in the area of drug abuse, where *all* citizens are likely to be affected by an epidemic of addiction and its legacy of unproductive individuals, ancillary crime, and shattered families. Assuming for the time being that psychotropic drugs are hazardous when abused, to prohibit the nonmedical use of these drugs is no more philosophically egregious than, for example, to prohibit the use of thalidamide by pregnant women.

Having said all of this, I should tell you that the conflict between the libertarian philosophy and the prevailing legal philosophy is largely academic. Although the law recognizes its right to punish individuals who choose to harm themselves by over indulging in drugs, Congress has chosen not to exercise this right. There is no federal criminal statute which prohibits the use of a controlled substance *(4).*

Rather, Congress has devised a scheme for the control of drug abuse that attempts to punish only those who *distribute* drugs to others. Its theory is to halt drug abuse by preventing the abusers from obtaining the drugs, not by punishing them as criminals. Furthermore, so as to intrude as little as possible into matters of primarily personal concern, Congress has chosen to control the distribution of only those drugs which realistically pose a danger to the welfare of the entire community. The only substances that may be regulated by the Attorney General are those that have a potential for widespread abuse and which, if abused, will result in psychological or physical dependence *(5).*

This regulatory scheme was adopted by Congress in 1970 after it had completed a rather extensive study into the drug problem in this country. Generally I try to avoid discussing the legislative history of any act of Congress. As a nobleman once remarked during the French Revolution, after observing a session of the national assembly: "Laws are like sausages. No one should see them being made." The enactments of Congress are no exception. However, because this particular act, the Comprehensive Drug Abuse Prevention and Control Act of 1970, imposes upon the medical profession a substantial role in the regulation of psychotropic drugs, it might be of some value for me to discuss some of its history with you.

During the 1960s a rise in the incidence of drug abuse prompted two presidents to appoint investigatory commissions to address that problem. In 1963 John F. Kennedy established the President's Advisory Commission on Narcotic and Drug Abuse, under the chairmanship of federal Judge E. Barrett Prettyman. In 1966 President Lyndon Johnson appointed Nicholas deB. Katzenbach to chair the President's Commission on Law Enforcement and Administration of Justice.

Many of the members of the Prettyman Commission were doctors. The Katzenbach Commission was primarily composed of lawyers. In spite of that fact, both commissions arrived at essentially the same recommendations. The report of the Prettyman Commission summarized those conclusions in three parts:

"I. The illegal traffic in drugs should be attacked with the full power of the Federal Government. The price for participation in this traffic should be prohibitive. It should be made too dangerous to be attractive.

II. The individual abuser should be rehabilitated. Every possible effort should be exerted by all governments–Federal, State, and local–and by every community toward this end. Where necessary to protect society, this may have to be done at times against the abuser's will. Pertinent to all, the causes of drug abuse must be found and eradicated.

III. Drug users who violate the law by small purchases or sales should be made to recognize what society demands of them. In these instances, penalties should be applied according to the principles of our present code of justice. When the penalties involve imprisonment, however, the rehabilitation of the individual, rather than retributive punishment, should be the major objective." See U.S. Code Cong. & Adm. News, 4575 (1970) (6).

Some of the recommendations of these commissions were implemented immediately. For example, in 1965 Congress enacted a statute that regulated the distribution and use of non-narcotic drugs capable of producing serious psychotoxic effects when abused *(7).* Then in 1966 Congress passed a law providing for increased federal efforts in the rehabilitation of narcotic addicts through civil commitment *(8).*

Nonetheless, until 1970 the federal approach to drug abuse control remained rather haphazard. In fact, the laws regulating narcotic drugs alone were strewn over at least a dozen different sections of the United States Code (9). The enforcement of those laws was charged to a variety of different federal agencies, including the Dept. of Health, Education and Welfare, the Internal Revenue Service, the Customs Service, and various agencies within the Dept. of Justice.

By 1970, several congressional committees had spent a good deal of time trying to overhaul these statutes, with notable assistance from the medical profession. The consensus of medical advice these committees received was that the drug abuse problem was reaching epidemic proportions and threatened not only the physical health, but also the mental health of the abusers (10).

The congressional response to this was the Comprehensive Drug Abuse Prevention and Control Act of 1970, which sought to attain three goals: to halt the spread in drug abuse by educating the public, to rehabilitate those who had already fallen into patterns of drug abuse; and to establish a system of regulation (backed up by stern criminal penalties) whereby the manufacture and distribution of dangerous drugs would be permitted only for legitimate, therapeutic purposes. The act attempted to realize the first two goals by providing authority to the Dept. of Health, Education and Welfare to increase its efforts in the rehabilitation, treatment, and prevention of drug abuse, through the funding of community mental health centers and public health service hospitals. Additional funds were authorized for drug abuse education activities, and for increased research and training under the auspices of the National Institute of Mental Health (11).

I am charged with the duty of effectuating of the third goal: enforcement of the regulatory scheme through criminal prosecution. The penal sections of the act appear in Title II of the bill–the Controlled Substances Act (12). Congress believed that the heart of the drug problem was the diversion of drugs out of legitimate channels into the illicit market. Its solution was quite simple: set up a "closed" system of drug distribution for legitimate purposes by regulating all manufacturers, distributors, and dispensers of certain controlled substances. Transactions outside the legitimate distribution chain were to become illegal.

As you know, all drugs subject to regulation have been classified in one of five schedules according to their medical usefulness and their susceptibility to contribute to serious addiction or abuse problems. Thus, for example, heroin, with no legitimate medical use and a high danger of physical and psychological dependence to the user is classified as a schedule I substance and carries the most severe penalties. The illegal manufacture or distribution of heroin (or for that matter any other narcotic substance in schedule I or schedule II) is punishable by up to 15 years in prison (13). Even stricter penalties apply to those offenders who supervise major narcotic distribution network (14), to those who are repeat offenders (15), to those who cause the distribution of narcotics to juveniles (16), and to those who may be otherwise shown to be highly dangerous to society (17).

As the potential for the abuse of any drug declines, it will be placed in a numerically higher schedule, and will incur lesser criminal penalties. Of course, none of these controlled drugs may be legally dispensed unless for a valid medical purpose, even the comparatively milder drugs in schedules III, IV, and V. However, the criminal justice system rarely deals with abuse of the drugs on these higher schedules. Virtually all federal drug prosecution involves the more abused and the more hazardous substances in schedules I and II. Within the last 5 years the old favorites of abuse–heroin, cocaine, LSD, PCP, and marihuana–have been receiving strong competition from several upstarts: notably dilaudid, percodan, seconal, tuinal, quaalude, desoxyn, preludin, and ritalin.

You will recognize immediately that each of the drugs on that long list is a prescription drug. Whereas a significant proportion of the prescription drugs available on the black market is counterfeit, the product of clandestine laboratories, a disturbingly high proportion is not. Clearly, the "closed" system of drug control that Congress devised a decade ago is being threatened by the illegal diversion of drugs *within* the system, as well as from the influx of illegally manufactured or imported drugs from outside the system.

This problem should be one of particular concern to each of you, not only because you are guardians of the public health, but also because some of your brethren in the medical profession are causing much of the illegal diversion of these prescription drugs. I can assure you that this is becoming a matter of particular concern to law enforcement authorities throughout the country. We are alarmed at the proliferation of clinics that employ doctors to write prescriptions for a steady stream of patients, ostensibly for weight control or some other medical reason, but without even taking medical histories or conducting physical examinations. We see enormous profits being made by doctors who sell blocks of prescriptions wholesale, and by pharmacists who fill the prescriptions knowing them to have been written illegally. I can safely predict that you are going to see, more and more, the prosecution of physicians, pharmacists, and clinic owners who bend to the temptation of windfall profit by abusing their privilege to prescribe and dispense controlled substances.

Let me conclude on much the same note that I began, with a comment about how important it is that the medical profession maintain a prominent and visible role in the resolution of questions about the effects of psychotropic drugs. One of the more curious legislative changes brought about by the passage of the Controlled Substances Act was to take the responsibility for designating controlled substances away from the Secretary of Health, Education and Welfare and to give that duty to the Attorney General. That change is curious inasmuch as the Dept. of Justice has never been noted for its expertise in psychopharmacology.

Perhaps in recognition of this, Congress has required that before the Attorney General may initiate proceedings to regulate or deregulate a drug, or to reschedule a drug, he must "gather the necessary data" from the Secretary of Health, Education, and Welfare. In turn, Health, Education, and Welfare is to consult with you in the medical and scientific communities, to help arrive at recommendations that will be binding on the Attorney General on questions about the likelihood of psychic, physiological, or other pharmacological effects of any drug, about the potential a drug poses for abuse, and about the history and current pattern for abuse of the drug (18). In a very real sense, it is to be the medical profession and not "the government" (and certainly not the Dept. of Justice) that has the leading role in the control of the abuse of psychotropic drugs. The public's conception about the fairness or unfairness of the drug laws is based less upon its opinion about all of the legal procedures that are established and carried out by lawyers, than it is upon its collective judgement that the drug laws either are well designed to protect society from a genuine health hazard, or instead are set up merely to superimpose overly rigid standards of morality upon society.

If drugs that are now subject to regulation should not be controlled, it is important that the medical profession may say so. If, on the other hand, the regulation of these drugs is necessary for the protection of society, it is equally (if not more) important for the profession to make this known. And not just to The Dept. of Health, Education, and Welfare or Dept. of Justice, but to the entire community.

Unless the public accepts the need for the control of psychotropic drugs–and it will not accept this just because *lawyers* tell them to–drug abuse legislation does not stand a chance. Only the medical profession can take the lead in this. A public acceptance of drug regulation based upon its respect for your medical judgement will increase the possibility that this regulation will result in its goal: reducing the incidence of drug abuse. Perhaps it might bring us closer to the day when there will be no need to philosophize about drug abuse and the law.

NOTES

1. Compare Grinspoon, *Marihuana Reconsidered*, Harvard University Press (1971) ("No amount of research is likely to prove that *Cannabis* is as dangerous as alcohol and tobacco") with Nahas, Marihuana–*Deceptive Weed*, Raven Press, p. 192 (1973) ("All of the major effects of *Cannabis* derivatives justify their classification ... among the 'psychodysleptic' compounds which 'disintegrate mental function'").

2. Forty years later the Supreme Court ruled that a State could not punish an individual simply because he had become addicted to drugs. *Robinson* v. *California*, 370 U.S. 660 (1962). The Court was concerned that the punishment of a condition such as drug addiction would throw us back to those days not too long ago when we herded the insane into dungeons, and beat them until they regained their reason. See *Action for Mental Health* (1961), p. 26. However, the Court adhered to its earlier holding that the police power permitted the State to regulate the sale and use of dangerous drugs. *Robinson* v. *California*, *supra*. 370 U.S., at 664.

3. Wilson, *Thinking About Crime*, Vanguard Press, p. 142 (1975).

4. There *is* a statute which makes it unlawful for any person simply to possess a controlled drug unless it was obtained from a practitioner directly or pursuant to a valid prescription. Title 21, United States Code, Section 844(a). However, this offense is designated as a misdemeanor, and a defendant's record of conviction for this offense may be expunged. Moreover, this statute has been virtually ignored by federal prosecutors. With few exceptions, the only drug possession infractions prosecuted are those involving the violation of a far stricter statute–Title 21, United States Code, Section 841–which prohibits the possession of controlled drugs with the intent to distribute them.

5. "If a drug creates no danger to the public health, it would be inappropriate to control the drug under this bill." U.S. Code Cong. & Adm. News, 4603 (1970).

6. Indeed, Congress recognized that possession of drugs with the intent to use may be more of a sickness than a crime. See U.S. Code Cong. & Adm. News, 4574–75 (1970).

7. The Drug Abuse Control Amendments of 1965, Title 18, United States Code, Section 1114, and Title 21, United States Code, Sections 321 et seq.

8. The Narcotic Addict Rehabilitation Act of 1966, Title 18, United States Code, Sections 4251–55, Title 28, United States Code, Sections 2901 et seq., Title 42, United States Code, Sections 3401 et seq.

9. Among these laws were The Narcotics Opiate Act, Title 19, United States Code, Section 1584, Title 21, United States Code, Sections, 171 et seq., and Title 26, United States Code, Sections 4701 et seq.; The Narcotics Registration Act, Title 18, United States Code, Section 1407; The Narcotics Manufacturing Act of 1960, Title 21, United States Code, Sections 501 et seq., and Title 26, United States Code, sections 4702, 4731; The Narcotic Drugs Importation and Exportation Acts, Title 21, United States Code, sections 171 et seq., and Title 31, United States Code, Section 529a; The Narcotic Control Act of 1956, Title 8, United States Code, Sections 1182, 1251, and Title 18, United States Code, Sections 1401 et seq.; and The Narcotic Addict Rehabilitation Act of 1966, *supra*, n. 7.

10. U.S. Code Cong. & Adm. News, 4572–73 (1970).

11. *Id*. At 4568–69.

12. Title 21, United States Code, Sections 801 et seq.

13. Title 21, United States Code, Section 841 (b)(1)(A).

14. Title 21, United States Code, Section 848.

15. Title 21, United States Code, Section 845.
16. Title 21, United States Code, Section 851.
17. Title 21, United States Code, Section 849.
18. U.S. Code Cong. & Adm. News, 4600 (1970).

66

Federal Regualtions for the Prescription of Controlled Substances
Drug Enforcement Administration (DEA)

John H. King

1. THE CONTROLLED SUBSTANCES ACT

Since its enactment in 1970, the Controlled Substances Act (CSA) has served as the legal foundation for Federal control of drugs of abuse. The CSA is a consolidation of numerous laws regulating the manufacture and distribution of narcotics, stimulants, depressants, hallucinogens, anabolic steroids and chemicals used in the illicit production of controlled substances. This act seeks, through appropriate regulation and criminal sanctions, to reduce the availability of drugs or other substances subject to abuse, while maintaining an adequate supply of these drugs or other substances for legitimate trade and industrial, medical or scientific use. There are five schedules (I through V), with Schedule I being the most restrictive, and Schedule V being the least restrictive.

The Act provides an administrative process for adding, deleting, or changing the schedule of substances under control. Since 1971, excluding anabolic steroids and listed chemicals, approximately 100 substances have been added to the CSA, and 33 substances have been rescheduled or removed from the CSA.

The criteria controlling or decontrolling any substance are based on medical use and safety, potential for abuse, and dependence profile. These criteria rely heavily on the integrity of scientific and medical data. In this respect, these criteria are similar to the Food and Drug Administration's (FDA) standards for finding a drug safe and effective. Each scheduling action must be based on scientifically verified and legally defensible data, and involve the review of available data by both the Drug Enforcement Administration (DEA) and the Department of Health and Human Services (HHS).

2. SCHEDULING CRITERIA

In order to understand how drugs are administratively placed in specific schedules, the criteria that determine that placement must be defined. The DEA must determine whether a substance meets the criteria for any of the schedules.

From: *Marihuana and Medicine*
Edited by: G. G. Nahas et al.   © Humana Press Inc., Totowa, NJ

In order for a substance to be placed into Schedule I, it must meet the following criteria:

1. The drug or other substance has a high potential for abuse.
2. The drug or other substance has no currently accepted medical use in treatment in the United States.
3. There is a lack of accepted safety for use of the drug or other substance under medical supervision.

Administrative control of substances in Schedules II through V require that they have currently accepted medical use in the United States. They range from high (Schedule II) to progressively lower (Schedule V) potential for abuse, dependence liability and regulatory oversight.

Substances placed in Schedule II must meet the following criteria:

1. The drug or other substance has a high potential for abuse.
2. The drug or other substance has a currently accepted medical use in treatment in the United States or currently accepted medical use with severe restrictions.
3. Abuse of the drug or other substances may lead to severe psychological or physical dependence.

The rescheduling of LAAM (levoacetylmethadol) gives you an example of how these criteria were utilized in a rescheduling process. LAAM was initially placed under Schedule I control (no currently accepted medical use and lacking medical safety). When HHS concluded that LAAM was safe and effective for the treatment of narcotic addiction and approved the use of LAAM for that indication, DEA was then able to make all the findings of Schedule II, including medical utility, and LAAM was rescheduled to Schedule II.

2.1. Potential for Abuse

The threshold finding for a substance to be administratively controlled under the CSA is abuse potential. Both Schedules I and II require the finding of a high potential of abuse and differ in their accepted medical use criteria. An examination of the working definition of these terms will help you understand how these determinations are made.

Although the term "potential for abuse" is not defined in the CSA, there is much discussion of the term in the legislative history of the Act. The following four items are indicators that a drug has a potential for abuse:

1. There is evidence that individuals are taking the drug or other substance in amounts sufficient to create a hazard to their health or the safety of others or to the community.
2. There is significant diversion of the drug or other substance from legitimate drug channels.
3. Individuals are taking the drug or other substances on their own initiative, rather than on the basis of medical advice from a practitioner qualified legally to administer such drug.
4. The drug or other substance is pharmacologically similar to a drug already under control, thus making it reasonable to assume it may have similar potential for abuse.

As you can see, the term encompasses both the actual abuse, trafficking, diversion, and health risks of a substance, as well as the potential for a substance to be involved in these activities.

2.2. Currently Accepted Medical Use

The term "currently accepted medical use" also is not defined in the CSA. Prior to 1988, the DEA interpreted the phrase "currently accepted medical use in treatment in the United

States" to mean that the substance may be lawfully marketed under the Food, Drug, and Cosmetic Act. This meant that only drugs lawfully marketed in the United States could be placed in Schedules II through V using the administrative scheduling process. Successful challenges to this interpretation in the United States Court of Appeals led to a clarification of the definition of the term by the DEA. The following five-part test for determining whether a drug meets the criteria of "currently accepted medical use" was developed and is in use today:

1. The drug's chemistry must be known and reproducible.
2. There must be adequate safety studies.
3. There must be adequate and well-controlled studies proving efficacy.
4. The drug must be accepted by qualified experts.
5. The scientific evidence must be widely available.

If a substance satisfies *each* of the five requirements, it has a currently accepted medical use; if one of the requirements is not satisfied, the substance does not have an accepted medical use for the purposes of the CSA.

3. ADMINISTRATIVE SCHEDULING

Scheduling under the CSA has been delegated by the United States Attorney General to the Administrator of the DEA, who, in turn, has redelegated this authority to the Deputy Administrator. Whereas there are several procedures that can be utilized to change the control status of drugs or other substances, the administrative scheduling process is the primary method. To help you explain how this process works, the major procedures that DEA must follow under the CSA are outlined below.

Administrative proceedings to add, delete, or change, the schedule of a substance may be initiated by the DEA, HHS, or through a petition from an interested party, such as the manufacturer of the drug, a medical society or association, a pharmacy association, a public interest group concerned with drug abuse, a state or local government agency, or an individual citizen. After a petition is received and accepted by DEA, the agency begins its own review of the drug.

3.1. Eight-Factor Analysis

Before making the decision that a drug or other substance meets the criteria for a specific schedule, the DEA is required to conduct a review that includes the consideration of the following eight factors:

1. Its actual or relative potential for abuse.
2. Scientific evidence of its pharmacological effects, if known.
3. The state of current scientific knowledge regarding the drug or other substance.
4. Its history and current pattern of abuse.
5. The scope, duration, and significance of abuse.
6. What, if any, risk there is to the public health.
7. Its psychological or physiological dependence liability.
8. Whether the substance is an immediate precursor of a substance already controlled under this subchapter.

After completing its initial review, the DEA forwards its findings to HHS and requests a scientific and medical evaluation, and a scheduling recommendation. The Assistant Secretary of Health then requests information from the Commissioner of the FDA, evaluations and recommendations from the National Institute on Drug Abuse (NIDA), and, on occasion, data from the general scientific and medical community. The HHS compiles the information and sends DEA a medical and scientific evaluation, and a recommendation as to whether the drug should be controlled, and in what schedule it should be placed.

The medical and scientific evaluations from HHS are binding on DEA. The scheduling recommendation is only binding if HHS recommends that the drug not be controlled. The DEA Deputy Administrator then evaluates all available data and makes a final decision based on the criteria of the individual schedules whether the drug should be controlled and into what schedule it should be placed.

When the DEA Deputy Administrator has determined that a drug should be controlled, decontrolled, or rescheduled, a notice of proposed rulemaking announcing his course of action is published in the *Federal Register.* The proposal invites all interested persons to file comments with DEA. Affected parties may also request a hearing with DEA. These procedures are governed by the Administrative Procedures Act.

If no hearing is requested, DEA will evaluate all the comments it received and publish a final order in the *Federal Register* to control the drug as proposed, or with modifications based upon the written comments if received. The order will set the effective dates for implementing the proposal under the CSA.

If a hearing is requested, it will be held before a DEA administrative law judge. At the conclusion, the judge will issue a recommended decision. That decision, along with the briefs filed by both parties, the transcript, and all evidence presented at the hearing will be submitted to the Deputy Administrator.

The Deputy Administrator reviews the documents and prepares his own findings of fact and conclusions of law (which may or may not be the same as those prepared by the Administrative Law Judge). The Deputy Administrator then publishes a final order in the *Federal Register,* either scheduling the drug or declining to do so.

Once the final order is published in the Federal Register, interested parties have 30 days to appeal to the United States Court of Appeals to challenge the order. The order imposing controls is not stayed during the appeal, unless so ordered by the court. Excluding marihuana, there have only been two hearings in the past 20 years involving the substances buprenorphine and 3,4-methlyenedioxmethamphetamine (MDMA).

As has just been illustrated, under the administrative process, DEA is required to follow specific procedures and meet criteria as established by law. However, Congress can place any substance under any level of control without regard to these criteria. When the CSA was initially enacted, Congress placed a number of substances under control. For example heroin, LSD, and marihuana were placed in Schedule I. Later, anabolic steroids were added to Schedule III through the legislative process.

4. OTHER FORMS OF SCHEDULING

4.1. International Treaty Obligations

The United States is party to the Single Convention on Narcotic Drugs of 1961 designed to establish effective control over international and domestic traffic in opiates, coca leaf, cocaine, and cannabis. A second treaty, the Convention on Psychotropic Substances of 1971, is designed to establish comparable control over stimulants, depressants, and hallucinogens. Congress ratified this treaty in 1980. Our treaty obligations under these conventions require that a drug or other substance be controlled under the CSA or be rescheduled if existing controls are less stringent than those required by the treaty. The DEA can place such a drug or other substance under control in the CSA without regard to the findings that are required by administrative procedures.

4.2. Temporary Scheduling and Controlled Substance Analogues

During the past three decades, the CSA has been amended by Congress and clarified by the courts. These actions have enabled the CSA to respond to the changing concerns of law enforcement, regulatory officials, and the public health community. Two of these amendments involve scheduling procedures and evolved in response to the proliferation of clandestinely produced drugs that were pharmacologically and chemically related to controlled substances, but not specifically listed under the CSA.

4.2.1. EMERGENCY SCHEDULING

The Comprehensive Crime Control Act of 1984 provided the DEA with emergency scheduling authority to place a substance into Schedule I on a temporary basis in order to avoid an imminent hazard to the public safety. The emergency scheduling provision may only apply to substances that:

1. Are not lawfully marketed in the United States.
2. Are not currently controlled in any other schedule of the CSA.
3. Have no active investigational new use status (IND) in effect.

The temporary placement of a substance into Schedule I is effective for one year with the possibility of a 6-month extension. Prior to invoking the emergency scheduling provision for a substance, the DEA is required notify the HHS and receive input from HHS with regard to the marketing and IND status. In order to keep a substance in Schedule I, the DEA must initiate traditional scheduling procedures and complete the action prior to the expiration of 18 months. Although this provision shortens the time required to control drugs that meet the above criteria, new designer drugs continue to enter the illicit market.

4.2.2. CONTROLLED SUBSTANCE ANALOGS

Despite the emergency-scheduling authority granted to the DEA, clandestine laboratory operators could synthesize new analogs of controlled substances faster than DEA could schedule them. As a consequence, the CSA was again amended by the Anti-Drug Abuse Act of 1986 to allow controlled substance analogs to be treated as Schedule I substances. To the extent intended for human use, a controlled substance analog is defined as a substance that:

1. Has a chemical structure substantially similar to a controlled substance in Schedule I or II.
2. Has a stimulant, depressant, or hallucinogenic effect on the central nervous system that is substantially similar or greater than that of a controlled substance in Schedule I or II.
3. A particular person represents or intends to have a stimulant, depressant, or hallucinogenic effect substantially similar to or greater than that of a controlled substance in Schedule I or II.

The term controlled substance analog does not include substances already controlled or substances that have an approved IND or are lawfully marketed in the United States. This amendment to the CSA provides a means to prosecute those individuals who attempt to circumvent existing drug laws by manufacturing and distributing substances with chemical structures that are only slightly different than those of controlled substances and that are likely to retain the psychoactive properties of the parent compound. Regulatory controls of Schedule I substances do not apply to controlled substance analogs; only criminal sanctions apply. To date, this provision of the CSA has been used on numerous occasions to prosecute individuals that are producing and trafficking controlled substance analogues that are intended for human use.

5. CONCLUSION

We recognize that drug scheduling actions are meant to protect the public health and safety, yet provide for the legitimate use and availability of needed medicines. Under the CSA, every step of the scheduling process—from the initial petition, the evaluations, and final rule—must meet the rigorous scientific and legal requirements established by Congress and the law.

67

FDA Regulation of Prescription of Controlled Substances

Nicholas Reuter

Abstract

The Federal Food, Drug, and Cosmetic Act requires the premarket approval of new drugs prior to their marketing. FDA accomplishes this through regulations that establish Investigational New Drug Applications (INDs) and New Drug Application (NDAs).

FDA IND regulations address phases of clinical investigations, from Phase I trials involving few subjects, to Phase III trials with thousands of subjects. Under these regulations FDA will not allow an investigation to proceed if human subjects would be exposed to unreasonable risks, investigators are not qualified, or if the investigation protocol is deficient. FDA also requires adequate animal toxicology studies to show it is reasonably safe to administer the drug to human subjects.

FDA drug approval regulations protect the public by ensuring that adequate scientific studies have been performed to provide a rational basis on which to conclude that the benefits of a drug outweigh its risks and by assuring that the product is accompanied by sufficient information to permit its accurate prescription. FDA regulations require that the marketing application (NDA) include adequate tests to show whether or not the drug is safe for use under the conditions prescribed, recommended or suggested in the labeling. In addition, there must be substantial evidence, consisting of adequate and well-controlled clinical investigations, that the drug product will have the effect it purports or is represented to have under the conditions prescribed, recommended or suggested in the labeling. Importantly, manufacturing methods and controls must be adequate to assure the identity, strength, quality, purity, stability, or bioavailability of the drug product.

FDA regulations set forth the "essentials of adequate and well-controlled clinical investigation," including requirements that the study design permits a valid comparison with a control (including, placebo, dose comparison, no treatment, active, and historical) to provide a quatitative assessment of drug effect.

From: *Marihuana and Medicine*
Edited by: G. G. Nahas et al.   © Humana Press Inc., Totowa, NJ

1. IND PHASES OF INVESTIGATIONS

FDA regulations address various phases of investigations that are conducted under INDs. However, before an investigation in human subjects can proceed, there must be approval by a local Institutional Review Board, or IRB. The IRB, among other human subject protection concerns, reviews informed consent forms.

Phase I: few subjects, determine "tolerable" dose.
Phase II: last a few years, several hundred subjects with condition, effectiveness investigated.
Phase III: thousands of subjects, four years or longer, dosing, effectiveness, safety information obtained.

FDA does not approve INDs. Instead, the investigation can proceed within 30 days of receipt of the IND, unless, during that time, after review, FDA places a clinical hold on the investigation.

FDA regulations establish narrow conditions for placing a clinical hold on an investigation that are tied to the phases of investigation just mentioned. FDA will invoke a clinical hold if:

1. Human subjects would be exposed to unreasonable risks.
2. Investigators are not qualified.
3. Part of the application is incomplete, including investigator brochure; or if there is insufficient information to assess the risk to subjects in the proposed study.
4. In phase II or III studies, if the protocol for the investigation is deficient to meet its objectives. Note that FDA regulations set forth requirements for protocols in seven areas, including study design (controls, and so on), dose determination, observations or measurements to be used to fulfill the study objectives, and so on).

In addition to IRB review, patient selection criteria, investigation protocols, blinding, and other investigator bias controls, FDA IND regulations require chemistry and manufacturing information to assure the proper identification, quality, purity, strength, and stability of the investigational drug. FDA also requires adequate animal toxicology studies to show it is reasonably safe to administer the drug to human subjects.

1.1. Preclinical Investigations

If information is contained in the IND application that is derived from animal studies, there must be an assurance that the animal studies were conducted in accordance with current Good Laboratory Practices regulations.

1.2. Reporting

IND holders must submit annual reports and periodic safety reports—the frequency of which are tied to severity of the adverse events encountered.

To get an approximate sense on the number of substances that are screened through the IND and NDA process, consider that for each 100 drugs with INDs: 70 complete phase I; 33 complete phase II; 25-30 complete phase III; and 20 are ultimately approved for market.

It should be noted that there is cross-referencing among DEA and FDA regulations on investigations that involve schedule I substances. DEA regulations recognize FDA authorization of an IND to verify the scientific merit of the protocol that must be supplied with a schedule I researcher registration application. In addition, FDA assesses the competence of the applicant for schedule I researcher registration procedures. Under DEA regulations, FDA must also evaluate the qualifications of the investigator and the merits of the protocol for non-IND, nonclinical research with schedule I substances.

2. REVIEW OF NEW DRUG APPLICATION

2.1. Purpose of Premarket Review

The FDA drug approval process protects the public by ensuring that adequate scientific studies have been performed to provide a rational basis on which to conclude that the benefits of a drug outweigh its risks and by assuring that the product is accompanied by sufficient information to permit its accurate prescription.

FDA regulations list at least 18 reasons for not approving an NDA. Rather than list all of these grounds for denial, it is appropriate to highlight some that are of particular interest. FDA will not approve a new drug application if:

- Manufacturing methods and controls are not adequate to assure the identity, strength, quality, purity, stability, or bioavailability.
- The application does not include adequate tests to show whether the drug is safe for use under the conditions prescribed, recommended, or suggested in the labeling. Or the submitted tests show the drug is unsafe under the labeling conditions.
- There is a lack of substantial evidence, consisting of adequate and well-controlled clinical investigations, that the drug product will have the effect it purports or is represented to have under the conditions prescribed, recommended or suggested in the labeling.

FDA regulations set forth the "essentials of adequate and well-controlled clinical investigation," including requirements that the study design permits a valid comparison with a control to provide a quantitative assessment of drug effect. FDA regulations address the use of:

- Placebo control—test of the article compared to inactive preparation.
- Dose comparison concurrent control—at least two doses are considered.
- No treatment concurrent control—objective measurements of effectiveness, when placebo effect negligible.
- Active control—intent to show similarity to test and control
- Historical control—treatment with test drug compared to experience derived historically from adequately documented natural history of disease or condition.

Many of these control groups can be combined into a single study.

A considerable portion of the NDA review process integrates what has been learned from clinical trials into what appears on the product labeling to guide the prescriber, including dosage and administration, indications (or approved uses), contraindications, warnings (including warnings about abuse and dependence in vulnerable populations). This conference includes a session on the treatment of pain. As part of the review process, the suggested use may relate to a more specific type of pain:

Acute
Postoperative
Traumatic
Inflammatory
Chronic
Neoplastic
Neuropathic
Chronic Intermittent (e.g., migraine)

In addition to the labeling and indication for use, there are other issues that need to be considered during the NDA review that relate to the abuse liability assessment. There are many types of routes of administration for a new drug product:

Oral (controlled, slow, immediate release)
IV (bolus or continuous)
IM
Inhaled
Transdermal
Transmucosal
Intrathecal
Epidural

3. ABUSE POTENTIAL ASSESSMENT

FDA NDA regulations require an abuse liability assessment for drugs with abuse potential. This permits the evaluation of a drug product's potential for abuse. Typically, an NDA will include:

Preclinical abuse liability tests.
Clinical abuse liability trials in special populations.
Trials that compare test drug to a prototype(s).

Often, sponsors will conduct postapproval monitoring for drug abuse outbreaks, dependence, withdrawal, and so on. These pre- and postmarket trials are important with new drug products because often there are limited or no epidemiological or actual experience data to reference. Information from these trials may result in a recommendation for scheduling, or appear in labeling as a warning, or both.

How long does it take FDA to review an NDA and approve or not approve a drug product for marketing? The agency has been subject to User Fees for NDA reviews. The act was recently modernized with new time-tables for actions on applications, along with other features to address the review process:

10-month turnaround on applications.
6-month turnaround for "impact" drugs.
Requirement for Development Plan.
Earlier industry-FDA meetings.
Agreements on study protocols at the phase II juncture.

In addition to premarketing approval, FDA has responsibilities in the review of substances for scheduling under the Controlled Substances Act (CSA). For drug products emerging from the NDA review, FDA initiates the scheduling of a drug product if appropriate. The agency often solicits advise from its Drug Abuse Advisory Committee on scheduling issues. For drug substances outside the NDA process, DEA typically initiates the scheduling review. After collecting information on the substance, or in response to a outside petition, DEA requests that FDA and NIDA provide scientific and medial evaluation and recommendation for control. FDA and the National Institute on Drug Abuse prepare an evaluation and recommendation in accordance with the criteria in the law:

Actual or relative potential for abuse.
Scientific evidence of its pharmacologic effect.
The state of scientific knowledge regarding the drug.
Its history and current pattern of abuse.
The risk to the public health.
Its psychic or physiological dependence liability.
Whether the substance is the immediate precursor to a known drug of abuse.

Upon receipt of recommendation, DEA proceeds via rulemaking to schedule the substance. The Department of Health and Human Services must forward a recommendation that includes a recommendation on the schedule for control among the five schedules. The department applies the criteria for scheduling recommendations that are in the CSA. These criteria relate to:

The drug products' relative potential for abuse (relative to substances currently controlled in the schedules).
Its capacity to produce psychological and physical dependence (mild, moderate, severe).
Its accepted medical use in treatment in the United States.

As discussed above, the determination of a new drug product's relative potential for abuse can be influenced by the dosage form and route of administration, particularly if these factors influence the onset of action of the active ingredient, or the availability of the drug product to the general population.

4. FDA–DEA INTERACTIONS

It is important to note that whereas the FDA and DEA reviews are independent to a certain extent, there is considerable interaction among the agencies to implement the drug-control laws and regulations discussed today. In addition, there are volumes of guidances and guidelines available that can accurately elaborate on this.

In conclusion, FDA enforces regulations that address the investigational use of drug substances and products in humans. These regulations are in place to assure, among other things, that human subjects are not exposed to inappropriate risks and that investigations conform with scientific standards. In addition, there are detailed regulations that address the requirements for NDAs for marketing approval. Finally, FDA applies procedures, along with regulations, standards, and guidelines in evaluating the abuse potential for substances in determining the appropriate control of substances and products under the CSA.

68

The Swedish Addiction Epidemic in Global Perspective

Nils Bejerot

Abstract

The Swedish epidemic of intravenous amphetamine injection that started in 1945, was surveyed annually in Stockholm from 1965 to 1987. During that period, approximately 250,000 arrestees were examined for needle marks from intravenous drug injections that they presented in their cubital regions. The progression or regression of the epidemic was gaged by calculating the percentage of addicts (marked with needle scars) among the population arrested for any kind of criminal or civil offense. This epidemiological study using an objective marker demonstrated that a permissive drug policy leads to a rapid spread of drug use. A restrictive policy not only checks the spread of addiction but brings about a considerable reduction in the rate of current consumption. The restrictive policy is based on a general consensus of social refusal of illicit drug use, and strict law enforcement. All countries that have adopted this model such as China, Japan, Korea, Singapore, and Taiwan have succeeded in controlling epidemics of amphetamine or heroin addiction. By contrast, Western industrialized nations that have accepted permissive policies have seen their epidemics of drug addiction grow steadily since World War II and erode their democratic institutions. The author concludes that such a trend may only be reversed by adopting a restrictive model validated by epidemiological and historical facts.

1. INTRODUCTION

Sweden was the first country in Europe to be afflicted by drug abuse of epidemic type immediately after the end of World War II. The Swedish epidemic has been extremely extensive, it has spread to neighboring countries and to the continent, and it has presented dramatic phases during its development. In addition it is probably the drug epidemic that has been most closely studied and documented. Therefore Swedish experience is of considerable international interest.

There are several types of drug abuse, regardless of the nature of the drug. It is important to differentiate between these types or patterns of abuse, since they differ fundamentally in regard to prevention and control.

From: *Marihuana and Medicine*
Edited by: G. G. Nahas et al.   © Humana Press Inc., Totowa, NJ

2. THERAPEUTIC TYPE

First we have the classical medical use of dependence-producing drugs that may give rise to abuse and addiction. Those affected are usually middle aged, socially stable people who developed a drug abuse as a result of an error in medical treatment. These people are ashamed of their drug abuse, try to keep it hidden–even from their physicians and relatives, and they rarely draw others into their abuse.

3. CULTURAL TYPE

The other main type of use and abuse is coupled to the culturally accepted consumption of certain inebriates–a consumption that often stretches back to prehistoric times. It is no breach of norms within a culture to enjoy these drugs, but severe cases of dependence may arise, even though the use is ritual in accordance with ancient rules and traditions. This cultural form of abuse may be exemplified by the coca chewing of South American Indians, Cannabis smoking in certain Muslim countries, opium smoking in the Far East, and alcoholism in the Christian world.

4. EPIDEMIC TYPE

The third type of drug dependence is epidemic abuse. Characteristically it arises in bohemian circles where small groups of romantic dreamers or risk-taking normbreakers experiment with exotic or new intoxicating drugs in the pursuit of novel experiences. After years or decades of use of the drug in isolated groups, the first phase of the epidemic, there is a spread in the second phase to new categories, often to other groups of norm-breakers, and then particularly to criminal circles. In the third phase, drug consumption spreads to broad groups of the normal population, first to those with the weakest impulse control and the least stable system of values, that is the youth. In the fourth phase the epidemic abuse tends to spread upwards through the age groups, and may begin to resemble drug use of cultural type: That is, it is no longer considered to be a breach of norms. A new, permanent drug problem has now been added to those already existing in the culture. Regardless of the country and the drug, these epidemics present a number of characteristics in common.

5. SPREAD

Spread of drug abuse occurs almost without exception through personal, psychosocial contact between an established abuser and a novice in very close friendship relation, often between sexual partners. Initiation usually occurs in an early phase of the initiator's abuse, during the period which is commonly called the honeymoon of addiction, before the negative physical, psychological, social, economic and legal complications have commenced. The honeymoon is short in the case of heroin, usually about a year, but far longer in *Cannabis* abuse. Initiation via pushers and incidental contacts is rare. Pushers enter the scene at a later stage, when they play a very destructive role in maintaining an established abuse or provide for a relapse.

6. EXPONENTIAL GROWTH

Epidemics of drug abuse often spread very rapidly. In most countries it has been possible to observe an exponential growth for long periods of time. For instance, intravenous abuse of amphetamine in Sweden doubled every thirtieth month during a period of 20 years, 1946–1965. In England the number of heroin addicts doubled every sixteenth month during a period of 10 years, 1959–1968.

Other characteristics for drug epidemics are their restriction by historic boundaries, and also, for long periods, within small coteries and by age, ethnic, geographical, and national boundaries.

7. YOUTH

Drug epidemics are for long periods checked by such boundaries, but when these barriers are broken through, the abuse spreads into new population strata. For instance the Jews lived side-by-side with *Cannabis*-smoking Muslims in the Middle East for 1000 years without any Jew smoking hashish. It was not until young American-Jewish *Cannabis* smokers came to visit Israel that Jewish youth began to smoke the drug *(1)*.

8. FASHION

Drug epidemics are extremely sensitive to fashion regarding the type of drug and method of administration, with sometimes rapid changes in the panorama of abuse. An example of this is cocaine, which, for a long period, was only consumed in the traditional way by chewing. With the production of pure cocaine, sniffing was introduced, later followed by intravenous injections, and finally by smoking the free base and coca paste.

The more drug epidemics spread in a society the more common will be the occurrence of mixed abuse with different drugs and varied mode of administration.

9. INTERACTION

Exposure and susceptibility interact in a predictable way.

The fact that there was no one in Europe before World War II who injected drugs intravenously was because of the same simple reason that we had no syphilis or tobacco smoking before Columbus. Nor was there any tuberculosis or alcoholism among the Eskimos before they were colonized by the Danes. There had been susceptible individuals before, but they had not been exposed to these factors.

10. MASSIVITY

The pressure of exposure, also called massivity, causes people to react differently: Some are affected immediately, others after a time, some only after the pressure from the drug culture has become very great, whereas many manage to resist throughout their whole lives, despite prolonged and intensive exposure. Thus, susceptibility varies between different individuals, but also in the same individual with age and a number of other factors.

We can now express the connection between exposure to drug culture (E), the susceptibility of the individual (S) and the risk that the individual will commence to use the drug, that is the psychosocial contagion (C): $C = S \times E$.

The susceptibility of the individual (S) is the result of a large number of individual factors such as sex, age, social situation, previous experience, and so on. Since exposure at one point also affects future susceptibility (fS) we can in general write the formula: $C = fS \times fE$.

Of all norm-breaking forms of drug abuse, intravenous administration is the one that is most suitable for scientific study, since the breach of norms here is distinct and important, and in addition injections leave clear, objective and characteristic diagnostic signs, that cannot be confused with medical injections *(2)*.

11. THE SWEDISH EPIDEMIC OF INTRAVENOUS DRUG ABUSE

The Swedish epidemic started through a few coincidental events. Intravenous drug abuse had been reported in the United States since 1926, but as far as I know, this did not initiate any drug epidemics in Europe until a young, adventurous Swede in 1946 learned the injection technique in the United States, and introduced it into a little bohemian coterie in Stockholm. In this group a few persons had become amphetaminists through medical treatment for alcoholism, and in this limited group an epidemic of intravenous abuse was established.

Up to 1949 there were a dozen cases within this bohemian coterie in Stockholm, but not a single case outside this group. In 1949 the epidemic spread out of this circle via a couple of artists models who were also prostitutes, and the epidemic thus gained a foothold in social problem groups. In the summer 1954, I diagnosed the first medically documented case of this type in Sweden.

In 1956 the epidemic of intravenous abuse spread to Gothenburg, when an addict of this category moved there, and for the rest of his life was a central figure in addict circles in the second largest city in Sweden. The Swedish amphetamine epidemic spread to Finland in 1965, to Denmark in 1966, to Norway in 1967, and to Germany in 1972.

In the study of the Swedish epidemic of intravenous abuse, I assumed that a breach of norms such as introducing a needle into a vein and injecting illicit drugs was so extreme that it would be expected to coexist with other severe breaches of norms such as traditional criminal conduct. I therefore initiated a study in 1965 in which nurses inspected the veins of the arms of persons brought to the central arrest premises in Stockholm. The first years of the study have been reported (2). From the study of representativity it is apparent that practically all active intravenous abusers are brought to the arrest premises sooner or later for one reason or another, and are included in the study.

The investigation is still continuing, and hitherto we have examined about a quarter of a million arrestees, many of them on several occasions.

12. CONTROL

When we have understood how individual and social factors interact to give rise to drug epidemics, we can begin to discuss how we should attack the problem.

Many studies have shown that the individual susceptibility factor is, unfortunately, not easily influenced, composed as it is of everything that has affected the individual up to the present. On the other hand the exposure factor, pressure from the addiction milieu and the drug market, have proved to be highly modifiable by means of certain strategies.

The rate of opiate addiction in the United States was reduced by about 90% between the years 1923 and 1939 (3), and this without any treatment or research to speak of. The instrument was a strict drug policy that reduced the exposure factors dramatically.

In the same way, an extensive cocaine epidemic in Germany was stopped in the late 1920s, and also a widespread amphetamine epidemic in Japan after World War II (4).

13. JAPAN

The Japanese epidemic deserves special attention. It arose when the Japanese military store of amphetamine went astray after capitulation. Abuse began among people who worked at night: Jazz musicians, artists, bohemians, and prostitutes, but it quickly spread to broad strata of the population.

The Japanese authorities introduced a number of countermeasures, but they did this too late and on too small a scale, and with too little energy: It was like operating on a growing cancer that could not be checked because the measures taken were not sufficiently radical.

The Japanese epidemic culminated in 1954, when it was estimated that two million of Japan's population of 100 million was abusing amphetamine tablets, and over half a million were taking intravenous injections. It was only then that a dramatic increase in the stringency of policy was introduced, with prison sentences of three to six months for possession, one to three years for drug pushing and five years for illicit manufacture of drugs. There was close surveillance when they were released from prison, and there was an immediate restriction on relapse.

During the first year of the campaign, 1954, 55,600 persons were arrested in Japan for amphetamine offenses of criminal nature. In 1958 the number was 271, and the epidemic was over. Altogether measures had been taken against 15% of the estimated number of intravenous abusers. The others stopped when the restrictive policy was applied. The campaign was drawn up on the basis of broad political consensus, and was carried out with the aid of massive public and media support *(5)*.

14. EXPERIENCE FROM CHINA

The Japanese had learned from the Chinese. In 1858, the legal trade of opium and the Opium Wars were imposed on China by British mercantilism. By 1900, 90 million Chinese were addicted to opium. It took a national revival at the turn of the century that stressed traditional Chinese values to stem the tide. The support of the US and the international community stopped the international opium trade. But it took 50 years of coercive measures for the country to become opium-free. Today, opium and other dependance-producing drugs are banned from China, as well as from Taiwan and Singapore *(6)*.

15. HISTORY AS A TEACHER

I have been unable to find any example of widespread drug abuse in any country that has been overcome without a general restrictive program directed to the drug market and its exposure, and this regardless of the level of development of the social system. Nor have I been able to find any example of a voluntary drug-free treatment program that has had more than a marginal effect on the extent of the problem. However we rarely learn from history.

16. BASIC EXPERIENCE

The period 1850–1950 was the age of prevention, when the mechanisms of most of the known infectious diseases were revealed and the great epidemics overcome, not so much by individual treatment as by preventive measures. Even alcohol and drug policy during this period were, in many countries, directed towards prevention. The advances made were often considerable, in Sweden they were epochmaking.

The period after 1950 is the age of therapy. Now preventive strategies and their social necessity have been forgotten, and we have instead an avalanche of different therapeutic schools and programs for the treatment of those already addicted. Most of these programs, unfortunately, have not given better results than no treatment at all.

17. NOT A DISEASE

Why is this so? Firstly because drug dependence is not a disease, and therefore, by definition, cannot be cured.

Caffeine and nicotine dependence, alcoholism, and heroinism are not diseases, even if all these dependence-producing substances may make the individual very ill. The physical dependence, or tolerance, and the very distressing abstinence symptoms following withdrawal of many drugs, are only incidental complications, whereas true dependence is a learned behavior in which craving for the drug has taken on the character and force of a natural drive. Theoretically, drug dependence is related to such conditions as gambling, pyromania, and kleptomania. The drug acts as a reinforcer.

Drug dependence is not a symptom of the factors that originally led to contact with the drug, consumption and dependence. Heavy nicotine dependence at 40 is not a late symptom of curiosity in the early teens, but an independent condition that is very difficult to handle.

A common factor in all types of drug dependence is an ambivalence of the addict towards his drug. He is anxious to obtain help for all the complications to his drug consumption, but he is not prepared to sacrifice the drug experience itself.

To combat drug epidemics by means of individual treatment is like attacking malaria by hunting mosquitos. It can occupy an enormous number of people, but the effect is negligible. What is required is drainage of the marshes.

18. THE LARGE AND THE SMALL DRUG MARKETS

Draining the drug marshes means breaking up drug traffic and reducing general exposure to illicit drugs in society. Enormous efforts have been made by the customs, police, and undercover agents all over the world. Despite this, the situation deteriorates very quickly and many countries are on the brink of giving up the fight.

Why were the advances so great in the antidrug campaign in Germany in the 1920s, the United States in the 1930s, and in China and Japan in the 1950s? And why have there been no decisive advances in the western world during the last two decades? I consider that this is largely because we have forgotten what is of primary and secondary importance on the drug market. The primary factor is not that nature produces plants such as the opium poppy or coca bush or that international crime syndicates take over the distribution of the drugs. The primary factor is that millions of people are prepared to break norms and laws in order to use these natural inebriates and also hundreds of synthetic preparations.

19. BREACH OF NORMS

It is thus the personal breach of norms that is the moral basis, and the personal possession of drugs the legal basis of the drug market, and not the international syndicates. These, in fact, are a late consequence of the emergence of a drug market.

Naturally the drug syndicates should be combatted just as actively as now, but we must open a new front if we are to win the war. If we were to destroy all the cultivations of narcotic drugs in the world, there would, none the less, still exist substances which are up to 40,000 times as strong as morphine and which can be produced synthetically.

We have to accept the painful fact that we cannot win decisive advances unless drug abuse, the abuser, and personal possession are placed in the center of our strategy.

"The junky merchant does not sell his product to the consumer, he sells the consumer to his product" said William S. Burroughs. I will quote another very astute remark from the foreword to his *Naked Lunch* from 1959 *(7)*:

> *"If you wish to alter or annihilate a pyramid of numbers in a serial relation, you alter or remove the bottom number. If we wish to annihilate the junk pyramid, we must start with the bottom of the pyramid: The addict in the street, and stop tilting quixotically for the "higher ups" so called, all of whom are immediately replaceable. The addict in the street who must have junk to live is the one irreplaceable factor in the junk equation. When there are no more addicts to buy junk there will be no junk traffic, as long as junk need exists, someone will service it."*

This is a brilliant summary of a difficult problem.

20. STRATEGY AND TACTICS

I consider that democratic, welfare states of western type ultimately stand and fall with the result of the fight against drug epidemics. To win that fight we must have realistic strategies and tactics. We must realize, and dare to affirm, that it is the drug addict who is the motor in the system. But the addict, who is extremely manipulative, and acts as the full-time defense lawyer for his or her dependence, has succeeded in duping so many honest and responsible but naive politicians and journalists, that during the last 20 years he or she has been practically scheduled as a protected monument. This I consider is the most important factor behind our failure.

21. THEY MUST BE PROSECUTED

This does not mean that I propose a return to the harsh American sentences of the 1930s for drug offenses. They were unrealistic and undermined their own purpose. We must, however, make it very uncomfortable to abuse illicit drugs if we are to reverse developments. The addict must learn to take the consequences of his or her behavior. In regard to Sweden, I have suggested a month clearing the forests for the first offence of possession of illicit drugs, two months for the second, and so on.

Society must clearly show that drug abuse is not accepted. We cannot blame the behavior of our youth on the mountain Indians in Colombia or the peasants in the Golden Triangle. We must, in the first place, put the blame on our own youth, and this may be difficult and painful. In the second place we should put the blame on ourselves for being duped into an inconsequent, permissive attitude with continual excuses and forgiveness.

22. POPULAR SUPPORT

No government in a democratic country can manage widespread drug epidemics without strong popular support. This must be achieved through broad political agreement and massive information that leads to something like a popular uprising against drug epidemics.

The near future will be decisive as to whether the western world will manage to overcome drug epidemics. With a one-sided supply-orientated strategy we will fight a war that we are doomed to lose. Only by opening a new front with a strategy oriented towards demand can development be reversed, and the fight against drugs be won. Otherwise developments will progress towards capitulation and a social chaos that may be the basis for a new period of fascism.

REFERENCES

1. Paigi, P. "The traditional role and symbolism of hashish among Moroccan Jews in Israel and the effect of acculturation," In: *Cannabis and Culture* (ed. Rubin, V.) pp. 147-172, Mouton, The Hague, 1975.
2. Bejerot, N. *Addiction and Society* (Springfield, IL: Charles C. Thomas, 1970). By the same author: *Addiction, an Artificially- induced Drive* (Springfield, IL: Charles C. Thomas, 1972), and "Drug abuse and drug policy," in *Acta Psych Scand.,* Suppl. 256 (Copenhagen: Munksgaard, 1975).
3. Harney, M. And Cross, J. *Narcotics Officer's Notebook,* Thomas, Springfield, 196 1.
4. Lewin, L. *Phantasica,* E.P. Dutton and Co., New York, 1964.
5. Brill, H. and Hirose, T., "The rise and fall of a methamphetamine epidemic: Japan 1945-1955" *(Seminars in Psychiatry,* Vol. 1, 1969, pp. 179-194). See also, Motohashi, N. *Addiction in Japan* (Tokyo: Ministry of Health, 1973)
6. Waley, A. *The Opium War Through Chinese Eyes,* (London: Allen & Unwin, 1958). See also, Willoughby, W. *Opium as an International Problem* (Baltimore, MD: Johns Hopkins University Press, 1930).
7. Burroughs, W. *Naked Lunch,* Grove Press, NY, 1959.

XI GENERAL CONCLUSIONS

69

The Medical Use of Marihuana and THC in Perspective

Nicholas Pace, Henry Clay Frick, Kenneth Sutin,
William Manger, George Hyman,
and Gabriel Nahas

Abstract

The curative properties attributed to marihuana for several thousand years have proved to be disappointing. The ancient oriental claims of marihuana as a pain soother and for the relief of muscle spasms, convulsions, rheumatism, epilepsy and migraine headaches were introduced into western medicine during the 19th century. The reason for the lack of success with marihuana remedies at that time was the same as the present observations encountered with THC and all of its novel applications: the variability and inconsistency of its effects associated with unwanted psychological and cardiovascular effects. The discovery of THC, the active ingredient of marihuana gave a new impetus for an intensive search for its potential therapeutic applications. THC and its psychoactive derivatives were proposed as analgesic, antidepressant, hypnotic tranquilizer, as a treatment for withdrawal symptoms, glaucoma, spasticity, nausea, vomiting, and to enhance the appetite. Marihuana smoke, in spite of its toxicity to the lung and immune system, was even advocated by some as a medically acceptable vehicle for THC. For many of these therapeutic applications, molecular pharmacologists have been able to tailor specific molecules targeted to receptor sites which control acute and inflammatory pain, nausea, vomiting, and glaucoma. These fundamental studies in molecular pharmacology have also provided for an explanation of the therapeutic inadequacy of THC. This cannabinoid deregulates the physiological signaling role of a receptor protein to which it binds and of the membrane bilipid layer which it permeates. This deregulation of membrane signaling will result in discordant and partial therapeutic effects coupled with unwanted side effects.

From: *Marihuana and Medicine*
Edited by: G. G. Nahas et al.   © Humana Press Inc., Totowa, NJ

HISTORY

The Chinese were the first to describe the medicinal properties of oral preparations of *Cannabis* in the *Pen-ts'ao Ching* 2,000 years ago, and they were the first to discard its use a few centuries later because the substance made one see "devils." Opium with other herbal remedies and acupuncture were preferred instead.

In India and Middle Eastern countries the medicinal properties of oral preparations of *Cannabis* were still widely used in the 19th century. At that time *Cannabis* was introduced to Western medicine by William O'Shaughnessy (1842) for use as an all-purpose medication. *Cannabis indica* (from India) became a wonder drug used to treat a wide variety of ailments ranging form menstrual cramps and convulsions to inflamed tonsils and migraine headaches. It was also used to increase uterine contractions and reduce childbirth pains. Even with the low dosage (1 to 6 grains, or 65 to 400 mg, administered by mouth) this medication allevi- ated many aches and pains without producing any of the signs of hashish intoxication described by Moreau in 1845 *(1)*.

However, many physicians were discouraged from using the drug because of the extreme variability of potency of different lots of *Cannabis* extracts and the difficulty of obtaining reproducible effects. With the advent of more specific and effective medications like aspirin, barbiturates, and anesthetic agents, hemp preparations rapidly fell into disuse and by 1932 were dropped form the British Pharmacopoeia.

Toward the end of the 19th century the burgeoning pharmaceutical industry attempted to develop more dependable and purified compounds from *Cannabis*, but without success. Oral preparations of cannabis were used with decreasing frequency in the first part of the 20th century, and they were eliminated from the United States Pharmacopoeia in 1942. In 1960, the World Health Organization Committee on Drug dependence advised the U.N. Commission on Narcotics that cannabis preparations are practically obsolete and there is no justification for their medical use. The recommendation led the United Nations Single Con- vention (in 1961) held in New York to classify the flowering tops of marijuana among the drugs with high abuse potential. These drugs are to be excluded by law from commerce and medical use.

MARIHUANA SMOKING AND THC

Marihuana as medicine regained popularity in the wake of widespread recreational smok- ing of marihuana smoking in the United States during the second part of the 20th century. To the old claims *(2,3)*, new applications were found for the old drug in the treatment of glau- coma, and of nausea and vomiting induced by cancer chemotherapy. Concurrently, the active ingredient of marihuana, THC delta 9-tetrahydrocannabinol, was isolated.

In addition to the cannabinoids, chemicals specific to the cannabis plant, the smoke of the crude marihuana drug contains 421 different chemicals, some toxic (carbon monoxide, acetaldehyde, phenol, creosol, naphthalene) and also twice as many carcinogens as a tobacco cigarette of the same weight. The inhalation of marihuana preparations carries an additional hazard: they may be contaminated with salmonella *(5)*, or with a fungus, *Aspergillus fumiga- tus*, which may cause severe pulmonary disease *(6)*. For therapeutic purposes, it is important to distinguish between the use of the crude marihuana smoke and its pharmacologically pure active compound THC: the potential therapeutic applications attributed to marihuana smoke have been traced to the effect of its main psychoactive ingredient, THC, which is available as an oral preparation.

1. INTRODUCTION

It is now possible to relate the therapeutic properties of marihuana preparations to their THC content THC, because of its oily nature cannot be given parenterally in man; its pharmacokinetics and the time course of its effects when administered orally are different from those of the inhaled form. Plasma THC concentration following oral administration reaches a more sustained steady-state level, twice as long as after smoking *(7)*. The overall pharmacological and psychoactive effects of the inhaled and oral forms of THC are similar, as well as the prolonged tissue retention of the drug which has a half-life of five to eight days.

Tolerance to the effects of marihuana and THC develops rapidly, and withdrawal symptoms similar to those of other sedative-hypnotic agents are present following abstinence after chronic use. Chronic treatment of animals with CBD or with THC have resulted in alteration of spermatogenesis *(8)*. Similar observations have been reported in humans after heavy marihuana smoking (oligospermia and abnormal forms of sperm) *(9)*.

Oral THC (dronabinol) is an approved medication in the United States as a 2.5–10 mg capsule in sesame oil for oral administration. Anecdotal accounts *(10)* have claimed that marihuana smoking is more effective than oral THC.

2. THERAPEUTIC APPLICATIONS OF CANNABINOIDS

The numerous pharmacological effects produced by THC led many investigators to seek some therapeutic application for this drug and other cannabinoids as well. Extensive research programs sponsored by the pharmaceutical industry (Abbott, Squibb, Lilly, and Pfizer) and by Federal agencies were initiated to establish the efficacy of THC and of its derivatives, of their mode of action, and of their main therapeutic indications. Several related synthetic molecules were designed and tested experimentally and clinically.

Among these derivatives, nabilone, a THC-like cannabinoid developed by Lilly laboratory, was approved for medical use in 1982 *(11)*. This drug has been used in the treatment of the nausea and vomiting associated with cancer chemotherapy, in doses of 1–2 mg/day, and in the treatment of muscle spasticity.

Another THC-like synthetic derivative, levonantradol *(12)*, was developed by Pfizer laboratory. It is a very potent substance with antalgic and antiemetic activity in the milligram dose *(13,14)*. Its marked side effects prompted the interruption of its clinical trials in 1982.

The potential therapeutic applications of THC and related cannabinoids were reported in eleven symposia and monographs published in the 1970s and 1980s *(15–25)*. As a result, several hundred reports were assembled in 1500 pages of text authored by organic, analytical, and pharmaceutical chemists; experimental and clinical pharmacologists, and physicians who had specialized in the chemistry, pharmacology, and therapeutic applications of the cannabinoids. The present review is an attempt to summarize, the main findings of this data reported by scientists from the United States, United Kingdom, Sweden, France, and Israel.

3. ANALGESIC EFFECT

The analgesic action of THC reported in the experimental animal *(26)* is equivocal in clinical trials. A double-blind study by Milstein et al. *(27)* observed a significant increase in pain tolerance among marihuana smokers. Noyes et al. *(28)* reported an analgesic effect of orally administered THC in cancer patients. These effects were associated with mental clouding and other psychoactive reactions. Hill et al. *(29)* failed to detect the analgesic activity after a dose of 12 mg THC given to 26 normal volunteers subjected to electrical stimulation of the fingers. Regelson et al. *(30)* also failed to observe analgesic effects of THC in cancer patients.

As pointed out by Clark *(31)*, the difficulty with classic threshold studies of experimental pain is that the pain threshold is influenced by both expectation and analgesia. The double-blind control is not sufficient since the psychoactive effects of marihuana may allow subjects to peak through the double-blind and distinguish between placebo and drug condition on the basis of subjective effects such as euphoria and clouding of consciousness.

Clark et al. confirmed the hyperalgesic effect of marihuana smoking reported previously by Hill et al. He recorded the effect of thermal pain in 16 heavy marihuana smokers studied in a controlled environment, evaluating the data by using a sensory decision analysis that differentiates between sensory input and subject perception. He concluded marihuana smoking has hyperalgesic activity and enhances the perception of pain (lower threshold) and increases pain-report criterion. These results are consistent with reports of heightened sensitivity or "sharpening" of perceptions produced by smoking marihuana.

4. NEUROLOGICAL DISORDERS

Consroe and Sandyk *(25)* have reviewed the potential therapeutic role of the cannabinoids (THC, its synthetic derivatives, CBD) in epilepsy, dystonia, movement disorders (Huntington's chorea, Tourette's syndrome, Parkinsonism, tardive dyskinesia), spasticity, migraine, and neuropathic pain.

They conclude that all of the clinical trials performed to treat these conditions with THC, its synthetic derivatives, or with CBD were inconclusive. They state "the realization of the potential benefits of cannabinoids in neurological disorders will depend upon a new breakthrough in research such as identification of an endogenous ligand, identification of subtypes of cannabinoid receptors, and of their selective antagonists—and agonist."

5. ANTIDEPRESSANT EFFECT

Moreau *(1)* was the first to assume that the "feeling of gaiety and joy" produced by *Cannabis* intoxication would be valuable to treat "the fixed ideas of the depressives." He treated several such cases of deep depression with increasing dosages of hashish, but with little effect. One hundred years later, a similar lack of effectiveness of *Cannabis* derivatives on the depressive state was observed. Whereas Regelson et al. *(30)* reported a significant reduction in self-related depressive symptoms in cancer patients treated with THC, Kotin et al. *(32)*, in a carefully controlled trial with four bipolar and four unipolar depressed patients, found no antidepressant activity. This latter study was confirmed by Ablon and Goodwin *(33)* who reported that THC was not effective in a group of depressed patients treated with 5–40 mg for one week, and caused dysphoria in subjects with unipolar depression.

6. ANXIOLYTIC AND SEDATIVE EFFECTS AND TREATMENT OF ALCOHOL AND OPIATE WITHDRAWAL

In normal subjects, Pillard et al. *(34)* did not find any effect of *Cannabis* (10 mg THC) on experimentally induced anxiety. Nabilone, a synthetic potent cannabinoid with THC-like activity *(35)*, was found to be less effective than diazepam in reducing induced anxiety in normal volunteers. *(36)* Furthermore, an unwanted side-effect of marihuana is to induce acute anxiety and panic attacks.

The alterations of THC on sleep EEG and its rebound effect *(37)*, its side effects before sleep induction, and its residual effects after awakening have contraindicated its clinical use as a sedative hypnotic.

It was suggested that *Cannabis* derivatives (pyrahexyl) and THC might be useful in treatment of withdrawal symptoms from alcohol. *(38,39)* A systematic evaluation failed to find *Cannabis* useful in treating this condition *(40)*. Epidemiological surveys report that the use of *Cannabis* and alcohol are combined and are frequently the gateway drugs to the usage of opiates and cocaine.

Early experimental reports suggested that *Cannabis* might be useful in alleviating the symptoms of opiate withdrawal *(41,42)*. These observations were not clinically documented.

In conclusion, THC has little therapeutic potential in treating common psychiatric disorders such as anxiety, depression, or insomnia. Currently, agents used in therapeutics are more effective, specific, and possess fewer unwanted side effects.

7. ANTIASTHMATIC EFFECT

The acute bronchodilator action of inhaled or oral *Cannabis* was observed in normal and asthmatic subjects *(43)*. However, Tashkin et al. *(44)* reported that chronic smoking of marihuana was associated with increased airway resistance and symptoms of irritation and inflammation of large bronchi. Such observations led other investigators to test oral THC. Abboud and Sander *(45)*, using a double-blind randomized crossover design, compared the bronchodilating effects of placebo and oral THC in normal subjects and asthmatic patients. They concluded that oral administration of THC would have doubtful therapeutic value in treating asthma because its bronchodilating action was mild, unpredictable, and associated with significant disturbing central nervous system effects.

8. ANTIEMETIC EFFECT

Several controlled studies have reported that THC in 15–20 mg oral dose exerts an antiemetic effect in cancer patients undergoing chemotherapy *(45,46)*. Some clinical trials have indicated that THC is more effective than prochlorperazine, the most commonly used antiemetic in the United States *(47–50)*, whereas others reported less effectiveness and more side effects *(51)*. However, THC is not as effective as metoclopramide against emesis produced by cisplatin therapy. Gralla et al. *(52)* and Carey et al. *(53)* made a critical review of 19 studies performed on 951 cancer patients between 1975 and 1982 to assess the antiemetic properties of THC, as compared to that of other medications, during chemotherapy. The authors concluded that the different studies showed "considerable inconsistencies," THC being claimed equal, superior, or inferior to other medications, and they recommended additional controlled trials. Subsequent studies indicated that a 5-HT$_3$ receptor antagonist (ondansetron) that is administered intravenously is the most effective antiemetic for cancer chemotherapy *(54)*. It is effective for high-dose cisplatin therapy with a global satisfaction of nausea and vomiting control of 85%. Another serotonin-receptor antagonist, granisetron (1 mg intravenously), results in a 93% complete control of nausea after cisplatin therapy.

In 1987 an oral preparation of THC, dronabinol (marinol) was declassified from schedule I to schedule II and made available to relieve the vomiting of cancer chemotherapy and as an appetite stimulant. After its commercial release, the Food and Drug Administration (FDA) formulated the following guidelines *(55)*.

Marinol is not indicated as first-line treatment for nausea and vomiting associated with cancer chemotherapy. (It is only indicated) in patients who have failed to respond adequately to conventional antiemetic treatments. Because of the limitations of its indication, comparisons of Marinol to conventional antiemetics are inappropriate. Marinol is not a therapeutic alternative to Compazine (prochlorperazine) or other conventional antiemetic treatments (metoclopramide, ondansetron).... Patients using Marinol should

be advised of possible changes in mood and other adverse behavioral or disturbing psy-
chotominetic reactions. ... Marinol is a medication with a potential for abuse. Physicians
and pharmacists should use the same care in prescribing and accounting for Marinol as
they would morphine or other (schedule II drugs) ... The risk/benefit ratio of Marinol use
should be carefully evaluated in the following types of patients ... patients with cardiac
disorders because of occasional hypotension and hypertension, syncope, or tachycardia;
patients with a history of substance abuse, including alcohol abuse or dependence;
patients with manic depression, or schizophrenia because Marinol may exacerbate these
illnesses; ... and patients receiving concomitant therapy with sedatives, hypnotics, or
other psychoactive drugs because of the potential for additive or synergistic (central ner-
vous system) effects.

These recommendations were issued because the promotional material for marinol contained "statements, suggestions or implications that (were) in the (FDA's) view, false and/or
misleading and in violation of the Federal Food, Drug and Cosmetic Act"

These conclusions of the FDA would also apply for the anecdotal reports of patients
"drinking marihuana tea against nausea and claiming that they have a better capacity to live
in the here and now" as reported by Neelman *(56)*.

In 1989 the Drug Enforcement Agency (DEA) rejected the reclassification of marihuana
smoking (for medicine) from schedule I to II, which in effect outlawed its medical prescription *(57)*. Its arguments were contained in an extensive scientific and medical analysis of all
of the available clinical data from recognized cancer specialists, ophthalmologists and neurologists. The opinion of the DEA. was supported by the American Cancer Society, the
American Medical Association, and by the FDA, which concluded:

There is inadequate scientific evidence to support a finding that marijuana is safe and effec-
tive for treating nausea and vomiting experienced by patients undergoing chemotherapy.

"Therapeutic" marihuana smoking could be especially hazardous for patients with the
acquired immunodeficiency syndrome (AIDS). Marihuana smoking impairs immunity and
lung macrophage function *(58)*, already compromised in AIDS patients who are vulnerable
to pulmonary infections. Prescribing marihuana to these patients as an appetite stimulant
should not be considered as a compassionate gesture extended to a patient at "death's door"
nor as a beneficial and proven therapy to maintain him alive *(59)*.

9. EFFECTS ON THE APPETITE

Cannabis was prescribed in Hindu medicine not only to stimulate appetite, as reported by
Snyder *(60)*, but also to deaden the need for food or beverages by concentrating the mind on
the eternal *(61)*. Greenberg et al. *(62)* reported an increase in body weight in marihuana
smokers studied while in the hospital, Hollister reported an inconsistent increase in appetite
from the drug in healthy subjects *(63)*. Mattes reported that THC in oral form had a variable
effect on appetite stimulation in normal men *(64)*. Some cancer patients receiving THC note
an increase in appetite *(13)*. Sallan et al. *(50)*, also reported that patients treated with THC as
an antiemetic during chemotherapy had an improved appetite.

In AIDS patients, oral THC has been observed to stimulate appetite but weight gain was
not significant *(65,66)*. Specific medication for controlled studies comparing THC with
megestrol acetate and human growth hormone have been suggested. The comparative effect
of oral THC with that of smoked marihuana could also be investigated.

The depressant effect of THC administration on immune mechanisms and that of marihuana smoke on pulmonary macrophages of AIDS patients should be a concern. The inter-

actions of THC with some of the other many medications taken by these patients should also be considered.

10. GLAUCOMA

A chance observation by Hepler *(67)* on subjects smoking marihuana (0.9–1.5% THC) showed a lowering of intraocular pressure. Subsequent studies *(68)* indicated that the smoking of *Cannabis* 1–2% THC decreased the intraocular pressure by 30%, and that this effect lasted four to five hour, and a ceiling effect was observed after two cigarettes (30 mg THC). There was no tolerance development to the lowering of intraocular pressure among marihuana smokers studied in a controlled environment during a period of 94 days. However, Dawson et al. *(69)* and Flom et al. *(70)* observed reduced intraocular pressure in smokers with little experience of use, but little or no change in subjects with extensive history of use. Dawson et al. compared 10 nonsmokers of marihuana with 10 matched subjects who had smoked marihuana for an average of 10 years or more. The smokers presented a *higher* intraocular pressure than the control group, along with a greater incidence of abnormalities of the anterior chamber of the eye.

The lowering of intraocular pressure by *Cannabis* smoking was attributed to THC or its 11-hydroxymethyl metabolite, which when infused intravenously to volunteers reduced ocular tension *(71)*. Nonpsychoactive cannabinoids have little effect. Smoking *Cannabis* (20–30 mg THC) reduced ocular tension *and* blood pressure in marihuana-naive, heterogeneous glaucoma subjects, and in subjects with open-angle glaucoma *(72,73)*. The reduction in blood pressure that reached basal levels, lasted four to five hours or longer. Associated hypotension may be severe; 6 of the 32 subjects experienced syncopal episodes. The systemic hypotensive effect is greatest in glaucoma subjects who are hypertensive. Oral administration of THC capsules significantly reduced ocular tension in healthy marihuana-naive volunteers only when administered in doses greater than 20 mg *(74)*. Marked side-effects were observed, including acute panic reactions, tachycardia, palpitations, depersonalization, and paranoia. These reactions were more common in subjects who were naive to marihuana.

In a randomized, double-blind study using 10 marihuana-naive nonsmokers with glaucoma, 5 and 10 mg THC administered per dose was not more effective than placebo in lowering intraocular pressure, although systematic hypotension was a problem.

Most antiglaucoma agents are administered topically and are effective by this route. This is not the case of THC *(75)*. Topical THC in light mineral oil vehicle (0.05–0.1%) when administered to six subjects with open-angle glaucoma was not more effective than placebo.

In summary, smoking THC containing *Cannabis* lowers intraocular pressure in glaucoma patients, producing unwanted psychoactive and cardiovascular side-effects, especially hypotension in older patients. The drug is ineffective when topically applied. Its oral administration is only effective in dosage associated with significant side-effects. There are many other effective preparations containing pilocarpine and beta-blockers that are available to treat glaucoma and have less systemic side-effects.

11. INTERACTIONS OF *CANNABIS* WITH SEDATIVES, OPIATES, AND HYPNOTICS

Dalton et al. *(76)* administered secobarbital, 150 mg/70 kg orally, to young males 50 minutes before a marihuana cigarette (THC, 25 µg/kg). The magnitude of the depressant effect of the drug combination on measures of standing steadiness and psychomotor and mental performance represented "additivity of the component effects." In addition, the subjective effects of the drug combination were greater than that produced by either drug alone. Similar additive effects of concurrent consumption of marihuana and ethanol have been reported (77).

Johnstone et al. (78) and Smith and Kulp (79) reported that injection of THC (27–130 µg/kg, intravenously) shortly after pentobarbital (100 mg/70 kg intravenously) induced profound subjective effects, including hallucinations and severe anxiety. The slight stimulant and depressant effects of pentobarbital and THC, respectively, on ventilation were mutually antagonized by the drug combination. Pentobarbital in conjunction with THC increased the heart rate and cardiac index and decreased total peripheral resistance.

Johnstone et al. (78) also observed that THC caused a dose-related enhancement of the sedation and ventilatory depression induced by oxymorphone (1 mg/70 kg, intravenously) Although oxymorphone had no influence on cardiovascular parameters, the concurrent injection of THC (134 µg/kg) increased the heart rate and cardiac index and decreased peripheral resistance. THC also augmented CNS and ventilatory depression caused by diazepam (5–20 mg/70 kg, intravenously) However, diazepam apparently counteracted the THC-mediated increase in heart rate and cardiac index (79).

These authors concluded that THC, because of its many interactions with currently used drugs during anesthesia, could not be recommended as a preanesthetic agent.

Inhalation of THC (150 or 500 µg/kg), in marihuana smoke, immediately before an oral dose of secobarbital (150 mg/70 kg), did not produce responses greater than those caused by barbiturate alone (80). Benowitz and Jones (81) reported that treatment of young men with THC (60–180 mg/day) for 14 days increased the half-lives of pentobarbital and antipyrine in the plasma and reduced the rate of absorption of barbiturate. Chronic marihuana use could alter the affects of other therapeutic drugs; after THC administration had ended, the metabolic clearance of pentobarbital was increased, suggesting that a metabolic cross-tolerance between the two drugs could occur. The evidence obtained to date indicates that there are significant interactions between Cannabis and drugs routinely used in anesthesia, such as opioids, benzodiazepines, and barbiturates. Such interactions should be known by physicians and anesthesiologists who may prescribe these drugs to habitual Cannabis users.

12. ORAL THC VERSUS INHALED THC VIA MARIHUANA SMOKE

An aerosol solution of THC that could be administered by inhalation, like antiasthmatic suspensions, has not been developed. THC is best tolerated and absorbed by the lung after pyrolysis of the crude plant material. It has been claimed that the inhaling of THC-containing marihuana smoke is superior to oral THC. This claim has not been scientifically documented.

In an open study (82), 74 patients were given marihuana smoke or oral THC to control nausea and asked for self-evaluation of the respective forms of medication. There was no randomized placebo control group. Eighteen patients dropped out of the study. Of the 56 remaining, 18 evaluated marihuana smoking as very effective, 26 as moderately effective, and 12 as not effective. There was no objective measurement of treatment success (number and length of emetic episodes.) This study was rebutted as insufficient evidence to prove the superiority of smoked marihuana over THC by the United States Court of appeals DC circuit in February, 1994. This decision supported the DEA refusal of rescheduling marihuana smoking from schedule I to schedule II (57).

Two surveys of oncologists have been performed to assess medical acceptance of marihuana smoking for medicine. In the first by Doblin and Kleiman (83), two nonphysicians specialized in "drug control policy," the majority (60%) of those surveyed did not respond and the survey could not be considered perfectly representative of oncologists at large. Among respondents, 44% acknowledged having used marihuana for at least one patient and 40% of the respondents had the "feeling" that marihuana smoking was more effective than oral THC.

In another survey *(84)*, oncologists were asked to state their drug of choice against emesis. Marihuana or THC was rated sixth and this survey was made before the availability of ondansetron, the current drug of choice, which would have displaced THC to the seventh rank. The cannabinoid antiemetic property, whatever the vehicle for THC might be, oral or inhaled, is only partially effective in cancer chemotherapy and it is ineffective in cisplatin therapy.

The pharmacokinetics of oral versus smoked THC in humans indicate that plasma levels of THC reach a more sustained level following oral administration *(7)*. Since a saturation of receptors in the chemoreceptor trigger zone (CTZ) of nausea and vomiting is the goal of the antiemetic medication, a more prolonged plasma and tissue concentration (four hours) following marinol should be more appropriate than the rapid short concentration peak (one hour) of smoked THC. It is unlikely that "smoking marihuana produces a rapid increase in the blood level of THC and is thus more likely to be therapeutic." On the basis of pharmacokinetics, the opposite should be true.

Additional studies to compare the respective efficacy of smoked marihuana versus THC delivered orally or in suppositories have been suggested. Such a comparison would have to take in account multiple confounding variables. The following factors would have to be controlled:

- Standardized marihuana cigarettes of known THC content sterilized in order to eliminate contaminants should be made available to all investigators. Several concentrations should be available in order to assess dose-response relationships.
- Measurements of the cannabinoids in body fluids, which present wide individual variations related to pharmacogenetics and method of inhalation (naive patients will have to be taught how to inhale marihuana smoke). Associated medications constitute another variable.
- The differences in pharmacological response related to previous exposure to the drug, (whether the subject is naive or tolerant to marihuana smoke).
- Objective measurements of drug response are only quantifiable in the case of vomiting (amount frequency and duration of episodes) or of glaucoma. For other conditions markers are missing or blurred.
- Independent evaluation of subjective responses would require groups treated with placebo in double-blind studies.

Methodological difficulties and statistical uncertainties would hamper an objective evaluation of such studies. How does one, for instance, perform a double double-blind study on the same subject between a placebo cigarette and a marihuana cigarette and one between a placebo pill and a marinol pill? How does one perform a crossover study from marihuana smoking to marinol ingestion? How does a physician evaluate the relief and well being reported by subjects after marihuana smoking against the toxic effects on lung and aveolar macrophage, which cannot be felt by the subject? Should a physician conform to the law?

13. CONCLUSION

The curative properties attributed to *Cannabis* oral preparations during the 19th century proved to be disappointing. Despite initial claims for its effectiveness as an analgesic, or for the treatment of tetanus, epilepsy, rheumatism, and many other ailments, *Cannabis* did not establish itself as a dependable remedy, unlike other dependence-producing drugs like opium or cocaine or over-the-counter drugs like aspirin.

The reason for the clinical lack of success of *Cannabis* as medicine in the 19th century was the same as the present difficulty encountered with THC in all of its potential therapeutic applications: the diversity and variability of its actions and its unwanted side effects. These are acute undesirable psychic and cardiovascular side-effects. THC tissue accumulation and development of tolerance during chronic administration constitute other limitations to prolonged use.

Today the use of oral THC, first proposed as an analgesic, antidepressant, hypnotic, anticonvulsant, tranquilizer, relaxant, a treatment for withdrawal symptoms, and glaucoma, has been narrowed down to an antiemetic in cancer chemotherapy and as an appetite stimulant for AIDS patients. In these conditions, their are other medications of equal or better effectiveness and without unwanted side effects.

The THC-containing marihuana smoke, resulting from the combustion of plant material, has not been proven more effective than its oral form, marinol. It contains toxic compounds (carbon monoxide, acetaldehyde, naphthalene) and carcinogens in amounts greater than tobacco smoke. It is damaging to the lung and pulmonary defense mechanisms. Marihuana smoke has not satisfied FDA guidelines for safety and efficacy of its claimed therapeutic properties.

The acceptance of marihuana smoking as a popular medication also could present the risk of a significant diversion of the drug for recreational use by children and adolescents. Their perception of marihuana as a harmless, soft drug has been related to an increase incidence of its smoking *(85)*.

The prospects of THC and marihuana as therapeutic agents described by Hollister in 1984 are worth recalling *(86)*.

> *"Cannabis and THC homologues should be treated like any other investigational new drug as the search for a clinical use in medicine goes on. We should expect neither less nor more in regard to the safety and efficacy than we would from other new agents. At present,* Cannabis *has not yet made its way back into the formularies. It is unlikely that it ever will. The ingenuity of pharmaceutical chemists in developing THC analogs may yet find a way to exploit some of these potential therapeutic uses without the side effects that make* Cannabis *itself undesirable."*

Fourteen years later, several hundred THC analogs, agonists and antagonists have been designed and tested experimentally. The G protein coupled receptor to THC has been identified as well as its natural ligand, arachidonyl-ethanolamine AEA ("Anandamide") *(87)*. Many synthetic agonists and antagonists of AEA have been experimentally tested *(88)*, but have not been proven to be of any clinical use. These studies have also shown that THC deregulates the physiological signaling role of G protein receptors and the membrane lipid bilayer *(89)*. The deregulation of membrane signaling by THC and cannabinoids explains their multiple partial and inconsistent therapeutic effects.

1. ACKNOWLEDGEMENTS

The authors wish to recognize the contributions of William Bennett M. D., Eric Voth M. D., Janet Lapey M. D., and Mark Gold M. D., as well as the editorial assistance of Gene Fisch, Jr.

REFERENCES

1. Moreau, J. J. (1845) Du Hachisch et de l'Alienation Mentale: Etudes Psychologiques. Libraire de Fortin, Masson, Paris. (English edition: Raven, New York 1972).
2. Mikuriya, T. H. (1969) Historical aspects of *Cannabis sativa* in Western medicine. *New Physician* **18**, 902–908.

3. Snyder, S. H. (1967) *The Uses of Marijuana* Oxford University Press, New York.

4. Mechoulam, R., Braun, P. and Gaoni, Y. A. (1967) stereospecific synthesis of (-)- [1]-and (-)- [116]tetrahydrocannabinols. *J. Am. Chem. Soc.* **89**, 4552–4554.

5. Taylor, D. N., Wachsmuth, I. K., Shangkuan, Y., et al. (1982) Salmonellosis associated with marijuana. *N. Engl. J. Med.* **306**, 1249.

6. Kagan, S. L. (1981) Aspergillus: an inhalable contaminant of marihuana. *N. Engl. J. Med.* **304**, 483.

7. Agurell, S., Lindgren, J., Ohlsson, A., Gillespie, H. and Hollister, L. (1984) Recent studies on the pharmacokinetics of delta-1-THC in man, In: *The Cannabinoids: Chemical, Pharmacologic, and Therapeutic Aspects* (Ahurell, S., Dewey, W. L., Willette, R. E. eds.) Academic, New York, pp. 165–183

8. Rosenkrantz, H. and Braude, M. C. (1976) Comparative chronic toxicities of delta-9-tetrahydrocannabinol administered orally or by inhalation in rat. In: *Pharmacology of Marihuana* (Braude M. C. and Szara S. eds.) Raven, New York. pp. 571–576.

9. Hembree, W. C. III, Zeidenberg, P. and Nahas, G. G. (1976) Marihuana's effect on human gonadal function. In: *Marihuana: Chemistry, Biochemistry and Cellular Effects* (G. G. Nahas and W. D. M. Paton eds.) Springer–Verlag, New York, pp.

10. Grinspoon, L. and Bakalar, J. B. (1993) *Marihuana the Forbidden Medicine*, Yale University Press, New Haven,

11. Archer, R. A., Hanasono, G. K., Lemberger, L. and Sullivan, H. R. (1981) Update on nabilone research: the relationship of metabolism to toxicity in dogs. In: *Treatment of Cancer Chemotherapy Induced Nausea and Vomiting* (Poster, D. S., Penta, J. S. and Bruno, S. eds.) Moser, New York, pp. 119–127.

12. Milne, G. M., Koe, B. K. and Johnson, M. R. (1979) Stereospecific and potent analgetic activity for nantradol: Astructurally novel, cannabinoid-related analgetic 1980. In: *Problems of Drug Dependence* (Harris, L. S. ed.) NIDA Research Monograph 27, Rockville, MD.

13. Cronin, C. M., Sallan, S. E., Belger, R., Lucs, V. and Laszlo, J. (1981) Antiemetic effect of intramuscular levonantradol inpatients receiving anticancer chemotherapy. *J. Clin. Pharmacol.* **21**, 43S–50S.

14. Diasio, R. B., Ettinger, D. S. and Satterwhite, B. E. (1981) Oral levonantradol in the treatment of chemotherapy-induced emesis; preliminary observations. *J. Clin. Pharmacol.* **21**, 81S–85S.

15. Therapeutic potential (1976) In 'Pharmacology of Marihuana' (Braude, M. and Szara, S., eds.) Raven, New York, pp. 747–837.

16. Cohen S. and Stillman R. (1976) *The Therapeutic Potential of Marihuana* Plenum, New York.

17. Lemberger L. (1980) Potential therapeutic usefulness of marihuana. *Ann. Rev. Pharmacolo. Toxicolo.* **20**, 151.

18. *Treatment of Cancer Chemotherapy-Induced Nausea and Vomiting* (Poster) (Penta J. S. and Bruno, S. eds.) Mason, New York.

19. *Therapeutic Progress in Cannabinoid Research* (Pfizer symposium) *Clin. Pharmacol.* **21**, Nos. 8–9 supplement p. 487.

20. Clinical and therapeutic aspects (1985) In: *Marihuana, 1984*, Oxford Symposium (Harvey, D., Paton, W. D. M. and Nahas, G. G. eds.) IRL Press, Oxford, pp. 673–724.

21. 'The medical use of cannabis' (1984) In: *Marihuana in Science and Medicine* (Nahas, G., Paris, M. and Harvey, D., eds.) Raven, New York, pp. 247–261

22. 'The cannabinoids, chemical, pharmacological and therapeutic aspects' (1984) (Agurell, S., Dewey W. L. and Willette, R. E., eds.) Academic New York.

23. Mechoulam, R., (1986) *Cannabinoids as Therapeutic Agents* CRC Press, Boca Raton, FL, p. 186.

24. Therapeutic and clinical effects of marihuana (1988) In: *International Research Report, Melbourne Symposium on Cannabis* (Consroe, P. and Musty, R., eds.) Australian Government Publishing Service, Canberra, pp. 119–167.

25. Consroe, P. and Sandy, R. (1992) 'Potential role of cannabinoids for therapy of neurological disorders'. In: *Marihuana/Cannabinoids, Neurobiology and Neurophysiology* (Murphy, L. and Bartke, A., eds.) CRC Press, Boca Raton, FL, pp. 459–524.

26. Sofia, R. D., Nalepa, S. D., Harakal, J. J. and Vassar, H. B. (1973) Anti-edema and analgesic properties of THC. *J. Pharmacol. Exp. Ther.* **186**, 646–655.

27. Milstein, S. L., MacCannnel, K., Karr, G. and Clark, S (1975) Marijuana-produced changes in pain tolerance. Experienced and nonexperienced subjects. *Int. Pharmacopsychiatry* **10**, 177–182.

28. Noyes, R., Brunk, S. F., Avery, D. H. and Canter, A. (1976) Psychologic effects of oral delta-9-tetrahydrocannabinol in advanced cancer patients. *Compar. Psychiatr.* **17**, 641–646.

29. Hill, S. Y., Goodwin, D. W., Schwin, R. and Powell, B. (1974) Marijuana: CNS depressant or excitant? *Am. J. Psychiatry.* **131**, 313–315.

30. Regelson, W., Butler, J. R. and Shulz, J. (1976) Delta-9-tetrahydrocannabinol as an effective antidepressant and appetite-stimulating agent in advanced cancer patients. In: *Pharmacology of Marihuana* (Braude M. C. and Szara, S. eds.) Raven, New York, pp. 763–776.

31. Clark, W. C., Janal, M. N., Zeidenberg, P. and Nahas, G. G. (1981) Effects of moderate and high doses of marihuana on thermal pain: a sensory decision theory analysis. *J. Clin. Pharmacol.* **21**, 299S–310S.

32. Kotin, J., Post, R. M. and Goodwin, F. K. (1973) Delta-9-Tetrahydrocannabinol in depressed patients. *Arch. Gen. Psychiatr.* **28**, 345–348.

33. Ablon, S. and Goodwin, Fr. (1974) High frequency dysphoric reactions to tetrahydrocannabinol among depressed patients. *Am. J. Psychiatr.* **131**, 448–453.

34. Pillard, R. C., McNair, D. M. and Fisher, S. (1974) Does marijuana enhance experimentally induced anxiety? *Psychopharmacologia* **40**, 205–210.

35. Fabre, L. F., McLendon, D. M. and Stark, P. (1978) Nabilone, a cannabinoid, in the treatment of anxiety; an open-label and double-blind study. *Curr. Ther. Res.* **24**, 161–169.

36. Nakano, S., Gillespie, H. K. and Hollister, L. E. (1978) A model for evaluation of antianxiety drugs with the use of experimentally induced stress: comparison of nabilone and diazepam. *Clin. Pharmacol. Ther.* **23**, 54–62.

37. Feinberg, I., Jones, R., Walker, J., Cavness, C. and Floyd, T. (1976) Effects of marihuana extract and tetrahydrocannabinol on electroenecephalographic sleep patterns. *Clin. Pharmacol. Ther.* **19**, 782–794.

38. Thompson, L. J. and Proctor, R. C. (1953) The use of pyrahexyl in the treatment of alcoholic and drug withdrawal conditions. *N. C. Med. J.* **14**, 520–523.

39. Scher, J. (1971) Marijuana as an agent in rehabilitating alcoholics. *Am. J. Psychiatr.* **127**, 971–972.

40. Rosenberg, C. M., Gerrein, J. R. and Schnell, C. (1978) Cannabis in the treatment of alcoholism. *J. Stud. Alcohol.* **39**, 155–158.

41. Hine, B., Friedman, E., Torrelio, M. and Gershon, S. (1975) Tetrahydrocannabinol-attenuated abstinence and induced rotation in morphine-dependent rats: possible involvement of dopamine. *Neuropharmacology* **14**, 607–610.

42. Bhargava, H. N. (1976) Effect of some cannabinoids on naloxone-precipitated abstinence in morphine-dependent mice. *Psychopharmacology* **49**, 267–270.

43. Shapiro, B. J., Tashkin, D. P. and Frank, I. M. (1973) Mechanism of increased specific airway conductance with marijuana smoking in healthy young men. *Ann. Int. Med.* **78**, 832–833.

44. Tashkin, D. P., Shapiro, B. J. and Frank, I. M. (1974) Acute effects of smoked marijuana and oral delta-9-tetrahydrocannabinol on specific airway conductance in asthmatic subjects. *Am. Rev. Respir. Dis.* **109**, 420–428.

45. Abboud, R. T. and Sanders, H. D. (1976) Effect of oral administration of delta-9-tetrahydrocannabinol airway mechanics in normal and asthmatic subjects. *Chest* **70**, 480–485.

46. Chang, A. E., Schiling, D. J., Stillman, R. C., Goldberg, N. H., Seipp, C. A., Barofsky, I., Simon R. M. and Rosenberg, S. A. (1979) Delta-9-tetrahydrocannabinol as an antiemetic in cancer patients, receiving high-dose methotrexate: a prospective, randomized evaluation. *Ann. Int. Med.* **91**, 819–824.

47. Sallan, S. E., Zinberg, N. E. and Frei, E. (1975) Antiemetic effect of delta-9-tetrahydrocannabinol in patients receiving cancer chemotherapy. *N. Engl. J. Med.* **293**, 795–797.

48. Herman, T. S., Einhorn, L. H., Jones, S. E. et al. (1979) Superiority of nabilone over prochlorperazine as an antiemetic in patients receiving cancer chemotherapy. *N. Eng. J. Med.* **300**, 1295–1297.

49. Lucas, V. S. and Laszlo, J. (1980) Delta-9-tetrahydrocannabinol for refractory vomiting induced by cancer chemotherapy. *JAMA* **243**, 1241–1243.

50. Sallan, S. E., Cronin, C., Zelen, M. and Zinberg, N. E. (1980) Antiemetics in patients receiving chemotherapy for cancer: a randomized comparison of delta-9-tetrahydrocannibinol and prochlor-perazine. *N. Engl. J. Med.* **302**, 135–138.

51. Frytak, S., Moertel, C. G., O'Fallon, J. R., Rubin, J., Creagan, E. T., O'Connell, M. J., Schutt, A. J. and Schwartau, N. W. (1979) Delta-9-tetrahydrocannabinol as an antiemetic for patients receiving cancer chemotherapy. A comparison with prochlorperazine and a placebo. *Ann. Int. Med.* **91**, 825–830.

52. Gralla, R. J., Itri, L. M., Pisko, S. E. and Young, C. W. (1981) Antiemetic efficacy of high-dose metoclopramide: randomized trials with placebo and prochlorperazine in patients with chemotherapy-induced nausea and vomiting. *N. Engl. J. Med.* **305**, 905–909.

53. Carey, M. P., Burish, T. G. and Brenner, D. E. (1983) Delta9-THC in cancer chemotherapy: research problems and issues. *Ann. Int. Med.* **198**, 106–114.

54. Markham, A. and Sorkin, E. M. (1993) Ondansetron; an update of its therapeutic use in chemotherapy-induced and postoperative nausea and vomiting. *Drugs* **45**, 931–952. [Published erratum in *Drugs*. Errors in dosage and in doses used in dose-finding studies.] 1993; **46**, 268.

55. Wojta, G. C. (1993) Important correction of drug information from Roxane Laboratories (requested by FDA) *N. Engl. J. Med.*, Dec. 23, 1993

56. Neelman, M. P. (1996) Marihuana, soft drug or medicine? *Pain Clinic* **9**, 243–248.

57. Denial of NORML marihuana rescheduling petition by DEA. Federal Register, December 29, 1989 vol. 54 No. 249.
58. Cabral, G. A. Burnette-Curley, D., Nahas, G. G. (1995) Marihuana-induced inhibition of macrophage cytolytic function. In *Drugs of Abuse and the Immune Response* (Friedman, H., Spector, S., Klein, T. W., eds.) CRC Press, Boca Raton, FL.
59. Kassirer, J. P. (1997) Federal foolishness and marijuana. *New. Eng. J. Med.* Jan. 30, 366.
60. Snyder, S. H. (1971) The uses of marijuana. Oxford University Press, New York.
61. Chopra, G. S. (1969) Man and marijuana. *Int. J. Addict.* **4**, 215–247.
62. Greenberg, I., Kuehnle, J., Mendelson, J. H. and Bernstein, J. G. (1976) Effects of marihuana use on body weight and caloric intake in humans. *Psychopharmacology* **49**, 79–84.
63. Hollister, L. E. (1971) Hunger and appetite after single doses of marihuana, alcohol and dextroamphetamine. *Clin. Pharmacol. Ther.* **12**, 44–49.
64. Mattes, R. D., Engelmann, K., Shaw, L. M. and Elsoholy, M. A. (1994) Cannabinoids and appetite stimulation. *Pharmacol. Biochem. Behavi.* **49**, 187–195.
65. Gorter, R. (1991) Management of anorexia-cachexia associated with cancer and HIV infection. *Oncology* **5 (suppl 9)**, 13–16.
66. Beal, J., Olsen, R., Shepherd, K. V. and Plasse, T. (1993) Effect of dronabinol on appetite and weight in AIDS; longterm followup. *Proc. IX International Conf. AIDS.* Berlin, June.
67. Hepler, R. S. and Frank, I. M. (1971) Marijuana smoking and intraocular pressure. *JAMA* **217**, 1392.
68. Hepler, R. S., Frank, I. M. and Petrus, R. (1976) Ocular effects of marijuana smoking. In: *Pharmacology of Marihuana* (Braude, M. C. and Szara, S. eds.) Raven, New York, pp. 815–824.
69. Dawson, W. W., Jimenez-Antillon, C. F., Perez, J. M. and Zeskind, J. A. (1977) Marijuana and vision-after ten years' use in Costa Rica. *Invest. Opthalmol. Vix. Sci.* **16**, 689.
70. Flom, M. C., Adams, A. J. and Jones, R. T. (1975) Marijuana smoking and reduced pressure in human eyes: drug actions or epiphenomena? *Invest. Opthalamol.* **14**, 52.
71. Perez-Reyes, M., Wagner, D., Wall, M. E. and Davis, K. H. (1976) Intravenous administration of cannabinoids and intraocular pressure. In: *Pharmacology of Marihuana* (Braude, M. S. and Szara, S., eds.) Raven, New York, pp. 829–832.
72. Crawford, W. J. and Merritt, J. C. (1979) Effect of tetrahydrocannabinol on arterial and introcular hypertension. *Int. J. Clin. Pharmacol. Biopharm.* **17**, 191–196.
73. Merritt, J. C., Crawford, W. J., Alexander, P. C., Anduze, A. L. and Gelbart, S. S. (1979) Effect of marijuana inhalation on the intraocular pressure and blood pressure in open angle glaucoma. *Ophthalmology* **86**, 45.
74. Merritt, J. C., Perry, D. D., Russell, D. N. and Jones, B. F. (1981) Topical delta-9-tetrahydrocannabinol and aqueous dynamics in glaucoma. *J. Clin. Pharmacol.* **21**, 467S–471S.
75. Green, K., Wynn, H. and Bowman, K. A. (1978) A comparison of topical cannabinoids on intraocular pressure. *Exp. Eye Res.* **27**, 239–256.
76. Dalton, W. S., Martz, R., Lemberger, L., Rodda, B. E. and Forney, R. B. (1975) Effects of marijuana combined with secobarbital. *Clin. Pharmacol. Ther.* **18**, 298–304.
77. Belgrave, B. E., Bird, K. D., Chesher, G. B. et al. (1979) The effect of THC alone and in combination with ethanol, on human performance. **64**, 243–246.
78. Johnstone, R. E., Lief, P. L., Kulp, R. A. and Smith, T. C. (1975) Combination of delta-9-tetrahydrocannabinol with oxymorphone or pentobarbital. *Anesthesiology* **42**, 674–684.
79. Smith, T. C. and Kulp, R. A. (1976) Respiratory and cardiovascular effects of delta-9-tetrahydrocannabinol alone and in combination with oxymorphone, pentobarbital, and diazepam. In: *The Therapeutic Potential of Marijuana* (Cohen, S. and Stillman, R. G., eds.) Plenum Medical Book Company, New York, pp. 123–135.
80. Benowitz, N. L. and Jones, R. T. (1977) Effects of THC on drug distribution and metabolism. *Clin. Pharmacol. Ther.* **22**, 259–268.
81. Benowitz, N. L. and Jones, R. T. Prolonged THC ingestion (1977) *Clin. Pharmocol. Ther.* **21**, 336–342.
82. Vinciguerra, V., Moore, T. and Brennan, E. (1988) Inhalation marihuana as an antiemetic for cancer chemotherapy. *NY State J. Med.* **88**, 525–527.
83. Doblin, R. and Kleiman, M. A. R. (1991) Marihuana as anti-emetic medicine; a survey of oncologists' attitudes and experiences. *J. Clin. Oncol.* **9**, 1275–1280.
84. Schwartz, R. H. (1994) Marihuana as an antiemetic drug—how useful is it today? Opinions from clinical oncologists. *J. Clin. Oncol.* **13**, 53–65.
85. (1996) The National Drug Control Strategy. The White House. Increased adolescent drug use 1991–1995. p. 19.
86. Hollister, L. (1984) Health aspects of cannbis use in: *The cannabinoids: Chemical, Pharmacologic, and Theraputic Aspects.* (Agurell, S., Dewey, W. L. and Willette, R. E. eds.) Academie, New York, p. 15.
87. Pertwee, R. (1995) *Cannabinoid Receptors.* Academic Press, New York.

88. Mechoulam, R., Hanus, L., Ben-Shabat, S., Fride, E. and Weidenfeld, J. (1994) The anandamides, a family of endogenous cannabinoid ligands—chemical and biological studies. *Neuropschychopharmacology* **10**, 145S–145S.

89. Nahas, G. G., Sutin, K., E., Turndorf, H., Cancro, R. (1998) Cannabinoids and regulation of membrane signal transduction. ACNP 37th Annual Meeting, Porto Rico.

70

Receptor and Nonreceptor Membrane-Mediated Effects of THC and Cannabinoids

Gabriel G. Nahas, David Harvey, Kenneth Sutin, and Stig Agurell

Abstract

A strict chemical nomenclature is first proposed. It is based on the definitions of cannabinoids, psychoactive (THC) and nonpsychoactive (CBD, CBN, and THC-11 oic acid), and of identified receptors (AEA and G protein) and their physiological ligands (arachidonyl ethanolamine [AEA] and arachidonyl diglycerol [2-AG]). THC is the only natural cannabinoid that interacts with a receptor protein in a stereospecific fashion, a property which is associated with its psychoactivity. Other natural, nonpsychoactive cannabinoids, CBN and CBD, vary over a wide range of concentration in marihuana preparations and antagonize the effects of THC. They also possess biological properties, activating membrane enzymes (phosphorylase and acyltransferase) that increase arachidonic acid biosynthesis.

When THC binds a specific G-protein receptor, a structural change is induced that modifies an effector mechanism (e.g., decreased adenylate cyclase activity). THC does not interact directly with neurotransmitters or neuromodulators, but alters their response in a dose-related fashion (e.g., enhancing the response of a catechol receptor and decreasing the response of an acetylcholine receptor or modulating the response of opioid [mu and delta] receptors). Also, THC permeates the lipid bilayer and influences the integral membrane proteins through alteration of the boundary lipid. This effect is distinct from the mechanism resulting from AEA-G protein binding.

It is proposed that AEA receptor interaction possesses a physiological function, which is to regulate the signaling between boundary lipids and the receptors or enzymes of the membrane in response to physiological stimuli. The boundary lipids surrounding the membrane proteins are the vehicles for the signals between the AEA receptor and the neurotransmitter receptors and their binding sites. The change of configuration of the AEA receptor modulates the signaling effect of the membrane on its enzymes and receptors. AEA, a by-

From: *Marihuana and Medicine*
Edited by: G. G. Nahas et al. © Humana Press Inc., Totowa, NJ

product of the membrane phospholipid, is an indirect signal modulator of membrane activity. THC can deregulate the physiological signaling role of the G protein and its boundary lipid bilayer, a fundamental feature of all living cells. This deregulation of membrane signaling by THC results in partial and discordant effects.

1. INTRODUCTION

Since the identification of Δ^9-THC (THC) by Gaoni and Mechoulam *(34)*, the multiplicity of the pharmacological and chemical effects of this cannabinoid have been described in over 6000 scientific and medical publications. Besides the brain, its principal target, THC has been reported to have acute and chronic interactions with neurotransmitters, neuromodulators, and steroids as well as lung, heart, immune, and reproductive functions.

Most of these effects were attributed to THC binding to a specific G-protein "cannabinoid" receptor identified by Devane (1988) and cloned by Matsuda *(58)*: CB_1 receptors in the brain, CB_2 in peripheral tissue, including spleen, pancreas, kidney, liver, lung, heart, adrenal glands, ovary, uterus, testis, and sperm *(1)*.

Endogenous ligands to these receptors were identified as phospholipid derivatives, arachidonyl ethanolamine (AEA), and arachidonyl diglyceride (2-AG).

It was postulated that most of the pharmacological effects and therapeutic properties of the cannabinoids were mediated by the interaction of THC with G-protein coupled receptor mechanisms *(72)*. However, membrane-mediated effects of THC and cannabinoids independent of a "cannabinoid" receptor have been known and described by investigators *(9,17,18,28,42,61,67,69)*, and some uncertainty remains concerning the primary role of the receptor modulating effects of cannabinoids. This uncertainty has been compounded by the general adoption of a new nomenclature to define cannabinoids, THC, their receptors, and their ligands *(60,73)*. This new nomenclature requires a critical analysis in order to define a common terminology based on chemical and pharmacological data.

2. DEFINING CANNABINOIDS, THEIR RECEPTORS, AND THEIR LIGANDS

Cannabinoids are a group of C_{21} compounds naturally occurring in the *Cannabis sativa* plant (which has about 60 different cannabinoids), their carboxylic acid analogs, and transformation products. Cannabinoids are three ring structures, which do not possess a nitrogen atom and have a pentyl side chain on the A ring, which confers lipid solubility. THC is one of the naturally occurring cannabinoid molecules, which possesses pharmacologic activity most clearly displayed in humans by its psychoactive effects. In 1973, Mechoulam *(59)* stated:

There are numerous biological and biochemical effects caused by THC and by other cannabinoids. The various effects are not necessarily caused by all cannabinoids. The best example is THC versus cannabidiol. Only the former causes the marijuana "high" but both are anticonvulsant; chemically both compounds are obviously cannabinoids. I suggest that the term "cannabinoids" be used only with reference to chemical structure and properties. As this term has no physiological or biochemical connotations, any use of the term cannabinoid to describe such biological properties should be discontinued.

It is incorrect to limit the "cannabinoid" designation to psychoactive cannabinoids. A case in point is THC-11 oic acid, a metabolite of THC and a cannabinoid, which has no psychoactive effects, but activates phosphorylase and inhibits cyclooxygenase-2 *(103)*.

Therefore, the colloquial terms "cannabinoid activity" or "cannabinoid-like" and "cannabimimetic" (literally "mimics cannabis" and coined by Weissmann (97) are ambiguous and their use should be restricted. Wittgenstein (99) emphasized a general rule of communication, which requires that words be clearly defined in the context of their etymology so that they may convey a consistent meaning to every one. In this paper terms will be used within their respective chemical or pharmacological context and etymology, as recommended by Mechoulam (59).

The same commentary may be addressed to the designation of "cannabinoid receptors," "CB1" and "CB2" to identify "G-protein" receptors, which bind in a stereospecific fashion psychoactive cannabinoids like delta^9-THC. The natural endogenous ligands of these receptors, which have been designated as "anandamides" or "endocannabinoids," are natural derivatives membrane phospholipids. The ligands presently identified are: arachidonyl ethanolamine (AEA) and arachidonyl diglycerol (2-AG); molecules that have the same binding sites as THC, but have different chemical structure, pharmacokinetics, and affinity. The term "endocannabinoid" used to designate natural ligands is a physiological and chemical misnomer.

Endogenous ligands AEA and 2-AG have a much lower affinity for their receptor, and much more rapid intracellular turnover. They play a physiological regulating function on membrane signaling, which is still undetermined. The homology of the endogenous G-protein receptor system predates the cannabinoids, since it has been identified in vertebrates (from the sea urchin to the ants) for over 300 million years, suggesting an integral membrane function quite different from that of other neuromodulator systems. The "AEA G-protein" receptor might be used until a proper designation is defined by the Receptor Nomenclature of the International Union of Pharmacology (96).

Most of the pharmacological properties of THC have been attributed to its stereospecific binding to a G-protein-coupled receptor, which inhibits adenylate cyclase. Other mechanisms are to be established. The most important mechanism is the physical interaction of the fat soluble cannabinoids with the lipid bilayer of the membrane. This membrane "expansion" effect is maximal for THC, "a partial anesthetic," and is less affected by nonpsychoactive cannabinoids that still may activate membrane-bound enzymes, controlling phospholipid metabolism and production of arachidonic acid and eicosanoids. This mechanism is not related to the G-protein-coupled "THC" receptor, and is induced by psychoactive and nonpsychoactive cannabinoids.

The respective contributions of these different molecular mechanisms and interactions of psychoactive and nonpsychoactive cannabinoids on protein receptors and double lipid bilayer of the membrane will now be considered to account for their pharmacological effects of THC which might lead to a unified hypothesis of cannabinoid action.

3. INTERACTIONS OF PSYCHOACTIVE AND NONPSYCHOACTIVE CANNABINOIDS

Membranes are fluid mosaics of lipids and proteins held together by noncovalent interactions that are cooperative (Fig. 1). Biological membranes are not homogeneous fixed structures; they are constantly in lateral motion and the membrane proteins are free to diffuse laterally in the lipid matrix unless restricted by special interactions. Their motion has been visualized by fluorescence microscopy, small angle X-ray neutron diffraction, and solid-state NMR, but results are not quantitatively expressed (56).

3.1. Physicochemical Interactions with Cell Membrane

Gill and Lawrence (36) used the electron-spin-resonance (ESR) technique of Hubbell and McConnell (48) to detect perturbation of the liposome membrane caused by cannabinoids.

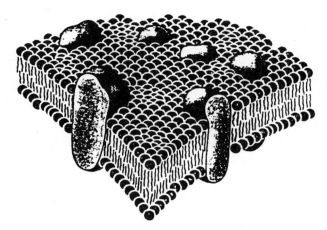

Fig. 1. The membrane is a two-dimensional solution of oriented lipids and protein molecules. The lipids, phospholipids, and glycolipids are arranged in a bilayer. This structure has a dual role, first as a permeability barrier and second as a solvent matrix for protein molecules, which are an integral part of the membrane. Membrane proteins may diffuse laterally unless restricted by special interactions. The lipid boundary of the lipid bilayer interacts with the protein and may be the site of a signaling mechanism that has never been clearly defined or measured. A physical signal from the protein (change in shape) may be transmitted laterally by the lipid bilayer. The lipid bilayer may have intrinsic dynamic physical properties. With permission from Stryer page 278 after S. J. Stryer, and G. L. Nelson. Copyright 1972 American Assoc Advancement of Science.

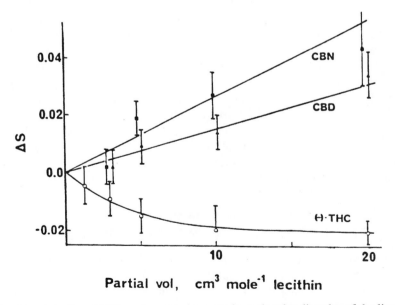

Fig. 2. At low concentration, THC produces an increase in molecular disorder of the liposome (measured by electron spin resonance). At higher concentration, THC effects level off and do not increase as molecular ratio of THC to lecithin is increased (partial anesthetic effect of THC). In contrast with THC, cannabinol (CBN) and cannabidiol produce an opposite effect, decreasing the molecular disorder of the lipid bilayer. Change in order parameter (S) of lecithin:cholesterol liposomes plotted against partial drug volume for cannabinol (CBN, solid square, molal volume 201 mL), canabidiol (CBD, solid triangle, molal volume 206 mL) and delta-1-THC ([−]-THC, empty circle, molal volume 203 mL). Each point is the mean of four and six readings ± SD (with permission *(36)*).

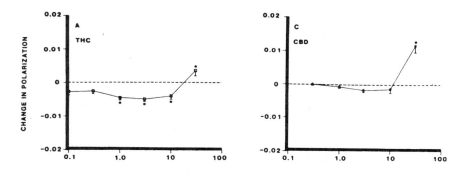

Fig. 3. Effects of psychoactive cannabinoid (THC) and nonpsychoactive cannabinoid (CBD) on fluorescence polarization of diphenylhexatranne (DPH) in rat brain synaptosomes. THC (1 and 3 μM) increases significantly (increased fluidization) while DPH fluorescence polarization CBD did not (with permission *(9)*).

Trudell et al. *(92)* using this ESR technique on liposomes had shown that volatile anesthetics, like halothane, cause a "fluidization" and expansion of the bilayer, and that this effect could be reversed, like anesthesia, by hyperbaric pressure *(92)*. Anesthesia occurs when the drug expansion of the cell membrane is equivalent to 10–20 cm^3/mol of lecithin. (Narcosis is considered a physical effect with very little biochemical interaction.) Using the same model, Gill and Lawrence observed that THC produces an increase in molecular disorder over a limited range. (This effect does not increase as the molecular ratio of THC to lecithin is increased.) THC solubility in the liposome bilayer is limited. The maximum degree of fluidization produced by THC does not approach that required to produce anesthesia in experimental animals, and THC has been designated a "partial anesthetic."

By contrast, in the same model the nonpsychoactive cannabinoids CBN and CBD produce an opposite effect to that of THC (Fig 2), decreasing the molecular disorder of the lipid bilayer. The liposomal membrane seems able to discriminate between psychoactive and nonpsychoactive cannabinoids in a way similar to the brain cell, and the protein-free liposomes exhibit a degree of molecular selectivity comparable to that of the neuron. Gill and Lawrence postulated that cannabinol and cannabidiol would be expected to antagonize in part the effect of THC in vivo, a prediction that has been documented by experimental and clinical observations.

The studies of Gill and Lawrence were supported by those of Bloom and Hillard *(9)* on synaptosomes. They studied the effects of 11 OH-THC, CBN, and CBD on synaptic plasma membranes using the fluorescence polarization method (Fig. 3); 1 and 3 μM THC produced significant decreases in DPH fluorescence polarization while CBD and CBN did not.

Bach et al. *(3)* and those of Tamir and Lichtenberg *(89)*, who used an 1-H-NMR spectra model of membranes, reported similar data. Makriyannis performed the most sophisticated investigations using X-ray diffraction and differential scanning calorimetry to study the interactions of THC on lipid bilayer organization *(56)*.

All of the foregoing data indicate that the pharmacological effects of THC and psychoactive cannabinoids may not be accounted for only by their "fluidizing" properties of the lipid bilayer of the membrane. The interaction of THC with the arachidonoid receptor must account for its psychoactive effects. However, a change in configuration of the arachidonoic receptor will also have an impact on the double lipid bilayer that surrounds it. The physical state of the layer (fluidity) should also influence the signal transmitted to contiguous neuro-

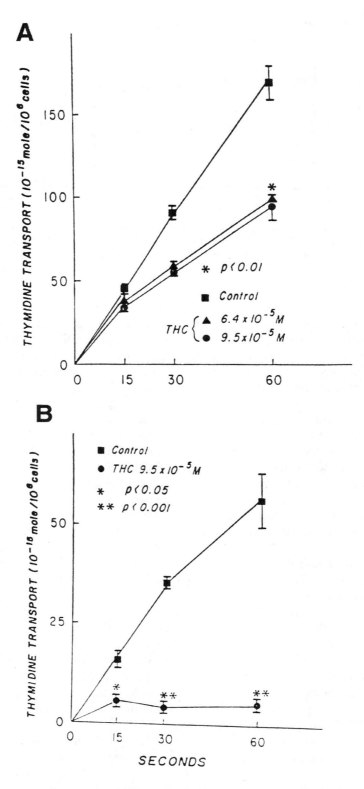

Fig. 4. **(a)** Inhibition of thymidine transport by THC (6.4 and 9.5×10^{-4} *M*) in L1210 lymphocytes incubated at 37°C (with permission *(28)*). **(b)** Inhibition of thymidine transport by THC (9.5×10^{-5} *M*) in PHA stimulated human lymphocytes incubated at 0°C (with permission *(28)*).

transmitter receptors in an allosteric fashion, but on a site that is located on another molecule. Effects of the interaction of the arachidonoid receptor with an altered lipid boundary on the signaling properties of the membrane is a matter of speculation, because they cannot be measured in a quantitative fashion with presently available techniques.

3.2. Cannabinoid and Membrane Transport Mechanisms

An interaction of cannabinoids with biochemical membrane mechanisms was reported in lymphocytes cultured in 20% BSA (67,68). Cannabinoids, in concentration of 10^{-6}–10^{-4} M exert an inhibitory effect on macromolecular synthesis of DNA, RNA, and protein in cultured lymphocytes. In this same model, ethanol in concentration of 10^{-1} M has no effect on thymidine uptake. In other studies (28) using the same model, it was observed that olivetol and its derivatives produced similar inhibitory effects on macromolecular synthesis of cultured lymphocytes. This effect was significantly correlated with the octanol–water partition coefficient of these molecules. The greater the lipid solubility, the greater the transport inhibition. Other authors reported similar inhibition of THC and other cannabinoids on DNA, RNA, and proteins in Tetrahymena, ameba, or HeLa cells (7,14,86,100,101).

Using the isotopic dilution technique in cultured lymphocyte cells, it was observed that THC decreases [^{3}H]thymidine uptake within 15 s after addition of the drug to the culture (Fig. 4). Experiments performed at 0°C indicate that THC had no action on thymidine binding to the carrier, an indication that the drug does not act on binding of thymidine to the carrier but in the transport function of the carrier (Fig. 5). This mechanism could account for the noncompetitive inhibition of THC on thymidine uptake (67). It was concluded that THC in micromolar concentration inhibits DNA precursor transport through a nonspecific alteration of membrane configuration, and that the liposolubility of the drug could induce conformational changes of membrane-bound transport enzymes, which would inhibit their function (28).

The concentration required to produce the observed inhibition indicates that the effect of THC is "nonspecific" and is related to its liposolubility in the lipid bilayer of the membrane (84). Similar inhibition of macromolecular synthesis in cultured lymphocytes has been observed with other psychotropic drugs in 10^{-6}–10^{-3} M concentrations (65). This inhibitory effect was correlated to the liposolubility of these drugs: the higher their octanol: water partition coefficient, the greater their cytotoxicity (65).

Like most lipophiles and psychotropic drugs, THC expands membranes and increases their resistance to hemolysis (22). The concentration of THC required to decrease in vitro hemolysis by 50% (AH_{50}) is similar ($10^{-5}M$) to the concentration of this drug that will inhibit by 50% (IC_{50}) thymidine incorporation in cultured human lymphocytes (65). Membrane expansion by THC could, as a result, produce conformational changes and inhibit membrane-bound enzyme carriers (61,84).

A nonspecific effect of THC is exerted with micromolar concentrations that might be reached in vivo only in heavy chronic consumption. By contrast, the acute psychotropic effects of this drug are exerted with nanomolar concentrations as a result of stereospecific interaction with receptor sites located in the central nervous system (69,83).

A similar dose-dependent inhibition by THC of [^{3}H]thymidine incorporation was observed in enterocytes of mice fed 10–100 mg/kg THC for 1–4 d. For a single dose, $p = 0.037$ for 100 mg/kg, $p = 0.033$ for 50 mg/kg, and $p = 0.10$ for 10 mg/kg. After 4 d of daily ingestion of 50 mg/kg inhibition is significant ($p < 0.03$). The inhibitory effects of THC thymidine incorporation were exerted on all parts of the small intestine. They would constitute a contraindication of its use in the treatment of the AIDS wasting syndrome, which is associated with an impairment of protein metabolism (55).

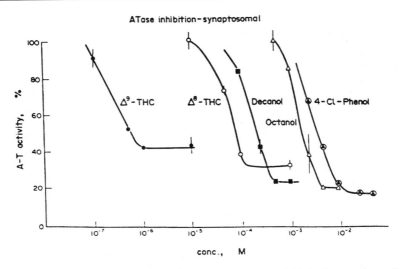

ATase inhibition-synaptosomal

Fig. 5. The inhibition of mouse brain synaptosomal lysophosphatidylcholine acyltransferase (AT) by cannabinoids and anesthetics in vitro. Values are expressed as percentages of controls and are given as means ± standard deviations (with permission (61)).

Other rapidly growing cells, such as sperm cells, are also affected by THC and cannabinoids, and decreased spermatogenesis has been observed in rodents treated with marihuana smoke (47) and in marihuana smokers (38). Arachidonoid receptors (arachidonyl diglyceride) to THC (dubbed CB_2) have been identified in the testis, sperm cells (82), on the ovum, on lymphocytes, and on most cells of the body.

3.3. Cannabinoids and Membrane-Bound Enzymes

Mellors (61) reported the inhibitory effects of cannabinoids on other membrane-bound enzymes. Lisophosphatidilcholine acyltransferase (LPC acyltransferase) from mouse splenic lymphocytes and brain synaptosomes is specifically inhibited by psychoactive cannabinoids in vitro (Table 1 (61)). The K_i for THC is 0.35 μM. The K_i of nonpsychoactive cannabinoid inhibited LPC acyltransferase is 30 times greater (10^{-4} M). In lymphocytes, basic lipid metabolism, calcium uptake, thymidine incorporation, and LPC acyltransferase activities were similarly inhibited in micromolar concentration by THC (0.3 μM) (Table 2 (61)).

Another membrane enzyme, lysophosphatidate (LPA) acyltransferase (which acylates LPA to form Phosphatidate PA), was also inhibited by THC in cultured lymphocytes. THC also inhibits mouse brain synaptosomal LPC acyltransferase in vitro (Figs 5,6) and in vivo (Fig. 7). The inhibition of LPC acyltransferase by 10 μM THC may account for the observed decreased turnover of membrane phospholipids and triglycerides at this concentration.

Some inhibition of synaptosomal LPC acyltransferase may be expected at in vivo dose levels of 1 mg/kg (61). Mellors (61) reported that calcium uptake, thymidine incorporation, and LPC acyltransferase activities in lymphocytes have a similar sensitivity to THC-induced inhibition. However, LPC inhibition by THC is specific for psychoactive cannabinoids, not for nonpsychoactive ones. Molar volume correlations indicate that the inhibition is much greater than that predicted for anesthetic action of similar hydrophobic molecules. THC inhibition of acetyltransferase, concluded Mellors, must therefore also be dependent on a stereospecific interaction with a hydrophobic region of the membrane.

Table 1
The Inhibition of Mouse Spleen Lymphocyte and Mouse Brain Synaptosome Lysophosphatidyl-choline Acyltransferase by Cannabinoids in vitro (61)

	K_i (M)	
Cannabinoid	Lymphocytes	Synaptosomes
Δ^9-THC	3.5×10^{-7}	3.0×10^{-7}
Δ^8-THC	1.3×10^{-5}	5.8×10^{-5}
Synhexyl	–	2.5×10^{-4}
11-hydroxy-Δ^9-THC	–	8.5×10^{-5}
Cannabinol	2.0×10^{-4}	5.5×10^{-4}
Cannabigerol	1.9×10^{-4}	2.6×10^{-4}

Table 2
The Inhibition of LPA and LPC by THC, and Effects of THC on Ca^{2+} Uptake and Thymidine Incorporation in Mouse Spleen Lymphocytes in vitro (61)

	K_i (M)
LPA Acyltransferase	6×10^{-6}
LPC Acyltransferase	3×10^{-7}
Ca^{2+} Uptake	3×10^{-7}
Thymidine Incorporation	2×10^{-7}

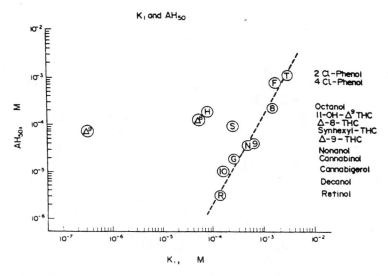

Fig. 6. Inhibition of mouse brain synaptosomal lysophosphatidylcholine acyltransferase (AT). (K_i) values compared to antihemolysis polenus (AH$_{50}$) for cannabinoids and other lipophilic compounds (with permission (61)).

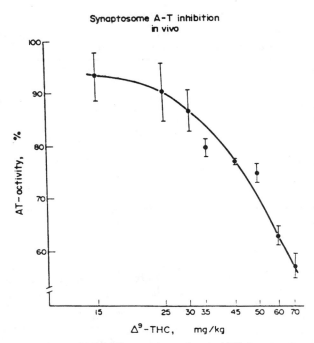

Fig. 7. The inhibition of lysophosphatidylcholine acyltransferase (AT) in synaptosomes from mice given single doses of delta-9-THC in vivo. Values are expressed as percentages of controls and are given as means ± standard deviations (with permission *(61)*).

These studies of Mellors confirm those of Gill and indicate that psychoactive cannabinoids have effects on neuronal membranes which are consistent with a specific stereochemical interaction with the membrane lipid bilayer, and are inconsistent with a simple alteration of membrane fluidity (i.e. an anesthetic effect).

3.4. In Vivo Interactions

In support of the studies of Gill and Lawrence and of Mellors, experimental observations have documented in vivo and in vitro the antagonistic effects of Δ^9-THC and of the two nonpsychoactive cannabinoids (CBD and CBN). In 1974, Borgen and Davis observed that CBD attenuates the depressant effect of THC on heart rate and temperature of rabbits *(12)*. CBD simultaneously administered with THC antagonizes the acute effects of THC on operant behavior of rodents *(102)* and monkeys *(13)*. CBD also blocks the epileptic seizures induced by THC in the genetically epileptic rabbit *(25)*.

Trouve and Nahas *(91)* reported that CBD and CBN antagonize the depressant effects of THC on coronary blood flow and force of cardiac contraction in the isolated heart (Fig. 8). CBD $10^{-6}M$ decreases by 50% cardiac microsomal calcium ATPase activity *(24)*. CBD, in equimolar concentration, neutralizes the depressant effect of THC on cardiac contraction. Nitrendipine, a calcium channel antagonist of the dihydropyridine type, has a similar effect, which would indicate that CBD has calcium channel antagonist properties.

THC chronically administered to rodents produces residual deficits similar to those observed after treatment with cannabis extracts, but of a greater magnitude *(87)*.

In humans CBD inhibits the increase in heart rate of THC when simultaneously administered with this drug *(52)*. Others *(26,44)*, using different protocols, failed to record such

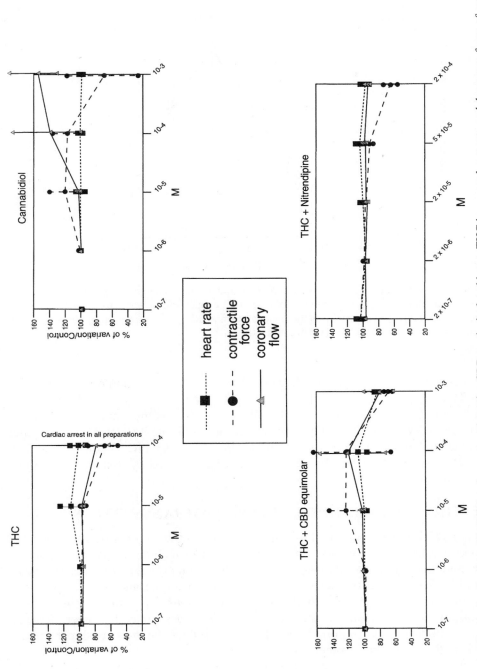

Fig. 8. Antagonistic effects of a psychoactive THC and a nonpsychoactive CBD on the isolated heart. THC increases heart rate and decreases force of contraction and coronary flow. CBD has no effect on rate but increases coronary flow and force of contraction. When CBD and THC are administered in equimolar concentration, cardioactive effects of CBD prevail with concentration of THC which will induce cardiac arrest. These positive effects of CBD are duplicated by a calcium antagonist, nitrendipine, which neutralizes the cardiac depressing effect of THC on coronary flow and cardiac contraction (with permission (91)).

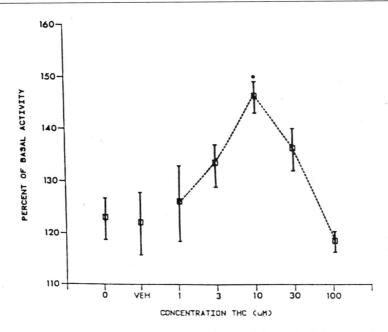

Fig. 9. Biphasic effect of delta-9-THC on isoproterenol stimulation of adenylate cyclase. All samples contained 30 μM, which had no effect on ISO stimulation. ISO concentration was 1 μM, which produced a 23% increase in basal activity. Each point is the mean and standard error of nine experiments ($p < 0.05$ when compared to vehicle treatment) (with permission *(9)*).

antagonistic effects, but all reported that CBD exerts an antagonistic action on the psychoactive effects of THC.

These results could account for the variability of effects of different cannabis preparations which contain markedly different cannabinoid concentration (Table 3 *(93)*). Most controlled observations made in humans were performed in the United States with cannabis of low CBD concentration. Results observed may be different from those caused by hashish preparations used in Africa and Asia.

4. THC, CANNABINOIDS, AND NEUROTRANSMITTERS

The effects of THC on behavior and biogenic amine neutrotransmitters was first reported in 1969 *(45)* and others reviewed the effects of various cannabinoids on dopaminergic, noradrinergic, and serotoninergic neurons. Bloom and Kiernan *(10)* reported that psychoactive cannabinoids increase the synthesis and turnover of dopamine and norepinephrine in brain slices while producing little or no change in endogenous levels of catechols. THC-induced increase of catechol synthesis was not caused by the associated hypothermic effect of the drug *(11)*. Bloom *(8)* also reported that THC increased the synthesis of dopamine and norepinephrine in the mouse brain synaptosomes.

THC also alters active uptake of catecholamine in brain synaptosomes *(4,39)* and the synaptosomal uptake of catecholamine precursors *(51)*. THC inhibits activity of $Na^+ - K^+$ ATPase, which indicates an active uptake of monoamine neurotransmitters *(10)*.

THC does not interact directly with neurotransmitters, but it will alter the binding of the neurotransmitter to its receptor (Table 4 *(9,11,31,35,37,74)*). THC changes the beta adrenergic binding in mouse cerebral cortex: suggesting that THC will alter the affinity of neuro-

Table 3
Cannabinoids Analysis by Dry Weight (% present) (93)

Cannabis Preparations[a]	CBD	CBC	CBGM	Delta-8-THC	Delta-9-THC	CBG	CBN
Marihuana (fiber type)	4.68	0.47	0.05	0.09	0.21	0.04	0.06
Marihuana (drug type)	0.01	0.15	0.06	0.09	2.11	0.10	1.12
Hashish (UN standard)	2.89	0.38	0.16	0.22	2.22	0.19	2.50
Marihuana (imed type)[b]	3.69	0.61	0.08	0.07	3.58	0.13	0.21
Marihuana (drug type)	0.02	0.27	0.04	0.05	4.40	0.21	0.47

[a]CBDV, cannabidivarin; THCV, tetrahydrocannabivarin; CBL, cannabicyclol; CBG, cannabigerol; CBGM, cannabigerolmonomethylether.
[b]Intermediate type; usually used in the preparation of hashish.

Table 4
Receptor-Mediated Interactions of THC with Neurotransmitters

		Effects	Reference
Acetylcholine	Muscarinic	↓	Domino et al. (31)
			Gessa et al. (35)
Dopamine	Receptor Channel	↑	Bloom et al. (9)
Epinephrine	β	↑	Bloom and Kiernan (11)
Gaba	Cl⁻ Channel	↑	Pryor et al. (74)
NMDA	Ca^{2+} Channel	↓	Hampson et al. (37)
Opioid	μ, δ	↓	Vaysse et al. (94)

transmitters for these receptors. THC selectively enhances the agonist binding to D_2 sites, while CBD does not (10). THC and its hydroxy derivative has a biphasic effect on [^{3}H]aloprenolol binding to the β adrenergic receptor, increasing it with 3 μM concentration and decreasing it with 30 μM concentration (Fig. 9). THC affects the ability of the neurotransmitter receptor ([^{3}H]DA) binding to discriminate between agonists and antagonists. Bloom concludes by stating that since THC alters the fluidity of the membrane, any effects of THC on "receptors" are due to "cannabinoid"-induced changes in the membrane environment and the receptors that are embedded within the membrane. Bloom and Kiernan reported that THC inhibited the binding of naloxone to opioid receptors but had no effect on D-ala D-leu enkephalin (DADL) binding (Fig. 10). Significant decreases were observed at concentration of 4 μM. THC can preferentially affect μ rather than delta opioid receptors.

Vaysse et al. reported that the treatment of brain membranes with THC decreased the *in vitro* binding of [^{3}H]dehydromorphine (μ opioid) in a dose-dependent noncompetitive fashion ($K_L = 3 \pm 1$ μM). They concluded that the allosteric modulation of the opioid receptor by THC results from a direct interaction with a receptor protein and is not merely the result of a perturbation of the lipid bilayer (94).

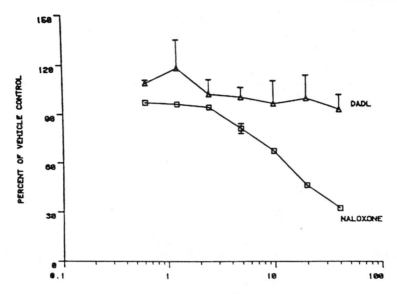

Fig. 10. Effects of delta-9-THC on the binding of [³H]Naloxone and [³H]-DADL (D-ala-D-leu-enkephalin) concentrations were 1 n*M*. Values shown are the mean and standard error of three separate experiments performed in triplicate (with permission *(9)*).

A dose-related decrease in acetylcholine utilization in the hippocampus of rats after THC administration has been reported by Domino *(30)*. This THC-induced decrease in acetylcholine hippocampal activity was inhibited by an antagonist of the THC receptor SR 141716A *(35)*, indicating that the THC receptor induces an allosteric change in the receptor site of the acetylcholine receptor.

It can also be hypothesized that the change in affinity of the neurotransmitter receptor caused by THC is related to the dual effect of the binding of the drug on the G-protein coupled receptor and of the physical effect of THC on membrane fluidity.

5. THC AND STEROIDS

A vast amount of literature *(79,80,98)* has documented that THC exerts profound effects on neuroendocrine targets in the brain and gonads. Numerous experimental studies on rats, mice, rabbits, hamsters, guinea pigs, and rhesus monkeys have documented that THC administration over a period of days and weeks induces cycle derangements, inhibition of ovulation, and interference with spermatogenesis. Modulation of these effects by alterations of gonadal and pituitary hormones and of releasing factors of the hypothalamus have also been reported.

In man, plasma testosterone changes as a result of acute or chronic marihuana smoking *(23,53)* have not been demonstrated convincingly, and there was no change in FSH or LH *(38,63)*. However, impairment of spermatogenesis as a result of chronic marihuana smoking is well documented in man *(53)*, as it has been in animal studies.

Effects on the gonadal function of female rodents and rhesus monkeys have been reported following daily or weekly administration of THC with alterations of LH, FSH, and prolactin *(2,75)*. In nonhuman primates, THC administered acutely for several weeks depresses FSH and LH, an effect that may be counteracted by LHRH *(85)*. As a result, anovulatory cycles were observed. However, monkeys develop tolerance to the disrupting effects of THC on the

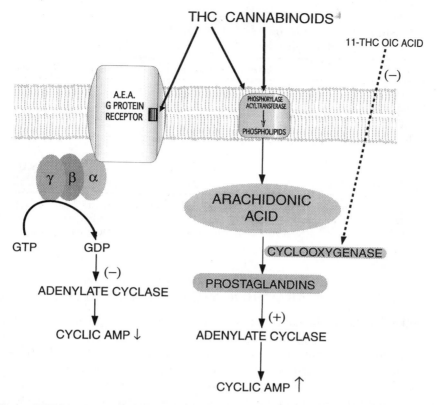

Fig. 11. Effects of THC and cannabinoids on phospholipid and arachidonic acid biochemical pathways.

menstrual cycle. A similar tolerance to chronic marihuana smoking in women was reported by Mendelson et al. *(62)*. Smith et al. reported that using cytosol preparations from the uterus of rhesus monkeys and humans failed to demonstrate any competition of THC with estradiol receptors. But studies of corticoid receptors in rat hippocampal cytosol have suggested that some affinity for THC existed in the brain *(32)*.

In animals, THC causes a release of corticosteroids in the rat *(29)*, which seems to be mediated by corticotropin releasing factor (CRF), so it appears that THC can mobilize CRF from the hypothalamus, as recently reported by de Fonseca et al. *(27)*. In contrast, marihuana smoking or THC does not produce any changes in corticol plasma levels in humans *(43)*.

The functional significance of binding of THC to glucocorticoids has yet to be defined *(46)*. All of the present experimental and clinical data indicates that THC has very limited interaction with steroid receptors in humans.

Steroid ligands (estradiol, progesterone, androsterone, and corticosterone) do not displace synthetic agonist of the AEA-G-protein receptor in rat membranes *(46)*. This lack of interaction between THC and steroid ligands is unexpected since steroids and cannabinoids share the same multiring structures with hydroxyl groups and are fat soluble. Gill and Lawrence *(36)* reported that the β hydroxy steroids, with little effect on lipid bilayer fluidity (like the endogenous steroids), have no anesthetic properties while the α isomer has anesthetic potential similar to that of halothane. Physicochemical properties of the endogenous steroids that have little effect on membrane fluidity differ from those of THC that increases fluidity.

Table 5
Effects of Cannabinoids (16.0 μ*M*) on Arachidonic Acid Formation from [^{14}C] Arachidonylphosphatidylcholine by Brain Synaptosomes *(49)*[a]

	Arachidonic Acid (dpm ± SD)	Change (%)
Vehicle (16.0 μM)	302 ± 14	–
Δ^1-THC (16.0 μM)	397 ± 38	31.3
7-Oxo-Δ^1-THC (16.0 μM)	351 ± 20	16.1
7-OH-Δ^1-THC (16.0 μM)	503 ± 26	66.5
Δ^1-THC-7-oic acid (16.0 μM)	364 ± 24	20.4
6α-OH-Δ^1-THC (16.0 μM)	360 ± 31	19.0
6β-OH-Δ^1-THC (16.0 μM)	308 ± 17	2.1 NS

[a]Synaptosomes (0.22 mg protein) were incubated with [^{14}C]arachidonylphosphatidylcholine (35,000 dpm) and cannabinoid or vehicle for 45 min. Results represent mean (dpm) ± SD, one tenth of sample, $N = 3$. Values were significantly different from the vehicle, $p < 0.0005$, determined by Student's t test; except NS, which was not significant.

6. CANNABINOIDS, ARACHIDONIC ACID, AND PROSTAGLANDINS

Psychoactive cannabinoids and some of their nonpsychoactive acid metabolites will release in a dose-dependent manner arachidonic acid from ^{14}C-labeled phosphatidylcholine in mouse synaptosomes, myelin, and mitochondria (Table 5 *(49)*). Hydrolysis of phosphatidylcholine was attributed to an activation of phospholipase A$_2$. *Nonpsychoactive cannabinoids are more effective than psychoactive ones (THC) in causing arachidonic acid release (18)*. In the same in vitro model, cannabinoid-generated arachidonic acid biosynthesis was inhibited by steroids, NSAIDs, aspirin, paracetamol, and indomethacin *(20)*.

While Burstein still suggests that arachidonic acid accumulation and resulting eicosanoid biosynthesis is mediated by the "CB1–CB2"-receptor-coupled G-protein mechanism *(21)*, Felder *(33)* states in a recent review that this mechanism remains controversial. It also should be pointed out that the cannabinoids, which do not effect the CB1 receptor, do mobilize arachidonic acid and prostaglandins.

A second mechanism for the increased arachidonic acid accumulations is the failure to reesterify free arachidonic acid in the phospholipid synthetic pathway, which requires acyl transferase activity (Fig. 11) *(61,76–78)*.

Reichman et al. *(76)*, who also reported that THC inhibits arachidonic acid acylation of phospholipid and triglycerides in guinea pig cerebral cortical slices, suggested this increased arachidonic acid accumulation may be entirely attributed to their ability to block lipid reacylation. As a result of this alteration of the phospholipid turnover, a decrease of phospholipid brain concentration has been reported.

Arachidonic acid mobilization by cannabinoids has been associated with a release of prostaglandins and other eicosanoids, such as leukotrienes and platelet activation factors (PAF). Burstein reported that THC and nonpsychoactive cannabinoids increased PGE$_2$ in human lung fibroblasts in an order of potency that correlated well with the magnitude of the [^{14}C]arachidonic acid accumulation *(15,16)*. A dose-related significant rise of PGE$_2$ and PGF$_{2\alpha}$ in the brain was reported by Bhattacharya 2 h following intraperitoneal injection of 2 mg/kg THC.

Burstein et al. *(20)* observed that the action of THC on prostaglandin biosynthesis was blocked by indomethacin and strongly inhibited by hydrocortisone (Table 6 *(20)*). Perez-Reyes et al. *(70)* reported in single blind placebo controlled study in four subjects that

Table 6
Indomethacin Inhibition of THC-Induced Prostaglandin E Release in Neuroblastoma (N2a) Cells (20)

	PGE Level (ng/ml ± SD)
Vehicle[a]	0.14 ± 0.02
Indomethacin[b]	<0.10
Delta[1]-THC[c]	4.99 ± 1.18
Delta[1]-THC + Indomethacin	0.46 ± 0.18

[a]Ethanol (10 µL).
[b]Added 15 min. Prior to THC. Concentration = 32 µM.
[c]Cells exposed for 60 min. Concentration = 32 µM.

indomethacin pretreatment significantly decreased prostaglandin plasma concentration, heart rate acceleration, and distortion of time perception produced by THC.

Burstein et al. (20) also observed that the action of THC on prostaglandin biosynthesis cells is blocked by indomethacin, a cyclooxygenase inhibitor, and is significantly inhibited by hydrocortisone. The same author showed that THC stimulatory activity on prostaglandin biosynthesis was inhibited by its own nonpsychoactive metabolite THC-11 oic acid (19). This same cannabinoid blocks the action of the platelet activation factor (PAF) (17) and suppresses cyclooxygenase activity in cell culture (19). These properties, comparable to those of NSAIDs, confer to a nonpsychoactive cannabinoid an antiinflammatory activity (103), which is enhanced by the addition of a dimethylheptyl side chain on the A-ring, a manipulation that increases the affinity of the cannabinoid for its molecular targets (Fig. 12). The synthetic nonpsychoactive cannabinoid, DMH-THC-11 oic acid, when administered orally (0.1 mg/kg) to mice and rats with experimentally induced acute or chronic inflammation, proved to be as effective as indomethacin in relieving inflammation and associated symptoms (103). DMH-THC-11 oic acid causes selective inhibition of cyclooxygenase-2, and is an effective antiinflammatory agent in experimental models. It is a nonpsychoactive cannabinoid that should reduce the pain of inflammation by a mechanism similar to that of the NSAIDS.

7. CANNABINOIDS, THC, AND ADENYLATE CYCLASE

Of all the cannabinoids, only THC has been related with alterations of adenylate cyclase activity.

7.1 THC and Stimulation of Adenylate Cyclase Activity

Administration of THC and of other psychoactive cannabinoids is related in humans with a dose-related increase in heart rate, the most consistently reported acute effect of THC. This tachycardia is not associated with an increase of plasma catechols and its entirely parallels the brain functional effects. This tachycardia is inhibited by propanolol (71). Bloom and Hillard (9) have reported that THC increases in a dose-related manner isoprenalin induced stimulation of adenylate cyclase (Fig. 12).

These authors suggest that changes of adenylate cyclase activity by THC could be caused "at least in part by drug induced alterations in the physical properties of the membrane" (9). It is further suggested in this paper that these membrane alterations by THC are caused by a deregulation of the AEA-G-protein receptor and of the signaling properties of the lipid bilayer.

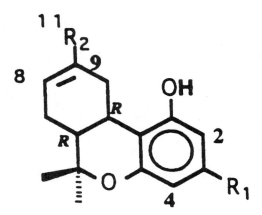

Fig. 12. Structures of the cannabinoids. R designates the absolute stereochemistry of the chiral centers in this series. THC = delta-9-THC. THC-11 oic acid = delta-8-THC-11 oic acid. DMH-11 C = 1',1' dimethylheptyl-delta-8-THC-11 oic acid (with permission *(103)*).

7.2 Cannabinoids, Prostaglandins, and Cyclic AMP

Prostaglandin biosynthesis, in response to cannabinoids, results in cyclic AMP accumulation. Psychoactive and nonpsychoactive cannabinoids increase free arachidonic acid concentration and the cascade of eicosanoid biosynthesis including prostaglandins (Fig. 11). Hillard and Bloom *(40)* proposed a role for prostaglandins after observing that in brain homogenates 10–30 μM THC, cannabidiol, or cannabinol stimulated adenylate cyclase above basal levels. This response to THC could be blocked by aspirin and indomethacin. Prostaglandin-induced increased cyclic AMP caused by cannabinoids may mitigate the adenylate cyclase G-protein inhibition of THC receptor binding. Increased cyclic AMP may become dominant because of their ubiquitous distribution of prostaglandins throughout the vascular system.

7.3 Inhibition of Adenylate Cyclase Activity by Psychoactive Cannabinoids

This inhibition has been attributed to a G-protein-receptor-mediated mechanism transduced by trimeric subunits to which it is coupled *(46)*. The AEA-G-protein-coupled arachidonoid receptor includes a seven-segment alpha-helical transmembrane structure with three extramembrane loops and a heterotrimeric alpha, beta, and gamma subunit located at the inner surface of the cell membrane. The latter components are coupled to adenylate cyclase and to other effector proteins or ion channels. The G protein is inhibited by pertussis toxin, which inactivates the alpha subunit of the G-protein complex. Activation of the arachinoid receptor, and its coupled G protein, will decrease cyclic AMP content within the neurons and thereby modify critical synaptic pathways *(73)*. Conversely, Bidault-Russell and Howlett *(6)* reported a G-protein "cannabinoid"-receptor-regulated cyclic AMP accumulation in rat striatum.

The inhibitory effect of THC on adenylate cyclase should be antagonized by the stimulatory effects of THC and other cannabinoids on cyclic AMP production.

8. RECEPTOR AND LIPID BILAYER MEDIATED SIGNAL TRANSDUCTION

While the mechanism of action of THC with the AEA-G-protein-coupled receptor has been investigated extensively, the physiological function of the natural ligand AEA to its

arachidonoid receptor is still undetermined. The mechanism of action of AEA has been identified with that of THC and of its synthetic analogs, involving G-protein dependent associated
mechanisms. On the basis of this analogy alone, one would expect that AEA should play a
major role in the regulation of membrane function and that the function of the AEA G-protein receptor is not limited to the binding of THC.

AEA is derived from membrane phospholipids. Phospholipase A_2, which hydrolyzes
phospholipids, generates highly active signal molecules or their immediate precursors like
arachidonic acid and eicosanoids (prostaglandins and leukotrienes) (88). AEA might play
the role of a signalling molecule in its interaction with the AEA-G-protein receptor
(Fig. 13).

AEA has a lower affinity than THC for the G-protein receptor. It occupies a smaller volume and has a briefer pharmacokinetic profile than THC and a very fast turnover and disposition (like most signaling and second messenger molecules). It is not stored in cells (41), it
accumulates in the brain following hypoxia or death of the neuron. AEA has properties one
would expect of an endogenous membrane phospholipid derived signaling molecule (AEA is
also reported to block gap junctions and astrocyte junctional conductance) (95).

Tolerance to THC, characterized by a decreased sensitivity to its effects and necessity to
increase dosage in order to obtain initial effects, does develop to a considerable degree with
this drug (66). An increase in the rate of metabolism of THC due to repeated administration
has been ruled out. A decreased sensitivity of the target cell is another mechanism.

This decreased sensitivity might be accounted for by the affinity (binding strength) of
THC and its staying power on the G-protein receptor, which accounts for the persistance of
the effects of THC. A single dose may last 24 h. As the AEA-G-protein receptors, which are
ubiquitous in the membrane of neuronal cells, become occupied in preferential areas of blood
flow distribution, one might speculate that larger doses of THC will be required to bind to the
AEA-G-protein receptors in contiguous areas. Since THC does not alter the sensitivity of the
AEA-G-protein receptor, it should alter distribution and possibly the turnover or density of
these receptors in the course of chronic use.

THC does not interact directly with the active sites of action the receptors of neuro transmitters proteins and does not compete with any ligands known to interact with these sites, but
THC and the psychoactive cannabinoids produce changes in the receptor sites of neurotransmitters. These are "allosteric" changes, which occur on neighboring receptors distinct from
the AEA-G-protein receptor. What is the nature of the signalling mechanisms between these
two classes of receptors? Could they be mediated by the double lipid bilayer in which the
receptor proteins are encased?

Sanderman (81) reported that the lipid environment (boundary lipids) surrounding membrane enzymes will influence enzymatic function. Jain and White (50) reported that
changes in the membrane lipid boundary could affect protein receptor function. Makriyannis (56) has summarized studies of the molecular mechanism of THC and its induced
membrane perturbation and linked its ability to perturb the lipid bilayer by its amphipathic
properties (owing to its hydrophobic and hydrophilic moieties). Alterations of the structural and dynamic properties of boundary lipids will affect the configuration of receptor
proteins. Membrane perturbation involves physical factors, which are caused by an
increase in the ratio of gauche:trans conformers in the phospholipid chain and a decrease
in cooperation between the chains. The critical interaction occurs at the membrane interface and is associated with a conformational change in the glycerol skeleton of the
membrane phospholipids (57). Some have even suggested the existence of specific
drug–membrane interactions (56), which indicate the sensitivity of lipid bilayer activity to
physical changes in its environment.

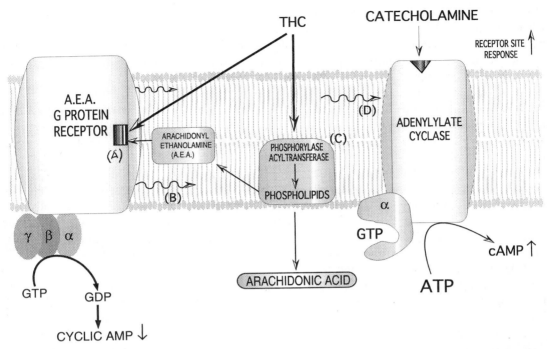

Fig. 13. Putative signal transduction changes generated by THC in the G-protein–AEA receptor and the lipid bilayer of the membrane. THC interacts simultaneously with **(A)** the G-protein–AEA receptor, which alters its configuration, and **(B)** the membrane phospholipid bilayer, which undergoes conformational changes and alteration of its signaling properties. As a result of the dual alterations of membrane signaling by THC, the following events might take place: **(C)** Alteration of the configuration of the membrane enzymes phosphorylase and acyltransferase, which control phospholipid metabolism, arachidonic acid, and arachidonyl ethanolamide (AEA) formation, and **(D)** an allosteric change of the conformation of adjacent neurotransmitter receptor site.

Koshland emphasized the fundamental role played by the protein molecule in controlling all living systems. The regulating function of the protein is not involved in a chemical reaction itself, but controls the activity of an enzyme by changing its shape or by inducing the same shape or form on an other (allosteric) site of the molecule. The simplest model of this regulatory function was described by Monod *(64)* for hemoglobin and by Koshland et al. *(54)* for enzymes. In both, the allosteric site is located on the same molecule.

This mechanism of allosteric change does not apply to the protein receptor embedded in the double lipid bilayer of the neuronal membranes. It is hypothesized that the signal imparted by THC to the AEA-G-protein receptor might be transmitted through the lipid bilayer to a contiguous receptor that would alter the configurations of its active site.

9. A PUTATIVE SIGNAL TRANSDUCTION ROLE FOR THE LIPID BILAYER OF THE MEMBRANE

It is proposed that AEA the (arachidonylethanolamine) receptor interaction possesses a physiological function, which is to regulate the signaling between boundary lipids and the receptors or enzymes of the membrane in response to physiological stimuli. The boundary lipids surrounding the membrane proteins are the vehicles for the signals between the AEA G-protein receptor and the neurotransmitter receptors and their binding sites. The change of configuration of the G-protein receptor would modulate the signaling of membrane on its enzymes and receptors. AEA, a by-product of the membrane phospholipid, would be an indirect signal modulator of membrane activity.

The arachidonyl ligand–G-protein receptor "physiological" interaction might maintain the membrane lipid bilayer in a "homeodynamic" equilibrium, associated with the transmission of instantaneous signaling to enzymes and neurotransmitter receptors in the lipid bilayer. The neurotransmitter receptor would be specific to the specialized neuronal structures where these neurotransmitter receptors are located.

The nature and physiological role of this signaling mechanism have not been identified, and there is no physical theory to account for such signaling that eludes any quantitative measurement. The lipid bilayer of the membrane is an exquisitely sensitive physical structure with an invisible fluid skeleton.

AEA has in common with the second messenger cyclic AMP an ubiquitous distribution in body cells. (One should note that cyclic AMP is not an effective therapeutic agent because of its multiple functional and pharmacological effects.) But the signaling function of AEA is fundamentally different from that of cyclic AMP, which has an intracellular mode of action. It is hypothesized that AEA-G-protein receptor signaling might be modulated through a physical change of its receptor configuration. This physical signal to the boundary lipid bilayer would be transduced to the membrane enzyme that initiates the phospholipid AEA cycle, thus completing an intramembranous physicochemical loop (Fig. 12).

This feedback loop could modulate the interaction of the double lipid bilayer with phospholipase and acyltransferase enzymes and thereby regulate by a process of "physicochemical" transduction the generation of AEA. Regulation of this process would depend on the interaction of AEA with its receptor, which, in turn, would modulate the signaling function of the double lipid bilayer in response to physiological stimuli. In order to perform its physiological signaling function, the physicochemical composition of the bilayer must preserve its physiological composition and physio-chemical structure.

The lipid bilayer is an "internal milieu" in which membrane receptors and enzymes are embedded. This milieu, as defined by Claude Bernard (5), is endowed with a constant composition; it has a unique physicochemical and structural organization independent from the composition of the extracellular fluid. It acts as a buffer and a permeability barrier between the extracellular fluid and the intracellular milieu.

THC will alter the physicochemical structure and composition of the membrane. THC is a xenobiotic surrogate ligand, which, instead of being recycled like AEA, must be entirely excreted from the body. THC deregulates the putative membrane signaling in two ways: first, by preempting AEA-G-protein receptor function; second, by altering the physicochemical organization of the boundary lipid bilayer in which it partitions. THC will deregulate the physiological signaling role of the lipid bilayer, a fundamental feature of all living cells. This deregulation of membrane signaling by THC results in multiple and partial therapeutic effects which lack consistency and effectiveness.

ACKNOWLEDGMENT

The contributions of David Michael Taylor in the composition, preparation, and formatting of this text as well as the creation of portions of graphic figure design for this manuscript are acknowledged with thanks.

REFERENCES

1. Abood, M. E. and Martin, B. R. (1996) Molecular neurobiology of the cannabinoid receptor. *Int. Rev. Neurobiol.* **39**, 197–221.
2. Asch, R., Fernandez, E., Smith, C. and Pauerstein, C. (1979) Precoital single doses of THC block ovulation in the rabbit. *Fertil. Steril.* **31**, 331–334.
3. Bach, D., Raz, A. and Goldman, R. (1976) The interaction of hashish compounds with planar lipid bilayer membranes. *Biochem. Pharmacol.* **25**, 1241–1244.
4. Banerjee, S. P., Snyder, S. H. and Mechoulam, R. (1975) Influence of neurotransmitter uptake in rat brain synaptosomes. *J Pharmacol. Exp. Ther.* **194**, 74–81.
5. Bernard, C. (1878) *Lecons sur Les Phenomenes de la Vie*, Paris.
6. Bidault-Russell, M. and Howlett, A. C. (1991) Cannabinoid receptor-regulated cyclic AMP accumulation in the rat striatum. *J. Neurochem.* **57**, 1769–1773.
7. Blevins, R. and Kegan, J. (1976) Delta-9-THC: Effects on macromolecular synthesis in human and other mammalian cells, in *Marihuana: Chemistry, Biochemistry and Cellular Effects* (G., Nahas, W. Paton and J. Idanpaan-Heikkila eds.), Springer-Verlag, New York, pp. 213–222.
8. Bloom, A. S. (1982) Cannabinoids and neurotransmitter receptors. *Brain Res.* **235**, 370–375.
9. Bloom, A. S. and Hillard, C. J. (1984) Cannabinoids, neurotransmitter receptors and brain membranes, in *Marihuana '84* D. J. Harvey, W. Paton, and G. G. Nahas, eds. Oxford, England, IRL Press, pp. 217–231
10. Bloom, A. S., Johnson, K. M. and Dewey, W. L. (1978) The effects of cannabinoids on body temperature and brain catecholamine synthesis. *Res. Commun. Chem. Path. Pharm.* **20**, 51–57.
11. Bloom, A. S. and Kiernan, C. J. (1980) Interaction of ambient temperature with the effects of delta-9-THC on brain catecholamine synthesis and plasma corticosterone levels. *Psychopharmacol.* **67**, 215–219.
12. Borgen, L. A. and Davis, W. M. (1974) Cannabidiol interaction with delta-9-tetrahydrocannabinol. *Res. Commun. Chem. Pathol. Pharmacol.* **7**, 633–670.
13. Brady, K. T., Balster, L R. (1980) The effect of delta-9-tetrahydrocannabinol alone and in combination with cannabidiol on fixed-interval performance in rhesus monkeys. *Psychopharmacol.* **72**, 21–26.
14. Bram, S. and Brachet, P. (1976) Inhibition of proliferation and differentiation of dictyostelium discoideum amoebae by tetrahydrocannabinol and cannabinol, *in Marihuana: Chemistry, Biochemistry and Cellular Effects* (G. Nahas, W. Paton, J. Idanpaan-Heikkila, eds.) Springer-Verlag, New York, pp. 207–211.
15. Burstein, S., Hunter, S. and Ozman, K. (1983) Prostaglandins and cannabis XII. The effect of cannabinoid structure on the synthesis of prostaglandins by human lung fibroblasts. *Mol. Pharmacol.* **23**, 121–126.
16. Burstein, S., Hunter, S., Sedor, C. and Shulman, S. (1982) Prostaglandins and cannabis IX. Stimulation of PGE-2 synthesis in human lung fibroblasts by delta-1-THC. *Biochem. Pharmacol.* **31**, 2361–2365.
17. Burstein, S. H., Audette, C. A., Doyle, S. A., Hull, K., Hunter, S. A. and Latham, V. (1989) Antagonism to the actions of platelet activating factor by a nonpsychoactive cannabinoid. *J. Pharmacol. Exp. Ther.* **251**, 531–535.
18. Burstein, S. H. and Hunter, S. A. (1978) Release of arachidonic acid from HeLa cells by cannabinoids. *Biochem. Pharmacol.* **27**, 1275–1280.
19. Burstein, S. H., Hunter, S. A., Latham, V. and Renzulli, L. (1986) Prostaglandins and cannabis-XVI: Antagonism of delta-1-tetrahydrocannabinol action by its metabolites. *Biochem, Pharmacol.* **35**, 2553–2558.
20. Burstein, S. H., Hunter, S. A., Ozman, K. and Renzulli, L. (1984) In vitro models of cannabinoid-induced psychoactivity in *Marihuana '84*. D. J., Harvey, W. Paton and G. G. Nahas, eds.), Oxford, England, IRL Press, 1984 pp. 399–406.
21. Burstein, S. H., Young, J. K. and Wright, G. E. (1995) Relationships between eicosanoids and cannabinoids. Are eicosanoids cannabimimetic agents? *Biochem. Pharmacol.* **50**, 1735–1742.
22. Chari-Bitron, A. (1976) Effects of THC on red blood cell membranes and on alveolar macrophages, in *Marihuana: Chemistry, Biochemistry and Cellular Effects* (G. Nahas, W. Paton, and J. Idanpaan-Heikkila, eds.), Springer-Verlag, New York, p. 273.
23. Cohen, S. (1976) The 94-day cannabis study. *Ann. NY Acad. Sci.* **282**, 211–220.
24. Collins, F. G. and Haavik, C. O. (1979) Effects of cannabinoids on cardiac microsomal ca++ATPase activity and calcium uptake. *Biochem. Pharmacol.* **28**, 2303–2306.
25. Consroe, P. F. and Wolkin, A. (1977) Cannabidiol-antiepileptic drug comparisons and interactions in experimentally induced seizures in rats. *J. Pharmacol. Exp. Ther.* **201**, 26–32.
26. Dalton, W. S., Martz, R., Lemberger, L., Rodda, B. E. and Forney, R. B. (1976) Influence of cannabidiol on delta-9-tetrahydrocannabinol effects. *Clin. Pharm. Ther.* **19**, 300–309.
27. de Fonseca, F., Carrera, M., Navarro, M., Koob, G. and Weiss, F. (1997) Activation of corticotropin-releasing factor in the limbic system during cannabinoid withdrawal. *Science.* **276**, 2050–2051.

28. Desoize, B., Leger, C. and Nahas, G. G. (1979) Plasma membrane inhibition of macromolecular precursor transport by THC. *Biochem Pharmacol.* **28**, 1113–1118.

29. Dewey, W., Yonle, L., Harris, L., Reavis, W. M., Griffin, E. D. J. and Newby, E. V. (1970) Some cardiovascular effects of trans-delta-9-THC. *Pharmacologist* **12**, 259.

30. Domino, E. (1981) Cannabinoids and the cholinergic system. *J. Clin. Pharmacol.* **21 suppl.**, 249S–255S.

31. Domino, E. F., Hardman, H. F. and Seevers, M. H. (1971) Central nervous system actions of some synthetic tetrahydrocannabinol derivatives. *Pharmacol. Rev.* **23**, 317–336.

32. Eldridge, J. and Landfield, P. (1990) Cannabinoid interactions with glucocorticoid receptors in rat hippocampus. *Brain Res.* **534**, 135–141.

33. Felder, C. C., Veluz, J. S., Williams, H. L., Briley, E. M. and Matsuda, L. A. (1992) Cannabinoid agonists stimulate both receptor- and non-receptor-mediated signal transduction pathways in cells transfected with and expressing cannabinoid receptor clones. *Mol. Pharmacol.* **42**, 838–845.

34. Gaoni, Y. and Mechoulam, R. (1964) Isolation, structure and partial synthesis of an active component of hashish. *J. Amer. Chem. Soc.* **86**, 1646–1647.

35. Gessa, G. L., Mascia, M. S., Casu, M. A. and Carta, G. (1997) Inhibition of hippocampal acetylcholine release by cannabinoids: reversal by SR 141716A. *Eur. J. Pharmacol.* **327**, R1–2.

36. Gill, E. W. and Lawrence, D. K. (1976) The physicochemical mode of action of THC on cell membranes, in *Pharmacology of Marihuana* (M. C. Braude and S. Szara, eds.), Vol. 1, Raven Press, New York, pp. 147–155.

37. Hampson, A. J., Bornheim, L. M., Scanziani, M., Yost, C. S., Gray, A. T., Hansen, B. M., Leonoudakis, D. J. and Bickler, P. E. (1998) Dual effects of anandamide on NMDA receptor-mediated responses and neurotransmission. *J. Neurochem.* **70**, 671–676.

38. Hembree, W. C., Nahas, G. G., Zeidenberg, P. and Huang, H. F. S. (1979) Changes in human spermatozoa associated with high dose marihuana smoking, in *Marihuana: Biological Effects. Analysis, Metabolism, Cellular Responses, Reproduction and Brain* (G. G. Nahas and W. D. M. Paton, eds.), Vol. 735–738, Pergamon Press, Elmsford, New York, pp. 643–657.

39. Hershkowitz, M., Goldman, R. and Raz, A. (1977) Effect of cannabinoids on neurotransmitter uptake, ATPase activity and morphology of mouse brain synaptosomes. *Biochem Pharmacol.* **26**, 1327–1331.

40. Hillard, C. J. and Bloom, A. S. (1983) Possible role of prostaglandins in the effects of the cannabinoids on adenylate cyclase activity. *Eur. J. Pharmacol.* **91**, 21–27.

41. Hillard, C. J. and Campbell, W. B. (1997) Biochemistry and pharmacology of arachidonylethanolamide, a putative endogenous cannabinoid. *J. Lipid Res.* **38**, 2383–2398.

42. Hillard, C. J., Edgemond, W. S. and Campbell, W. B. (1995) Characterization of ligand binding to the cannabinoid receptor of rat brain membranes using a novel method: application to anandamide. *J. Neurochem.* **64**, 677–683.

43. Hollister, L., Moore, F., Kantor, S. and Noble, E. (1970) Delta-1-THC, synhexl and marijuana extract administered orally in man: catecholamine excretion, plasma cortisol levels and platelet serotonin content. *Psychopharmacologia* **17**, 354–360.

44. Hollister, L. E. and Gillespie, L. E. (1975) Interactions of delta-9-THC and CBD. *Clin. Pharmacol. Ther.* **18**, 80–84.

45. Holtzman, D., Lovell, R. A., Jaffe, J. H. and Freedman, D. X. (1969) 1-delta-9-THC: Neurochemical and behavioral effects in the mouse. *Science* **163**, 1464–1467.

46. Howlett, A. C. (1995) Cannabinoid compounds and signal transduction mechanisms, in *Cannabinoid Receptors* (R. G. Pertwee, ed.), Academic Press, London, pp. 167–204.

47. Huang, M. F. S., Nahas, G. G. and Hembree, W. C. (1979) Effects of marihuana inhalation on spermatogenesis of the rat, in *Marihuana: Biological Effects* (G. G. Nahas and W. D. M. Paton, eds.), Pergamon Press, Oxford.

48. Hubbell, W. L. and McConnell, H. M. (1971) Molecular motion in spin-labelled phospholipids and membranes. *J. Am. Chem. Soc.* **93**, 314–326.

49. Hunter, S. A., Burstein, S. and Renzulli, L. (1984) Cannabinoid modulated phospholipase activities by mouse brain subcellular fractions, *Marihuana '84* D. J. Harvey, W. Paton, and G. G., Nahas, eds.), Oxford, England, IRL Press, pp. 245–251.

50. Jain, M. and White, H. (1977) Long-range order in biomembranes. *Adv. Lipid Res.* **15**, 1–60.

51. Johnson, K. M., Dewey, W. L. (1978) effects of delta-9-THC on the synaptosomal uptake of 3-H-tryptophan and 3-H-choline. *Pharmacology* **17**, 83–87.

52. Karniol, I. G., Shirakawa, I., Kasiniski, N., Pfeferman, A. and Carlini, E. A. (1974) Cannabidiol interferes with the effect of delta-9-tetrahydrocannabinol in the rat. *Eur. J. Pharmacol.* **28**, 172–177.

53. Kolodny, R., Masters, W., Kolodner, R. and Toro, G. (1974) Depression of plasma testosterone levels after chronic intensive marihuana use. *N. Engl. J. Med.* **290**, 872–874.

54. Koshland, D., Nemethy, G. and Filmer, D. (1966) Comparison of experimental binding data and theoretical models in proteins containing subunits. *Biochemistry* **5**, 365–385.

55. Kotler, D., Tierney, A., Wang, J. and Pierson, R. (1989) Magnitude of body cell-mass depletion and the timing of death from wasting in AIDS. *Am. J. Clin. Nutr.* **50**, 444–447.

56. Makriyannis, A. (1995) The role of cell membranes in cannabinoid activity, in *Cannabinoid Receptors* (R. Pertwee, ed.), Academic Press, New York, pp. 87–115.

57. Makriyannis, A., Yang, D. and Mavromoustakos, T. (1990) The molecular features of membrane perturbation by anesthetic steroids: a study using differential scanning calorimetry, small angle X-ray diffraction and solid state 2-H NMR, in *Steroids and Neuronal Activity, Ciba Foundation Symposium No. 153* (M. Simmonds, ed.), Wiley, Chichester, pp. 172–189.

58. Matsuda, L. A., Lolait, S. J., Brownstein, M. J., Young, A. C. and Bonner, T. I. (1990) Structure of a cannabinoid receptor and functional expression of the cloned cDNA [see comments]. *Nature* **346**, 561–564.

59. Mechoulam, R. (1973) *Marijuana, Chemistry, Pharmacology, Metabolism and Clinical Effects.* Academic Press, New York.

60. Mechoulam, R., Feigenbaum, J., Lander, N., Segal, M., Jarbe, T. and Consroe, P. (1988) Enantiomeric cannabinoids: stereospecificity of psychotropic activity. *Experientia* **44**, 762–764.

61. Mellors, A. (1979) Cannabinoids and membrane-bound enzymes, in *Marihuana: Biological Effects* (G. Nahas and W. D. M. Paton, eds.), Vols. 22 & 23, Pergamon Press, New York, pp. 329–342.

62. Mendelson, J., Ellingboe, J., Kuehnle, J. and Mello, N. (1978) Effects of chronic marihuana use on integrated plasma testosterone and luteinizing hormone levels. *Pharmacol. Exper. Ther.* **207**, 611–617.

63. Mendelson, J., Kuehnle, J. and Babor, T. (1974) Plasma testosterone levels before, during and after chronic marihuana smoking. *N. Engl. J. Med.* **291**, 1051–1055.

64. Monod, J. (1963) Allosteric proteins and cellular control systems. *J. Mol. Biol.* **6**, 306–329.

65. Nahas, G., Desoize, B. and Leger, C. (1979) Effects of psychotropic drugs on DNA synthesis. *Proc. Soc. Exp. Biol. Med.* **160**, 344–348.

66. Nahas, G. G. (1984) Toxicology and pharmacology, excerpt, in *Marihuana in Science and Medicine*, Raven Press, New York, pp. 196–206.

67. Nahas, G. G., Morishima, A. and Desoize, B. (1977) Effects of cannabinoids on macromolecular synthesis and replication of cultured lymphocytes. *Fed. Proc.* **36**, 1748.

68. Nahas, G. G., Suciu-Foca, B. and Desoize, B. (1974) Inhibition of cellular-mediated immunity in marihuana smokers. *Science* **185**, 541.

69. Paton, W. D. M., Pertwee, R. J. and Temple, D. M. (1972) The general pharmacology of cannabinoids, in *Cannabis and its Derivatives: Pharmacology and Experimental Psychology* (W. D. M. Paton and J. Crown, eds.), Oxford University Press, Oxford, pp. 50–74.

70. Perez-Reyes, M., Burstein, S. H., White, W. R., McDonald, S. A. and Hicks, R. E. (1991) Antagonism of marihuana effects by indomethacin in humans. *Life Sci.* **48**, 507–515.

71. Perez-Reyes, M., Lipton, M. A., Timmons, M. C. et al. (1973) Pharmacology of orally-administered delta-9-tetrahydrocannabinol. *Clin. Pharmacol. Ther.* **14**, 48–55.

72. Pertwee, R. (1995) Pharmacological, physiological and clinical implications of the discovery of cannabinoid receptors: an overview, in *Cannabinoid Receptors* (R. Pertwee, ed.), Academic Press, Manchester, England, pp. 1–34.

73. Pertwee, R. G. (1995) Cannabinoid Receptors. Academic Press, London.

74. Pryor, G., Larsen, P., Carr, J., Carr, E. and Braude, M. (1977) Interactions of delta-9-THC with penobarbitol, ethanol and chlordiazepoxide. *Pharmacol. Biochem. Behav.* **7**, 331–345.

75. Raine, J., Wing, D. and Paton, W. (1978) The effects of delta-1-THC on mammary gland growth, enzyme activity and plasma prolactin levels in the mouse. *Eur. J. Pharmacol.* **51**, 11–17.

76. Reichman, M., Nen, W. and Hokin, L. E. (1988) Delta-9-THC increases arachidonic acid levels in guinea pig cerebral cortex slices. *Mol. Pharmacol.* **34**, 823–828.

77. Reichman, M., Nen, W. and Hokin, L. E. (1991) Delta-9-THC inhibits arachidonic acid acylation of phospholipids and triacylglycerols in guinea pig cerebral cortex slices. *Mol. Pharmacol.* **40**, 547–555.

78. Reichman, M., Nen, W. and Hokin, L. E. (1987) Effects of delta-9-THC on prostaglandin formation in the brain. *Mol. Pharmacol.* **32**, 686–690.

79. Rosenkrantz, H. (1984) Cannabis components and responses of neuroendocrine-reproductive targets: an overview, in *Marihuana '84* (D. Harvey, ed.), IRL Press, Oxford, pp. 457–505.

80. Rosenkrantz, H. (1976) The immune response and marihuana, in *Marihuana: Chemistry, Biochemistry and Cellular Effects* (G. Nahas, ed.), Springer-Verlag, New York, pp. 441–456.

81. Sanderman, H. (1978) Regulation of membrane enzymes by lipids. *Biochim. Biophys. Acta* **515**, 209–237.

82. Schuel, H., Goldstein, E., Mechoulam, R., Zimmerman, A. and Zimmerman, S. (1994) Anandamide (arachidonylethanolamide), a brain cannabinoid receptor agonist, reduces fertilizing capacity in sea urchins by inhibiting the acrosome reaction. *Proc. Natl. Acad. Sci.* **91**, 7678–7682.
83. Seeman, P. (1977) *Biochem. Pharmacol.* **26**, 1741.
84. Seeman, P. (1972) The membrane action of anesthetics and tranquilizers. *Pharmacol. Rev.* **24**, 583.
85. Smith, T. C. and Kulp, R. A. (1976) Respiratory and cardiovascular effects of delta-9-tetrahydrocannabinol alone and in combination with oxymorphine, pentobarbital and diazpeam, in *The Therapeutic Potential of Marijuana* (S. Cohen and R. C. Stillman, eds.), Plenum Medical Book, New York, pp. 123–135.
86. Stein, G., Mon, J., Haas, A. and Jansing, R. (1979) Cannabinoids: The influence on cell proliferation and macromolecular biosynthesis, in *Marihuana: Biological Effects* (G. Nahas and W. Paton, eds.), Pergamon Press, New York, p. 171.
87. Stiglick, A. and Kalant, H. (1983) Behavioral effects of prolonged administration of delta-9-THC in the rat. *Psychopharmacol.* **80**, 325–330.
88. Stryer, L. (1995) *Biochemistry*, 4th ed., W. H. Freeman and Co., New York.
89. Tamir, I. and Lichtenberg, D. (1983) Correlation between the psychotropic potency of cannabis and their effect on the 1-H-NMR spectra of model membranes. *J. Pharm. Sci.* **72**, 458–461.
90. Trouve, R. (1985) Effects and interactions of natural cannabinoids on the isolated heart. *Proc. Soc. Exp. Bio. Med.* **180**, 312–316.
91. Trouve, R. and Nahas, G. (1985) Cardiac dynamics of the Langerdorff perfused heart. *Proc. Soc. Exp. Biol. Med.* **180**, 303–311.
92. Truddell, J. R., Hubbell, W. L. and Cohen, E. N. (1973) The effect of two inhalation anaesthetics on the order of spin-labelled phospholipic vesicles. *Biochim. Biophys. Acta.* **291**, 321–327.
93. Turner, C. (1984) Marijuana and cannabis: research. Why the conflict?, in *Marihuana '84* (D. Harvey, ed.), IRL Press, Oxford, pp. 31–36.
94. Vaysse, P. J., Gardner, E. L. and Zukin, R. S. (1987) Modulation of rat brain opioid receptors by cannabinoids. *J. Pharmacol. Exp. Ther.* **241**, 534–539.
95. Venance, L., Piomelli, D., Glowinski, J. and Giaume, C. (1995) Inhibition by anandamide of gap junctions and intercellular calcium signalling in striatal astrocytes. *Nature* **376**, 590–594.
96. Watson, S. and Girdlestone, D. (1994) 1994 receptor and ion channel nomenclature supplement. *TiPS.* **Suppl.** 1–51.
97. Weissmann, A. (1981) On the definition of cannabinoids: Botanical? chemical? pharmacological? *J. Clin. Pharmacol.* **21 (8–9)**:159S–165S.
98. Wenger, T., Croix, D., Tramu, G. and Leonardelli, J. (1992) Effects of THC on pregnancy, puberty and the neuroendocrine system, in *Marihuana/Cannabinoids: Neurobiology and Neurophysiology* (L. Murphy and A. Bartke, eds.), CRC Press, Boca Raton, pp. 539–560.
99. Wittgenstein, L. (1962) *Tractatus Logico-Philosophicus*, in Routledge & Kegan Paul, London.
100. Zimmerman, A., Padilla, G. and Cameron, I. (1973) *Drugs and the Cell Cycle*, Academic Press, New York.
101. Zimmerman, A. M. and Zimmerman, A. B. (1976) The influence of marihuana on eukaryote cell growth and development, in *Marihuana: Chemistry, Biochemistry and Cellular Effects* (G. Nahas, W. Paton, and J. Idanpaan-Heikkila, eds.), Springer-Verlag, New York, pp. 195–206.
102. Zuardi, A. W., Finkelfarb, E., A, B. O. F., E, M. R. and Karniol, I. G. (1981) Characteristics of the stimulus produced by the mixture of cannabidiol with delta-9-tetrahydrocannabinol. *Arch. Int. Pharmacodyn.* **249**, 137–146.
103. Zurier, R. B., Rossetti, R. G., Lane, J. H., Goldberg, J. M., Hunter, S. A. and Burstein, S. H. (1998) Dimethylheptyl-THC-11 oic acid: a nonpsychoactive antiinflammatory agent with a cannabinoid template structure. *Arthritis Rheum.* **41**, 163–170.

71 Marihuana and Medicine
From Human to Molecule

Gabriel G. Nahas

Cannabinoids, the specific chemicals of marihuana, and their metabolites can be classified into two major categories corresponding to particular chemical structures and pharmacological effects. The psychoactive cannabinoids, Δ^9-tetrahydrocannabinol (THC), Δ^8-THC, and their 11-hydroxy-derivatives which bind stereospecifically to receptors in nanomolar concentrations. The non-psychoactive cannabinoids, comprise natural biochemical precursors and degradation products such as cannabidiol (CBD), cannabinol (CBN), and the acidic metabolites of THC such as Δ^9-THC-11-oic acid, which, while not psychoactive, nevertheless possess other biological activities. As first emphasized by Paton, the target of THC is the neuronal membrane which comprises a complex assembly of contiguous integral receptors embedded in a functional lipid bilayer. The membrane bilayer and receptors are closely interacting and may only be considered separate entities at the molecular level.

THE INTERACTION OF CANNABINOIDS
WITH THE MEMBRANE LIPID BILAYER

The solubility of THC in the lipid bilayer is limited and the maximum degree of fluidization produced by THC does not approach that required for anesthesia and THC has been classified as a "partial anaesthetic." By contrast, the nonpsychoactive cannabinoids, CBN and CBD, produced an opposite effect to that of THC, decreasing the molecular disorder of the lipid bilayer. The membrane seems able to discriminate between psychoactive and non-psychoactive cannabinoids in a way similar to the brain cell, and the protein-free liposomes exhibit a degree of molecular selectivity comparable to that of the neurone. It was also postulated that CBN and CBD would be expected to antagonize, in part, the effect of THC in vivo, a prediction that has been documented by experimental observations. These results could account for the variability of effects of different cannabis preparations that contain markedly different cannabinoid concentrations. In spite of these interactions with cell membranes, which appeared to explain many of the actions of the cannabinoids, it was concluded that, while THC altered, in a specific fashion, the physicochemical organization of the membrane, this effect was only partial and could not account for the stereospecific psychoactive properties of this cannabinoid, which are exerted with nanomolar concentrations. Such effects are more typical of drugs acting at specific receptors.

From: *Marihuana and Medicine*
Edited by: G. G. Nahas et al.   © Humana Press Inc., Totowa, NJ

INTERACTION OF THC WITH SPECIFIC RECEPTORS

The first THC receptor (CB_1) was identified in rat brain and exhibited the characteristics for a neuromodulator receptor associated with a guanine nucleotide regulatory (G) protein. This receptor is unevenly distributed with highest concentrations in the globus pallidus, substantia nigra, pars reticulata, cerebral cortex, striatum, and the molecular layers of the cerebellum and hippocampal gyrus. A second receptor (CB_2) showed 44% sequence homology with the first and also appeared to belong to the G protein-linked receptor superfamily. Although the CB_2 receptors appear to be confined to the periphery, CB_1 receptors are found both centrally and peripherally.

FUNCTIONAL CORRELATES OF THC RECEPTOR BINDING AND SIGNALING ALTERATIONS

The binding of THC to its CB_1 or CB_2 G protein coupled receptors is associated with changes in the signaling functions of the brain, the immunity system, and the reproductive organs. In the brain, the binding of THC to CB_1 receptors is associated with marked functional changes of sensory perception. These changes were first described in 1845 by Moreau, who emphasized alterations of visual, auditory, and "body image" perceptions. Subsequently, these self-reported alterations were correlated with functional markers used to estimate visual, auditory, and somatosensory perceptions. Cannabis intoxication induces a binocular depth inversion that represents an illusion of visual perception, which is also observed in unmedicated schizophrenia. It is also associated with a delay in the P_{300}-related response to auditory cues, a dysfunction that may persist for weeks. Distortion of somatosensory perception reported by Moreau was also observed in a controlled clinical setting. Lowering of thermal pain perception was measured in heavy marihuana smokers. Such perceptual alterations may be related to the persistent binding of THC to the CB_1 receptors in areas of the brain where sensory perceptions are transduced into neuronal signaling.

Binding of THC to peripheral CB_2 receptors will induce alterations of signaling in the two major peripheral systems of intercellular communication: the immunity system and reproductive organs. CB_2 receptors are present on the surface of lymphocytes and macrophages and binding of THC to these receptors are associated with functional alterations. Sperm cells and ovum present THC receptors on their membrane surface, and the binding of THC to this CB_2 receptor interferes with important signaling functions of these gametes: acrosomal reaction, fertilization, and ovum implantation. These signaling alterations could account for the clinical and experimental observations reporting a decreased spermatogenesis, decreased sperm motility, and increase of abnormal forms of sperm in rodents and humans exposed to marihuana smoke or THC.

ENDOGENOUS MEMBRANE-DERIVED LIGANDS OF THE "THC" RECEPTOR

An endogenous lipid and a ligand, arachidonylethanolamide (AEA), that had an agonist action at the THC receptor was first isolated. It was named "anandamide" after the Sanskrit word ananda meaning bliss. It has a much lower affinity for the G protein receptor than THC, a briefer pharmacokinetic profile and a very fast turnover and disposition (like most signaling and second messenger molecules). It is not stored in cells and has been found to accumulate in brain following hypoxia or death of the neurone. Like THC, AEA has also been found to fluidize the cell membrane. The mechanism of action of AEA has simply been identified with that of THC and its synthetic analogs, involving G protein-dependent associated mechanisms. On the basis of this analogy alone, one might expect that AEA should play a major fundamental role in the regulation of membrane function and that the function of the AEA–G protein receptor is not limited to the binding of THC. A second ligand of both CB_1 and CB_2 receptors has subsequently been identified as 2-arachidonylglycerol (2-AG). Its affinity for the receptors parallels that of anandamide (AEA).

EFFECTS OF CANNABINOIDS ON NEUROTRANSMITTER RECEPTORS

THC does not interact directly with neurotransmitters but will alter the binding of a neurotransmitter to its receptor in an allosteric fashion: effects of acetylcholine, NMDA, and opiods are decreased, while those of catecholamines, are increased or present a biphasic pattern. Bloom concludes that since THC alters the fluidity of the membrane, its effects on constituent receptors are due to changes in the membrane environment which, in turn, affect the various receptor conformations. Although some differences undoubtedly exist in interactions with specific proteins, the fact remains that cannabinoids affect a wide range of membrane-bound neurotransmitter receptor molecules, suggesting a direct influence by the membrane lipid bilayer.

EFFECT OF CANNABINOIDS ON PHOSPHOLIPID ENZYMES AND ARACHIDONIC ACID BIOSYNTHESIS

A phospholipid messenger system is one of the major functions of the lipid bilayer and involves a signal-mediated hydrolysis of phospholipids within the membrane. The best characterized of these systems is that originating from arachidonic acid, which is released from phospholipids following activation by a phospholipase. Psychoactive cannabinoids and some of their nonpsychoactive acid metabolites will release, in a dose-dependent manner, arachidonic acid from phosphatidylcholine. Arachidonic acid, released by cannabinoids, has been associated with formation of prostaglandins and other eicosanoids such as leukotrienes and platelet activation factors (PAF). Cannabinoid-generated arachidonic acid biosynthesis has been shown to be inhibited by steroids, NSAIDs, (aspirin, paracetamol, and indomethacin). A cyclooxygenase inhibitor, significantly decreased prostaglandin concentration in plasma, heart rate acceleration and time-distortion produced by THC. The THC-stimulatory effect on prostaglandin synthesis is inhibited by its nonpsychoactive metabolite, THC-11-oic acid which suppresses cyclooxygenase activity.

A PUTATIVE SIGNAL TRANSDUCTION ROLE FOR THE LIPID BILAYER

It is proposed that AEA and 2-AG protein receptor interaction possesses a physiological function that regulates the signaling between boundary lipids and the receptors or enzymes of the membrane. The boundary lipids surrounding the membrane proteins are the vehicles for the signals between the AEA and 2-AG G protein receptor and the neurotransmitter receptors. The change of configuration of the G protein receptor catalyzed by the lipid mediators would modulate the signaling effect of the membrane on its constituent enzymes and receptors in an allosteric fashion. AEA and 2-AG, by-products of the membrane phospholipids, would, thus, be indirect signal modulators of membrane activity. THC deregulates the putative membrane signaling in two ways, first, by persistent binding to the AEA and 2-AG receptors and second, by altering the physicochemical organization of the boundary lipid bilayer into which it partitions.

PHYSIOLOGICAL IMPLICATIONS FOR MEDICINE
AND THERAPEUTICS

As a result of the deregulation of this ubiquitous membrane signaling system, marihuana and THC alters, *in a time- and dose-related fashion,* functions of the brain and cerebellum impairing visual, auditory, somatosensory perceptions, coordination, memory and consciousness.

In binding to central and peripheral receptors and displacing their natural ligands, THC alters central and peripheral mechanisms of cardiovascular regulation inducing tachycardia and vasodilatation.

A similar interaction of THC with this membrane signaling system affects spermatogenesis, fertilization and ovum implantation. THC is gametotoxic and fetotoxic. THC also interacts with the signaling function of lymphocytes and macrophages. Marihuana smoke, which is more damaging to the lungs than tobacco smoke, is not a proper therapeutic vehicle for THC.

The main therapeutic properties of the cannabinoids (analgesic, antiemetic, antiglaucoma) have been attributed to natural psychoactive Δ^9-THC, Δ^8-THC, and to their 11-hydroxy metabolites which bind stereospecifically to the AEA-G protein-coupled receptor complex. The synthetic analogues of THC, namely nabilone and levonantradol have a similar mode of action. In the treatment of vomiting for cancer chemotherapy, of glaucoma and of pain relief, these compounds have proven to be much less effective than other specific medications with less noxious effects.

The therapeutic properties of psychoactive cannabinoids are associated with adverse psychoactive and cardiovascular effects and it has not been possible to dissociate their therapeutic properties from the undesirable side effects. Prolonged storage in tissues and slow release and elimination is influenced by genetic polymorphism, which results in marked individual variability of plasma concentration and precludes dose-response effects. Development of tolerance further compounds the difficulty of administering uniform amounts. THC is also an addictive substance. All of these factors are associated with the deregulation of membrane signaling by THC and result in partial, inconsistent and discordant therapeutic effects.

Marihuana or THC do not qualify as safe and effective medications which aim at restoring or maintaining physiological function of cells, organs and organisms. They have no place in modern Pharmacopeia from which cannabis was eliminated in the first part of the century.

However, the experimental use of THC and of its synthetic analogues in molecular physiology ahs provided invaluable information leading to a better understanding of membrane signal transduction. As a result, the relationship between allosteric receptor responsiveness, molecular configuration of proteins and regulations of cellular function may be better understood.

INDEX